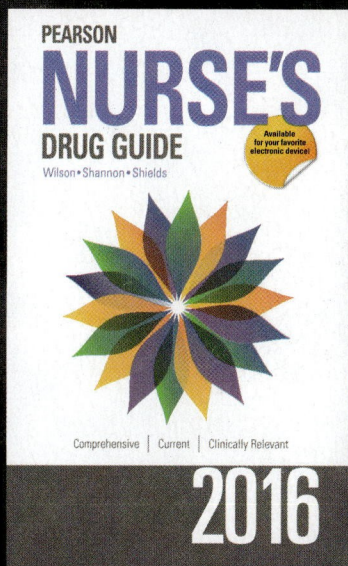

Clinical Nursing Skills
Basic to Advanced Skills

Ninth Edition

Sandra F. Smith, MS, RN
President, National Nursing Review; Los Altos, California

Donna J. Duell, RN, MS, PhD ABD
Consultant to Deans and Directors of Nursing; California

Barbara C. Martin, RN, BSN
Professor of Nursing, The University of Tulsa; Tulsa, Oklahoma

Michelle L. Aebersold, PhD, RN, FAAN
Clinical Associate Professor, Director Clinical Learning Center, University of Michigan School of Nursing; Ann Arbor, Michigan

Laura Gonzalez, PhD, ARNP, CNE
Assistant Professor of Nursing, University of Central Florida; Orlando, Florida

PEARSON

Boston   Columbus   Indianapolis   New York   San Francisco   Hoboken
Amsterdam   Cape Town   Dubai   London   Madrid   Milan   Munich   Paris   Montreal   Toronto
Delhi   Mexico City   Sao Paulo   Sydney   Hong Kong   Seoul   Singapore   Taipei   Tokyo

Publisher: Julie Levin Alexander
Editorial Coordinator: Sarah Henrich
Executive Editor: Lisa Rahn
Editorial Assistant: Bianca Sepulveda
Development Editor: Rachel Bedard
Program Manager: Kevin Wilson
Project Manager: Michael Giacobbe
Director, Product Management Services: Etain O'Dea
Team Lead, Program Management: Melissa Bashe
Team Lead, Project Management: Cynthia Zonneveld
Manufacturing Buyer: Maura Zaldivar-Garcia
Art Director: Maria Guglielmo Walsh
Cover and Interior Designer: Beth Paquin

Vice President of Sales & Marketing: David Gesell
Vice President, Director of Marketing: Margaret Waples
Senior Product Marketing Manager: Phoenix Harvey
Field Marketing Manager: Debi Doyle
Marketing Specialist: Michael Sirinides
Marketing Assistant: Amy Pfund
Media Production Product Manager: Amy Peltier
Media Production Project Manager: Lisa Rinaldi, Karen Bretz
Full-Service Project Manager: Vicki Rowland
Composition: Lumina Datamatics, Inc.
Printer/Binder: RR Donnelley/Menasha
Cover Printer: Lehigh-Phoenix Color
Cover Images: Patrick Watson

Credits and acknowledgments borrowed from other sources and reproduced, with permission, in this textbook appear on appropriate page within text.

Cataloging-in-Publication data on file with the Library of Congress.

Notice: Care has been taken to confirm the accuracy of the information presented in this book. The authors, editors, and the publisher, however, cannot accept any responsibility for errors or omissions or for consequences from application of the information in this book and make no warranty, express or implied, with respect to its contents.

The authors and the publisher have exerted every effort to ensure that drug selections and dosages set forth in this text are in accord with current recommendations and practice at time of publication. However, in view of ongoing research, changes in government regulations, and the constant flow of information relating to drug therapy and drug reactions, the reader is urged to check the package inserts of all drugs for any change in indications of dosage and for added warnings and precautions. This is particularly important when the recommended agent is a new and/or infrequently employed drug.

The authors and publisher disclaim all responsibility for any liability, loss, injury, or damage incurred as a consequence, directly or indirectly, of the use and application of any of the contents of this volume.

10 9 8 7 6 5 4 3 2 1

ISBN 10:   0-13-408792-5
ISBN 13: 978-0-13-408792-4

Acknowledgments

The authors express their thanks to the many people who assisted with the editorial and production phases of this edition of *Clinical Nursing Skills*, with special thanks to Lisa Rahn, Nursing Editor, and the team at Lumina Datamatics, Inc. We especially wish to thank our Developmental Editor, Rachel Bedard, for support, guidance, and editorial advice. We thank our contributors to this edition, Brian Busk and Janis Laiacona. We also thank our photographer for this edition, Patrick Watson, and the many models involved in our most recent photo shoot. A huge thanks to Sharon Decker and her assistant Marissa Cisneros at Texas Tech University Health Sciences Center in Lubbock, Texas, for their assistance and the use of their wonderful facility for our photo shoot. We appreciated your generous assistance and support throughout the process.

Thanks to our families and friends for their encouragement and support while we were preparing this new edition.

Thank You

A special thank you to all of the nurse educators and practicing nurses who have spent their time reviewing and contributing to this new edition.

CONTRIBUTORS TO CURRENT AND PREVIOUS EDITIONS

Theresa Britt, RN, MSN
Director of Nursing, Lab and Clinical Assessment
University of Tennessee Health Science Center
Memphis, TN

Brian Busk, MSN, RN
Faculty and Assistant Director of Nursing, College of the Siskiyous
Yreka, CA

Shirley S. Chang, RN, MS, PhD
Professor, Evergreen Valley College
San Jose, CA

Janet W. Cook, RN, MS
formerly Assistant Professor, University of North Carolina
Greensboro, NC

Deborah Denham, RN, MS, PhD
Critical Care
Sequoia Hospital
Redwood City, CA

Jacqueline Dowling, RN, MS
Professor, University of Massachusetts
Lowell, MA

Lou Ann Emerson, RN, MSN
Assistant Professor, University of Cincinnati
Cincinnati, OH

Rachel Faiano, RN, MS
Clinical Simulation Coordinator, Salinas Valley Memorial Healthcare System
Salinas, CA

Janis Laiacona, MSN, RN, PMHCNS-BC
Director of Accreditation and Clinical Support, John Muir Behavioral Health Center, Concord, CA
Nursing Programs Assistant Director, College of the Siskiyous
Weed, CA

Patricia J. Rahnema, RN, MSN, FNP
Nurse Practitioner, Southwest Cardiovascular Associates
Bullhead City, AZ

Sally Talley, RN
ET Specialist in Enterostomal Therapy
San Jose, CA

Jean O. Trotter, RN, C, MS
Assistant Professor, University of Maryland
Baltimore, MD

REVIEWERS

Patricia Ahearn, BS, MSN
Saint Peter's University
Jersey City, NJ

Traci Ashcraft, BSN, RN, BC
Ruby Memorial Hospital
Morgantown, WV

Lawrette Axley, PhD, RN, CNE
University of Memphis
Memphis, TN

Katherine Balkema, MM, BSN, BA, RRT, RN, CMSRN
Holland Hospital
Holland, MI

Mitzi Bass, MSN, RN
Baltimore City Community College
Baltimore, MD

Michelle Beckford, BSN, MSN, DMH
Saint Peter's University
Jersey City, NJ

Billie E Blake, EdD, MSN, BSN, RN
St. John's River Community College
Orange Park, FL

Cynthia M. Bork, EdD, RN
Winona State University
Winona, MN

Staci M. Boruff, PhD, RN
Walters State Community College
Morristown, TN

Katherine Brashears
University of Central Oklahoma
Edmond, OK

Cody Bruce, MSN, RN
Texas A&M
Bryan, TX

Michelle Bussard, MSN, RN, ANCS-BC, CNE
Firelands Regional Medical Center
Sandusky, OH

Barbara Callahan, MEd, RN, NCC, CHSE
Lenoir Community College
Kinston, NC

Barbara Celia, EdD, RN, MSN
Drexel University
Philadelphia, PA

Victor Ching, MD, MBA, FACS
Loma Linda School of Medicine
Loma Linda, CA

Ann-Marie Cote, MSN, RN, CEN
Plymouth State University
Plymouth, NH

Melissa Culp, MSN-Ed, BSN, RN
University of South Florida
Tampa, FL

Mary Davis, RN, MSN, MPA, CRNI
Hartnell College
Salinas, CA

Michelle DeLima
Delgado Community College
New Orleans, LA

Erin Heleen Discenza, MSN, RN
Cuyahoga Community College—Metropolitan
Cleveland, OH

Denise R. Doliveira, RN, MSN
Community College of Allegheny County—Boyce
Monroeville, PA

Bernadette Dragich, PhD, RN
Bluefield State College
Bluefield, WV

Mary Farrell, MSN-Ed, RN
Huron School of Nursing
East Cleveland, OH

Cindy Fong, RN, MSN
Loma Linda Hospital
Loma Linda, CA

Mary A. Gers, MSN, CNS, RNC
Northern Kentucky University
Highland Heights, KY

Theresa A. Glanville, RN, MS, CNE
Springfield Technical Community College
Springfield, MA

Jeanine Goodin, MSN, BSN
University of Cincinnati
Cincinnati, OH

Susan Growe, DNP, RN, COI
Nevada State College
Henderson, NV

Jennifer Hatley, RN, MSN
Vernon College
Vernon, TX

Katherine Houle, RN, BSN, CNS
Gillette Children's Specialty Healthcare
St. Paul, MN

Kathleen Hudson, RN, MSN
Illinois Eastern Community College
Olney, IL

Paula Hutchings, MSN, RN
Hill College
Lamar Hillsboro, TX

Denise Isibel, RN, MSN
Old Dominion University
Norfolk, VA

Kathleen C. Jones, MSN, RN, CNS
Walters State Community College
Morristown, TN

Fran Kamp, RN, MSN
Mercer University
Atlanta, GA

Patricia Ketcham, MSN, RN
Oakland University
Rochester, MI

Vicky Keys, MSN, DNP
Texas A&M University
Bryan, TX

Susan M. Koos, MS, RN, CNE
Heartland Community College
Normal, IL

Cheryl M. Lantz, PhD, RN
Dickinson State University
Dickinson, ND

Lori Lioce, BSN, DNP
University of Alabama
Huntsville, AL

Carol List, RN, BSN
Hutchinson Community College
Hutchinson, KS

Rosemary Macy, PhD, RN, CNE, CHSE
Boise State University
Boise, ID

Kathleen McManus, RN, MSN, CNE
Central Maine Community College
Auburn, ME

Joshua Meringa, MPA, MHA, BSN, RN, ONC
Spectrum Health Hospitals
Grand Rapids, MI

Juleann H. Miller, RN, PhD
St. Ambrose College
Davenport, IA

Patricia Novak, RN, BSN, MSN
Gateway Community College
New Haven, CT

Linda Olsen, BSN, MSN
Mid-State Technical College
Wisconsin Rapids, WI

Rebecca Otten, EdD, MS, BA
Mount Saint Mary's University
Los Angeles, CA

Amanda Pierce, DNP, RN
Texas Tech University
El Paso, TX

Janice Ramirez, MSN, BS, ADN, CCRN, RN-BC, CNE
North Idaho College
Coeur d'Alene, ID

Nancy Renzoni, RN, MS
Trocaire College
Buffalo, NY

Mark Reynolds, MSN, RN
University of Alabama
Huntsville, AL

Kathy Rogers, MSN, RN, CNE
Ursuline College
Pepper Pike, OH

Shielda Glover Rodgers, PhD, RN
The University of North Carolina
Chapel Hill, NC

Deanna Schaffer, MSN, RN, CNE, ACNS-BC
Drexel University
Philadelphia, PA

Vicki Simpson RN, MSN, CHES, PhD
Purdue University
West Lafayette, IN

Kristen Smith, MSN, RNC-NC
Northern Michigan University
Marquette, MI

Charlotte Stephenson, RN, DSN, CLNC
Texas Woman's University
Houston, TX

Patricia Taylor, RN, MSN Ed
Kapiolani Community College
Honolulu, HI

Jennifer M. Thayer, MS, ARNP, PNP-BC
University of South Florida
Tampa, FL

Elaine Tobias, RN, BSN, IBCLC
The Women's Place at Heart of Lancaster
Regional Medical Center
Lititz, PA

Cheryl Tveit, RN
Gillette Children's Specialty Healthcare
St. Paul, MN

Donna Woshinsky, RN, MSN, CNE
Springfield Technical Community College
Springfield, MA

PHOTO CONSULTANTS

June Brown, RN, BSN
Arnold Failano, RN, BSN
Wendy Ogden, RN, MS

Cathy Patton, RN, BSN, MA
Diana Soria, RN, BSN

Constance Troolines, RN, BSN
Virginia Williams, RN, MS

Preface

Our primary goal in writing *Clinical Nursing Skills* is to produce a relevant, useful, and comprehensive text that is flexible for various education programs and learning needs of students. *Clinical Nursing Skills*, a highly acclaimed skills book since its first edition in 1982, applies to all levels of nursing education. It is also used as a procedure manual by many hospital systems. Current with both the National Council Test Plan for RN and the NCLEX®, this textbook offers faculty a format for teaching nursing skills content that is both progressive and innovative. Content flows from basic to more complex skills and teaches the student how to assess the client, formulate nursing diagnoses, perform the procedure according to accepted and safe protocols, evaluate the outcomes, and document pertinent data.

The content continues to be organized around the nursing process and offers both a theoretical overview and step-by-step practical skills. Within the chapters, skills are grouped together into units. Nursing process data is then provided for each unit. Unlike other skill textbooks, *Clinical Nursing Skills* conceptualizes the nursing process data for each unit so that it does not have to be repeated with every skill. Each numbered skill includes a list of necessary equipment, associated preparation, and step-by-step nursing interventions. Critical steps include relevant rationales for nursing actions. This streamlined approach continues with Unit Documentation and Evaluation, giving students a feel for categories of skills and the similarities when documenting them. Units conclude with sets of Unexpected Outcomes and Alternative Actions. These charts not only provide more information for students, but they also reinforce how evaluation can lead to further action within the nursing process.

Chapter Wrap-Ups provide information specific to the older adult population. They also supply Management Guidelines for assistance in delegating tasks and in maintaining appropriate interprofessional communication to support quality care. They offer Case Study Applications, a set of clinical scenarios for students to use to practice decision making and planning. They provide 10 NCLEX® questions per chapter for student review, plus a new QSEN activity to promote awareness and adherence to nursing standards.

The clear, newly numbered format of the ninth edition enables the student to easily access key material for immediate reference in the clinical area. Extensive color photographs and drawings within each unit illustrate the concepts presented and enable students to visualize steps that must be performed.

Ninth Edition Highlights

- **New!** Updated design for fast access to content and features!
- **New!** QSEN Activities to give students practice aligning nursing care with QSEN standards.
- **Expanded!** Evidence-Based Nursing Practice boxes presenting specific scientific studies that validate the skills protocols. Research studies emphasize new information related to improving client care.
- **More than 550 new and updated skills** with the most up-to-date nursing techniques recommended by current standards of practice.
- **Documentation and Evaluation,** with succinct teaching about each unit of skills. To give students a broader understanding of how to document, Documentation sections list *data to record for each category of skills.* They compare Expected Outcomes with Unexpected Outcomes and then offer Alternative Actions the nurse might take when client goals are not met.
- **Critical Thinking and the Nursing Process chapter** integrating critical thinking into the steps of the nursing process.
- **New skills** Determining Gastric pH and NovaCath Integrated IV System.
- **Legal Alerts** that help nurses recognize legal pitfalls and actions that constitute legal malpractice when performing procedures.
- **New Trends** feature presenting equipment and systems that are being incorporated in 21st-century nursing care.
- **Practice Guidelines** boxes, with attention to maintaining standards of care.
- **Case Study Applications** at the end of each chapter to help students apply critical thinking principles to clinical situations.
- **NCLEX® questions** with rationales for all distractors.

Hallmark Features

Clinical Nursing Skills' all-inclusive, clear, and concise format teaches the student to:

- Learn each skill from basic to advanced in a contextual framework.
- Understand the theoretical concepts that serve as a foundation for skills.

- Apply this knowledge to a clinical situation with a "client need" focus.

- Use critical thinking to assess and evaluate the outcome of the skill and consider unexpected outcomes.

- Appreciate cultural diversity principles as they apply to client situations.

- Validate clinical skills by applying evidence-based nursing practice data and studies.

- Function in, and adapt to, the professional role by understanding management responsibilities.

Educator Resources

- Instructor's Manual, which provides teaching and learning strategies for lecture and lab, writing assignments and activity suggestions, and critical thinking exercises

- Skills Checklists featuring editable checklists of procedures found in each chapter

- Image library that showcases photos and art from the textbook to enhance "in-the-moment" teaching

- Test Item File offering over 700 questions that you can use to create assignments

- NCLEX®-style questions with complete rationales for both correct and incorrect answers.

We believe faculty will find this textbook a valuable teaching tool and reference for clinical practice.

The Only Skill Resource You'll Need . . .
Complete Coverage of over 550 Skills in a Clear, Time-Saving Format!

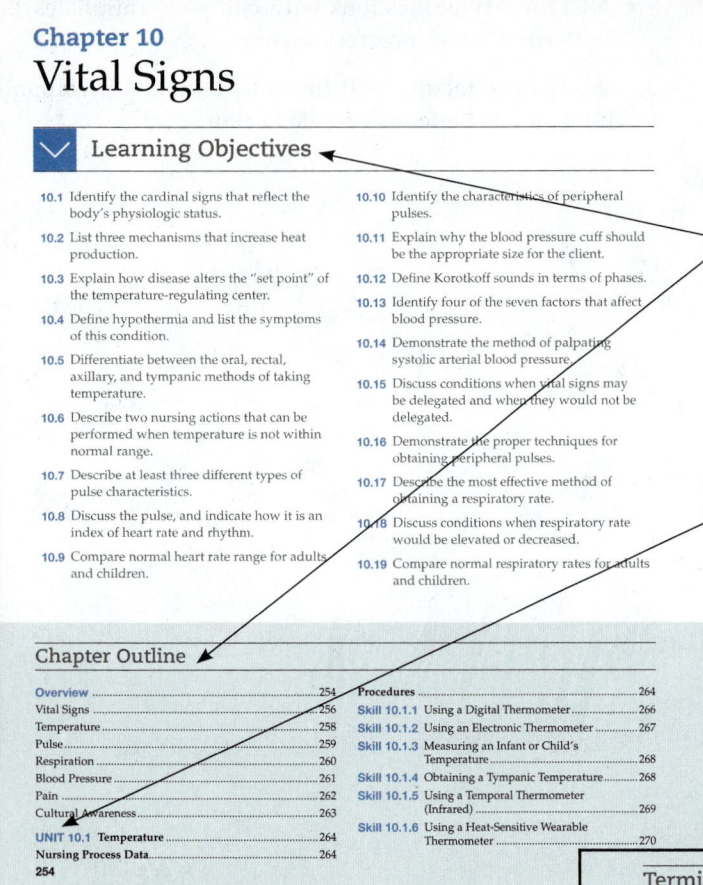

Chapter 10
Vital Signs

Learning Objectives

10.1 Identify the cardinal signs that reflect the body's physiologic status.

10.2 List three mechanisms that increase heat production.

10.3 Explain how disease alters the "set point" of the temperature-regulating center.

10.4 Define hypothermia and list the symptoms of this condition.

10.5 Differentiate between the oral, rectal, axillary, and tympanic methods of taking temperature.

10.6 Describe two nursing actions that can be performed when temperature is not within normal range.

10.7 Describe at least three different types of pulse characteristics.

10.8 Discuss the pulse, and indicate how it is an index of heart rate and rhythm.

10.9 Compare normal heart rate range for adults and children.

10.10 Identify the characteristics of peripheral pulses.

10.11 Explain why the blood pressure cuff should be the appropriate size for the client.

10.12 Define Korotkoff sounds in terms of phases.

10.13 Identify four of the seven factors that affect blood pressure.

10.14 Demonstrate the method of palpating systolic arterial blood pressure.

10.15 Discuss conditions when vital signs may be delegated and when they would not be delegated.

10.16 Demonstrate the proper techniques for obtaining peripheral pulses.

10.17 Describe the most effective method of obtaining a respiratory rate.

10.18 Discuss conditions when respiratory rate would be elevated or decreased.

10.19 Compare normal respiratory rates for adults and children.

Chapter Outline

Each chapter opens with **Learning Objectives** and a **Chapter Outline** for easy reference and review of chapter contents.

Skill procedures within each chapter are grouped together in **Units** and organized around a Nursing Process Framework.

Key **Terminology** is provided at the beginning of the chapter for easy review.

Terminology

Antipyretic an agent that reduces febrile temperatures.

Apex the pointed end of a cone-shaped part or organ (e.g., lower heart, upper lung).

Arteriosclerosis an arterial disease characterized by inelasticity and thickening of the vessel walls with lessened blood flow.

Atherosclerosis a form of arteriosclerosis in which there are localized accumulations of lipid-containing material within the internal surfaces of blood vessels.

Atrial pertaining to the atrium, the upper cardiac chamber that receives blood from the lungs and systemic circulation.

Atrial fibrillation atrial arrhythmia characterized by rapid, random contractions of the atrial myocardium causing a rapid, irregular ventricular rate.

Autoregulation the intrinsic ability of an organ or tissue to maintain blood flow despite changes in arterial pressure.

Axilla armpit.

Bigeminal pulse a regularly irregular pulse where every

Cardiac output the amount of blood ejected by the heart or the stroke volume (SV) times the heart rate (CO = SV × HR).

Cardiogenic originating in the heart itself.

Chemoreceptor a sense organ or sensory nerve ending that is stimulated by and reacts to chemical stimuli.

Contractility having the ability to contract or shorten muscle tissue or cells.

Core temperature the body's interior deep tissue temperature (e.g., the abdominal cavity).

Diastole the period in which the heart dilates and fills with blood; the period of relaxation.

Doppler a type of ultrasound stethoscope or probe that uses an ultrasound beam to detect blood flow.

Febrile feverish, increased body temperature.

Fibrillation quivering, involuntary contraction of individual muscle fibers.

Hypertension blood pressure that is considered to be higher than the normal range.

Multicultural Health Care

In the twenty-first century, demographic shifts are occurring that will change the direction of health care. As of the 2012 census, Asians are the fastest growing race or ethnic group in the United States. This is due mostly to international migration. Hispanics remain the second largest race or ethnic group, representing 17% of the nation. Five states have a majority-minority, meaning that the prevailing minority group is now more than half the population (Brown, 2014).

Because of this change in the U.S. population demographics, there are emerging barriers to health care for many groups of people. Perhaps the greatest barrier is language, and since communication is an essential component of providing nursing care, it is important to consider language under the topic of communication. Other barriers

Cultural Awareness

It is important for nurses to understand the impact of various cultures on healthcare practices if they are to become culturally competent. As more and more people immigrate to this country, nurses will be faced with challenges related to **cultural diversity** when administering health care. Cultural diversity implies the range of differences in values, beliefs, customs, folklore, traditions, language, and patterns of behavior for the various cultural groups. For example, people from different cultures define personal space differently. Some may prefer closer personal contact, while an individual moving into their personal space offends others. The nurse needs to be aware that personal space is related to culture, gender, and group behavior. Because all of these aspects potentially affect how an individual experiences,

◄ **Cultural Awareness** sections remind nurses of issues surrounding diversity and providing culturally responsive client care.

LEGAL ALERT
Nurses' Negligence
The client had transthoracic vagotomy. The doctor ordered vital signs q 15 minutes × 1 hour and q hour for 10 hours. Vital signs were recorded four times for 1 day. The next day the client's temperature was 102°F (38.9°C) and it remained there until the day after, when it was 105°F (40.6°C). The nurse administered aspirin when it rose to 106°F (41°C). The nurse then contacted the doctor who found signs of serious wound infection. The client suffered organic brain syndrome as a direct result of the continued high temperature. The court found that the nurses breached standard of care when they failed to notify the doctor of the client's high temperature.

◄ **Legal Alert** boxes highlight legal pitfalls and make nurses aware of legal malpractice.

New Trends boxes present new equipment and systems that are being incorporated in 21st-century nursing care. ▶

Box 10-8 NEW TRENDS: ELECTRONIC STETHOSCOPE
A new electronic stethoscope is now available. It measures a client's blood pressure via Bluetooth-enabled Cardioscan and sends the results directly into the client's computer record for immediate evaluation.

Nursing Diagnoses

The following nursing diagnoses may be appropriate to include in a client care plan when the components are related to establishing and maintaining a nurse–client relationship.

NURSING DIAGNOSIS	RELATED TO . . .
Impaired Communication: Verbal	Psychologic barrier, inability to speak dominant language, impaired **cognition**, lack of privacy
Powerlessness	Perceived lack of control resulting in dissatisfaction
Impaired Social Interaction	Lack of motivation, anxiety, **depression**, lack of self-esteem, disorganized thinking, delusions, hallucinations
Social Isolation	Hospitalization, terminal illness

Source: Herdman, T. H. & Kamitsuru, S. (Eds.) Nursing Diagnoses – Definitions and Classification 2015-2017. Copyright © 2014, 1994–2014 by NANDA International. Used by arrangement with John Wiley & Sons Limited. Companion website: www.wiley.com/go/nursingdiagnoses. In order to make safe and effective judgments using NANDA-I nursing diagnosis it is essential that nurses refer to the definitions and defining characteristics of the diagnoses listed in this work.

◄ **Nursing Diagnoses** for each chapter give quick and clear guidelines for appropriate use of nursing diagnoses in client care plans.

Unit 10.2
Pulse Rate

Nursing Process Data

ASSESSMENT Database

- Assess appropriate site to obtain pulse.
- Check pulse with health status changes, as ordered by healthcare provider, or before administering certain medications.
- Assess for rate, rhythm, volume, and quality.
- Assess an apical pulse on clients with irregular rhythms or those on cardiac medications.
- Obtain baseline peripheral pulses with initial assessment or in any client undergoing cardiac or vascular surgery. Also obtain pulse for medical clients with diabetes, arterial occlusive diseases, **atherosclerosis**, or aneurysm, or any color or temperature changes in the periphery.
- Obtain an apical–radial pulse when deficits occur between apical and radial measurements.
- Assess the need to monitor pulses with an ultrasound or electronic device.

PLANNING Objectives

- To determine whether the pulse rate is within normal range and if the rhythm is regular
- To evaluate the quality (amount of blood pumped through peripheral arteries) of arterial pulses
- To determine whether peripheral pulses are equal in amplitude when compared with corresponding pulses
- To determine presence of peripheral pulses with ultrasound device when palpation is ineffective
- To monitor and evaluate changes in the client's health status
- To determine apical pulse rate before heart medications are administered

IMPLEMENTATION Procedures

- **Skill 10.2.1** Palpating a Radial Pulse 273
- **Skill 10.2.2** Taking an Apical Pulse 274
- **Skill 10.2.3** Taking an Apical–Radial Pulse 275
- **Skill 10.2.4** Palpating a Peripheral Pulse 276
- **Skill 10.2.5** Monitoring Peripheral Pulses With a Doppler Ultrasound Stethoscope 277

Note: See also Skill 30.3.2, Using Pulse Oximetry, page 1187

DOCUMENTATION AND EVALUATION

Expected Outcomes

- Pulse is palpated without difficulty.
- Pulse rate is within normal range and rhythm is regular.
- All peripheral pulses are equal in amplitude when compared bilaterally and when compared with the next proximal site.
- Apical pulse is easily detected and counted.

Unexpected Outcomes/Alternative Actions

Pearson Nursing Student Resources

Find additional review materials at **nursing.pearsonhighered.com.** Prepare for success with NCLEX®-style practice questions and Skill Checklists.

◄ Within each chapter, **Units** open with a complete overview of the Nursing Process Data that applies to the Procedures.

Online Nursing Student Resources for each unit contain competency checklists for each procedure. (Visit nursing.pearsonhighered.com.)

Step-by-Step Skills. More than ► 1,100 full-color photographs, line drawings, charts, and tables depict step-by-step nursing procedures. Clear, concise skills with helpful rationales enable nurses of all levels to visualize, perform, and evaluate skills in any clinical setting.

11. Check to see that client is comfortable.
12. Perform hand hygiene and clean stethoscope.
13. Document apical pulse rate, rhythm, and intensity.

CLINICAL ALERT

The best practice for taking a pulse for infants or children is to listen to the heart itself, rather than palpating the pulse. Too much pressure may obliterate it, and inadequate pressure may not detect it.

❶ Accurate apical pulse is found in fifth intercostal space, left of sternum at midclavicular line or mitral area.

accurate readings are obtained over 1 minute, especially if pulse is irregular.
c. Determine if pattern is regular, regularly irregular, or chaotic. ➤ *Rationale:* This finding helps describe the rhythm disturbance.

EVIDENCE-BASED PRACTICE
Effect of Music on Vital Signs
One hundred and fifteen clients who were scheduled to undergo ophthalmic procedures and who were exposed to live classical piano music showed a statistically significant decrease ($P < 0.0001$) in blood pressure, heart rate, and respiratory rate.
Source: Camara, Ruskowskis, & Worak, (2008)

Skill 10.2.3 | Taking an Apical–Radial Pulse

Equipment
Watch with sweeping second hand
Stethoscope
Another nurse to assist with procedure (optional)

Procedure
1. Gather equipment.
2. Perform hand hygiene.
3. Clean stethoscope bell and diaphragm with alcohol swab or equivalent.
4. Check two forms of client ID. Introduce self.
5. Provide privacy.
6. Explain procedure to client, especially if two nurses are taking the pulse. ➤ *Rationale:* Clients may be apprehensive

when two nurses are at the bedside, so a full explanation helps allay fears.
7. Assist client to a supine position and expose chest area.
8. Place watch where clearly visible to both nurses. ➤ *Rationale:* Both nurses count pulse rates within the same time span, preferably using one watch.
9. Warm stethoscope in palm of your hand. ➤ *Rationale:* This prevents startling the client with cold stethoscope.
10. Locate radial pulse. The second nurse locates apical pulse at the fifth intercostal space left of sternum at the midclavicular line and firmly places diaphragm of stethoscope on the site. ❶ ➤ *Rationale:* Firm application helps transmit high-pitched heart sounds.

❶ A. Auscultate apical pulse and **palpate** radial pulse simultaneously. B. This can also be done by two nurses.

(continued)

Clinical Alerts and **Safety Alerts** call attention to safety issues, essential information, nursing judgment, and actions that require critical decision making.

Skill 10.1.5 | Using a Temporal Thermometer (Infrared) *(continued)*

EVIDENCE-BASED PRACTICE
Accuracy of Temporal Artery Thermometers
A recent study by Emergency Nurses Association (ENA) on temporal artery thermometer accuracy found that among the pediatric participants (*N* = 52), temporal artery temperatures were within the acceptable range set by the experts to use as a noninvasive substitute for core body temperatures (Reynolds et al., 2014).

❷ After releasing scan button, note the reading in the window.

◄ **Expanded! Evidence-Based Practice** boxes present specific scientific studies that validate skill protocols.

10.4 Documentation and Evaluation

DOCUMENTATION for Blood Pressure

- Two phases of Korotkoff sounds (e.g., 120/80) and site
- Three phases of Korotkoff sounds (e.g., 130/110/80) and site
- Response to alternative nursing actions
- Response to position changes
- Document vital signs in chart, in addition to attaching digital readouts

EVALUATION/Critical Thinking

Expected Outcomes
- Blood pressure readings provide information regarding the overall health status of the client.
- Major changes from prior assessments are documented.
- Accurate readings are taken by using the correct cuff size and procedure.
- Beginning and disappearance of Korotkoff sounds during a blood pressure reading are evaluated and documented.
- The presence of factors that can alter blood pressure readings is identified.

Unexpected Outcomes	Alternative Actions
Blood pressure reading is abnormally high without apparent physiologic cause.	• Check if arm was unsupported. • Check if cuff was not snug. • Check if cuff was deflated too slowly or reinflated during deflation, causing venous engorgement and abnormally high diastolic readings. • Ask if client has pain, was anxious (white coat syndrome), or had just exercised, eaten, or smoked. Recheck pressure as indicated. • Check blood pressure on both arms. The normal difference from arm to arm is usually no more than 5 mmHg. • Check if insufficient rest before assessment.
Blood pressure reading is very low and there are no significant clinical indicators.	• Assess if cuff is too wide. • Check if client's arm was above heart level. • Check if inflation was too slow. This reduces intensity of Korotkoff sounds. • Assess if Korotkoff sounds were barely audible. Raise client's arm, and then recheck. Sounds should be louder. • Identify if stethoscope was misplaced and was not on brachial artery. • Take blood pressure 3 minutes after client rises from supine to standing if postural hypotension is suspected.
Blood pressure cannot be measured on upper extremity due to casts or other causes of inaccessibility.	• Use lower extremity to obtain blood pressures.

(continued)

Each unit ends with **Documentation and ▶ Evaluation.**

- The **Documentation** section focuses on important data to record regarding the skills, outcomes, and client responses.

- The **Evaluation/Critical Thinking** section reviews Expected Outcomes and provides Alternative Actions to take when Unexpected Outcomes occur.

Chapter Wrap-Up Helps Tie Everything Together!

Chapter Wrap-Up

GERONTOLOGIC Considerations

Cardiac Status—Changes

- Changes in cardiovascular status with aging are often insidious and may become apparent when system is stressed and there is increased demand for cardiac output (which may occur with illness and hospitalization). Nursing care assessment should focus on client's cardiovascular status, even when diagnosis does not include a cardiac condition.
- Blood pressure measurement should take age into account. If client has severe joint stiffness, pseudohypertension may be present. If this is suspected, raise the cuff pressure above the systolic blood pressure and, if the radial pulse remains palpable, the reading may show 10–15 mm Hg in error.
- Postural hypotension is common in the older adult (positional drop of less than 20 mm Hg); nurses should take note when helping a client out of bed. Hypertension is also common in this age group.
- A rise in blood pressure may be associated with reduced cardiac output, vasoconstriction, increased blood volume, or fluid overload.
- Pulse changes, particularly an irregular pulse, can be related to hypoxia, airway obstruction, or electrolyte imbalance.
- The arteries in older adult clients may feel stiff and knotty due to decreased elasticity. Excessive pressure to site when taking pulse may obliterate it. The normal rate is 60–90 beats/min.
- If pulses are not palpated, a Doppler may need to be used.

Respiratory Status—Changes

- Changes in the respiratory system may be subtle and gradual with the older adult: Oxygen saturation is decreased to 93%–94%; there is often poor cough response and incomplete lung expansion—all of which leads to increased risk of pulmonary infection when the older adult client is hospitalized.
- Slightly irregular breathing patterns are not unusual in the older adult.

Temperature—Changes

- With the older adult, temperature may be as low as 95°F (35°C). Because they may be easily dehydrated with increased temperature, nursing assessment should include baseline temperature at admission and continued monitoring during hospitalization.
- Older adults with acute infections may have a subnormal temperature.
- Increased temperatures can lead to increased metabolism, thus increasing the body's demand for oxygen. This causes the heart to work harder.
- Oral temperatures are the preferred method for obtaining the older adult client's temperature.

Gerontologic Considerations help nurses consider special adaptations for care of older adults.

Management Guidelines include two sections. A **Delegation** section teaches nurses to delegate tasks within safe, legal, and appropriate parameters. An **Interprofessional Communication** section helps nurses prioritize and communicate relevant client information to members of the healthcare team, in order to ensure consistent quality of care.

MANAGEMENT Guidelines

Each state legislates a Nurse Practice Act for RNs and LPN/LVNs. Healthcare facilities are responsible for establishing and implementing policies and procedures that conform to their state's regulations. Verify the regulations and role parameters for each healthcare worker in your facility.

Delegation

- Taking vital signs for clients may be assigned to any healthcare worker provided they have been assessed for competency in the procedure. This includes LPN/LVN, unlicensed assistive personnel (UAP), and EMT.
- The registered nurse must identify parameters for which the healthcare worker is to notify the nurse (i.e., blood pressure above or below a certain reading, pulse rate, or irregular pulse).

- The nurse must provide detailed explanations and/or demonstrate alterations in the procedure or specific methods of obtaining the vital signs to UAP, or EMTs.
- Obtaining peripheral pulses by use of the Doppler is the responsibility of the RN or LPN/L responsible for using the Doppler.
- The UAP may monitor blood pressure sive monitoring device; however, the U sible for initiating the procedure or sett

Interprofessional Communication

- Directions must be given to healthcare mentation procedures. Do they com record, enter data into the EHR, write

vital sign sheet at the nurses' desk, or give the results to the nurse?
- The registered nurse must evaluate all abnormal or changed vital signs identified by the healthcare workers. The nurse maintains total responsibility for client care

even though someone else performs the task of taking the vital signs.
- The registered nurse must ensure that the healthcare workers know the parameters for reporting unusual vital signs. Periodic checks with the workers may be necessary.

Case Study Applications provide case scenarios that help nurses develop clinical reasoning skills.

CASE STUDY Applications

Scenario 1

Mr. Trager (age 92) has been admitted to your unit with a temperature of 103°F (39.4°C), BP 140/90, P 114, and R 30 and labored. He reports a history of 3 days of diarrhea and fever and asks you for something to drink.

1. From your analysis of the admission data, determine the following:
   a. Appropriate nursing diagnosis in order of priority for this client.
   b. The metabolic effects of fever on pulse and respiration.
   c. Age factors that contribute to the existing problem.
2. What are the other assessment findings indicative of the diagnosis established from primary admitting data?
3. Develop a plan of care for this client.
4. Describe the evaluative outcomes for problem resolution.

Scenario 2

Mr. Sondheim is admitted to the hospital with unstable hypertension for evaluation. He has a family history of

hypertension and heart disease. The nurse will complete a physical exam and a history.

1. What information is missing in the family history that the nurse will want to elicit from the client?
2. Which questions regarding lifestyle would be appropriate to ask?
3. Which aspects of client teaching would the nurse want to cover before Mr. Sondheim is discharged?

Scenario 3

You are caring for a client, and when checking his vital signs, you are unable to palpate his radial pulse.

1. What would be your follow-up intervention?
2. When you still cannot find a pulse clear enough to document, what would be your next intervention?
3. What parameters of the pulse will you pay attention to when assessing and recording a client's pulse?

NCLEX® Review Questions

Unless otherwise specified, choose only one (1) answer.

1. During a shift assessment, the nurse notes that the client's peripheral pulses are absent. What would the next intervention be?
   A. Palpate the peripheral pulse.
   B. Use a Doppler to assess peripheral pulse.
   C. Notify the healthcare provider.
   D. Administer O₂ as ordered.

2. When a pulse deficit is detected in a client, what would the nurse expect the client is experiencing?
   A. Premature ventricular beats
   B. Bradycardia
   C. Tachycardia
   D. Heart block

3. A client's temperature remains elevated despite the administration of antipyretic drugs. What would be the first intervention after determining this condition?
   A. Administer a cool bath.
   B. Assess all remaining signs.

   C. Request orders for a cooling blanket.
   D. Obtain an order for a blood culture.

4. When taking a client's blood pressure that has been within normal limits, the nurse gets a reading that is very low without any significant clinical indicators. Which intervention would be appropriate?
   A. Assess if the BP cuff is too narrow.
   B. Assess if the BP cuff is too wide.
   C. Assess if the client's arm was positioned below heart level.
   D. Notify the healthcare provider.

5. When taking a client's blood pressure, the nurse finds the reading very different from previous readings recorded on the chart. What is the first intervention?
   A. Recheck the blood pressure with different equipment.
   B. Notify the healthcare provider.
   C. Validate the reading with another nurse.
   D. Check the client's circulatory status.

NCLEX® Review Questions

Unless otherwise specified, choose only one (1) answer.

1. Which intervention is most useful when communicating with an aphasic client?
   A. Use correct medical terminology when teaching or explaining.
   B. Ask open-ended questions to obtain information.
   C. Repeat the same word until the client understands.
   D. Provide frequent praise and encouragement.

2. A psychiatric client rapidly improves and is scheduled to be discharged tomorrow. Which of the following responses demonstrates that the nurse has a good understanding of termination of a relationship?
   A. "You have worked really hard the last three weeks. Good-bye and good luck."
   B. "Stop by and let us know how things are going."
   C. "You've done some good work here. I hope you are able to follow through with it."
   D. "Good-bye and good luck. Hopefully, we won't be seeing you here again."

3. One characteristic of a nurse–client relationship is that it is a professional one. What does this imply about the nurse?
   A. The nurse should be primarily concerned with implementing the policies of the hospital.
   B. The nurse views the client's needs as her or his primary concern.
   C. The nurse maintains a distance between self and client.
   D. The nurse establishes boundaries, formulate goals, and maintain the boundaries of a professional relationship.

4. One day a client with terminal cancer says to the nurse, "Well, I've given up all hope. I know I'm going to die soon." Which is the most therapeutic response?
   A. "Now, one should never give up hope. We are finding new cures all the time."
   B. "We should talk about dying."
   C. "You've given up all hope?"
   D. "Your doctor will be here soon. Why don't you talk to him about your feelings?"

5. Which of the following statements would be best to stimulate conversation with a client about his or her social history?
   A. "Are you married?"
   B. "Do you have any children?"
   C. "Tell me about your family."
   D. "Is your role in the family important?"

6. A client is admitted to CCU with a diagnosis of anterior myocardial infarction. Shortly after admission, he states: "I might as well have died because now I won't be able to do anything." Which is the most appropriate response by the nurse?
   A. "Don't worry, everything will turn out all right."
   B. "What do you mean, not able to do anything?"
   C. "Take one day at a time and it will all work out."
   D. "You shouldn't be thinking like this, because you are doing well now."

7. A male client is becoming increasingly angry and verbally abusive. Which of these is the appropriate intervention?
   A. Send the client back to his room.
   B. Ask the healthcare provider for an order for restraints.
   C. Summon assistance from a male staff member.
   D. Set firm limits on the abusive behavior.

8. Which of the following components would you include in a cultural assessment?
   Select all that apply.
   A. Cultural background
   B. Nutritional practices
   C. Beliefs and perceptions of health
   D. Age of the client
   E. Belief in God
   F. Communication patterns
   G. Health practices, including alternative

9. A client you are assigned to care for is hearing impaired. Which is the most effective way to communicate with this client?
   A. Use a writing pad and gestures.
   B. Speak clearly and slowly.
   C. Use nonverbal communication.
   D. Describe loudly and carefully what you are doing.

10. Which nursing intervention would be the highest priority when caring for a client who is depressed?
    A. Form a good nurse–client relationship.
    B. Encourage the client to talk about his feelings of depression.
    C. Suggest that the client do an activity.
    D. Assess the client frequently for potential suicide.

◀ **NCLEX® Review Questions.** NCLEX®-style questions have been included at the end of each chapter and reflect the Practice Analysis of newly Licensed Registered Nurses upon which the NCLEX® is based. Answers with complete rationales are in the Answers Appendix.

QSEN Activity These activities help train students to think about the knowledge, skills, and attitudes that are integral to Quality and Safety Education for Nurses. ▶

Bibliography Opportunities for further research are provided at the end of each chapter. ▶

QSEN Activity

Domain: Communication
KSA: Attitude
Activity:

Have student(s) identify a particular clinical situation where the communication was not very effective, and perhaps the student wished it had gone another way. The scenario can be any dyad:

- Student nurse and client
- Student nurse and family member
- Student nurse and preceptor
- Student nurse and provider

Have the group reflect on how it could have been more effective. Role-play effective communication within the classroom using the techniques identified within the chapter.

Bibliography

Agency for Healthcare Research and Quality (AHRQ). (n.d.). TeamStepps: National implementation. Retrieved from http://teamstepps.ahrq.gov/

Amato-Vealey, E. J., Barba, M. P., & Vealey, R. J. (2008, Nov.). Hand-off communication: A requisite for perioperative patient safety. *AORN Journal, 88* (5), 763–770.

Baker, D. P., Gustafson, S., Beaubien, J. M., Salas, E., & Barch, P. (n.d.). Medical team training programs in health care. Retrieved from http://www.ahrq.gov/professionals/quality-patient-safety/patient-safety-resources/resources/advances-in-patient-safety/vol4/Baker.pdf

Blumenthal, J. A., Smith, P., & Benson, H. (2012, Jul.–Aug.). Opinion and evidence: Is exercise a viable treatment for depression? *ACSM's Health & Fitness, 16* (4), 14–21. doi: 10.1249/01.FIT.0000416000.09526.eb

Brown, A. (2014). U.S. Hispanic and Asian populations growing, but for different reasons. Pew Research Center. Retrieved from http://www.pewresearch.org/fact-tank/2014/06/26/u-s-hispanic-and-asian-populations-growing-but-for-different-reasons/

Census. (2012). http://www.census.gov/newsroom/releases/archives/population/cb13-112.html

Chen, K., Ku, Y., & Yang, H. (2012, Mar.). Violence in the nursing workplace—A descriptive correlational study in a public hospital. *Journal of Clinical Nursing, 22*(5–6), 798–805. doi:10.1111/j.1365-2702.2012.04251

Downey, L., Zun, L., & Burke, T. (2012). What constitutes a good hand off in the emergency department: A patient's perspective. *International Journal of Healthcare Quality Assurance, 26* (8), 760–767.

Office of Minority Health. (2012). National Standards for Culturally and Linguistically Appropriate Services (CLAS standards). Retrieved from https://www.thinkculturalhealth.hhs.gov/CLAS/Clas_Overview.asp

Schenker, Y., Karter, A. J., Schillinger, D. Warton, E. M., Adler, N. E., Moffet, H. H., & Fernandez, A. (2010, Nov.). The impact of limited English proficiency and physician language concordance on reports of clinical interactions among patients with diabetes: The DISTANCE study. *Patient Education and Counseling, 81*(2), 222–228.

Spector, R. E. (2013). *Cultural Diversity in Health and Illness* (8th ed.). Hoboken, NJ: Prentice Hall.

Contents

Chapter 1
Professional Nursing

 ## Learning Objectives

1.1 Discuss what is meant by the concept "professional role of the nurse."

1.2 Discuss the ANA Code of Ethics.

1.3 Define professional nursing.

1.4 Define the term *accountable*.

1.5 Identify the guidelines that will assist the nurse to convey nursing competence to the clients.

1.6 Define the purpose of "A Code of Academic and Clinical Conduct."

1.7 List three ways you can assist the client to assume and adapt to the client role.

1.8 Describe Core Measures, the Joint Commission Standards, and National Patient Safety Goals and how they are developed and utilized in practice.

1.9 Describe the purpose of the Nurse Practice Act.

1.10 Discuss major sections of the Nurse Practice Act.

1.11 Define the term *nurse licensure*.

1.12 State four functions of the Board of Registered Nursing.

1.13 Discuss four grounds for licensure revocation for professional misconduct.

1.14 Explain the legal issues of drug administration.

1.15 Discuss the role of HIPAA in health care.

1.16 Describe what is meant by clients' rights and the Patient Care Partnership brochure.

1.17 Explain what is meant by advance directives.

1.18 List four actions or guidelines that you need to complete to prepare for daily client care.

1.19 Describe the steps of planning for client care.

Chapter Outline

Terminology

Accountable answerable for one's own behavior and the nursing care one provides or delegates.

Advance directive a medical directive related either to treatment (such as a living will) or to appointment of a legal representative (such as durable power of attorney for health care). It allows clients to make legal decisions about future medical treatment. It is written and signed before care becomes necessary and takes effect when the client becomes incapacitated.

Asepsis prevention of infection; medical asepsis ("clean technique") is absence of pathogens; surgical asepsis ("sterile technique") is absence of all organisms.

Client chart information about a client contained on forms or computer screens, depending on the documentation systems used in the healthcare facility.

Code of ethics set of formal guidelines that assist decision making and choice of actions; a set of values, beliefs, goals, and obligations of an organization or profession.

Core Measures a common set of measurement specifications to use at healthcare facilities as an improvement tool to track evidence-based, scientifically researched standards of care.

Durable power of attorney for health care legal document, prepared and signed while the client is competent, giving power to make healthcare decisions to a designated individual in the event the client is unable to make competent decisions.

HIPAA the Health Insurance Portability and Accountability Act, enacted to protect the individual's health information and to set standards to control how health information is used and disclosed.

Living will advance directive that indicates the client's wishes regarding prolonging life using life support measures, refusing or stopping medical interventions, or making decisions about his or her medical care when diagnosed with a terminal or permanent unconscious condition.

Malpractice professional misconduct that is an unreasonable lack of skill or fidelity in professional duties; bad, wrong, or injurious treatment of a client resulting in injury, unnecessary suffering, or death whether caused by lack of skill or criminal intent.

National Patient Safety Goals (NPSGs) national standards set by The Joint Commission to promote improvement in client safety in healthcare settings.

Negligence failure to act as a reasonable and prudent individual (or nurse) would act under similar circumstances; negligence consists of the following elements: a duty owed to the client, a breach of that duty, damages to the client, and a causal relationship between the damages and the breach of duty.

Nurse licensure the right to practice nursing of an individual who holds an active nursing license issued by the state in which she or he intends to work.

Nurse Practice Act state law that defines professional nursing practice and recommends actions the nurse can practice independently and actions that require a physician's order before completion; Nurse Practice Acts vary greatly by state.

Professional Role

As you enter the profession of nursing, you will experience some of the most frustrating and some of the most rewarding situations of your life. To decrease the frustrations and increase the positive experiences, this chapter introduces you to the role of the nurse. Emphasis is placed on those procedures that will assist you to become a functioning member of the healthcare team, even with limited experience.

The information in this chapter will help you through the first few critical days of your clinical experience. In addition, legal aspects of the nursing profession are discussed to help you become aware of the far-reaching consequences of nursing actions. Clients' rights and the Nurse Practice Act (also called the Nursing Practice Act in some states) are also presented for your information.

Ethics is an integral part of the foundation of nursing. Nursing is concerned with the welfare of the sick, injured, and vulnerable as well as with social justice. Nurses provide health care to both individuals and the community by preventing illness, alleviating suffering, and promoting, protecting, and restoring health for individuals, families, groups, and communities. A **code of ethics** describes the primary goals, values, and obligations of the profession.

Nurses must function within the nurses' Code of Ethics. The Code of Ethics is a set of formal guidelines for governing professional action. It assists the nurse in problem solving where judgment is required. More emphasis is now being placed on the professional organizations to uphold the Code of Ethics and to admonish those nurses who violate the code. The Code of Ethics was revised in June 2008 by the American Nurses Association (ANA) (Box 1-1 ■). The Code should be reviewed as you progress in the program. The National Student Nurses' Association, Inc., also developed a Code of Academic and Clinical Conduct in April 2001 and updated it in 2009. The Code (discussed later) provides guidance for nursing students in the personal development of an ethical foundation as both a nurse and human being.

Definition of Professional Nursing

The American Nurses Association in 2003 defined professional nursing as the protection, promotion, and optimization of health and abilities, prevention of illness and injury, alleviation of suffering through the diagnosis and treatment of human responses, and advocacy in the care of individuals, families, communities, and populations.

Box 1-1 AMERICAN NURSES ASSOCIATION: CODE OF ETHICS FOR NURSES

1. The nurse in all professional relationships practices with compassion and respect for the inherent dignity, worth, and uniqueness of every individual, unrestricted by considerations of social or economic status, personal attributes, or the nature of health problems.

2. The nurse's primary commitment is to the client, whether an individual, family, group, or community.

3. The nurse promotes, advocates for, and strives to protect the health, safety, and rights of the client.

4. The nurse is responsible and accountable for individual nursing practice and determines the appropriate delegations of tasks consistent with the nurse's obligation to provide optimum client care.

5. The nurse owes the same duties to self as to others, including the responsibility to preserve integrity and safety, to maintain competence, and to continue personal and professional growth.

6. The nurse participates in establishing, maintaining, and improving healthcare environments and conditions of employment conducive to the provision of quality health care and consistent with the values of the profession through individual and collective action.

7. The nurse participates in the advancement of the profession through contributions to practice, education, administration, and knowledge development.

8. The nurse collaborates with other health professionals and the public in promoting community, national, and international efforts to meet health needs.

9. The profession of nursing, as represented by associations and their members, is responsible for articulating nursing values, for maintaining the integrity of the profession and its practice, and for shaping social policy.

Source: Fowler (2008)

ANA's Nursing's Social Policy Statement, second edition (American Nursing Association, 2010), identifies six essential features of professional nursing. These features include the following:

- Provision of a caring relationship that facilitates health and healing
- Attention to the range of human experiences and responses to health and illness within the physical and social environments
- Integration of assessment data with knowledge gained from an appreciation of the client or the group
- Application of scientific knowledge to the processes of diagnosis and treatment through the use of judgment and critical thinking
- Advancement of professional nursing knowledge through scholarly inquiry
- Influence on social and public policy to promote social justice
- Assurance of safe, quality, and evidence-based practice

Assuming the Nursing Role

Your actions and words as a professional influence the way the client will judge your level of competence and the role of nurses as professionals. This, in turn, will influence the client's ability to adapt to the healthcare facility. Assuming a professional role means that you behave as a professional. Following the guidelines below will assist you to convey nursing competence, not only to clients, but also to your peers and other nursing staff.

- Always dress neatly in appropriate, clean attire, and follow the dress code of your school or facility.
- Cover visible tattoos and body piercing with clothing or dressing according to nursing program policies and procedures.
- Keep hair off collar and cut fingernails short. Wear clear nail polish, not colored polish. Synthetic nails are discouraged as potential sites that could harbor bacteria and fungus.
- Speak in correct English without slang or inappropriate language, using medical terminology appropriate to the situation.
- Relate to the clients as worthwhile individuals who deserve respect and consideration. Call the client by his or her surname, and use the appropriate title (Mr., Ms., Miss, Mrs.). Do not use first names or nicknames (such as "grannie" or "sweetie").
- Do not "talk down to" or patronize the client. Remember that the client knows more about his or her own body, symptoms, feelings, and responses than anyone else. Listen and pay attention to what the client says about himself or herself or the underlying feelings that are not expressed in words.
- Remain in a professional role at all times. Do not socialize with the clients. Clients should view you as a knowledgeable professional who brings healing, caring, and teaching roles to the relationship.
- Use yourself as a therapeutic tool to convey caring and healing. Use body language to reinforce honest and direct verbalization, not to contradict it.
- Be **accountable** (answerable for your behavior and nursing actions and the nursing care you are expected to provide). If you do not understand what is expected, seek assistance from a staff member or your instructor. Your responsibility is to remain reliable, honest, and trustworthy in administering nursing care.
- Maintain client confidentiality. Do not talk about clients in public areas. Follow HIPAA standards (see HIPAA section later in this chapter).

The National Student Nurses' Association, Inc., has developed a Code of Academic and Clinical Conduct (Box 1-2 ■). The Code is based on an understanding that to practice nursing as a student is an agreement to uphold the trust that society has placed in the student. Students have a responsibility to learn the academic theory and clinical skills needed to provide nursing care. The clinical setting presents unique challenges and responsibilities to nurses caring for clients in a variety of healthcare environments.

Box 1-2 **A CODE OF ACADEMIC AND CLINICAL CONDUCT**

As students are involved in the clinical and academic environments, we believe that ethical principles are a necessary guide to professional development. Therefore, within these environments, we:

1. Advocate for the rights of all clients.

2. Maintain client confidentiality.

3. Take appropriate action to ensure the safety of clients, self, and others.

4. Provide care for the client in a timely, compassionate, and professional manner.

5. Communicate client care in a truthful, timely, and accurate manner.

6. Actively promote the highest level of moral and ethical principles and accept responsibility for our actions.

7. Promote excellence in nursing by encouraging lifelong learning and professional development.

8. Treat others with respect and promote an environment that respects human rights, values, and choice of cultural and spiritual beliefs.

9. Collaborate in every reasonable manner with the academic faculty and clinical staff to ensure the highest quality of client care.

10. Use every opportunity to improve faculty and clinical staff understanding of the learning needs of nursing students.

11. Encourage faculty, clinical staff, and peers to mentor nursing students.

12. Refrain from performing any technique or procedure for which the student has not been adequately trained.

13. Refrain from any deliberate action or omission of care in the academic or clinical setting that creates unnecessary risk of injury to the client, self, or others.

14. Assist the staff nurse or preceptor in ensuring that there is full disclosure and that proper authorizations are obtained from clients regarding any form of treatment or research.

15. Abstain from the use of alcoholic beverages or any substances that impair judgment in the academic and clinical setting.

16. Strive to achieve and maintain an optimal level of personal health.

17. Support access to treatment and rehabilitation for students who are experiencing impairments related to substance abuse and mental or physical health issues.

18. Uphold school policies and regulations related to academic and clinical performance, reserving the right to challenge and critique rules and regulations as per school grievance policy.

Source: National Student Nurses' Association, Inc. (2009)

The Client Role

Assisting the client to adapt to hospitalization and ensuring that the client is as comfortable as possible will assist him or her to be less anxious and more open to receiving treatment during hospitalization. The nurse can assist in adaptation by understanding that all clients have individual needs, concerns, and perceptions that require discussion and planning as they take on the role of client in the healthcare setting. You must accept the client's perceptions of his or her new surroundings. If possible, try to accommodate client's wishes, assess previous concepts of illness and hospitalization, and discuss previous experiences. Be aware that anxiety is a natural reaction to an unfamiliar setting, to new procedures, and to new people. If, for example, a client is extremely fatigued or overwhelmed by traveling to the hospital and the admission procedure, you can help him or her adapt to the surroundings, regain a sense of control and identity, and accept the changed circumstances.

Another way to assist the client to retain his or her identity and uniqueness is to communicate with the client as an individual (Figure 1-1 ■). Ask questions and observe verbal responses as well as nonverbal cues. Provide ways to care for a client's personal possessions, clothing, and physical comfort so that the client adapts more easily to the change in environment and feels more secure and in control.

Be aware that the medical condition is only one part of the client's life and that the changes that have led up to admission affect other areas of his or her well-being. Clients may have concerns about new routines, financial matters, their families, or their future. By responding to clients' total needs at the time of admission, you can help them establish a positive attitude toward their total care.

Acknowledge and accept any statements or behavior the client uses to adapt to his or her new surroundings. Even though various cultures and groups differ in their response to illness and some responses may differ from your personal beliefs, acknowledge the client's individuality. These specific groups often utilize their own identified and respected traditional healthcare providers. Concepts of illness, wellness, and health are part of the client's total belief system and must be recognized by the nurse as part of what makes

FIGURE 1-1 Relate to clients as worthwhile individuals who deserve respect and consideration.

the client an individual. Support the client's beliefs and behavior as long as they do not increase the risk of injury or illness. Be sensitive to any past healthcare experiences that may influence the client's feelings at the time of admission. A prior experience in the hospital may determine how a client responds to the current environment and how he or she accepts treatment. If they are present and the client is negative or fearful, allow time for the client to discuss these feelings. Try to answer questions they may have about this hospitalization in light of earlier admissions.

Standards and Statutes

Legal issues and regulations play a dominant role in nursing practice today. The law provides a framework for establishing nursing actions in the care of clients. Laws determine and set boundaries and maintain a standard of nursing practice. The Joint Commission sets standards that are the basis of an objective evaluation process to help healthcare organizations measure, assess, and improve performance. The standards focus on important client, individual, or resident care and organizational functions that are essential to providing safe, high-quality care. The standards are developed with input from healthcare professionals and each provides expert data, research, and documentation.

Two of the major standards that relate to safe, effective care are the **National Patient Safety Goals (NPSGs)** and the Core Measure Sets. In 2002, the Joint Commission established the first set of NPSGs. Updated NPSGs are available on the Joint Commission website. They are summarized in Chapter 7, Table 7-1, National Patient Safety Goals.

Core Measure Sets were established in 1999. The Joint Commission worked with the Centers for Medicare and Medicaid Service (CMS) to create one common set of measurement specifications to use as an improvement tool. **Core Measures** track a variety of evidence-based, scientifically researched standards. Data are collected among hospitals for clients with specific reportable conditions. This information assists the Hospital Board of Directors and the community to track the quality of care being provided by hospitals.

The initial data researched for core measurement areas for hospitals included acute myocardial infarction (AMI) and heart failure (HF) (Nix, 2009). Core measures are being studied in both adult and pediatric clients. The CMS is not requiring the submission of a core set of clinical quality measures (CQMs). Instead, they are encouraging professionals to report from the recommended core set by selecting the CQMs appropriate to the scope of their practice and client population (Nix, 2009).

The Nurse Practice Act

The **Nurse Practice Act** defines professional nursing practice and recommends those actions that the nurse can practice independently and those actions that require a physician's order before completion. Individual states allow

other healthcare providers with prescriptive rights to write orders; these include nurse practitioners, physician assistants, dentists, and so on.

Each state has the authority to regulate and administrate healthcare professionals. Although the provisions of Nurse Practice Acts are quite similar from state to state, it is imperative that the nurse know the licensing requirements and the grounds for license revocation defined by the state in which he or she works.

Legal and ethical standards for nurses are complicated by a myriad of federal and state statutes and the continually changing interpretation of them by the courts of law. Nurses are faced today with the threat of legal action based on negligence, malpractice, invasion of privacy, and other grounds. This chapter covers the basic legal issues and topics, from clients' rights and nurses' liability in the administration of drugs to grounds for proceedings to address professional misconduct.

The Nurse Practice Act is a series of statutes enacted by a state to regulate the practice of nursing in that state. Subjects covered by Nurse Practice Acts include definition of the scope of practice, education, licensure, and grounds for disciplinary actions. Nurse Practice Acts are quite similar throughout the United States, but the professional nurse is held legally responsible for the specific requirements for licensure and regulations of practice as defined by the state in which she or he works.

The responsibilities of the professional nurse involve a level of performance for a defined range of healthcare services. These services include assessment, planning, implementation, and evaluation of nursing action, as well as teaching and related services, such as counseling. Skills and functions that professional nurses perform in daily practice include:

- Providing direct and indirect client care services.
- Performing and delivering basic healthcare services.
- Implementing testing and prevention procedures.
- Observing signs and symptoms of illness.
- Administering treatments per physician's order.
- Monitoring treatment reactions and responses.
- Administering medications per physician's order.
- Monitoring medication responses and any side effects.
- Observing general physical and mental conditions of individual clients.
- Observing client and family teaching.
- Acting as a client advocate when needed.
- Documenting nursing care.
- Supervising allied nursing personnel.
- Coordinating members of the healthcare team.

Nurse Licensure

The authorization to practice nursing is defined legally as the right to practice nursing by an individual who holds an active license issued by the state in which she or he intends to work. The **nurse licensure** process is administered by the Board of Registered Nursing, frequently called the BRN (or BON) (Box 1-3 ■). This board may also grant endorsement or reciprocity to an applicant who holds a current license in another state. The applicant for RN licensure must have attended an accredited school of nursing, be a qualified nursing professional or paraprofessional, or have met specific prerequisites if licensed in a foreign country. Paraprofessionals can sit for the NCLEX if they meet all the requirements (one example is a medic, in some states).

Standards of Clinical Nursing Practice

The American Nurses Association first published Standards of Clinical Nursing Practice in 1973. The standards were revised in 1991 and updated in 2010 (Box 1-4 ■). The standards of practice consist of two segments: ten Standards of Care, which describe the standards of clinical nursing practice based on the nursing process, and nine Standards of Professional Performance. These nine standards describe a competent level of behavior in the professional role. Within the guidelines of professional performance, the central theme is caring for clients from every aspect. Based on the guidelines, the nurse can further define his or her role as the one individual who has the ability to assist clients in increasing their mental and physical wellness by coordinating, educating, and working with cohorts to promote a caring and supportive environment.

These standards have shaped nursing practice and have helped both nurses and others understand what nursing is and does (see example in Box 1-5 ■). The standards describe a competent level of professional nursing care and professional performance common to all nurses engaged in clinical practice. This includes descriptions of the responsibility and accountability of the professional.

The standards apply to all registered nurses working in clinical practice regardless of clinical specialty, practice setting, or educational preparation. Nurses in specialty nursing practice, such as critical care nursing or neonatal nursing, practice under standards that further define the responsibilities in these settings. The nursing specialties and appropriate groups, with the American Nurses Association, determine these standards.

Nurses practicing at an advanced level are accountable for meeting and maintaining the basic standards of clinical nursing practice in addition to the Scope and Standards of Advanced Practice Registered Nursing.

Liability and Legal Issues

Each state defines and regulates the grounds for professional misconduct. Even though many states have similar standards, the practicing nurse must know how his or her state defines professional misconduct. The penalties for professional misconduct include probation, censure and reprimand, suspension of license, or revocation of license. The state's Board of Registered Nursing (BRN/BON) has the authority to impose any of these penalties for professional misconduct. Any one of the following actions would be considered professional misconduct:

- Obtaining an RN license through misrepresentation or fraudulent methods
- Giving false information on application for license
- Practicing in an incompetent or gross negligent manner
- Practicing when ability to practice is severely impaired
- Being habitually under the influence of drugs and/or alcohol
- Furnishing controlled substances to himself or herself or to another individual
- Impersonating another certified or licensed practitioner or allowing another individual to use his or her license for the purpose of nursing
- Being convicted of or committing an act constituting a crime under federal or state law
- Refusing to provide healthcare services on the grounds of race, color, creed, national origin, religion, or beliefs different from your own
- Permitting or aiding an unlicensed individual to perform activities requiring a license
- Practicing nursing while license is suspended
- Practicing medicine without a license
- Procuring, aiding, or offering to assist a criminal abortion
- Holding oneself out to the public as a "nurse practitioner" without being certified by the BRN/BON as a nurse practitioner

Drugs and the Nurse

In their daily work, most nurses handle a wide variety of drugs. Failure to give the correct medication or improper handling of drugs may result in serious problems for the nurse due to strict federal and state statutes relating to drugs. The Comprehensive Drug Abuse Prevention Act of 1970 provides the fundamental federal regulations for compounding, selling, and dispensing narcotics, stimulants, depressants, and other controlled items. Each state has a similar set of regulations for the same purpose (Box 1-6 ■).

Noncompliance with federal or state drug regulations can result in liability. Violation of the state drug regulations or licensing laws is grounds for the Board of Registered Nursing to initiate disciplinary action.

Negligence/Malpractice

The doctrine of **negligence** rests on the duty of every individual to exercise due care in his or her conduct toward others from which injury may result. Negligence includes doing something that the reasonable and prudent individual would not do. Anyone, including nonmedical individuals, can be liable for negligence. Professionals (nurses) are held to a higher standard of care than nonprofessionals. The

Box 1-6 GUIDELINES FOR DRUG ADMINISTRATION

- Nurses must not administer a specific drug unless allowed to do so by the particular state's Nurse Practice Act.
- Nurses must not administer any drug without a specific healthcare provider's order.
- Nurses are to take every safety precaution in whatever they are doing.
- Nurses are to be certain that employer's policy allows them to administer a specific drug.
- Nurses must not administer a controlled substance if the physician's order is outdated.
- A drug may not lawfully be administered unless all the above items are in effect.
- Nurses are not permitted to fill prescriptions and in most states cannot write prescriptions, except in the case of nurse practitioners in some states.
- General rules for drug dispensing:
  - Check two forms of client identification before administering medications. Use Bar Code Administration System, if available.
  - Never leave prepared medicines unattended.
  - Always report errors immediately.
  - Send labeled bottles or packages that are unintelligible back to the pharmacist for relabeling.
  - Store internal and external medicines separately if possible.

doctrine of negligence consists of the following elements: a duty owed to the client, a breach of that duty, damages to the client, and a causal relationship between the damages and the breach of duty. To find liability, it is necessary to identify a breach of duty to act with care, or a failure to act as a reasonable and prudent individual (or nurse) would act under similar circumstances.

The standards referenced above form the basis for negligence or malpractice. **Malpractice** addresses a professional standard of care as well as the professional status of the caregiver. To be liable for malpractice, the individual committing the civil wrong must be a professional. Courts define malpractice as any professional misconduct, unreasonable lack of skill, or fidelity in professional or judiciary duties that results in unnecessary suffering, injury, or death to the individual.

Gross negligence is the intentional failure to perform a duty in reckless disregard of the consequences affecting the client. It is viewed as a gross lack of care to such a level as to be considered willful and wanton. Gross negligence can be due to improper use of restraints, client falls, or medication errors that lead to a client injury.

Criminal negligence also consists of a duty on the part of the nurse and an act that is the proximate cause of the injury or death of a client. This type of negligence is usually defined by statute and as such is punishable as a crime. The punishable act represents a flagrant and reckless disregard to the safety of others and/or a willful disregard to the injury liable to follow so as to convert the act into a crime when it results in personal injury or death. One is not "negligent" unless he or she fails to exercise the degree of reasonable care that would be exercised by an individual of ordinary prudence under all the existing circumstances in view of probable danger of injury. The death or serious injury of a client after a medication or IV error can result in criminal negligence.

Malpractice is any professional misconduct that is an unreasonable lack of skill or fidelity in professional duties. In a more specific sense it means bad, wrong, or injurious treatment of a client resulting in injury, unnecessary suffering, or death to a client, proceeding from ignorance; carelessness; lack of professional skill; disregard of established rules, protocols, principles, or procedures; neglect; or a malicious or criminal intent.

Civil Law	Criminal Law
Contract	Assault
Unintentional tort	Battery
Intentional tort	Murder
Negligence	Manslaughter

Malpractice is a cause of action for which damages are allowed.

It is the nurse's legal duty to provide competent, reasonable care to clients. To ensure that this occurs, the nurse must know the standards of care, develop consistent patterns of practice that meet the standards, and reflect his or her action in accurate and complete documentation. Legal action against nurses has been increasing over the last decade. Nursing actions that constitute a breach of a standard of care that can lead to injury of a client include such actions as not inserting a Foley catheter correctly, not taking appropriate steps to decrease a client's temperature, not reporting unusual or worsening condition of the client to his or her physician, and not preventing falls. All of these situations can lead to malpractice suits.

Most lawsuits against nurses are for alleged violations of tort law. A tort is defined as an action or omission that harms someone. Malpractice refers to a tort committed by a professional acting in his or her professional capacity.

Legal doctrine holds that an employer may also be liable for negligent acts of employees in the course and scope of employment. Physicians, hospitals, clinics, and other employers may be held liable for negligent acts of their employees. This doctrine does not support acts of gross negligence or acts that are outside the scope of employment.

HIPAA

The Health Insurance Portability and Accountability Act (**HIPAA**), enacted into law in 1996, requires the Secretary of Health and Human Services (HHS) to devise standards to improve Medicare and Medicaid programs and the efficiency and effectiveness of the healthcare system. It ensures continuing healthcare insurance if the client has had existing group insurance and the client either changes or loses his or her job, proposes standards for electronic transactions and security signatures, and ensures privacy of individual health information.

The privacy rule component went into effect on April 14, 2003. The Privacy Rule applies to health plans, to healthcare clearinghouses, and to any healthcare provider who transmits health insurance information in electronic form. This is based on adopted HIPAA standards. A major purpose of the Privacy Rule is to define and limit the circumstances in which an individual's protected health information may be used or disclosed by the entities listed above. Information is disclosed only if allowed by the Privacy Rule.

Under this act, the client can request copies of his or her medical record and request that corrections be made if he or she identifies errors. The act specifies that personal healthcare information may not be used for any purpose not related to health care. The act also provides for client information to be given only to the client, or his or her representative, unless directed to do otherwise.

Compliance with HIPAA regulations is mandatory. Noncompliance can lead to civil penalties up to $25,000 per calendar year for multiple violations of a single standard. There are also penalties from $50,000 to $250,000 and/or imprisonment up to 10 years for other violations of the act.

For additional information on HIPAA, refer to HIPAA Guidelines on the United States Department of Health and Human Services website.

Medicare Prescription Act

The Medicare Prescription Drug Improvement and Modernization Act of 2003 was signed into law on December 8, 2003, although it was not enacted until 2005. This law brings affordable health care and prescription drug coverage to all Medicare recipients, older adults, low-income individuals, and individuals with disabilities; expanded health plan options; improved healthcare access to rural Americans; and preventative care services such as mammograms. A prescription drug plan was made available in 2006 for low-income individuals. This is the first innovative change to the Medicare program since its inception in 1965. There are still proposed changes regarding the legislative healthcare tax credits and expansion of tax-free medical savings accounts. The Affordable Care Act makes some changes in Medicare but does not replace it.

Clients' Rights and Responsibilities

State and federal regulations governing healthcare facilities mandate that certain rights be afforded to clients receiving health care. Hospitals and healthcare facilities must have established policies that discuss clients' rights and how staff members are to adhere to them. The American Hospital Association (AHA) distributes "The Patient Care Partnership" brochure to all clients (Box 1-7 ■). This brochure describes what to expect during the hospital stay, the client's rights and privacy, and a short definition of a **living will** and **advance directives**. The AHA directs clients to the individual healthcare facility for further information.

Because clients' rights may conflict with nursing functions, nurses should be familiar with the key elements of these rights. It is important to remember that within a healthcare system, all clients retain their basic constitutional rights, such as freedom of expression, due process of law, freedom from cruel and inhumane punishment, equal protection, and so forth. Clients also have the right to know the identity of all healthcare providers and others involved in their care, including student nurses. All healthcare workers must wear a name badge indicating their title (e.g., Jane Doe, Student Nurse). The name of the nursing program is also included on the name badge. Most badges include a photo ID in addition to the name.

Under the "The Patient Care Partnership" brochure, hospitals must provide a foundation for understanding and respecting the rights and responsibilities of clients, their families, physicians, and other caregivers. The hospital must ensure and respect the role of clients in decision making about treatment choices and other aspects of their care. There must be a sensitivity to cultural, racial, linguistic, religious, age, and gender differences. In addition, the needs of individuals with disabilities must be considered when providing healthcare services. Each hospital is encouraged to tailor its bill of rights to its particular community and client population. Individualization to the community ensures that the families and their specific rights are considered when the bill of rights is written.

Clients have a responsibility for their role in utilizing healthcare facilities. Their responsibilities include providing the physician with a complete history, relevant clinical manifestations, current medications, and herbal remedies. The client is responsible for asking questions and informing the physician of changes in clinical manifestations or general medical situations. Clients also need to respect the hospital personnel and treat hospital property and equipment with respect.

Consent to Receive Health Services

There are two major forms of consent signed by clients in a healthcare facility. The first consent is completed at the time of admission; the client signs the form in the admissions office or in the emergency department, wherever the admission is initiated. This agreement usually indicates that the client has agreed to such things as medical treatment, x-ray examinations, blood transfusions, and injections. The second type of consent is for invasive testing procedures, such as a liver biopsy, surgery, special studies involving contrast media, or other treatments in which there are risks associated with the procedure.

Consent is the client's approval to have his or her body touched by specific individuals, such as doctors, nurses, and laboratory technicians. Informed consent refers to the process of providing information before asking the client to agree to treatment, such as tests and surgery. Informed consent ensures that the client understands the intended outcome and the potential harmful results. Once informed consent is given, the client may still rescind consent either verbally or in writing.

The authority to sign a consent form must be given by a mentally competent adult. Adults must give permission for children under 18 years of age. Court-authorized individuals may give consent for mentally incompetent adults. In emergency situations, if the client is in immediate danger of serious harm or death, action may be taken to preserve life without the client's consent.

The practitioner who will perform the procedure is legally responsible for obtaining the client's informed consent. The nurse's liability in terms of consent is to ensure that the client is fully informed before being asked to sign a consent form. The physician, nurse, or other healthcare personnel must inform the client of any potentially harmful effects of the treatment. If this is not done, it may result in the nurse being held personally liable. The nurse must respect the right of a mentally competent adult client to refuse health care; however, a life-threatening situation may alter the client's right to refuse treatment. In life-threatening emergencies, informed consent may not be required, because the law assumes a client will want treatment to save his or her life. The practitioner therefore intervenes appropriately to save the client's life regardless of whether informed consent was obtained.

Confidentiality

As stated earlier, clients are protected by law (invasion of privacy) against unauthorized release of personal clinical data, such as symptoms, diagnoses, and treatments. Nurses, as well as other healthcare personnel, may be held personally liable for invasion of privacy, should litigation arise from the unauthorized release of client data. Advances in technology, including computerized medical databases, the Internet, and telehealth, pose potential (unintentional) breaches of confidentiality and privacy. Changes in technology have changed not only the delivery of health care, but also the system used to record and retrieve health information.

The computer, fax machine, and phone calls between facilities and agencies leave the client at risk for information dissemination to unintended sources. Information is readily available to anyone walking by a fax machine or a computer. Confidential information, however, may be released with the client's consent. Information release is mandatory when ordered by a court or when state statutes require reporting child abuse, communicable diseases, or other incidents. Nurses have a legal and ethical responsibility to become familiar with their employer's policies and procedures regarding protection of clients' information.

Medical records are the key written account of such client information as signs and symptoms, diagnosis, treatment, and responses to treatment. Not only do these records document care given to clients, but they also provide effective means of communication among healthcare personnel. These records contain important data for insurance and other expense claims and are used in court in the event of litigation.

Healthcare professionals are becoming more aware of the implications of clients' rights as society in general becomes more aware of every human being's basic rights. Although there are still gaps in the legal process, many states are beginning to grapple with the status of laws applicable to clients who are hospitalized. It is essential that nurses be aware of the particular state's laws and statutes affecting clients and themselves. Nurses as well as physicians are accountable for their actions, and the threat of civil and criminal prosecution is becoming more prevalent. The American Nurses Association has developed a position statement supporting the principles of client privacy and confidentiality as a commitment to client advocacy. This statement is part of the Code of Ethics for Nurses (Privacy and Confidentiality Interpretive Statements 3.1 and 3.2).

Patient Self-Determination Act

The Patient Self-Determination Act of 1991 (PSDA) is a federal law that applies to all healthcare institutions receiving Medicaid funds. It imposes on the state and providers of health care, such as hospitals, nursing homes, hospices, home health agencies, and prepaid healthcare organizations, certain requirements concerning advance directives and an individual's rights under state law to make decisions concerning medical care. This includes the right to accept or refuse medical or surgical care. The act informs clients about existing rights but does not create new rights or change existing state law. The act did serve as an incentive for many states to pass **durable power of attorney for healthcare** statutes. It does not require clients to execute advance directives, but it does require that they be apprised and educated about advance directives. It also requires that assistance be offered in the execution of the advance directives if the client elects to do so. The PSDA defines an *advance directive* as a written instruction, such as a living will or durable power of attorney,

for health care. A competent adult can communicate preferences about future medical treatment through the advance directive. Clients must be provided written documentation regarding their rights to formulate advance directives. Clients must be made aware of their rights to make decisions about these issues on admission to all healthcare facilities and health maintenance organizations (HMOs); however, they are not required to sign an advance directive if they do not choose to do so. Client education regarding advance directives should be accomplished outside the acute care setting. The directives allow clients to control their own healthcare decisions, even if they become incapacitated in the future.

Advance Medical Directives

Advance medical directives (Box 1-8 ■) are of two types: treatment directives (such as living wills), and appointment directives (such as a durable power of attorney for health care). An advance medical directive is a document that allows clients to make legal decisions about how they wish to receive future medical treatment. It is written and signed before any such care becomes necessary. The document takes effect only when the client becomes incapacitated. The directives may be in the form of a living will or durable power of attorney. Within this document, the client may indicate the individual or individuals he or she wishes to make medical decisions in situations in which the client is unable to do so. An advance directive does not need to be written, reviewed, or signed by an attorney. It must, however, be signed and witnessed by two individuals, and the witnesses should not be hospital employees, relatives, or heirs to the estate. Copies of the document should be kept on file in the physician's office and the hospital. Advance directives vary among states, and therefore the nurse must be knowledgeable about the use and type of directives in the state in which he or she practices. Advance directives do not expire but should be evaluated frequently to ensure they are accurate. The directives need to follow HIPAA rules. If the directives were written before 2006, they should be reviewed and made up to date with current information.

Living Will A living will is a type of advance directive that indicates the client's wishes regarding prolonging life

---

Box 1-8 **ADVANCE DIRECTIVES**

An advance directive allows the client to participate in the following decisions:

- Choosing healthcare providers such as physicians and nurses
- Deciding who may have access to medical records
- Choosing the type of medical treatments the client desires
- Consenting to or refusing certain types of medical treatments
- Choosing the agent who will make decisions about the client's health care when the client is unable to do so

using life support measures, refusing or stopping medical interventions, or making decisions about his or her medical care when the client is diagnosed as having a terminal or permanent unconscious condition. It does not apply to any other healthcare decisions. Living wills are executed while the client is competent and able to make sound decisions. As conditions change, a living will needs to be evaluated for relevance. (States differ in their acceptance of living wills as legal documents.)

Durable Power of Attorney for Health Care   This legal document must be prepared and signed while the client is competent. The document gives power to make healthcare decisions to a designated individual (agent) in the event the client is unable to make competent decisions for himself or herself. The designated individual is obligated to follow the directives outlined in the document. The document gives the client's agent specific healthcare decisions or the authority to make any and all healthcare decisions the client would make if able. Decisions regarding withdrawing or using life support, organ donation, or consent to treatment or procedures are included in the directive. As long as the client is competent, the agent does not have the authority to make treatment decisions.

The major difference between living wills and the durable power of attorney is that the durable power of attorney is more flexible. A living will is used only if the client's condition is terminal or he or she is in a permanently unconscious state. A living will only allows the client to direct that life-sustaining treatments be withheld or withdrawn. The durable power of attorney is not limited to terminal or permanent unconscious conditions. It also addresses all types of healthcare decisions, including life-sustaining treatments.

Clients should be encouraged to carry a card in their wallet indicating that they have a living will and/or durable power of attorney on file. The name of their agent should be listed.

Do Not Resuscitate

Healthcare facilities must provide written information to clients concerning their right to make decisions regarding their care.

A "Do Not Resuscitate" (DNR; sometimes called "Do Not Attempt to Resuscitate" [DNAR]) order is another type of advance directive. A DNR is a request to not have cardiopulmonary resuscitation (CPR) if the client ceases to breathe or is unable to sustain a heartbeat. An advance directive form can be signed at any time before or during hospitalization. When signed, the physician places a DNR notation in the client's medical chart. (See Chapter 34.) In some facilities these orders are reviewed every 48 to 72 hours.

If a terminally ill client without a DNR order states that he or she does not want to be resuscitated in a crisis, document this information and state the client's level of orientation. Notify the physician and administration, legal services, or social services of the client's wishes.

Clinical Practice

Legal Issues

As a student nurse, you need to maintain a high standard of practice and protect yourself against legal problems. Most legal actions against nurses result from a claim that the nurse breached a standard of care that results in injury to the client. In order to prevent legal problems, the nurse must always do the following:

- Follow the steps of the nursing process.
- Administer medications following the seven rights of medication administration.
- Continually assess the client, clearly communicate changes in the client's condition to the appropriate individual, and then document findings on proper forms or computer screens (the medical record is a legal document).
- Follow hospital policies and procedures.
- Understand and use equipment safely and appropriately.

Constantly refer to these guidelines to protect the client from harm and to protect yourself from potential lawsuits.

Before your first clinical experience, you should review the most essential components of client care to enable you to practice safe and efficient nursing care. Laws in each state vary in relationship to how the law applies to your practice and the medical record; therefore, check that you are familiar with your individual state laws. Box 1-9 ■ lists classifications of law related to nursing.

Guidelines for clinical practice, the parts of a **client chart** or computer printout, communication techniques, principles of medical asepsis, a basic nursing assessment, and protocols for nursing care procedures are presented here to give you confidence and background information in providing nursing care.

Guidelines for Safe Clinical Practice

Before attempting to provide client care, you need to familiarize yourself with all aspects of the care the client requires. The following guidelines will assist you in this preparation. Usually, you will complete the preparation the night before you go to the clinical setting. If this is not possible, you need

---

Box 1-9 CLASSIFICATIONS OF LAW RELATED TO NURSING

Classification	Example
Constitutional	Clients' rights to equal treatment
Administrative	Licensure and the state BRN
Labor relations	Union negotiations
Contract	Relationship with employer
Criminal	Handling of narcotics
Tort	Reasonable and prudent client care
Medical malpractice	Warranty on medical equipment

to identify those aspects of preparation that will render you a safe practitioner.

- Obtain the clinical assignment in sufficient time to be able to prepare for safe practice.
- Read the client's chart or computer data and obtain information necessary to assist you in client care. This usually encompasses the following items: history and physical, physician's progress notes, graphic sheet, medication record, laboratory findings, nurses' notes or flow sheets or both, admissions database, client care plan, computer plan of care or Kardex card, and physician's orders. These documents are illustrated later in this chapter.
- Review all procedures that you will provide for the client. Use your skills and fundamentals books for your review.
- Research the medical diagnosis so that you are more aware of signs and symptoms the client may exhibit. Identify alterations from normal such as altered laboratory values, vital signs, and so forth.
- Research nursing diagnoses identified on the chart or potential diagnoses you identify from review of the chart. Your client care will focus on the nursing diagnoses and interventions associated with collaborative care.
- Research all medications you will administer to the client. Many instructors require that medication cards or documents be completed on all medications before administration.
- Plan your day's schedule by developing a time management plan to help keep you organized and to enable you to complete client care in a timely manner.
- Practice charting the procedures you will be administering so that you can identify appropriate vocabulary and include necessary information. Pertinent charting information is included with each procedure described in this text.
- Complete a clinical prep sheet as required by the instructor. The sheet usually has a section for all pertinent data.

Military Time The use of 24-hour or "military time" is common in healthcare facilities today (Figure 1-2 ■). One advantage of using this time frame is that the confusion of whether something is ordered or documented in the a.m. or p.m. is avoided. Military time describes time as a 24-hour clock rather than the standard 12-hour clock like your watch.

Midnight is identified as 2400, 1:00 a.m. is 0100, 3:00 p.m. is 1500, and so on. Review both the 24-hour clock and the chart to acquaint yourself with this method of keeping time.

Use of Electronics in the Clinical Setting

Students are generally adept in the use of electronic devices such as digital notebooks, tablets, and smartphones, especially as they have pocket drug guides, diagnostic test guides, and clinical calculators contained within them. Increasingly, facilities have computers at the client's bedside for entering data. Students should ensure that electronic devices and the computer they are using are compatible.

HIPAA (see section about HIPAA in this chapter) requires that healthcare workers recognize and protect oral, written, and electronic information that could reveal a client's identity and health-related information. This information is referred to as PHI (protected health information).

HIPAA has developed guidelines for using electronic devices safely. HIPAA recommends that the client's name or any identifying data not be input into the device. Personal demographics or client identifiers such as history and physical findings, lab data, physical data, and phone numbers must be input using passwords only. If identifying data must be input into the device, the nurse needs to utilize the "security" feature, which requires a password to enter the system. Most nursing students will not use this type of data entry. It is more usual for a home health nurse to need the personal identifiers.

Providing Client Care

Students prepare for clinical practice before coming to the nursing unit. Information regarding client needs and care is provided through shift report and an individualized, in-depth client report by the team leader or preceptor. Each hospital has a method for presenting the report. In some facilities, the offgoing shift tapes a report that is listened to by the oncoming staff. Other nursing units give a verbal report in which they review the information obtained by the previous shift. Facilities where primary nursing is practiced have a one-to-one report between the oncoming nurse and the offgoing nurse for a specific group of clients. At this time, a worksheet is completed that lists times for treatments and medications.

Following the report, the team leader or the preceptor nurse goes over all aspects of the care the student will deliver for the client. This is the time to ask questions regarding policy or procedure for the nursing unit or the client.

Essential Nurse Actions

The following outline of client care will assist you in planning your nursing care for the day. Before you begin client care, you need to review the client's profile or computer plan of care and check that all medications are available in the computer workstation on wheels (WOW), Pyxis medication management system, or medication cart.

24-HOUR CLOCK

12-hour clock	24-hour clock
12 midnight	2400
1:30 AM	0130
1:59 AM	0159
12 noon	1200
2:18 PM	1418
7:30 PM	1930
9:00 PM	2100

3:30 PM standard time or 1530 military time.

FIGURE 1-2 Clock showing 24-hour designation.

FIGURE 1-3 Electronic health record showing computer-generated client profile.

Source: From Cerner electronic health record. © Cerner corporation. Pearson has restricted permission to reproduce and distribute this copyrighted work. Further reproduction or distribution is strictly prohibited without written consent of Cerner Corporation.

1. Perform hand hygiene.
2. Gather equipment, such as a stethoscope, sphygmomanometer, thermometer, and linen.
3. Check two forms of client identification. There are three accepted client identifiers: client's name, client's date of birth, and medical record number. Two of these must be used to identify a client.
4. Introduce yourself to the client and explain the nursing care you will be giving.
5. Check if the client has any preference for the order in which the care is to be given when possible.
6. Complete a nursing assessment. You may use the basic nursing assessment outlined in this chapter as a guide if your instructor does not have one she or he prefers you to use.
7. Document your findings as you are completing the physical assessment, and enter them in the nurses' notes section of the chart or on the flow sheet or in the computerized documentation system.
8. Take vital signs if it is the policy of the unit. In some facilities, nursing assistants take vital signs, while nursing staff receives report.
9. If using a handheld device to enter client data, follow HIPAA guidelines specific to such devices.
10. Don gloves (if appropriate) and complete all nursing interventions, and document the findings immediately after completion.
11. Administer all medications, including checking two identifiers, according to policies and procedures in the healthcare facility. If gloves were used, remove and wash hands.
12. Document medication administration in the appropriate place, and observe for signs of side effects or unusual findings.
13. During your nursing care, practice good communication techniques.
14. Complete all charting per facility policy.
15. Terminate the interaction with the client.
16. Report off to the appropriate individual.
17. Perform hand hygiene after providing nursing care and before leaving the nursing unit.

Client's Forms

Become familiar with each form or computer screen, its placement in the chart or computer, and the information that it contains. Brief examples of some computer screens are included in this chapter, and examples of these forms are included in Chapter 3.

Day 3 POD 2	Day 4 POD 3	Day 5 POD 4
• **q 8 hr.** ✓ Basic assessment, CMS, Drsg, I&O, SPO₂, VS, IV site, skin assessment. • ✓ Homan sign. HV dc'd. • Oxygen protocol.	• **q 8 hr.** ✓ Basic assessment, CMS, Drsg, I&O, past or present IV site healing, skin assessment, Homan sign. • Oxygen protocol.	• **q 8 hr.** ✓ Basic assessment, skin, assessment, CMS, Drsg, I&O, Homan sign. • Oxygen protocol. • ✓ past or present IV site healing.
• ↑ gait training. • Ambulate BID if able.	• Ambulate BID. • PT/Nursing.	• Ambulate BID. • PT/Nursing.
• TED/SCD, I.S., TCDB, Foley remains if needed or until Epidural dc'd. • Hip Precaution for hemiarthroplasty only	• TED/SCD • DC Foley. • TCDB, especially prior to SpO₂. • Hip Precaution for hemiarthroplasty only	• TED/SCD. • TCDB. • Hip Precaution for hemiarthroplasty only
• Stool softener, Iron supp. BID (hold if GI upset). Cathartic if no BM. • Anticoagulant.	• Stool softener, Iron supp. BID (hold if GI upset). • Anticoagulant.	• Stool softener, Iron supp. BID (hold if GI upset). • Anticoagulant.
• IV TKO, IVL, or DC if not needed (leave IVL until Epidural dc'd.)	• IV dc'd.	
• Diet as tolerated.	• DAT.	• DAT.
• If PCA or Epidural taper dose & give PO pain meds.	• Taper and DC PCA; give PO pain meds. ✓ SpO₂ × 1. SpO₂ reading.	• PO pain meds, reassessing pain level.
• Analgesia method.	• Analgesia method, Pharmaceutical & non-pharmacological pain control. • Discharge plan reinforced.	• Understands Ortho inst, risk of DVT/PE, Hip precautions. • Reinforce any instruction given. • Answer any questions patient may have.
• BCP CN or RN to notify MD if platelet count shows 100,000 drop in past 24 hr.	• BCP CN or RN notify MD if platelet count shows 100,000 drop in past 24 hr.	• As indicated.
• PT BID. • Chaplain Services & Dietary consult PRN.	• PT. Chaplain Services & Dietary consult PRN.	• PT. Chaplain Services & Dietary consult PRN.
• SS assess if needed for SNF transfer (notify SS if min. assist needed).	• Discharge decision, S.S. assess if needed and not done.	• Arrange equipment needed for home. • Complete transfer sheet or discharge instructions.

Shift			Circle Yes (Y) or No (N)	Shift			Circle Yes (Y) or No (N)	Shift			Circle Yes (Y) or No (N)
7-3	3-11	11-7		7-3	3-11	11-7		7-3	3-11	11-7	
Y N	Y N	Y N	Ambulation started (PT).	Y N	Y N	Y N	Voiding without Foley.	Y N	Y N	Y N	Discharge plan reinforced (RN).
				Y N	Y N	Y N	SS note re. discharge plan (SS).*	Y N	Y N	Y N	Discharged to appropriate care level (RN).
				Y N	Y N	Y N	BM passed (RN).				
				Y N	Y N	Y N	Pain managed with PO medicine (RN).*				

11-7	11-7	11-7
11-7	11-7	11-7
7-3	7-3	7-3
7-3	7-3	7-3
7-3	7-3	7-3
3-11	3-11	3-11
3-11	3-11	3-11
3-11	3-11	3-11

FIGURE 1-4 Sample clinical pathway.

Kardex/Client Profile The Kardex card or Client Profile represents the "hub" for all client activities. Physician's orders are transcribed on the Kardex card or computer. Laboratory tests, medications, and activity levels are just a few items documented in designated areas of the Kardex, electronic record (Figure 1-3 ■), or profile.

The computerized plan of care has replaced the Kardex card in many facilities. The same information is contained in the electronic version, but in many cases, the information is more up to date.

Care Plan Client care plans vary among healthcare facilities. The older individualized handwritten care plan has largely been replaced by preprinted standardized care plans, computerized care plans, or critical pathways. Regardless of the type of care plan used, the purpose does not change. Care plans are written guidelines for client care that all healthcare workers use to deliver individualized care. Most care plans today are termed *Multidisciplinary Care Plans* because all health team providers document treatments and observations on one form. Pertinent data regarding client care needs can be communicated to all providers using the multidisciplinary care plan. Client teaching is frequently detailed on the same form.

Critical or Clinical Pathway You may see either of these terms used to describe an approach to deliver collaborative, outcome-driven health care to clients. These documents are another approach to providing individualized care to clients. Interventions and outcomes are progressively outlined within the pathway as illustrated (Figure 1-4 ■).

Client's Chart

Client information is contained on several forms or computer screens, depending on documentation systems used in the healthcare facility. These forms or computer screens are important to your preparation and administration of nursing care. Be sure to familiarize yourself with the specific forms or screens in the healthcare facility where you have your clinical experience. The following forms are intended as examples only. Refer to Chapter 3 for a complete description of forms or screens.

Nurses' Notes *Nurses' notes* are documents that contain clinical observations and nursing interventions. Many facilities have limited the narrative charting format (Figure 1-5 ■) and increased the use of flow sheets and checklists, termed *Patient Care Records* or *Multidisciplinary Team Records*. This type of charting decreases the time it takes nurses to document and promotes comprehensive documentation.

Many facilities have computerized charting systems that facilitate a more thorough mechanism for data input. In-service education programs on use of the computer for charting and data retrieval need to be completed before clinical experience is begun, to ensure that you can obtain all the necessary information to provide safe care for the client. Hospitals with paper charting may have developed their own documentation system; it is crucial to become familiar with the system before beginning to document.

Medication Records Medication records are usually similar to those illustrated in Figure 1-6 ■. All medications should be documented on a medication record. Electronic health records have medication screens for recording information. Some facilities chart routine medications on one medication sheet and PRN and one-time only medications on another sheet. Check the institution's policy for each record's use.

Graphic Records Vital signs are recorded on the graphic sheet (Figure 1-7 ■); see Chapter 3 for the information on blood pressure, pulse, respirations, temperature, and pain level. Most facilities have included the pain scale on the graphic record because pain is referred to as the fifth vital sign. Weight is also included on this form. Intake and output results may be recorded on this record or on a separate form, depending on the facility.

Physician's Orders Depending on the facility, physician's orders may be computerized, preprinted, or written on forms with copies attached. If copied, the original is retained in the client's chart and copies can be sent to the pharmacy and to the lab. Computerized orders can be easily utilized by all hospital departments.

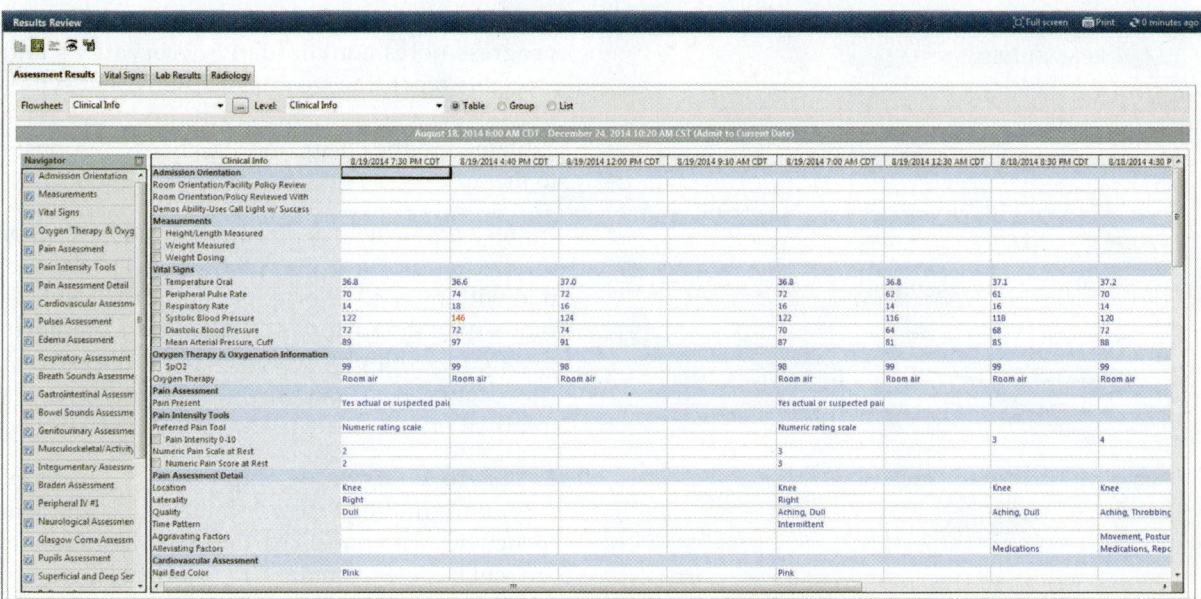

FIGURE 1-5 Sample flow sheet.

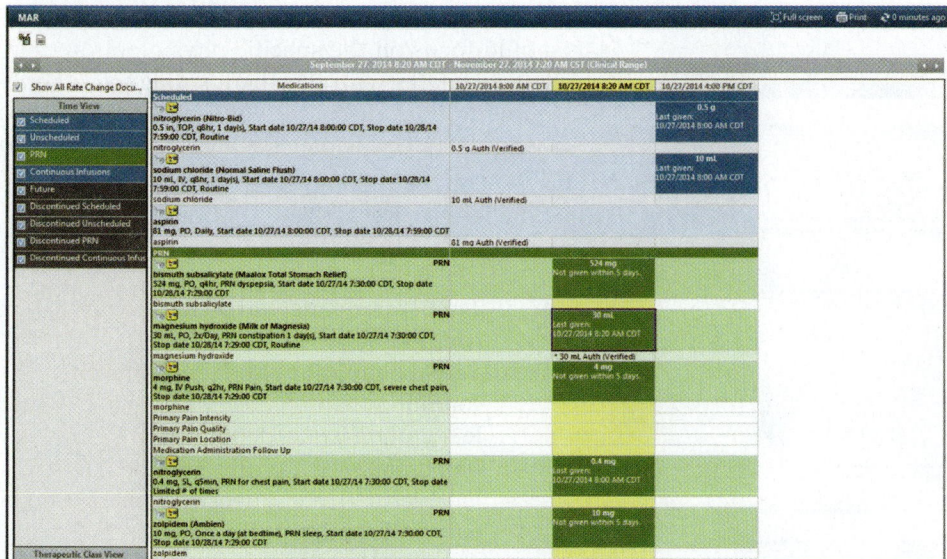

FIGURE 1-6 A medication administration record (MAR).

Source: Images this page from Cerner Electronic Health Record. © Cerner Corporation. Pearson has restricted permission to reproduce and distribute this copyrighted work. Further reproduction or distribution is strictly prohibited without written consent of Cerner Corporation.

FIGURE 1-7 Graphic chart.

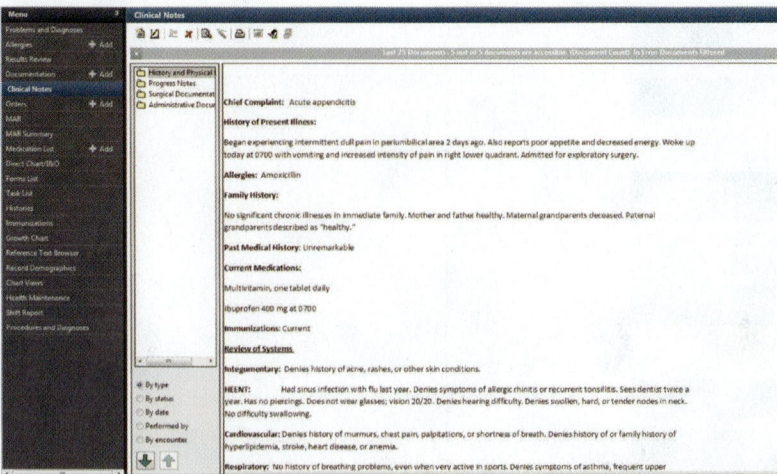

FIGURE 1-8 Physician's history and physical record.

Source: Images this page from Cerner Electronic Health Record. © Cerner Corporation. Pearson has restricted permission to reproduce and distribute this copyrighted work. Further reproduction or distribution is strictly prohibited without written consent of Cerner Corporation.

Physician's Progress Notes Physician's progress notes contain daily observations and thoughts regarding treatments, signs, and symptoms experienced by the client, operative risks explained to the client, and the client's responses to therapy.

History and Physical The physician's report of his or her assessment is written on a special section within the EHR or a special form. Most hospitals type the history and physical from notes dictated by the physician (Figure 1-8 ■). When this occurs, it may be several days before this information is available.

Laboratory Forms Computerized reports of laboratory findings have become more common. In facilities with paper charting, laboratory results are sent back to the unit on the original laboratory order form (Figure 1-9 ■). The information from each form may be transcribed to a laboratory data flow sheet (Figure 1-10 ■) that provides an overview of all laboratory results.

Basic Nursing Assessment

Each nurse develops her or his own routine for completing a basic nursing assessment. There is no right or wrong way, although it should be consistent and complete. The following outline for basic assessment is a simple approach to the assessment and one you may wish to adopt until you have established a good system for yourself.

The basic assessment is completed at the beginning of each shift (usually a complete assessment is done once per day and focus assessments at the beginning and end of the other shifts). You should focus on the specific physiologic system that correlates with the client's diagnosis. For a more in-depth discussion of each system in the assessment, see Chapter 11, Physical Assessment.

The following outline will assist you in completing a basic physical assessment.

1. Vital signs:
   a. Temperature (method dictated by condition)
   b. Radial or apical pulse (depending on condition)
   c. Respirations: rate, depth, and rhythm
   d. Blood pressure: Korotkoff sounds
   e. Pain: location and intensity of pain; use pain scale to determine pain level.

2. Response to medications if given
3. Emotional responses: client behavior, reactions, and demeanor; general mood (crying, depression)

FIGURE 1-9 Laboratory order form.

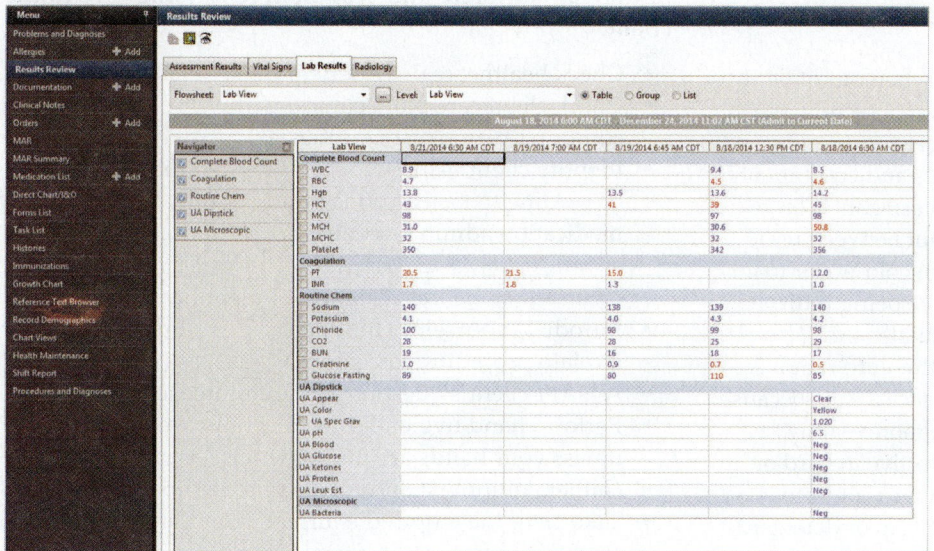

FIGURE 1-10 Laboratory results flow sheet.

Source: Images this page from Cerner Electronic Health Record. © Cerner Corporation. Pearson has restricted permission to reproduce and distribute this copyrighted work. Further reproduction or distribution is strictly prohibited without written consent of Cerner Corporation.

4. Skin, hair, and nails
   a. Skin: presence or absence of abrasions, contusions, tears, erythema, pressure ulcers, incision line, color, turgor, temperature, edema
   b. Hair: distribution, thickness or thinness, texture, and amount
   c. Nails: curvature and angle, texture, color, and surrounding tissue
5. Musculoskeletal: activity level, general mobility, gait, range of motion
6. Neurologic system: pupils (size, response, equality); hand grips; strength and sensation of all extremities; ability to follow commands; level of consciousness
7. Respiratory system: breath sounds; sputum color and consistency; cough (productive or nonproductive)
8. Cardiovascular system: heart sounds; presence of pulses; edema; observe presence of hair on extremities (lack of hair indicates poor circulation)
9. Gastrointestinal system: bowel pattern and sounds; presence of nausea or vomiting; abdominal distention; consumption of diet
10. Genitourinary system: voiding; color, odor, and consistency of urine; dysuria; vaginal drainage or discomfort; penile discharge

If any unusual findings are assessed, complete a more in-depth assessment of the particular system affected. Throughout the day, continue to assess changes in the client's condition by paying particular attention to the alterations from normal that you identified in the initial assessment. At the end of the shift, make a notation of any changes in the client's condition.

Medical Asepsis Principles

Microorganisms are found everywhere in nature. Pathogenic microorganisms, or pathogens, cause disease; nonpathogenic microorganisms, or nonpathogens, do not cause disease. Some microorganisms are nonpathogens in their normal body environment. An example of this is *Escherichia coli*, which is normally present in the intestinal tract and does not cause a problem until it inhabits another environment such as the urinary tract.

The spread of microorganisms is prevented by the use of two forms of **asepsis**: medical asepsis and surgical asepsis. Medical asepsis occurs when there is an absence of pathogens. Surgical asepsis occurs when there is an absence of all organisms. Medical asepsis is often referred to as "clean technique," whereas surgical asepsis is termed "sterile technique." A discussion of surgical asepsis can be found later in this book. This chapter discusses medical asepsis as it affects nursing care.

Principles of medical asepsis are used in all aspects of client care. In fact, the use of medical asepsis begins before you report to the nursing unit. To ensure protection for the client, you begin practicing medical asepsis by limiting jewelry to only a wedding band and perhaps small earrings for pierced ears when administering client care. Fingernails are short and in good repair. Your hair is off your collar and under control to prevent contaminating sterile fields and falling into client's food or wounds. While providing client care, the following principles should be kept in mind:

- Linen rooms or carts are considered clean; therefore linen not used for client care cannot be returned.
- Utility rooms are designated as areas for clean and dirty supplies. Cross-contamination must be avoided by not placing articles in the wrong area.
- Linen and articles are carried away from your uniform and are not held close to your body.
- Articles dropped on the floor are considered contaminated and must be discarded appropriately. If linen is accidentally dropped on the floor, it is placed in a soiled linen hamper.
- Clients are to wear slippers or shoes when out of bed.
- Paper tissue is used for removing client's secretions. Tissues are discarded in the trash basket.
- Each client has his or her own supplies and equipment, which are not used by other clients. Sterilization or disinfection of equipment is carried out between uses.
- Equipment is cleaned and rinsed with cold water to remove secretions or substances before being returned to the central supply area. Heat coagulates the substances and makes them more difficult to remove.
- Soap and water are considered the best cleansers because they help break down soil so it can be more readily removed. Detergents may be more effective in hard or cold water; however, tissue damage can result from their use. Germicides, when added to soap or detergent, increase the effectiveness of the cleansing agent.
- Chlorhexidine gluconate is used in bath wipes to prevent bacteria from remaining on the skin.
- Friction is used to facilitate soil removal. A brush, sponge, or cloth may be used to produce the friction.
- When aseptic technique is used, cleaning is conducted from the cleanest to the least clean area. For example, always clean the incision area from the center of the incision to the periphery of the skin.
- If you are not feeling well, you should not report for clinical experience. If you are running a temperature or have a cold and a runny nose, call the appropriate individual and report that you are ill.

Hand Hygiene

The single most effective medical aseptic practice is hand washing. When you first arrive at the nursing unit and before beginning nursing practice, you should complete a medical hand-washing procedure. The important concept to remember is that you thoroughly soap and rinse your hands twice before providing any nursing care to the client. Hands are washed before all procedures and between clients. Alcohol-based hand rub is usually used between clients if hands are not visibly dirty. The specific step-by-step hand-washing procedure is covered in Chapter 14, Infection Control.

Clean, nonsterile gloves are worn when touching, or there is a potential for touching, blood, body fluids, secretions, excretions, and contaminated items. Gloves are discarded immediately after use in an appropriate container. Gloving decreases the risk of cross-contamination between clients and between clients and healthcare workers. Hand washing is completed before donning and after removing gloves.

Protocol for Procedures

Each procedure in this textbook follows a basic protocol. **These steps *must be followed in every procedure* in order to deliver complete and responsible nursing care to the client.**

- Check healthcare provider's orders.
- Check client care plan, clinical pathway, client computer plan of care, or Kardex.
- Identify client using two forms of identification (according to facility policy, and not only for medication administration). *Use client name, client date of birth, or client medical record number. Do not use the client's room number* as a form of identification.
- Introduce yourself to the client, if first time in room.
- Explain procedure to be done.
- Answer client's questions and reinforce teaching.
- Perform hand hygiene using alcohol-based solution unless your hands are dirty; then use soap and water.
- Gather equipment and fill out charge slips.
- Take all of the required equipment and linens to the room.
- Provide privacy for the client by drawing curtain or screen around bed.
- Raise bed to HIGH position.
- Lower side rail nearest you.
- Drape client (if appropriate).
- Don gloves (if appropriate).
- Perform procedure according to the protocol.
- Clean client as necessary.
- Remove drape and position client for comfort.
- Remove gloves.
- Raise side rail to UP position.
- Lower bed.
- Replace call bell.
- Pull back curtain or remove screen.
- Remove equipment and clean, dispose of, and disperse used equipment.
- Perform hand hygiene using alcohol-based solution unless your hands are dirty; then use soap and water.
- Document or chart findings.

Chapter Wrap-Up

MANAGEMENT Guidelines

Each state legislates a Nurse Practice Act for RNs and LVN/LPNs. Healthcare facilities are responsible for establishing and implementing policies and procedures that conform to their state's regulations. Verify the regulations and role parameters for each healthcare worker in your facility.

Delegation

- As an RN you will be held accountable and responsible for your actions. When delegating client care, you must know the healthcare worker's level of client care tasks that can be assigned to each category of worker. The Nurse Practice Act for both RN and LVN/LPN must be adhered to when assigning client care. The skill level and scope of practice of unassisted licensed personnel must be evaluated before assigning client care.

- The RN must abide by and function within the American Nurses Association Code of Ethics for Nurses. The RN is responsible for the appropriate delegation of nursing tasks to others in order to provide safe, competent client care.

- Legal issues and regulations must be followed in order to establish appropriate client care standards when delegating to other healthcare workers. The RN has a responsibility for a level of performance that must be carried out and cannot be delegated, including healthcare teaching, initial assessment, and the administration of IV medications.

- The signing of a consent form for surgery or an invasive procedure may be delegated to the LVN/LPN, and in some facilities a ward clerk may obtain the consent. Informed consent is the responsibility of the physician; however, most facilities allow nurses and other healthcare workers to witness the client's signature on the consent form after an explanation has been provided by the physician. Some facilities require that a physician obtain the signed consent form. The signature of the witness indicates only that he or she obtained the client's signature on the form. The RN is still responsible for ensuring that the client understands what the procedure is, including potential complications. If the client is unsure of the procedure, the physician needs to be notified to re-explain the procedure until the client understands.

Interprofessional Communication

- Each member of the nursing unit should be given appropriate directions on the tasks to be completed, keeping in mind the legal issues surrounding delegation. Assign only those tasks the healthcare worker is legally responsible to carry out.

- The RN must ensure that proper consent forms are signed by the client prior to invasive procedures or surgery. Even when the task of witnessing a consent form signing is delegated, the RN is responsible for ensuring it is completed and placed in the client's chart. Ask the witness to inform you when all paperwork is completed for the procedure in order for you to check the forms.

- Ensure that all healthcare workers are aware of DNR orders. Make sure the plan of care or Kardex adequately states the DNR order, and provide that information during report.

- Give specific directions to healthcare workers regarding the client information you wish reported and how you wish to receive it (i.e., written or verbal).

- Provide current information to healthcare workers in a timely manner as it impacts their care of the client (i.e., changes in activity or diet orders).

- Ensure that all forms of documentation are completed in a timely manner; if computerized charting is utilized in the facility, all healthcare workers have the responsibility to complete particular forms.

CASE STUDY Applications

Scenario 1

As a new student you are going into the hospital to prepare for the clinical experience tomorrow morning. There are two stages of preparation. The first stage is obtaining all the necessary information you will need to provide safe care. The second stage is reviewing your textbooks and lecture notes to gain an understanding of the client's diagnosis, medications, lab values, and diagnostic tests that will be done during his or her hospitalization.

- If you have only a limited time to review the client's chart, what sections of the chart will provide you with sufficient information to render you safe to care for the client?

- In preparing for clinical practice, what information is essential to review in addition to the data you have obtained from the clinical record? Where is the most appropriate place to find this information?

- List the priority interventions you will carry out within the first hour of the clinical experience. Explain the rationale for your answers.

Scenario 2

As a student nurse you have been assigned to complete an activity where you compare and contrast legal/ethical issues related to nursing practice. You are assigned to research the ANA Standards of Clinical Nursing Practice, The Nurse Practice Act in your state, and the Code of Academic and Clinical Conduct from the National Student Nurses' Association, Inc.

- Briefly describe the primary purpose/function of each of these nursing regulations or guidelines.
- Select one of the above nursing regulations/guidelines and describe how the regulation/guideline will impact your role as a professional nurse.
- The National Student Nurses' Association developed the Code of Academic and Clinical Conduct. How do you plan to incorporate the code into your practice as a student nurse? How will this practice prepare you for the Registered Nurse profession?

NCLEX® Review Questions

Unless otherwise specified, choose only one (1) answer.

1. According to the American Nurses Association, which statement best defines nursing as a profession?
   A. Cares for clients in all types of settings
   B. Protects, promotes, and optimizes health and abilities of clients
   C. Provides client care as ordered by the physician
   D. Assists clients in activities of daily living and prepares them for home care

2. The National Student Nurses' Association has formulated a code for nursing students. What is the most important rationale for adhering to this code?
   A. It encompasses ethical principles that guide professional behavior.
   B. It governs nursing behavior in the clinical setting.
   C. It lets the student know what is acceptable behavior.
   D. It gives guidelines for administering medications.

3. Guidelines for clinical preparation include which of the following activities?
   A. Ensure your uniform is similar to the staff nurse uniform.
   B. Begin the nurse–client relationship using a more social communication to place the client at ease.
   C. Address the client by first name to make him or her feel comfortable.
   D. Listen to client's statements and feelings regarding their clinical manifestations because he or she is more familiar with his or her bodily functions.

4. The Nurse Practice Act regulates the practice of nursing in each state. Which skills and functions are included?
   Select all that apply.
   A. Delegate registered nursing responsibilities to an LVN/LPN who has many years of practice.
   B. Instruct the CNA to obtain the vital signs and health history on a newly admitted client.
   C. Complete a client care plan on a newly admitted client.

   D. Refer a client to the discharge planning nurse.
   E. Administer IV medications ordered by the physician.
   F. Observe and document client's responses to medications and treatments.

5. Which statement best describes the Standards of Clinical Nursing Practice?
   A. They apply only to nurses in specialty practice or those who function under a physician.
   B. They do not apply to nurses who are advance practice nurses as they are not accountable for maintaining the basic standards of clinical practice.
   C. They describe a competent level of professional nursing care and professional performance common to all categories of nurses.
   D. They apply to nurses employed in acute care and long-term care settings only.

6. Which of the following are possible penalties for professional misconduct?
   Select all that apply.
   A. Probation
   B. Revocation of license
   C. Imprisonment for practicing without a license
   D. Compensation to facility for costs accrued from criminal act
   E. Reprimand

7. When can the nurse be charged with gross negligence?
   A. There is an act that causes the death of a client.
   B. The nurse demonstrates a reckless disregard for client safety.
   C. There is an improper use of restraints.
   D. The nurse refuses a client assignment before the shift begins.

8. What functions does the nurse complete before providing client care?
   A. Gather appropriate equipment.
   B. Ask the RN what order of care the client usually likes.

C. Check the computerized plan of care record or Kardex to determine the order of care for the client.

D. Identify the client by using his or her name.

9. What is the purpose of studying Core Measures in hospitals?

A. To align specific client diagnoses with other facilities for the purpose of promoting research studies

B. To collect client data to determine appropriate treatments

C. To study clinical data on specific diagnoses for the purpose of developing an improvement tool

D. To collect data on reportable conditions among hospitals to provide a uniform reimbursement plan

10. Which option is included in the principles of medical asepsis?

A. Placing soiled linen only on the bottom of the linen cart

B. Cleaning (with alcohol) equipment that has been dropped on the floor

C. Using equipment from another client providing it is cleaned with 2% chlorhexidine before and after use

D. Cleaning equipment with cold water before returning it to central supply according to facility policies

QSEN Activity

Verbal and Nonverbal Actions for Conveying Confidence to the Client

Domain: Patient Centered Care

KSA: Knowledge

Activity:

Discuss the verbal and nonverbal actions the nurse must perform to convey nursing confidence in the care of the client. Work in groups (number in group is dependent on number of students in class). Each student identifies an action and explains how he or she would relate this to the client or how he or she would present himself or herself in front of the client. For example, "Do not talk down to a client."

Bibliography

American Hospital Association. (2003). *The Patient Care Partnership: Understanding Expectations, Rights, and Responsibilities*. Atlanta, GA: AHA Services.

American Nursing Association. (2010). *Scope and Standards of Practice* (2nd ed.). Silver Spring, MD: Author.

Fowler, M. (Ed.) (2008). *American Nurses Association, Guide to the Code of Ethics for Nurses: Interpretation and Application*. Silver Spring, MD: American Nurses Association.

National Student Nurses' Association, Inc. (2009). *A Code of Academic and Clinical Conduct*. Washington, DC: Author.

Nix, Ella. (2009). Core Measures 101. Retrieved from http://www.clinical-insights.com/resources-Apr09CoreMeasures.html

The Center for Bioethics and Human Dignity. End of life resources. Retrieved August 7, 2014 from https://cbhd.org/resources/advance-directive

The Health Insurance Portability and Accountability Act (HIPAA). (2003, Apr.). *The Privacy Rule*. Washington, DC: United States Department of Health & Human Services.

The Joint Commission. National Patient Safety Goals. (2014). Retrieved from www.jointcommission.org/standards

The Joint Commission. (n.d.). Sentinel Event Glossary of Terms. http://www.jointcommission.org/SentinelEvents/se_glossary.htm

Chapter 2
Critical Thinking and the Nursing Process

 Learning Objectives

2.1 Define the term *critical thinking*.

2.2 Define the term *nursing process*.

2.3 Explain how critical thinking is used in each step of the nursing process.

2.4 Describe how the nursing process relates to nursing.

2.5 Discuss the term *assessment*, and describe how it influences the nursing process.

2.6 List the components of the assessment step.

2.7 Describe the primary purpose of the analysis phase of the nursing process.

2.8 Define the term *nursing diagnosis*.

2.9 Define outcome planning and identification, and give an example of this step in the nursing process.

2.10 Define what is meant by the implementation phase of the nursing process.

2.11 Explain evaluation and include your understanding of why it is an important step in the nursing process.

2.12 Differentiate nursing diagnosis from medical diagnosis.

2.13 Define NIC and NOC and their role in standardizing nursing language.

2.14 Compare and contrast the two-part and three-part Nursing Diagnosis Statement.

2.15 State two examples of nursing diagnoses.

2.16 Define evidence-based nursing practice.

Chapter Outline

TERMINOLOGY

Assessment first step in the nursing process that establishes a database for each client by collection and clustering of subjective and objective data

Best practices nursing interventions that have been proven effective in promoting positive client outcomes or in reducing overall costs to the client or facility

Critical thinking process of identifying and questioning assumptions, determining what is important in each situation, and examining alternatives before making an informed decision

Evaluation examination of the outcome of nursing actions or the extent to which the expected outcomes or goals were achieved

Evidence-based practice application in clinical practice of the best available empirical evidence from recent research findings in order to aid clinical decision making

Implementation priority nursing action or intervention performed to accomplish a specified goal

NIC nursing interventions classification; a system that provides an element of uniformity to nursing actions; each intervention has a label name and a set of activities that are identified as steps to carry it out

NOC nursing outcomes classification; a comprehensive, standardized classification of client outcomes developed to evaluate the effects of interventions provided by nurses or other healthcare professionals

Nursing diagnosis analysis and naming of distinct client problems that nurses are licensed to treat

Nursing process a systematic, problem-solving approach, based on reasoning and scientific knowledge, that guides the nurse in client care and that commonly is described as having the following steps: assessment, analysis/nursing diagnosis, planning, implementation, and evaluation

Outcome a measurable state, behavior, or perception that is observed along a continuum and is responsive to nursing interventions

Planning phase of the nursing process involving identification of nursing actions to achieve goals or desired outcomes of nursing care

Reflection recalling earlier clinical situations to determine what worked or didn't work and whether previous experience can be applied in the current situation

Critical Thinking

Critical thinking is an important element in all professional fields. It involves the careful acquisition and interpretation of information and use of it to reach a well-justified conclusion. It is sometimes referred to as "thinking about thinking." All nurses are required to use critical thinking skills as they provide nursing care for clients. Nurses are expected not only to master nursing content from many disciplines, but to think creatively, solve problems, communicate, and use judgment in nursing practice. Critical thinking involves higher-level thinking. It employs interpretation, analysis, evaluation, and inference. Critical thinking requires understanding of abstract concepts, consideration of the context in which a situation exists, and openness to new ideas. This means asking questions, analyzing, and examining one's own thinking as well as that of others.

Critical thinking focuses on judgment, because each clinical situation nurses encounter is unique. Effective critical thinking and problem solving depend on relevant knowledge and previous experience. An important aspect of critical thinking is the ability to use reflection and language properly. **Reflection** is the action of thinking back

or recalling an earlier clinical situation, remembering nursing actions that worked or didn't work, and determining whether this information is helpful in the current situation.

The ability to use language is associated with the ability to think meaningfully. To become a critical thinker, the nurse must use language accurately. Without appropriate terminology, communication with the client and other healthcare workers is likely to be impaired.

Critical thinking skills assist the nurse to look at all aspects of a situation and then arrive at a conclusion. Critical thinkers identify and question assumptions, determine what is important in each situation, and examine each alternative before making an informed decision. When critical thinking is employed in a clinical situation, the nurse examines ideas, beliefs, principles, assumptions, conclusions, statements, and inferences before coming to a conclusion. Because the conclusions and decisions made by nurses affect clients' lives, they must be guided by precise, disciplined thinking. Nurses must be critical thinkers, using scientific reasoning, the nursing process, and decision-making processes.

Critical thinking skills assist nurses during the assessment process. Through the use of critical thinking, nurses can question, evaluate, and reconstruct the nursing care process by challenging the established theory and practice. These skills assist nurses to problem solve, reflect, and make a conclusive decision about a current situation facing them. Critical thinking skills create new possibilities for the development of nursing knowledge. Due to the sociocultural, environmental, and political issues that are affecting healthcare delivery, it would be helpful to incorporate new techniques in nursing.

Nurses who are considered critical thinkers are those who use logic, creativity, and good communication and are flexible and competent in delivering client care. They exhibit open-mindedness, empathy, realism, and cooperation in being team players.

To acquire critical thinking skills, the nurse must first develop a sound theoretical knowledge base. This means studying the concepts appropriate to each clinical discipline (e.g., pathophysiology related to medical diagnoses or disease states, pharmacology, growth and development, nutrition, and psychology, as well as client problems in each area of nursing practice). This knowledge is transferred to clinical situations. With each clinical situation, the nurse gains immeasurable experience in identifying clients' problems. Over time, the nurse is able to select the best solution for assisting clients to resume a healthy state.

Nurses use critical thinking skills as they relate theory to practice and apply the nursing process in client care.

Nursing Process

Nursing process, a familiar term in nursing, is a way of organizing nursing actions in healthcare delivery. It is a systematic, problem-solving approach and is considered a critical thinking competency that assists the nurse to intervene in client care. The nurse's actions are based on reasoning and scientific knowledge. The nursing process—assessment, analysis/nursing diagnosis, planning, implementation, and evaluation—provides an organized structure and framework for the delivery of nursing care in all settings: The nursing process is used to diagnose and treat human responses to health and illness (American Nurses Association, 2015). Although the steps can be described separately and in logical order, in practice they overlap, and events may not always occur in the order listed here.

This chapter presents, defines, and illustrates the steps of the nursing process and assists you in integrating this framework into your mastery of nursing content. It also demonstrates how critical thinking is linked to each step of the process.

Assessment

Assessment is the first step in the nursing process because it establishes a database for a client. Assessment requires skilled observation, reasoning, and a theoretical knowledge

---

Box 2-1 ASSESSMENT

Gather Data: Objective and Subjective

Verify data.

Confirm observations.

Organize data.

Make inferences from data.

Communicate data.

Observe—Interview—Examine

Identify client needs.

Be aware of staff reactions to clients.

Assess sources of data:

Client history

Data from family

Client status—physical and emotional

Signs and symptoms

Test results and findings.

Recall stored knowledge.

---

base to gather and differentiate, verify and organize data, and document the findings (Box 2-1 ■). The nurse gathers information about a client's psychological, physiological, sociological, and spiritual status from a variety of sources and then assigns meaning to these data. Nurses conduct a client interview and perform a physical examination, obtaining a client's health history and family health history during this examination. While performing the examination, the nurse will also complete a general observation to gather additional assessment data. Assessment is a critical phase, because all the other steps depend on the accuracy and reliability of the information obtained. Assessment is based on concepts of physiology, pathophysiology, psychology, and social adjustment.

Critical Thinking in Assessment A leading cause of error in making clinical judgments or decisions is collection of inaccurate or incomplete data during the assessment phase. The data collection or assessment step of the nursing process assists the nurse to predict, detect, prevent, and control client problems. A nurse with good critical thinking skills develops a systematic approach to obtain and validate data. This includes using all sources for data collection (i.e., reviewing the client's chart, asking pertinent questions, and completing the assessment in a systematic manner). If an assessment tool is used, ensure that thought goes into the way the data are recorded; don't just write information down in a rote manner. Review the assessment form to determine whether additional or more in-depth information is required. Ask yourself, "Is this information relevant?" and "Do I need to assess anything else?" Listen to the client. Clients provide important subjective data to add to objective information. Once all of the data are collected, validate to ensure that data are not missing and that existing data are correct. Cluster similar information to help form a picture of the client's problems and strengths and to identify whether patterns of behavior or responses exist. Clustering

Analyze and synthesize collected data.
Examine defining characteristics, both major and minor.
Determine clusters of clues.
Identify related factors.
Identify potential nursing diagnoses.
Develop nursing diagnoses appropriate to the client problem.

data helps distinguish relevant from irrelevant data as well as gaps in information. It also pinpoints cause-and-effect relationships. Once the clustering is completed, inferences may be formulated.

Nursing Diagnosis

Nursing diagnosis is an integral component of the nursing process, an educated judgment about potential or actual health problem or problems of a client (Box 2-2■). The nursing diagnosis describes something nurses are independently qualified to treat. It may include an actual description of the problem or risk for developing the problem. It is derived from the systematic collection of data and their analysis. It is a clinical judgment about a designated client, family, or community that provides the basis for completion of the nursing process. Nursing diagnosis provides the foundation for each individual client's therapeutic plan of care, and once it is established, the nurse is accountable for actions that occur within the scope of this nursing diagnosis framework.

The nurse must use critical thinking and decision-making skills when determining nursing diagnoses.

Critical Thinking in Nursing Diagnosis Use of critical thinking skills is essential in the nursing diagnosis step of the nursing process. As you cluster data, you are applying the scientific principle of classifying information in order to determine whether relationships exist among the data and whether data are relevant or irrelevant. Inconsistencies among the collected data may prompt additional assessment. Determining when additional information is needed for an accurate diagnosis prevents the nurse from making a very common critical thinking error—making a judgment based on incomplete information.

Once the completed data are clustered, the nurse begins to organize defining characteristics into meaningful patterns. Identifying patterns requires critical thinking skills associated with a sound scientific knowledge base. The nurse must differentiate normal from abnormal findings and identify risk factors for abnormal patterns of functioning. Nursing diagnosis reference books can help clarify data relevant to defining characteristics or risk factors related to the client's clinical manifestations. Usually, the presence of two to three defining characteristics validates the nursing diagnosis.

During this step of the nursing process, actual client problems are identified, potential problems are predicted,

and priorities are established. Establishing nursing diagnoses is an important independent action of the nurse but nursing diagnoses are not treated in isolation. Medical diagnoses must be considered as well. Collaborative problem identification and treatment with other healthcare workers form the basis of a holistic approach to client care.

Planning and Outcome Identification

This phase of the nursing process refers to identification of nursing actions for achieving goals or desired outcomes of nursing care (Box 2-3■). The **planning** and outcome phases are directly related to solving or alleviating the problems identified in the nursing diagnosis. The plan includes short- and long-term, client-centered goals, strategies for goal outcomes, and nursing measures for the delivery of care. During this phase, the nursing diagnoses are prioritized to meet the client's immediate needs. **Outcomes** must be measurable, time specific, quantifiable, and realistic.

During the planning phase, systems like Nursing Outcomes Classification (NOC) can be utilized. **NOC** is a comprehensive, standardized classification of client outcomes developed to evaluate the effects of interventions provided by nurses or other healthcare professionals. An outcome is a measurable individual, family, or community state, behavior, or perception that is measured along a continuum and is responsive to nursing interventions. The outcomes are used to follow client's status throughout hospitalization, long-term care, or home care. Each outcome provides a definition and list of indicators that can be used to evaluate the client's status.

Standardized outcomes are necessary for electronic records, for use in clinical information systems, for the development of nursing knowledge, and for education of professional nurses. Nursing Outcomes Classification (NOC), developed and maintained by the University of Iowa College of Nursing, is one of several standardized systems for documenting outcomes (Moorhead, S., et al., 2013).

Client involvement in the planning phase is crucial to ensure that the client's and the healthcare team members'

Identify short- and long-term goals and outcomes that are measurable, time specific, quantifiable, and realistic.
Prioritize nursing diagnoses.
Develop a plan based on goals and outcomes, including a teaching plan.
Anticipate needs of client and family based on priorities.
Select nursing actions needed to accomplish goals.
Specify deadlines for completion of plan.
Coordinate care and community resources.
Consider contingencies for modifying the plan.
Record relevant information.

goals are congruent. If clients are not engaged in the planning process, they may not be motivated to achieve established goals. Planning focuses on the development of a plan of care individualized for each specific client.

Planning is based on the client's healthcare needs, selected goals, and strategies directed toward goal achievement. It is a plan of care in which the appropriate nursing actions and the client's desires are considered and chosen to achieve a goal. Clear documentation of a comprehensive plan provides the basis for the later step of evaluation.

Critical Thinking in Planning and Outcome Identification

Defining realistic goals that are acceptable to the client requires critical thinking. A prioritized plan of care is developed during this phase of the nursing process. Long-term outcomes or goals are usually based on what is expected by the time of discharge from a nursing unit or a facility. In acute care facilities, short-term outcomes are based on time frames as short as by the end of the shift, within 24 hours, etc. The long-term goal or expected outcome for discharge should be determined before other outcomes and interventions are initiated.

There are two critical thinking skills inherent in this step. One is listing the client problems and determining whether there are relationships between the problems, and the other is ordering the problems by highest priority. These critical thinking skills require sound scientific principles and scientific method, clinical judgment, reasoning skills, and goal-directed thinking.

When listing the actual and potential problems identified by the assessment data, critical thinking is used to identify which problems need immediate intervention and which ones are underlying causes of the client's problems. The situations identified as causing the problem must be assigned the highest priority. After listing the problems, determine whether there are relationships among the problems. If relationships exist, critical thinking is used to explore how one problem affects another. Maslow's Hierarchy of Human Needs is employed by many nurses to determine prioritization of problems. Maslow lists problems with survival needs (food, fluids, oxygen) as the highest priority. These needs must be addressed first in the plan of care for the client's well-being.

To write specific, realistic, client-centered outcomes, the problems must be stated clearly. Outcomes are derived directly from the problem statement, and the subject of the problem statement is the client. Remember, problem statements are written as nursing diagnoses, such as "Deficient Knowledge: Insulin Administration" for a client newly diagnosed with diabetes. An example of a client outcome utilizing a nursing diagnosis is this: "The client will demonstrate accurate administration of insulin according to the guidelines established by the diabetic educator within 24 hours of admission." Notice there is a time-specific statement included within the outcome statement. This time frame assists the nurse to evaluate outcome achievement and the need to reevaluate the plan of care.

Implementation

The fourth phase in the nursing process is the **implementation**, or intervention, phase. This phase refers to the priority nursing actions or interventions performed to accomplish a specified goal. It explicitly describes the action component of the nursing process (Box 2-4 ■). This phase involves initiating and completing those nursing actions necessary to accomplish the identified client goals and outcomes. Nursing actions must be appropriate, individualized for the client, and based on safe nursing practice; they should be formulated on scientific principles, classifications systems such as NOC Standards, and principles of the problem-solving process. Finally, the interventions must be congruent with the total medical and nursing treatment plans. Implementation involves giving direct care to the client to accomplish the specified goal.

Implementation is based on accurate and complete assessment, interpretation of data, identified client needs, goals and outcomes, analysis, nursing diagnosis, and strategies to achieve goals.

Critical Thinking in Implementation

Nursing interventions are specific strategies developed to achieve positive client outcomes. These interventions are determined by using the critical thinking skills of generalizing, explaining, and predicting outcomes. After consideration of all identified possible actions, nursing interventions are chosen and implemented.

Identifying appropriate nursing actions requires critical thinking skills. These skills include the ability to identify specific actions, predict and monitor the client's response to those actions, and weigh risks and consequences of each. By examining the risks and consequences of an action, a nurse can determine the most beneficial and least harmful approach to client care. When interventions are clearly delineated on the plan of care, the likelihood of the actions being carried out is enhanced. The more specific the intervention, the greater chance there is that the outcome will be

---

Box 2-4 **IMPLEMENTATION**

Utilize the client care plan by giving direct care based on goals, outcomes, and NOC Standards.

Perform actions or interventions and procedures in accordance with client needs.

Counsel and teach client, family, or both.

Use preventive, palliative, or emergency measures for client's welfare.

Encourage independence and self-care.

Motivate and maintain optimum wellness.

Communicate appropriately to client and client's family.

Record data.

Continue assessment process.

successful. If increasing fluid intake is the intervention, specifics about fluid likes and dislikes of the client should be addressed. For example, "Client prefers noncarbonated beverages at room temperature." Another example of a specific intervention is, "Ambulate the client after his bath, before lunch, and before dinner." This would be appropriate for the client goal of ambulating the length of the hall by discharge. Putting times for interventions or distances for ambulation increases the likelihood of compliance with the intervention by all healthcare workers.

Evaluation

The final phase of the nursing process is evaluation. **Evaluation** is the examination of the outcome of nursing actions or the extent to which the expected outcomes or goals were achieved.

To evaluate, the nurse asks several questions. Was the goal achieved? Were the client outcomes met? If they were not met, what parts of the goal were not achieved? Was client behavior modified? Evaluation is a necessary phase to complete the nursing process. It allows the nurse to continue to identify goals in the overall treatment plan and to alter the current plan to adapt to the client's needs.

Evaluation is based on the previous phases of the nursing process (assessment, analysis, planning and outcome identification, and implementation). The evaluation phase completes the process and examines the outcome (Box 2-5 ■).

The nursing process has provided the framework for the immense amount of nursing content that is contained in this textbook. The rationale for choosing this framework is that it provides a way to organize and present nursing knowledge, and it is also an essential component of providing quality client care.

Critical Thinking in Evaluation   During the final phase of the nursing process, the nurse critically analyzes each of the client outcomes. If the client need (goal or objective) was not met, the plan is revised. Clear documentation of the care plan provides the basis for effective evaluation. Review of client progress toward outcome achievement assists the nurse in evaluating the effectiveness of the overall plan. A critical thinking question during this phase of the nursing process is: "How well did the client accomplish the goal?" The nurse might also ask: "What could have been done differently?"

Box 2-5 EVALUATION

Determine effects of nursing actions.
Determine extent to which goals and outcomes were achieved.
Examine appropriateness of nursing actions.
Investigate effect and degree of compliance for client and family.
Reassess care plan—judge if goal modification is necessary.
Consider alternative nursing actions.
Record client responses.

Nursing Diagnosis: Uses, Types, and Components

Nursing Diagnosis Versus Medical Diagnosis

An important implication of nursing diagnosis is that it refers to a health problem or condition that nurses are legally licensed to treat. Nursing diagnoses help to demonstrate nursing as a profession with its own body of knowledge, education, and experience. The list of nursing diagnoses identified by the North American Nursing Diagnosis Association (NANDA International) provides a common set of labels to identify client problems. Such standardization of language is especially useful as electronic health records become the norm. Using standardized terminology, such as Nursing Diagnosis, Nursing Interventions Classifications (**NIC**), and Nursing Outcomes Classifications (NOC), will allow for systematic collection of nursing data across all healthcare organizations. Collecting data in this manner provides for analysis and audit of a large volume of information at minimal cost. Standardized terminology more effectively meets client needs while ensuring client safety.

The term *nursing diagnosis* is not the same as *medical diagnosis* (Box 2-6 ■). Medical diagnoses by a physician focus on illness, injury, or disease. Nursing diagnoses focus on the response of the client to actual or potential health problems or life processes, illness, change in lifestyle, and so on. Medical diagnoses do not vary until treatment is completed, but nursing diagnoses change as the client's condition or response to treatment changes.

The nurse is not legally able to intervene and treat a medical diagnosis without specific physician's orders. In contrast, the nurse is legally qualified and prepared to intervene and treat a condition for which a nursing diagnosis is established. So, for example, the nurse cannot intervene independently to treat the medical diagnosis of *pneumonia*, but can establish the nursing diagnosis of *Ineffective Breathing Pattern* and can institute nursing interventions to assist the client with that problem.

Nursing diagnoses provide a consistent vocabulary to use in communication with all healthcare workers regarding the client's status. They offer a means of synthesizing and communicating nurses' observations and judgments to all members of the healthcare team. The classification of nursing diagnoses, now known as Taxonomy II, groups diagnostic data within the following concepts:

- Health promotion
- Nutrition
- Elimination/Exchange
- Activity/Rest
- Perception/Cognition
- Self-perception
- Role relationship

Box 2-6 COMPARISON OF MEDICAL AND NURSING DIAGNOSES

Medical Diagnosis	Nursing Diagnosis
Cancer of liver	Acute Pain
Heart failure	Excess Fluid Volume
Chronic obstructive pulmonary disease	Ineffective Breathing Pattern

---

- Sexuality
- Coping/Stress tolerance
- Life principles
- Safety/Protection
- Comfort
- Growth/Development

Types of Nursing Diagnoses

NANDA International states that a nursing diagnosis can be written as an "actual" or as a "risk for" statement, and there are also "possible," "syndrome," or "health promotion" statements. Many diagnoses are further qualified by terms such as effective, ineffective, impaired, imbalanced, readiness for, disturbed, and decreased.

Actual: The nurse has validated an actual nursing diagnosis using clinical judgment, and the client has presented with specific defining characteristics. The client could benefit from nursing care.

Risk for: Based on clinical judgment, the client is more vulnerable to develop the problem than others in similar circumstances. This may also be referred to as a "potential problem." Risk diagnoses include risk factors.

The term *possible diagnosis* is not considered a true diagnosis. Writing a nursing diagnosis as "possible" alerts other nurses that some data are present to confirm the diagnosis, but the data are incomplete or insufficient to support the diagnosis as yet. Further data collection is needed to confirm or deny the diagnosis.

The term *syndrome* is a clinical judgment describing a specific cluster of nursing diagnoses that occur together and are best addressed together and through similar interventions.

A *health promotion* diagnosis focuses on the client's progress or potential progress toward healthier behaviors rather than focusing on a problem.

Diagnostic Statements

The diagnostic statement describes the health status of the client and the factors that have contributed to the status. More than 230 nursing diagnoses have been endorsed by NANDA International. With the increased use of computers for documentation, a standardized language for describing client problems is mandatory. NANDA International

diagnoses provide a consistent terminology for a variety of clinical settings. NIC also can be used both with electronic documentation systems and older, paper-based documentation systems. Table 2-1 ■ describes nursing diagnosis care plan data.

With the implementation of electronic health records (EHRs), standardized nursing languages such as NANDA International (NANDA-I) will be used to provide a broad base of nursing knowledge at the point of care. Although implementation of electronic medical records has been hampered by technical and financial issues and has not occurred universally, more than 80% of hospitals have agreements in place to adopt a certified EHR.

Components of a Nursing Diagnosis

There are basically two formats used to write the nursing diagnosis: the two-part statement and the three-part statement.

The two-part statement is the most common type of format used in practice (Box 2-7 ■). The first component is the *Diagnostic Label* or problem statement. This describes the client's response to an actual or risk health problem. The second component, *Etiology*, is the cause or contributing factor to the problem. The two components are linked by the *related to (r/t)* term.

There are several approaches to formulating a three-part statement of nursing diagnosis. The PES system (for problem, etiology, and signs and symptoms) was developed by Marjory Gordon and is used by many schools of nursing throughout the United States.

Box 2-7 EXAMPLES OF NURSING DIAGNOSIS COMPONENTS

Actual Nursing Diagnosis, written as a two-part statement:

DIAGNOSTIC LABEL (Problem)	Impaired Walking
CONTRIBUTING FACTOR (Etiology or Cause)	Related to long-leg cast secondary to fractured femur

An *Actual Nursing Diagnosis*, written as a three-part statement:

DIAGNOSTIC LABEL (Problem)	Impaired Transfer Ability
CONTRIBUTING FACTOR (Etiology or Cause)	Related to inability to move left side
CLINICAL MANIFESTATIONS (Defining Characteristics)	As evidenced by flaccid paralysis of left side

Risk-for Diagnosis, written as a two-part statement, when there are no defining characteristics:

DIAGNOSTIC Label (Problem)	Risk for Infection
RISK FACTORS	Traumatic wound with embedded debris

Table 2-1 Nursing Diagnosis Care Plan Data

Each nursing diagnosis care plan includes the following data:
• Definition of the individual nursing diagnosis
• Defining characteristics as cues describing client behavior
a. Objective data, observed or gathered through other sources such as assessment findings by the nurse
b. Subjective data, verbalized by the client
c. Meaningful patterns that identify potential client problems
d. Two to three problems that verify an actual or potential nursing diagnosis
• Related factors or risk factors
a. "Related to" indicates what should change for the client to return to optimal health.
b. Related factors are stated as: "related to," "associated with," or "contributing to" the diagnosis. They are classified as:
1. Environmental (external; e.g., hypothermia, moisture, physical immobilization)
2. Somatic (internal; e.g., alterations in fluid status, altered circulation)
3 Developmental factors (e.g., extremes in age)
c Risk factors lead to potential nursing diagnoses.
• Suggestions for use: how to use the diagnosis appropriately or differentiating it from similar diagnosis
• Suggested alternative diagnosis
a. Similar diagnosis that can be considered when identifying client's problems
b. Diagnosis that can be substituted for one that only partially matches client data
• NOC outcomes
a. Client outcomes that reflect client states or behaviors that nursing care can affect
b. Outcomes are not goals but can be used to set goals.
• Goals and evaluation criteria
a. Goals represent measurable or observable criteria that indicate whether the client problems have been resolved.
b. Use NOC outcomes, indicators, and measuring scales to establish goals.
c. Documented times and dates for meeting goals are stated.
d. Documentation of progress toward meeting goals is set according to client's condition and standards set by facility for documentation.
• NIC Interventions
a. Guide for selecting appropriate interventions
b. Each intervention has a label name and a set of activities that are identified as steps to carry out the intervention.
• Nursing activities taken by the nurse related to the nursing diagnosis
a. Assessments
b. Nursing interventions
c. Client/family teaching
d. Collaborative activities with other healthcare team members

P refers to the *problem*, or state of health, of the individual, family, or community. This problem is expressed as clearly as possible; for example, "Skin Integrity, Impaired."

E describes the *etiology*, or probable cause, of the health problem. This may refer to many factors that include client behaviors, environmental components, or the interaction of both. The etiology is combined with the problem statement by using the words "related to"; for example, "related to prolonged bed rest."

S signifies the relevant *signs and symptoms*—usually a summary of the objective assessment findings (signs) and subjective data reported by the client (symptoms). The phrase that connects this part of the statement is "as evidenced by (aeb) or as manifested by (amb)"; for example, "Impaired Skin Integrity, related to prolonged bed rest, as evidenced by a 2 × 2 cm circular red lesion or erythematous macules with moderate serosanguineous drainage."

Evidence-Based Practice

The term *evidence-based practice (EBP)* has been used since the late 1970s. Even though nursing has recognized the importance of research as an essential basis for its development, it is becoming more prevalent in nursing practice as a response to calls for quality and efficiency in client care. Nurses should make clinical decisions using the best available research and other evidence that is reflected in approved policies, procedures, and clinical guidelines in a particular healthcare agency. Use of evidence-based data promotes a consistent approach to client care that results in less care-quality variability as groups of nurses provide care to groups of clients. Other health-related disciplines have long relied on this type of empirical data when making clinical decisions.

Evidence-based nursing practice is defined as the application to clinical practice of the best available empirical evidence that applies recent research findings, in order to aid clinical decision making.

Evidence-based nursing practice, or evidence-based practice (EBP), is differentiated from research in several key ways. Basing nursing practice on evidence entails locating the latest research and other evidence, synthesizing results, and translating the evidence into protocols or guidelines that can be used to guide practice. Research is systematic investigation aimed at generating new knowledge or refining existing knowledge. Evidence-based nursing practice and research involve some of the same tasks, but the purposes of the tasks differ in the way they achieve their goals. Research generates new knowledge; evidence-based nursing practice applies the knowledge to practice.

The levels of evidence vary among researchers. Some researchers believe that the synthesis and use of scientific information comes from randomized clinical trials. Others look at the process more broadly and include information gleaned from case reports and expert opinion to guide healthcare decisions.

EBP emerges from evidence-based medicine (EBM). EBM rigorously integrates individual clinical expertise with evidence from systematic research. Systematic reviews are comprehensive in scope and quality of research, and they use mostly randomized clinical trials as the gold standard by which evidence is judged.

EBP boxes can be found throughout this book. EBP will provide you with a framework for determining the effectiveness of selected nursing skills and practice issues. As you proceed through your nursing program, you will be exposed to additional EBP research and its effect on clinical practice.

In developing evidence-based nursing practice, nurses begin not just reading research articles but also critically examining the content of articles and questioning current practice. The steps for developing a research project are provided in Box 2-8 ■.

Asking the right question is a difficult skill to learn; however, it is fundamental to the evidence-based decision-making process. The question includes four parts, referred to as PICO (some refer to it as PICOT, with T indicating the time frame for data collection).

P refers to identifying the client problem or chief complaint. This phase should also identify the disease or health status of the client, age, race, sex, previous ailments, and current medications.

I is intervention and the second step of the process. It is critical that you identify what plans are discussed for this client. It may include the use of a specific diagnostic test, treatments, adjunctive therapy, medication or the other procedures. This phase is the main consideration for the client.

C, the third phase of the process, refers to the alternative plan that is being considered. It should be specific and limited to one alternative choice in order to facilitate an effective computerized search.

O is outcome and the final phase of the PICO question. It identifies what the plan is to accomplish, improve, or affect and should be measurable. Outcomes should consist of relieving or eliminating specific symptoms, improving or maintaining function, or enhancing aesthetics.

Specific outcomes will yield better search results and allow you to find evidence-based studies that focus on the outcomes you are looking for. In order to accomplish this, you need to describe *how* the intervention is more effective, not just state that the intervention is effective. After you have identified a specific client problem and defined the question you are researching, using PICO will assist you in finding the most current valid evidence (PICO, n.d.).

Once research data are available, nursing must consider making changes in clinical practice based on the findings. In many facilities, this involves research teams that review current literature and then make appropriate recommendations

Box 2-8 EVIDENCE-BASED RESEARCH PROJECT

When completing an evidence-based research project you need to perform the following steps:

Step 1: Create the question.

The first step in implementing EBP in nursing is to identify the clinical problem and form a question. It may be a simple question related to a standard nursing procedure that has been done a certain way for many years. It may be a new way of completing a procedure. Review the medical problem and the interventions that have been in place to treat the client.

Step 2: Gather research.

Once the medical question is in place, gather the evidence (information). The primary purpose of this step is to gather information that will help solve the treatment question. Do a literature search, use the Internet, and review medical and nursing studies reported in journals that relate to your subject of interest.

Step 3: Analyze the findings.

Analyze and assess the evidence. Did it come from a valid source? Who did the study, and how was the study actually conducted? Some medical sources are more reliable than others. You must evaluate the sources of information, types of research done, and currency of the information. The information must be valid and relevant to the current treatment question.

Step 4: Implement treatment.

Based on research findings, use the information you have researched to treat the client. Everyone involved in treating the client will use the research information to create a plan of care. The plan must be based on research findings, and it must be formally implemented.

Step 5: Reexamine the process.

Obtain feedback from individuals involved in the research. Review all previous actions. Reevaluate the EBP process to determine if the plan was effective. If the treatment plan was not effective, further research or modifications may need to be done.

Step 6: Analyze and report.

Analyze and report the outcome resulting from the research project. Reporting a change in practice that improves nursing procedures will encourage others to make changes in practice settings as well.

for clinical practice. Evidence-based nursing practice can strengthen client outcomes, improve client safety, promote effective nursing practice, and increase nursing's credibility with other healthcare professionals and the general public. It should be considered another step in developing nursing's theory base.

A note of caution when reading about evidence-based practice: It should not be confused with best practices. These terms are sometimes used interchangeably, but they do not mean the same thing. **Best practices** is a term used to describe nursing interventions that have been proven effective in promoting positive client outcomes or in reducing overall costs to the client or facility. Best practices are nursing practices that are based on the best evidence available from nursing research. The goal of best practices is to apply the most recent, relevant, and helpful nursing interventions, based on research, in real-life practice. "Best practice" is a generic or general phrase for a process of infusing nursing practice with research-based knowledge.

Chapter Wrap-Up

MANAGEMENT Guidelines

Each state legislates a Nurse Practice Act for RNs, LVNs or LPNs, and advanced nurse practitioners. Healthcare facilities are responsible for establishing and implementing policies and procedures that conform to their state's regulations. Verify the regulations and role parameters for each healthcare worker in your facility.

Delegation

- The RN's responsibility when delegating client care tasks is to ensure that the care plan is followed for each client. Information contained on the care plan is reported to each healthcare worker assigned to client care.

- The RN is responsible for implementing the nursing process in all aspects of client care. LVN/LPNs may be assigned to carry out tasks within the nursing process, such as assessing clients after the initial assessment and executing interventions based on the client care plan. The RN, however, is ultimately responsible for client care, developing the plan of care, and ensuring that the plan is followed.

- The LVN/LPN may assist the RN in planning and updating the plan of care, but may not be responsible for these actions.

- Assistive personnel, such as unlicensed assistive personnel (UAP) and certified nursing assistants (CNAs), are delegated client tasks, but do participate in the actual development of the plan of care. Their input is valuable and should be considered when changes in the plan of care are necessary.

- Critical thinking processes are used by all team members as they provide client care. The RN has a more expanded scientific knowledge base and experience in utilizing these skills to provide the leadership necessary for effective and safe client care. The RN must use these skills when assigning client care and delegating activities.

Interprofessional Communication

- The RN synthesizes client data and determines the most appropriate healthcare worker to provide care to each client in her/his assignment.

- Each healthcare worker is given a report on activities to be completed during the shift.

- Dissemination of client care information is based on the client's plan of care.

- Directions are given to all healthcare workers indicating the type of client information the nurse needs immediately and information that can be given during report times. For example, if a client has a fever, the RN may want to know the temperature as soon as it is obtained.

CASE STUDY Applications

Scenario 1

You have been assigned to care for Mr. Peters, a 76-year-old widower who was admitted with the diagnosis of heart failure. He has lived alone for the last 2 years since his wife died. His children live about 1 hour away and visit him once a month. The children ordered Meals on Wheels for him, but he refused to eat the food that was delivered. "I can do my own cooking, I am not an invalid," was the answer when the nurse asked why he didn't like the Meals on Wheels program. He had not seen the physician for at least 6 months. At the last visit, the physician prescribed a moderately low-sodium diet, furosemide (Lasix) 40 mg daily, verapamil (Calan), and multiple vitamins. His admitting vital signs were BP 180/90, P 98, R 22. His weight indicated a gain of 10 pounds since the last visit. His physical assessment indicated rales in the lung bases, 3+ edema of the ankles, and difficulty breathing in the supine position and with the least amount of exertion.

- How will you use the nursing process to determine an accurate assessment database?
- What information is missing that might be important to the nurse to assist in planning care for this client? What is the best approach for obtaining the information?
- Identify at least four nursing diagnoses that are relevant for this client's plan of care. Write a two-part

and a three-part diagnostic statement for each nursing diagnosis.

- Using a nursing diagnosis book, identify NIC and NOC statements for the four nursing diagnoses listed in question 3.
- Identify the priority nursing diagnosis, and provide the rationale for your decision.
- Develop a very brief nursing care plan using the nursing process format as outlined in the text.

Scenario 2

8 a.m. You are assigned to a 22-year-old male client who was in a motorcycle crash yesterday. He sustained a compound fracture of the right fibula and tibia. He states his pain is 9/10 and it is throbbing. He is nauseated all the time. He is scheduled for surgery later in the day. You assess his wound area and notice there is a large amount of serosanguineous drainage in the dressing. You reinforce the dressing.

- Determine priority nursing diagnoses and provide rationales for your decision.
- Based on the information provided in the scenario, identify two priority nursing interventions.
- Using a nursing diagnosis textbook, develop a client care plan incorporating NIC and NOC data.

NCLEX® Review Questions

Unless otherwise specified, choose only one (1) answer.

1. Place the steps of the nursing process in sequence.
   A. Evaluation
   B. Planning
   C. Implementation
   D. Assessment
   E. Nursing diagnosis

2. Nurses who are considered critical thinkers exhibit which of the following attributes?
   Select all that apply.
   A. Possess good communication skills and are flexible
   B. Use logic and creativity
   C. Are structured in their delivery of nursing care
   D. Use a systematic method for providing care in the same order for each client
   E. Relate theory to practice

3. Which one of the following examples accurately describes a properly stated nursing diagnosis?
   A. Poor airway exchange r/t mucus accumulation in the alveoli
   B. Client exhibits pain as a result of coughing as evidenced by grimacing.

   C. Deficient knowledge r/t inadequate understanding of diabetes as evidenced by lack of regular blood glucose testing
   D. Pneumonia r/t inadequate ventilation during surgery

4. Which of the following diagnoses are considered nursing, not medical, diagnoses?
   Select all that apply.
   A. Acute pain
   B. Heart failure
   C. Cancer of the liver
   D. Ineffective breathing pattern
   E. Pulmonary edema
   F. Excess fluid volume

5. How is evidence-based nursing practice research used?
   A. To aid in clinical decision making
   B. To determine the most often used method to provide nursing care
   C. To develop new techniques for providing nursing care
   D. To differentiate nursing diagnosis from medical diagnosis

6. What is the major role of assessment, the first step of the nursing process?
   A. To develop a nursing diagnosis after collecting client health data
   B. To collect the client data and establish a database
   C. To identify short- and long-term goals based on the client's verbal statements regarding health needs
   D. To evaluate sources of client data to determine accuracy prior to implementing client care

7. How does effective client care planning promote compliance?
   A. It ensures all healthcare needs are identified.
   B. It develops the plan within 1 hour of admission.
   C. It involves the client and family with the healthcare team to develop congruent healthcare goals.
   D. It includes a teaching plan as part of the overall short-term goals.

8. During the implementation phase of the nursing process, what does the nurse do?
   A. Gathers all data and prioritizes client needs
   B. Determines clusters of clues from collected data
   C. Provides education to client and/or family
   D. Considers contingencies for modifying care plan

9. Why are systems such as the Nursing Interventions Classification (NIC) used with nursing diagnoses?
   A. They state the diagnosis more clearly in nursing terminology.
   B. They are not easily confused with medical diagnoses.
   C. They can only be used as a paper-based documentation system.
   D. They can be sent to national and regional databases.

10. In which situation can responsibilities be delegated by the nurse to other healthcare members?
   A. Asking the unlicensed assistive personnel to assist in the development of the client's plan of care
   B. Assigning the certified nursing assistants to clients who require completion of care-plan goals before discharge
   C. Asking the LVN (LPN) to assist in revising the care plan
   D. Requesting that the LVN (LPN) complete the initial care plan after admitting the client

QSEN Activity

Research Topic on Client Care

Domain: Evidence-Based Practice

KSA: Skills

Activity:

Identify a clinical problem you are interested in researching to determine the most appropriate nursing interventions that should be implemented. Follow the PICO guidelines for setting up the process: Formulate a question; gather research information that will discuss and answer the question; analyze the findings; implement the treatment; re-examine the process; and analyze the results from the research.

Bibliography

Academy of Medical-Surgical Nurses. (2014). Evidence-based practice. Retrieved from https://www.amsn.org/practice-resources/evidence-based-practice

American Nurses Association. (2015). The nursing process. Retrieved from http://www.nursingworld.org/EspeciallyForYou/StudentNurses/Thenursingprocess.aspx

Herman, T. H. & Kamitsuru, S. (Eds.). (2014). *NANDA International. Nursing Diagnoses: Definitions and Classifications, 2015–2017*, (10th ed.). Oxford: Wiley Blackwell.

Moorhead, S., Johnson, M., Maas, M. L., & Swanson, E. (2013). *Nursing Outcomes Classification (NOC)*, (5th ed.). St. Louis: Mosby.

PICO: Asking a Good Question (PICO). (n.d.). Retrieved from http://www.usc.edu/hsc/ebnet/ebframe/PICO

Riva, J. J., Malik, K. M. P., Burnie, S. J., Endicott, A. R., & Busse, J. W. (2012). What is your research question? An introduction to the PICOT format for clinicians. *Journal of the Canadian Chiropractic Association*, 56(3): 167–171. Retrieved from http://www.ncbi.nlm.nih.gov/pmc/articles/PMC3430448/

Chapter 3
Managing Client Care: Documentation and Delegation

 Learning Objectives

3.1 Describe the components of the client care plan.

3.2 Explain the method for individualizing the care plan when a standard care plan is used.

3.3 Define the term *client problem or need*.

3.4 State the most important reason for using nursing diagnoses in care planning.

3.5 Define the use of deadlines and checkpoints in the client care plan.

3.6 Compare and contrast a clinical pathway and a client care plan.

3.7 Explain at least three purposes of charting.

3.8 Describe at least three major components of accurate charting.

3.9 Complete a charting exercise in any of the charting systems using a simulated situation.

3.10 List the four items that should be charted for every client.

3.11 Define the terms *subjective data* and *objective data* in SOAP and other documentation.

3.12 Describe the legal ramifications for completing unusual occurrence reports.

3.13 Discuss specific client activities requiring consent forms.

3.14 Discuss the legal risks of computer charting.

3.15 Discuss the RN's role in delegating client care.

3.16 Complete a data collection tool based on a clinical situation.

3.17 Develop a time-management worksheet for client care.

Chapter Outline

Cross Reference: See discussion of the nursing process in Chapter 2. At the end of each chapter, see Delegation as it applies to that chapter's skills.

Terminology

Acuity system a method for determining staffing requirements based on the assessment of client needs

Client care plan a plan of care, usually written, that meets the special needs of each client

Charting a process of recording information about a client concerning the progress of his or her disease and treatment

Charting by exception (CBE) documenting only exceptions to predetermined nursing standards in a narrative format

Clinical pathways, *also called* critical paths or care paths; interdisciplinary client care plans using specific assessments, interventions, and outcomes for specified health-related conditions

Computer-assisted charting entering client information into the computer for storage and retrieval at a later time

Delegation transferring to a competent individual the authority to perform a selected task in a selected situation

EHR electronic health records

EMR electronic medical records

Flow sheets client data recorded or graphed to show patterns or alterations in findings

Focus charting charting on one "specific" area using DAR format (data, action, response)

HIPAA health insurance portability and accountability act; legislation that describes privacy requirements in the healthcare industry

HIT health information technology

Kardex a method of paper documentation that uses a convenient and readily accessible file of cards containing current client information

NIC nursing interventions classification; a system of standardized nursing interventions that nurses perform; used for clinical documentation and communication across disciplines

NOC nursing outcome classification; a system of standardized nursing outcomes for evaluating the effects of interventions provided by nurses or other healthcare professionals

Nursing informatics a specialty area in which nurses develop, customize, and evaluate information technologies for adaptation to their particular facility's needs

Point-of-care (POC) documentation charting that is completed while interacting with the client, preferably immediately after care has occurred

Problem-oriented medical record (POMR) a client record that is organized according to the individual's specific health problems

Report an account of something that has been seen, heard, done, or considered

SBAR situation, background, assessment, and recommendations; a tool that standardizes a "handoff communication" when one nurse turns a client over to another nurse

SOAP subjective, objective, assessment, plan; pattern for organizing nursing notes consistently by what the client feels subjectively (S), what the nurse observes objectively (O), how the nurse assesses the situation (A), and what the nurse plans (P)

Source-oriented charting information in the chart organized according to its source; for example, healthcare provider's progress notes, nurses' notes

Unusual occurrence record of an unusual happening or event that could affect client or staff safety; also commonly referred to as variance or incident report

Client Care Plans

Documentation is a major component of the nurse's role. Importance is based on several factors: evaluation of planned client care, communication to other healthcare professionals, The Joint Commission and client safety regulations, reimbursement from the federal government, and legal implications. If a treatment, medication, or activity has not been documented in the chart, legally it is very difficult to prove that the client actually received the care. Contact with the client and care delivered to the client must be documented. One of the most useful tools to provide this care is the client care plan.

Client care plans are an integral part of providing nursing care. Without them, quality and consistency of client care may not be obtained. Client care plans provide a means of communication among nurses and other healthcare providers. Plans should serve as a focal point for client care assignments and making **report**.

Each client must have an individualized care plan; the client or family must be involved in the development of the care plan, and it must be interdisciplinary.

Some facilities still require that nurses develop standardized or individualized care plans. These care plans require ongoing modification to ensure they include multidisciplinary planning and interventions. Computerized nursing care plans have had a positive impact because of the variety of nursing diagnoses to choose from and the increase in documentation of signs and symptoms, related factors, and nursing interventions for any nursing problem. They have improved overall documentation and completeness.

All care plans must include the following information: client's needs or problems (both actual and potential), expected outcomes or short-term goals, nursing interventions or actions, and discharge criteria or long-term goals. There is an ongoing movement to ensure that care plans, while personalized to meet individual client goals, include standardized components and benchmarks based on evidence-based practice, such as guidelines for care of the client with an acute myocardial infarction (AMI).

Once the goals of client care are established, each step in meeting these goals is detailed, including specific observations and how often the observations are made. Step-by-step directions are included for difficult problems, such as lengthy and involved dressing changes. Individualized client teaching programs are described on the care plan. All of this information is essential in providing continuity of client care.

Components of a Care Plan

Individualizing Care Plans All clients must have an individualized plan of care even when a standard care plan (SCP) is used (Figure 3-1 ■). To individualize the care plan, space is generally provided at the end of the preprinted or electronic form to allow the nurse to identify unusual problems or needs. SCPs are individualized by activating the problems that pertain to the client (Figure 3-2 ■). The nurse may add another problem to the bottom of the form to further individualize the care plan.

Initiating the Plan The client plan of care is formulated after the assessment phase of the nursing process. The nurse, after completing the nursing history and assessment, determines whether an SCP is available for the client's medical diagnosis or if an individualized care plan must be generated. If an SCP is available, the nurse need only circle, date, and initial the needs that are relevant for that client. When an individualized care plan is being generated, the nurse translates client needs into nursing diagnoses and enters them into the computer or writes them on the care plan. Nursing diagnoses are recognized descriptions of client needs.

Note: An overview of the nursing process is provided in Chapter 2.

EVIDENCE-BASED PRACTICE
Standardized Care Plans
In one study, nurses reported that the use of an SCP facilitated their daily work, especially for new employees, and worked well as a checklist ensuring the quality of care. The documentation was experienced as easy and less time consuming, with less redundant information. However, even though 90% reported a positive attitude toward working according to an SCP, it was also sometimes experienced as inflexible (Jakobsson & Wann-Hansson, 2012).

Identifying Client Problems or Needs A client problem or need is a condition that requires assistance or intervention from a healthcare team member to return the client to a healthy state. The client problem is identified as any unmet need. It can be as basic as the need for adequate comfort or nourishment or can address more complex psychosocial needs. (See Chapter 2.)

Expected Outcomes or Goals After the problems have been identified, the nurse sets goals or expected outcomes for client care that are congruent with the goals of the client or significant other. The electronic client care plan (see Figure 3-2) shows several examples of a client-centered goal and the nursing interventions necessary to attain each goal.

Nursing Outcomes Classification NOC is a comprehensive research-based standardized classification of client and client outcomes developed to evaluate the effects of interventions provided by nurses or other health care professionals. An outcome is an observable physical or behavioral state that is measured along a continuum. Each outcome has a definition and a list of indicators that can be used to rate the status of the client in relation to the outcome.

Interventions After problems and expected outcomes are identified on the care plan, the nurse determines appropriate nursing interventions that meet the goals of care. The activated plan of care will specify the exact nursing actions to be carried out or provide explicit instructions on how care is to be delivered, including time and frequency of the intervention. In most instances, there is an opportunity to free-text additional personalized caring interventions in the chart.

Nursing Intervention Classification NIC is a comprehensive, research-based standardized classification of interventions that nurses perform. It is useful for clinical documentation and communication across disciplines. The classification includes interventions nurses do on behalf of the client. To date, there are over 550 recognized interventions separated according to domains, such as Family, Communication, and Behavioral. The American Nurses Association and The Joint Commission recognize the NIC system as a standardized nursing set.

Checkpoints and Deadlines SCPs include checkpoint (CP) and deadline (DL) columns. The electronic version of a care plan typically includes alerts and/or messages that prompt the nurse to address DL and CPs. In some instances, electronic messages are sent to the nurse inbox as a reminder to follow up with client care plan. The CP indicates how often the action or intervention should be checked, observed, or carried out and therefore how often it should be charted. The DL column indicates the time when the goal should be met or the action is no longer necessary. It is important to document the exact time and date when the nursing action should be completed to communicate this information to the entire nursing staff.

Updating Care Plans

To ensure that client care plans are current and relevant, they should be reviewed on a daily basis and updated at

(Text continues on p. 39.)

Pneumonia - CAP (Planned)
Last updated on: 4/10/2015 1:06 PM CDT   by: Murray, Phyllis

⊿ Vital Signs			
☐		Vital Signs	q8hr
☐	+1 day	Vital Signs	QID
☑		Pulse Oximetry	q8hr
⊿ Activity			
☐		Ambulate	Constant order
☐		Bedrest	Constant order
☐		Up ad Lib	Constant Order, with assistance
☐		Up to Chair	3 times a day
⊿ Diet			
☐		NPO	
☐		Regular Diet	Start Meal: Breakfast
☐		Therapeutic Diet	1500 kcal
⊿ Patient Care			
Assessment			
☐		Cardiac Monitoring	Constant Order
☐		Height/Length	Once
☐		Intake and Output	q8hr
☐		Weight	Once
General			
☐		Notify Provider	
Interventions			
☐		Below the Knee Graduated Compression Stocking	Constant Order
☐		Below the Knee Intermittent Pneumatic Compression Device	Constant Order
☐		Peripheral IV Insertion	
☐		Urinary Catheter Insertion	External
☐		Education General	Constant order
⊿ IV Solutions			
☐		Dextrose 5% with 0.45% NaCl	
☐		Sodium Chloride 0.45%	
☐		Sodium Chloride 0.9%	
⊿ Medications			
Analgesics: Combination Analgesics			
☐		acetaminophen-oxycodone (Percocet 5/325)	1 tab(s), Oral, q6hr, PRN Pain
☐		acetaminophen-hydrocodone (Vicodin ES)	1 tab(s), Oral, q6hr, PRN Pain
Analgesics: Non-Opioids			
☐		acetaminophen	650 mg, Oral, q4hr, PRN Pain
☐		ibuprofen	400 mg, Oral, q4hr, PRN Pain
Analgesics: Opioids			
☐		morphine	1 mg, IV, q4hr, PRN Pain
Antimicrobials			
☐		gentamicin	10 mg/kg, IV, q24hr
☐		tobramycin	10 mg/kg, IV, q24hr
Cephalosporins			
☐		cefotaxime	750 mg, IV, q4hr
Immunizations: Influenza			
☐		influenza virus vaccine, inactivated	0.5 mL, IM, Once
Immunizations: Pneumococcal			
☐		pneumococcal 23-valent vaccine	0.5 mL, IM, Once
Smoking Cessation Medications			
☐		buPROPion	150 mg, Tab-ChewER, Oral, QID, 3 day(s)
⊿ Laboratory			
Chemistry Panels			
☐		Electrolyte Panel	Blood, AM Draw collect
☐		Hepatic Function Panel	Blood, AM Draw collect
☐		Basic Metabolic Panel	Blood, AM Draw collect
⊿ Consults			
☐		Consult to Home Health	Routine
☐		Consult to Respiratory Therapy	Routine
☐		Consult to Social Services	Routine

FIGURE 3-1 Template of care plan for client with pneumonia.

Source: From Cerner Electronic Health Record. © Cerner Corporation. Pearson has restricted permission to reproduce and distribute this copyrighted work. Further reproduction or distribution is strictly prohibited without written consent of Cerner Corporation.

	Offset		Component	Status	Details	
Pneumonia - CAP (Initiated)						
Last updated on: 4/10/2015 1:21 PM CDT by: Murray, Phyllis						
◢ Vital Signs						
✔			Vital Signs	Ordered	04/10/15 13:20:00 CDT, q8hr	
✔	+1 day		Vital Signs	Ordered	04/11/15 13:20:00 CDT, QID	
✔			Pulse Oximetry	Ordered	04/10/15 13:20:00 CDT, q8hr	
◢ Activity						
✔			Ambulate	Ordered	04/10/15 13:20:00 CDT, Constant order	
✔			Up to Chair	Ordered	04/10/15 13:20:00 CDT, Stop Date 04/10/15 13:20:00 CDT, …	
◢ Diet						
✔			Regular Diet	Ordered	04/10/15 13:20:00 CDT, Start Meal: Breakfast	
◢ Patient Care						
Assessment						
✔			Cardiac Monitoring	Ordered	04/10/15 13:20:00 CDT, Constant Order	
✔			Height/Length	Ordered	04/10/15 13:20:00 CDT, Once, Stop Date 04/10/15 13:20:00 …	
✔			Intake and Output	Ordered	04/10/15 13:20:00 CDT, q8hr	
✔			Weight	Ordered	04/10/15 13:20:00 CDT, Once, Stop Date 04/10/15 13:20:00 …	
Interventions						
✔			Peripheral IV Insertion	Ordered	04/10/15 13:20:00 CDT	
✔			Education General	Ordered	04/10/15 13:20:00 CDT, Constant order	
◢ IV Solutions						
✔			Dextrose 5% with 0.45% NaCl 1,000 mL	Ordered	Total volume (mL): 1,000, Infuse at: 125 mL/hr, Start da…	
◢ Medications						
Analgesics: Combination Analgesics						
✔			acetaminophen-oxycodone (Percocet 5/325)	Ordered	1 tab(s), Oral, q6hr, PRN Pain 1 day(s), Start date 04/10/15 …	
Analgesics: Non-Opioids						
✔			ibuprofen	Ordered	400 mg, Oral, q4hr, PRN Pain, Start date 04/10/15 13:20:00 …	
Analgesics: Opioids						
✔			morphine	Ordered	1 mg, IV, q4hr, PRN Pain, Start date 04/10/15 13:20:00 CDT, …	
Antimicrobials						
✔			gentamicin	Ordered	840 mg, IV, q24hr, Start date 04/10/15 13:20:00 CDT, Stop …	
Cephalosporins						
✔			cefotaxime	Ordered	750 mg, IV, q4hr, Start date 04/10/15 14:00:00 CDT, Stop …	
Immunizations: Influenza						
✔			influenza virus vaccine, inactivated	Ordered	0.5 mL, IM, Once, Start date 04/10/15 14:00:00 CDT, Stop …	
Immunizations: Pneumococcal						
✔			pneumococcal 23-valent vaccine	Ordered	0.5 mL, IM, Once, Start date 04/10/15 14:00:00 CDT, Stop …	
◢ Laboratory						
Chemistry Panels						
✔			Hepatic Function Panel	Ordered	AM Draw collect, 04/11/15 5:00:00 CDT	
✔			Basic Metabolic Panel	Ordered	AM Draw collect, 04/11/15 5:00:00 CDT	
◢ Consults						
✔			Consult to Home Health	Ordered	04/10/15 13:20:00 CDT, Routine	
✔			Consult to Respiratory Therapy	Ordered	04/10/15 13:20:00 CDT, Routine	

FIGURE 3-2 Activated care plan for client with pneumonia. Note that only applicable interventions have been ordered.

least every 24 to 48 hours. There are several ways to update a care plan.

Computerized Client Care Plans

The format used in most electronic health or medical records (**EHRs** or **EMRs**) individualizes client care plans according to each healthcare facility's specifications. Electronic format decreases preparation time for writing individualized care plans, as do standardized plans developed and written by clinical experts using evidence-based guidelines, but the nurse must always determine the relevance and appropriateness of the care plan for each individual client. The care plan for each client is updated daily by the EHR.

Kardex or Nurses' Notes

Some facilities that have not migrated to an electronic healthcare system still use the **Kardex** system, which is a tool to organize the nurses' daily activities. In this system, the "update" column is used when the original deadline is reached but the problem persists. A new deadline must then be established. If the problem exists beyond the third postoperative day, a new time frame for goal achievement is determined and documented in the update column.

Paper Care Plans

Activating Paper Care Plans

When SCPs are used, a systematic approach to activation and deactivation must be understood by all nursing personnel. As already stated, a common approach is to circle, date, and initial problems that are relevant for the individual client. Any problem that is not circled remains inactivated and should not be assessed, treated, or documented. From the example, you can see that the client has two of the problems listed, an ineffective breathing pattern and a knowledge deficit regarding discharge medication. Items 1 and 3 are circled. In the date column, the date, time, and initials of the nurse activating the problem are entered. The second problem is not activated; therefore, a circle is not placed around the number.

Inactivating Paper Care Plans

To inactivate the problem using a paper–pencil SCP, a single line through the problem or intervention with a black pen can be made. In the update/DC column, the date, time, and nurse's initials should be placed next to the crossed out, inactivated information. If only one of the interventions is not necessary, a line is drawn through that intervention and initials placed next to it in the initial column. The other interventions are left current and active.

Evaluating Care Plans

The evaluation of how well the client care plan was individualized to meet the needs of the client is tested at discharge. If the care plan was appropriate, the discharge criteria are met. The nursing interventions and problems are then inactivated or discontinued. Frequently, there are clients who, on discharge, have not met the discharge criteria for various reasons. The documentation should reflect those problems that still exist, the extent to which the problem is being resolved, and additional information to indicate which plans were formulated for goal achievement.

Care Plan Formats in the form of electronic health records are gradually replacing the paper–pencil format for documentation. This workplace redesign is transforming how we deliver nursing care. The type and method of nursing care plans available is also changing. The Joint Commission's requirements are becoming more flexible and are allowing new ways to document client care. Critical paths, protocols, and standardized nursing care plans are used with or are replacing the more traditional care plans.

Critical Paths (Clinical Pathways)

Critical pathways use an interdisciplinary approach. It routinely utilizes a nursing information system (NIS), a technology that supports collaboration and improves healthcare decision making at the point of care, which can ultimately improve healthcare outcomes. In this system, traditional nursing care plans do not exist. A critical path, or **clinical pathway**, is a standardized multidisciplinary plan of care developed for clients with common or prevalent conditions. It is a tool developed using best practice guidelines by all health team members to achieve client outcomes in a predictable and established time frame. It is used on each shift to direct and monitor client care. These plans indicate the actions and interventions achieved at designated times in order to meet the criteria for reimbursable length of stay. For example, a client with a total hip replacement has a critical path that states time frames for getting out of bed, gait training, and ambulation listed under the physical activity section of the form. On the second postoperative day, the client should move from bed to chair with assistance. Nursing diagnoses are not always incorporated in the critical path.

Documentation of nursing activities completed in response to the critical path varies according to facility policies and guidelines. Some facilities initial each day's completed tasks on the critical path document; others use flow charts and narrative **charting**. In the EHR, the actions and interventions highlighted in the clinical pathway are identified as "Tasks." This term is a reminder to the nurse to ensure these activities are performed.

If the client does not achieve the expected outcome in the specified time, a "variance" occurs (Figure 3-3 ■), and an individual plan of care is developed that may then incorporate a nursing diagnosis. For example, if a client is unable to ambulate by Day 3, a nursing diagnosis can be used to individualize the client's variance from the critical path expectations. An individualized care plan is initiated and charting continues on the variance until it is resolved.

In addition to the pathway and multidisciplinary problem record, the more sophisticated clinical pathways also include an admitting assessment, nursing history including risk factors for falls and skin, nutrition risk evaluation, and social or cultural variables. An ongoing admission database is included in the packet. Also, this section contains a discharge planning risk assessment and multidisciplinary team conference section.

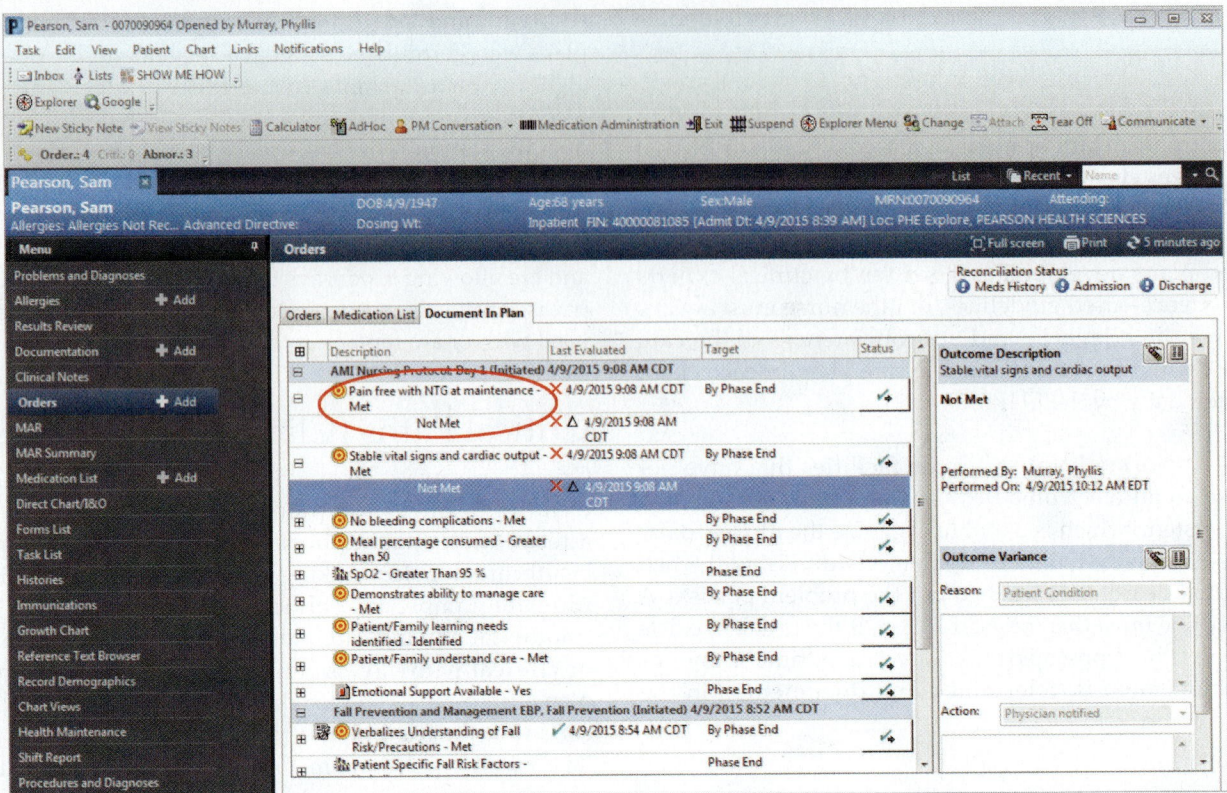

FIGURE 3-3 Sample of variance charting.

Source: From Cerner Electronic Health Record. © Cerner Corporation. Pearson has restricted permission to reproduce and distribute this copyrighted work. Further reproduction or distribution is strictly prohibited without written consent of Cerner Corporation.

There are several advantages for using critical or clinical pathways, including continuity of care among all healthcare workers—discharge planning is begun on admission, and teaching plans are initiated early in the hospitalization. Clinical or critical pathways have been proven to reduce length of hospital stay, complications, and costs. Client satisfaction has also increased with the use of pathways. However, not all clients can be placed on pathways. For more complex cases, those requiring specialized care, or clients experiencing complications, individualized care plans are more appropriate.

Protocols   A protocol is a series of actions that are nurse driven and that may be implemented to manage a client's clinical course. It is based on specific interventions (to include medications) to be decided by the nurse as long as the client meets certain criteria. There are several uses for protocols within various healthcare settings. Protocols can be used with specific disorders, such as hyperglycemia. The glycemic management protocol requires ongoing nursing assessment and intervention. Protocols identify specific actions to be taken to ensure accurate and safe care of clients requiring specialized equipment or treatments.

Protocols are sometimes used in place of care plans, particularly in emergency departments, outpatient surgery, labor and delivery, postanesthesia departments, and operating rooms. Protocols for client care in each of these areas are practical, because clients have common needs. For example, all clients in the postanesthesia care unit (PACU) must have their respiratory status monitored, fluid balance maintained, and level of consciousness assessed. These clients must also meet certain criteria for discharge from the

unit. In these settings, there is no real requirement for individualized plans of care. The time spent in these specialty areas is usually very limited and the service very specific. Protocols can be used in conjunction with SCPs, individualized care plans, and critical paths. The use of protocols decreases the amount of documentation required on the care plan, because actions and interventions are described in detail on the protocol. Using protocols in these situations promotes safety and has been shown to improve client care outcomes and to decrease client length of stay (Figure 3-4 ■).

Documentation (Charting)

Next to direct client care, documentation is one of the nurse's most important functions. Documenting is the process of recording vital information about a client, describing the care or service provided to that client. It serves many important purposes:

- Documentation communicates information, such as facts, figures, and observations, to other members of the client's healthcare team.
- Documentation assists supervisory personnel to evaluate the staff's performance on a day-by-day basis for specific clients.
- Documentation provides a permanent record for future reference that may become a legal document in the event of litigation or prosecution.
- Documentation helps management to establish an **acuity system** to maintain adequate staff levels based on client acuity.

Pearson, Sam				

Pearson, Sam
DOB:4/9/1947 | Age:68 years | Sex:Male | MRN:0070090964
Allergies: Allergies Not Recorded | Advanced Directive: | Dosing Wt: | Inpatient FIN: 4000081085 [Admit Dt: 4/9/2015 8:39 AM] Loc: PHE Explore, PEARSON HEALTH SCIE

Menu

Problems and Diagnoses
Allergies ✚ Add
Results Review
Documentation ✚ Add
Clinical Notes
Orders ✚ Add
MAR
MAR Summary
Medication List ✚ Add
Direct Chart/I&O
Forms List
Task List
Histories
Immunizations
Growth Chart
Reference Text Browser
Record Demographics
Chart Views
Health Maintenance
Shift Report
Procedures and Diagnoses

Orders

✚ Add | Document Medication by Hx | Reconciliation ▾ | Check Interactions

Orders | Medication List | Document In Plan

View

Orders for Signature
Plans
  Document In Plan
  Medical
    AMI Protocol
      Day 1 (Planned Pending)
      Day 2 (Planned Pending)
      Day 3 (Planned Pending)
      AMI Medical OrderSet (Planned Pending)
  Nursing
    AMI Nursing Protocol
      Day 1 (Planned Pending)
      Day 2 (Planned Pending)
      Day 3 (Planned Pending)
      Fall Prevention and Management EBP
        Fall Prevention (Initiated)
        Post-Fall Care (Planned)
        Fall Seen AND Has No Injury Risk Factors (Planned)
        Fall Not Seen OR Has Injury Risk Factors (Planned)
  Suggested Plans (0)
Orders
  Protocol
  Non Categorized
  Condition
  Vital Signs
  Activity
  Diet
  ☑ Patient Care
  IV Solutions
  Medications
  Laboratory
  Diagnostic Tests

	Component	Status	Details
	AMI Nursing Protocol, Day 1 (Planned Pending)		
	Outcomes		
☑	Pain free with NTG at maintenance - Met		By Phase End
☑	Stable vital signs and cardiac output - Met		By Phase End
☑	No bleeding complications - Met		By Phase End
☑	Meal percentage consumed - Greater than 50		By Phase End
☑	SpO2 - Greater Than 95 %		During Phase
☑	Demonstrates ability to manage care - Met		By Phase End
☑	Patient/Family learning needs identified - Identified		By Phase End
☑	Patient/Family understand care - Met		By Phase End
	Interventions		
☑	Cardiac Monitoring		
☑	Intake and Output		
☑	Emotional Support Available - Yes		During Phase
	AMI Nursing Protocol, Day 2 (Planned Pending)		
	Outcomes		
☑	Patient/Family understand care - Met		By Phase End
☑	Pain free with NTG at maintenance - Met		By Phase End
☑	SpO2 - Greater Than 95 %		During Phase
☑	Stable vital signs and cardiac output - Met		By Phase End
☑	Meal percentage consumed - Greater than 50		By Phase End
☑	Demonstrates ability to manage care - Met		By Phase End
	Interventions		
☑	Cardiac Monitoring		
☑	Intake and Output		
	AMI Nursing Protocol, Day 3 (Planned Pending)		
	Outcomes		
☑	Pain free with NTG at maintenance - Met		By Phase End
☑	Stable vital signs and cardiac output - Met		By Phase End
☑	No bleeding complications - Met		By Phase End
☑	Pain free with NTG at maintenance - Met		By Phase End
☑	Discharge medications initiated - Met		By Phase End
	Interventions		
☑	Cardiac Monitoring		

FIGURE 3-4 Example of protocol triggered by assessment data in EHR. Notice the circled indication about initiated actions.

Source: From Cerner Electronic Health Record. © Cerner Corporation. Pearson has restricted permission to reproduce and distribute this copyrighted work. Further reproduction or distribution is strictly prohibited without written consent of Cerner Corporation.

Documentation—A Method of Communication

Complete and accurate documentation is essential to protect both the client and the nurse. In communicating observations and actions, the nurse helps to ensure both quality and continuity of health care for clients. (Frequently, a client's reaction time is nearly as important as the reaction itself, so accuracy of time observations is an integral part of the charting process.) Recorded information provides a valuable database for nurses on subsequent shifts (Figure 3-5 ■). As they resume responsibility for the client, they can determine what events occurred during prior time periods.

FIGURE 3-5 Charting is completed immediately following client care, either at the bedside or nurses' station.

Other personnel interested in the chart include the client's attending physician, the infection control nurse, discharge coordinator, utilization review personnel, and other hospital staff specialists who are checking on the client's progress or lack of positive reaction to treatment.

It is important to communicate the needs of the client as identified by each member of the healthcare team. Since nurses have the greatest amount of direct client contact, it is appropriate for them to coordinate the important function of documentation.

EVIDENCE-BASED PRACTICE
Nurse–Physician Communication

A recent study, focused on challenges to nurses in retrieving, documenting, and communicating client care information, found that nurse–physician communication accounted for only 1%–5% of the nurse's time, despite the importance of interprofessional communication (Keenan, Yakel, Lopez, Tschannen, & Ford, 2013).

Charting provides one means for assessing the quality and effectiveness of nursing care. Nurse managers, team leaders, and supervisors use nurses' notes as a basis for staff evaluations. Because charts are documented descriptions of nursing actions, the quality of nursing care may be evaluated on the basis of the quality of charting notes.

Since charting describes nursing interventions and their outcomes, other healthcare personnel can determine whether subsequent treatment should be changed.

A client's record includes all charting and becomes part of a legal document. Should a client's hospital record be introduced in court, the notes become a legal record of the care provided by each healthcare provider. Legally, care that is not recorded is considered to be care that was not provided. It is necessary therefore to chart all care that you *do* provide, as well as any care that you *do not* provide.

The legal requirement for documentation is found in state laws and professional requirements. As a new nurse, you should be aware of the state regulations regarding documentation in the state in which you practice.

The Joint Commission states its requirements for documentation in its nursing care standards. Examples of the documentation standards include an admission assessment performed and documented by a registered nurse that includes consideration of biophysical, psychosocial, cultural, environmental, self-care, educational, and discharge planning; nursing care based on identified nursing diagnoses or client care needs and client care standards; needs that are consistent with the therapies of other disciplines; interventions identified to meet the client's needs; the actual client care provided while hospitalized; educational information provided; and the ability of the client or family to manage the continuing care on discharge.

Charting Format

The format of the client health record, whether electronic or paper, varies from hospital to hospital. Most important is the content. First, documentation should include the assessment completed at the beginning of the shift. This information provides a baseline for changes that may occur later in the client's condition. If there are no such changes, this fact should be entered as the final entry. Some hospitals require that all parts of the assessment be documented; others require that only abnormalities be documented.

As the shift progresses, certain items should always be included in documentation, including changes in the client's emotional, medical, or mental condition. Nurses are generally attuned to medical changes, such as shock, hemorrhage, or a change in level of consciousness; however, they must also observe for subtle or overt emotional changes. Anger, depression, or joy should be documented, because these emotions often indicate the client's response to the illness. Recording these changes enables other nurses to act appropriately during subsequent shifts. It is also important to document if *no* changes occurred in the client's condition so that treatments can be modified as necessary. Normal aspects of the client's condition should be noted as well.

Whenever possible, **point-of-care (POC) documentation** is highly recommended. POC documentation is the documentation of clinical information *while* nurses are interacting with and delivering care to clients. POC documentation is recommended to ensure accurate and timely entries.

Reactions to any unscheduled or PRN medications must be documented. Because each medication is given to meet a specified need, the client's response or lack of response must be recorded to document whether the need was met. To complete this part of the entry, note the time the medication was given, the problem for which the medication was given, and the expected solution. For example: "7 a.m. c/o moderate RUQ abdominal incisional pain, 7 on pain scale. Roxanol, 30 mg, PO for pain." When the effects of the medication are known, write another note: "8 a.m. States pain tolerable at 3 on pain scale."

Finally, client teaching and the client's response to teaching are important to document. Notes may describe return demonstrations, verbalization of learning, or resistance to instruction. Because most teaching takes place over a period of days, documentation includes both what was taught and how the client responded. Then other nurses will know whether to repeat the previous instructions, reinforce them, or start a new topic.

Frequently, repetitive aspects of nursing care, such as vital signs and intake and output, are documented on **flow sheets**. If flow sheets are used, the information does not need to be repeated in the nursing notes. The exception is an abnormal measurement that is a part of a larger assessment. For example: *"c/o sharp abd. pain. BP 78/50. P 136. Skin cold & diaphoretic. NG tube draining bright red bloody fluid with small clots. Reported to Dr. Jones."*

Avoiding Legal Problems in Documentation

- Use facts. If you chart "healthcare provider notified," include time called, facts you gave, and his or her response.
- Do not use pat phrases. Be specific and use individual assessment parameters. Do not chart global assessments such as "IV running."
- Be professional when you chart. Do not make interpretations; state what happened; for instance, "suggested to healthcare provider that client requires heart monitor" and healthcare provider responded "case does not warrant a monitor." If this client were later to be involved in a lawsuit, these notes indicate that the nurse was observant, alert, and aware that the client might be in danger.
- Do not use words such as *mistake* or *accident*; write specifically what incident occurred and what actions were taken.
- Do not use tentative or vague statements such as *appears* or *apparently*.
- Use correct language and medical terms. Do not use slang or abbreviations that are not generally accepted.
- Use correct grammar and spelling.
- Do not chart for someone else.
- Do not chart ahead of time. Charting should be done at point of care. Do not wait until the end of the shift.
- Do not alter a medical record. Draw a single line through an incorrect entry and initial and date the error.
- Write in late entries when you think about them; do not try to go back into earlier charting and insert the information. Label the information as "late entry" and put the time it actually happened in the entry.

- Countersign care given by assistive staff only if the facility allows you to countersign, and then do so only after you review the entry and are familiar with the care provided to the client.
- Chart potentially serious situations; include observations, reports to the healthcare provider and supervisor, and whether any action was taken. Be precise; add quotes or specific communication. This is the only kind of charting that holds up in court.
- Report problems to appropriate authorities, such as suspected child or elder abuse, to social services.
- Provide the best care you are capable of giving; then precisely chart your observations, interventions, and communications. This is the best deterrent to later legal problems.
- When using an electronic health record, never cut and paste clinical notes from a previous encounter.

Forensic Charting

The content of nurse's notes may affect the outcome of criminal investigations; when charting, especially in the ER, OR, or suspected assault cases, nurses must document exactly and carefully. Forensics is not only linked to criminal investigations; it is the connection between medical data and the legal process. Nurses must be aware that their documentation may be involved in a future legal case.

LEGAL CONSIDERATIONS

The client was admitted with a fractured right femur. Physician orders were to turn the client every 2 hours. While hospitalized, the client developed several pressure ulcers, one severe enough to cause her right leg to be amputated. From examination of the documents, the court determined the client was turned 18 times and should have been turned 117 times.

Most cases will be judged on the basis of "if it was not documented, it was not done." Good documentation is critical for the nurse's defense.

Source: Hurlock v. Parklane Medical Center (1985)

Informatics

Nurses are at the hub of client health information, so it is increasingly important for nurses to master technology (Figure 3-6 ■). **Nursing informatics** is a specialty area in which nurses develop, customize, and evaluate various information technologies for adaptation to their particular facility's needs. Nurse informaticists' major responsibilities are to develop systems and act as communication liaisons for their care facility.

According to the office of the National Coordinator of Health Information Technology (**HIT**), as of 2012, 44% of hospitals in the United States had adopted a basic EHR (a system with basic functionality such as clinician notes). Furthermore, more than 85% of hospitals had agreements in place to adopt a certified EHR. Approximately 34.5% of U.S.

FIGURE 3-6 RN informatics tech specialist helps to update and maintain the electronic database.

hospitals use bar code technology for medication administration. These numbers will increase, as there is a more determined effort to adhere to safety regulations.

Electronic Charting

With the advent of the American Reinvestment & Recovery Act (ARRA) enacted in 2009, more hospitals are integrating **electronic health record** systems as a way of improving client care and utilizing nurses' time more efficiently. Electronic information systems are moving documentation of client care from handwritten charting into the computer. With these systems, client data can be input and retrieved with the click of a mouse. Data can be input and a new assessment generated within minutes. These electronic systems improve client care, reduce health disparities, improve care coordination but are also purported to save nurses' time. Nursing organizations and accrediting agencies are placing more and more emphasis on electronic documentation. Some disadvantages include limitations on software to communicate the personal aspects of nursing care. Narrative text boxes have character limitations; this forces the nurse to parse the documentation to conform to the space available.

Computer-assisted charting can be implemented by itself, or, as in most cases, it is a component of a facility medical information system. There are so many constraints on time and resources that this type of system is becoming a necessity for healthcare agencies today. Inaccurate documentation has a significant impact on quality of client care, costs, and revenues. Redundant information input wastes valuable nursing time. Missing or incomplete documentation is costly and frustrating. If supplies or treatments are not documented, payment cannot be obtained.

NISs can manage clinical data in a variety of inpatient and outpatient healthcare settings (Box 3-1 ■). These systems allow nurses to provide and access accurate and timely information. This type of charting allows the nurse to select content phrases on a screen that automatically builds a comprehensive record without inputting all the individual pieces of information.

FIGURE 3-7 Charting at nurses' station.

Box 3-1 **TIGER INITIATIVE**

The Technology Informatics Guiding Educational Reform (TIGER) initiative is a grassroots effort started in 2006 dedicated to preparing the clinical workforce to use health information technology and informatics in the delivery of health care. The TIGER initiative identified a set of recommended competencies that all nurses in health care should have: basic computer skills, information literacy, and clinical information management.

Source: The TIGER Initiative (n.d.)

Computerized charting can be accomplished in a nurses' station or at the bedside (Figure 3-7 and 3-8 ■). Most of the necessary documentation can be done at the bedside if the equipment is available. This includes vital signs, admission assessment, nursing assessment, intake and output records, client education records, and client care plans.

Once the information is entered into the computer, it can be disseminated to different reports without the nurse's intervention. This type of charting constantly updates information from many sources. For example, physiologic measurements are documented and updated on the computer terminal instantaneously. The information is easily retrievable by the nursing personnel as questions arise (Figure 3-9 ■). Reference material and clinical decision support (CDS) for common nursing problems ensure quick reference and easily retrieved information to provide safe nursing care. When the client is to be discharged, the nursing discharge summary is completed. The electronic discharge summary includes not only the client's physical condition, but also the status of client teaching and follow-up plans.

In addition to making the documentation of client care and the communication between departments much simpler and less time-consuming, many EHRs contain NISs, which are technologies that support collaboration and clinical decision making. EHRs such as Cerner contain drug databases that give nurses up-to-date information about medications. In addition, they include evidence-based protocols built in with direct links to the evidence. Safety features include triggers and alerts to remind the nurse to include certain aspects of the initial assessment. For example, if the nurse documents the client is bedridden and incontinent, immediately the EHR will prompt the nurse to complete a Braden Skin Assessment.

Bedside E-Documentation   Electronic documentation
is becoming more familiar in hospitals and clinics. Tablets, workstation on wheels (WOWs), and smart devices have the following advantages:

- Data are entered into the client's chart immediately.
- This method saves nurses' time.
- Entry may be more accurate, because it is entered immediately after the intervention.

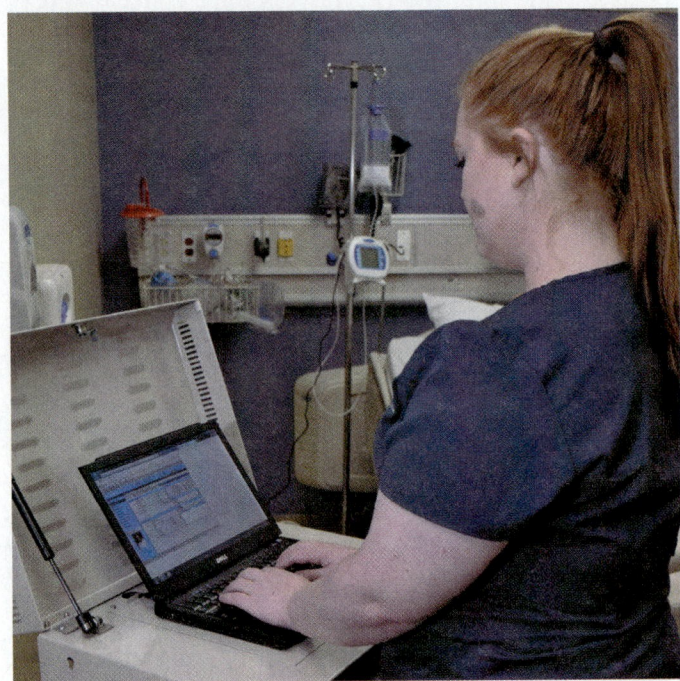

FIGURE 3-8 Bedside electronic documentation is becoming more accessible to nurses in hospital settings.

FIGURE 3-9 Computer-generated client data can be accessed from many locations.

- Charges to the client are automatic.
- Portable bedside computer unit facilitates client charting.

Alternative Documentation Systems

To date, there still exist some alternative charting methods such as *source-oriented*, *problem-oriented*, *focused*, *charting by exception*, and *narrative* methods. **Source-oriented charting** is so named because the information is organized and presented in separate sections according to its source (e.g., provider's progress notes, nurses' notes, and respiratory therapists' notes). To obtain a complete "picture" of the client, one must read through all sections and piece together the separate bits of data. This is time-consuming, and the result may not produce an accurate or complete assessment of the client. Narrative charting is found in this type of charting system.

A system for chart organization is the **problem-oriented medical record**. In this system, the chart is based on a problem list—all problems, present or potential, that are identified with a particular client. Using the problems as reference points, each individual who provides care adds progress notes on the same sheets. In this way, assessment of a specific incident by everyone concerned (e.g., healthcare provider, RN, dietitian, enterostomal therapist) is in the same location, and the client's overall picture can be easily seen.

Focus charting makes client needs or problems the focus of care in the progress notes. This method moves away from labeling client status a problem because it includes the client's condition, nursing diagnosis, signs or symptoms, or a significant client event or change in status (need for surgical intervention). The focus is not necessarily written as a nursing diagnosis. The progress notes are organized using the DAR format: data, action, and response. Data include the information that supports the focus, action is the nursing intervention used to treat the problem, and response is how the client responds to the intervention and the outcome. The following is an example:

D: Client found grimacing, hands clenched, and body rigid. Verbalized pain at 9 on pain scale.
A: Administered 15 mg morphine sulfate IV push. Called healthcare provider to request PCA for client.
R: Pain moderately relieved after 35 minutes. Able to understand instruction in use of PCA.

Charting by Exception (CBE) is a system that focuses only on significant findings or deviations from the norm. It reduces time spent documenting and reduces multiple data entries in the record. It uses flow sheets, protocols and standards of practice, nursing diagnosis, care plans, **SOAP** (subjective, objective, assessment, plan) progress notes, and a nursing database. Only changes or findings significantly different from the norm are documented. Nurses chart only when the client does not meet the predetermined standard or norm. All exceptions to the standards must be documented narratively. When nurses see entries in the chart, it alerts them that something unusual has occurred with the client. An additional advantage in CBE charting is that all flow sheets are kept at the bedside, which eliminates the need to transcribe information from a work sheet to the permanent record. Some legal or reimbursement issues, such as admissibility in court, may be related to charting by exception, since at this time, the rule "if it wasn't charted, it wasn't done" is still the prevailing attitude in legal issues.

Narrative Charting Another system of charting, less common, is source-oriented narrative charting. This form is based on chronology rather than systems. When using narrative charting, an assessment should be performed at the beginning of the shift and as needed thereafter. When assessment is the initial entry in narrative charting, subsequent entries are more understandable. A combination of assessment and narrative charting helps ensure that adequate information about the client is documented for all personnel who use nurses' notes.

Rules for Documenting Client Care

Note: Most rules apply when documenting in either an electronic or a traditional paper format.

1. Document from firsthand knowledge—if you chart for other caregivers, you may have errors or inaccurate data. An exception to this rule is when you are responsible for documenting for nonprofessional personnel.
2. If using paper documentation, write clearly and legibly in black or blue ink, not felt pen or pencil.
3. Give clear, concise, and unambiguous information. Go back to the client to clarify or validate if information is incomplete. Avoid vague expressions or clichés in charting (i.e., slept well).
4. Select neutral terms and describe observed behaviors, rather than making value judgments or generalizations. For example, use "noted alcohol odor on breath and speech was slurred" rather than "client was drunk."
5. Mistaken entries are automatically captured in the EHR as corrections are made. On paper charts, correct errors by drawing a single line through the error, writing the words "mistaken entry" or "ME" above it, and then initialing the error. The error must be readable. Ink eradication, erasures, and use of occlusive materials are not acceptable. The word *error* is no longer advised because juries tend to associate the word *error* with an actual nursing care mistake.
6. When documenting electronically, the "save & sign" function automatically signs the entry with the user name. In paper documentation, sign each entry with your first initial, last name, and status; for example, "SN" for student nurse, "LVN" for licensed vocational nurse, or "RN" for registered nurse. Script, not printing, is used for the signature. Each signature should appear at the right-hand margin of the nurses' notes.
7. In paper charting, notes should appear on each succeeding line. Lines should not be omitted in the

nurses' notes. A horizontal line is drawn to "fill up" a partial line. Continuous charting is done for each entry unless a time change occurs. You may or may not use a new line for each new idea or statement, depending on agency protocol.

8. In the EHR, every entry is time stamped. In paper documentation, the date is entered in the data column on the first line of every page of nurses' notes and whenever the date changes. Time is entered in the time column whenever a new time entry occurs. Time changes are not placed in the text of the nurses' notes. If only one time is entered for block charting, enter the last time you were with the client.

9. Chart objective facts, not interpretations. For example, chart "ate 100%," not "good appetite." If the client complains, place the complaint in quotation marks to indicate that it is his or her statement. For example, "c/o chest pain radiating down left arm."

10. Document any refusal of medications and treatments. In paper charting, place a circle around the time the medication or treatment should have been given in the appropriate area of the chart. Enter an explanation regarding the reason the medication was not given in the nurses' notes.

11. When using an EHR, sign and save all entries. With paper documentation, do not leave any entry unsigned. If all the charting is completed for the shift at one time, place a single signature at the end of the charting.

12. Chart only those abbreviations and symbols approved by the facility. Information can be misinterpreted or misleading when unfamiliar abbreviations are used. (*See* the listing at the end of Chapter 18 for examples of commonly used abbreviations and those to avoid.)

13. Spell correctly, using proper terminology and grammar.

14. Do not use the word *client* in the chart. The chart belongs to that client.

15. Do not double chart. If something appears on a flow sheet, it does not need to appear on the nurses' narrative record unless there is an alteration from normal. Within the EHR, data automatically populate related fields.

16. When using paper charting, do not squeeze information into a space because you forgot to chart it earlier. Add the information on the first available line. Write in the time the event occurred, not the time you entered the information. Insert the words *late entry* before the charting.

17. Never leave an EHR open; always log off before leaving the workstation or terminal.

18. Include the following information when documenting:
   a. Healthcare provider's visits
   b. Times the client leaves and returns to the unit, mode of transportation, and destination
   c. Medications (chart immediately after given). Include dosage, route of administration (if parenteral, where given), whether pain was relieved (if pain medication), and side effects
   d. Treatments (chart immediately after given)

Technology at the Bedside The "smart" device such as the iPhone has the ability to share information with a host or central computer. Nurses can use the device as a clinical resource for medication doses and calculations, as well as drug side effects. This device can also be used to access diagnostic test results, evaluate lab tests, and review treatments and interventions. It may also assist the nurse to review medical diagnoses and the steps of procedures. In addition, unlicensed assistive personnel (UAP) are using the devices to document point-of-care at the bedside (e.g., vital signs), which will be instantly transmitted to the RN. With all of these attributes, the smart devices have the potential to improve nursing care, save nurses' time, and promote client safety.

HIPAA Guidelines for Using a Smart Device The **HIPAA** Privacy Rule establishes standards to protect the confidentiality of individually identifiable health information maintained or transmitted electronically. The security rule adopts standards for the security of electronic protected health information. This rule is comprehensive in that it includes 19 standards and 42 specifications. Healthcare providers must check with their employers to be sure that they are compliant with the electronic standards for security.

Protected Health Information (PHI) is a component of the HIPAA guidelines. It is recommended that the client's name or any identifying data *not be* entered into the smart device. Personal demographics or client identifiers such as history, physical findings, data, and phone numbers must be input using passwords only. If identifying data must be input, the healthcare provider should use the "security" feature, which requires a password to enter the system.

Assistive Devices

Other assistive devices also deserve mention.

- The AccuNurse is a voice-enabled speech recognition system that has the ability to interface with the EHR. This system prioritizes interventions and enables nurses to dictate documentation into the electronic medical record. The software is a voice-activated system and can alert the nurse about a new order.

- Smart devices (Figure 3-10 ■) or iPhones are also being considered to assist nurses working at the bedside. Information and software in the form of applications (apps) can be downloaded to these devices to include such information as procedures, lab values, medication information, calculations, medical terminologies, healthcare provider's preferences, and much more, including a rhythm strip comparing the client's strip with a normal one. In fact, the application of the iPhone may be preferable to a computer because it allows the nurse to access information any time, any place, whereas the computer is at the client's bedside.

FIGURE 3-10 Nurse using smart tablet for capturing data.

FIGURE 3-11 Robot delivering medication to a nurse assigned to the client.

- Robotic technology (Figure 3-11 ■) is becoming more available. Designed to take over certain clinical activities, robots can save the nurse's precious time. They have telescopic vision and the technology to transfer vital information, such as a live image, a client's ECG tracings, urine output, heart sounds, etc. This aspect allows nurses off-site to teach, mentor, or help with client monitoring.

Minimizing Legal Risks of Computer Charting

The American Nurses' Association, the American Medical Record Association, and the Canadian Nurses' Association offer guidelines and strategies for computer safety in charting.

- Your personal password or computer signature should not be given to anyone: neither another nurse on the unit, a float nurse, nor a healthcare provider. The hospital issues a short-term password with access to certain documents for infrequent users such as students.
- Do not leave a computer terminal unattended after you have logged on. Most computers do have a timing device that shuts down a terminal when it has not been used for a certain length of time.
- Do not leave computer information about a client displayed on a monitor where others have access to it. Also, do not leave printed files unattended.
- A positive diagnosis of human immunodeficiency virus (HIV) or hepatitis B virus (HBV) is part of the client's confidential record. Disclosure of this information to unauthorized people may have legal implications. If the diagnosis is entered as any other diagnosis, take steps to follow your hospital's confidentiality procedures. Check your state's special protocols for treatment of a client's HIV or HBV status.

Legal Forms of Documentation

Unusual Occurrence, Variance, or Incident Report

Unusual occurrence, also called incident report (IR), or unexpected occurrence, serves three main purposes: to help document quality of care, to identify areas where in-service education is needed, and to document the details of an incident for possible legal reference.

With some staff nurses, unusual occurrence forms have a poor reputation. When something goes wrong and a nurse is told to "make out a report," it may be interpreted as a form of punishment. Although these forms are, on occasion, used as a form of reprimand, they should be neither more nor less than what their title suggests: a report of an incident. As such, they should be completed regularly when any unusual occurrence happens.

As a tool for documenting quality of care, **unusual occurrence** forms direct the quality assurance coordinator and the head nurse to areas of practice on the unit that need improvement. For example, there may be an increase in the number of clients who fell out of bed. Further research may show that because the census is up, the staff is very busy and is forgetting to reposition clients' overbed tables. In their attempts to get water or tissues, for example, more clients are falling out of bed. The solution to the problem may be to speak with the staff about the consequences of this action, and as a group find a mutually acceptable way of preventing this type of incident from recurring.

Unusual occurrences also suggest and document the need for in-service education. For example, when an unusual number of reports are written related to a new piece of equipment, the head nurse may conclude that the staff, especially those on evening and night shifts, needs instruction on operating this equipment properly and effectively. If reports are made showing that IVs are behind or ahead of schedule, this might indicate that the nurses do not know how to regulate the IV pump correctly. A solution to this problem is to conduct a series of classes for all shifts in which the operation of the IV pump is discussed and hands-on practice is given. Such classes could be given by someone in the hospital's in-service education department or by a representative of the manufacturer of the IV pumps.

Unusual occurrences may also document the details of an occurrence for possible legal use. In some hospitals, unusual occurrences cover any situation that prevented the client from having a normal recovery. These incidents could include nonnursing actions such as returning to surgery for control of bleeding or having chest tubes inserted for a pneumothorax.

When completing an unusual occurrence form with possible legal implications, it is very important to document all details of the incident. Frequently, lawsuits are not filed for months or even years after an incident, when it will not be easy to recall details of care. It is essential to document important details promptly on the form.

Information to document on the unusual occurrence form includes general details of the incident, the client's response, your action or reaction to the incident, and a list of other personnel who were aware of the details of the incident. Often there is space on the form to document the healthcare provider's report of the client's condition after the incident. To fill in the section regarding the healthcare provider's report, the nurse later copies the doctor's progress notes from the chart onto the form. At no time is the unusual occurrence form given to the healthcare provider. It is a written document between the hospital and its insurance carrier, not the healthcare provider.

On completion, unusual occurrence forms are forwarded to the unit manager or head nurse and then to nursing administration. Information from the report that is of interest for in-service education or quality assurance can be obtained at this time. Ultimately, the unusual occurrence form is passed along to the hospital's legal department to be retained indefinitely in the event that legal action is later initiated on behalf of the client.

Consent Forms

When an individual enters a hospital, some of his or her basic legal rights are affected. So that these rights are not violated, the client must give permission (informed consent) for all treatment (Figure 3-12 ■). If consent is not obtained, the hospital, healthcare provider, or nurse may be charged with committing "battery" against the client. *Battery*, as defined by law, is an "offensive touching" of the client. This could include an injection or any breaking of the skin's surface, use of x-rays, or insertion of tubes, for example.

This does not mean that consent needs to be signed for routine procedures like taking a blood pressure. Routine nursing care is "consented to" when the client signs the "conditions of admissions" form. Also, certain procedures, such as injections, intubations, and dressings, are treatments ordered by the healthcare provider and agreed to by the client. If the client has listened to the explanation of a specific procedure and has agreed to allow the procedure to be carried out, he or she is giving implied consent. However, the client has the right to refuse any treatment, including changing his or her mind about a procedure previously agreed to. In that case, the healthcare provider must be contacted regarding alternative actions.

When discussing the formal written or explicit consents, the two key nursing activities are obtaining and witnessing consent. Initiating consent is not a nursing function because it includes the explanation of what is to be done, the risks of the procedure to that client, alternative procedures, and probable outcomes, information that should be given by the doctor. The nurse may clarify the information to be sure the client understands.

The nurse's role is to witness the signing of the consent. When the consent form is presented to the client, it should be explained, and the client should be encouraged to read it thoroughly before signing. Under ordinary circumstances, only one witness to signing the consent is necessary. The witness does not have to be an RN, just someone over the age of 18 years.

Occasionally, a nurse is asked to explain or expand upon the healthcare provider's presentation. Acceptable practice is for the nurse to clarify, define a medical term, or add more details to the healthcare provider's initial information. If the nurse feels that the client does not really understand what is going to occur, it is the nurse's responsibility to notify the doctor to give further explanation before the client signs the consent. An easy way to determine what the client understands is to ask him or her to repeat the healthcare provider's explanation.

There are many rules and regulations governing consents. If you have questions about them, consult the consent manual for your hospital or a supervisory person. There are several important situations in which more information may be needed. One relates to the client's mental competency. Generally, the client must sign personally, and spouses are unable to sign for the client. Permanent incompetence usually involves legal action to assign someone else as conservator. Temporary incompetence may be the result of hospital treatments, such as drugs or anesthetics. When a narcotic or sedative has been given, at least 4 hours of elapsed time is recommended before the client is considered competent to sign a consent.

NAME:

MRN:

BIRTHDATE:

CSN:

ENTER PATIENT INFORMATION or APPLY PATIENT LABEL TO ALL PAGES

1. I have spoken with my doctors. They have explained my diagnosis and condition (listed on page 3).

2. My doctors have recommended the procedures listed on page 3 to diagnose or treat my condition. They have explained the **POTENTIAL BENEFITS** of these procedures. They also have explained the **RISKS OF REFUSING** the procedures.

3. My doctors have explained the **RISKS OF THE PROCEDURES** and I understand them. The major risks are listed on page 3.

4. I understand the planned location of my procedures may be marked on my body before the procedures. It may also be marked on the diagrams on page 3.

5. I understand that if I am given **ANESTHESIA OR SEDATION ANALGESIA** there will be other risks. These risks include severe blood loss, infection, damage to teeth, mouth, throat, or vocal cords, nerve or eye damage, drug reaction, slowing or stopping of breathing, failure of the anesthetic or sedation analgesia, cardiac arrest, risks that cannot be predicted, permanent disability or even death. There may be other unknown risks. I understand these risks and I consent to the use of any anesthetic or sedation analgesia that my doctors or the anesthetists believe is necessary.

6. I understand that **blood and urine specimens** may need to be collected in order to determine my care. If I am a woman of childbearing age, this may include a **pregnancy test**.

7. My doctors have explained the **ALTERNATIVES** to the recommended procedures and their risks. I want to have the recommended procedures.

8. I understand that sometimes during a procedure or afterwards (for example if I am in an intensive care unit), my doctors may decide that **RELATED OR ADDITIONAL PROCEDURES** are also necessary. I request and authorize the University   and the providers responsible for my treatment to perform any necessary additional procedures.

9. I **DONATE** and authorize the University   to own, use, retain, preserve, manipulate, analyze, or dispose of any **excess tissues, specimens, or parts of organs** that are removed from my body during the procedures described above and are not necessary for my diagnosis or treatment. The University   may use or retransfer these items to any entity for any lawful purpose, including education and retrospective research on anonymous specimens.

10. I request and authorize the University   and any **doctors, nurses, medical residents and other trainees, technicians, assistants or others** who may be assigned to my case to participate in my diagnosis and treatment. I understand that **representatives of companies** that sell equipment used in my procedures may also be present and participate. I also understand that the University   is a teaching institution. Medical and other students can and do participate in procedures as part of their education. By signing this form, I agree to allow these students to participate in my procedures. This may include performing **exams under anesthesia** that are relevant to my procedures.

11. I understand that unexpected events may happen before or during a surgery or procedure. This may require changing the providers originally scheduled to perform or supervise my procedures.

12. I understand that the practice of medicine, surgery and dentistry is not an exact science. I have been told about the probability of success of the procedures. **NO PROMISES OR GUARANTEES** have been made or can be made to me about the success, outcomes, or side effects of the procedures.

13. I have been given a chance to ask questions about the procedures and this form and my questions have been answered.

List any exceptions under the Exceptions section located on page 3.

Page 1 of 3

| 30-10000 | VER: A/13
HIM: 04/13 | Original – Medical Record
Copy – Patient/Family | | Request and Consent to
Medical, Surgical, Radiological or Other Procedures |

NOTE: Image ALL PAGES or send ALL PAGES to Health Information Management – including pages without a signature section

---

infection, transfer failure, or two surgical sites.

(2) **Allograft** – tissue obtained from a human donor. Risks include communicable disease such as hepatitis, HIV/AIDS, or CJD (the human form of mad cow disease), infection, or implant failure.

(3) **Synthetic materials** – artificially prepared human and non-human based. Risks include communicable disease such as hepatitis, HIV/AIDS, or CJD (the human form of mad cow disease), infection, possible blood thinning medication, or foreign material rejection.

(4) **Xenograft** – animal tissue. Risks include infection, immune rejection, or viral infection.

3. I understand that   uses tissue obtained from Food and Drug Administration registered tissue establishments which must screen donors and perform testing for communicable disease.   does not do its own testing and makes no guarantees about the tissue implants.

4. I understand the risks and potential benefits of a tissue implant. I want to receive any medically necessary tissue implants during my course of treatment.

Provider: List any exceptions under the Exceptions section located on page 3.

Page 2 of 3

| 30-10000 | VER: A/13
HIM: 04/13 | Original – Medical Record
Copy – Patient/Family | | Request and Consent to
Medical, Surgical, Radiological or Other Procedures |

NOTE: Image ALL PAGES or send ALL PAGES to Health Information Management – including pages without a signature section

---

patient is a minor or unable to sign)

Printed Name of Legally Authorized Representative (if patient is a minor or unable to sign)

Relationship: ☐ Spouse ☐ Parent ☐ Next-of-Kin
☐ Legal Guardian ☐ DPOA for Healthcare

Consent Obtained, Explained and Witnessed by:

Date: _____   Time: _____ A.M. / P.M.
        (mm/dd/yyyy)

Excluded sites are as follows:
- Mid-line sternotomy for a non-sided organ (e.g., CABG)
- Cesarean deliveries
- Surgery through a body orifice that does NOT involve laterality of the organ (e.g., Cystoscopy)
- Laparotomy, laparoscopy that does NOT involve laterality of the organ (e.g., splenectomy, laparoscopic cholecystectomy)
- Interventional procedures for which the site of insertion is NOT predetermined, such as cardiac catheterization procedures, angiography, and dialysis catheters
- Breast biopsy with wire localization
- Intra-oral and dental procedures
- Premature infants, for whom the mark may cause a permanent tattoo
- Marking for superficial cosmetic procedures using lasers (or similar energy-based devices) or injectables (such as neurotoxins and soft tissue fillers) when there are multiple sites and/or when marking would be impractical or pose a potential adverse outcome to the procedure.

Page 3 of 3

| 30-10000 | VER: A/13
HIM: 04/13 | Original – Medical Record
Copy – Patient/Family | | Request and Consent to
Medical, Surgical, Radiological or Other Procedures |

NOTE: Image ALL PAGES or send ALL PAGES to Health Information Management – including pages without a signature section

FIGURE 3-12 Example of a consent form.

A second situation concerns the client who is a minor. The age of consent varies by state and also according to specific situations, such as emancipation (being away from the family and self-supporting) and the type of medical problem (reportable diseases or pregnancy). An associated problem may arise when deciding who can legally sign for a minor.

Reporting/Handoff: A Component of Documentation

There are various ways to conduct a handoff. In some facilities, a verbal report is given; in others, a recorded report is given. There has been increasing emphasis for handoffs to occur at the bedside. Bedside handoffs have been shown to improve the quality of care and promote client-centered care. A shift-to-shift report or handoff should be given from the client care plan. It does not need to review such activities as dressing changes that are outlined on the care plan. A simple statement to the effect that the procedure is listed on the care plan is all that is necessary. This decreases both time and repetition of information.

To avoid confusion from shift to shift, specific times for treatments and for activities of daily living (ADLs) are indicated. For example, it is noted on the care plan that the client prefers his bath before 8 a.m. This avoids having to ask the client again every day. This consistency promotes a feeling of confidence in the nursing staff and alleviates fear.

Intrashift Reports

Reporting your observations and interventions to other health team members is as essential as documenting them on the client's chart. Intrashift reports are usually verbal reports relayed to team members, team leaders, or charge nurses to keep them informed of changes in the client's conditions. Examples of findings that need to be communicated to other health team members include significant changes in vital signs, unusual responses to treatments, medications, or changes in the client's physical or emotional condition.

Intershift Reports

Intershift reports disseminate client information between shifts. This may be accomplished through a verbal report or by tape recording the information. The intershift report should include the following data: client's name, room number, healthcare provider's name, diagnosis, and date of surgery when appropriate. In addition, it should include unusual findings based on the nursing assessment, response to treatments or medications, unusual occurrences, laboratory results, laboratory studies, tests to be completed on the next shift, and any physical or psychosocial problems that exist.

SBAR (situation, background, assessment, and recommendations) is a technique that nurses use to communicate with other members of the healthcare team about the client's condition. When the nurse is making an inter- or intrashift report, this technique provides the critical elements that must be transferred from one healthcare team to another. It is meant to be succinct and specific.

Healthcare Provider Notification

Healthcare providers should be notified whenever treatment or nursing care parameters are exceeded, significant alterations occur in physical assessment findings, or abnormal laboratory findings and test results are obtained.

Before calling the healthcare provider, have all data available to allow you to answer questions. It is best to use the SBAR technique to organize your thoughts. Include current vital signs, laboratory results, when medications were given last, and what your recommendation is. It is a good idea to have the entire chart with you. When calling the healthcare provider, identify yourself by name, your status (RN or SN), nursing unit, and the client's name. State the exact reason you are calling. Give pertinent and succinct information. Remember you are the eyes and ears of the healthcare provider. Based on your report, clinical decisions will be made.

Nurse Manager Reports

Written or verbal reports are given to nurse managers, nursing supervisors, or clinical coordinators during each shift. The report includes information on all critically ill clients, those with unusual occurrences or complications, and clients with conditions that are difficult to manage. It is also a good idea to alert the supervisor to problems with families, healthcare providers, or other health disciplines so she or he can assist you in the problem solving.

Client Care Conferences

Client care conferences and care plan meetings play an integral role in planning and delivering health care for difficult or unusual problems. The client care conference can focus on developing the care plan or on identifying difficult problems. A conference can be scheduled to plan appropriate interventions and to inform all health team members of the goals for that client's care.

Delegating Client Care

Client care assignments should be based on careful analysis of each client's needs and goals of care. The care plan may be consulted for an effective use of healthcare team members to their best advantage, as well as for the client's welfare. A client requiring extensive sterile dressing changes, frequent assessments, and IV medications is more appropriately assigned to a professional nurse. A client who is convalescing after a stroke and requires mainly bathing and ambulation assistance can usually be assigned to another member of the health team such as a UAP.

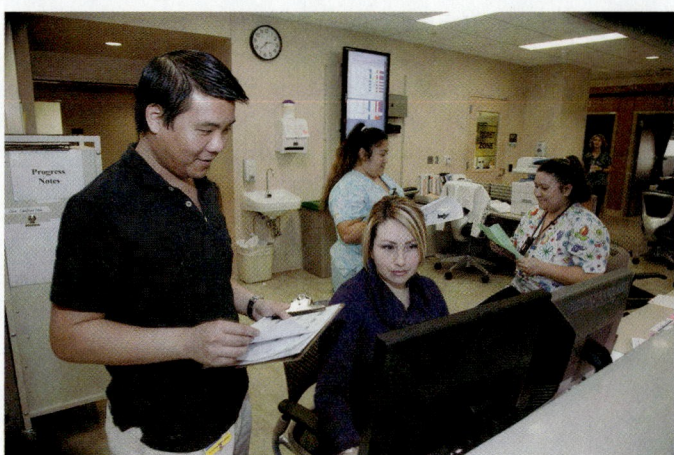

FIGURE 3-13 Client care assignments are delegated based on client acuity and competence of the healthcare worker.

In most healthcare facilities, delegating client care to healthcare workers has become a financially driven reality. RNs have less responsibility for actual direct care activities such as hygienic care, ambulation, and feeding. However, delegation of these tasks is under the jurisdiction of the RN (Figure 3-13 ■). To delegate appropriate tasks, the nurse must be familiar with the Nurse Practice Act for RNs and Licensed Practical Nurses/Licensed Vocational Nurses (LPN/LVNs) in their state and with the hospital's job descriptions for each level of healthcare worker.

More UAP are being employed by facilities as a method of cost containment. The goal is still to deliver service to the clients. This classification of healthcare UAP includes many titles, such as client-focused care technician, client care technician, and clinical nurse assistant. This level of healthcare worker provides basic care functions and can be a help to the overburdened nurse. UAPs must receive training in the skills they are to perform before client care is assigned. The RN retains responsibility for the care that is provided by this category of healthcare worker. Because of this, many state boards of nursing have developed position statements and guidelines to help RNs delegate activities safely. Guidelines vary among states, so you need to check your state's guidelines. Also, there are general guidelines that should be followed regardless of the state in which you practice. According to the National Council of State Boards of Nursing (NCSBN), tasks that involve nursing judgment and the need to assess the client's responses to the plan of care must not be delegated to any other level of worker than an RN. Any nursing intervention that requires independent, specialized nursing knowledge, skill, or judgment can only be delegated to an RN, according to the American Nurses Association.

RN Delegation

Delegation is defined as "transferring to a competent individual the authority to perform a selected nursing task in a selected situation" (National Council of State Boards of Nursing). State licensing laws designate that nurses are legally accountable for quality of care and for direct client care. For example:

- RNs decide which tasks to delegate and under what circumstances.
- RNs must know what is safe delegation of nursing care tasks.
- RNs must supervise (monitor and evaluate) outcomes for all delegated tasks. The RN retains accountability for the delegation.

RNs must know the legal scope of practice of other licensed providers. They must also know competency of licensed and unlicensed personnel as well as the tasks, which may be delegated.

- Some states identify tasks that may *never* be delegated (such as a sterile dressing to unlicensed personnel).
- RNs may *not* delegate assessment, evaluation, or nursing judgment functions.

RNs and LPN/LVNs must check with their own states' laws and regulations to determine which activities may *not* be performed by UAP.

Examples are as follows:

- Administration of medications or IV drugs
- Venipuncture or intravenous therapy
- Parenteral or tube feedings
- Any invasive procedures such as NG tube insertion, catheters, or suctioning
- Assessment of the client's condition
- Educating client or family concerning healthcare problems
- Reporting on laboratory tests

RN Responsibilities That Cannot Be Delegated

- Initial health assessments
- Checking advanced directives in client's chart
- Formulating nursing diagnoses through observation of the client's physical condition and behavior, and through interpretation of information obtained from the client and others, including the health team
- Formulating a care plan, in collaboration with the client, which ensures that nursing care services provide for the client's safety, comfort, hygiene, and protection, and for disease prevention and restorative measures
- Performing skills essential to the kind of nursing action to be taken, explaining the health treatment to the client and family, and teaching the client and family how to care for the client's health needs
- Carrying out pain management activities (epidural narcotic analgesia done only by RN)
- Delegating tasks to subordinates based on the legal scope of practice of the subordinate and on the preparation and capability needed in the tasks to be delegated and effectively supervising nursing care given by subordinates

- Data entry into client's charts for all unlicensed personnel to whom tasks are delegated
- Care plan objectives—checked by RN if completed by LPN/LVN
- Review of data obtained by other healthcare workers
- Receiving reports of client conditions and any unexpected findings from delegated activities
- Identifying parameters for which delegatee is to notify nurse
- Evaluating the effectiveness of the care plan through observation of the client's physical condition and behavior, signs, and symptoms through communication with the client and health team members, and modifying the plan as needed
- Acting as the client's advocate, as circumstances require, by initiating action to improve health care or change decisions or activities that are against the interests or wishes of the client and by giving the client the opportunity to make informed decisions about health care before it is provided
- Completing referral form for additional client services
- Client teaching
- Completing the discharge teaching plan

Activities That May Be Delegated to LPN/LVN   The RN is legally responsible for client care. As such, the nurse must determine which task may be delegated. These decisions are based on the client's diagnosis, what the state allows the LPN/LVN to do, the amount of judgment and experience needed to complete the task, and whether the assistant is capable of performing and completing the task. Following are guidelines for delegation:

- After the RN completes the initial assessment, the LPN/LVN documents assessment changes.
- The LPN/LVN may reinforce client teaching, but the RN must initiate the teaching and evaluate the results.
- LPN/LVNs, depending on the individual state standards, may or may not add medications to the IV. They may add vitamins and minerals in most states. After completing an IV course, LPN/LVNs may initiate IV therapy.
- Organ donation—RN or LPN/LVN is responsible for carrying out hospital policies.

Delegation Regulations of Unlicensed Assistive Personnel (UAP)   This term refers to a group of workers who are trained and/or certified, but not licensed. These workers cannot be assigned tasks in lieu of a registered nurse. The nurse must determine which tasks may be performed by a UAP.

How to delegate to a UAP:

- The assistant's areas of competence must be judged against the specific needs of the client.
- The nurse must give specific instructions and do active monitoring during the assignment.

- Progress in client care through feedback and evaluation of outcomes should occur frequently.
- The nurse must be sure that the appropriate delegation is made: Can the assistant legally do this task, has the worker been trained to perform this task, has the worker demonstrated that they can complete the task, and is the client response predictable?
- When performing the task, can the worker obtain the same result as the RN?

Duties Most Often Delegated to Unlicensed Assistive Personnel

- Taking vital signs and charting results
- Obtaining height and weight
- Repositioning a client or assisting a client to bed
- Bathing a client and making the bed
- Transferring a client between units
- Escorting a client out of the hospital
- Documenting drainage from an NG tube
- Serving food trays and feeding a client
- Obtaining a specimen that is nonsterile and noninvasive
- Performing range-of-motion activities after instruction
- Initiating CPR after certification
- Working with a dying client
- Completing postmortem care

Standards of Competent Performance

- A registered nurse shall be considered competent when he or she consistently demonstrates the ability to transfer scientific knowledge from social, biological, and physical sciences in applying the nursing process.
- *Incompetence* means lacking possession of or failure to exercise that degree of learning, skill, care, and experience ordinarily possessed and exercised by a competent registered nurse.

Parameters of Delegation

Many state boards of nursing have identified the parameters of delegation. Examples of these "Rights of Delegation" are:

Right Task—a task that can be legally delegated to an LPN/LVN or UAP. Check the state nurse practice act to determine whether the caregiver is trained to perform the task. Judge whether the UAP or LPN/LVN is competent to perform the task.

Right Circumstances—the LPN/LVN or UAP understands the elements of the procedure and the RN is assured that the UAP can perform the procedure safely in an appropriate setting. Caregiver is able to collect the right supplies to perform the procedure.

Right Person—the right person (RN or LPN/LVN) delegates the right task (legally can be delegated to a UAP) to the right person (legally can perform the task) on the right client (stable with predictable outcomes).

Right Direction/Communication—person delegating the task (RN or LPN/LVN) has described the task clearly, including directions, special steps of the task, and the expected outcomes. Then, the delegator must trust those they are delegating to, supporting the right to make certain decisions.

Right Supervision/Evaluation—the RN or LPN/LVN delegating the activity answers the UAP's questions and is available to problem solve, if necessary. Evaluation of the task is ongoing.

Source: Smith (2016)

Student Clinical Planning

Preclinical Planning

To assist students with client care planning prior to and during the clinical experience, many nursing programs have developed student clinical preparation forms. Forms such as these help focus the student's attention on the information necessary to ensure safe nursing practice. Most forms include information related to the client's biographical data, history and physical assessment findings, medical diagnosis, nursing diagnosis, medications including IVs, and nursing interventions.

Time Management

Implementing time management techniques during your student clinical experience will assist you not only in organizing client care management, but also in completing your assignment efficiently. Some techniques you may find helpful are listed below.

- Design a time management work sheet you can follow.
- Collect the appropriate information you will require to identify client care tasks (e.g., RN report, care plan, Kardex, medication record).
- Identify specific tasks of client care and the time frame needed for completion in consultation with your preceptor or instructor.
- Prioritize tasks included in the client care plan.
- Make an initial visit to assess your client's status early in the shift.
- Revise priorities based on your assessment.
- Plan nursing interventions in sequence.
- Group and sequence client care activities for completion in the same time frame. Allocate sufficient time to complete client assignment.
- Consider client's wishes for completing nonpriority tasks, such as bathing and grooming.
- Identify tasks for which you will require assistance.
- Notify the appropriate colleague to assist you (e.g., ambulating your client).
- Identify and collect necessary equipment for task completion.
- Complete client care, implementing the prioritized plan of action (POA) using your time management work sheet.
- Allocate appropriate time to interact with your client.
- Mark off tasks on the time management sheet as you complete them, leaving a record for giving verbal report to the nurse when leaving the unit.
- Document client care as soon as feasible, or at least every 2 hours, on the appropriate records.

Chapter Wrap-Up

MANAGEMENT Guidelines

Interprofessional Communication

- Information relative to client care is provided both in written and verbal communication. Written information is found on the EHR, client care plan, or critical pathway. Verbal communication consists of the shift and team report and directions provided to the workers throughout the shift. When assigning client care to healthcare workers, the RN uses both communication processes. When directions are given to healthcare workers, the care plan or pathway is the foundation for client information. This information is provided in a verbal report at the beginning of the shift. Two-way communication is encouraged throughout the shift, as client's needs change or new orders are written for client care.
- Verbal reports can be given individually or to a group of healthcare workers. It depends on the type of healthcare delivery system that is employed in the facility.
- Specific information regarding client care must be provided to each healthcare worker. This information includes activity level, vital sign times, diet, ability to perform ADLs, procedures or treatments that will be conducted during the shift and the approximate time this will occur, specimens needing collection as well as any safety precautions necessary, visual and hearing deficits, dentures, and specific tasks to be completed by the healthcare worker.

- Communicate with all members of the healthcare team through the multidisciplinary care plan. Ensure they follow the plan of care and document to the care plan.
- After receiving report from UAPs, the RN must complete the charting except where flow sheets are used.
- The RN is responsible for the accuracy of all documentation, including information contained in the flow sheet; therefore, it should be checked each shift.
- Licensed nursing staff should review the documentation for the past 24 hours before beginning nursing care. The chart will provide details on the client's status, including assessment findings, response to pain medication, and client's response to treatments. Continuity of care can be provided when client information is known.
- The RN should review necessary data, obtained by reading the chart, with the unlicensed personnel to provide for continuity of care.
- RNs should review principles of charting with personnel if guidelines for charting are not being followed. The records are permanent and reflect the care provided to the client while hospitalized. The chart can be subpoenaed if a lawsuit is filed.

CASE STUDY Applications

Scenario 1

Determine appropriate delegation of client activities for a staff team on a unit. This scenario does not take into consideration the acuity of the client, only the nursing tasks needed for the day shift. Each facility and state have differing policies regarding personnel; therefore, these policies need to be reviewed before this activity is completed.

The team consists of one RN, one LPN/LVN, and one UAP. There are 10 clients and two unoccupied beds. There is a charge nurse and ward clerk assigned to the nursing unit. There are two other teams, and these three teams make up the medical–surgical nursing unit.

RM 601A Mr. Rodriguez, 98, admitted 24 hours earlier
Diagnosis: congestive heart failure
Bed rest, bed bath and assistance with oral hygiene, daily weight, I&O
Vital signs every 4 hours, low sodium diet, restricted fluids to 1500 mL
IV #2 1,000 mL D5/.2NS with 20 mEq KCl at 50 mL/hr—800 mL remaining
IV medications: furosemide 40 mEq BID
Oral medications: digoxin 0.25 mg daily, vitamin supplement

RM 601B Mr. Jamisen, 69, admitted this a.m.
Diagnosis: coronary artery disease
Surgery at 10 a.m.: triple bypass—will go to ICU following surgery
Pre-op checklist and client teaching has been completed
Pre-op meds on call to OR
IV medications
IV #1 1,000 mL D5/.2 NS at 75 mL/hr

RM 602A Mrs. Jones, 59, admitted 2 days ago
Diagnosis: cholelithiasis
Surgery 2 days ago: Laparoscopic cholecystectomy
Ambulate ad lib, self-care
Oral medications for pain

IV discontinued at 8 a.m.
To be discharged today with discharge teaching

RM 602B Not occupied

RM 603A Mrs. Henderson, 38, admitted yesterday
Diagnosis: metastatic cancer to the brain
CT scan scheduled for 12 noon
IV #2 1,000 mL D5W with 20 mEq potassium chloride at 50 mL/hr
Assist with ADLs
Vital signs and neuro checks every 4 hours, I&O
Oral medications for pain

RM 603B Miss Johnson, 70, admitted 3 days ago
Diagnosis: pancreatic cancer with metastasis to the lungs
Chair three times a day, and ambulate to bathroom
Vital signs every 4 hours
Spirometry every 4 hours with RT
Deep breathing and coughing exercises every 4 hours
Nasotracheal suction PRN
IV #5 1,000 mL D5W at 50 mL/hr
PCA pump for pain medication
Chemotherapy IV daily

RM 604A Mr. Scott, 64, admitted this a.m.
Diagnosis: benign prostatic hypertrophy
Surgery for TURP at 1 p.m.—to return to the nursing unit
Needs pre-op teaching and a surgical checklist completed

RM 604B Mr. Jackson, 37, admitted last night
Diagnosis: torn ACL
Surgery this a.m. at 7:30—will return to unit by 10:30 a.m.
Continuous passive motion (CPM) ordered postop

RM 605A Mrs. Price, 89, admitted 1 week ago

Diagnosis: terminal heart failure, semi-comatose

Complete ADLs, keep comfortable, turn and position every 2 hours

Vital signs every 8 hours, I&O

Indwelling urinary catheter to drainage

IV #8 D5/0.45 NS with 40 mEq potassium chloride at KVO (keep vein open) rate

RM 605B Not occupied

RM 606A Mrs. Fellipe, 28, admitted last evening

Diagnosis: gastroenteritis for past 4 days

Ambulate to bathroom, chair as tolerated

Independent in ADLs

Vital signs every 4 hours, NPO, I&O

IV #3 1,000 mL NS with 40 mEq potassium chloride at 125 mL/hr

RM 606B Mrs. Blake, 48, admitted yesterday

Diagnosis: sickle cell crisis

Bed rest until pain subsides

Vital signs every 4 hours, I&O, diet as tolerated

Oral medications: folic acid, nonsteroidal anti-inflammatory drug

Narcotic analgesic medication for pain

IV #3 1,000 mL D5/0.2 NS with 40 mEq potassium chloride at 125 mL/hr

- Determine the appropriate staff assignment for this client roster. What information do you need to complete this assignment?
- How would you as team leader make client assignments for each individual staff member?
- How do the theory of delegation and the facility/state policies of delegation impact on your assignment?
- What additional factors would you need to consider in making these assignments?

Scenario 2

You are assigned to provide nursing care for Mr. Fred Smith, 39 years of age. He is admitted to the hospital for severe dehydration due to the effects of chemotherapy. On your initial rounds at 7:30 a.m., you find him sleeping. His respirations are labored and stertorous. His color is ashen, eyes sunken, and skin dry. At 8 a.m., you enter the room and find him awake. He complains of being very thirsty and wants a glass of water. He cannot tolerate oral fluids and is receiving IV fluids with potassium chloride (KCl) added because of his nausea and vomiting on admission the day before. After taking his vital signs (T: 100.6; P: 100; R: 32), you give him his bath and make his bed. You notice he has reddened areas over his coccyx and on his elbows and heels, each area about the size of a quarter. His skin is dry and peeling. Drainage from his urinary catheter is a dark amber color with a very strong odor. You measure the urine at 8 a.m. The total is 75 mL. The last output was measured at 6 a.m.

- How would you chart the information obtained from the simulated situation? What would be appropriate forms to use?
- What assessment information (that you just charted) would require nursing interventions? If you were assigning this client to a team member, who would be most appropriate—RN, LPN/LVN, or CNA?

Scenario 3

You have just received your client care assignment. There are two stages of preparation. The first stage is obtaining all the necessary information you will need to provide safe care. The second stage is reviewing your reference materials to gain an understanding of the client's diagnosis, medications, lab values, and diagnostic tests that will be done during his or her hospitalization.

- If you have only a limited time to review the client's chart, what sections of the chart will provide you with sufficient information to render you safe to care for the client?
- In preparing for clinical practice, what information is essential to review in addition to the data you have obtained from the clinical record? Where is the most appropriate place to find this information?
- List the priority interventions you will carry out within the first hour of the clinical experience. Explain the rationale for your answers.

NCLEX® Review Questions

Unless otherwise specified, choose only one (1) answer.

1. Charting is an important nursing activity. Which of the following functions does client charting fulfill?
   Select all that apply.
   A. It communicates information to members of the health team.
   B. It is a legal document.
   C. It reminds nurse of the treatments to be performed for the client.
   D. It assists supervisors to evaluate staff performance.
   E. It provides a permanent client record.
   F. It protects both client and nurse in terms of quality and continuity of health care.

2. Hospitals are rapidly adopting electronic charting programs. What are some advantages of using this system? *Select all that apply.*
   A. It allows nurse to document more client details quickly.
   B. It limits the ability to communicate personal aspects of care.

C. It gives the nurse more time to spend on client care.

D. It provides instant test results and information.

E. It relieves the nurse of having to make report.

3. The nurse finishes documenting on a client's paper chart and notices that the information has been written in the wrong chart. What is the next action to take?

A. Notify the team leader to correct it.

B. Completely cross out the writing so it is not visible.

C. Cross out the entry with a single line, write "mistaken entry" and "wrong chart" above it, and initial the entry.

D. Draw a red line through the incorrect entry, write "wrong entry" and initial.

4. What is necessary to record when completing an unusual occurrence (incident report)?

A. Major details of the incident

B. Only the actual nursing interventions made

C. All of the details of the incident

D. General details with focus on client's reactions

5. Your hospital has implemented the use of standard clinical pathways as the major type of documentation. What is one of the advantages of this type of documentation?

A. It allows for individual plans of care.

B. There is continuity of care among all healthcare workers.

C. It includes history, assessment, and risk factors.

D. It allows for clients with complex problems to receive specialized care.

6. A bedridden Islamic client asks the nurse to bring a basin of water every morning and evening. The unit is understaffed and extremely busy. How would you resolve this issue?

A. Explain to the client that you are too busy to bring him water today.

B. Bring him the water regardless of the busy schedule.

C. Delegate the task to the UAP.

D. Tell him that you will try to do it, but it may be late.

7. When planning client care assignments in team nursing, which action could lead to instability and inadequate care?

A. Changing assignments frequently

B. Considering the job description of the team members

C. Considering the physical location of the clients on the unit

D. Considering the acuity level of the clients

8. Which of the following actions will help a nurse manager increase leadership skills through the process of delegation?

A. Close supervision, thereby not allowing any errors

B. Clearly making all decisions about how a task is to be completed

C. Delegating responsibility in such a way that the worker is capable of handling responsibility

D. Delegating those tasks that are distasteful to the nurse manager

9. Which of the following is implied when a nurse witnesses a client signing a surgical consent form?

A. The nurse saw the client sign the consent form.

B. The nurse knows the client understands the proposed procedure.

C. The nurse believes the client to be competent.

D. The nurse believes the client is able to tolerate the procedure.

10. Delegation is an important nursing function. Of the following statements, which one is not applicable?

A. RNs decide which tasks to delegate.

B. RNs must supervise outcomes for all delegated tasks.

C. All nursing tasks may be delegated if an RN takes responsibility.

D. RNs must know the legal scope of practice of other licensed providers.

QSEN Activity

Domain: Informatics

KSA: Knowledge

Have class work in groups and identify examples of how technology and information management are related to the quality and safety of care.

Bibliography

Bulchek, G., Butcher, H., Dochterman, J., & Wagner, C. (2013). *Nursing Interventions Classification (NIC)*, (6th ed.). St Louis, MO: Elsevier. Retrieved from http://www.nursing.uiowa.edu/cncce/nursing-interventions-classification-overview

Centers for Disease Control and Prevention. (2012). *Meaningful Use*. Retrieved from http://www.cdc.gov/ehrmeaningfuluse/introduction.html

Hurlock v. Parklane Medical Center NO. WD 36288. (1985). Missouri Court of Appeals, Western District. Readopted May 30, 1986. Retrieved from http://leagle.com/decision/19851581709SW2d872_11526.xml/HURLOCK%20v.%20PARK%20LANE%20MEDICAL%20CENTER,%20INC

Jakobsson, J., & Wann-Hansson, C. (2012, Dec.). Nurses' perception of working according to standardized care plans: A questionnaire study. *Scandinavian Journal of Caring Sciences, 27*(4), 945–952.

Keenan, G., Yakel, E., Lopez, K.D. Tschannen, D., & Ford, Y.B. (2013, Mar.–Apr.). Challenges to nurses' efforts of retrieving, documenting and communicating client care information. *Journal of The American Medical Informatics Association, 20*(2), 245–251. doi: 10.1136/amiajnl-2012-000894

Kerr, D., Lu, S., & McKinlay, L. (2013, Jul.–Sep.). Bedside handover enhances completion of nursing care and documentation. *Journal of Nursing Care & Quality, 28*(3), 217–225. doi: 10.1097/NCQ.0b013e3182aa6e0

King, C. D., Patel, V., & Furukawa, M. F. (2013). Adoption of electronic health record systems among U.S. non-federal acute care hospitals 2008–2012. *ONC Data Brief, no 9*. Washington, DC: Office of the National Coordinator for Health Information Technology.

McEwen, D., & Dumpel, H. (2013, May). Narrative documentation: Protecting your clients, practice and license in the information age. *National Nurse, 109*(4), 20–31.

McPeck, P. (2006, May 8). Beyond illegible scrawl: Computerized order entry. *Nurse Week*, California ed., San Jose, CA.

National Association for Healthcare Quality. (2004, March–April). Client safety: A case study in team building and interdisciplinary collaboration. Retrieved from www.nahq.org/Journal/ce/article_ID=171

Ray, J. D., & Overman, A. S. (2014). Hard facts about soft skills. *American Journal of Nursing, 114*(2), 64–68.

Reeves, S., Perrier, L., Goldman, J., Freeth, D., & Zwarenstein, M. (2013, Mar. 28). Interprofessional education: Effects on professional practice and healthcare outcomes (update). *Cochrane Database of Systematic Reviews 3*, 1–49.

Smith, S. F. (2016). *Sandra Smith's review for NCLEX-RN* (13th ed.). Burlington, MA: Jones & Bartlett Learning, LLC.

Technology Informatics Guiding Education Reform (TIGER). (n.d.). The TIGER initiative: The national health information technology agenda, a TIGER collaborative report. Retrieved from http://www.thetigerinitiative.org/docs/TigerReport_NationalHITAgenda_000.pdf

The Joint Commission. (2011). Meditech: Health care information system. Retrieved from http://meditech.com/Industrynews/pages/jcaho.htm

U.S. Department of Health & Human Services. (2013). Doctors and hospitals use of health IT more than doubles since 2012. Retrieved from http://www.hhs.gov/news/press/2013pres/05/20130522a.html

Chapter 4
Communication and Nurse–Client Relationship

 ## Learning Objectives

4.1 Define the term *communication*.

4.2 Explain why communication is an important concept in nursing.

4.3 Describe what is meant by the term *confidentiality*.

4.4 Discuss four factors that affect communication.

4.5 List five examples of therapeutic communication.

4.6 List five examples of barriers to communication.

4.7 Explain why multicultural health care is important and discuss the term *cultural diversity*.

4.8 List three components of a cultural sensitivity assessment.

4.9 List two questions that would elicit information about the client's spiritual issues.

4.10 Demonstrate the steps for beginning a client interaction.

4.11 Explain why it is therapeutic to encourage the client to express feelings and thoughts.

4.12 Describe the phases of a nurse–client relationship.

4.13 List three components for maintaining a nurse–client relationship.

4.14 Describe the rationale for discussing termination at the beginning of the relationship.

4.15 Practice assisting a client to communicate with his or her healthcare provider.

4.16 List at least three cues you would observe if a client were depressed, anxious, or angry.

4.17 Discuss two interventions you would make if one of your assigned clients was depressed, anxious, or angry.

Chapter Outline

Terminology

Acceptance favorable reception; basic acknowledgment.

Agitation excessive restlessness and increased mental and especially, physical activity.

Anxiety a state of uneasiness and distress; diffuse apprehension or dread of the future.

Assistance aid, help, or support.

Attitude a state of mind or feeling with regard to some matter; disposition.

Behavior the actions or reactions of individuals under specified circumstances.

Clarify to make clear or easier to understand.

Clichés stereotyped responses; trite or overused expressions or ideas.

Cognition the mental process or faculty by which knowledge is acquired.

Communication the exchange of thoughts, information, or messages.

Confusion disorder; jumble; distraction; bewilderment.

Congruence agreement; conformity.

Consent to agree; to be of the same mind.

Convey to communicate or make known; to impart.

Coping mechanisms he means by which to adjust or adapt to disequilibrium; defense mechanisms against anxiety.

Counseling to give support or to provide guidance.

Cultural diversity differences among people with respect to their values, beliefs, language, customs, and general patterns of behavior.

Cultural sensitivity being aware of and accepting diversity among people.

Depression a mental state characterized by dejection, lack of hope, and absence of cheerfulness.

Emotions any strong feelings, as of joy, hate, sorrow, or love.

Empathy ability to readily comprehend the feelings, thoughts, and motives of another individual.

Esteem to consider as of a certain value; regard; respect.

Evaluate to examine and judge; to appraise.

Expressions manifesttions or communications; ways of making things known.

Feedback the return of information to the place of origin.

"Handoff" Communication *See* SBAR definition.

Helping relationship an interaction of individuals that sets the climate for movement of the participants toward common goals.

HIPAA Health Insurance Portability and Accountability Act, enacted into law in 1996 to improve Medicare and Medicaid programs and efficiency of healthcare system.

Maladaptive inability to, or faulty adjustment or adaptation.

Noncompliance failure or refusal to go along with a plan or program.

Nonverbal communication aspects of communication that are not content (such as body language or gestures) but still convey meaning.

Overdependence the state of needing or relying on someone or something too much.

Perceptions the processes of receiving and interrupting sensory impressions.

Rapport a feeling of mutual trust experienced by individuals in a satisfactory relationship.

Refer to send or direct someone for action or help.

Relationship an interaction of individuals over a period of time.

SBAR a tool that standardizes a "handoff communication" when one nurse turns a client over to another nurse indicating the following: **s**ituation, **b**ackground, **a**ssessment, and **r**ecommendations.

Self-esteem a sense of pride in oneself; self-love.

Situational awareness ability to gather the right information, analyze it, and make projections as it relates to client care.

Social having to do with involvement with communities and other individuals.

Spiritual assessment assessing a client's religious or spiritual beliefs and values.

Support to lend strength or give assistance to.

Termination the end of something; a limit or boundary; conclusion or cessation.

Therapeutic having medicinal or healing properties; a healing agent.

Understanding to perceive and comprehend the nature and significance of; to know.

Validate to substantiate or verify.

Verbal communication the words, content, or information conveyed in the message.

Communication

Communication is the process of sending and receiving messages by means of symbols, words, signs, gestures, or other actions. It is a multilevel process consisting of the content, or information, part of the message and the part that defines the meaning of the message. Messages sent and received define the relationship between people. From the point of view of a learned skill, communication is intended to accomplish a defined goal. It is the transmission of facts, feelings, and meaning through the communication process.

The communication process forms one of the primary bases for administering all skills. Without clear communication, the nurse cannot assess, administer, or **evaluate** his or her actions in performing the skill. The principles of **therapeutic** communication also form a basis for interviewing and **counseling** skills.

Communication is a vital element in nursing. Everything that occurs within the nurse–client interaction involves some form or mode of communication, whether it includes listening to an upset family member, assisting a client in health teaching, or performing a nursing procedure. Without communication, the nurse could not give nursing care.

The communication process includes both verbal and nonverbal **expressions** and is affected by the intrapersonal framework of the individual, the relationship between the participants, and the purpose of the sender. The content of the message and the context also influence the communication process. The manner in which the message is sent and the effect on the receiver also play a role in the eventual outcome of the communication process. As you can see, the communication process can be very complex. As a beginning practitioner, however, the most important factor to remember is that *what* you say and *how* you say it have a very great influence on your client.

One of the most important skills you must master is to be able to talk therapeutically to clients and to be able to listen to them. Nurse–client communication is an integral component of nursing care. In fact, the initial step in the nursing process—assessment—comprises observation, interview, and examination. The interview involves talking and listening to the client. Initially, it may be difficult for you to concentrate on both talking and listening, since you have not yet mastered the basic skills, such as a bed bath or taking vital signs. As you gain experience, however, these skills will become more familiar and you can focus on the communication-interaction process with the client.

Confidentiality (Client's Right to Privacy)

Clients are protected by law (invasion of privacy) against unauthorized release of personal clinical data such as symptoms, diagnoses, and treatments. Confidential information may be released with the **consent** of the client. Information release is mandatory when ordered by the court or when a state statute requires reporting child abuse, communicable diseases, or other specific incidents.

Nurses, as well as other healthcare providers and their employers, may be held personally liable for invasion of privacy (as well as other torts) should litigation arise from the unauthorized release of client information. Nurses have a legal and ethical responsibility to become familiar with their employers' policies and procedures, as well as the new aspects of **HIPAA**, regarding reproduction of client information.

Health Insurance Portability and Accountability Act (HIPAA)

This act, enacted into law in 1996 and phased in gradually, requires the Secretary of Health and Human Services to devise certain standards. This act improves the efficiency and effectiveness of Medicare and Medicaid programs, ensures continuing healthcare insurance if the client has had existing group insurance, and ensures the privacy of individual health information. One of the most important components of HIPAA is the privacy rule, which became effective in April 2003.

This act requires healthcare providers to protect clients against unauthorized disclosures of personal medical information. HIPAA requires client consent for any information dispersed to others. It states that clients must receive written notice of privacy practices and their rights. Clients may access personal medical records more freely than previously.

Guidelines That Influence Effective Communication

- An individual cannot *not* communicate. This idea is basic to communication. We have an inherent need to communicate, whether it be verbal or nonverbal. Even silence is a form of communication.
- There is a content, or informational, value to messages sent and received that explains what the message is about and expresses how the sender regards the receiver.
- The message sent is not necessarily the meaning received.
- Communication becomes dysfunctional when an individual does not assume responsibility for his or her communication. Dysfunctional communications result from failing to learn to communicate properly and leaving the responsibility for communicating to others.

Learning to talk with clients and listening to them is the beginning of a nurse–client relationship. Some of you come to nursing with many of these basic communication skills already mastered. Others experience shyness, hesitancy, and awkwardness in relating to clients. Try to keep in mind that you are being educated to be a professional individual—a nurse—and as such you have a great deal to give to your clients. They will learn to respect your skill, value your presence, and depend on you when they are ill. One of the most rewarding aspects to nursing is experiencing a communication between you and your client. If you do feel shy or hesitant, remember that communication skills can be learned. Begin by practicing or role-playing with your classmates until you feel comfortable in the initial phases of a relationship.

All communication between nurse and client should be therapeutic, whether it involves obtaining information for an assessment, interacting with the client during a bed bath, or doing client teaching. The difference between therapeutic communication and a therapeutic relationship is that a relationship has a beginning, middle, and end with specified goals for each phase. Therapeutic communication techniques should be used in all forms of communication.

Guidelines for Communicating With Clients

When establishing nurse–client communication, some basic guidelines should be remembered.

- Accept the client as a valued and worthwhile individual, for this **acceptance** is a prerequisite for a nurse–client relationship.
- Be aware of the total client, not just his or her physical needs. The client's **social**, emotional, and spiritual needs are also important.

- Understand your own needs, feelings, and reactions so that they do not interfere with the therapeutic process with the client.
- Be prepared to feel some degree of emotional involvement with your client, evidencing caring and concern for his or her welfare. At the same time, however, it is necessary to maintain objectivity.
- Remember that the nurse–client interaction is a professional one. As such, you as the nurse possess the skills, abilities, and resources to relieve the other individual's pain and discomfort, and your client seeks comfort and **assistance** for alleviation of some existing problem.
- A nurse–client relationship does not require a long-term agreement or formal meetings between nurse and client to be effective. You may still meet the objectives of such a relationship in a short clinical experience.
- Take an active role and guide the conversation if the client is overly hesitant. For example, "I'm here to listen to any concerns you might have, Mr. Smith. You were mentioning having trouble understanding. . . ."
- Give broad opening statements and ask open-ended questions to help the client describe what is happening to him or her. Pick up cues and follow through with the subject that the client introduces to provide continuity.
- Use body language to **convey empathy**, interest, and encouragement to facilitate communication.
- Use silence as a therapeutic tool, as it allows the client to pace and direct his or her own communications. Long periods of silence, however, may increase the client's **anxiety** level, so use this technique wisely.

New Trends in Communication

Text messaging nurse to nurse or nurse to healthcare provider allows the individual receiving the text to instantly learn the critical nature of the text. For example, texting "please review these critical lab values," or "please call back STAT referencing client X." While this method of communication is very quick and efficient, it should only be allowed when using a HIPAA secure text-messaging app such as Doc Halo or TigerText.

The Joint Commission Safety Goal 2: Improve Effectiveness of Caregiver Communication

The National Patient Safety Goals identified in 2003 by The Joint Commission (formerly JCAHO) are updated every year. One important safety goal targets good communication because poor communication between caregivers can cause errors and risk client safety. The Joint Commission, to improve the effectiveness of this goal, has identified four requirements that apply to nurses:

1. "Read back" is a reminder to take the steps needed to verify a verbal telephone order or if the nurse is notified of a critical test result. In these situations, the nurse

should write down the information, enter it into the computer, read it back to the individual with whom he or she is speaking, and then confirm what was read back.

2. Develop a list of abbreviations, acronyms, symbols, or dose designations that cannot be used in the facility because they are often misread or confused. (See Abbreviation Alert on page 627.)

3. Critical test results must be reported immediately. These are test results that are abnormal and for client safety may require an immediate intervention.

4. **"Handoff" communication** means that a nurse must pass off crucial information about a client—status, his or her condition, recent changes, or ongoing treatment—to the next clinical caregiver. A tool available that standardizes handoff is the **SBAR** technique. This is a technique that covers situation, background, assessment, and recommendations for the client that is being handed off.

"Handoff" Communication

"Handoff" communication is a system or process that includes all relevant (especially critical elements) information about a client when one member of a healthcare team is "handing off" a client to another member. Using this technique increases client safety and implements a continuum of care.

SBAR is particularly important when you are handing off a client between preoperative and intraoperative areas (Box 4-1 ■). The transition of care must summarize critical

---

Box 4-1 **SBAR**

The SBAR mnemonic communication technique is a standardized, focused method of communicating essential client information when members of the health team are transitioning from one member or team to another. This technique consists of four parts.

1. Situation: Identify yourself and the client and state the primary problem.

2. Background: Give the background of the client and be ready to answer any questions the other care provider may have.

3. Assessment: Give the essential assessment parameters of the client's current state (e.g., BP, P, R).

4. Recommendations: Make suggestions for continued care of the client in a priority framework.

Adhering to this format when one nurse is handing off a client to another caregiver will help to minimize safety risks for the client as well as assist the new health team members to give the best care possible. This method also provides a framework that directs a focus on a critical situation, if present, so that an immediate intervention may be made.

Source: Amato-Vealey, Barba, M., & Vealey (2008)

---

client data, and SBAR provides a framework to accomplish this goal. Further, TJC's universal protocol is now included in the 2009 Hospital National Patient Safety Goals, which state that there must be three aspects of this protocol:

- Active communication among all members of the surgical team
- Involvement of the client or the client's legal representative
- Requirement for site marking and prevention of the wrong site, wrong procedure, and wrong individual

Therapeutic Communication Techniques

Communication includes the totality of the human individual and reflects what is happening within and outside of us. Body sensations, thoughts, feelings, **emotions**, ideas, **perceptions**, judgments, previous experiences, and memories are all part of how and what we communicate. Effective, functional communication occurs only when what is happening within is congruent with what we share with the outside. It is important to be a therapeutic as well as a functional communicator and not to disturb the communication process by using nontherapeutic techniques or blocks to communication (Figure 4-1 ■).

EVIDENCE-BASED PRACTICE

Improving Communication in the Emergency Department
Emergency departments have the highest rate of preventable errors. Communication failures between providers and clients have been cited in 65% of sentinel events. Results of a recent study (Downey, Zun, and Burke, 2012) found that when providers in a busy emergency department used a formal handoff approach, such as "IPASBATON" (which follows), it resulted in an improved sense of communication. When clients had an opportunity to ask and respond to questions, they were more satisfied with their treatment and more likely to comply with medical instructions.

I. Introduction: introduce yourself.

P. Patient: Name, identifiers, age, gender, location

A. Assessment: The problem, procedure, or issue, so far in the process

S. Situation: Current status/circumstances, uncertainty, recent changes

B. Background: Comorbidities, previous episodes, current medications, family

A. Actions: What actions to take and brief rationale

T. Timing: Urgency, explicit timing, prioritizing actions

O. Ownership: Who is responsible (individual/team), including client/family

N. Next: What happens next?

Source: Downey, Zun, & Burke (2012)

FIGURE 4-1 Example of nontherapeutic communication. Note how the nurse's focus is not on the client.

FIGURE 4-2 Within the interpersonal framework, nurses share part of who they are with the client.

Therapeutic communication techniques assist the flow of communication and always focus on the client. Nontherapeutic communication techniques block or hinder communication and generally focus on the nurse and meet the nurse's needs. The major therapeutic and nontherapeutic techniques are listed below.

Acknowledgment   Acknowledging the client without inserting your own values or judgments (Figure 4-2 ■). Acknowledgment may be simple and with or without **understanding**, verbal or nonverbal.

Example: In the response "I hear what you're saying," the nurse acknowledges a statement without agreeing with it.

Example: "Yes, go on." "Uh huh."

Clarification   Clarifying the client's message. Check out or make clear either the intent or hidden meaning of the message, or determine if the message sent was the message received.

Example: "I don't understand. Can you say it in a different way?"

Example: "Are you saying . . ." (Repeat meaning of client's message as understood by you.)

Feedback   Using **feedback** to relay to the client the effect of his or her words. This method helps keep the client on course or alters the course. It involves acknowledging, validating, clarifying, extending, and altering.

Example: "You changed the bag on your colostomy very well."

Example: "When you say that, it makes me feel uncomfortable." (If the client is making personal comments about the nurse.)

Focus   Focusing or refocusing on the client's statement. Pick up on central topics or "cues" given by the client.

Example: "You were telling me how hard it is to talk to your doctor."

Example: "You said the Doppler test tomorrow is frightening."

Incomplete Sentences   Encouraging the client to continue.

Example: "Then your life is . . ."

Listening   Consciously receiving the client's message.

Example: Listening eagerly, actively, responsively, and seriously.

Minimum Verbal Activity   Keeping your own verbalization minimal and letting the client lead the conversation.

Example: "You feel . . .?" "Go on."

Mutual Fit or Congruence   Creating harmony of verbal and nonverbal messages.

Example: A client is crying, and the nurse says, "I'll sit with you awhile," and puts his or her hand on the client's shoulder.

Example: A client tells the nurse he or she feels fine, but the client's body language indicates that he or she is in pain. "You say you feel fine, but you look like you are in pain."

Nonverbal Encouragement   Using body language to communicate interest, attention, understanding, **support**, caring, and listening to promote data gathering.

Example: The nurse nods appropriately as the client talks.

Example: The nurse leans forward.

Open-Ended Questions   Asking questions that cannot be answered with a simple "yes" or "no" or "maybe." Generally ask questions requiring an answer of several words to broaden conversational opportunities and to help the client communicate.

Example: "How is your PCA working?" rather than "Is the pain gone?"

Reflection   Identifying and sending back a message acknowledging the feeling or repeating the last few words the client said. (Conveys acceptance and great understanding.)

Example: "... distrust your diagnosis?"

Restatement   Repeating the client's statement as encouragement for him or her to continue.

Example: "You said that you can't bear to look at your stoma."

Validation   Verifying the accuracy of the sender's message.

Example: "Yes, it is confusing when so many staff are in the room."

EVIDENCE-BASED PRACTICE
Healthcare Team Performance

There is evidence to suggest that outcomes in health care depend on effective healthcare team performance. As a member of the healthcare team, you will be working alongside physicians, nurse practitioners, pharmacists, technicians, and other health professionals. You will be a unique contributing member. Health care is not a solitary event but an interprofessional exercise. Working with others as a team, you can ensure greater client safety and fewer errors. Teams who know their individual roles and responsibilities have fewer overall errors. As a student, you may have opportunities to interact with other healthcare discipline students. These interactions will assist you in being a contributing member of the interprofessional team.

Among teams, there is a concept referred to as **situational awareness**: being able to gather the right information, analyze it in a timely manner, and make projections from it as it relates to client care. This can occur only when the team is aware of the environment and is able to communicate effectively. Many healthcare organizations are training their employees on the TeamSTEPPS approach provided by the USDHHS Agency for Healthcare Research and Quality. This is an evidence-based approach that has been found to improve communication and teamwork skills among healthcare professionals. Its steps include: (1) a pretraining, readiness assessment, (2) training for on-site trainers and healthcare staff, and (3) implementation and sustainment. It has also been found to empower nurses to speak up if they feel there is something missing or just not right about a particular clinical situation.

Source: Baker, Gustafson, Beaubien, Salas, & Barch (n.d.)

Barriers to Communication

Changing the Subject   Introducing new topics inappropriately, a pattern that may indicate anxiety.

Example: The client is crying and discussing his or her fear of surgery when the nurse asks, "How many children do you have?"

False Reassurance   Using **clichés**, pat answers, "cheery" words, advice, and "comforting" statements in an attempt to reassure the client. Most of what is called "reassurance" is really false reassurance.

Example: "It's going to be all right."

Example: "Don't worry. This pain medication always works."

Giving Advice   Telling the client what to do. Giving your opinion or making decisions for the client implies he or she cannot handle his or her own life decisions and that you are accepting responsibility for him or her.

Example: "If I were you...."

Example: "You should try some alternative treatments."

Incongruence   Sending verbal and nonverbal messages that contradict one another; two or more messages, sent via different levels, seriously contradicting one another. The contradiction may be between the verbal/nonverbal content or time/space content.

Example: "I'd like to talk to you" (but I'm just too busy), said while nurse is turning away from the client.

Assumptions   Making an assumption about the meaning of someone else's **behavior** that is not validated by the other individual.

Example: The nurse finds the suicidal client smiling and tells the staff he's in a cheerful mood and much better.

Invalidation   Ignoring or denying another individual's presence, thoughts, or feelings.

Example: Client: "Hi, how are you?" Nurse: "I can't talk now, I'm on my way to lunch."

Overloading   Talking rapidly, changing subjects, and giving more information than can be absorbed at one time.

Example: "I see you're 48 years old and were admitted yesterday. Have you had a physical assessment? Where do you come from?"

Social Response   Responding in a way that focuses attention on the nurse instead of the client.

Example: "This sunshine is good for my roses. I have a beautiful rose garden."

Underloading   Remaining silent and unresponsive, not picking up cues, and failing to give feedback.

Example: Nurse asking, "I hope your pain is better" as he or she smiles and walks away.

Value Judgments   Giving one's own opinion, moralizing, or implying one's own values by using words such as *nice*, *good*, *bad*, *right*, *wrong*, *should*, and *ought*.

Example: "I think he's a very good doctor."

Example: "I think it's good that you decided to have the blood transfusion."

Multicultural Health Care

In the twenty-first century, demographic shifts are occurring that will change the direction of health care. As of the 2012 census, Asians are the fastest growing race or ethnic group in the United States. This is due mostly to international migration. Hispanics remain the second largest race or ethnic group, representing 17% of the nation. Five states have a majority-minority, meaning that the prevailing minority group is now more than half the population (Brown, 2014).

Because of this change in the U.S. population demographics, there are emerging barriers to health care for many groups of people. Perhaps the greatest barrier is language, and since communication is an essential component of providing nursing care, it is important to consider language under the topic of communication. Other barriers may be living in urban, poor neighborhoods; poor prevention practices such as poor nutrition; and beliefs that affect how certain cultural groups understand illness and respond to treatment. Perhaps the greatest barrier for many ethnic groups is poverty. Those in the lower socioeconomic group have reduced access to health care, including health insurance, availability and location of health facilities, transportation, and so on.

Cultural Awareness

It is important for nurses to understand the impact of various cultures on healthcare practices if they are to become culturally competent. As more and more people immigrate to this country, nurses will be faced with challenges related to **cultural diversity** when administering health care. Cultural diversity implies the range of differences in values, beliefs, customs, folklore, traditions, language, and patterns of behavior for the various cultural groups. For example, people from different cultures define personal space differently. Some may prefer closer personal contact, while an individual moving into their personal space offends others. The nurse needs to be aware that personal space is related to culture, gender, and group behavior. Because all of these aspects potentially affect how an individual experiences, copes with, and responds to illness, nurses must be aware of these cultural differences (Box 4-2 ■).

Cultural Competence

Within the literature, you will find the terms **cultural sensitivity**, *cultural awareness*, and *cultural competence*. They are oftentimes used interchangeably. However cultural awareness is more the perception of the individual in the context of the aesthetics of a culture, such as the dress and the arts. Cultural sensitivity has more to do with personal **attitude** and the desire to *not* be offensive when caring for someone of another culture or ethnicity. Awareness and sensitivity are

---

Box 4-2 CULTURAL ASSESSMENTS

When completing a total assessment on a client, the individual cultural components that are important to include are:

- Cultural background and orientation
- Communication patterns (based on culture)
- Nutritional practices
- Family relationships
- Beliefs and perceptions relating to health, illness, and treatment modalities
- Values relating to health practices
- Education
- Issues affecting the delivery of health care

---

just two of the elements of cultural competence, which also includes linguistic competency (Box 4-3 ■). Cultural competence is defined as the ability of the nurse and the healthcare organization to respond effectively to the cultural and linguistic needs of the client (Spector, 2013).

Diversity in Health Care

Diversity is a key to delivering competent and safe nursing care because U.S. population projections beyond 2012 show that Hispanics, Asian Americans, and African Americans will outnumber non-Hispanic Whites. These diverse cultural groups will present all healthcare workers with a challenge: a challenge to make appropriate ethical decisions based on the unique cultural values, beliefs, and practices of each group.

Diversity awareness can be viewed in three parts: how people are different, recognizing the unique needs of others, and sensitivity (recognizing personal biases) so that they do not interfere with giving professional and safe nursing care.

Spiritual Assessment

When you are completing a total client assessment, it is important to include a **spiritual assessment**. This need not be invasive or intrusive. The purpose of such an assessment is to open the channels of communication so that the client will feel comfortable in discussing spiritual issues. If the client experiences no opening from the nurse, he or she may conclude that the nurse does not wish to discuss spirituality; therefore, just asking a few pertinent questions during a general assessment may accomplish the goal of opening communication (Table 4-1 ■).

Relationship Therapy

Nurses are given the unique opportunity to share part of who they are with others who have asked directly or indirectly for assistance. It is within this interpersonal framework that the nurse–client relationship begins to develop and take on its individual characteristics.

Both individuals bring into the relationship their thoughts, feelings, sense of self or self-worth, behavior patterns, abilities to adapt and cope, belief systems, and points of view about life and how they interact with it. Within all

---

Box 4-3 PRACTICE GUIDELINES

Cultural Competence

The Office of Minority Health (OMH) (2012) released the enhanced National Standards for Culturally and Linguistically Appropriate Services (CLAS) in health and health care. This blueprint is available free of charge to all healthcare providers. The blueprint is intended to "ensure care and services are respectful of and responsive to the cultural and linguistic needs of all individuals."

Table 4-1 Religious Diversity Considerations for Client Care

Religious Orientation	Baptism	Death Rituals	Health Crisis	Diet
Adventist	Opposed to infant baptism	No last rites	Communion or baptism may be desirable.	No alcohol, coffee, tea, or any narcotic; dietary restrictions. Vegetarianism is common.
Baptist	Opposed to infant baptism	Clergy supports and counsels.	Some believe in healing and laying on of hands. Some sects resist medical help.	Condemn alcohol; some do not allow coffee and tea.
Islam	No baptism	Prescribed procedures by family for washing body and shrouding after death	No faith healing Ritual washing after prayers every day	Prohibit alcohol and pork
Buddhist	Rites are given after child is mature.	Send for Buddhist priest last rite chanting.	Family should request priest to be notified.	Alcohol and drugs discouraged; some are vegetarian.
Christian Scientist	No baptism	No last rites No autopsy	Deny the existence of health crises Many refuse all medical help, blood transfusions, or drugs.	Alcohol, coffee, and tobacco are viewed as drugs and not allowed.
Episcopalian	Infant baptism mandatory	Last rites not essential for all members	Medical treatment acceptable	Some do not eat meat on Fridays.
Jehovah's Witness	No infant baptism	No last rites	Opposed to blood transfusions	Do not eat anything to which blood has been added.
Judaism	No baptism but ritual circumcision on eighth day after birth	Ritual washing of body of dead	All ill people seek medical care. Treatment supersedes dietary restrictions.	Orthodox observe kosher dietary laws, which prohibit pork, shellfish, and the eating of meat and milk products at the same time.
Methodist	Baptism encouraged	No last rites	Medical treatment acceptable	No restrictions
Mormon	Baptism eight years or older	Baptism for the dead can be done by proxy.	Do not prohibit medical treatment, although they believe in divine healing	Alcohol, caffeine, tobacco, tea, and coffee not allowed
Roman Catholic	Infant baptism mandatory	Last rites required	Sacrament of the sick	Most ill people are exempt from fasting.

Note: There may exist circumstances that require a court order to supervene religious practices (e.g., a blood transfusion to save the life of a child).

these complex variables, there is a commonly shared point at which the nurse relationship begins.

This relationship may be defined as the interaction between the nurse and a client with shared therapeutic goals and objectives. Characteristics of the relationship include acceptance, honesty, understanding, and empathy of the nurse toward the client who is willingly or unwillingly seeking help. Generally, it is important for the nurse to view the client as a unique individual who is responsible for his or her own feelings, actions, and behaviors and who is an active participant in a healthcare program. The relationship is more effective if the client shows a willingness to accept responsibility and actively participates in the therapeutic relationship. This is not always possible, and the nurse must begin the relationship by accepting the level at which the client is able to participate. This, at times, is a difficult and frustrating process. The goal of relationship therapy is to assist the client to identify and meet his or her own needs (Figure 4-3 ■). The nurse may assist the client in reaching the goals by demonstrating acceptance so that the client may experience the feeling of being accepted as

FIGURE 4-3 Relationship therapy includes bringing the family together to discuss client care needs.

an individual; by developing mutual trust through consistent, congruent nursing behaviors; by providing corrective emotional experiences to increase **self-esteem**; and finally by creating a safe, supportive environment. Some degree of emotional involvement and honest, open communication is essential throughout the relationship. The nurse must encourage the client to express his or her feelings, concerns, expectations, fears, and the like within safe limits.

Relationship Principles

Principles underlying a **helping relationship** include:

- Awareness of the total client, including emotional, physical, cultural, and spiritual needs
- Some degree of emotional involvement while maintaining objectivity
- The setting of appropriate limits and consistency in behavior while caring for the client
- Open, honest, and clear communication
- Encouragement of the expression of feelings
- Focus on "here and now"

Dangers to the relationship include overemotional involvement and judgmental attitudes on the part of the nurse and the staff.

Phases in Nurse–Client Relationship Therapy

There are three phases in a traditional nurse–client relationship.

Initiation, or Orientation, Phase In the initial interaction with the client, you introduce yourself and establish the boundaries of the relationship. It is also the phase in which you identify problems, expectations, and relevant issues (cultural and spiritual) that need to be addressed during the relationship. It is at this stage in the relationship that you would identify any impairment, such as hearing, speaking, developmental, or psychologic, that must be taken into account so that adjustments in the relationship may be made.

Continuation, or Active Working, Phase This is the phase in which you would develop a working relationship, and in conjunction with meeting the client's needs, begin resolving the client's problems; for example, working with the client to handle his pain; teaching the client to care for a new device, such as a colostomy; or implementing a plan to increase the client's independent functioning.

Termination Phase At this final phase, when the client is soon to be discharged, you would follow the plan that you began when the client was admitted; for example, anticipate problems the client will face when he or she goes home, complete discharge planning and teaching, and deal with client's fears about being on his or her own after leaving the hospital.

Nursing Diagnoses

The following nursing diagnoses may be appropriate to include in a client care plan when the components are related to establishing and maintaining a nurse–client relationship.

NURSING DIAGNOSIS	RELATED TO . . .
Impaired Communication: Verbal	Psychologic barrier, inability to speak dominant language, impaired **cognition**, lack of privacy
Powerlessness	Perceived lack of control resulting in dissatisfaction
Impaired Social Interaction	Lack of motivation, anxiety, **depression**, lack of self-esteem, disorganized thinking, delusions, hallucinations
Social Isolation	Hospitalization, terminal illness

Source: Herdman, T. H. & Kamitsuru, S. (Eds.) *Nursing Diagnoses – Definitions and Classification 2015-2017*. Copyright © 2014, 1994–2014 by NANDA International. Used by arrangement with John Wiley & Sons Limited. Companion website: www.wiley.com/go/nursingdiagnoses. In order to make safe and effective judgments using NANDA-I nursing diagnosis it is essential that nurses refer to the definitions and defining characteristics of the diagnoses listed in this work.

Unit 4.1
Therapeutic Communication

Nursing Process Data

ASSESSMENT Database

- Determine client's ability to process information at the cognitive level.
- Assess mental status data to establish baseline for intervention.
- Assess client's ability to communicate on a verbal level.
- Observe what is happening with the client here and now.
- Identify client's developmental level so interaction expectations will be realistic.
- Assess client's anxiety level because anxiety interferes with communication.
- Assess client's cultural background.
- Teach clients to communicate with their healthcare providers.
- Assess cultural preferences.
- Assess spiritual issues.
- Assist a client to describe personal experiences.
- Encourage a client to express needs, feelings, and thoughts.
- Use communication to increase a client's sense of self-worth.

PLANNING Objectives

- To assist client to meet his or her own needs
- To assist client to experience the feeling of being accepted
- To increase client's self-esteem
- To provide a supportive environment for change
- To institute therapeutic rather than casual or non–goal-oriented communication
- To affect or influence the client's physical, emotional, and social environment
- To be sensitive to client's cultural orientation

IMPLEMENTATION Procedures

DOCUMENTATION AND EVALUATION
Expected Outcomes

- Client develops the ability to assess and meet his or her own needs.
- Communication becomes clearer, more explicit, and centered on problem areas.
- A supportive environment is created so that the client can reduce the level of anxiety and experience change.
- Cultural diversity is accepted by the healthcare team.
- Cultural preferences and spiritual issues are addressed.
- Clients are able to communicate effectively with their healthcare providers.

Unexpected Outcomes/Alternative Actions

Pearson Nursing Student Resources

Find additional review materials at
nursing.pearsonhighered.com.
Prepare for success with NCLEX®-style practice questions and Skill Checklists.

Skill 4.1.1 | Introducing Yourself to a Client

Procedure

1. Obtain client assignment.
2. Read chart and review healthcare provider's orders.
3. Check client care plan. **Clarify** any questions about client assignment.
4. Perform hand hygiene.
5. In client's room check client ID with two forms of identification.
6. Introduce yourself to the client. (Example: "Good morning, Mr. Jones. My name is Miss Barnes. I am a student nurse from the Bellington School of Nursing, and I will be caring for you today.")
7. If the client is blind, introduce yourself as you come into the room: Tell exactly what you are doing and when you are leaving. ➤ *Rationale:* Blind clients become anxious when they hear someone enter the room who does not speak.
8. Begin to establish a nurse–client relationship using clear, open communication.

Skill 4.1.2 | Beginning a Client Interaction

Procedure

1. Following hand hygiene, introduction, and identification of the client using two identifiers, relate the purpose of interaction.
2. Tell client specifically what you will be doing in terms of his or her care.
3. Ask if the client understands or has any questions (Box 4-4 ■).
4. Encourage client to describe how he or she is feeling at the time (especially focusing on the pain level).
5. Encourage client to participate in his or her care—both verbally and nonverbally. In certain instances, the client may feel more comfortable with a family member or close friend in attendance. ❶
6. Pay attention to communication as well as the procedure you are administering. ➤ *Rationale:* Often, your best database is drawn from observation.
7. Assess nonverbal behavior and determine if it fits (is congruent) with **verbal communication**, especially when you are evaluating pain level (Table 4-2 ■).
8. Complete communication by asking client for feedback.
9. Complete interaction by telling client when you will return.
10. Follow through on agreed-upon meeting time to build client trust.

❶ When interacting with a client, the nurse may include friends and family members as important elements in client's support system.

Box 4-4 COMMUNICATING WITH THE HEARING IMPAIRED

If your client is hearing impaired, it is very important to establish a method of communication (pen and pencil, sign language, speaking loudly and clearly). Other factors to take into consideration when communicating with the hearing impaired are to pay attention to the client's nonverbal cues, decrease background noise such as television, and always face the client when speaking. It is also important to check with the family regarding how they communicate with the client. Finally, it may be necessary to contact the appropriate department resource individual for this type of disability.

Table 4-2 Communication Deficits and Interventions

Deficit	Intervention
Language/Culture	Determine client's level of fluency in English and understanding. Use an interpreter or translator. Pay attention to **nonverbal communication**. Learn client's cultural values. Be aware of client's cultural preferences that may affect etiquette (personal space, use of touch, eye contact). Avoid jargon or slang—select words you use carefully.
Sensory—Hearing, Seeing	Speak slowly, clearly, and directly to the client; do not use a loud voice. Use gestures to clarify or drawings to illustrate. Describe carefully the care you are giving to the client. Provide alternate means of communication: writing pad, gestures, etc. Work out a code with client for answers to basic questions; for example, "Are you in pain? For yes, blink once."
Cognitive	Orient to reality frequently (day, year, etc.). Use the same staff as much as possible. Introduce yourself repeatedly; explain aspects of care simply. Speak in clear, simple sentences.
Verbal Communication	Speak directly to clients and treat them with dignity and respect, even if they are nonverbal. Ask specific questions that require a yes or no, not open-ended questions. Recognize a client's facial expressions as well as his or her gestures. If a client's behavior changes drastically, look for an acute illness, such as an infection. Try flash cards or a chalkboard for a response. Use nonverbal techniques yourself, such as touch. Include client in the conversation even though there is no response.

Skill 4.1.3 | Teaching Clients to Communicate With Their Healthcare Providers

Preparation

1. Introduce self and identify client using two forms of identification.
2. Wash hands.
3. Explain the procedure.

Procedure

1. Practice with client how to formulate and verbalize direct (vs. indirect) questions.
2. Role-play with client how to extract the specific information he or she wish to receive from the healthcare provider. ➤ *Rationale:* Receiving the information will increase client satisfaction and lower anxiety.
3. Verify directly (clarify) the information the client receives from the healthcare provider. ➤ *Rationale:* This will decrease client's anger and anxiety.
4. Assist client to ask about functional status of the disease and symptoms. ➤ *Rationale:* Increases client's sense of control over his or her condition.
5. Assist client to ask the healthcare provider purpose and expected outcomes of treatments. ➤ *Rationale:* Increases adherence and compliance to treatment.

Note: It is a good idea to recommend to your clients to keep a notepad and a list of the things they want to mention when they see their provider. This way, all their concerns can be addressed.

CLINICAL ALERT

Beginning in 2006, The Joint Commission requires hospitals to document the client's language and communication needs in the medical record. The Joint Commission is implementing this because research shows that differences in language and culture can have a major impact on quality and safety in client care.

EVIDENCE-BASED PRACTICE

Impact of Client–Provider Language Concordance

Providing care that is both respective and responsive of client preferences is recognized by the Institute of Medicine as a goal of quality health care. Language barriers found by clients with limited English proficiency have been found to complicate client–physician interactions. Expanding access to language-concordant providers (providers who speak an individual's language) improves clinical interactions and improves outcomes. Having access to a language-concordant provider encourages quality interactions and may improve the client's overall health and sense of well-being.

Source: Schenker et al. (2010)

Skill 4.1.4 | Assessing Cultural Preferences

Procedure

1. Review client history related to cultural orientation to determine if adequate information pertaining to cultural preferences is included. ➤ *Rationale:* A complete history will detail cultural diversity patterns.

   a. Ethnic heritage and language
   b. Family organization and role of members
   c. Dietary practices and knowledge about nutrition
   d. Education, formal and informal
   e. Healthcare practices and beliefs

2. Introduce self to client, identify client with two identifiers, and perform hand hygiene.
3. Determine client's perception of illness based on cultural beliefs.
4. **Validate** verbal and nonverbal communication from client based on cultural understanding. ➤ *Rationale:* When the client's cultural background is different from the nurse's, communication problems may result.

5. Consider using an interpreter if communication seems unclear. ➤ *Rationale:* An interpreter will facilitate communication and reduce stress on the client.
6. Examine expectations of health care based on the client's cultural influences. ➤ *Rationale:* Health care should be congruent with the client's expectations or a positive outcome of treatment may be in jeopardy.

> **CLINICAL ALERT**
> Never use a child or minor to interpret for a parent or elder. Placing a child or minor in this situation creates an unjust burden on the translator. In addition, the parent or adult may not feel comfortable providing the child or minor with potentially personal information.

Skill 4.1.5 | Assessing Spiritual Issues

Procedure

1. Introduce self to client, identify client with two identifiers, and wash hands.
2. Ask the client relevant questions concerning spiritual issues.
   ➤ *Rationale:* If the nurse never broaches this subject, the client will not feel free to discuss spiritual issues.

   a. Do you have a spiritual component in your life?
   b. If so, how will this help you during your illness?
   c. Is there any particular individual or spiritual advisor that you would like me to contact for you?
   d. Is there anything that I (as your nurse) can do to support your spiritual beliefs?

3. "Are there any spiritual issues that you would like to discuss? If so, let's arrange a time to talk about these issues."
   ➤ *Rationale:* This approach will open communication and notify the client that you are willing to discuss these issues.

Skill 4.1.6 | Assisting a Client to Describe Personal Experiences

Procedure

1. Introduce self to client, identify client with two identifiers, and wash hands.
2. Encourage client to describe his or her perceptions and feelings.
3. Focus on communication as well as body reactions.
4. Don't dominate the conversation. ➤ *Rationale:* The less you say, the more you encourage spontaneity and verbalization from the client.

5. Assist client to clarify feelings.
6. Maintain an accepting, nonjudgmental attitude.
   ➤ *Rationale:* Making value judgments, even nonverbal ones, negatively affects the nurse–client relationship.
7. Give broad opening statements, and ask open-ended questions. ➤ *Rationale:* This open approach enables the client to describe what is happening.

Skill 4.1.7 | Encouraging a Client to Express Needs, Feelings, and Thoughts

Procedure

1. Within every interaction, focus on feelings rather than superficial topics during interactions.
2. Assist client to identify thoughts and feelings.
3. Pick up on verbal cues, leads, and signals from the client.
4. Convey attitude of acceptance and empathy toward the client. ➤ *Rationale:* Being aware of your own feelings and attitudes and separating them from the client's contributes to acceptance.
5. Note what is said as well as what is not said.
6. Assist the client to become aware of differences between behavior, feelings, and thoughts.
7. Give honest, nonjudgmental feedback to the client.

| **Skill 4.1.8** | Using Communication to Increase a Client's Sense of Self-Worth |

Procedure

1. Within every procedure, use body language as well as verbal communication to convey empathy. ➤ *Rationale:* Sitting down at the client's bedside or not acting as if you are in a hurry encourages communication.
2. Respect the client's need for emotional privacy, but be available to the client.
3. Be nonjudgmental (see example of making judgmental responses).
4. Mutually identify goals to meet the client's individual needs.
5. Keep all agreements with the client.
6. Become the client's advocate.
7. Give the client positive feedback when appropriate.

> **LEGAL ALERT**
>
> A neonate receiving an IV in his right foot showed discoloration and edema at the injection site. The infiltration was noted on a transfer sheet as the baby was being transferred to another unit. It was not noted in the medical record. When the parents questioned the injury, they were told that it was just a "blister." In time, the infiltration led to scarring and loss of motion. The nurse who originally noted the infiltration was sued.
>
> This is an example of poor or inadequate communication when "handing off" a client.

Unit 4.1 Documentation and Evaluation

DOCUMENTATION for Therapeutic Communication

- Identification of client needs
- Explicit goals of interaction
- Communication patterns of client
- Emotional state of client
- Expressed feelings and thoughts if relevant
- Cultural issues if relevant
- Spiritual issues if relevant

EVALUATION/Critical Thinking

Expected Outcomes

- Client develops the ability to assess and meet his or her own needs.
- Communication becomes clearer, more explicit, and centered on problem areas.
- A supportive environment is created so that the client can reduce the level of anxiety and experience change.
- Cultural diversity is accepted by the healthcare team.
- Cultural preferences and spiritual issues are addressed.
- Clients are able to communicate effectively with their physicians.

Unexpected Outcomes

- Therapeutic communication is not achieved.

Alternative Actions

- Eliminate barriers to communication from interaction style. If a barrier does occur, recognize it. Move to correct communication by using therapeutic modes of communication.
- Evaluate your own process of communication during and after interaction.
- If client needs to verbalize and you cannot help him or her do so, contact another nurse or the social worker.

Unexpected Outcomes	Alternative Actions
• Client's demanding behavior interferes with the therapeutic communication process.	• Do not ignore demands; they will only increase in intensity. • Attempt to determine causal factors of behavior, such as high anxiety level. • Set limits to response patterns when client is demanding. Control own feelings of anger and irritation. • Teach alternative means to getting needs met.
• Cultural preferences/issues were not recognized, so communication was hindered.	• Complete a cultural assessment before revising a plan of care. • Bring in a translator to converse with the client to establish baseline communication. • Evaluate values, beliefs, preferences, and expectations related to health care.
• Spiritual issues were not discussed until the client asked for a priest, minister, rabbi, imam, or shaman.	• At this time, assess the client's spiritual beliefs and ask if there is any way you can assist him or her in this area.
• Client remains uncomfortable in talking to healthcare provider.	• Continue to work with client by role-playing with nurse taking role of healthcare provider. • Be present when client is questioning healthcare provider and give support. • Encourage client to write down concerns.

Unit 4.2
Nurse–Client Relationship

Nursing Process Data

ASSESSMENT Database

- Determine the purpose of establishing a nurse–client relationship.
- Consider the overall condition of client to determine if he or she can benefit from a nurse–client relationship.
  - A specific relationship could feed into secondary gains of attention.
  - An individual with chronic organic brain disorder cannot benefit from a relationship per se.
- Identify client expectations of a therapeutic relationship to determine if you can meet these needs.
- Examine your own feelings and expectations to evaluate potential effect on such a relationship.

PLANNING Objectives

- To provide an environment in which client can feel secure enough to alter behavior patterns
- To allow a client to experience a positive, satisfying relationship
- To enable client to test more adaptive ways to handle anxiety
- To provide a climate conducive to raising the client's self-esteem
- To allocate enough time to complete planned process of interaction
- To terminate relationship successfully

IMPLEMENTATION Procedures

DOCUMENTATION AND EVALUATION

Expected Outcomes

- Principles of therapeutic communication are used.
- Boundaries of professional relationship are maintained.
- The appropriate environment for interaction is established.
- **Termination** of the relationship is completed successfully.

Unexpected Outcomes/Alternative Actions

Pearson Nursing Student Resources

Find additional review materials at
nursing.pearsonhighered.com.
Prepare for success with NCLEX®-style practice questions and Skill Checklists.

Skill 4.2.1 | Initiating a Nurse–Client Relationship

Procedure

1. Read client's chart and be familiar with history, medications, and status.
2. Identify client with two forms of client ID.
3. Perform hand hygiene.
4. Approach client and introduce self.
5. Assess client's symptoms and problems, and communicate a willingness to help alleviate these discomforts.
6. Establish a beginning relationship. ➤ *Rationale:* Open, honest, congruent communication and consistent behavior help lay the groundwork for trust in a relationship. ❶
7. Establish mutual goals as a basis for the relationship.
   ➤ *Rationale:* Goals mutually set and agreed on are more easily accepted by both parties in the relationship.
8. Be consistent in your behavior; do what you say you will do, and only make promises you are willing to keep. ➤ *Rationale:* The most important element is the beginning of trust. Without trust, the nurse–client relationship is ineffective.
9. Encourage client's participation in his or her care.
   ➤ *Rationale:* This focus enhances compliance to treatment.
10. Approach client in a warm, accepting manner during interactions. ➤ *Rationale:* The client may interpret a cool, aloof manner as lack of interest.

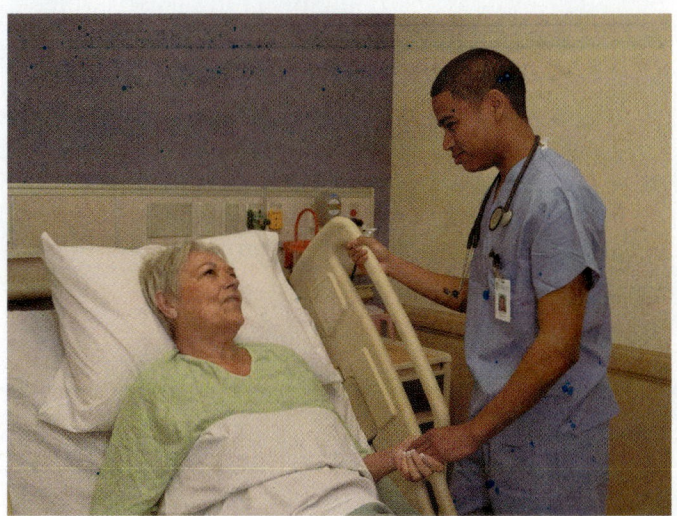

❶ Initiating a relationship is an important component of client care.

Skill 4.2.2 | Facilitating a Nurse–Client Relationship

Procedure

1. In every interaction, assume the role of facilitator.
2. Accept client as having value and worth as an individual.
   ➤ *Rationale:* Basic acceptance is a fundamental prerequisite of a relationship.
3. Provide a safe environment conducive to client's willingness to share.
4. Maintain the relationship on a professional level.
   ➤ *Rationale:* Responding on a professional rather than a social level defines the relationship.
5. Keep interaction reality-oriented, that is, in the here and now. ➤ *Rationale:* Discussion of past or future experiences does not contribute to a change in behavior now.
6. Listen actively; that is, respond to the client's cues. ❶
7. Use nonverbal communication to support and encourage client.
   a. Recognize meaning and purpose of nonverbal communication, especially in assessing pain.
   b. Keep verbal and nonverbal communication congruent.
8. Focus content and direction of conversation on client's cues, not on social or superficial topics.
9. Interact on client's intellectual, developmental, and emotional level.
10. Focus on "how," "what," "when," "where," and "who" rather than "why." ➤ *Rationale:* Asking "why" places the

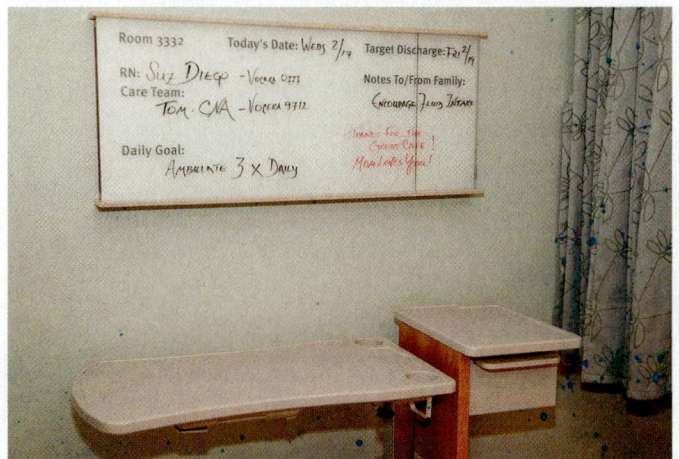

❶ Communication to and from the client can be verbal as well as written.

client on the defensive because it requires justification of behavior.
11. Assist client to identify, express, and cope with feelings.
12. Help client develop alternative **coping mechanisms** that are more adaptive.

Skill 4.2.3 | Terminating a Nurse–Client Relationship

Procedure

1. Work closely with the client in discharge planning and in planning the termination of the relationship from its beginning. ➤ *Rationale:* This approach promotes the client's independence and increases his or her sense of self-esteem.
2. Anticipate problems of termination and plan for their resolution. ➤ *Rationale:* Saying goodbye is often uncomfortable and difficult for both the client and the nurse.

3. Be aware that the client's behavior may reflect fear that he or she cannot cope at home, **overdependence**, depression, and withdrawal. ➤ *Rationale:* Allowing this behavior to be expressed helps the client to work it through.
4. Do not terminate the relationship too abruptly or allow it to persist beyond the client's needs.
5. Complete a satisfactory termination of the relationship. ➤ *Rationale:* This enables the client to move on.

Unit 4.2 Documentation and Evaluation

DOCUMENTATION for Nurse–Client Relationship

- Primary goals of nurse–client relationship and identified client needs
- Ongoing process of relationship therapy, including client's expressed feelings, thoughts, and so forth

- Client's behavior and changes in behavior, both positive and negative
- Cues to other team members on how best to relate to this particular client
- Elements of discharge planning

EVALUATION /Critical Thinking

Expected Outcomes
- Principles of therapeutic communication are used.
- Boundaries of professional relationship are maintained.
- The appropriate environment for interaction is established.
- Termination of the relationship is completed successfully.

Unexpected Outcomes	Alternative Actions
• Client refuses to participate in a nurse–client relationship.	• Comply with client's request, and do not force or impose relationship therapy. • Continue to offer relationship therapy at intervals. • Suggest that another team member attempt to establish a relationship.
• Nurse–client relationship frequently degenerates into a social conversation.	• Reevaluate the goals for the relationship, and remind client of terms originally established. • Set firm limits, and continually reexamine progress.

Unexpected Outcomes	Alternative Actions
• Termination of the nurse–client relationship is not successful.	• Reexamine the process of termination (termination should begin at the beginning of the relationship).
	• Devote more interaction time to this aspect of the relationship.
	• Attempt to elicit feelings about termination from the client as well as examining your own feelings.
• Nurse–client relationship cannot be established due to cultural differences.	• Allow the client's behavior to be expressed without making value judgments, and assist the client to discuss his or her feelings.
	• The nurse may make a special effort to understand the cultural preferences of the client.
	• Consider finding another nurse to establish the relationship—one with a similar background.

Communication in Special Situations: Depression, Anxiety, Anger, and Denial

Nursing Process Data

ASSESSMENT database

- Observe for behaviors that do not fit expected reactions to illness or hospitalization.

  Depression: *verbal cues* (expressing feelings of sadness, hopelessness, helplessness); *physical cues* (loss of motivation, vegetative, frequent crying episodes, bodily complaints, psychomotor retardation, weight loss); *emotional cues* (low self-esteem, preoccupation with inner thoughts, thoughts of suicide)

  Anxiety: *psychologic symptoms* (**confusion**, dread, **agitation**, difficulty making decisions, rumination); *physical symptoms* (tremors, dyspnea, palpitations, tachycardia, sweating, sleep disturbance); stages of anxiety (mild, moderate to severe)

  Aggression/anger: *verbal expressions* (voicing anger in loud voice, yelling, cursing); *physically acting out* (clenching fists, throwing objects, refusing treatments, threatening actions)

  Denial: *verbal expressions (expressing denial of the client's condition or diagnosis)*

PLANNING Objectives

- To recognize client's behavior that fits special situations of depression, anxiety, anger, or denial
- To intervene therapeutically when special circumstances exist
- To provide a supportive climate for the client to work through feelings of depression, anxiety, or anger
- To assist client to develop more adaptive ways of handling feelings

IMPLEMENTATION Procedures

DOCUMENTATION AND EVALUATION

Expected Outcomes

- Client's unhealthy responses were recognized and identified, and planned interventions were made.
- Verbal, physical, and emotional cues indicating depression, anxiety, anger, or denial decreased.
- Nurse's therapeutic interventions resulted in more adaptive behaviors. Clients developed new coping mechanisms to handle feelings.

Unexpected Outcomes/Alternative Actions

Pearson Nursing Student Resources

Find additional review materials at
nursing.pearsonhighered.com.
Prepare for success with NCLEX®-style practice questions and Skill Checklists.

Skill 4.3.1 | Communicating With a Depressed Client

Procedure

1. Within interactions, Identify cues that client is depressed.
2. Establish a nurse–client relationship. ➤ *Rationale:* A relationship provides the framework for therapeutic intervention.
3. Ask if client is feeling "down," sad, or upset. ➤ *Rationale:* The answer will validate nurse's perceptions or behavioral cues.
4. Remain with client, but it is not useful to encourage client to talk at length about feeling depressed; he or she will become even more depressed as conversation progresses. ➤ *Rationale:* Depression is best handled by mobilizing client, not talking.
5. Respond to client by suggesting activity, exercise, and involvement with another client. ➤ *Rationale:* Activity lifts mood and focus outside client's feelings and decreases depression.
6. Give client positive feedback for decisions, actions, and independent behavior. ➤ *Rationale:* Depressed clients have difficulty in making decisions.
7. Convey to client you care by spending time talking or participating in activities. ➤ *Rationale:* Knowing someone cares helps to lift depression.
8. Focus away from somatic complaints. ➤ *Rationale:* Depressed people often focus on somatic problems, but discussing them only increases depression.
9. Assess if client is considering suicide and intervene appropriately.

EVIDENCE-BASED PRACTICE

Exercise and Depression

Experts have found physical exercise can be an effective treatment against depression. The findings suggest exercise is comparable to psychotherapy and pharmacotherapy. Research is still needed to better quantify the exact amounts and types of exercise. However, the researchers agree that exercise is a low-risk option for many clients suffering with depression.

Source: Blumenthal, Smith, & Benson (2012)

Skill 4.3.2 | Communicating With an Anxious Client

Procedure

1. During interactions, identify cues that client is anxious (see Assessment Database) and degree of anxiety.
2. Establish nurse–client relationship. ➤ *Rationale:* Anxious clients may have difficulty relating to others.
3. Identify anxiety in self and maintain a calm, quiet approach. ➤ *Rationale:* Anxiety in the nurse will be transmitted to the client.
4. Assist client to identify anxiety and describe feelings and reactions. ➤ *Rationale:* Identifying presence and/or source will help to relieve anxiety.
5. Provide physical outlet for anxiety if possible (i.e., pacing).
6. Remain with anxious client, answering questions, supporting, etc. ➤ *Rationale:* This will help to prevent anxiety escalating, especially if client is in critical condition.
7. Provide a structured, nonstimulating environment. Give clear, firm directions, and information.

Skill 4.3.3 | Communicating With an Aggressive or Angry Client

Procedure

1. During interactions, observe client for cues of anger or aggression getting out of control (see Assessment Database).
2. Intervene immediately when loss of control is imminent (Box 4-5 ■).
3. Use a nonthreatening approach to client. ➤ *Rationale:* This approach will help to defuse situation.
4. Set firm limits and give specific expectations concerning behavior.
5. Avoid engaging in arguments or provoking client.
6. Calm client so that he or she may regain control.
7. Use problem-solving focus. ➤ *Rationale:* Discussion of feelings, and examining causal factors and client's response will help to defuse situation.
8. Responses to verbally abusive behavior: Do not respond in kind; do not take abuse personally; do not reject client; help client calm down by remaining calm, give feedback concerning your response to comments, and teach alternative ways for client to express feelings.

Box 4-5 PRACTICE GUIDELINES

Aggression

It is an unfortunate truth that violence does occur to nurses in the hospital environment. Most violence tends to occur in the emergency room. Nurses interact very closely with clients and their families. This oftentimes causes physical and emotional stress resulting in nurse–client (or family) conflicts. This type of

encounter can escalate and turn into a source of violence against nursing staff.

- Most violence is verbal in nature.
- All incidences should be reported.
- Violence at the workplace can affect job satisfaction.

Source: Chen, Ku, & Yang (2012)

Skill 4.3.4 | Communicating With a Client in Denial

Procedure

1. While establishing a relationship with the client, determine that the client is using the coping mechanism of denial—that is, denying the diagnosis or condition. (Denial is a defense mechanism whereby the ego protects itself from pain or conflict by denying reality.)
2. Do NOT confront client that he or she is in denial.
   ➤ *Rationale:* This is a protective defense mechanism the client needs at this time.
3. Be aware that denial may be a phase the client will pass through and eventually be able to cope with reality of the condition.
4. Discuss client's condition honestly and the options for treatment. ➤ *Rationale:* This focus may enable client to move more rapidly through the denial phase.
5. Offer to spend time with the client and respond to cues that he or she is ready to discuss feelings, but do not force client to confront issues before he or she is ready.

Unit 4.3 Documentation and Evaluation

DOCUMENTATION for Communication in Special Situations

- Description of specific cues of client's behavior evidencing depression, anxiety, or anger
- Interventions completed and client's response
- Instructions for other team members on how best to relate to client

EVALUATION/Critical Thinking

Expected Outcomes

- Client's unhealthy responses were recognized and identified, and planned interventions were made.
- Verbal, physical, and emotional cues indicating depression, anxiety, anger, or denial decreased.
- Nurse's therapeutic interventions resulted in more adaptive behaviors. Clients developed new coping mechanisms to handle feelings.

Unexpected Outcomes

- Client remains depressed, anxious, or angry; interventions do not bring about change in behavior.

- Client has thoughts of suicide and is identified as a suicide risk.

- Client remains angry and abusive to staff and others.

Alternative Actions

- Transfer to another nurse to work with client or request mental health consultant.

- Notify healthcare provider.
- Place client on suicide precautions.

- Try to change source of anger or aggressive behavior by identifying source, changing staff, and relocating client to another room or a private room.

Chapter Wrap-Up

GERONTOLOGIC Considerations

Physical Changes That Affect Communication

- Hearing changes (e.g., presbycusis, tympanic membrane atrophy, and distorted sounds) may make communication difficult. The nurse must speak clearly, loudly, and in view of the client. Use simple sentences and request feedback to validate understanding.
- Visual changes, such as presbyopia, and pupil, cornea, and lens impairment may diminish visualization. The nurse should be aware of eye changes and check that client sees clearly enough to perform required activities.

Psychosocial Changes That Affect Communication

- Relationships change with age. There is a loss of nurturing functions within the family. The nurse may need to perform this function with the older adult.
- Role changes within and outside the family occur—loss of spouse and loss of support systems. Older adults may require more support from caregivers.
- Older adults have fears of physical dependency, chronic illness, and loneliness. Caregiver may need to address these fears and work with client through communication and relationship to reduce them.

MANAGEMENT Guidelines

Each state legislates a Nurse Practice Act for RNs and LVN/LPNs. Healthcare facilities are responsible for establishing and implementing policies and procedures that conform to their state's regulations. Verify the regulations and role parameters for each healthcare worker in your facility.

Delegation

- Evaluation of cultural diversity and spiritual issues should be completed by the RN.
- A full history should be completed by the RN. This is an exclusive RN task that is not to be delegated to LPNs/LVNs.
- Care plan objectives relating to communication, spiritual issues, and cultural differences should be completed by the RN or checked by the RN if completed by the LVN.

Interprofessional Communication

All staff caring for the client from a different cultural heritage should be informed of special needs of the client based on cultural diversity theory.

- The unit manager should include special needs of the client based on communication patterns and cultural background when making staff assignments. (For example, is there a nurse from the same cultural background or who speaks the same language as the client who can be assigned to that client's care?)
- Assign a nurse who is comfortable dealing with spiritual issues if the initial assessment indicates the client wishes to discuss these issues.

CASE STUDY Applications

Scenario 1

A 25-year-old male comes to the emergency department. He has a bleeding wound on his arm, and he refuses surgical intervention when told he must remove his clothes and jewelry.

1. What effect would this client response have on the initial nursing plan of care?
2. What is your understanding of this client response? What are some questions you might ask the client?
3. Describe the strategies and goals you would devise to solve this problem.
4. Describe the measures you would implement to resolve this situation.

Scenario 2

A client has just been admitted with a diagnosis of rectal cancer. He is scheduled for surgery the next day. When you are completing an assessment and you ask about spiritual beliefs, the client says, "I'm a washed-out Catholic and I don't think I'm going to live, so what's the sense in talking about it?"

1. What would be the consequence of not responding to the client's comments about spiritual beliefs?
2. How would the goals of establishing a nurse–client relationship and assessing spiritual beliefs overlap in this situation?
3. Describe the actions you would take to engage this client in a discussion about these issues.

NCLEX® Review Questions

Unless otherwise specified, choose only one (1) answer.

1. Which intervention is most useful when communicating with an aphasic client?
   A. Use correct medical terminology when teaching or explaining.
   B. Ask open-ended questions to obtain information.
   C. Repeat the same word until the client understands.
   D. Provide frequent praise and encouragement.

2. A psychiatric client rapidly improves and is scheduled to be discharged tomorrow. Which of the following responses demonstrates that the nurse has a good understanding of termination of a relationship?
   A. "You have worked really hard the last three weeks. Good-bye and good luck."
   B. "Stop by and let us know how things are going."
   C. "You've done some good work here. I hope you are able to follow through with it."
   D. "Good-bye and good luck. Hopefully, we won't be seeing you here again."

3. One characteristic of a nurse–client relationship is that it is a professional one. What does this imply about the nurse?
   A. The nurse should be primarily concerned with implementing the policies of the hospital.
   B. The nurse views the client's needs as her or his primary concern.
   C. The nurse maintains a distance between self and client.
   D. The nurse establishes boundaries, formulate goals, and maintain the boundaries of a professional relationship.

4. One day a client with terminal cancer says to the nurse, "Well, I've given up all hope. I know I'm going to die soon." Which is the most therapeutic response?
   A. "Now, one should never give up hope. We are finding new cures all the time."
   B. "We should talk about dying."
   C. "You've given up all hope?"
   D. "Your doctor will be here soon. Why don't you talk to him about your feelings?"

5. Which of the following statements would be best to stimulate conversation with a client about his or her social history?
   A. "Are you married?"
   B. "Do you have any children?"
   C. "Tell me about your family."
   D. "Is your role in the family important?"

6. A client is admitted to CCU with a diagnosis of anterior myocardial infarction. Shortly after admission, he states: "I might as well have died because now I won't be able to do anything." Which is the most appropriate response by the nurse?
   A. "Don't worry, everything will turn out all right."
   B. "What do you mean, not able to do anything?"
   C. "Take one day at a time and it will all work out."
   D. "You shouldn't be thinking like this, because you are doing well now."

7. A male client is becoming increasingly angry and verbally abusive. Which of these is the appropriate intervention?
   A. Send the client back to his room.
   B. Ask the healthcare provider for an order for restraints.
   C. Summon assistance from a male staff member.
   D. Set firm limits on the abusive behavior.

8. Which of the following components would you include in a cultural assessment?
   Select all that apply.
   A. Cultural background
   B. Nutritional practices
   C. Beliefs and perceptions of health
   D. Age of the client
   E. Belief in God
   F. Communication patterns
   G. Health practices, including alternative

9. A client you are assigned to care for is hearing impaired. Which is the most effective way to communicate with this client?
   A. Use a writing pad and gestures.
   B. Speak clearly and slowly.
   C. Use nonverbal communication.
   D. Describe loudly and carefully what you are doing.

10. Which nursing intervention would be the highest priority when caring for a client who is depressed?
    A. Form a good nurse–client relationship.
    B. Encourage the client to talk about his feelings of depression.
    C. Suggest that the client do an activity.
    D. Assess the client frequently for potential suicide.

QSEN Activity

Domain: Communication

KSA: Attitude

Activity:

Have student(s) identify a particular clinical situation where the communication was not very effective, and perhaps the student wished it had gone another way. The scenario can be any dyad:

- Student nurse and client
- Student nurse and family member
- Student nurse and preceptor
- Student nurse and provider

Have the group reflect on how it could have been more effective. Role-play effective communication within the classroom using the techniques identified within the chapter.

Bibliography

Agency for Healthcare Research and Quality (AHRQ). (n.d.). TeamStepps: National implementation. Retrieved from http://teamstepps.ahrq.gov/

Amato-Vealey, E. J., Barba, M. P., & Vealey, R. J. (2008, Nov.). Hand-off communication: A requisite for perioperative patient safety. *AORN Journal, 88* (5), 763–770.

Baker, D. P., Gustafson, S., Beaubien, J. M., Salas, E., & Barch, P. (n.d.). Medical team training programs in health care. Retrieved from http://www.ahrq.gov/professionals/quality-patient-safety/patient-safety-resources/resources/advances-in-patient-safety/vol4/Baker.pdf

Blumenthal, J. A., Smith, P., & Benson, H. (2012, Jul.–Aug.). Opinion and evidence: Is exercise a viable treatment for depression? *ACSM's Health & Fitness, 16* (4), 14–21. doi: 10.1249/01.FIT.0000416000.09526.eb

Brown, A. (2014). U.S. Hispanic and Asian populations growing, but for different reasons. Pew Research Center. Retrieved from http://www.pewresearch.org/fact-tank/2014/06/26/u-s-hispanic-and-asian-populations-growing-but-for-different-reasons/

Census. (2012). http://www.census.gov/newsroom/releases/archives/population/cb13-112.html

Chen, K., Ku, Y., & Yang, H. (2012, Mar.). Violence in the nursing workplace—A descriptive correlational study in a public hospital. *Journal of Clinical Nursing, 22*(5–6), 798–805. doi:10.1111/j.1365-2702.2012.04251

Downey, L., Zun, L., & Burke, T. (2012). What constitutes a good hand off in the emergency department: A patient's perspective. *International Journal of Healthcare Quality Assurance, 26* (8), 760–767.

Office of Minority Health. (2012). National Standards for Culturally and Linguistically Appropriate Services (CLAS standards). Retrieved from https://www.thinkculturalhealth.hhs.gov/CLAS/Clas_Overview.asp

Schenker, Y., Karter, A. J., Schillinger, D. Warton, E. M., Adler, N. E., Moffet, H. H., & Fernandez, A. (2010, Nov.). The impact of limited English proficiency and physician language concordance on reports of clinical interactions among patients with diabetes: The DISTANCE study. *Patient Education and Counseling, 81*(2), 222–228.

Spector, R. E. (2013). *Cultural Diversity in Health and Illness* (8th ed.). Hoboken, NJ: Prentice Hall.

Chapter 5
Admission, Transfer, and Discharge

 ## Learning Objectives

5.1 Explain the steps of admitting a client to the hospital.

5.2 List client data that are included in documentation when admitting a client to the hospital, including the plan of care, goals, and outcome criteria.

5.3 Describe the disposition process for safeguarding client's valuables.

5.4 State what is meant by advance directives.

5.5 List documents that may be included in the client's admission record (Patient's Care Partnership brochure, Advance Directives, etc.).

5.6 Propose two solutions for clients who are unable to adapt to the hospital environment.

5.7 Identify essential "handoff" information to be communicated when client care is transferred to another caregiver, setting, or home.

5.8 Describe the process and rationale for medication reconciliation across the continuum of care.

5.9 Outline steps for transferring a client to another unit within the hospital or to the home.

5.10 Discuss discharge procedures when a client leaves the hospital.

5.11 Describe expected outcomes for clients being discharged from the hospital, including meeting criteria in the initial plan of care.

5.12 Complete discharge documentation including client's achievement of criteria established in the initial plan of care.

5.13 Describe three solutions for clients leaving the hospital against medical advice.

5.14 Outline discharge procedures that must be completed when a client leaves the hospital against medical advice.

Chapter Outline

Terminology

Adaptation ability to adjust to a change in environment.

Admitting the process of signing a client into the hospital.

Ambulation ability to walk, not confined to bed.

Assessment critical evaluation of information; the first step in the nursing process.

Behaviors an individual's total activities—actions or reactions, especially conduct—that can be observed.

Caring thoughtful attentiveness accompanied by responsibility.

Client care plan a plan for care of a specific client or one designed especially for one client.

Comfort to ease physically; relieve, as of pain.

Communication transmission of knowledge, information, or messages to another individual.

Diagnostic test a test used to determine a diagnosis or to determine the cause and nature of a pathologic condition.

Disability a disabled state or condition; incapacity.

Discharge to let go, as in discharging a client from the hospital.

DME durable medical equipment.

DRG diagnosis-related group. A system to classify all types of clients to determine how much Medicare pays the hospital, since clients within each category are similar clinically and are expected to use the same level of hospital resources.

Empathy the vicarious experience of another's situation.

Handoff transfer of information during a transition in care; it includes a transfer of authority and responsibility and an opportunity to ask questions and clarify information.

Home care nursing care given in the client's home.

Identification band a band, usually worn on a client's wrist, with the client's name and medical record number.

Limitation the state of being limited or restricted.

Maladaptation inability to adjust to a change in environment.

Potential possible but not yet realized.

Procedure a particular way of accomplishing a desired result.

Reconcile to resolve discrepancies.

Stress a state of agitation that renders the body out of balance.

Supervise to direct or inspect performance; to oversee.

Termination the spatial or temporal end of something; a limit or boundary.

Therapeutic having healing or curative powers.

Transfer to convey or shift from one individual or place to another.

Transition the process or an instance of changing from one form, state, activity, or place to another.

Verbalize to express in words (written or spoken).

Volunteer an individual who performs or gives his or her services of his or her own free will.

Admission, Transfer, and Discharge

Admission to the hospital can be a positive event if handled with attention and **empathy**. On the other hand, it can be a negative experience if it is impersonal or mechanized.

   Because impressions formed by clients during the admission process can affect their attitude and their ability to adapt to the total hospital experience, the nurse should consider this an important aspect of client care. The same holds true for transferring clients. Clients and families can feel lost if **transfers** from one unit to another are badly handled or not properly communicated, particularly when they are transferring from a high level of care to a less intensive environment. The **discharge** process begins at the time of admission, as the nurse collects data to work with clients to plan their care.

Admission to the Hospital

The process of **admitting** a client to a healthcare facility varies among institutions, such as nursing homes, clinics, and hospitals. Regardless of the size or type of facility, the admission process assists in the provision of safe, effective care (Figure 5-1 ■). Because the nurse–client relationship begins with admission, the nurse should have a thorough understanding of the standard admission process for the particular facility (Box 5-1 ■).

FIGURE 5-1 The client may be admitted to the hospital in a wheelchair.

Box 5-1 **ADMISSION PROTOCOL**

- Advance directives are made available to clients.
- The *Patient's Care Partnership* brochure is presented to each client.
- The admission **assessment** is completed by a registered nurse within a specified time after admission.
- All clients must be clearly identified by a legible **identification band**.
- When consent forms are required (for invasive **procedures**), they must be signed by an adult or guardian who is mentally competent. The adult must give voluntary consent, understand the risks and benefits of the treatment, and have the opportunity to ask questions.

Clients who present to the emergency department (ED) are stabilized, transferred to another facility, discharged, or admitted to the hospital by a licensed practitioner permitted by the state to admit clients. In some cases, the nurse calls the admitting healthcare provider for these orders.

Initial laboratory procedures and diagnostic testing are often completed before admission. The client may be provided a copy and/or explanation of an admission plan outlining the client's projected clinical course. If a client enters the hospital in an emergency situation, he or she may feel insecure or fearful because there has been little time to make plans concerning family, travel, finances, or employment. When a client enters the hospital for elective treatment or surgery, both the nurse and client have more time for orientation and preparation for the hospital experience. The initial contact with the nurse leaves a lasting impression, so it should be conducted in an unrushed, organized, and respectful manner.

When the elective client arrives at the hospital, the first contact is usually with the admitting receptionist, who assigns a medical record number and interviews the client. If preadmission forms were mailed to the client, the information is verified by the receptionist at this time; otherwise, the client must answer questions about age, address, financial or insurance status, next of kin, religion, employment, and consent for treatment. If the client cannot answer these questions because of age or condition, a relative usually gives the information. A parent or guardian must do this for a child. At this time, the client receives an identification band. This identification band includes the client's name, medical record number, the client's birth date, and a bar code. The band is used to identify clients accurately and meets The Joint Commission National Patient Safety Goal (2014) for improving the accuracy of client identification.

Admission to the Nursing Unit

Most clients are not admitted directly to the nursing unit but are generally admitted after their procedure (surgery or other) or from the ED. When a client is admitted in this way, the nurse must review the medical record carefully for any treatment or **diagnostic test** the client has received, because these may indicate the need for follow-up assessment or intervention. Within a specific time, a registered nurse performs a more thorough history and physical assessment (Figure 5-2 ■), determines a priority of needs, and initiates an individualized plan of care.

The client is informed about telephone use, clergy availability, recreational area and lounge use, mealtimes, visiting hours, and other hospital schedules. Some hospitals have printed booklets or television channels describing this information. The client is also familiarized with the immediate environment, including the space for belongings, the bathroom, and operation of the nurse call system inside the bathroom. The nurse also demonstrates operation of the bedside nurse call system, television, radio, and bed controls. The

FIGURE 5-2 Vital signs are obtained during the admission procedure.

more information the client receives, the more control he or she has over the environment.

Clients are discouraged from bringing items of monetary or sentimental value to the hospital (e.g., money, credit cards, jewelry, photographs, documents). If they are brought, the client may send them home with a family member or friend or place them in the agency vault per security personnel, or the client may retain them, assuming total responsibility and signing a "Release from Responsibility" form. Some facilities may have a safe or locker where valuables may be stored. Prosthetic devices such as hearing aids, dentures, and glasses are also considered to be valuables, but these are retained by the client.

Upon admission, a comprehensive list of the client's home medications is obtained (prescribed, OTC medications, and supplements), including route, dose, and frequency of use. A list of allergies to foods, drugs, devices, and materials is also obtained. This is required to meet The Joint Commission Patient Safety Goal (2014) of maintaining and communicating accurate client medication information. The healthcare provider then orders continuation or discontinuation of home medications during hospitalization. Any medications or supplements the client brings to the hospital should be sent home with the family or stored in a locked area. If it is determined a client's own medication will be administered, the medication is verified by pharmacy and given with a healthcare provider's order according to agency policy. No medication should be kept at the client's bedside.

Because clients may not be sure of their role while in the hospital, many hospitals have adopted versions of the American Hospital Association's *Patient's Care Partnership* brochure (see Box 1-7 in Chapter 1, page 9). Partnership includes the client's rights to obtain information about the illness or injury, to refuse medication or treatment, to participate in his or her own care, to know the rationale and risks of the treatment, and to receive courteous care.

The *Patient Self-Determination Act* requires all Medicare and Medicaid recipient hospitals to provide clients with information regarding their rights to reject medical treatment and to complete advance directives. An advance directive is a document the client creates that reflects goals, values, and preferences for health care. Advanced directives, sometimes called "Living Wills," specify medical treatments the client wants or does not want at the end of life (e.g., feeding tube, mechanical ventilation). When advance directives apply to appointing legal representation, they are called "durable power of attorney for health care." This directive designates an individual who will make decisions for the client when the client is unable to make them. Copies of living will and durable power of attorney are placed in the client's chart. These documents vary from state to state.

Additionally, many states mandate that an agency inquire about a client's requests concerning resuscitation. Competent clients who have been informed about their diagnosis and prognosis may be asked to execute a "Do Not Resuscitate (DNR)" directive at the time of admission. Following such a request, the healthcare provider attaches an order to the client's record, and the order is then reevaluated according to agency policy. (See Chapter 1 for more information about advance directives.)

Client Acuity Systems

State law, such as Title 22 of the California Code of Regulation, provides information on how staffing is determined in hospitals within that state. Title 22 states the following regulations regarding staffing.

> There shall be a method for determining staffing requirements based on assessment of client needs. This assessment shall take into consideration at least the following:
>
> 1. The ability of the client to do self-care
> 2. Degree of illness
> 3. Requirements for special nursing activities
> 4. Skill level of personnel required in delivery care
> 5. Placement of the client in the nursing unit
>
> There shall be documentation of the methodology used in making staffing determinations. Such documentation shall be part of the records of the nursing service and be available for review.

Various systems to determine staffing patterns have been used for many years. With the advent of diagnosis-related groups (**DRG**s), acuity systems for planning staffing needs have been used in many hospitals. This system provides information to assist in planning client care delivery. Categories of nursing care are identified, and a numerical value is assigned to each category. These categories of care include areas such as activities of daily living (ADLs), **ambulation**, client teaching, and medication administration. The numerical values assigned to each category are based on a point scale. For example, using a scale of 1 to 5, a score of 1 indicates the client can function independently in certain tasks and a score of 5 indicates complete dependency on a caregiver for that category.

The scores from all categories are totaled; this score is divided by the number of categories in the acuity system. The final score is designated as the client's acuity level, which is determined for each 8-hour shift. Every nursing unit has a predetermined number of client care hours assigned for each acuity level. For example, a client acuity level of 4.0 on the day shift is allotted 2.8 hours of nursing care for that shift.

After all clients in the nursing unit are assigned an acuity level, the total client care acuity number is used to determine the number of nursing staff required for the next shift. Then, the acuity level of individual clients is used to plan care assignments for the staff. A nurse may be able to care safely for a total acuity of 16. This method seems equitable, since each staff member is assigned to clients based on acuity. Thus, instead of assigning the nursing staff to clients based on room location or number of clients, the acuity level is used to allocate staff resources. Staffing patterns based on the acuity system have often been found to be a practical, equitable, and manageable solution.

Transfer to Another Unit

Clients may be transferred from one unit to another within the same facility as their condition changes. When a client is moved, all medications, belongings, and personal hygiene and special equipment are transferred with him or her. A complete **handoff** report is given to the receiving unit's nursing staff. The new unit's receiving nurse has an obligation to validate all information relayed about the client, to perform an independent client history and physical assessment, and to handle the client's transfer as a "new admission" to the receiving unit (Box 5-2 ■). The client also has a right to receive an orientation to the new setting just like that provided in the previous setting. Sometimes clients are transferred within the same unit (e.g., from a semiprivate to a private room or vice versa) for various reasons. Similarly, when the client goes off the unit for tests or other procedures, the nurse needs to provide a "handoff" to transport personnel and when the client returns, the nurse must consider any intervening events that occurred (e.g., medications administered) that may influence care decisions. This information, as well as any special instructions for client care, is included on the "handoff" **communication** form.

In an electronic health record, the transfer of clients from one location to another is entered into the system and the new location is immediately visible. In the situation where a paper medical record is still being used, processes must be in place to inform other departments when clients are transferred to ensure that timely delivery of medications and other care needs are met.

Discharge From the Hospital

Discharge planning begins at the time of admission. Discharge goals are identified and members of the healthcare team identify ongoing needs and make arrangements for the client's reintegration into the community setting. This discharge planning process takes into consideration the physical, emotional, and psychosocial needs of the client, family, and caregiver. Sometimes hospitalization introduces the client to a lifelong need to chronically adapt to declining physical health and to chronically affiliate with the healthcare system. The nurse must be empathetic to the client's response at discharge and approach the client with all possible options for continued care, educational and financial resources, and any other services to assist the client to adapt to a chronic situation. The final responsibilities of the discharge process are to terminate the nurse–client relationship and evaluate the discharge process.

Discharge Against Medical Advice

If, for a variety of reasons, a client decides to leave the hospital against medical advice (AMA), it is imperative that the nurse notify the healthcare provider, especially if the client is still undergoing diagnosis and ongoing treatment. Most hospitals have AMA protocols that include a mental status evaluation to determine if the client is competent and has the capacity to understand and make a rational decision about his or her care needs. If there is a question about this, it may require a psychiatric consult.

A competent client, of course, has the right to refuse treatment, but the nurse must still advocate for the client by attempting to determine the reason for the client's decision to leave and explaining that diagnosis and/or treatment have not been completed. An AMA discharge form should be signed by the client and witnessed. This form usually includes a place to document the specific risks and benefits of the treatments being proposed, the specific consequences of leaving AMA, the clients' understanding of the consequences for refusing treatment, and what discharge instructions were given to the client such as when to seek medical care and show any self-care activities.

Box 5-2 **"HANDOFF" PROCESS**

One effective strategy to improve handoffs uses the acronym SHARE. SHARE refers to the following steps:

- **S**tandardize critical content—include key information and synthesize content.
- **H**ardwire within your system—use standard forms and tools.
- **A**llow opportunity to ask questions—exchange contact information for follow-up questions.
- **R**einforce quality and measurement—monitor use of standard forms and hold staff accountable.
- **E**ducate and coach—teach staff what constitutes successful handoffs.

Source: Adapted from Blouin (2011)

See Chapter 6 (Client Education and Discharge Planning) for further information on discharging clients to home or another healthcare facility.

Adaptation to Home Care

The home healthcare industry has experienced drastically reduced payments and fewer reimbursable visits as a result of the Balanced Budget Act of 1997. Now home healthcare agencies are required to complete data collection information forms. The Outcome and Assessment Information Set (OASIS) was instituted in February 1999, and the newest form, OASIS C, was implemented in January 2010. (See the Medicare website for more information on OASIS C.)

The OASIS items were designed to enable systematic measurement of client home healthcare outcomes, with appropriate adjustment for client risk factors affecting those outcomes. The items have specific definitions used to measure changes in client's health status between two or more time points.

In addition to measuring client outcomes, OASIS data have the following uses:

- Client assessment and care planning for individual adult clients
- Agency reports on various client characteristics such as demographic, health, or functional status at the start of care
- Internal Home Health Agency (HHA) performance improvement

The information collected through OASIS is much more comprehensive, particularly in the area of the client's health history.

Legal Issues in Home Care

Home health nurses are at risk for **potential** legal liability. Nurses work alone in the **home care** setting and do not have the advantage of calling on a colleague to collaborate on a client situation. This situation leaves the nurse vulnerable to legal risks. Home health nurses must be extremely skilled in handling equipment of all types, as well as performing specialized procedures without the assistance of another nurse. It is critical that these nurses attend workshops, keep abreast of new equipment and procedures, and continue to read nursing journals on a regular basis. If home equipment is not functioning properly, the nurse should inform the client, call the medical equipment provider, fill out an incident report, and not use the equipment.

Home health nurses are also responsible for delegating tasks to unlicensed assistive personnel. It is the responsibility of the nurse to know the competence level of the staff and to use critical thinking and professional judgment when delegating. The American Nurses Association

(ANA) and the National Council for State Boards of Nursing (NCSBN) have a joint statement on delegation that includes a decision tree that provides clear guidance on delegation.

It is extremely important to maintain open communication with healthcare providers and professionals in other disciplines who provide care to clients in the caseload. Cell phones, email, and electronic health records allow for quick response time and improved communication.

Another legal issue is the need for appropriate client documentation that supports the need for home care services. If documentation is not accurate, timely, and complete, the client's reimbursement may be denied. This can lead to hours of time attempting to recover the costs of service, or it could lead to legal repercussions. Maintaining appropriate client records protects the nurse, client, and agency in cases under investigation. As electronic health records become more prevalent, nurses can enter data as they provide care.

The purpose of the unit "Admission to Home Care" in this chapter is to present clinical skills appropriate for the home setting. Many of these skills are exactly the same as those presented in other sections of this book. Some skills require minor change for **adaptation** to the home environment.

The use of the nursing process is just as important in home care as it is in the hospital. Nursing care plans are required by Medicare regulations and are also used as a justification for skilled nursing services by private insurers. Information regarding admission to home care is presented in the nursing process format to assist in organizing nursing actions and evaluating health care.

Plan of Treatment

A plan of care for home health care is based on previous hospitalization admission findings. Centers for Medicare and Medicaid Services (the federal office that administers the Medicare program) requires that all agencies certified to provide home health care to Medicare clients complete the OASIS forms and the home health certification and plan of treatment forms. These forms must be completed on admission to home health care and be signed by a healthcare provider. The plan of treatment is effective for 60 days. If the client's condition changes, an updated plan must be signed and submitted to the Medicare office every 60 days.

Documentation

Charting must follow the nursing care plan and cover the areas listed in the OASIS C documentation system. OASIS C is an assessment instrument used to collect specific information when an individual is receiving Medicaid or Medicare and requires the services of an HHA. OASIS C is a key component of Medicare's partnership with the home care

Nursing Trends

DISEASE Management

A current trend in delivering health care specifies a goal of reducing complications associated with chronic diseases. Designed to incorporate healthcare interventions based on standard practice guidelines, this system is a cost-saving, empowering approach for clients. Studies show that 90 million U.S. citizens live with chronic diseases, which are responsible for 7 out of 10 deaths in the United States

Disease management is a process that begins when the group paying for the health care identifies a client with a targeted chronic disease, including such diseases as cancer, chronic obstructive pulmonary disease (COPD), asthma, diabetes, or depression.

A nurse contacts the client, asks his or her permission to enter him or her in the program, and does an initial assessment. Following this, the nurse discusses recommended medical care to the client. The nurse then discusses lifestyle **behaviors** proven to improve the chronic conditions. All are based on evidence-backed practice guidelines. Self-care efforts have proved to be significant in altering the course of the disease.

Most programs involve telephone communications from a registered nurse, although home visits may be arranged.

industry to foster and monitor client outcomes and assist with quality improvement. Oasis C data items include sociodemographic, environmental, support system, health status, and functional status attributes of adult clients. Data are collected at the start of care, 60 days after initial care, and at discharge. Information gathered in the OASIS C form is forwarded to the state, where it goes to the Centers for Medicare and Medicaid Services. There, the information is used for reimbursement purposes for the specific HHA. This prospective payment system went into effect in October 2000. Several forms must be completed for each client.

An in-depth assessment identifies areas in which client status differs from optimal health or functional status and is used as the basis of client care planning. Many agencies use standardized care plans and individualize them for each client.

Since interventions are implemented by the client, family, and part-time caregivers, all are involved in the treatment plan. The nurse or the case manager is responsible to coordinate and evaluate the care. The physical therapist can assume the role of case manager when the client is receiving rehabilitation services only.

Because home health aides provide care without direct daily supervision of a nurse, agencies usually hire only experienced nursing assistants (in most states, those who have worked in a hospital or nursing home). Home health aide certification is voluntary in some states and required in others. In many states, the training is completed after nursing assistants have obtained a CNA certificate.

Medicare requires the nurse to make a home visit at least every 14 days to reassess client and family needs and to revise the care plan. One visit each month is to discuss the treatment plan with the family. The nurse also accompanies the home health aide once a month for a **supervised** visit.

Home health nurses must meet the national standards of care as published by the ANA. The best preparation for home health nursing continues to be a sound base of nursing skills coupled with a broad knowledge of agency procedures and protocols.

Cultural Awareness

In 2010, The Joint Commission published a Roadmap for Hospitals to advance effective communication, cultural competence, and client- and family-centered care. Within this set of guidelines are specific recommendations targeted at the initial point of contact the client has with the hospital admission. These recommendations include several that focus on developing an awareness of client's preferences, values, and beliefs. Specifically, identify the client's preferred language for discussing health care and then make sure this is noted in the electronic health record. Arrange for interpreter services if needed. Determine if the client needs assistance completing admission forms due to health literacy challenges.

Collect client race and ethnicity data in the medical record to help identify needs of individual clients and to collect data to help eliminate health disparities. Ask the client if there are any additional needs that may affect his or her care and communicate information about unique client needs to the healthcare team. These can include religious or spiritual needs as well as cultural needs.

Nursing Diagnoses

The following nursing diagnoses may be appropriate to include in a client care plan when the components are related to admission, transfer, and discharge of a client.

NURSING DIAGNOSIS	RELATED TO . . .
Anxiety	Actual or perceived threat to self-concept, threat to biologic integrity, unfamiliar environment and treatments, change in socioeconomic status
Fear	Known or unknown outcome of hospitalization, medical or surgical diagnosis, and treatments
Grieving	Loss of function, change in lifestyle, lack of social support system, change in social role or economic status
Powerlessness	Actual or perceived lack of control over situation, imposed regimens, lack of privacy
Social Isolation	Hospitalization, chemical dependency, altered appearance

Source: Herdman, T. H. & Kamitsuru, S. (Eds.) *Nursing Diagnoses – Definitions and Classification* 2015-2017. Copyright © 2014, 1994–2014 by NANDA International. Used by arrangement with John Wiley & Sons Limited. Companion website: www.wiley.com/go/nursingdiagnoses. In order to make safe and effective judgments using NANDA-I nursing diagnosis it is essential that nurses refer to the definitions and defining characteristics of the diagnoses listed in this work.

Admission and Transfer

Nursing Process Data

ASSESSMENT Database

- Determine client's understanding of reason for hospitalization.
- Observe and record client's physical, emotional, and mental status.
- Observe and record client's ability to adapt to the hospital environment.
- Observe for disabilities or **limitations.**
- Obtain a list of medications client is currently taking (prescribed, OTC, and supplemental), including dose, route, and frequency of use.
- Identify any food, drug, device, or device material allergies.
- Assess the client's level of comfort.
- Assess client for potential discharge needs.
- Assess condition prior to transfer.
- Obtain a thorough "handoff" report of client's progress and status at shift report, when receiving from another unit, or when returning from any test or procedure.

PLANNING Objectives

- To obtain a preliminary nursing history/assessment
- To assist client to adapt to hospital environment with minimal distress
- To encourage the client to participate in his or her own plan of care
- To provide a comfortable and aesthetically pleasing environment for the client
- To provide the client with some control over his or her immediate environment

- To provide the client with an opportunity to **verbalize** his or her feelings about hospitalization
- To facilitate safe and individualized continuity of care at all **transition** points throughout the continuum of care

IMPLEMENTATION Procedures

- **Skill 5.1.1** Admitting a Client 93
- **Skill 5.1.2** Transferring a Client 94

DOCUMENTATION AND EVALUATION

Expected Outcomes

- Client adapts to the hospital environment.
- Client participates in the individualized plan of care.
- Client understands rationale for and accepts transfer to a new care unit.
- Client is transferred to a new unit without complication.

Unexpected Outcomes/Alternative Actions

Pearson Nursing Student Resources

Find additional review materials at **nursing.pearsonhighered.com.**
Prepare for success with NCLEX®-style practice questions and Skill Checklists.

Skill 5.1.1 | Admitting a Client

Equipment

Admission kit with personal hygiene articles (if indicated)

Hospital gown

Thermometer

Blood pressure cuff and stethoscope (or automated unit)

Hospital Nursing History and Assessment form (if using a paper documentation system) ❶

Computer workstation to access electronic health record

Labeled containers for client's dentures or other items

Procedure

1. Perform hand hygiene.
2. Introduce yourself to the client and begin to establish a **therapeutic** nurse–client relationship.
3. Verify client's identity using two client identifiers.
4. Refer to client's electronic medical record to determine reason for hospitalization and note any orders to be initiated immediately (e.g., oxygen administration). ➤ *Rationale:* Timely initiation of tests or treatments reduces hospitalization time and costs.
5. Notify healthcare provider of client's admission and obtain orders if not already done.
6. Orient client to hospital room, various controls, and routines. ➤*Rationale:* This reduces anxiety about hospitalization.
7. Provide labeled container for client's prosthetic items (e.g., dentures).
8. Assist client to don hospital gown if client is not already in a hospital gown.
9. Perform preliminary data collection (e.g., vital signs, height, weight). These may be obtained by a delegate.
10. Obtain client's health history and complete the physical assessment (performed by the registered nurse) (Box 5-3 ■).
11. Complete assessments for fall and pressure ulcer risk status.
12. Obtain a complete list of medications client is currently taking (prescribed, OTC, and supplements) including dose, route, and frequency. ➤*Rationale:* The healthcare provider **reconciles** this list by continuing or discontinuing each medication and by ordering new ones.
13. Place allergy and other alert bands on client's wrist per agency protocol.

CLINICAL ALERT

The Institute of Medicine (2011), The Joint Commission, and The U.S. Preventive Services Task Force (2013) have recommended and/or required screening and counseling for "interpersonal and domestic violence" for women and others. This is often done as part of the admission process.

A

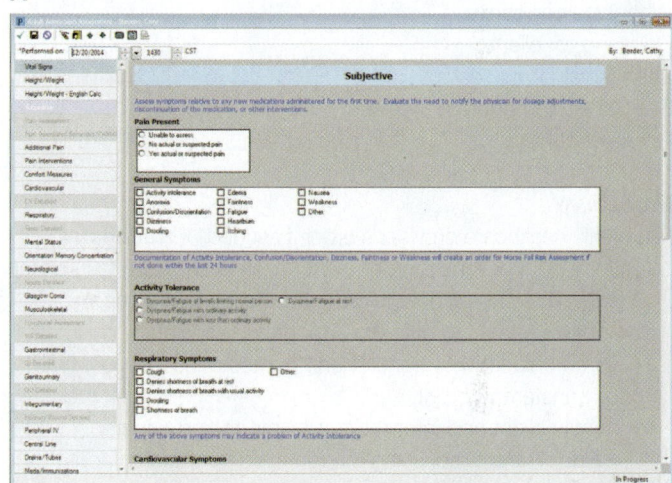

B

❶ **A.** Sample adult client history form. **B.** Sample adult admission assessment form. *Source:* From Cerner Electronic Health Record. © Cerner Corporation. Pearson has restricted permission to reproduce and distribute this copyrighted work. Further reproduction or distribution is strictly prohibited without written consent of Cerner Corporation.

14. Initiate client's care plan: Identify individual client's problem areas and needs.
15. Reassess client's level of **comfort** and ability to adapt to hospitalization.
16. Complete client teaching for all unfamiliar procedures or interventions.
17. Document information on appropriate forms in electronic medical record.

(continued)

Skill 5.1.1 | Admitting a Client *(continued)*

Box 5-3 OBTAINING A HEALTH HISTORY

- Past medical history or health problems, including those for which client was not hospitalized
- Signs and symptoms of current problems according to client's perceptions
- Client's knowledge of illness (understanding of present illness) and expectations of care
- Lifestyle patterns: diet, elimination pattern, exercise, habits (i.e., smoking, alcohol intake), sleep patterns
- Relationships and social support systems; emergency contacts

- Values, beliefs, religious or spiritual practices
- History of food, drug, device, or device materials allergies and nature of reaction
- Medications (prescribed and OTC) and supplemental products including dose, route, and frequency used
- Risk analysis for discharge (anticipated needs)
- Special database for older adult client: level of independence, ability to complete ADLs, side effects of medications, history of recent loss of loved one, and management of chronic conditions

Skill 5.1.2 | Transferring a Client

Equipment
Wheelchair or gurney
Covering for client
Client's valuables receipt
Special equipment (e.g., walker)
Personal belongings

Procedure
1. Verify healthcare provider's order if needed. ►*Rationale:* Healthcare providers order client transfers from and to hospital units. They do not always order transfers within a unit.
2. Contact admitting office to arrange for transfer.
3. Communicate with transfer unit to determine the best time for transferring client.
4. Identify client and inform client of impending transfer. ►*Rationale:* Discussing the rationale for transfer facilitates adjustment to the new unit.
5. Gather equipment and belongings.
6. Obtain necessary staff assistance for transfer.
7. Perform hand hygiene.
8. Transfer client to wheelchair or stretcher unless he or she is remaining in bed for the transfer. Use protective belts and rails as indicated. ❶
9. Cover client to provide warmth and to avoid exposure during transfer.
10. Notify receiving nurse when you arrive on the unit.
11. Introduce client to new staff who will be **caring** for the client that day.
12. Give complete report to staff, using the electronic medical record. Give information concerning client's current status, individualized care needs (e.g., bed alarm), client problems or alerts, and when next medications or treatments are due. Note any completed or pending test results. If necessary, give phone report to receiving nurse. ►*Rationale:* Complete "handoff" communication maintains continuity of care after transfer and promotes client safety.

❶ Clients may be admitted or transferred on a stretcher.

13. Notify healthcare provider when client's transfer is completed.
14. Enter transfer in the electronic medical record or initiate appropriate processes if using a paper-based documentation system.

CLINICAL ALERT
Healthcare facilities must accurately and completely record and pass along correct information about a client's medication and compare those to new medications given to him or her (NPSG.03.06.01).

Source: The Joint Commission (2014)

LEGAL CONSIDERATIONS

Misidentification of Clients Does Not Ordinarily Occur in Absence of Negligence

This client underwent an apparently uncomplicated hysterectomy. She was placed in Bed B of a semiprivate room to recover.

Several hours later, the client occupying Bed A in the same room was moved elsewhere in the facility, but hospital staff failed to note the move in its records. Two shifts of nurses also failed to note the move.

The next day, the nurses on the unit directed the orderly to the room to find the woman who had previously been in Bed A to transport her to the lab for an ultrasound.

The hysterectomy client in Bed B, who wore a traditional hospital ID bracelet and whose name was posted on her bed, protested that she had just come from surgery, had been instructed not to move without direction, and that she knew of no scheduled test. Nevertheless, the orderly persisted without checking the client's identity.

The client testified that she felt excruciating pain and nearly passed out, but the orderly proceeded to take her to the lab. The lab commenced the procedure, and after client complaints, finally determined her true identity and returned her to her room, but failed to notify the attending nurse of the mistake.

The client suffered an incisional dehiscence and hernia, necessitating further surgery. Based on evidence at trial, the jury found the hospital had a "lackadaisical attitude" toward client identification procedures, evincing a "reckless and wanton disregard of the rights of the client." Potentially, this would allow an award of punitive damages in excess of actual damages determined.

Source: Scribner v. Hillcrest Medical Center (1992)

Unit 5.1 Documentation and Evaluation

DOCUMENTATION for Admitting and Transferring

- Admission procedures/orientation provided
- Adaptation to hospitalization
- Client's health history and physical assessment including risk assessment
- Individualized care plan and progress toward goal achievement
- Client-signed documents added to the chart (e.g., advance directive)
- Inventory and dispensation of client's valuables and home medications
- Transfer time, destination, mode of transfer, transporter's name, and client's status
- Name of receiving unit's staff to whom report was given

EVALUATION/Critical Thinking

Expected Outcomes

- Client adapts to the hospital environment.
- Client participates in the individualized plan of care.
- Client understands rationale for and accepts transfer to a new care unit.
- Client is transferred to new unit without complication.

Unexpected Outcomes

- Client has difficulty adapting to the hospital environment.

Alternative Actions

- Assess physiologic, emotional, or cultural basis for difficulty.
- Consult case manager, interpreter, clergy, or other assistant to facilitate client's adaptation.

(continued)

Unexpected Outcomes	Alternative Actions
• Client appears depressed, refuses to participate in the plan of care.	• Understand client's values and beliefs and personal goals for care. • Consider referral to social work for evaluation. • Emphasize essentials of care and discharge planning as many feel the hospital is a place to die. • Allow client as much control over environment as possible.
• Client is anxious about transfer.	• Orient client to new setting and elicit client's perception of reason for transfer. • Correct misperceptions regarding transfer and continuity of care. • Explain that transfer decision is based on client's clinical progress and that new unit will be appropriate to provide client's current care needs.
• Upon transfer, client's personal belongings are lost.	• Check with transferring unit for retained items. • Check with security personnel for client's registered items. • File a variance report if belongings are not located.

Unit 5.2
Height and Weight

Nursing Process Data

ASSESSMENT Database

- Check the need for daily or weekly body weight measurements.
- Determine appropriate method for obtaining client's weight (standing scale, bed scale).
- Determine client's ability to stand for height measurement.
- Obtain previous height and weight measurements to compare with expected norms or to establish a base for identifying trends.

PLANNING Objectives

- To identify excess or deficit of fluid balance
- To establish baseline data to monitor response to drug therapy (e.g., diuretic)
- To determine weight-based drug dosages
- To determine nutritional status in relation to body requirements

IMPLEMENTATION Procedures

- **Skill 5.2.1** Measuring Height and Weight 98

DOCUMENTATION AND EVALUATION

Expected Outcomes

- Height and weight are obtained and recorded.
- Client's weight, depending on disease state and therapy, shows expected losses, gains, or stabilization.

Unexpected Outcomes/Alternative Actions

Pearson Nursing Student Resources

Find additional review materials at
nursing.pearsonhighered.com.
Prepare for success with NCLEX®-style practice questions and Skill Checklists.

Skill 5.2.1 | Measuring Height and Weight

Equipment

Balance beam scale (for clients who are able to stand without assistance)

Bed scale (for clients who are confined to bed or who are unable to stand) or

Bed scale (built into the bed)

Floor scale (for clients in wheelchairs) ❶

Paper towel

Preparation

1. Perform hand hygiene, introduce self, and verify client identification using two client identifiers.
2. Weigh client in the morning before breakfast. Ask client to void before weighing. ❷
3. Use the same scale each time you weigh the client.
   ➤ *Rationale:* For consistency in weight from day to day, keep variables the same as possible.
4. Make sure the client wears the same type of clothing (e.g., gown or robe) for each weighing.
5. If bed scale is used, account for weight of linens, etc.
   ➤ *Rationale:* Extraneous variables, such as linens, extra pillows, etc., result in inaccurate client measurements. ❸

6. Change wet gown or heavily saturated dressings before weighing the client.

❷ Weigh client in the morning, before eating or drinking, using the same scale each time.

❶ Scales accommodate wheelchairs for weighing clients.

❸ Bed scale is used to weigh clients who are on complete bed rest.

Source: Voisin/Phanie/Science Source

Note: See Chapter 8 for specialty beds that include scale capability.

Table 5-1 Body Mass Index

Measurement Units	Formula and Calculation
Kilograms and meters (or centimeters)	Formula: weight (kg) / [height (m)]^2 With the metric system, the formula for BMI is weight in kilograms divided by height in meters squared. Because height is commonly measured in centimeters, divide height in centimeters by 100 to obtain height in meters. Example: Weight = 68 kg, Height = 165 cm (1.65 m) Calculation: $68 \div (1.65)^2 = 24.98$
Pounds and inches	Formula: weight (lb) / [height (in)]^2 x 703 Calculate BMI by dividing weight in pounds (lbs) by height in inches (in) squared and multiplying by a conversion factor of 703. Example: Weight = 150 lbs, Height = 5'5" (65") Calculation: $[150 \div (65)^2]$ x 703 = 24.96

Body Mass Index Interpretation for Adults	
BMI	**Weight Status**
Below 18.5	Underweight
18.5 – 24.9	Normal or Healthy Weight
25.0 – 29.9	Overweight
30.0 and Above	Obese

Source: CDC (2015)

4 Instruct client to stand erect to measure height.

Procedure

1. Transport client to scale or bring scale to bedside.
2. Balance scale so that weight is accurate. (See Table 5-1 for a body mass index table.)
3. Place a clean paper towel on scale and ask client to remove shoes.
4. Assist client to stand on scale.
5. Move weights until the weight bar is level or balanced.
6. Record weight on appropriate record.
7. Ask client to face front so back is toward scale's balancing bar.
8. Instruct client to stand erect. **4**
9. Place L-shaped sliding height bar on top of client's head.
10. Read client's height as measured.
11. Record height on appropriate record. **5**
12. Discard paper towel (if used) and assist client back to room.
13. Perform hand hygiene.

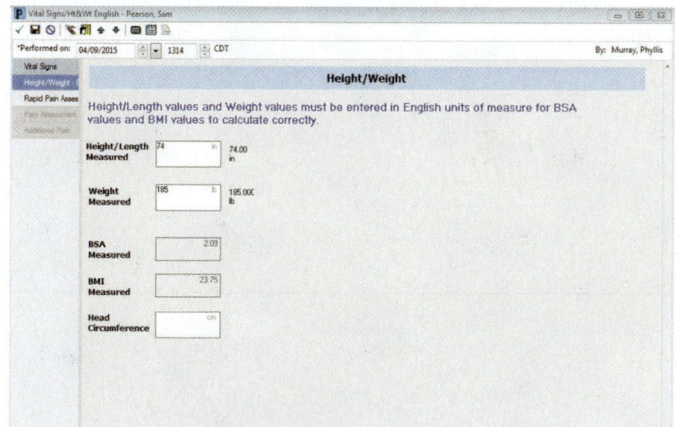

5 Document height and weight in appropriate chart.
Source: From Cerner Electronic Health Record. © Cerner Corporation. Pearson has restricted permission to reproduce and distribute this copyrighted work. Further reproduction or distribution is strictly prohibited without written consent of Cerner Corporation.

Unit 5.2 Documentation and Evaluation

DOCUMENTATION for Height and Weight

- Time of day height and weight were measured
- Client's height and weight measurement recorded on client's chart and Medication Administration Record (MAR)

- Type and identifying number of scale used for weighing
- Weight of any attached equipment, shoes, or clothing that adds to client's actual weight

EVALUATION/Critical Thinking

Expected Outcomes
- Height and weight are obtained and recorded.
- Client's weight shows expected losses, gains, or stabilization.

Unexpected Outcomes	Alternative Actions
• Client cannot be weighed accurately because of attached mechanical devices.	• Analyze unexpected weight loss or gain by assessing other factors, such as fluid intake and urinary output, presence of edema, lung sounds. • Remove attached device momentarily to obtain accurate weight.
• Client's weight varies more than expected from one day to the next.	• Check time of day weight was measured. • Check if same scale was used for both weighings. • For equipment reliability, check client's weight with another scale and compare findings. • Check what clothing or linen was on the client when weighed on both days. • Check MAR for medications that alter fluid balance (e.g., diuretics). • Check Intake & Output (I & O) record for sources of fluid loss or gain.

Nursing Process Data

ASSESSMENT Database

- Verify order for client's discharge.
- Identify discharge destination (home, rehabilitation unit, etc.).
- Assess client's feelings about discharge.
- Review care plan to determine client's progress toward goal achievement during hospitalization.
- Identify client's teaching needs for discharge and report findings to multidisciplinary team.
- Assess for any unaddressed need for healthcare assistance in the home.
- Determine that discharge needs have been addressed by case manager, dietitian, occupational or physical therapist, social worker, or members of the multidisciplinary team.
- Verify that client is ready for discharge.
- Try to determine reason for client's intent to leave the hospital AMA.

PLANNING Objectives

- To collaborate with the multidisciplinary team
- To prepare client for discharge and complete discharge planning
- To assist in the discharge of a client whose condition necessitates lifestyle changes or care at another facility
- To allow the client to verbalize feelings about discharge and to identify the client's strengths and needs

- To inform client of risks involved in leaving the hospital AMA

IMPLEMENTATION Procedures

DOCUMENTATION AND EVALUATION

Expected Outcomes

- Client understands discharge process and is not exhibiting anxiety.
- Client remains in the hospital until discharged by the healthcare provider.

Unexpected Outcomes/Alternative Actions

Pearson Nursing Student Resources

Find additional review materials at **nursing.pearsonhighered.com.**
Prepare for success with NCLEX®-style practice questions and Skill Checklists.

Skill 5.3.1 | Discharging a Client

Equipment

Client's record

Hospital Discharge Instructions form

Copy of discharge medication order list and any new healthcare provider's written prescription

Educational pamphlets/instructions

Telephone numbers and information regarding follow-up appointments or special referrals

Adaptive aids (e.g., walker, toilet seat extender) needed on discharge (may be dispensed by the hospital)

Client's home medications retained, hospital dispensed liquids, MDIs (metered dose inhalers), if continuation is prescribed

Materials for dressing changes (if indicated), antiembolic stockings, or any additional items previously dispensed for individual client use

Transport vehicle for discharge

Preparation

1. Determine that healthcare provider's discharge orders have been written.
2. Notify client's interdisciplinary team of discharge order.
3. Along with care team, determine that client is ready for discharge.
4. Ensure that all laboratory work, diagnostic test, treatments, and procedures are completed before discharge.
5. Determine that client understands instructions for self-care, including medications and follow-up arrangements.
6. Complete client teaching if applicable.
7. Notify client's caregiver to arrange transportation.
8. Obtain adaptive aids or other supplies that can be dispensed by the hospital (e.g., dressings, potty extender) or arrange for follow up with medical equipment supplier.
9. Provide opportunities for client to discuss impending discharge.

(continued)

Skill 5.3.1 | Discharging a Client *(continued)*

Procedure

1. Perform hand hygiene, introduce self, and verify client's identity using two client identifiers.
2. Review details of discharge with client (see Discharge Planning unit in Chapter 6).
3. At discharge, the client's list of medications received during hospitalization is reconciled by the healthcare provider and prescriptions are written or entered into the electronic system for new medications to be taken if indicated. The healthcare provider should document reasons for discontinuing or omitting certain medications upon discharge from the hospital, such as a beta blocker and aspirin for the post–myocardial infarction client.
4. Review any teaching and answer questions about medications, diet, bathing, any activity restrictions (e.g., lifting, sexual activity, driving), physical/wound care, use of special equipment or supplies, and follow-up appointments.
5. Explain how to recognize complications and what to do if they occur.
6. Print out discharge instruction from the electronic health record and other client education materials appropriate for the client's condition.
7. Have client sign Discharge Instructions form and provide the client with a copy per agency protocol.
8. Assist client to retrieve safeguarded valuables per hospital policy.
9. Terminate relationship with client. ➤ *Rationale:* Providing an opportunity for the client to express feelings and impressions contributes to a positive **termination**.

10. Follow hospital procedure for client discharge, including time and method of leaving hospital unit. ❶
11. Document time and method of client's discharge, destination, individual accompanying, and any supplies, prescriptions, and forms sent with client.
12. Notify appropriate departments of client's discharge.

❶ In many hospitals clients are discharged in a wheelchair for their safety.

Skill 5.3.2 | Discharging a Client Against Medical Advice (AMA)

Equipment
Client's record
Form for discharge AMA

Procedure

1. Immediately notify healthcare provider and nurse manager if client insists on leaving the hospital prematurely. ➤ *Rationale:* If the nurse judges that the client is endangered by leaving AMA, the healthcare provider should be notified immediately.
2. Ascertain why the client wants to leave the hospital prematurely and ask the client to wait until the healthcare provider arrives to meet the client. ➤ *Rationale:* It is important for the healthcare provider to determine the client's level of competence and capacity to understand the risks of leaving AMA.
3. If the healthcare provider is unavailable, explain reasons that continued hospital care is necessary (e.g., diagnosis, treatment).
4. If the healthcare provider is unavailable, explain risks of leaving hospital AMA (e.g., incomplete testing or treatment).

5. Request client to sign the AMA form if he or she still insists on leaving AMA. The nurse witnesses and cosigns the document.
6. Place signed AMA form in client's electronic health record per agency protocol and provide a copy to the client along with prescriptions, self-care, and follow-up instructions, etc. per agency protocols.
7. *If the client refuses to sign the AMA form,* write this on the form, have it witnessed, and notify appropriate hospital personnel. ➤ *Rationale:* This documents the conditions upon which the client left and indicates that the nursing staff explained the risks to the client.
8. Document client's verbatim statement in nurses' notes indicating reason for leaving.
9. Notify client's caregiver and hospital security if there is concern for the client's welfare or safety.
10. Notify appropriate people when the client leaves (healthcare provider, case manager, nursing supervisor, risk management personnel).

Unit 5.3 Documentation and Evaluation

DOCUMENTATION for Discharging a Client

- Discharge education plan including teaching and return demonstration and achievement of discharge goals
- Discharge instructions, discharge medications, and client teaching/instructions provided
- Discharge data (time, destination, how discharged, and accompanied by whom)
- Client's own medications, healthcare provider–written prescriptions, special equipment taken home by client

- Discharge criteria not met and reason criteria were not met as identified on client's care plan
- Client's signed Release from Responsibility for Discharge (AMA) form, instructions provided, name of individual accompanying client out of the hospital, and client's telephone number and address for follow-up call or visit by social worker
- Individuals notified of client's discharge AMA

EVALUATION/Critical Thinking

Expected Outcomes

- Client understands discharge process and is not exhibiting anxiety.
- Client remains in the hospital until discharged by the healthcare provider.

Unexpected Outcomes

- Client is anxious about discharge to an extended care unit.

Alternative Actions

- Reinforce healthcare provider/hospital's recommendation for extended care.
- Provide time for client and caregiver to recognize that the goal is to increase client's strength and independence.

- Client wants to leave the hospital AMA.

- Attempt to identify client's reasons for wanting to leave AMA.
- Notify client's healthcare provider.
- Consult hospital policy and procedures regarding AMA before releasing client.
- Negotiate possible alternative to leaving hospital (e.g., child care arrangements, employment concerns).
- Encourage discussion about risk of leaving/benefits of remaining hospitalized.
- Notify charge nurse, or supervisor, case manager and social worker, or clergy to discuss situation with client.
- In case of a minor or client with mental incompetency, contact hospital attorney ASAP.
- Have client sign hospital AMA form.
- If client will not sign AMA form, have another nurse witness refusal, and chart details of discharge.

Admission to Home Care

Nursing Process Data

ASSESSMENT Database

- Assess client's financial eligibility for home care service.
- Observe client's physical, emotional, and intellectual status.
- Observe client's ability to adapt to the home setting.
- Assess the client's level of comfort.
- Determine client's understanding of the health status and any limitations.
- Assess home condition and safety factors prior to client returning home.
- Examine equipment for safety features.
- Assess nurse's safety for making home visits.

PLANNING Objectives

- To assist client to adapt to home care with minimal distress
- To encourage client and family to participate in the plan of care
- To provide a comfortable and safe environment for the client
- To maximize client's outcomes after discharge from hospital
- To provide the necessary and appropriate home care treatment modalities
- To provide a safe environment for the nurse

IMPLEMENTATION Procedures

Note: See Chapter 7 for Adaptation to Home Care.

DOCUMENTATION AND EVALUATION

Expected Outcomes

- Client adapts to home setting with minimal difficulties.
- Client and family participate in the plan of care.
- Safe environment is provided for client.
- Nurse's safety is maintained during home visits.

Unexpected Outcomes/Alternative Actions

Pearson Nursing Student Resources

Find additional review materials at
nursing.pearsonhighered.com.
Prepare for success with NCLEX®-style practice questions and Skill Checklists.

Skill 5.4.1 | Nurse's Role in Home Care

Equipment
Discharge Planning Records
OASIS C Forms
H485 Forms
Consent Forms
Agency Forms

Preparation
1. Obtain appropriate documents from healthcare facility.
   a. History and physical examination
   b. Diagnosis
   c. Treatments
   d. Medications
   e. Subjective and objective discharge notes
   f. Physical or occupational therapy during home care
   g. Hospital follow-up care appointments
   h. Caregiver status (i.e., family member or home health)
2. Obtain all OASIS C documents to be completed during initial visit.
3. Contact discharge planner at facility to determine date, time of discharge, method of transfer to home, and availability of health caregiver when client reaches home.
4. Contact client, health caregiver, or family to arrange time for initial visit (Box 5-4 ■).

Procedure
1. Introduce self to client, family, and health caregiver.
2. Describe services that will be provided, including time frames and use of ancillary personnel, including role of each member of the health team.
3. Assess home for safety issues (see Chapter 7).
4. Determine client's eligibility for services.

5. Complete OASIS C forms and CMS-485 forms, in addition to relevant forms based on assessment (pressure ulcer forms, mental status, sensory status, etc.). Develop **client care plan**.
6. Review client's or caregiver's responsibility for care during absence of agency staff.
7. Provide telephone numbers for agency, emergency services, and, if appropriate, the RN (will vary among agencies).
8. Review medication names, doses, and time of administration and side effects that should be reported to the healthcare provider.
9. Review and have client or caregiver demonstrate any treatments that will be completed when agency personnel are not in home.
10. Develop a nurses' worksheet and care plan to be reviewed each visit. ➤ *Rationale:* To ensure all activities have been completed and documented.

Note: Worksheet to include assessment findings, flow sheets (ADLs, pain assessment, medications, etc.), vital signs, education provided, IVs. Care plan update.

Box 5-4 GUIDELINES FOR GIVING HOME CARE

- Take as little with you into the home as possible.
- Use appropriate nursing protocols in home setting.
- Perform hand hygiene on entering and leaving home.
- Maintain clean technique in the home.
- Know CDC infection control guidelines.
- Review state and federal guidelines and protocol for reimbursement.

Skill 5.4.2 | Identifying Eligibility for Medicare Reimbursement

Procedure
1. Complete OASIS C forms.
   a. Integrate information with CMS-485 data.
   b. Complete all sections of document. ➤ *Rationale:* Denial of service can result if documentation incomplete.
   c. Complete forms within required time frame.
   d. Ensure information from forms is transcribed accurately onto CMS-485 forms. ➤ *Rationale:* To prevent denial of service
2. Check required criteria for Medicare coverage eligibility.
   ➤ *Rationale:* This prevents administering care for which reimbursement will not be received.

3. Identify client as homebound.
   a. Client's condition severely restricts leaving the home.
   b. Leaving the home requires considerable effort and assistance of another individual.
   c. Special transportation is necessary.
   d. Absences from the home are infrequent and short.
4. Check that home service is considered skilled. To be skilled, service must be under the supervision of a registered nurse or a physical therapist.
5. Provide supplemental services from home health aide, social worker, or occupational therapist; care is reimbursed

(continued)

Skill 5.4.2 | Identifying Eligibility for Medicare Reimbursement *(continued)*

by Medicare only when one of the three skilled services is required.

6. Provide care that is part-time and intermittent.

7. Check that plan of treatment is authorized by healthcare provider and recertified every 60 days.

   a. Centers for Medicare and Medicaid Services form (CMS-485) is standardized for plan of treatment. This form is used by all home health agencies for Medicare clients.

8. Assess that care is medically reasonable and necessary.

   a. Entire plan of care must correlate with client's medical problems and client's clinical status.

b. Each service's goals (client outcomes) must be clearly stated and realistic for the client.

> **CLINICAL ALERT**
>
> The Outcome and Assessment Information Set (OASIS-B1) and the Discharge Form in the OASIS paperwork is more extensive than previously gathered information on documentation forms. Be careful to complete all sections of the form.

Skill 5.4.3 | Completing Admission Documentation

Procedure

1. Complete all sections of the OASIS C document.

   a. Demographic data: address, referring healthcare provider, payment source, etc.

   b. Present history

   c. Present illness

   d. Living arrangements

   e. Supportive assistance

   f. Physical assessment/review of systems

   g. ADLs

   h. Medications

   i. Equipment management

   j. Homebound status

   k. Therapy modalities required

   l. Unmet needs

   m. Lack of Knowledge section

   n. Treatment/procedures performed

   o. Response to teaching/training performed

   p. Client rights and responsibilities

   q. Coordination of client services

   r. Discharge planning

2. Signed consent forms

   a. IV therapy

   b. Consent for treatment

   c. Consent for service

3. Signed HIPAA form

4. Signed Advance Directive document

5. Signed Patient's Rights document

6. Billing Database

7. Discipline Specific Evaluation, if therapy was instituted

8. Plan of Care

9. CMS-485 Worksheet

10. Aide Assignment and Duties, if appropriate

11. Healthcare provider Plan of Care

12. Home Health Plan of Care

13. Nurses' Notes as necessary

14. Identify if prehospital "Do Not Resuscitate" form has been signed.

Skill 5.4.4 | Maintaining Nurse's Safety

Procedure

1. Evaluate safety of nurse before the visit.

   a. Call the client before the visit to determine convenient time.

   b. Confirm directions to home.

   c. Determine whether household pets are present; if so, ask that they be secured during visit.

   d. Check neighborhood to determine need for assistance from police to make home visit.

2. Wear identifying name badge. Most agencies request that the nurse wear a lab coat.

3. Wear flat shoes to allow you to walk quickly or to run if necessary.

4. Maintain personal safety while traveling in the car.

   a. Keep car in good working order and stocked with necessary equipment.

   b. Keep gas tank at least half full at all times.

   c. Obtain automobile club membership for emergency use. ➤ *Rationale:* Membership allows the nurse to call for assistance with car problems.

   d. Keep a windshield cover with CALL POLICE sign available. ➤ *Rationale:* The sign will alert neighbors that you need immediate assistance.

   e. Have cell phone available and charged at all times, and keep a car charger in the car.

f. Keep blanket in car. ➤ *Rationale:* A blanket will keep you warm in the winter if you need to wait for assistance.

g. Keep a bottle of water in the car at all times.
   ➤ *Rationale:* Water is protective if you need to wait for assistance in hot weather.

h. Keep doors locked and windows up at all times.

i. Park in full view of neighbors, preferably directly in front of home.

j. Lock all personal items in the car trunk before leaving home or office.

k. Keep all equipment in the car trunk.

l. Restock the nurses' bag before the visits for the day. Keep nurses' bag on front seat.

m. Place all valuable objects out of direct sight in car (i.e., laptop computers, phone). Place these under the seat if possible. ➤ *Rationale:* Keeping valuables out of sight helps to prevent car break-in and theft.

5. Maintain personal safety while walking on the street.

   a. Keep one arm and hand free when walking from car to house.

   b. Walk directly to client's residence.

   c. When approaching a group of strangers, cross the street or walkway, if appropriate.

   d. When leaving a residence, keep keys in your hand with the pointed end of the key facing outward. ➤ *Rationale:* The keys can be used as a weapon if necessary.

   e. Carry a chemical spray and whistle within easy reach.

CLINICAL ALERT

If your safety is in jeopardy, use one of the following defensive strategies: Scream or yell *FIRE* or *STRANGER*. Kick the individual in the shin or groin. Bite or scratch the individual. Use chemical spray or blow a whistle. If you feel your personal safety is in question, do not make a visit or stay in the residence.

6. Maintain personal safety when making home visit.

   a. Use common walkways or hallways. Do not park behind a building or in a dark area.

   b. Knock on the door and wait for permission to enter.

   c. Keep a clear pathway to the door if the situation is potentially unsafe.

   d. Observe home environment for safety hazards (i.e., weapons).

   e. Make a joint visit with another agency staff member or ask for an escort if there is a potentially unsafe situation.

   f. Call for police support if the visit is essential and the situation is unsafe. ➤ *Rationale:* There may be times when a visit is essential, but it is unsafe for one individual to make a visit.

   g. Make a visit in the morning when good visual support exists if neighborhood is unsafe.

   h. Close the case if the nurse feels the situation is unsafe and there are no alternative actions that can guarantee nurse's safety.

Skill 5.4.5 | Assessing for Elder Abuse

Procedure

1. Assess client for indications of neglect: failure to provide adequate food, clothing, medical assistance, or assistance with ADLs. Check body for signs of cleanliness. Determine whether emotional abuse is present. Ask about threats, intimidation, or isolation (Box 5-5 ■).

2. Identify whether financial abuse has occurred, such as misuse of finances or property.

3. Assess for signs of physical abuse: signs of restraining; hitting, biting, burning; black and blue marks on trunk, abdomen, buttocks, upper thighs; scars; and abrasions. Bilateral bruises or parallel injuries may indicate forceful restraining; shaking may cause parallel injuries of upper arms. Accidental injuries affect knees, back of hands, forehead, and elbows.

4. Assess for signs of malnourishment or dehydration.

5. Check skin for pressure ulcers.

6. Assess for signs of sprains or dislocations from pulling or pushing the client.

7. Ask about visits to the hospital ER. Ask why client sought medical care, and how much time elapsed between injury and visit to ER.

8. Assess for signs of emotional abuse. Observe if client is fearful of strangers, becomes quiet when caregiver enters room, and craves attention and socialization.

Box 5-5 **QUESTIONS TO ASK IF ABUSE IS SUSPECTED**

- Who cares for you at home?
- Did someone hurt you?
- Are you happy with where you live?
- Tell me about your daily routine.
- Who assists you with ADLs?
- Do you feel safe living here?
- Who manages your money?
- How did the injury (or bruises) occur?
- Did you receive medical attention?
- Has this type of injury happened before?

Unit 5.4 Documentation and Evaluation

DOCUMENTATION for Admission to Home Care

- All required forms (i.e., OASIS C, CMS-485, agency-specific forms) complete
- Safety issues occurring within house
- Mental status of client and ability to care for self
- Teaching activities for client or caregiver
- Nursing care plan update
- Medication side effects and referral to healthcare provider
- Changes in client status
- Notification of healthcare provider

EVALUATION/Critical Thinking

Expected Outcomes
- Client is acclimated to home environment and is able to provide care after a period of support from agency staff.
- Safe environment provides for client safety in home.
- Nurse's safety is maintained during home visit.

Unexpected Outcomes	Alternative Actions
• Client is noncompliant with treatments, safety procedures, and taking medications at home.	• Explain rationale for following home care plan. • Discuss reason with client, caregiver, and family members to determine whether change in plan would increase compliance. • Remind client that if he or she refuses to follow plan, he or she will be taken off services. • Document appropriately on all forms indicating noncompliance issues. • Notify healthcare provider.
• Client is in an abusive environment.	• Assess for signs of elder abuse or neglect. • Notify healthcare provider. • Take appropriate steps according to agency protocol. • Make a joint visit with another agency staff member. • Call for police support if the visit is essential. • Make the visit during the safest time of the day.

Chapter Wrap-Up

GERONTOLOGIC Considerations

U.S. Demographics Affect Hospital Admissions

- The average life expectancy has increased.
- The number of older adults will double by 2020.
- Healthcare services are used by older adults more than any other age group.
- Three of four older adults die of heart disease, cancer, or stroke.

Older Adult Clients Admitted to the Hospital Require Special Consideration

- Fatigue and pain may be pronounced; admission procedures may need to be altered.
- Repeated orientation may be indicated due to short-term memory deficit, confusion, or sensory impairment.
- Special problems associated with age must be anticipated and nursing care planned appropriately (e.g., risk for falls).

MANAGEMENT Guidelines

Each state legislates a Nurse Practice Act for RNs and LVN/LPNs. Healthcare facilities are responsible for establishing and implementing policies and procedures that conform to their state's regulations. Verify the regulations and role parameters for each healthcare worker in your facility.

Delegation

- Delegation for the admission of a new client may be divided into three task areas:
  1. An unlicensed assistive personnel (UAP) may assist the client into bed, place client's personal items in a designated area, describe the room environment including the use of telephone, television, and nurse summon controls, visiting hours, mealtimes, and other hospital routines. The UAP may also take vital signs and obtain height and weight measurements.
  2. The LVN/LPN may complete a health history form, obtain admission data required by the hospital, witness consent forms, and complete the same tasks identified above.
  3. The RN is responsible for the complete health history and reviewing the data obtained by other healthcare workers, initiating the client care plan (nursing diagnosis, goals, and interventions), and beginning the discharge plan in collaboration with the healthcare team.
- An LVN/LPN may complete discharge teaching following the established discharge teaching plan.

- Escorting a client out of the hospital can be delegated to a **volunteer**, UAP, or LVN/LPN. Many facilities have escort services that utilize volunteers.

Interprofessional Communication

- Clients being admitted to the hospital are usually frightened and unsure of the events that will take place. It is important to communicate their needs to and collaborate with all staff members involved in the client's care. This will provide a team approach for comprehensive care.
- A complete report on the newly admitted client must be given to all team members. If an LVN/LPN or UAP assisted in the admission process, he or she must provide immediate feedback to the RN manager regarding their findings.
- A client care plan must be established within a designated time frame. The time is determined by the facility in accordance with The Joint Commission guidelines.
- "Handoff" shift report must contain a brief history: reason for admission, overview of the client's assessment, current status, and any special needs. Diet, specific treatments, procedures, test results or those pending, and any alerts (e.g., DNAR, isolation) should be included. The handoff process (including audiotaped reports) must allow opportunity for asking and receiving answers to questions relevant to safe client care.

CASE STUDY Applications

Scenario 1

Mr. Moore has been told by his cardiologist that his coronary arteriogram indicates he has three-vessel disease and he is a candidate for coronary artery bypass surgery. The surgery is scheduled and Mr. Moore is welcomed at the facility's preadmission testing unit one week before admission for preliminary blood work and preoperative instructions. At this time he receives information about his expected clinical course, which includes a multidisciplinary plan of care.

1. What is the advantage of providing the client with information this far in advance of surgery?
2. What is included in the plan of care?
3. Who participates in the development of the plan of care?
4. How does the plan of care facilitate the client's admission, transfer, and discharge processes? Are there drawbacks?

Scenario 2

Marilyn James, age 45, has been admitted to the hospital for corrective back surgery for a herniated disc. She was expected to be discharged the next day. During surgery, she experienced a complication (dural tear) and is required to be on bed rest for an extended period of time, delaying her discharge by several days.

After hearing the news, she says she is going to leave the hospital AMA. She "wasn't prepared for prolonged hospitalization" and has to go home to care for her 3-year-old granddaughter and elderly mother who live with her.

1. What right does a client have to leave the agency prematurely, AMA?
2. What should the nurse's initial response to this client be?
3. How can the nurse advocate for this client?
4. What are the usual procedures involved in discharging a client AMA?
5. How is this process documented in the client's record?

NCLEX® Review Questions

Unless otherwise specified, choose only one (1) answer.

1. Who makes DNR decisions?
   A. Client's family
   B. Advance directive counselor
   C. Client
   D. Client's healthcare provider

2. Who is responsible for inquiring if the client has an advance directive?
   A. The hospital chaplain
   B. The admitting nurse
   C. The hospital attorney
   D. The client's healthcare provider

3. During the admission process, when does the client receive an identification band?
   A. Upon arrival to the area where care is initially received
   B. Upon arriving on the nursing unit
   C. After the initial assessment has been completed
   D. Upon receipt of admitting healthcare provider's orders

4. What essential information must the identification band contain besides the client's name?
   Select all that apply.
   A. Client's room number
   B. Admitting healthcare provider's name
   C. Client's date of birth

D. Client's medical record number
E. Name of the hospital

5. During the admission process, the client is oriented to the hospital unit, including use of various control systems. What is the purpose of this orientation?
   A. To save time for the nursing staff
   B. To provide client control over the environment
   C. To release the hospital from liability in case the client falls
   D. To prevent the client's abuse of expensive equipment

6. What information should be included in the client's orientation to the hospital environment?
   Select all that apply.
   A. Mealtimes
   B. Use of emergency call system
   C. Visiting hours
   D. Use of nurse call system
   E. Healthcare provider visit times

7. Personal safety is important when visiting a client's home. What precautions should the home care nurse take?
   Select all that apply.
   A. Wear a name badge.
   B. Carry a cell phone at all times.
   C. Park in front of the home.
   D. Keep valuables locked in the trunk of the car.
   E. Restock supplies between each visit.

8. What elements are used to calculate the client's body mass index (BMI)?
   A. Height and waist measurement
   B. Age and weight
   C. Height and weight
   D. Gender and waist measurement

9. Which of the following activities can be delegated to the UAP during discharge?
   A. Teaching the client about discharge medication
   B. Assessing if the client met discharge goals
   C. Escorting the client off the unit
   D. Teaching a client what complications to look for

10. When a client intends to leave the hospital prematurely, against medical advice, what should the nurse do first?
    A. Have the client sign the hospital AMA form.
    B. Try to identify the reasons why the client wants to leave AMA.
    C. Notify the client's healthcare provider.
    D. Inform the client about risks of leaving AMA.

QSEN Activity

Domain: Teamwork and Collaboration

KSA: Follow communication practices that minimize risks associated with handoffs among providers and across transitions in care.

Activity:

You are a nurse working on a unit that routinely transfers clients to other units in your hospital. You are concerned about making sure that the receiving units have all the information they need to provide excellent care to your clients. You remember reading about the SHARE process for ensuring a smooth handoff process. Create a checklist that includes elements of SHARE for the staff to use when transferring clients to other units.

Bibliography

Alfandre, D. (2013, Dec.). Reconsidering against medical advice discharges: Embracing patient-centeredness to promote high quality care and a renewed research agenda. *Journal of General Internal Medicine, 28* (12), 1657–1662.

American Nurses Association (ANA) and the National Council of State Boards of Nursing (NCSBN). (n.d.). *Joint statement on delegation.* Retrieved from https://www.ncsbn.org/Delegation_joint_statement_NCSBN-ANA.pdf

Blouin, A. S. (2011, Apr.–Jun.). Improving hand-off communications: New solutions for nurses. *Journal of Nursing Care Quality, 26* (2), 97–100.

Centers for Disease Control. (2015). *Assessing Your Weight.* Retrieved from http://www.cdc.gov/healthyweight/assessing/bmi/adult_bmi/index.html

Devitt, P. J., Devitt, A. C., & Dewan, M. (2000, Jul.). An examination of whether discharging patients against medical advice protects physicians from malpractice charges. *Psychiatric Services, 51*(7), 899–902.

Institute of Medicine. (2011, Dec.). *Clinical preventive services for women: Closing the gaps.* Retrieved from http://www.iom.edu/Reports/2011/Clinical-Preventive-Services-for-Women-Closing-the-Gaps.aspx

Levy, F., Mareiniss, D. P., & Iacovelli, C. (2012, Sep.). The importance of a proper against-medical-advice (AMA) discharge: How signing out AMA may create significant liability protection for providers. *The Journal of Emergency Medicine, 43* (3), 516–520.

NHLBI Obesity Education Initiative Expert Panel on the Identification, Evaluation, and Treatment of Obesity in Adults (US). (1998, Sep.). *Clinical Guidelines on the Identification, Evaluation, and Treatment of Overweight and Obesity in Adults: The Evidence Report.* Bethesda, MD: National Heart, Lung, and Blood Institute. Available from: http://www.ncbi.nlm.nih.gov/books/NBK2003/

The Joint Commission. (2010). *Advancing effective communication, cultural competence, and patient- and family-centered care: A roadmap for hospitals.* Oakbrook Terrace, IL: Author.

The Joint Commission. (2014). *The Joint Commission National Patient Safety Goals.* Retrieved from http://www.jointcommission.org/standards_information/npsgs.aspx

U.S. Preventive Services Task Force. (2013). *Intimate partner violence and abuse of elderly and vulnerable adults: Screening.* Retrieved from http://www.uspreventiveservicestaskforce.org/uspstf12/ipvelder/ipvelderart.pdf

Chapter 6
Client Education and Discharge Planning

 Learning Objectives

6.1 Describe the purpose of client and family education.

6.2 Describe the challenges to providing client education.

6.3 Discuss the application of Adult Learning Principles (Knowles) to client education.

6.4 Outline the process of collecting client data to determine learning needs.

6.5 Explain the application of the nursing process to client education.

6.6 Discuss the meaning of the term *discharge planning*.

6.7 List two factors to consider when determining an appropriate teaching strategy.

6.8 List and describe specific teaching strategies appropriate for clients and families.

6.9 Define cultural competence.

6.10 Identify assessments to determine readiness to learn.

6.11 Identify one strategy to determine readability level of written material.

6.12 Describe how to develop an evaluation tool.

6.13 List three risk factors that require discharge planning.

6.14 Identify the steps necessary to complete a discharge summary.

6.15 Describe documents required to accompany client to home.

6.16 Identify appropriate referral for Home Health Team.

Chapter Outline

Terminology

Assessment the first step in identifying client's knowledge base; it is used to set meaningful learning goals and strategies.

Client education the process of influencing behavior and teaching the client self-care techniques so that he or she can resume responsibility for certain aspects of health care following discharge from the health facility.

Compliance follow-through on advice and direction by medical personnel to promote wellness and rehabilitation.

Comprehensive health care a total system of health care that takes the whole individual into account.

Counseling giving support or providing guidance.

Culture characteristic patterns of attitudes, values, beliefs, and behaviors shared by members of a society or population. Cultural attitudes can affect a client's receptivity to an educational process and willingness to accept information and incorporate it into his or her lifestyle.

Cultural competence a set of congruent behaviors, attitudes, and policies that enables nurses and other healthcare workers to work effectively in a cross-cultural situation.

Discharge to release from care; done by a physician, nurse, or medical care facility.

Discharge planning systematic process of planning for client care following discharge; includes client needs, goals of care, and strategies for implementation.

Evaluation tool a test, questionnaire, or direct observation that evaluates the effectiveness of the teaching.

Learning the process of conceptual change, within the framework of the client's perceptions, that leads to modifications in behavior.

Maladaptive unable to change to adjust to circumstances.

Readiness to learn a component of the learning process; referring to the psychological state of being open and accepting of new information and the learning process.

Relationship an interaction of individuals over time.

Resistance inability to listen and participate in discussion of health behavioral changes.

Support to lend strength or give assistance to.

Therapeutic having medicinal or healing properties; a healing agent.

Transfer to convey or shift from one individual or place to another.

Transitional care the process of facilitating the transition or move between hospital and home to maintain continuity of health care.

Understanding to perceive and comprehend the nature and significance of; to know.

Validate to substantiate or verify.

Client Education

In current health care, **client education** is a client's right and a healthcare provider's responsibility. The goal of client education has changed from telling the client the best actions to take, to now assisting clients in **learning** about their health care to improve their own health. The U.S. government efforts regarding health and client education are outlined in the *Healthy People* initiatives.

The current initiative (2010) outlines the participation in health promotion and disease prevention through exercising, appreciating better health and fitness, avoiding workplace injuries, immunizing children against disease, and participating in preventive screening programs. *Healthy People 2020* expands the goals for health promotion and client teaching and learning by incorporating specific health objectives for various races and ethnicities. It also expands the definition of the concept of health equality in relation to health risks caused by various genetic differences and predispositions to diseases or disorders.

Historically, client education has been one of the most important responsibilities of the professional nurse. With advances in medical science and an increasing number of clients with progressive chronic illness, the role of client education can directly affect the client's health, adaptation to illness, and recovery. While a number of healthcare consumers are more informed and active in making healthcare decisions, there still remain those who lack "health literacy," or lack the ability to read, comprehend, and act on medical information. These factors contribute to the increasingly difficult task of providing appropriate and comprehensive client education (Box 6-1 ■). In addition, the influx of clients from various diverse **cultures**, different languages, availability of educational materials written at appropriate readability levels and/or languages, lack of time, and shorter hospital stays present challenges for nursing.

Box 6-1 CHALLENGES TO PROVIDING CLIENT EDUCATION

- Various cultures
- Various languages
- Lack of time
- Lack of reimbursement
- Lack of appropriate readable materials
- Lack of literacy-appropriate materials
- Lack of training in providing client education or in the development of materials

---

The purpose of client and family education is for them to gain knowledge, skills, and behavior changes necessary to meet the client's healthcare needs. Client education should be individualized, specific, and understandable. Clients have a right to know about their illness, medications, and any procedures being performed. Client education is an expected standard for nursing practice.

Two important principles for providing client education are simplicity and reinforcement. *Simplicity* refers to the content being presented to the client in a readily understandable format. Health information can be very difficult to understand. It is best to start the teaching by first assessing what the client knows. Never assume the client needs to be taught everything about the topic. It is not necessary to over-teach the information. It is best to identify the most important information the client needs to know at the time. If possible, the topic should be covered from the simpler concept to the more complex. *Reinforcement* is review of the content and should be done at the end of a session or at the start of the next teaching session. When the client understands the concepts, you can proceed to the next concepts.

The Joint Commission has mandated that client and family education be part of comprehensive care and devised Patient and Family Education (PFE) standards for accredited agencies.

The Joint Commission (2014) set the following goals for client and family teaching:

- Education that supports client and family participation in care decisions and processes
- Educational needs assessed and recorded in the client's record
- Assessment of client and family's ability and willingness to learn
- Education methods that respect client and family's values and preferences and allow enough interaction for learning to occur
- Collaboration among health professionals to provide education

The Joint Commission reviews for evidence of three major processes involved in client education: the hospital's internal focus on education, direct education of the client and family, and evaluation of how well the education program achieves the identified goals. The Joint Commission stresses the need for a multidisciplinary approach to planning and implementing client education. Nurses are the principal providers of care and have legal responsibility for client education, as outlined in each state's Nurse Practice Act and emphasized in documents published by the American Nurses Association and many specialty associations. As such, nurses usually provide the leadership role in directing the educational plan for the client and family. Nurses provide the communication link between the multidisciplinary team members to ensure the client's goals are met in a timely manner.

The cultural beliefs and practices of the client have a major influence on healthcare behaviors, beliefs, and willingness to learn. Client education must be sensitive to these beliefs. For example, if teaching a Chinese client with diabetes, the nurse must consider the food the client likes to eat, as well as the social values. Eating is not merely for nutrients, but is also a gesture of politeness and social interaction. It is important that nurses gain an awareness of the various cultures in order to provide *culturally competent* care.

The goal of client and family education is to promote optimal client health. To achieve this goal, clients and families must learn in a way that is meaningful and acceptable to their concept of self and in **relationship** to the illness. Thus learning is a process of conceptual change within the framework of the client's perceptions that leads to behavioral change.

To be effective and facilitate the teaching/learning process, the nurse must utilize excellent listening and communication skills to establish rapport (Box 6-2 ■). Determining learning needs, preferred learning style, and learning readiness are all requirements included in the The Joint Commission's Standards for Patient & Family Education. Once a client has received a new diagnosis or new information about his or her condition, the nurse must assess three areas: (1) what they already know, (2) what they need to know, and (3) how best to assist with learning. Clients need to be able to identify and understand what the illness is, effects of the treatment, whether it is acute or chronic, and short- and long-term care needs and outcomes. Discussing possible outcomes of the illness will help the client accept the condition, be open for new ideas or teaching, and be motivated to learn and make appropriate health behavior changes. The client must recognize any gaps in knowledge

---

Box 6-2 TIPS TO FACILITATE CLIENT-FOCUSED EDUCATION

- Get to know the client, his or her knowledge level, perception, current practices, and preferences.
- Determine client's goals and **readiness to learn**, and individualize ways to achieve goals.
- Take into account client's goals, learning style, special skills, cultural beliefs, and developmental level.
- Utilize simple language and interact at client's level with empathy and concern.
- Utilize a variety of materials and methods that encourage active learning and participation.
- Plan for right time and right place to maximize client and family learning.
- Follow up at another time to clarify information and reassess learning.

---

and misconceptions and then assimilate new information for possible actions. When the client and family assist in goal setting and the information is presented based on their preferences, learning becomes more meaningful. Increased client and family involvement in health care represents an important part of quality improvement in all healthcare organizations. Clients' participation in healthcare **assessment** and education has been associated with better health outcomes.

The client education plan is a component of the total nursing care plan, which is part of the nursing process. Thus the same principles of the nursing process apply to client education: assess the learning needs, and plan appropriate teaching, implementation, and evaluation. Client education, when viewed as a process rather than the simple action of imparting information, helps the client to actively participate in his or her health plan for wellness. Individualized to the specific client needs and included as part of a total care plan, client education contributes to continuity of care following **discharge**. In addition to the actual teaching, effective educational materials will assist the client in **understanding** medical complexities, thus reducing anxiety and increasing **compliance** with instructions. Client education resources have the ability to change communication into actions and to improve health.

Principles of Client Education

Malcolm Knowles (1970), author of a seminal work called *The Modern Practice of Adult Education*, discusses strategies for adult learning. He suggests that adult learning and readiness to learn are influenced by developmental tasks. Knowles formulated the still-current "Adult Learning Principles," which include the following:

- Adults learn best when there is a perceived need. In order for learning to occur, the client must understand why they need to know about a subject. Therefore, the nurse must ensure that the client understands the underlying health issue that is to be prevented or the illness that is to be resolved before teaching.
- Teaching plan is considered a part of client care plan.
- Teaching of adults should progress from the known to the unknown. Assess what they already know; do not reteach the things they already know.

- Teaching of adults should progress from the simpler concepts to more complex topics.
- Adults learn best using active participation. Asking the client to restate what has been discussed will encourage learning and provide for clarification.
- Adults require opportunities to practice new skills. When acquiring new manual skills, such as drawing up or injecting insulin, it is essential that the client be allowed to practice the skill. It is important to observe a return demonstration in order to evaluate the effectiveness of the teaching.
- Adults need behavior reinforced. An example of reinforcing behavior would be to allow the client to draw up and give his or her insulin each time it is required.
- Immediate feedback and correction of misconceptions increase learning.

Similar to Knowles's principles of adult learning, simplicity and reinforcement are essential in providing client education. An understanding of these principles is essential for individuals who teach adults in the healthcare setting.

Resistance to Change   Most nurses recognize that the client may resist learning and cannot be forced to learn; the nurse can only assist the client, encourage him or her, and facilitate learning. To master information, the client must have internalized some form of motivation to learn; for example, the client realizes that to control diabetes adequately and feel better, he or she must understand the relationship of insulin and food to body needs.

Many clients appear to resist change, even when changing would result in a positive outcome. When this occurs, the process of learning is blocked. As a nurse educator, you are functioning as an agent of change, and dealing with **resistance** to change is a necessary task (Table 6-1 ■). There are several reasons underlying resistance; one of the most common is that change is frightening, even when an individual consciously wishes to alter his or her behavior. If an individual perceives change as a possible threat, he or she may resist. Another cause of resistance is inaccurately perceiving the reason for or effect of change. Other sources of resistance include psychological inflexibility, cultural practices, inability to tolerate change, and not believing that change will have a positive effect.

Table 6-1 Strategies for Dealing with Barriers to Change

Barriers to Change	Nursing Approaches
Perceived threat or fear of change	Identify specific fears or threats and impart accurate information that may reduce fears. Focus on the positive outcome of change.
Inaccurate perceptions of effect of change	Clarify client perceptions. Impart accurate information, and discuss results of behavior change.
Disagreement that change is positive	Work to agree on mutual goals and demonstrate positive outcomes so client views change as positive rather than negative.
Psychological resistance or perceived loss of freedoms or behaviors	Focus on discussion of client's perceived loss of freedom and demonstrate willingness to alter plan or adapt to client's needs.
Inability to tolerate change	Recognize that low tolerance is often caused by fear—allaying fear through developing trust, being supportive when client attempts to change, and giving positive feedback decreases fear of change.

The nurse is both an educator and an agent of change. If the client resists change (the teaching process), the nurse may better accomplish the goals of client education by identifying the reason for that resistance and altering the teaching approach accordingly.

Client education is more than imparting information to a client; it is the process of influencing behavior. As such, it needs to be directed toward the client's thinking to facilitate meaningful behavioral changes. When goals are mutually agreed on and clearly stated, the learner understands what is expected, the nurse understands his or her role and can evaluate it, and the results can more easily be measured. Because of the need to control costs and the current practice of discharging clients earlier, a more extensive teaching plan must be developed and implemented.

Readiness to Learn   Assessing the client's readiness to learn is an essential component of client education. Readiness to learn can be limited by physical and psychosocial demands caused by illness, such as pain and fatigue. For many clients, the postacute or recovery phase and desire to return to normalcy act as an incentive to learning.

Methods of Teaching   The methods of client teaching may include:

- One-to-one education: most common methodology used in hospitals, clinics, and physician offices
- Group teaching: most often utilizes videotapes or similar technology, such as CDs or DVDs
- Computer-aided instruction: used in clinics, hospitals, and physician offices or for client to learn at home
- Internet: can increase the client's understanding of symptoms, conditions, and treatments—key to Internet use is choosing appropriate health websites

Regardless of the methodology chosen, selection of educational materials and resources should be appropriate for age, developmental level, cognitive level, culture, and language.

Discharge Planning

Recent changes in healthcare delivery systems, as an attempt to contain rapidly rising costs, have altered client care. The number of hospital days for clients in acute care hospitals has decreased, with the average hospital stay now being 2 to 3 days. Frequently, clients are discharged still requiring care, and this care is frequently delivered in the home setting. Most clients, especially those who are high risk, benefit from the process of **discharge planning**. Discharge planning is defined as the systematic process of planning for client care after discharge from the hospital. The emphasis and goal of discharge planning are to meet client needs through continuity of care—from an acute care setting to a discharge facility.

To comply with The Joint Commission requirements related to discharge planning, initial assessment at admission, ongoing assessments, and referrals must be documented (Box 6-3 ■).

Hospitals must have a discharge planning process that applies to all clients. Policies and procedures must be specified in writing. Newer terminology refers to *transition planning* or *community care transition*. These terms are preferred by some because they shift the focus from primarily the clients' hospitalization to other client care settings as well. See Section 1861 (ee) of the Social Security Act.

Box 6-3 THE JOINT COMMISSION STANDARDS FOR CLIENT EDUCATION

- Hospitals perform a learning needs assessment for each client that includes cultural and religious beliefs, emotional barriers, desire and motivation to learn, physical or cognitive limitations, and barriers to communication.
- Client receives education and training specific to the client's assessed needs, abilities, learning preferences, and readiness to learn as appropriate to the care and services provided by the hospital.
- Hospital plans for and supports the provision and coordination of client education activities.
- Hospital identifies and provides the resources necessary for achieving educational objectives.
- Education process is coordinated among appropriate staff or disciplines who are providing care or services.
- Client is educated, based on assessed needs, about how to safely and effectively use medications according to law and regulation and the hospital's scope of services, as appropriate.
- Client is educated about nutrition interventions, modified diets, or oral health, when applicable.
- Hospital ensures that the client is educated about how to safely and effectively use medical equipment or supplies, as appropriate.
- Client is educated about pain and managing pain as part of treatment, as appropriate.
- Client is educated about habilitation or rehabilitation techniques to help him or her become more functionally independent, as appropriate.
- Client is educated about other available resources, and when necessary, how to obtain further care, services, or treatment to meet his or her identified needs.
- Education includes information about client's responsibilities in his or her care.
- Education includes self-care activities, as appropriate.
- Discharge instructions are given to client and those responsible for providing continuing care.
- Academic education is provided for a hospitalized child or adolescent, either directly by the hospital or through other arrangements, when appropriate.

Source: Adapted from the Joint Commission (2014)

Table 6-2 Comparison of Katz and Lawton ADL Scales

Activities of Daily Living	Instrumental Activities of Daily Living
(Katz ADL)	(Lawton IADL)
Feeding	Using the telephone
Continence	Shopping
Transferring	Preparing food
Toileting	Housekeeping
Dressing	Doing laundry
Bathing	Using transportation
Handling medications	Managing own medications
—	Handling finances

Source: Graf (2008a, Apr.)

It is not uncommon for clients discharged from inpatient hospital settings to be readmitted within a short period of time for a related condition. Some readmissions are unavoidable, while others are related to a poor discharge planning process. Reducing the number of preventable hospital readmissions is a major priority for client safety. Multiple factors contribute to high rates of preventable readmissions. Jencks, Williams, and Coleman (2009) identified that 19.6% of Medicare fee-for-service beneficiaries were rehospitalized within 30 days of discharge and 34% within 60 days. The readmissions may result from poor quality care or poor transitions between different providers and care settings.

When the client is admitted and the care plan formulated, discharge planning should be initiated. The process includes an assessment of the client and family's anticipated needs; physical, emotional, and psychosocial status; home environment; and family and community resources. Two common assessment instruments measuring physical and cognitive function are frequently given to at-risk clients at the time of admission. The Lawton Instrumental Activities of Daily Living (IADL) and Katz Activities of Daily Living (ADL) scales provide useful information when developing discharge plans. Comparison of the two scales is provided in Table 6-2 ■.

Discharge planning requires a multidisciplinary approach with participation by all members of the healthcare team, including the client and family (Box 6-4 ■). Many of the larger hospitals have discharge planners or coordinators, who orchestrate the discharge planning. This is especially important when the client is considered high risk. Physicians must order the client's release from the hospital, particularly Medicare clients (Box 6-5 ■). The nursing staff still plays a major role in assessing discharge needs and preparing the client and caregivers to assume responsibility for care after hospital discharge. With the assistance of social workers or community-based nurses, the nurse identifies and anticipates client needs and formulates a plan for meeting these needs after discharge from the hospital.

Box 6-4 DISCHARGE PLAN

Basic Steps

Evaluation of the client by qualified personnel
Discussion with client or his or her representative
Planning for going home or to **transfer** to another facility
Determining if caregiver training or other **support** is required
Referrals to home health agency and/or appropriate community agencies
Arranging for follow-up appointment or tests and transportation

High-Risk Indicators

- Age (older adults)
- Multisystem disease process
- Major surgical procedure
- Chronic or terminal illness
- Emotional or mental instability
- Inadequate or inappropriate living arrangement
- Lack of transportation
- Financial insecurity
- Unsafe features in the home

Successful discharge planning includes:

1. A transitional plan of care from the acute care setting to home or another healthcare facility
2. Appropriate teaching for family and client in self-care
3. Knowledge and skills necessary for self-care and emergency procedures
4. Appropriate agencies involved in transition to the home care setting

Another approach to discharge planning is **transitional care** using transition specialists. These practitioners facilitate the transition from hospital (where discharge planning is initiated) to recovery (in the home). The transition

---

Box 6-5 FEDERAL REQUIREMENTS FOR DISCHARGE PLANNING PROCESS

- Hospitals must identify at an early stage of hospitalization all clients who are likely to have adverse health consequences on discharge if there is no planning.
- The hospital must provide a discharge planning evaluation.
- A registered nurse, social worker, or other qualified individual must develop or supervise development of the evaluation.
- Discharge planning must include an evaluation of the likelihood of needing posthospital services and of the availability of the services.
- The evaluation must include the client's capacity for self-care or the possibility of the client being cared for in the environment from which the client entered the hospital.
- The evaluation must be completed on a timely basis so that appropriate arrangements for posthospital care are made before discharge.
- The discharge planning evaluation must be in the client's medical record.

specialist meets with the family and client in the acute setting, begins discharge planning, and usually makes a home visit before the client is discharged. After discharge to the home, this specialist is available to the client and family. This type of transitional care and coordination has proven to be cost-effective and has improved the quality of client care.

Communication between the client, family, and healthcare agencies is essential for effective discharge planning (Box 6-6 ■). According to HIPAA, discussing client information with the family members or friends is only permitted if it directly affects them and the client agrees. The information reflecting client approval needs to be documented in the client's record. Family members involved in discharge planning are helpful, as they can inform the healthcare team about cultural traditions, financial issues, unsafe living conditions, and support for the client at home. The nurse establishes a dialogue between these various people and coordinates the discharge plan before the client leaves the hospital. When referrals to other agencies are necessary, these are initiated before the client is discharged. The nurse, if there is no discharge planner available, is responsible for coordinating such referrals—including signed physician's orders for specific care, treatments, or medications.

Adaptation to Home Care

Home Care Definition

The term *home health care* refers to all services that promote, maintain, or restore physical, social, or emotional health to clients in the home setting. Home care is provided in the individual's residence. For a smooth transition from hospital

---

Box 6-6 CARE TRANSITIONS: BEST PRACTICES AND EVIDENCE-BASED PROGRAMS IN CARE TRANSITION

Best practices in care transitions are based on effective programs focusing on transitions from the hospital to home. There is little research on transitions from the hospital to other settings. Poorly coordinated care transitions from the hospital to other care settings cost an estimated $12 billion to $44 billion per year. Poor transitions also often result in poor health outcomes. The most common adverse effects associated with poor transitions are injuries due to medication errors, complications from procedures, infections, and falls.

Elements described as best practices include:

- Comprehensive discharge planning
- Complete and timely communication of information
- Medication reconciliation
- Client–caregiver education using the teach-back method
- Open communication between providers
- Prompt follow-up visit with an outpatient provider after discharge

Research strongly suggests that these best practices create a strong foundation for high-quality, cost-saving transitions from the hospital to home.

Source: Center for Healthcare Research & Transformation. (2014)

---

to home, the home care coordinator communicates with the family members and the home health nurse. Home care is also provided to clients in long-term care or residential care facilities in which there are no or limited staff members.

A variety of health workers are needed to provide comprehensive home care services to clients and families. Table 6-3 ■ presents an overview of healthcare providers

Table 6-3 Home Health Team

Healthcare Provider	Major Responsibilities
Registered Nurse	Performs as a case manager. Initiates physician-ordered plan of care; performs assessment, planning, and interventions for needed home care skills and teaching. Assists in evaluating treatment regimens for all services.
Home Care Aide	Performs hygienic care, skin care, exercise, ambulation, dressing, and elimination skills. Some may prepare and serve meals. Assists in maintaining a clean, safe, client environment (e.g., client's bedroom).
Homemaker	Maintains the home environment, shops for and prepares meals, transports client, and runs errands.
Social Worker	Assists in planning for home care needs, instructs in use of social and community services and resources. Provides information relative to long-term planning and respite care in the home.
Physical Therapist	Evaluates environment in preparation for client's return home. Assists with safety adaptations for the home, instructs in exercise program, gait training, and use of special adaptive equipment.
Occupational Therapist	Instructs in activities of daily living, grooming, upper extremity strengthening, function activities, and use of adaptive equipment.
Speech Therapist	Evaluates swallowing and chewing ability; memory; assists with increasing communication techniques for client, family, and healthcare provider; and provides speech reeducation program.
Registered Dietician	Evaluates and provides for nutritional needs of client. Plans and instructs in appropriate diet.
Physician	Prescribes medical plan of treatment. Writes specific prescriptions for medications, diet, supplies, nursing interventions, and therapist parameters.
Licensed Practical or Vocational Nurse	Provides skilled nursing care similar to a Home Care Aide under RN supervision. They are not used by all agencies because of limited independent activities allowed.

and their major responsibilities. The list and responsibilities are not inclusive; consult an additional home care reference for more detailed information.

Referral to Home Care

It is necessary for nurses in all settings to be aware of the referral process and the type of client who should be referred for home care services. Although most home care clients have been hospitalized, it is not a prerequisite for service. Physicians, individual clients, families, residential care administrators, and friends may refer a client by calling a home health agency and requesting service. A physician's approval is needed for reimbursement. An evaluation visit is made by the RN or PT, who acts as case manager, to determine if service is needed. If it is needed, an appropriate plan of care is established. Speech therapists are not allowed to do initial evaluations in most states.

Most hospitals have a designated protocol for making referrals, which is described in the hospital policy manual. In most hospitals it is the discharge planner, case manager, or social worker who makes the referral. The nurse may alert the appropriate individual to the client's need for home care. It is essential that the nurse provides complete and thorough information about the client's condition, including physical and psychosocial needs. This information is documented on a standard referral form or on an official form from the Department of Health and Human Services and sent to the home health agency. Accurate information and orders are needed to facilitate a smooth transition from hospital to home. Incomplete or inadequate communication could mean a lapse in service and inadequate care for the client.

All age groups use home health services. The criteria for referral depend on various factors, such as client need, agency protocol, and insurance criteria. Since the older adult on Medicare represents the largest segment of the population using home care services, it is important that all nurses know Medicare eligibility criteria for home visits. This ensures that accurate information is given to the client and family. In addition to eligibility criteria, many regulations govern the type and frequency of care. Since these regulations are subject to change and interpretation by the fiscal intermediaries who administer Medicare insurance, frequent review of Medicare regulations should be done. Eligibility for another funding agency, Medicaid, differs from state to state. It is the nurse's responsibility to be familiar with these policies. Each individual insurance company reimburses for services at different rates and for different levels of service. Each insurance plan needs to be reviewed to determine reimbursement.

Transition From Hospital to Home

A smooth transition from hospital to home depends on an appropriate discharge plan. The shorter duration in-hospital stay requires a thorough, efficient discharge plan that must be initiated at the time of hospital admission. Identifying the client's needs and resources before planning for discharge results in a realistic plan. Since any illness causes additional stress in the family and necessitates an adaptive coping response, the needs of the family or significant other must be included in the teaching and discharge plan. Discharge planning is completed during meetings of the interdisciplinary healthcare team. Representative members of each discipline discuss the client's progress and individual needs for discharge. In addition, accurate and comprehensive documentation must accompany the physician's plan of treatment to ensure a smooth transition. A description of the client at discharge should be provided; include physical assessment findings, ability to assist in ADLs, adaptive devices needed for care, and a brief summary of hospitalization. These data greatly assist in the transition from hospital to home.

Home Health Care Changes

Home health care, a rapidly growing field of health care, has developed in response to recent changes in political and social forces in the United States. These changes have demanded that nurses expand their knowledge about home care and acquire skills needed to provide safe, competent care to clients in the home setting.

Several factors have contributed to the emergence of home health care as a primary delivery system. The fastest growing segment of the American population is 85 years of age or older. These older adults constitute the largest proportion of population currently using home healthcare services. Nine percent of those 65 to 74 years of age and 25% of those 75 years and older require some type of home care service. Many younger clients are receiving home care visits as a direct result of early discharge from hospitals. Home care visits are funded by private insurance companies and are a cost-effective measure for providing nursing care.

Another factor is the changing structure and role of the American family. Traditionally, women have provided health care for the family members at home. With more women working outside the home, the demand for home health services has increased.

Political factors have had an effect on healthcare delivery patterns. A cost-containment measure initiated by the federal government in 1983 to curb rising costs of hospitalized Medicare clients drastically altered the extent of care administered in the hospital setting. A prospective payment system (diagnostic-related groups or DRGs), rather than a retrospective payment system, was implemented. This resulted in shorter hospital stays for Medicare clients. With the shorter stays came a dramatic increase in the need for professional services to care for high-acuity clients in the home. Additional types of services have also had to be added to the home care system to meet the needs of these clients. Even more changes occurred with healthcare reform in the 1990s. Health maintenance organizations (HMOs) and reimbursement policies directly affected the home healthcare agencies.

Documentation using Outcome and Assessment Information Set (OASIS) is regulated by the Health Care

Financing Administration. The OASIS system was developed by The Center for Health Policy Research in Denver, Colorado. The information set contains data items for measuring client outcomes for the purpose of performance improvement in home health care. OASIS data items address sociodemographic, environmental, support system, health status, functional status, and health service utilization characteristics of the client. Medicare certified home care agencies are required to conduct client-specific comprehensive assessments at specified times.

OASIS C, a newer version, has added 30 process measures that will affect outcomes. The new client assessment information was also used to develop a prospective payment system for home health agencies, which went into effect October 2000. Home visits for maternity clients and children under 18 do not require completion of these forms.

Client Teaching

Client teaching is an essential component of both hospital and home care. Since clients are discharged earlier and with a higher acuity level, the client and his or her family are expected to accept more responsibility for follow-up care. It is essential for client teaching to begin in the hospital and provide a description of the disease or condition and the treatment regimen. The client and family should be instructed in skills and treatments necessary to restore health and prevent other illness or complications. The home health nurse builds on the teaching plan, with the main emphasis on adapting care in the home environment. Continuity of care depends on comprehensive communication between the discharging and home care agencies.

Adapting Care to the Home Setting

The client is often a passive recipient of care in the hospital. In the home setting, on the other hand, the client is in control—it is his or her environment. That is, the environment is determined by the client and family according to their needs, desires, values, and resources. The nurse is a guest in this environment, which requires flexibility in adapting to a variety of situations.

In the hospital, equipment is readily available. Nurses perform procedures or treatments and provide 24-hour-a-day coverage of nursing care. In the home, equipment must be ordered or improvised, and the emphasis is on teaching the client or caregiver self-care activities. The home care nurse must become very creative in adapting and improvising equipment and techniques.

When a client referral is received by a home health agency, a nurse or physical therapist makes an initial admission visit. This visit includes a thorough assessment of the client, family, and home environment. The home environment is evaluated for safety, and the client and family are assessed for knowledge of safety and emergency procedures. Assessment of the client includes physical, emotional, psychological, and economic status. The home is assessed

for any adaptations that must be made to enable the client to function optimally in his or her environment. Family members are assessed for understanding of the client's illness or needs; cultural, ethnic, and health beliefs and values; ability to cope with (being adaptive or **maladaptive** to) the current situation; the physical, emotional, and spiritual needs of family members; financial resources; and knowledge of how to use community resources. A complete list of assessment parameters for each of these areas is included on the initial assessment form.

Cultural Awareness

The Developmental Disabilities and Bill of Rights Act of 2000 defined culturally competent services as services that are (a) provided in a manner responsive to the beliefs, interpersonal styles, attitudes, language, and behaviors of individuals; and (b) provided in a manner that demonstrates respect for individual dignity, personal preference, and cultural differences.

It is essential to remember that all client teaching plans and strategies must consider cultural aspects in the planning phase. Cultural differences affect clients' open-mindedness to client education and their willingness to listen to the teaching and then be compliant with the changes that need to occur. Cultural differences affect clients' attitudes about illness, healthcare workers, and treatment modalities. The Joint Commission has mandated that there must be greater awareness of diversity, attention to the needs of special populations, and staff training to meet their needs.

When taking **cultural competence** into account, nurses should consider the following to make client teaching more effective:

- Be aware of own cultural biases and prejudices.
- Become familiar with the core cultural values of client groups.
- Whenever possible, use a translator to convey information.

All cultures have health beliefs about illness: what causes it and what cures it, as well as who they will allow to treat them. It is important for nurses to understand each culture's differences, as it will impact the client teaching process. Table 6-4 ■ summarizes cultural beliefs that may have an effect on health care and client teaching.

Included in the discharge plan is a discharge summary. This summary includes an overall review of hospitalization activities and the client's learning needs. There is a statement indicating how well the learning needs have been met, the client teaching completed, short- and long-term goals of care, referrals made, and coordinated care plan to be implemented after discharge.

Since 1988, hospitals have been mandated by federal requirements to provide a discharge planning process for all Medicare clients. These same requirements now apply to all clients within hospitals in the United States.

Table 6-4 Cultural Beliefs Affecting Client Teaching

Ethnic Group	Cultural Beliefs
Asian–Pacific Islander	Extended family has large influence on client. Older family members are honored and respected, and their authority is unquestioned. Oldest male is decision maker and spokesman. Strong emphasis on avoiding conflict and direct confrontation. Respect authority and do not disagree with healthcare recommendations—but they may not follow recommendations.
Chinese	Chinese clients will not discuss symptoms of mental illness or depression because they believe this behavior reflects on family; therefore, it may produce shame and guilt. Use herbalists, spiritual healers, and physicians for care.
Japanese	Believe physical contact with blood, skin diseases, and corpses will cause illness. Believe improper care of the body, including poor diet and lack of sleep, causes illness. Believe in healers, herbalists, and physicians for healing, and energy can be restored with acupuncture and acupressure. Use group decision making for health concerns.
Hindu and Muslim	Indians and Pakistanis do not acknowledge a diagnosis of severe emotional illness or mental retardation because it reduces the chance of other family members getting married.
Vietnamese	Vietnamese accept mental health **counseling** and interventions, particularly when they have established trust with the healthcare worker.
Hispanic	Older family members are consulted on issues involving health and illness. Patriarchal family—men make decisions for family. Illness is viewed as God's will or divine punishment resulting from sinful behavior. Prefer to use home remedies and consult folk healers known as *curanderos* rather than traditional Western healthcare providers.
African American	Family and church oriented. Extensive extended family bonds. Key family member is consulted for important health-related decisions. Illness is a punishment from God for wrongdoing, or is due to voodoo, spirits, or demons. Health prevention is through good diet, herbs, rest, cleanliness, and laxatives to clean the system. May wear copper and silver bracelets to prevent illness.
Native American	Oriented to the present. Value cooperation. Value family and spiritual beliefs. Strong ties to family and tribe. Believe state of health exists when client lives in total harmony with nature. Illness is viewed as an imbalance between the ill individual and natural or supernatural forces. Use medicine man or woman known as a shaman. Illness is prevented through elaborate religious rituals.

Nursing Diagnoses

The following nursing diagnoses are appropriate to include in a client care plan when the components are related to establishing and maintaining a client teaching and discharge planning.

NURSING DIAGNOSIS	RELATED TO . . .
Impaired Communication: Verbal	Cognitive impairment, auditory impairment, language barrier
Denial	Attempt to disavow need to alter lifestyle by avoiding client teaching
Ineffective Health Maintenance	Cultural and religious beliefs, information misinterpretation, lack of education, lack of motivation, inadequate health care services
Deficient Knowledge	Inadequate understanding of condition, misinformation, language differences
Noncompliance	Impaired ability to perform tasks, poor self-esteem, lack of motivation
Relocation Stress Syndrome	Changes associated with transfer between facilities or facility and home, effects of losses associated with moving, stress in family members
Ineffective Role Performance	Change in self-perception of role; change in others' perception of role as a result of an altered health status, which leads to denial of learning need

Source: Herdman, T. H. & Kamitsuru, S. (Eds.) *Nursing Diagnoses – Definitions and Classification 2015-2017*. Copyright © 2014, 1994–2014 by NANDA International. Used by arrangement with John Wiley & Sons Limited. Companion website: www.wiley.com/go/nursingdiagnoses. In order to make safe and effective judgments using NANDA-I nursing diagnosis it is essential that nurses refer to the definitions and defining characteristics of the diagnoses listed in this work.

Nursing Process Data

ASSESSMENT Database

- Assess high-risk criteria for client education.
- Determine the need for a client teaching program.
- Identify client's learning style and preferences.
- Assess knowledge and skill level of the client.
- Assess motivation to learn.
- Assess readiness to learn.
- Identify physical or emotional barriers that may affect client's ability to participate in teaching plan.
- Identify health beliefs and practices.
- Assess developmental and educational level of client.
- Determine appropriate methodology for client teaching sessions.
- Identify appropriate adjunctive materials, such as audiovisual aids, to enhance learning process.
- Assess appropriate setting for the individual client.
- Determine family members or significant others who will be involved in client education.

PLANNING Objectives

- To develop a plan using the nursing process framework and adult learning principles
- To determine learning needs and establish learning objectives
- To select appropriate teaching strategies
- To increase client's knowledge to promote compliance with health regimen
- To encourage client participation in goal selection and implementation program
- To encourage client to acknowledge individual responsibility for health behaviors and health status
- To improve client's ability to make informed decisions affecting health status
- To facilitate behavioral changes that are conducive to optimum health status
- To provide continuity of care when the client is moving from one healthcare setting to another

IMPLEMENTATION Procedures

DOCUMENTATION AND EVALUATION

Expected Outcomes

- Client's knowledge regarding his or her health status has increased.
- Client's ability to make informed and effective health-related decisions, based on accurate information and awareness of self, has improved.
- Effective use of the healthcare delivery system has been promoted.
- Continuity of care and information exchange has occurred between health agencies or between the hospital and client's home and family.
- The nurse has evaluated his or her teaching effectiveness and revised the plan, teaching style, and content as necessary.
- Increased compliance to medical regimen as demonstrated by client's ability to manage condition or disease process.

Unexpected Outcomes/Alternative Actions

Pearson Nursing Student Resources

Find additional review materials at
nursing.pearsonhighered.com.
Prepare for success with NCLEX®-style practice
questions and Skill Checklists.

Skill 6.1.1 | Collecting Data and Establishing Rapport

Equipment

Client teaching plan

Room or suitable setting to complete assessment

Adjunct materials, such as audiovisual equipment, charts, and illustrations

Written materials, such as outlines or other handouts in client's language and level of understanding

Equipment for demonstration and return demonstration

Documentation forms: Kardex, client's chart, electronic forms

Preparation

1. Develop a client teaching plan utilizing the following information: assessment findings, expected learning outcomes, teaching strategies, teaching materials, education methods. ❶

   a. Use adult (and/or age-appropriate) learning principles. ❷

   b. Use communication and interpersonal relationship skills. Ask the client how he or she prefers to receive information, for example, by reading, listening, or viewing. ➤ *Rationale:* This encourages client's participation in the plan.

   c. Speak in plain language and avoid using technical terms or medical jargon. Include examples when possible.

   d. Use a nonjudgmental approach. Refrain from asking the client, "Do you understand?" ➤ *Rationale:* A nonjudgmental attitude assists client to be honest with feelings.

      i. Use "how" questions to facilitate communication. ➤ *Rationale:* "How" is more effective than "why"

❷ When collecting data to determine learning needs and strategies, use age-appropriate materials.

in a question, as "why" tends to set up a defensive reaction to the question. "How would you withdraw the insulin to promote sterility?" is preferable to, "Why did you withdraw the insulin that way?"

      ii. Use verbal and nonverbal behavior and congruency of behavior to build a relationship with the client.

   e. Use assessment (observation) skills. ➤ *Rationale:* This establishes a baseline for client teaching.

   f. Request demonstration of a skill previously learned or currently used (e.g., giving self an insulin injection). ➤ *Rationale:* Client's ability to demonstrate the skill helps you evaluate both ability to perform and mastery of previous teaching principles.

2. Develop an evaluation plan that determines extent of client learning goals.

Procedure

1. Identify personal characteristics.

   a. Age, gender, developmental level

   b. Educational level

   c. Marital status

   d. Family composition and living situation

   e. Ethnic group and cultural practices pertinent to language skill and preference

2. Identify resources available, both personal and community.

3. Identify values and attitudes toward self and others having his or her particular disease or condition.

4. Assess baseline knowledge—anatomy and physiology (normal and disease-related) and the disease process—by asking specific questions.

5. Assess current knowledge and ability to perform specific skills.

❶ Obtain data from the client profile to prepare the teaching plan.
Source: From Cerner Electronic Health Record. © Cerner Corporation. Pearson has restricted permission to reproduce and distribute this copyrighted work. Further reproduction or distribution is strictly prohibited without written consent of Cerner Corporation.

(continued)

Skill 6.1.1 | Collecting Data and Establishing Rapport *(continued)*

6. Assess patterns of coping.

   a. Past experiences of self and others in relation to the disease
   b. Perception by client of how ill he or she is at this time
   c. Reactions to stress and ways of managing anxiety
   d. Current level of self-management
   e. Willingness of client to change behavior

Skill 6.1.2 | Determining Readiness to Learn

Procedure

1. Determine client's physiologic readiness.

   a. Degree of physical comfort of client (level of pain), level of alertness, ability to concentrate, degree of interest
   b. Acuteness of the illness and its influence on client's ability to learn
   c. Environmental factors that may affect client's degree of readiness
   d. Safety issues and need for supervision

2. Evaluate client's psychological readiness.

   a. State of client's feelings and their influence on receptivity to learning. ➤ *Rationale:* An angry and hostile client is not going to absorb information until his or her anger is acknowledged or worked through.
   b. Psychological barriers (e.g., the presence of denial) and their influence on the learning process
   c. Client's intellectual capacity and level of comprehension

3. Assess client's willingness to make changes and be compliant with the teaching plan.

4. Assess family's ability and willingness to participate in teaching. ❶

   a. Determine willingness to participate in actual hospital instruction.
   b. Determine cognitive ability to understand instruction.
   c. Evaluate the extent of time and active participation of the family during instruction.
   d. Assess the interaction of the client and family during client teaching. ➤ *Rationale:* This will provide data on potential compliance and noncompliance issues related to the teaching plan.

5. Assess the extent of support and actual care the family members will provide for the client at home. ➤ *Rationale:* This will determine the extent of the instruction necessary for the family.

> **CLINICAL ALERT**
> The Joint Commission's Standards for Patient and Family Education require that client's learning needs, preferred learning styles, literacy level, educational level, language spoken and understood, and learning readiness are assessed.

❶ Include the family in teaching, particularly if they will play a role in caring for client.

Skill 6.1.3 | Assessing Learning Needs

Procedure

1. Assess if client has learning needs related to diagnosis, hospitalization, surgical procedures, or treatments.

   a. Ask specific questions relative to what physician has told client related to specific learning need(s).
   b. Ask client what he or she is most interested in learning about specific learning need(s).
   c. Ask client to tell you in his or her own words what they know about specific learning need(s).

2. Interview client to determine what his or her daily life is like.
   ➤ *Rationale:* The information will assist you in determining impact of changes in client's lifestyle brought on by illness or condition. This will help you determine how to approach the teaching plan.

   a. Ask client to describe his or her usual daily routine.
   b. Determine whether anything has changed with this pattern since illness began.
   c. Describe hobbies or sports activities in which the client participates.
   d. Describe a normal workday and what activities are involved with employment, if still working.
   e. Describe usual family responsibilities. Will the family be involved with his or her care (Box 6-7 ■)?

Box 6-7 FAMILY ASSESSMENT FOR TEACHING AND CLIENT CARE

Family assessment is an integral part of planning an effective teaching plan if family members will be affected by, or part of, client care. Include the following information in the assessment:

- Which family members will be involved with care of client?
- What is the most available time for the family member to participate in the teaching?
- Has client approved that family members be given confidential medical information?
- Can family members provide necessary care or will additional support be necessary?
- Does home environment support client's care needs?
- Are any changes to home necessary to provide a safe environment?
- Do family members speak English and have basic literacy skills?
- Are there any cultural belief conflicts that could inhibit adequate care in home?
- Do family members interact in a supportive manner with the client?
- What do family members know about the client's condition? Do they need additional teaching?

3. Determine client's age and developmental level.
   ➤ *Rationale:* Knowing client's developmental level is necessary to provide the most effective teaching strategies.
4. Determine client's learning style. ➤ *Rationale:* This will assist in selecting the most appropriate teaching strategy for client education.
   a. Ask questions related to what time of day he or she learns best.
   b. Determine whether he or she learns best by reading, listening, hands-on learning, or a combination of styles.
   c. Use a commercial learning style inventory, if available.
5. Complete a cultural assessment. ➤ *Rationale:* This helps the nurse develop a culturally responsive teaching plan based on client's beliefs.
   a. Determine client's belief about illness.
   b. Determine how strong the client's belief system is relative to his or her traditional culture.
   c. Determine whether he or she uses folk medicine practices and uses a traditional healer. Clients from Asia, Africa, and South America are more likely to maintain this cultural component of their former country.
   d. Identify whether traditional dietary habits are practiced in the home. If so, these should be included in the teaching plan, particularly nutritional counseling.
6. Determine client's educational and literacy levels (Box 6-8 ■).
   ➤ *Rationale:* Clients may seem disinterested in learning

Box 6-8 DETERMINING READING GRADE LEVEL

Rapid Estimate of Adult Literacy in Medicine—Short Form

The Rapid Estimate of Adult Literacy in Medicine—Short Form (REALM-SF) is a seven-item word recognition test to provide clinicians with a valid quick assessment of client health literacy. The REALM-SF has been **validated** and field tested in diverse research settings, and has excellent agreement with the 66-item REALM instrument in terms of grade-level assignments (Arozullah et al., 2007).

Note: This quick tool was developed with AHRQ funding, independently of **REALM-R**, created by the developers of **REALM** at Louisiana State University.

REALM-SF FORM

Client name _____ Date of birth _____
Reading level _____ Date _____
Examiner _____ Grade completed _____

Word	
Menopause	☐
Antibiotics	☐
Exercise	☐
Jaundice	☐
Rectal	☐
Anemia	☐
Behavior	☐

Instructions for Administering the REALM-SF

Give the client a laminated copy of the REALM-SF form and score answers on an unlaminated copy that is attached to a clipboard. Hold the clipboard at an angle so that the client is not distracted by your scoring. Say:

"I want to hear you read as many words as you can from this list. Begin with the first word and read aloud. When you come to a word you cannot read, do the best you can or say, 'blank' and go on to the next word."

If the client takes more than 5 seconds on a word, say "blank" and point to the next word, if necessary, to move the client along. If the client begins to miss every word, have him or her pronounce only known words.

Scores and Grade Equivalents for the REALM-SF

0	Third grade and below; will not be able to read most low-literacy materials; will need repeated oral instructions, materials composed primarily of illustrations, or audio- or videotapes
1–3	Fourth to sixth grade; will need low-literacy materials, may not be able to read prescription labels
4–6	Seventh to eighth grade; will struggle with most client education materials; will not be offended by low-literacy materials
7	High school; will be able to read most client education materials

Source: Agency for Healthcare Research and Quality (2014)

(continued)

Skill 6.1.3 | Assessing Learning Needs *(continued)*

when in fact they do not understand what is being said and are embarrassed to ask. This can lead to missed physician appointments, noncompliance with treatment or medication usage, and even disability.

   a. Determine client's reading level by measuring his or her reading and comprehension skills.
   b. Use a test of reading and comprehension to obtain a client profile before beginning teaching process.
      ➤ *Rationale:* This helps determine the most appropriate written material for the client.

7. Assess client's ability to speak and read English.

   a. Determine whether client requires an interpreter during assessment of learning needs and teaching process.
   b. Ensure that words you use in client's language are correct for the situation.
   c. Do not use slang that could be misunderstood.
   d. Use simple words and phrases to allow interpreter to relate the intent of your statement.

8. Use assessment data and assessment instrument to jointly determine client's learning needs: educational, physical, psychosocial, and financial needs.
9. Formulate needs as goals.
10. Prioritize learning needs or goals.

11. Review with client alternative resources available to accomplish goals.
12. Determine ability of facility, family, staff, or multidisciplinary team to meet goals or learning needs.
13. Identify potential barriers to learning.

   a. Physical: visual or auditory, pain level, literacy level, reading level
   b. Emotional barriers: stress or anxiety, inability to focus on information
   c. Language or culture: ability to understand and speak English, beliefs about health, folk practices, or communication style differences

14. Obtain verbal or written contract with client for educational program.
15. Refer client to other resources or agencies when appropriate.

> **CLINICAL ALERT**
> Agencies contract with telephone language lines to provide interpreter services. These services are available through AT&T Language Line Services and Pacific Interpreters Inc. on a 24-hour basis and in over 140 languages.

Skill 6.1.4 | Determining Appropriate Teaching Strategy

Procedure

1. Consider the following factors when determining appropriate strategy (Box 6-9 ■):

   a. Input from client about how he or she learns best ❶
   b. Specific task or nature of the content to be transmitted and how it is best learned
   c. Client attention span and retention ability
   d. Reading level of client
   e. Teaching materials and resources available. Electronic material is available for client education; it is used particularly for medications, diagnostic tests, and diagnoses.
   f. Availability, skills, and abilities of staff; appropriate use of paraprofessional and professional staff
   g. Participation by members of other healthcare disciplines as part of a team
   h. Determination of most appropriate time for teaching

❶ Determine which teaching strategy will be most effective for the client.

Box 6-9 **COMPONENTS OF A TEACHING PLAN**

- Client learning needs
- Expected learning outcomes
- Teaching content organized from simple to complex
- Teaching methods and tools
- Barriers to learning and readiness to learn
- Evaluation tools

2. Use appropriate reading material for the individual client.

   a. Determine reading level of written material.
   b. Use a readability formula to determine most appropriate written information for the client.
   c. Use brochures, handouts, and written material written at a sixth-grade level if client has low literacy skills.
      ➤ *Rationale:* Seventy-five percent of the adults in the United States should be able to read the material.

d. Provide written materials in client's native language, if non-English speaking.

e. Use short, common words in written material. ➤ *Rationale:* Medical terminology may be misunderstood.

f. Make sentences 10 words or less and written in active voice.

g. Make paragraphs short with one focus.

h. Use large type (fonts) and lowercase letters.

➤ *Rationale:* Large font size is easier for clients with visual impairments or older adult clients, and lowercase letters are easier to read.

i. Use diagrams and photos whenever possible to make a point.

j. Set realistic goals and only one or two objectives for each teaching session. ➤ *Rationale:* Overloading client with information will not allow him or her to master information necessary for compliance.

k. Ensure client completes a return demonstration, if appropriate. ➤ *Rationale:* This assists you to determine the extent to which client understands information presented. The greater the understanding and ability to perform a particular skill, the greater the compliance to treatment.

3. Determine which type of teaching strategy will be effective in a given situation.

a. Group process: use of principles from group dynamics, mental health, or other related fields to enhance learning or behavior changes in a small group setting

b. Lecture–discussion: presentation of content in a didactic fashion with opportunity for questions and interaction during or at the conclusion of the presentation

c. Demonstration–return demonstration: demonstration (videotape) by the instructor with practice by the learner and return demonstration of mastery of the skill

d. Role playing: assumption of roles by various participants or learners for the purpose of clarifying various aspects of a situation

e. Games: structured (age-appropriate) game situation with rules designed for the learner to accomplish specific educational objectives

f. Use of tablet or computer programs if available and demonstration of ability to use equipment

4. Select appropriate teaching adjuncts based on developmental level, learning style, and reading literacy.

a. Videotape or videocassette programs

b. Films; slide and tape presentations

c. Diagrams, charts, and illustrations

d. Programmed instruction materials, that is, computer or Internet ❷

e. Books

f. Pamphlets and other written handouts

5. Provide language-specific material for non-English-speaking clients.

a. Photos

b. Models of specific body parts

c. Audiotapes in specific language

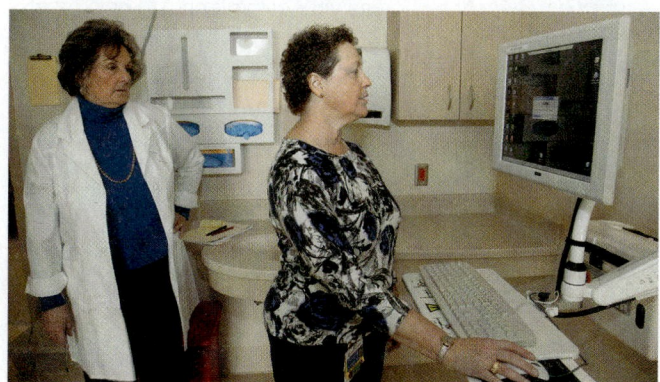

❷ Client education using computerized program assists nurse in providing information that is relevant to client's needs.

Skill 6.1.5 | Selecting the Educational Setting

Procedure

1. Choose an appropriate setting based on selected teaching strategy and available facility space.

2. Evaluate types of setting most appropriate to individual client and family learning needs.

3. Consider an informal setting.

a. Spontaneous teaching interactions between nurse and client can occur at any time in any setting.

b. Usually no formal plan or **evaluation tool** is used.

4. Consider a formal setting.

a. Teaching is carried out in a specified area of the facility such as an in-service classroom.

b. Teaching can occur independently, such as with audiovisual programmed instruction modules, or in a group setting. ❶

c. Formal plan for the teaching program includes written goals, objectives, teaching strategies, content, and evaluation method.

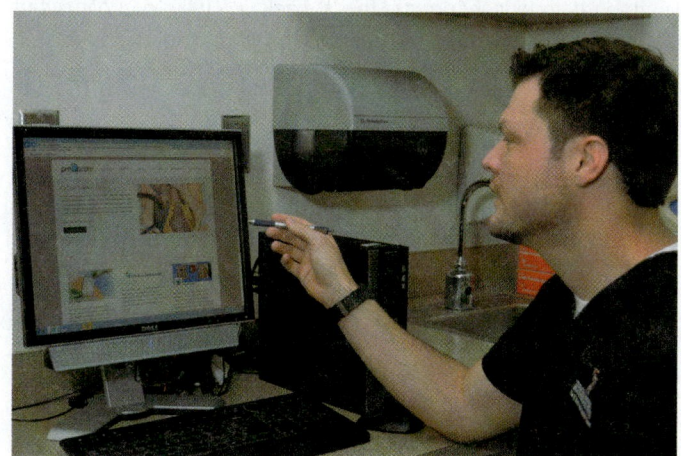

❶ Preoperative teaching using computerized module.

Skill 6.1.6 | Implementing the Teaching Strategy

Procedure

1. Gather teaching materials appropriate for client's learning needs and teaching strategy. Introduce self; identify client.
2. Sit with client in designated setting, and establish a warm and accepting relationship. ➤ *Rationale:* This is conducive to teaching and assists client in learning.
3. Specify previously established mutual goals and behavioral objectives of the program. ➤ *Rationale:* Mutually agreed-on goals promote acceptance of teaching strategy by the client.
4. Clarify or reclarify contract, agreements, or expected outcomes with individual or group. ➤ *Rationale:* Beginning at the level of understanding of individual or group facilitates the process.
5. Assess teaching situation for any modifications needed and adjust plans accordingly.
6. Teach content or components of the plan to client. ❶
   ➤ *Rationale:* Sticking to the plan and not deviating or going off on a tangent reinforces your commitment to help client master the content.
7. Use appropriate communication skills throughout session.
   ➤ *Rationale:* **Therapeutic** communication techniques enhance the learning environment.
8. Request feedback (evaluation interchange) during teaching process. ➤ *Rationale:* Feedback lets you know how the client is understanding content and allows for modification as indicated.
9. Plan for short teaching sessions on a frequent basis.
10. Adhere to agreed-upon starting and ending times; negotiate any changes. ➤ *Rationale:* This encourages the client to trust you.
11. Provide closure to teaching situation by summarizing and reiterating agreements made, actions to be taken, or subsequent events to follow.

❶ Demonstration is an important component of teaching strategy.

12. Provide positive reinforcement if not done previously.
    ➤ *Rationale:* This approach increases self-esteem and encourages learning in client.
13. Terminate teaching session by establishing time for next client contact.
14. Do postassessment of your own participation, and plan for corrections and improvements in presentation.
    ➤ *Rationale:* Ongoing evaluation assists in final step of nursing process evaluation.
15. Reinforce teaching throughout hospitalization.

    a. Use return demonstration of skills frequently throughout hospital stay (Box 6-10 ■).

Box 6-10 THE TEACH-BACK METHOD

Studies have shown that 40–80% of the medical information clients receive is forgotten immediately and nearly half of the information retained is incorrect. Teach-back is a way to confirm that you have explained to the client what he or she needs to know in a way in which he or she understands. Suggested approaches when using teach-back include:

- "I want to be sure that I explained your medication correctly. Can you tell me how you are going to take this medicine?"
- "We covered a lot today about your diabetes, and I want to make sure that I explained things clearly, so let's review what we discussed. What are three strategies that will help you control your diabetes?"
- "What are you going to do when you get home about controlling your diabetes?"

Teach-back method (practice):

- Start slowly. Initially, you may want to try it with the last client of the day.

- Plan your approach. Think about how you will ask the client to teach-back information based on the information you will be reviewing. Not all situations will be appropriate for using this technique.
- Use handouts or tablet or computer programs. Review the material to reinforce the teaching points. This will assist the client in understanding the content.
- Clarify. If clients cannot remember or accurately repeat what you asked them, clarify the information or directions and allow them to teach it back again. This needs to be done until clients correctly describe in their own words what they are going to do, without just parroting what you said.
- Practice. It may take time getting used to this technique, but studies indicate that once established as part of a routine, it does not take long to perform.

b. Review teaching content through use of videotapes and reading material.

c. Provide positive reinforcement for changes in behavior.

d. Discuss teaching content and written information by asking pertinent questions and providing answers to client's questions.

16. Send teaching plan and written materials home with client and family. Computer-generated written material (medications, tests, diagnosis, etc.) should be discussed verbally, in addition to providing written material.

17. Place copy of written instructions in chart for documentation. Instructions must be signed by client. This stays in chart.

18. Provide copy of teaching plan and written material to home health agency if referral has been made for visiting nurse. ➤ *Rationale:* This promotes consistency in information dissemination and reinforces teaching provided to client while hospitalized.

19. Document your teaching on specific client teaching forms or electronic forms.

   Documentation should include:

   a. Educational assessment and comprehension level

   b. Knowledge and skill level of learning need(s)

c. Motivational level (interaction during teaching session)

d. Learning barriers (language, speech, vision, hearing)

e. Overall goal achievement

EVIDENCE-BASED PRACTICE

Computer-Generated Client Education

Computer-generated client education has been studied several times. Leaffer and Gonda found that clients taught how to use the Internet to retrieve health information were still using it 90 days later, and 66% of them were taking the information they found on the Internet to their healthcare providers when they had a scheduled visit. More than 50% of the clients stated that using the Internet made them feel more knowledgeable, and thus they were more satisfied with the treatment they received.

Source: Leaffer & Gonda (2000)

Baker et al. surveyed 4,764 individuals, and the results indicated that 40% stated they had used the Internet for information or advice about health or health care during the last year. Sixty-seven percent stated that using the Internet improved their understanding of symptoms, conditions, or treatments.

Source: Baker, Wagner, Singer, & Bundorf (2003)

Skill 6.1.7 | Evaluating Teaching/Learning Outcomes

Procedure

1. After demonstrating skill(s), ask client to complete a return demonstration. Evaluate client's ability to perform tasks. ❶

2. Ask client and/or family to explain demonstration using own words.

3. Ask client and/or family specific questions regarding information provided. ➤ *Rationale:* Determine necessity of reinforcing or reteaching information.

4. Develop a simple pre- and post-test to determine client's knowledge base.

5. Develop hypothetical situations for client to problem solve. ➤ *Rationale:* This will help determine client's understanding of disease or condition.

6. Use an evaluation tool, if appropriate. ➤ *Rationale:* Evaluating with a specific tool focuses the evaluation phase better. ❷

   a. Evaluate forms, format, and types of tools available for evaluation.

      1. Pretest–post-test: measures changes in areas such as knowledge level, attitudes, and values

      2. Questionnaire: completed by client to report attitudes, certain behaviors, and, most frequently, level of satisfaction with the teaching program

❶ Request a return demonstration to evaluate client understanding.

(continued)

Skill 6.1.7 | Evaluating Teaching/Learning Outcomes *(continued)*

3. Physiologic tracers: determined before teaching episode to be the criterion of measurement of success (e.g., changes in blood pressure values after teaching program for hypertensive clients)

4. Direct observation of behavior changes: report of level of performance during return demonstrations

b. Choose an evaluative tool based on goals and objectives of the teaching program. ➤ *Rationale:* The purpose is to achieve goals, thus the evaluative tool should be based on goals.

❷ Multidisciplinary teaching record.

Source: From Cerner Electronic Health Record. © Cerner Corporation. Pearson has restricted permission to reproduce and distribute this copyrighted work. Further reproduction or distribution is strictly prohibited without written consent of Cerner Corporation.

Unit 6.1 Documentation and Evaluation

DOCUMENTATION for Client Education

- Client's learning needs
- Client's learning objectives and goals set by client and staff

- Topics or subjects covered as a part of client education process, such as medications, procedures, dietary plan, activity restrictions, or follow-up care

- Teaching strategies used
- Degree of client's participation in the teaching activity
- Client's reading level
- Client's learning style preference

- Progress in meeting the expected outcomes of teaching
- Client's emotional response to the learning process
- Information or equipment sent home with client
- Client's developmental level

EVALUATION/Critical Thinking

Expected Outcomes

- Client's knowledge regarding his or her health status has increased.
- Client's ability to make informed and effective health-related decisions, based on accurate information and awareness of self, has improved.
- Effective use of the healthcare delivery system has been promoted.
- Continuity of care and information exchange has occurred between health agencies or between the hospital and client's home and family.
- The nurse has evaluated his or her teaching effectiveness and revised the plan, teaching style, and content as necessary.
- Increased compliance to medical regimen as demonstrated by client's ability to manage condition or disease process.

Unexpected Outcomes

- Client's health status or treatment compliance has not improved as a result of the teaching program.

Alternative Actions

- Reevaluate nursing care plan according to the nursing process.
- Reassess client for barriers to learning.
- Assess client's reading and developmental levels.
- Assess client's ability to understand English or evaluate other language skills.
- Reevaluate testing tool.
- Review client's learning style preference.
- Determine readability level of written material.
- Problem solve with client as to next step to take.
- Request assistance from in-service consultant for determining which aspects of the teaching program were not successful and why.
- Assist in revising parts of the program and restructure for individual client needs.

- Client is hostile to teaching program.

- Attempt to determine underlying reason for hostility.
- Terminate this session of teaching program, but tell client you will return tomorrow or at a later time.
- Bring another nurse along to assist you in teaching as well as to help you evaluate reason for hostility.

(continued)

Unexpected Outcomes

- Client's ability to make informed and effective health-related decisions, based on accurate information and awareness of self, has not improved.

Alternative Actions

- Assist client to take realistic responsibility for ineffective decisions without guilt and shame attached.
- Assist client to identify those areas in which he or she is willing to make changes and support development of a plan of action.
- Refer to other resources such as groups with like conditions (e.g., cancer, diabetes).

- Client is unable to understand client teaching due to language barrier.

- Identify a volunteer or family member who can be used as an interpreter.
- Use the AT&T Language Line.
- Obtain teaching material in client's native language.
- Use photos or models, or make drawings that depict task to be performed.

Discharge Planning

Nursing Process Data

ASSESSMENT Database

- Determine client discharge planning needs.
- Determine if client is in a high-risk category.
- Assess special needs of client for individualized planning.
- Assess need for multidisciplinary healthcare workers.
- Determine information needed for compiling discharge summary.

PLANNING Objectives

- To complete a discharge risk factor assessment when admitting a client
- To determine healthcare workers needed for discharge planning
- To make appropriate referrals for client discharge
- To complete discharge teaching
- To develop a discharge plan
- To complete a discharge summary

IMPLEMENTATION Procedures

DOCUMENTATION AND EVALUATION

Expected Outcomes

- Client's discharge plan is initiated upon admission.
- Client's discharge teaching is completed before discharge.
- Client's plan for discharge is based on identified long-term goals.

Unexpected Outcomes/Alternative Actions

Pearson Nursing Student Resources

Find additional review materials at
nursing.pearsonhighered.com.
Prepare for success with NCLEX®-style practice questions and Skill Checklists.

Skill 6.2.1 | Preparing a Client for Discharge

Procedure

1. Obtain admission history, physical, and hospital progress notes.
2. Determine risk factors for discharge planning at time of admission.
3. Refer high-risk clients to discharge coordinator or social service department, if appropriate.
4. Develop discharge plan (if not already completed) including short- and long-term goals in conjunction with physician and client. ❶ Plan components should include:

   a. Diet
   b. Medications
   c. Treatments

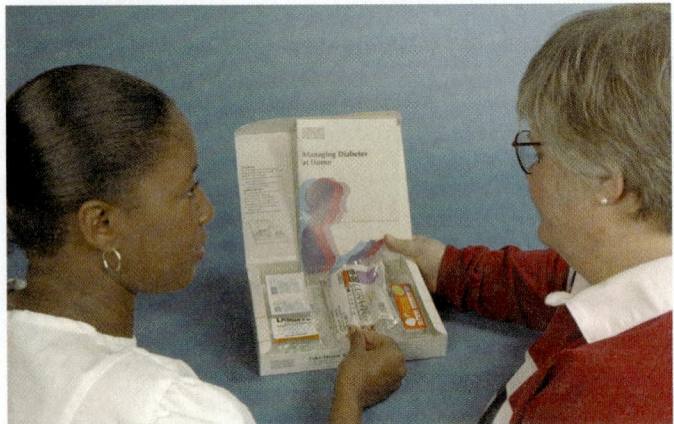

❶ Discharge teaching is an important component of the discharge plan.

   d. Physical activity limitations
   e. Signs and symptoms to report
   f. Follow-up medical care
   g. Equipment
   h. Appropriate community resources

5. Evaluate degree to which client education plan was implemented; reinforce aspects that were incomplete or refer to home agency.
6. Identify need for follow-up care after discharge in conjunction with physician. Physicians must order the release from the hospital but the actual process can be completed by a healthcare worker.
7. Make appropriate agency referrals.
8. Complete a discharge referral form, and communicate directly with referral agency about client.

Note: Healthcare agency may prefer its own discharge form to be completed rather than documentation in the nurses' notes.

9. Develop written discharge instructions for client and family, including medication administration times, dose, and side effects; treatments to be carried out at home or in a facility, potential side effects or complications from treatments or surgery; when to notify physician regarding symptoms; etc.
10. Update client care plan, and send copy to referral agency.
11. Send client teaching plan and materials to referral agency.
    ➤ **Rationale:** This helps maintain consistency in client teaching.
12. Document discharge summary.

Skill 6.2.2 | Completing a Discharge Summary

Procedure

1. Document a complete physical and psychosocial assessment at time of discharge.
2. Review vital sign ranges, and state latest vital signs.
3. Identify activity level of client.
4. Describe use of adaptive devices or equipment needs.
5. Review client teaching plan. ❶ Provide explanation of areas where teaching was adequate and where additional reinforcement is required.
6. Identify prescribed medications, dosage, and administration times. Provide information on client's knowledge of medication.
7. Describe goal achievement based on client care plan. Describe action taken if goal not achieved.

8. Identify referral agencies contacted.
9. Provide information regarding instructions on physician office visits, appointments to healthcare agencies, or support services.
10. Describe client's condition at time of discharge.
11. Document discharge instructions provided to client and family.
12. Describe method of discharge (e.g., wheelchair) and individual accompanying client at discharge.
13. State means of discharge transportation (e.g., private car, ambulance).
14. Specify discharge facility where client is going.

Note: Many facilities have developed forms that combine discharge summaries and client instructions.

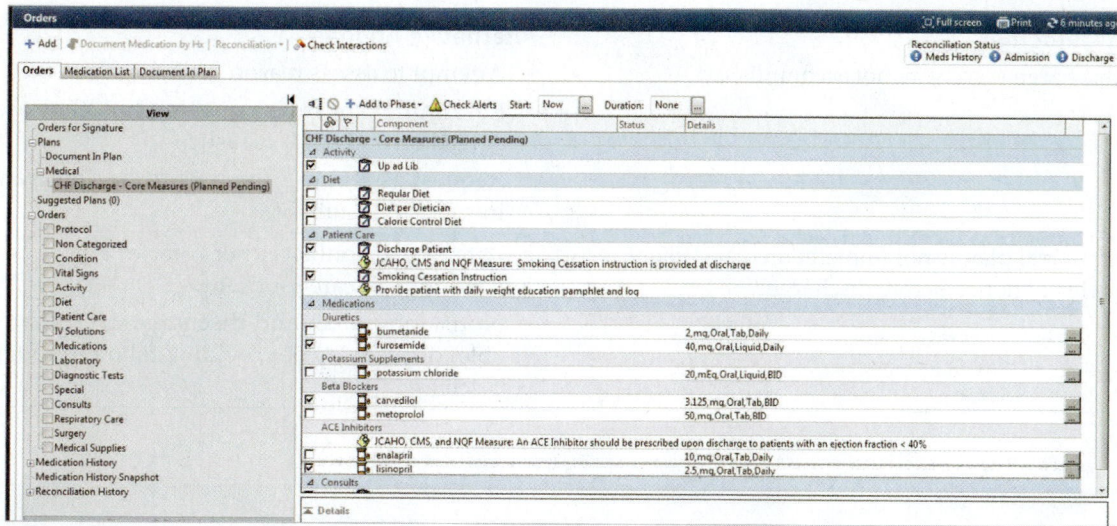

❶ Sample discharge plan form.

Source: From Cerner Electronic Health Record. © Cerner Corporation. Pearson has restricted permission to reproduce and distribute this copyrighted work. Further reproduction or distribution is strictly prohibited without written consent of Cerner Corporation.

Unit 6.2 Documentation and Evaluation

DOCUMENTATION for Discharge Planning

- Discharge teaching completed, and additional teaching need(s) necessary after discharge
- Discharge plan completed, including risk factors, short- and long-term goals, and degree to which plan was implemented
- Summary of client care during hospitalization, client interventions provided

- Need for follow-up after discharge
- Referral agencies contacted
- Discharge summary form completed; discharge instructions including medications, treatments, etc.
- Client's condition at time of discharge
- Date, time, location, and mode of discharge

EVALUATION/Critical Thinking

Expected Outcomes

- Client's discharge plan is initiated upon admission.
- Client's discharge teaching is completed before discharge.
- Client's plan for discharge is based on identified long-term goals.

Unexpected Outcomes

- Client is discharged before discharge plan is completed.

- Discharge plan does not contain adequate data.

Alternative Actions

- Continue to complete discharge plan, and send to referral agency.
- Verbally communicate to referral agency and discuss discharge needs of client.

- Reassess parameters of a discharge plan, and revise accordingly.
- Elicit assistance from another nurse or supervisor to revise discharge plan.

(continued)

Unexpected Outcomes	**Alternative Actions**
• Goals of discharge plan were not accomplished.	• Attempt to assess reason goals were not met. • Reformulate or revise goals so that they are mutually agreed on and more realistic. • Request assistance from expert healthcare workers or in-service consultant.
• Discharge referral plan is not implemented and client receives no referral notice before discharge.	• Attempt to contact other referral agencies to provide continuity of care for client. • Notify physician and discharge coordinator (if available) of necessity of providing follow-through care after discharge.

Chapter Wrap-Up

GERONTOLOGIC Considerations

Teaching Strategies

Memory changes occur with the older adult population.

- There is better short-term memory with auditory rather than visual presentation of information.
- Structure should be brief and simple.
- Repetition is important.
- Older clients learn better by doing, using multiple senses, than by reading instructions.
- Memory is better for things considered important.
- Clients remember best what is told *first*.
- Declining mentation is not inevitable with aging, but some memory loss is usual.

Retention facts that underlie teaching strategies. People remember:

- 5% to 10% of what they read.
- 10% to 20% of what they hear.
- 30% to 50% of what they hear and verbalize.
- 70% of what they verbalize and write.
- 90% of what they say as they perform a task.

Interventions for teaching the older adult:

- Speak distinctly and sit close to the learner.
- Face the learner so that lip reading can supplement hearing.
- Use visual aids and verbal teaching.
- Decrease extraneous noise.
- Use printed materials with large type and high contrast.
- Limit use of blue, green, and violet illustrations. Use red.
- Avoid totally dark room for audiovisual presentations.

- Increase time allowed for psychomotor skills, and allow time for repetition.
- Slow the pace of presentation.
- Give small amounts of information at one time.
- Use analogies and examples to explain information. Mnemonic devices are helpful to compensate for imperfect memory.
- Establish attainable short-term goals.
- Encourage participation in goal setting and planning.
- Integrate new behaviors with previously learned ones.
- Focus on problem solving, not just delivery of facts.
- Apply teaching to the present situation.
- Bolster self-esteem and self-confidence in self-care.
- Stress the "why" of what is presented.
- Recognize that the older adult client may prefer to be alone when learning.
- Make follow-up phone calls, if indicated, to check on the client, reinforce teaching, or to clarify any misunderstanding.

Discharge Planning

A discharge plan for the older adult contains some of the same components as a plan for a younger adult; at every step in the plan, however, the coordinator must remember that this is an older adult individual and he or she must be evaluated for the ability and resources to manage at home. Include family and/or caregiver in discharge planning. This is especially so if the older adult individual lives alone or with another older adult individual. Following are several issues that the discharge planner must consider when formulating the plan:

- Was the individual functioning independently at home before hospitalization, and is it realistic to expect him or her to do so again?
- Does this individual have capable family or friend resources to assist with functioning in the home (in addition to the necessary professional resources)?
- What is the baseline health status of the individual (assuming he or she recovers from the current hospitalization), and does this status allow for independent functioning after hospitalization?
- What are the long-term financial resources of the older adult individual and do special measures need to be initiated for coverage?
- If the older adult individual cannot return to the facility he or she was in before hospitalization, what special arrangements need to be made?

- Special considerations the discharge planner must take into account when coordinating a plan for an older adult individual. For example:
  1. Does the individual have a hearing or visual impairment that interferes with learning?
  2. Does the teaching need to be done in written form (not just verbal)?
  3. Would a return demonstration of care procedures by the home health nurse be beneficial after the client has returned home?
  4. Will the anxiety level of the client to be discharged interfere with understanding and learning?
  5. Is the health status of the client a way of gaining attention? If so, this need should be separated from the needs of self-care after discharge. It is important to convey this need to the follow-up caregiver.

MANAGEMENT Guidelines

Each state legislates a Nurse Practice Act for RNs and LVN/LPNs. Healthcare facilities are responsible for establishing and implementing policies and procedures that conform to their state's regulations. Verify the regulations and role parameters for each healthcare worker in your facility.

Delegation

- RNs must develop the teaching and discharge plans based on the assessment of client needs. The Nurse Practice Act sets the standards for who assesses and plans client care. Multidisciplinary team input is critical and a major component of both plans. The nurse is usually the coordinator of most client care plans and teaching plans.
- Once the teaching and discharge plans have been developed, other members of the healthcare team may participate in implementing them.
- LVN/LPNs follow the guidelines established in the teaching plans. They can assist with the discharge plans;

however, an RN must write the discharge referral summary and communicate with the referring agency.

Interprofessional Communication

The teaching plan should be developed in concert with the client and family. Mutually acceptable goals should be established with realistic time frames.

- The teaching plan is initiated early in the hospitalization. It must be written because it is a permanent part of the client record. It is updated as goals are achieved.
- Team members are kept apprised of the progress toward meeting the teaching goals by updates during shift report.
- Client information is disseminated between referral agencies and the hospital through a written discharge summary and/or referral sheet. The data in the summary include pertinent information on the hospitalization and the condition at discharge, the medications and treatments the client is to continue to take, and specific equipment required for client care.

CASE STUDY Applications

Scenario 1

Mr. John Johanson, age 58, was admitted to the medical unit with a diagnosis of heart failure. He is African American, 5'7", and weighs 260 pounds. He is a cross-country truck driver. He lives alone when not working. He usually watches TV and eats fast foods or frozen dinners. This is his second hospital admission in the last month. His vital signs are BP 230/108, P 108 and irregular, R 36. He has bibasilar rales and a 3+ pitting edema of the lower extremities. His point of maximal impulse (PMI) is at the sixth intercostal space (ICS), midaxillary line. He states he is short of breath

and has had difficulty ambulating the last few days. He states he has tried to lose weight but even after dieting, he gains more weight back. When asked about his smoking habits, he states he knows he is not supposed to smoke and he has tried to stop, but with his work it is too difficult because he is alone so much. He states he is on blood pressure drugs, but unsure of the name.

1. Identify the current nursing diagnoses by priority and provide rationale for answers.
2. From these data, identify the teaching needs by priority and develop a teaching plan for Mr. Johanson.

3. Are there any cultural considerations that need to be taken into account when considering his teaching plan? If so, identify actions you will take relative to the cultural considerations.

4. Briefly outline how you will determine when it is appropriate to initiate the teaching plan.

5. Describe the discharge plan you might develop for Mr. Johanson.

Scenario 2

A very young mother brings a 6-month-old child to the emergency room and tells the triage nurse that she does not know what is wrong with her child, but the child does not seem to be "normal." The child is assessed by the pediatrician and is admitted for further testing. The pediatrician's admitting diagnosis is *failure to thrive*. The child's weight is only 5 pounds over birth weight (7 lb 2 oz), and the child is still not turning over from back to front. As the admitting nurse, you need to begin the discharge plan and the teaching plan. Based on the limited information from the physician and the admitting diagnosis, complete the following scenario:

1. What information will you need to obtain before you can plan for discharge?

2. What information is necessary to obtain before you can develop a teaching plan?

3. What approach will you take with the mother in order to obtain the necessary information for both the discharge and teaching plan?

4. Describe the nurse's role in client teaching for this mother.

NCLEX® Review Questions

Unless otherwise specified, choose only one (1) answer.

1. Which healthcare team member (HCT) usually assumes the leadership role in directing the educational plan for the client and/or family?
   A. Physician
   B. Healthcare member whose role represents the greatest teaching need requiring education
   C. Discharge planner
   D. Nurse

2. Which client with high-risk factors at discharge usually requires specific instructions?
   A. Client living alone
   B. Client with multisystem issues
   C. Small child
   D. Client with a job requiring immediate return to work

3. Data for which one of the personal characteristics below are least necessary to obtain when planning for client teaching?
   A. Educational level
   B. Family composition and living situations
   C. Ethnic group
   D. Employment/occupation

4. It is imperative the client's family participate in teaching activities. What actions would *not be used* to determine their ability and willingness to participate?
   A. Assessment of cognitive ability to understand instructions
   B. Assessment of how long and how often they visit the client
   C. Evaluation of the extent of active participation of family during instruction
   D. Evaluation of interactions between client and family

5. You have been assigned to develop a teaching plan for a client being discharged after a laparoscopic procedure for gallbladder removal. What is your priority intervention?
   A. Assess the home environment for specialized equipment needs.
   B. Determine when the client plans to return to work.
   C. Determine who will be at home with the client after discharge.
   D. Assess the client's usual lifestyle and daily activities.

6. You are developing the strategy for an initial teaching plan for a 24-year-old client admitted with newly diagnosed acute leukemia. Which factor is *least* important as you develop the initial teaching plan?
   A. Attention span and retention ability
   B. Reading level
   C. Input from client on how he or she learns best
   D. Support for client at home

7. How do nurses evaluate the effectiveness of teaching strategies?
   Select all that apply.
   A. Ask the client to do a return demonstration of the skill being discussed.
   B. Have the client take a post-test of the teaching content.
   C. Ask pertinent questions relative to the teaching content.
   D. Summarize the teaching content they presented.
   E. Clarify misinformation after each teaching session.

8. A client becomes very agitated and hostile when you approach him to begin client teaching for discharge. Which one of the actions would *not* be an appropriate action by the nurse?
   A. Begin the teaching and explain you are required to complete the teaching.
   B. Attempt to determine the reason for the agitation and hostility.

C. Do not begin the teaching program but explain that you will return later.

D. Ask another nurse to assist you in assessing the reason why the client is refusing the teaching.

9. In documentation for discharge, which of the following would you include?

Select all that apply.

A. Summary of vital signs during hospitalization, including latest vital signs

B. Description of the activity level of the client during hospitalization

C. Summary of the teaching plan and client's response to teaching

D. Summary of nursing interventions provided during hospitalization

E. Intake and output findings during hospitalization

10. Gerontologic considerations for client education should include which one of the following concepts for older clients?

A. Older adults learn best by reading material.

B. They remember 30% to 50% of what they read.

C. Older adults need extraneous noises decreased while teaching is being presented.

D. Older adults learn best in group settings.

QSEN Activity

Domain: Safety

KSA: Role-Play Knowledge

Activity:

Engage the client and appropriate family member (one who will care for client at home) in discharge planning conference. The client fell at home and has been hospitalized; following the fall, she sustained a fractured hip. The client refused to go to the rehabilitation facility. She is being discharged home after seven days in the hospital. She must use a walker at home.

- Outline the necessary information required for client discharge with emphases on safety.
- Discharge information should concentrate on safety factors: house changes that need to be made for safety, physical therapy activities, bathing activities, use of walker in house, and medication administration.
- Provide rationale for discussing this content in discharge planning meeting.

Bibliography

Agency for Healthcare Research and Quality. (2014, Nov.). Health literacy measurement tools (revised): Fact sheet. Rockville, MD: Author. Retrieved from http://www.ahrq.gov/professionals/quality-patient-safety/quality-resources/tools/literacy/index.html

American Hospital Association. (2006–2009). *Understanding expectations: The patient care partnership.* Chicago: AHA Press.

Arozullah, A. M., Yarnold, P. R., Bennett, C. L., Soltysik, R. C., Wolf, M. S., Ferreira, R. M., … Davis, T. (2007, Nov.). Development and validation of a short-form, rapid estimate of adult literacy in medicine. *Med Care 2007,* 45(11): 1026–1033. PMID: 18049342

Artz, M., Conant, R., & Lennox, C. (2006, Jan.). The politics of caring: The Patient Safety Act of 2005 is reintroduced. *American Journal of Nursing,* 106(1), 36.

Baker, L., Wagner, T. H., Singer, S., & Bundorf, M. K. (2003). Use of the Internet and e-mail for health care information: Results from a national survey. *JAMA,* 289(18), 2400–2406.

Carroll, P. (2008, Jun.). The transition to home care. *NurseWeek, West* 5(14), 28–31.

Center for Healthcare Research & Transformation. (2014, Jan. 15). Care transitions: Best practices and evidence-based programs: CHRT policy paper.

Chaboyer, W., James, H., & Kendall, M. (2005). Transitional care after the intensive care unit. *Critical Care Nurse,* 25(3), 16.

Chapman, L. (2007, May). Discharge planning: A family affair. *Nursing,* 37(5), 56hn12–56hn14.

Craig, K., & Hopkins-Pepe, L. (2006). Understanding the new AHA guidelines, part II. *Nursing,* 36(5), 52.

Effective Patient Teaching. Retrieved from http://uuhsc.utah.edu/pated/authors/teaching.html

Family Caregiver Alliance: National Center on Caregiving. (2009). Hospital discharge planning: A guide for families and caregivers. Retrieved from https://caregiver.org/hospital-discharge-planning-guide-families-and-caregivers.

Graf, C. (2008a, Apr.). The Lawton instrumental activities of daily living scale. *American Journal of Nursing,* 108(4), 52–62.

Graf, C. (2008b, Aug.). The hospital admission risk profile. *American Journal of Nursing,* 108(8), 62–71.

Jencks, F. J., Williams, M. V., & Coleman, E. A. (2009). Rehospitalization among patients in the Medicare fee-for-service program. *The New England Journal of Medicine,* 360 (14), 1418–1428.

Knowles, M. (1970). *The modern practice of adult education: Andragogy versus pedagogy.* New York: The Association Press.

Leaffer T. & Gonda B. (2000). The internet: An underutilized tool in patient education. *Computers in Nursing* 18(1):47-52.

Mascioli, S., Laskowski-Jones, L., Urban, S., & Moran, S. (2009). Improving handoff communication. *Nursing,* 39(2), 52–55.

Ray, L. (2009). A ticket to ride protects patients off the unit. *Nursing,* 39(5), 57–58.

The Joint Commission. (2008). Hand-off communications. NPSG.02.05.01

The Joint Commission. (2010a). National patient safety goals. Retrieved from http://jointcommission.org/PatientSafety/NationalSafetyGoals

The Joint Commission. (2010b). Provision of care, treatment, and services. Retrieved from http://www.jointcommission.org/AccreditationPrograms/BehavioralHealthCare

The Joint Commission. (2014). *Comprehensive accreditation manual for hospital: The official handbook. JCAHO patient and family education (PFE) 2015 standards.* Oakbrook Terrace, IL: Author.

Ward, J. (2013, May). Patient education: A guide for nurses. Retrieved from http://www.nursetogether.com/patient-education-guide-nurses#sthash.9VKWXiAI.dpuf

Chapter 7
Safe Client Environment and Restraints

 Learning Objectives

7.1 Define the term *adaptation*.

7.2 Describe three characteristics that influence adaptation.

7.3 Outline four sociocultural dimensions of environmental adaptation.

7.4 State two nursing diagnoses relevant to maintaining a safe environment.

7.5 Outline the objectives for providing a safe environment.

7.6 Describe how client-centered care (QSEN competencies) supports client safety.

7.7 Describe The Joint Commission National Patient Safety Goals and application in nursing practice.

7.8 Identify clients who are at high risk for falls.

7.9 Demonstrate two methods of client evacuation when a fire occurs in a nursing unit.

7.10 List the guidelines for providing safety when clients are receiving radioactive materials.

7.11 Describe nursing actions for clients with seizure activity.

7.12 List and briefly describe at least four guidelines for using restraints to prevent mechanical injuries.

7.13 Demonstrate the application of wrist restraints.

7.14 Demonstrate the application of a torso/belt restraint.

7.15 List the components that should be included when charting for application of restraints.

7.16 Describe the Home Assessment Checklist.

Chapter Outline

Terminology

Adaptation ability of an organism to adjust to a change in environment.

Ambiance the pervading atmosphere of the surrounding environment.

Ambulation to move from place to place by walking.

Arousal state of responsiveness to sensory stimulation or excitability.

Aseptic sterile; free from bacteria and infection.

Assessment critical evaluation of information; the first step in the nursing process.

Awareness condition of being alert and cognizant of one's surroundings and external activity as well as one's personal state.

Behavior an individual's total activity—actions or reactions; especially conduct that can be observed.

Chemical restraint use of a sedating psychotropic drug to manage or control behavior.

Contaminated waste radioactive waste, which, if improperly disposed of, may be harmful or cause a radiation hazard.

Decibel a unit for measuring difference in acoustic signals; a unit of intensity and volume of sound.

Ecosystem the biological and physical dimensions of the environment that refers to all living and nonliving elements.

Epidemiologist one who studies the causes, distribution, and frequency of disease outbreaks in a human community.

Healthcare-acquired infection (HAI) (formerly termed nosocomial) infection or disease originating in a hospital.

Homeostasis a state of equilibrium of the internal environment.

Hygiene pertinent to a state of health and its preservation.

Licensed independent practitioner (LIP) an individual licensed by the state or institution who is permitted to provide and monitor conscious sedation to clients and order restraints or seclusion. This practitioner is either a healthcare provider, dentist, advanced nurse practitioner, or physician's assistant.

Limitation the state of being limited or restricted.

National Patient Safety Goals (NPSGs) national standards to promote client safety in healthcare settings. Goals change in response to Joint Commission findings and recommendations from national healthcare stakeholders.

Nosocomial formerly used term for infection or disease originating in a hospital (now called hospital-acquired infection).

Physical restraint any manual method or physical or mechanical device that restricts freedom of movement or normal access to one's body, material, or equipment, attached to or adjacent to the client's body that he or she cannot easily remove. Holding a client in a manner that restricts his or her movement.

Physiologic relating to or characteristic of the normal functioning of a living organism.

Psycho prefix referring to the mind or mental processes of an individual.

Psychosocial a term that refers both to psychological and social factors.

QSEN an acronym for Quality and Safety Education in Nursing.

Restraint any involuntary method (chemical or physical) of restricting an individual's freedom or movement, physical activity, or normal access to the body.

Root cause analysis a process for examining the reasons an error occurs and suggesting changes to the system that can prevent the incident from happening again in the future.

Seclusion the isolation of a client in a special room to decrease stimuli that might be causing or exacerbating the client's emotional distress, free from objects that could cause the client harm.

Sentinel event any unexpected occurrence involving death or serious physical or psychological injury or the risk thereof.

Sociocultural a term that refers both to society and culture.

Stress any emotional, physical, social, economic, or other factor that requires a response or change.

Therapeutic having healing or curative powers.

Thermal pertaining to using, producing, or caused by heat.

Orientation to the Client Environment

Maintaining Homeostasis

As a nurse, one of your primary responsibilities is to make sure your clients have a safe and comfortable health-care environment. It is your responsibility to help clients adapt to this environment as well as to their health care in general.

From a holistic view, the term *environment* can generally be explained as the total of all conditions and influences, both external and internal, that affect the life and development of an organism. As human beings we are constantly exposed to changing physical, biological, and social conditions. To survive, we continually assess our relationship to our changing surroundings. We also learn how to make adjustments that help us control and improve our environment. This complex process is called **adaptation**.

Adaptation includes psychological and **physiologic** adjustments. People in most situations are able to control or adapt to their immediate surroundings. Although no two people respond to the environment in exactly the same way, common principles related to adaptation can be found in all human beings:

- All adaptations are attempts to maintain optimum physical and chemical states, or **homeostasis**.
- Individuals retain their own identity and uniqueness regardless of the degree of adaptation required.
- Adaptation affects all aspects of human existence.
- Human beings have limits in the process and degree of their adaptation.
- Adaptation is measured in relationship to time.
- Adaptive responses to the environment may or may not be adequate or appropriate.
- Adaptive attempts may be stressful.
- The degree and process of adaptation varies from individual to individual.
- Adaptation is an ongoing process about which the individual may be consciously or unconsciously aware.

Each of us adjusts to our immediate environment in a way that is unique to us. When this environment changes suddenly, for instance when we are hospitalized, we may not be able to adapt independently to our immediate surroundings safely and comfortably. It is at this point that assistance must be provided.

Characteristics That Influence Adaptation

The characteristics that make all people unique also provide information about the process of adaptation to the environment. These factors must be considered when assessing clients' needs and abilities to safely adjust to their immediate surroundings.

Age

A client's age is a critical factor in the **assessment** process. Because terms such as *elderly* and *young* can be interpreted in many different ways, the nurse may need to look at the client's developmental stage (physical and mental growth) rather than at the client's chronologic age.

As people develop, sensory receptors help process day-to-day events. Human beings learn how to protect themselves and how to adjust to changing needs through experiencing these events. During the learning process, young children may require entirely different protection than teenagers. Even a 30-year-old man who has learned through experience how to protect himself in a routine environment may not have adequate skills in an unfamiliar atmosphere.

The older adult often requires special assistance. Sensory and motor changes, such as slowness of movement, postural instability, decreased vision or hearing, and even diminished acuity for taste and touch, are not uncommon. These changes can result in an altered ability to sense and adapt to harmful environmental stimuli. The older adult may not see or hear an approaching car, detect the taste of spoiling food, or move quickly enough to avoid falling.

Experiences of hospitals and health care vary significantly among individuals. Perception of health care and ability to adapt may be influenced by previous experiences, such as seeing a family member in the hospital, or past outcomes from illness.

Mental Status

The ability to perceive and react to environmental stimuli is closely related to mental status. Adapting to a new or different environment requires learning through experience and possessing a cognitive **awareness** of the immediate surroundings. Making adjustments to the environment requires stimuli to travel over the sensory pathways of nerves to the central nervous system. To respond to stimuli, such as avoiding a burn from a hot object, motor neurons carry impulses to muscles to cause an involuntary reflex action, such as withdrawing the hand from hot water. Sensory impulses traveling to the cerebral cortex of the brain inform the individual that this stimulus is potentially harmful. Voluntary movement then provides additional adaptation.

Consciousness is the state in which individuals are aware of themselves and their relationship to their surroundings. Consciousness is sometimes described as two components: awareness and **arousal**. Unconsciousness indicates a lack of awareness and inability to cognitively respond to the environment. Levels of consciousness range from fully conscious to nonresponsive. Difficulty in adapting to the immediate environment due to alterations in mental status can manifest itself in a variety of ways:

- Confused clients often view their environment in a distorted way. This condition can lead to extreme behavioral changes, injury, or combativeness.
- Neurologically injured clients may have decreased perception of stimuli such as heat, cold, pain, or friction. In extreme cases, they may have no perception of any stimuli.

- Paralysis inhibits movement and is accompanied by a loss of position sense (dangling limbs or poor body alignment).
- Alterations in communication, sight, or hearing are barriers to identifying hazards and sharing fears or concerns with others.
- Fluctuating levels of consciousness create difficulty in promoting self-care and self-image.

Continuous assessment of changes in the client's ability to relate and adapt to the environment is essential. Ability to adapt to the environment or illness influences the type and amount of assistance the client needs, especially while in less than familiar surroundings.

States of Illness

Illness or injury causes an individual to focus more intensely on himself or herself. The very nature of disease or trauma (psychological and physical) requires the individual to use physical and mental energy to adapt to the situation and to become more egocentric. A client often cannot perform even the simplest daily activity. Fatigue or pain may render clients helpless. Assistance with activities, such as bathing, eating, skin care, and elimination, may be necessary.

Similarly, family members may also become increasingly focused on the client's condition because of fear, financial and scheduling challenges, and additional responsibilities. Ability or willingness to provide support or assistance to the client may vary as circumstances and stressors change. The client may or may not be aware of the family's responses and concerns, since both parties may find it difficult to communicate.

Some medications produce such side effects as drowsiness, which prevent the individual from adequately assessing the environment. Perceptions may be distorted, and the client is more vulnerable to hazards.

Emotional **stress** and anxiety can be mild to severe and acute or chronic. Although mild anxiety very often increases perceptual awareness, severe anxiety reduces perceptual awareness.

Because an individual is able to focus only on a specific amount of stimuli at one time, additional stimuli that may be equally important are not perceived. Potential environmental dangers are not processed. The client whose energy is focused on pain may not even hear instructions from the nurse. Depressed clients also require assistance. Depression often results in slower than normal responses to stimuli, decreased ability to concentrate, and impaired memory. Alcohol, a central nervous system depressant, also causes dull, slow reactions to stimuli.

When pain, anxiety, illness, injury, weakness, medications, or even lack of sleep cause a decrease in sensory acuity, awareness of potential hazards is altered. The client may not be able to make the necessary biological, physical, or emotional adjustments to adapt to the immediate environment. Any of these conditions necessitates immediate assessment and action.

Physical and Biological Dimensions

The influences that make up an environment include the basic categories of biological and physical conditions, and the third dimension termed **sociocultural**. The biological dimensions of our environment covered in this section include all living things, such as plants, animals, and microorganisms. Water, oxygen, sunlight, organic compounds, and other components in which living things exist and develop make up the physical dimensions of an environment.

As the nurse becomes more aware of the factors that affect environmental adaptation, a safe and comfortable atmosphere for the clients becomes a greater challenge. As you assess your clients and help them adapt to the environment of a healthcare facility, you should consider the following essential elements: space, lighting, humidity, temperature, ventilation, sound levels and volume and amount of noise including talking, surfaces and equipment, safety, food, water, and waste disposal.

Adequate Space

Everyone needs space in which to grow and develop. This space may consist of a room or an area as small as a shelf or corner. No matter what form space takes, individuals need to feel they have control over it—that they can arrange it or decorate it to their liking (Figure 7-1 ■).

Providing space for clients encourages stimulation and experimentation. Toddlers need the space of an area like a recreation room for discovery and motor skills, since playtime is their primary source of development. Adults often enjoy the social activities of a lounge but may also require well-defined personal areas, even if these areas are as simple as a bedside table or a bulletin board.

FIGURE 7-1 Provide a comfortable environment with space for personal effects.

Natural and Artificial Light

Light, like space, is necessary for growth and development. The production of vitamin D, a critical component of bone metabolism, occurs from ultraviolet radiation on the skin. Natural light also assists in wound healing. In a hospital setting, natural light can be used to decrease feelings of isolation and to encourage clients to continue their normal routine, including sleep patterns.

Whether natural or artificial, adequate light is essential for the preservation of sight, for safety, and for accurate assessments and nursing care. Because eye strain, as well as nervousness and fatigue, can result from improper lighting, care should be taken to avoid glare, sharp contrast, and flickering lights. For the older adult, night lights promote safety and orientation to the environment, as does the availability of personal assistive devices such as canes, glasses, or magnifying glasses.

Humidity and Temperature

The ability to adapt to changes in humidity or temperature is directly related to comfort. Most people in this country are comfortable at a room temperature of between 18.3° and 25°C (65°–77°F) with the humidity at 30% to 60%. People in other cultures function equally well at lower or higher readings.

Conditions that may inhibit an individual's ability to adjust to high temperatures include excessive physical work, dehydration, many medical conditions, extremes in age (the very young and very old), decreased physical fitness, and inappropriate clothing. An individual who has difficulty adapting to high temperatures may experience a rapid rise in pulse rate, cramps, nausea, and vomiting. Severe inability to adapt to heat can result in heatstroke and death.

An individual who has difficulty adapting to lower temperatures may experience a change in behavior, depressed vital signs, and eventual unconsciousness. Hypothermia, or abnormally low body temperature, occurs when there is an imbalance between heat loss and heat production.

Extremes of heat or cold increase the incidence of infection and add to discomfort. Temperatures in healthcare institutions can be regulated with air conditioners and dehumidifiers, although care should be taken to avoid drafts and excessive moisture or dryness. As hospitals are being redesigned, clients are being provided the opportunity to manage their own room temperature.

Ventilation

Particular attention should be given to assessing the movement of air within a client's immediate environment. An adequately ventilated room should contain a comfortable amount of moisture; be free of irritating pollutants, odors, or noxious fumes; and be at a tolerable temperature.

Adequate ventilation is especially important when more than one client is in a room. Other areas requiring optimum ventilation are operating rooms, delivery rooms, nurseries, isolation rooms, and sterile supply rooms.

A properly functioning ventilation system reduces airborne contaminants by regulating the amount of air movement within an enclosed area. When ventilation cannot be maintained by using doors and windows, mechanical devices, such as fans or air conditioners, may be used. However, personal use fans carry the risk of dispersing microorganisms and drying the environment.

Clients requiring airborne isolation are placed in private rooms where the ventilation system is a directional air flow negative-pressure ventilation system. Six to 12 air exchanges per hour occur with this system.

Comfortable Sound Levels

Noise can be defined as any undesirable sound. The intensity and kind of noise that is comfortable is highly individual and related to past experiences. A businessman who lives on a busy street in a city may not adjust well to the quiet he may experience at night in a hospital room. On the other hand, a farmer from a rural community may be disturbed by the slightest sound. Infants often sleep peacefully in an atmosphere of loud noise and activity.

Decibel is the unit for measuring the intensity of noise. At close range, noise produced from heavy traffic, for example, has a decibel measure of 90, whereas a whisper at 3 feet has an intensity of 20 decibels.

At certain levels noise is considered hazardous. Temporary or permanent hearing loss or damage can occur when noise is present for a prolonged time at intensities over 90 decibels. Other effects of sustained loud noise are muscle tension, increased blood pressure, blood vessel constriction, pallor, increased secretion of the adrenal hormone, and nervous tension.

The pitch, quality, and duration of noise may also affect the client's environment. Unwanted sounds produced by sirens, traffic, and aircraft are often beyond the control of the nurse. But noise within a hospital setting, such as television, call systems, careless handling of dishes and other equipment, visitors, excessive conversation at the nurses' station or outside client rooms, and some care-related sounds (e.g., beeping monitors) can be controlled.

Nursing personnel should always be aware of the noise level and its effects on the clients' well-being. Very ill individuals are often more sensitive to excessive or meaningless stimuli. Certain sounds can be reassuring because they represent activity or assistance to the client.

Furniture: Bed Safety

Today, most healthcare facilities are designed to be attractive, orderly, efficient, and clean. Since an individual's outlook is strongly influenced by the surroundings, careful attention to appearance and cleanliness can assist with adjustment to the healthcare environment. Although it is essential to assess the routines and standards of cleanliness of each client, the nurse may also have to teach the client how to organize and clean up. In some cases, instruction to the client may be critical to maintaining or improving a healthcare condition.

The standards and routine cleaning procedures of the hospital are generally not a nursing function now because hospital housekeeping has become a specialized occupation. Maintaining an organized, clean environment, however, requires coordination by all healthcare providers.

Furnishings should be arranged to be physically safe, comfortable, aesthetically appealing for the client, and easily cleaned. Hospital furnishings are being designed for ease of cleaning by incorporating flat surfaces with few crevices. Adequate cleaning of the room should be done at a time of day that is coordinated with the client's needs so that the resulting sense of security adds to the client's ability to adapt adequately to the surroundings. Cleanliness and a feeling of order contribute to the client's sense of well-being (Figure 7-2 ■).

Hospital beds are adjustable in height from the floor; when the bed is in LOW position, the client can more easily and safely get in or out of it; when it is in HIGH position, the nursing staff can more efficiently render care. The head and sometimes the knee areas of the bed can be elevated or lowered; this is accomplished by electric controls. The electric controls are found on the foot, the side of the bed, or on the side rails. When placed at the side, the client can more easily control bed positions. Bed wheels are equipped with locks and kept in locked position.

For many years, side rails have provided what everyone thought was safe nursing care, protecting clients from injury as a result of falling out of bed. Changes have occurred in both long-term care and acute-care settings regarding the use of side rails. The Center for Medicare and Medicaid Services (CMS), the Food and Drug Administration (FDA), and the Joint Commission (TJC) have established guidelines and standards to decrease the routine use of side rails which in some cases are considered a form of **restraint**. There is still controversy over the safety of side rails. Appropriately placed half-rails function as assistive devices, helping clients transfer from bed to chair or wheelchair. Older adult clients

and those with altered mental status are at high risk for injury when side rails are routinely used. Many falls occur as clients attempt to climb over side rails. As a result, many beds are equipped with alarm systems that alert staff that clients are getting out of bed. However, due to the potential for alarm fatigue of staff, bed alarms may not always be effective.

A half- or quarter-length upper side rail is not considered a restraint if the client uses it as an aid for moving in and out of bed. A full-length or four half-length rails are not considered restraints if the client requests them in order to feel more secure and if he or she is able to lower them by himself or herself before getting into or out of bed (Figure 7-3 ■).

Nurses must assess appropriateness for side rail use for each client and inform both client and family of benefits and risks for their use. These assessments must be completed according to hospital policies and procedures to ensure that client is not at risk for injury if they are in use.

Additional Furniture

The overbed table is adjustable in height and slides over the bed to provide space for self-care activities or additional working surface for the nurse. The overbed table may also be used when the client sits in a chair. Small bed trays are sometimes convenient when the overbed table cannot be used.

The bedside table, similar to a nightstand, holds the client's personal possessions in drawers. A cabinet section in the table can be used to store bathing or toiletry equipment, and the top provides space for the client's familiar items, such as pictures or books.

A chair with firm back and arm supports should always be a part of the client's furnishings. Chairs should be made of durable, easily cleanable materials, such as plastic or other synthetic material. The client should be instructed to avoid contact between skin surfaces and the chair when sitting in a chair. A small towel or blanket can be placed under the client for this purpose.

A signaling system is also essential for the client to call for assistance (Figure 7-4 ■). A signaling system may be an

FIGURE 7-2 In the client's room, a pleasant environment promotes a sense of well-being.

FIGURE 7-3 Half-length side rails can be requested by clients to use as an assistive device.

FIGURE 7-4 Ensure that call light or other summoning device is within easy reach of client to provide access to nursing staff.

intercom, buzzer, electric light, or hand bell. Whatever device is available must be within the client's reach and ability to use.

Food and Water

Fresh, nourishing food and clean water are vital to recovering and maintaining health and must be planned for and provided in appropriate amounts in healthcare facilities. A client's well-being can be positively affected by the ingestion of the correct number of calories, fat, proteins, carbohydrates, minerals, vitamins, and water, but it is well known that many people have nutritional habits that can negatively affect their well-being. A careful nutritional assessment and referral for dietary evaluation (if indicated) is a critical step in helping the client adjust to the environment.

Hazardous Products and Waste Management

All waste products, whether contaminated equipment, blood or body fluid, **contaminated waste**, garbage, soiled dressings, refuse, or hazardous products, must be handled and disposed of in a way that prevents risk for injury or illness.

Nurses must be aware of potential dangers to themselves as well as to their clients when handling and disposing of hazardous materials. Just a few of the hazardous chemicals that nurses and other healthcare workers may be exposed to include disinfectants, such as isopropyl alcohol and iodine; sterilizing agents, such as formaldehyde and ethylene oxide; and anesthetic waste gases, such as nitrous oxide and halothane (Fluothane). Antineoplastic agents used in cancer treatment may also pose a hazard even when proper prevention policies and procedures are in place.

The OSHA Hazard Communication Standard requires that chemical manufacturers, distributors, and importers provide Safety Data Sheets (formerly Material Safety Data Sheets) for each hazardous chemical to "downstream" users to communicate information about hazards. Safety Data Sheets (Table 7-1 ■) contain much of the same information as Material Safety Data Sheets but utilize a 16-section standardized format that is user friendly. Some sections establish consistency with the UN Globally Harmonized System of Classification and Labeling of Chemicals. The Safety Data Sheets contain information such as identification, first aid measures, and handling and storage requirements. They must be readily available for employees to access. Figure 7-5 ■ shows a safety plan in the EHR.

Table 7-1 Safety Data Sheets

Section Number and Title	Section Description
Section 1: Identification	Product identifier on label, manufacturer, etc.; information, recommended use of chemical
Section 2: Hazard(s) Identification	Hazard classification; flammable, liquid Hazard statement and precautions Pictogram
Section 3: Composition/Information on Ingredients	Chemical name and common names, concentration of ingredients; Health risks associated with concentration levels
Section 4: First Aid Measures	First aid by routes of exposure
Section 5: Firefighting Measures	Recommendations for fighting a fire caused by the chemical
Section 6: Accidental Release Measures	Responses recommended for spills, leaks, or releases
Section 7: Handling and Storage	Safe handling practices and safe storage
Section 8: Exposure Controls/Person Protection	Exposure limits and personal protective measures to minimize worker exposure
Section 9: Physical and Chemical Properties	Examples of information in this section: pH, flammability, solubility, and odor
Section 10: Stability and Reactivity	Reactivity hazards and chemical stability information
Section 11: Toxicological Information	Health effects of chemicals, for example, symptoms and impact of short- and long-term exposure
Section 12: Ecological Information	Environmental impact of a chemical
Section 13: Disposal Considerations	Guidance for proper disposal
Section 14: Transport Information	Guidance for shipping by road, air, rail, and sea
Section 15: Regulatory Information	Regulatory specific information not addressed elsewhere
Section 16: Other Information	When SDS was last revised and what changes have been made

Source: U.S. Department of Labor (n.d.)

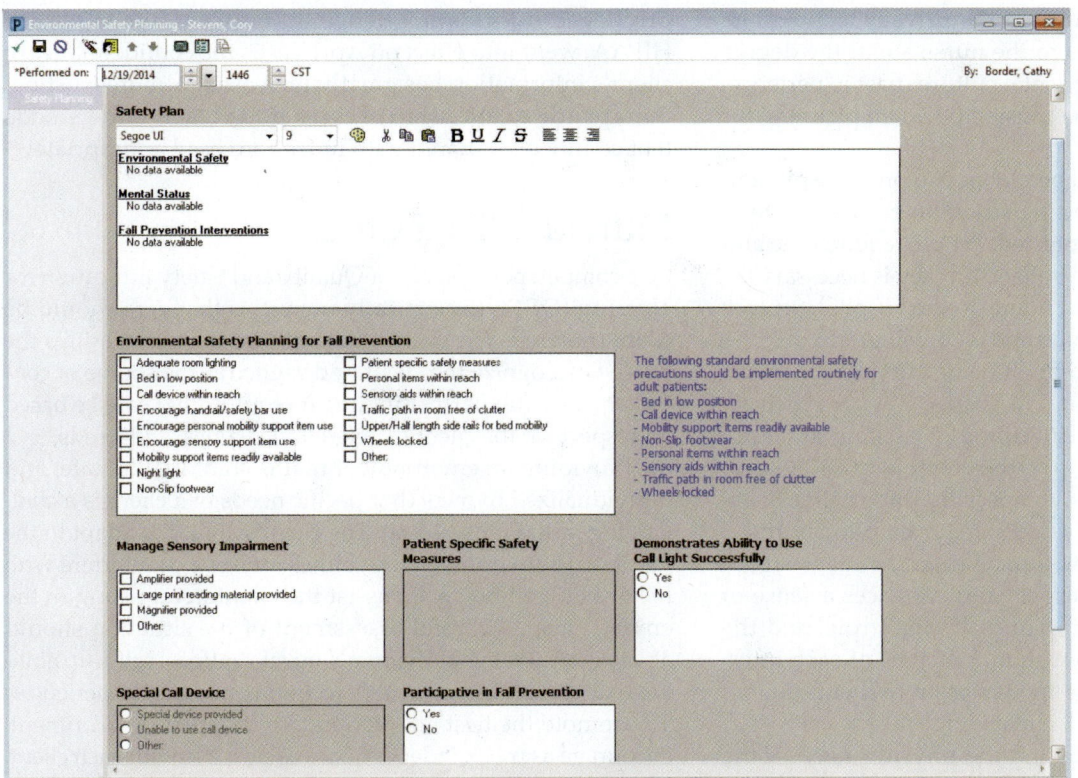

FIGURE 7-5 Safety plan. *Source:* From Cerner Electronic Health Record. © Cerner Corporation. Pearson has restricted permission to reproduce and distribute this copyrighted work. Further reproduction or distribution is strictly prohibited without written consent of Cerner Corporation.

OSHA requires hospitals to educate employees about chemical hazards and to train them in safety precautions before they work in an area where toxic agents are used. Training about hazardous chemicals is part of required initial staff development and ongoing educational updates.(Refer to Chapter 14, Infection Control, for more details on handling hazardous material.)

All hospitals identify an individual, often a nurse, responsible for infection prevention and control. That individual gathers data on the type and frequency of various infections found in the hospital and participates in infection prevention activities. Data collected helps locate the source of a problem, predict its spread, and identify the best method of preventing its recurrence. Many **healthcare-acquired infections (HAIs)** can be traced to inadvertent transmission by care providers. Each nurse plays a significant role in establishing a safe environment for the client by using standard precautions in client care and by handling and disposing of biohazards appropriately. Annual infection prevention education is required for all healthcare providers.

The infection prevention nurse plays a major role in identifying the "no pay" adverse events in hospital-acquired conditions. The identified events listed by CMS will not be reimbursed by Medicare-Medicaid. Therefore, the nurse must ensure they do not occur.

Sociocultural Dimensions

The first two dimensions of the environment, the biological and physical, or **ecosystem**, refer to all living and nonliving elements. The third dimension of an environment is sociocultural, which includes both past and present influences from the people and the culture surrounding the individual. Customs, religious and legal systems, and economic and political beliefs are all part of this environment. This dimension also involves responses and adjustments to the ideals, concepts, beliefs, activities, and pressure of various groups, such as social clubs, peer groups, or colleagues.

Organization of Time

How clients perceive and deal with time and the passing of time depends on their age, immediate situation, culture, and past experiences, as well as their present physical and emotional condition. To a mother waiting for her child to return from surgery, hours seem like days. Small children generally do not have a well-developed sense of time. A 3-year-old may act out feelings of abandonment when separated from a parent for just a few minutes. In an intensive care unit, time can be severely disrupted, since healthcare activities continue around the clock. The ability to organize time is a critical element in adaptation. Helping clients assess and plan their time is one of the most important ways you can help them cope with their new surroundings.

Privacy

Many people who enter a healthcare facility fear exposure and loss of identity. Providing privacy for a client is more than a luxury or a mere courtesy. It is necessary and vitally important to the individual's attitude toward health care.

Clients should be given as much privacy as possible. Most individuals give clues to the nurse about the degree of privacy they need. The client's culture, past experience, values, and age should all be considered when planning for privacy.

Hospital routines should be planned to promote privacy. If an embarrassing or upsetting situation occurs, the feelings of the client must be protected. People require time and space to think, organize, and reflect. Privacy is necessary for human development, even at home. In the hospital, privacy is critical to the client's attitude and well-being.

Privacy can be promoted by drawing curtains or screens (Figure 7-6 ■). Doors and window shades may also be used. Signs stating "Do Not Enter Without Checking at Desk" posted on room entrances give the client a sense of security from disturbances. This is especially important during physical examinations, personal care, or emotional upset. Knocking or asking for permission to enter the client's room or area promotes mutual respect and enhances a sense of emotional space. Introducing oneself, one's role, and the reason for entering the room should be part of each interaction. In rooms where there are two or more clients, nurses must support the needs of all clients.

Privacy also extends beyond the physical need of the individual. Health status, conversation, and records are privileged information. Since the privacy rule, a part of HIPAA, went into effect on April 2003, the confidentiality of client's information has greatly increased. A more trusting, **therapeutic** relationship evolves if the client understands that confidences shared with nurses are used appropriately.

Individualized Care

One competency domain of Quality and Safety Education for Nursing (**QSEN**) specifically identifies that care should be client centered. The client-centered care domain requires the nurse to recognize the client or designee as the source of control and as a full partner in care. It requires that care be based on respect for the client's preferences, values, and needs.

Providing an environment that is comfortable, safe, and individualized to meet the specific needs of a client is a challenging task (Figure 7-7 ■). The client's ability to adapt to the immediate environment can either improve or interfere with his or her well-being. To assist the client in adjusting to the environment, a careful assessment of the situation should always include the individual's usual routines, self-care abilities, cultural beliefs, current perceptions, and past experiences. To promote the best adaptation to a different environment, encourage as much independence as possible with each client. You may be required to use your resourcefulness, imagination,

FIGURE 7-6 Clients should be given as much privacy as possible by drawing curtains or using screens.

FIGURE 7-7 Providing an environment that is both safe and individualized is a challenging task for the nursing staff.

and ingenuity to assist the client through difficult periods. Ongoing assessment and open communication between client and staff is essential if positive adaptation is to occur.

Hospitalized clients also need emotional space. This form of space is that psychological area where the individual can experience a sense of self. This is particularly difficult to achieve in a hospital setting when caregivers exercise control over many of the activities of daily living. It is important that the staff be aware of this psychological need so that they can provide adequate privacy, quiet, and freedom of choice over all of the areas that the client can control. The staff must also be aware that the client rarely needs to relinquish total responsibility for his or her care.

Information and Teaching

The amount of information the client has about the environment and immediate situation directly affects his or her ability to adjust safely and comfortably. When the individual is given information and explanation about strange equipment, diagnostic procedures, or unfamiliar healthcare personnel, fears and feelings of helplessness can be reduced and a shared sense of responsibility enhanced. The client becomes more capable of asking questions and expressing concerns if prepared for unfamiliar occurrences and supports the model of client-centered care.

Providing the client and his or her family, if appropriate, with information about the client's environment is the responsibility of the nurse. As more people assume the role of consumers of health care, there is more demand for knowledge about aspects of health care. Including the client (and family) in planning and caring for himself or herself promotes a sense of responsibility, independence, and self-respect.

Teaching the client about various aspects of health care is one method of information sharing. Over the years, the focus

has changed from the professional staff doing everything for the client to helping the client be more independent. This change enables the client to adapt to the environment with guided assistance from nurses. As the client learns about his or her own health care and becomes involved in meeting his or her particular needs, a sense of trust, responsibility, and usefulness develops and the client participates more fully in promoting healing, health promotion, and illness prevention.

A Safe Environment

TJC and CMS are taking the lead in attempting to ensure that Americans are better protected from unsafe health care. Nurses are expected to carry a major responsibility in preventing medical errors, as they are the managers of client care. TJC is committed to improving safety for clients and residents in healthcare organizations. Many of TJC standards are directly related to safety. TJC has standards that address restraints and seclusion, environment of care (fire drills, medical equipment monitoring), physical environment, and infection-control policies, to name only a few.

TJC's mission statement indicates it is continuously trying to improve the safety and quality of care provided to the public through its accreditation standards. In 2009, **National Patient Safety Goals** (NPSGs) were published by TJC. Since then, the NPSGs have changed a number of times. The 2015 NPSGs designate which NPSGs apply for specific healthcare sites such as hospitals, ambulatory care settings, behavioral health settings, and laboratories. Hospital NPSGs include using at least two client identifiers (not the room number) when providing care in these and other healthcare situations: administering medication, identification of patients at risk for suicide, and improving communication among caregivers. Table 7-2 ■ outlines the patient safety goals that directly affect hospitals.

Table 7-2 Hospital National Patient Safety Goals 2015

Goal 1—Improve the accuracy of patient identification.
- Use at least two patient identifiers when providing care, treatment, and services (NPSG.01.01.01).
- Eliminate errors in medication and blood and blood product administration. Label specimens in presence of the client. Room number is not an acceptable identifier.

Goal 2—Improve the effectiveness of communication among caregivers.
- Report critical tests and critical results in a timely manner (NPSG.02.03.01).

Goal 3—Improve the safety of using medications.
- Label medications in procedural settings (NPSG.03.04.01).
- Reduce harm from anticoagulation therapy (NPSG.03.05.01).
- Maintain and communicate accurate client medication information (NPSG.03.06.01).

Goal 6—Reduce the harm associated with clinical alarm systems.
- Improve the safety of clinical alarm systems (NPSG.06.01.01).

Goal 7—Reduce the risk of healthcare-associated infections.
- Comply with hand **hygiene** guidelines (NPSG.07.01.01).
- Implement evidence-based practices to prevent healthcare-associated multidrug-resistant organism infections (NPSG.07.03.01).
- Prevent central line–associated bloodstream infections (NPSG.07.04.01).
- Implement evidence-based practices to prevent surgical site infections (NPSG.07.05.01).
- Prevent catheter-associated urinary tract infections (NPSG. 07.06.01).

Goal 15—The hospital identifies safety risks inherent in its patient population.
- Identify individuals at risk for suicide (NPSG.15.01.01).

Note: Client safety goals that directly affect hospitals. Goals no longer on the current NPSG list have become "Standards of Care." For complete description of Home Care National Patient Safety Goals, refer to the list available on The Joint Commission website.

In addition to NPSGs, TJC has introduced the Universal Protocol for Preventing Wrong Site, Wrong Procedure, and Wrong Person Surgery. Goals no longer on the current NPSG list have become "Standards of Care."

Sentinel Events

In 1996, TJC implemented a policy to address sentinel events. TJC defines a **sentinel event** as "an unexpected occurrence involving death or serious physical or psychological injury, or the risk thereof" and includes serious injuries such as loss of limb or function (Box 7-1 ■). Sentinel events can occur in facilities across the healthcare spectrum from psychiatric hospitals to emergency departments to long-term care facilities to office-based surgeries (Table 7-3 ■). Most reporting of sentinel events to TJC is voluntary. Organizations have policies about sentinel events that require immediate investigation and response including a root cause analysis to identify systems and processes that contributed to the event (Box 7-2 ■). A **root cause analysis** examines the reasons the error occurred and suggests changes to the system that can prevent the incident from happening again in the future. The majority of sentinel events usually have multiple root causes including leadership issues such as organizational planning and prioritization, communication and human factors, assessment, physical environment, and information management.

Box 7-1 THE JOINT COMMISSION SENTINEL EVENTS

According to TJC, the following events are considered sentinel events:

- Incidents that involve unexpected death or major permanent loss of function not related to the natural course of the client's condition
- Any of the following incidents, even if the outcome was not death or major permanent loss of function:

  1. Suicide of a client receiving around-the-clock care or within 72 hours of discharge
  2. Unanticipated death of a full-term infant
  3. Abduction of any patient receiving care, treatment, and services
  4. Discharge of an infant to the wrong family member
  5. Medication error resulting in major permanent loss of function or death
  6. Rape, assault (leading to death or permanent loss of function), or homicide of any patient receiving care, treatment, and services

7. Rape, assault (leading to death or permanent loss of function), or homicide of a staff member, **licensed independent practitioner**, visitor, or vendor while on site at the healthcare organization
8. Hemolytic transfusion reaction involving administration of blood or blood products having major blood group incompatibilities
9. Invasive procedure, including surgery, on the wrong patient, wrong site, or body procedure
10. Unintended retention of a foreign object in a patient after surgery
11. Severe neonatal hyperbilirubinemia (bilirubin >30 mg/dL)
12. Prolonged fluoroscopy with cumulative dose >1,500 rads to a single field or any delivery of radiotherapy to the wrong body region or >25% above the planned radiotherapy dose

Source: The Joint Commission (2014)

Table 7-3 Most Frequently Reviewed Sentinel Event Categories by Year

2011	2012	2013
Unintended retention of a foreign body	Unintended retention of a foreign body	Delay in treatment
Wrong-patient, wrong-site, wrong-procedure	Wrong-patient, wrong-site, wrong-procedure	Wrong-patient, wrong-site, wrong-procedure
Delay in treatment	Delay in treatment	Unintended retention of a foreign body
Op/Post-op complication	Suicide	Suicide
Suicide	Op/Post-op complication	Fall
Fall	Fall	Other unanticipated event*
Other unanticipated event*	Other unanticipated event*	Op/Post-op complication
Criminal event	Criminal event	Criminal event
Medication error	Medication error	Medication error
Medical equipment-related	Perinatal death/injury	Perinatal death/injury

*Other includes: unexpected additional care, extended care, and psychological impact. Note that the reporting is voluntary and represents only a small portion of actual events.
Source: Data from The Joint Commission (n.d.)

Table 7-4 Estimates of Healthcare-Associated Infections Occurring in Acute Care Hospitals, 2011

Type of Healthcare-Associated Infection	Estimated No.
Pneumonia	157,500
Gastrointestinal illness	123,100
Urinary tract infections (wards and critical care units)	93,300
Primary bloodstream infections	71,900
Surgical-site infections from an inpatient surgery	157,500
Other types of infections	118,500
Estimated total number of infections in hospitals	721,800

Source: Magill et al. (2014)

"Never Events"

The use of the term "Never Events" was first discussed in 2001 by the National Quality Forum (NQF). Since the inception, the term has expanded to include 29 events grouped into six categories (Surgical, Product or Device, Patient Protection, Care Management, Environmental, Radiological, and Criminal) that can lead to serious error, indicating a problem with the safety of a health care facility. It has been estimated that medical errors cost billions of dollars annually and account for thousands of deaths and additional hospital days (Haberly, 2009).

As of October 2008, the CMS has ceased reimbursing hospitals for costs associated with specific events, such as serious hospital-acquired pressure ulcers and infections it considers preventable. Catheter-associated urinary tract infection (CAUTI) is one of the most common preventable infections and can be directly related to care that is not evidence based. It is estimated that implementation of evidence-based practice will result in improved client outcomes during hospitalization. Estimates of HAIs in 2011 (Magill et al., 2014) are shown in Table 7-4 ■.

Providing a safe environment involves a number of people, including the clients, visitors, and healthcare providers (Figure 7-8 ■ and Box 7-3 ■).

Clients who are moved from their usual environment into one that is unfamiliar and often frightening may act

FIGURE 7-8 Providing a safe environment involves instructing the client, family, healthcare providers, and visitors in safety measures. Providing protection from hazardous situations and education about safety precautions is one of the most important responsibilities of the nurse.

Box 7-3 **SMOKING POLICIES**

TJC standards require hospital smoking policies be disseminated and enforced throughout hospital buildings. All hospitals in the United States are required to be smoke-free facilities. Clients and families should be given instruction about smoking policies.

- Directives on smoking policy should be conveyed to each client on admission.
- Smoking is prohibited throughout the hospital.
- A physician may write orders for an exception to this policy for an individual client.
- A designated smoking area may be made available for family or visitors. (See Chapter 30 for safety measures for clients receiving oxygen therapy.)

in ways that are very different from their usual behavior. A threatening situation can interfere with the individual's adaptation to the immediate surroundings.

The design and decor of the client's room must satisfy two needs: comfort and safety. Tasteful, unobtrusive colors help to normalize the hospital room. Interesting color combinations and patterns generally appeal more to the senses than do the traditional white or green choices. Pictures, flowers, cards, colorful linens, and curtains can add variety and familiarity to a room.

Safety Precautions

The client's age and health status influence the specific safety precautions that need to be taken to provide a safe environment. Parents and caregivers should be included in safety discussions. For example, infants require constant supervision, since they may attempt to put anything in their mouths or noses. Infants, toddlers, and sometimes preschool children are placed in cribs, many of which have protective tops to prevent climbing. Electronic banding is often used in young children for locating them if necessary. All hospitals have identified overhead paging codes to alert personnel if a child cannot be located.

Preschool-aged children can be taught more detailed aspects of safety. Fire precautions and guidelines for bathing should be stressed.

Elementary school-aged children can usually protect themselves from hazards. They do, however, require instruction on how to operate mechanical equipment as well as information about fires and emergency exits.

Client Falls

Falling is a common cause of morbidity and the leading cause of nonfatal injuries and trauma-related hospitalization. Falls are the leading cause of fatal and nonfatal injuries in older adults. Complications that occur from falls include soft tissue injury, bone fractures, the fear of falling again, head trauma, and death. More than 90% of hip fractures result from falls, most occurring in individuals over 70 years of age. It is estimated that one third of individuals over 65 years of age and more than half of individuals over 80 years of age will fall at least one time each year. Two thirds of those who fall will fall again within six months.

All hospitals are required by TJC to assess and manage clients' risk for fall (Box 7-4 ■). It has been shown that most of the falls in the hospital have occurred from or near the client's bed. Other common areas where falls occur include the bathroom and corridor.

Even though much research has been done on falls and fall prevention, it is still a major problem for healthcare organizations. Clients at risk for falls include those with impaired mental status due to confusion, delirium, disorientation, impaired memory, and inability to understand; those taking medications that affect mental status and the cardiovascular system; those with chronic illness; individuals who have deficits in balance, strength, coordination, and vision; and those with a history of falls. In addition to physical injury, falls result in substantial psychological and social consequences, such as anxiety, loss of independence, and increased rate of nursing home placements.

A fall risk assessment is now part of the admission assessment of all clients, including children. If the client is at high risk for falling, appropriate interventions are implemented immediately. (See Fall Risk Assessment Form in Skill 7.1.1.)

Older adults are especially at risk for injury from falls. Decreased sensory acuity, decreased balance and postural instability, acute confusion, or chronic physical problems such as arthritis contribute to the high risk for falls among older adults. Specialized safety equipment, such as toilet and bathtub railing and modified seats, are often used in geriatric units to decrease risk of injury during bathroom use (Figures 7-9, 7-10, and 7-11 ■).

Box 7-4 CLINICAL GUIDELINES FOR THE PREVENTION OF FALLS AND INJURIES IN THE OLDER ADULT

- Brief assessment of all clients will identify those who should be referred for a comprehensive fall evaluation.
- Assessments may be done by all healthcare professionals.
- Because of the many factors associated with falls, one test cannot identify individuals at risk for falls. Several tests assessing for risk factors should be utilized.
- **Clients at risk for falls include older clients with the following:**
  Medical needs, and who have experienced one or more falls
  Reported recurrent falls
  Abnormalities in gait or balance
- **Comprehensive clinical risk assessment usually consists of the following:**
  A review of falls, history, and circumstances
  Assessing home for hazards
  Identifying medications routinely taken
  Assessing gait, balance, mobility, and muscle weakness
  Identifying risk for osteoporosis
  Evaluating perceived functional ability and fear of falling
  Assessing visual impairment and effects of corrective eyewear
  Presence of urinary incontinence
  Assessing acute and chronic health problems, joint function, and basic neurologic function
- **Fall prevention interventions include the following:**
  Utilize exercise programs.
  Implement behavior changes.
  Review medications.
  Treat contributing health conditions.
  Use assistive and protective devices.
  Modify house to prevent injury.
  Educate client and family in ways to prevent falls.

Source: American Geriatrics Society (2004)

FIGURE 7-9 Rails next to the toilet assist in preventing client falls.

FIGURE 7-10 Shower chairs provide for client safety.

FIGURE 7-11 Safety features such as handrail on bathtubs assist in preventing client falls.

It is sometimes difficult to balance the need for client safety with that for autonomy. Surveillance by agency personnel or family members, use of alarm systems, or special monitoring devices provide alternatives to use of restraints in promoting client safety. Adequate hydration, monitoring of orthostatic vital sign changes, medication review, and physically locating client near nurses' station will facilitate nurse monitoring of client. In addition, early identification of fall risk, use of appropriate footwear and assistive devices, physical therapy, and dietary referrals are possible nursing actions to prevent falls.

Use of Restraints

Restraints are defined as any physical or chemical means used to restrict a client's movement or activity or access to his or her body. **Physical restraints** or **chemical restraints**

Table 7-5 Root Cause Information for Restraint-Related Events Reviewed by The Joint Commission

(Resulting in death or permanent loss of function) 2004 through 2Q 2012 (*N* = 115)	
The majority of events have multiple root causes	
Human Factors	93
Communication	79
Assessment	73
Leadership	72
Special Interventions	72
Physical Environment	46
Information Management	23
Care Planning	23
Medication Use	17
Continuum of Care	13

Source: The Joint Commission (n.d.)

may be used in medical surgical, obstetrical, pediatric, and rehabilitation settings to directly support medical healing. Restraints may also be employed in alcohol and drug treatment centers and in long-term care. Restraints should not be used unless they are necessary for the safety of the client (TJC, 2013). Restraints may also be used in mental health emergency care when there is dangerous behavior. For many years, restraining a client or placing a client in **seclusion** was considered a way to protect the client or the staff from injury. After much research into the subject, it has been determined that use of restraints is very problematic and actually can lead to severe client injury and even death (Table 7-5 ■).

Because of client injury or potential injury from use of restraints or seclusion, both TJC and the CMS, have developed regulations regarding use of restraints in hospitals and long-term acute care, long-term care, psychiatric settings, and in surgical specialty areas (Box 7-5 ■). The situations in which standards apply are dependent on the reason for restraint use. Devices and immobilization that are considered protective interventions but not "restraint" interventions include arm boards for IV stabilization, procedural immobilization such as the temporary use of soft restraints to prevent a client from interfering with a related treatment, or soft restraints and tabletop chairs that are used as a temporary preventative measure. Healthcare workers who intervene with restraints and seclusion must undergo special training. The rights of clients must be protected and guarding safety must be paramount. All healthcare facilities are accountable for appropriate use of restraints and seclusion.

If restraints are used for nonbehavioral health purposes, a physician or licensed independent practitioner (LIP) must write an order. If a client's condition changes rapidly, a nurse may initiate use of restraints but then notify the LIP or physician immediately. Time frames for orders may vary depending on facility accreditations and licensures. The nurse must be knowledgeable about facility-specific policies and understand the safety issues associated with use of restraints.

Box 7-5 **RESTRAINT GUIDELINES**

Review hospital policy for the use of restraints. Requires a physician's order.

Use restraints for the client's protection and to prevent injury only if all other less restrictive measures are not effective.

- Use the least amount of restraint possible.
- Allow clients as much freedom of movement as possible. Use slipknots for quick release. Do not use square knots or bows. Many restraints use Velcro. Behavioral health units sometimes use leather restraints with key locks.
- Always explain the purpose of the restraint to the client and family. Afford as much dignity to the client as possible.
- Remember that restraints can cause emotional, mental, and physical deterioration and increase the risk of injury. The client is unable to protect himself or herself by sitting up if choking, pulling away from the pain source, or moving to avoid injury.
- Remember that circulation and skin integrity can be affected by restraints. Always monitor circulation distal to the restraint and skin integrity beneath and adjacent to the restraint.
- Use a wedge pillow if needed to elevate the client's upper body to prevent aspiration and difficulty breathing.
- Place the client in a supine position unless there are specific contraindications.
- Observe the client every 15 minutes. In some cases, clients must be continuously observed.
- Release restraints every 2 hours for at least 5 minutes to inspect tissues and provide joint range of motion and position change to prevent circulatory impairment. When a client is combative, release only one restraint at a time and have a colleague present or nearby. If restraints have been used to prevent danger to self or others, have adequate personnel present during restraint removal.
- Assess and provide for client's fluid and elimination needs, pain management, and position change every 2 hours.
- Pad bony prominences, such as wrists and ankles, beneath a restraint.
- Attempt to make restraints as inconspicuous as possible for the sake of the client's relatives and friends, who may be upset by seeing restraints.
- Clearly document rationale and precautions taken for client safety.
- Notify family, significant other, or guardian if restraints are necessary.
- Enlist support of family members or significant other to sit with client rather than implement restraints.

When restraints are used in behavioral health situations, it is primarily to protect against injury to self or others from imminent risk. Orders for restraints can be written for up to 4 hours for an adult. The order can be renewed every 4 hours, up to a total of 24 hours. TJC allows that after an assessment by an RN, restraints may be implemented, and then the physician must be contacted within a specified time frame. Continued use of restraints must be reevaluated every 4 hours for clients over 18 years of age, every 2 hours for clients 9 to 17 years of age, and every hour for children under 9 years. No standing orders or PRN orders are allowed for restraints. Facilities may choose to be more restrictive, but they cannot be less restrictive in the time frame for renewal of orders.

Documentation of the client's symptoms that lead to the implementation of restraints must include both subjective and objective data and derived from a clinical evaluation. All less restrictive interventions utilized must be documented as well.

When restraints are employed, they must be an appropriate method of restraint and be used in the least restrictive manner. In some situations, the family, significant other, or guardian must be informed immediately when restraints are required. Many hospitals use one-to-one supervision in place of restraints for clients whenever possible. In nonbehavioral health settings, family members may be called on to sit with the client as well.

Adaptation to Home Care

The home environment should be evaluated for safety issues before the client is discharged from the hospital. The National Home Care Patient Safety Goals should be followed at home in order to improve the client's safety while recuperating. The following safety goals should be discussed with the client, family, and healthcare provider.

1. Identify clients correctly. Use at least two ways to identify clients. Use the client's name and date of birth. Street address should be confirmed. Label specimens in the presence of the client.
2. Maintain and communicate accurate client medication information.
3. Prevent infection.
   - Use the hand-cleaning guidelines from the World Health Organization or Centers for Disease Control and Prevention.
4. Decrease risk of falls.
   - Determine which clients are most likely to fall. Take action to prevent falls in these clients including environmental assessment of the home; for example, area rugs, playful pets, extension cords, and presence or absence of assistive devices including grab bars.
5. Identify safety risks inherent in the client population.
   - Identify any risks associated with home oxygen treatment; for example, fires in the client's home due to smoking materials and open flames. Evaluate for presence of smoke detectors. Educate about risk for fires.
6. Other nursing activities that support client safety in the home include confirming that the correct treatments and procedures are being done, reading back telephone orders written on the patient's record, conveying important test results to the right individual in a timely

manner, checking client medications and assessing ability to self-administer, and monitoring carefully when anticoagulation therapy is prescribed. Confer with the client's pharmacist or primary care provider if there are questions about medication compatibility. Provide education regarding medications, equipment, and strategies to promote health and prevent complications or deterioration in condition. Confirm that equipment is functioning appropriately. Prevent infection from invasive devices by following evidence-based and best-practice guidelines for nursing actions requiring medical and surgical asepsis. Assist with appointments if needed. Listen to the client and family.

Note: For complete description of Home Care National Patient Safety Goals, refer to the list available on TJC website.

Nursing Diagnoses

The following nursing diagnoses may be appropriate to include in a client care plan when the components are related to maintaining a safe environment.

NURSING DIAGNOSIS	RELATED TO . . .
Injury, Risk for	Motor, sensory, or cognitive alterations; elimination urgency; bleeding tendency; physiologic instability due to medications, aging, illness, environmental hazards
Impaired Tissue Integrity	Chemical, thermal, or mechanical factors, decreased mobility, nutritional deficiency
Self-Mutilation, Risk for	Labile affect and unpredictable behavior, depression, guilt, inadequate coping, loss of control over problem-solving situations

Source: Herdman, T. H. & Kamitsuru, S. (Eds.) *Nursing Diagnoses – Definitions and Classification* 2015-2017. Copyright © 2014, 1994–2014 by NANDA International. Used by arrangement with John Wiley & Sons Limited. Companion website: www.wiley.com/go/nursingdiagnoses. In order to make safe and effective judgments using NANDA-I nursing diagnosis it is essential that nurses refer to the definitions and defining characteristics of the diagnoses listed in this work.

Nursing Process Data

ASSESSMENT Database

- Identify client's age, previous or chronic sensory impairments, previous level of mobility, ambulatory aids used, and general health history.
- Assess the client's reliability as an accurate health historian.
- Identify any alteration of sensory or motor abilities or emotional adaptation due to illness, injury, or hospitalization.
- Observe and record client's present level of consciousness, orientation, mobility, gait, balance, any sensory or motor restrictions, and need for adaptive devices.
- Evaluate client's ability to comprehend instruction about how to use potentially dangerous equipment.
- Evaluate client's ability to make judgments.
- Assess need for specific precautions to promote a safe environment.
- Assess type of fire extinguisher needed for specific types of fires or use ABC extinguisher.
- Assess the need for protection while administering care to clients with radioactive implant.
- Assess prodromal signs and symptoms (aura) for potential seizure activity.
- Assess home for environmental safety.

PLANNING Objectives

- To provide protection when states of illness decrease the individual's ability to receive and interpret environmental stimuli
- To assist client to interpret environmental stimuli relevant to his or her safety
- To determine safety equipment necessary to promote a safe environment
- To place all personal articles and call light within easy reach of client
- To enhance degrees of mobility in a safe environment
- To determine that all electrical equipment is intact and operated safely
- To determine the protective devices needed when caring for clients receiving radioactive material
- To provide a safe environment for a client with seizure activity
- To determine that home environment is safe

IMPLEMENTATION Procedures

DOCUMENTATION AND EVALUATION

Expected Outcomes

- Client's environment is safe from potential mechanical, chemical, and fire or electrical hazards.
- All personal articles and call light are within easy reach of the client.
- All electrical equipment is intact and operated safely.
- If oxygen is used, appropriate safety measures are in effect.
- Personnel are protected from radioactive material.
- Client is free of injury after seizure.
- Client does not experience sequelae from seizure activity.

Unexpected Outcomes/Alternative Actions

Pearson Nursing Student Resources

Find additional review materials at
nursing.pearsonhighered.com.
Prepare for success with NCLEX®-style practice questions and Skill Checklists.

Skill 7.1.1 | Preventing Client Falls

Equipment
Side rails, handrails
Alarm systems
Restraints
Locks for movable equipment, such as beds, wheelchairs, and gurneys

Procedure
1. Perform hand hygiene.
2. Identify client using two identifiers.
3. Introduce yourself to the client and explain the procedure that will be performed.
4. Assess all clients for risk factors for falls (Boxes 7-6 and 7-7 ▪).

Box 7-6 ASSESS CLIENTS FOR RISK FACTORS FOR FALLS

Older clients are more prone to falls. There are intrinsic and extrinsic factors involved with the falls. Risk for falls increases each year as older adults age.

1. Intrinsic factors involved in falls:
   a. Deceased vision and other senses
   b. Weakness and alterations in mobility/gait and balance problems. Alterations in 4-Stage Balance Test, 30-Second Chair Stand Test, and Timed Up and GO (TUG Test)
   c. Urinary incontinence
   d. Chronic illness and confusion
   e. Polypharmacy, the use of five or more medications, especially medications that affect the cardiovascular or neurologic systems
   f. Alcohol consumption
   g. Chronic pain
   h. Orthostatic hypotension
   i. Length of stay in hospital
   j. Fear of falling and history of falls

2. Extrinsic factors related to the physical environment:
   a. Lack of grab bars
   b. Poor condition of floor surfaces
   c. Inadequate or improper use of assistive devices
   d. Reaching for articles out of the way

Box 7-7 RISK ASSESSMENT TOOLS FOR FALLS

- CDC Fall Risk Checklist—STEADI (Stopping Elderly Accidents, Deaths, and Injuries)
- Falls Efficacy Scale—measurement of how confident the individual is when performing activities of daily living
- Morse Fall Scale Assessment
- Balance Self-Perception Test
- Berg Balance Scale
- Tinetti Mobility Assessment
- The Mini Mental State Examination—for assessing cognition

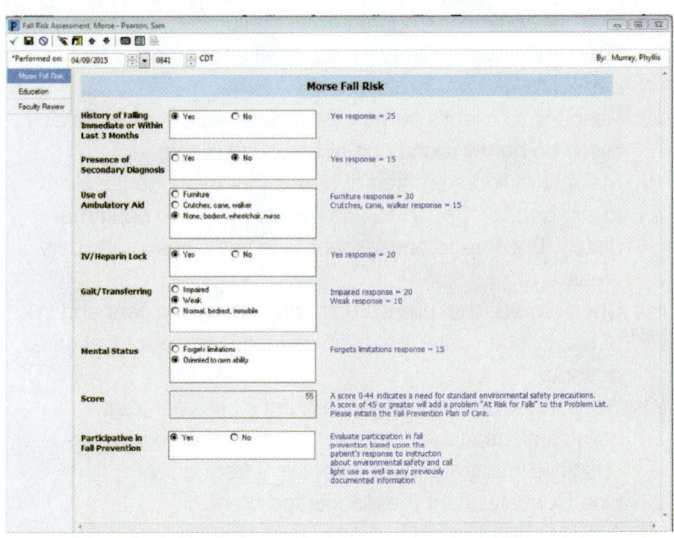

❶ Fall Risk Assessment Form.

Source: From Cerner Electronic Health Record. © Cerner Corporation. Pearson has restricted permission to reproduce and distribute this copyrighted work. Further reproduction or distribution is strictly prohibited without written consent of Cerner Corporation.

5. Complete a comprehensive interview to determine potential for falls. ❶ Determine how many falls the client experienced in the last 6 months. Ask how he or she fell, backward or forward? Determine if medications are taken correctly and any dietary supplements the client is taking. Discuss client's diet: What foods and fluids does he or she eat and drink?
6. Determine psychosocial status. ➤ *Rationale:* This provides insight into how the client will react to necessary changes in his or her daily routine or changes in his or her home necessary to prevent falls.
7. Orient new clients to their surroundings, including use of call light.
8. Instruct ambulatory client in use of toilet and shower controls and emergency signals in bathroom.
9. Determine client's ability to safely use mobility aids.
10. Place bed in low, locked position when you are not providing direct client care.
11. Determine appropriateness for side rail use.
12. Keep half side rails up for all heavily sedated, older adults, confused, and immediate postsurgical clients according to hospital policy.
13. Place articles such as call light, remote controls, cups, and water within the client's reach.
14. Pad bed rails for client with high risk for seizures.
15. Remind client and hospital personnel to lock beds, wheelchairs, and gurneys and to release the lock only after client is secure for transport.
16. Tell clients who are weak, sedated, in pain, or who have had surgery to ask for assistance before getting out of bed.

(continued)

Skill 7.1.1 | Preventing Client Falls (continued)

17. Use two staff members to transport client on gurney or wheelchair when nonattached equipment, such as chest-tube system or IV poles, must accompany client in transport.
18. Respond to client's summons as soon as possible. Proactively, do hourly rounds on all assigned clients.
19. Make sure floors are free of debris that might cause clients to slip and fall. Spilled liquids should be wiped up immediately. Encourage housekeepers to use signs for slippery areas.
20. Check to see that client's unit and hallway are neat and free of hazardous obstacles, such as footstools, electrical cords, or shoes.
21. Respond to acute changes in client's behavior (e.g., hallucinations, abrupt disorientation, or altered responses or cognitive impairment). Monitor client frequently.
22. Continuously orient the disoriented client.
23. Assess and respond to fluid and elimination needs every 2 hours.
24. Employ bed, chair, and exit or "wander" alarms (Box 7-8 ■). Bed alarms involve placing a sensor on the client's bed or activating an integrated bed alarm. When a change in position or loss of contact with the sensor occurs, an alarm alerts the nurse. Ambualarm devices are placed on the client's leg and signal an alarm when the legs are in a dependent position, indicating the client is trying to get out of bed.
25. Use a low-rise bed to decrease height of fall.

26. Apply hip protectors on clients at risk for a fractured hip if they fall (i.e., clients with osteoporosis). Soft foam pads are held in place at the hips with specially designed removable briefs.
27. Assign aides or elicit the assistance of healthcare assistants for one-to-one supervision or family to monitor the high-risk client; make certain they inform you when they leave the client's side.
28. Relocate high-risk client to room near nurses' station.
29. Utilize a recliner chair for client safety.
30. Place absorbent pad next to bed. ➤ Rationale: This prevents severe injury if client falls out of bed.
31. Keep intercom open between client's room and nurses' station.
32. Obtain physician's specific orders if restraints are deemed absolutely necessary.

> **CLINICAL ALERT**
> **Risk Factors for Falls for the High-Risk Client**
> There is a tendency for multiple fallers to repeat the type and location of the fall on successive falls (e.g., use of commode). Studies have identified a variety of fall risk factors that have led to the development of a number of fall risk assessment tools. Clients at high risk for fall generally demonstrate more than one of the following:
>
> - History of falls
> - Advanced age
> - Sensory or motor impairment
> - Urgent need for elimination
> - Postural blood pressure instability

Box 7-8 EXIT ALARMS

Posture indicator:	Adhesive transmitter patch is applied to thigh and to a receiver alarm box. When client attempts to get up, alarm goes off.
Pressure release:	Pads, mats, or other devices are placed on the floor or chair. They sense changes in weight and pressure.
Pressure-sensitive:	Pad or mat is placed on the floor by bed or chair and sounds when stepped on.
Clip-on alarms:	Alarms are activated by pulling a detachable tab from the unit, a small box attached to the bed, chair, or wheelchair. A clip is attached to client's clothes. When client gets up, tab detaches from box and sounds an alarm.
Beam or motion detector alarms:	Alarms sound when motion is detected or if beam is interrupted.

EVIDENCE-BASED PRACTICE
Are Hospital Bed Rails Safe for Patients?
Regulators Investigate

Current guidelines for bed rails are voluntary. Federal agencies have launched an investigation into the safety of hospital bed rails, which injure at least 4,000 clients per year, the *New York Times* reports. A Consumer Product Safety Commission (CPSC) review of death certificates and Emergency Room visits found that about 150 adults died from being trapped in their bed rails from 2003 to May 2012. In addition, 36,000 clients were treated in the ER for a bed rail injury during the same time period. The FDA and CPSC feel that the data probably underestimate the problem. In 2011, 27 clients died of bed rail–related incidents.

Source: The Advisory Board Company (2012)

Methods of Preventing Falls

To prevent at-risk clients from falling out of bed, consider using one of the following interventions:

- Use a mattress with raised edges; use body-length pillows, rolled blankets, or "swimming noodles" (foam flotation aids) under mattress edges.
- Place mat on floor next to bed.
- Place client in a very low to ground bed (7 to 13 inches above floor).
- Use bed alert alarms.
- Use half or three-fourth length side rails.
- Identify high-risk clients and implement a plan of action to prevent falls.
- Place high-risk client near nurses' station.
- Monitor high-risk client frequently; make rounds at least every hour.
- Educate staff in fall prevention programs.
- Decrease environmental risks, obstacles, and clutter.
- Install grab bars in bathroom and ensure that bed rollers are locked.
- Support client's elimination needs.
- Monitor client's reaction to medications.
- Assist clients with mobility.
- Ensure client wears nonskid slippers.

- Monitor client's mental status.
- Institute interventions to prevent falls from bed.
- Use safety straps or seat belts when in wheelchairs or geri-chairs.
- Involve family members in client prevention program.
- Do a bedside report.

Client Falls

Even though client falls are second only to medication errors in untoward events that happen to clients in hospitals, it does not mean that fault will be assessed against healthcare providers.

If it can be proved that the nursing staff used poor judgment in preventing client falls, liability will be assessed against the staff. In *Williams v. Covenant Medical Center*, a client was noted to be at high risk for falls but even with this data, was not placed on fall prevention interventions.

In a second case, *Sullivan v. Edward Hospital*, 2004, the court found that the institution had taken appropriate measures to safeguard a client who fell and developed a subdural hematoma.

Source: Guido (2006)

Skill 7.1.2 | Preventing Thermal/Electrical Injuries

Equipment
Fire extinguishers

Procedure

1. Make sure that all electrical apparatuses are routinely checked and maintained. Look for safety inspection expiration dates on biomedical equipment.
2. Have all electrical appliances brought to the hospital by client (radios, electric razors, hair dryers, etc.) inspected by hospital maintenance staff. Once inspected and approved for use, equipment should be labeled as inspected with date. It is best to discourage use of nonhospital equipment.
3. Make sure water in the tub or shower is not more than 100°F (37.8°C) or 95°F (35°C) for those with circulatory insufficiency. Monitor client often during sitz bath. Water should be cooler for children and clients over 65.
4. When heating pads or hot compresses are used, check the client frequently for redness. Never apply direct heat.

Maximum temperature should not exceed 105°F (40.6°C) or 95°F (35°C) for those with circulatory insufficiency.

Infants, children, older adults, and clients who are comatose or have diabetes are especially vulnerable to **thermal** injuries.

5. Hospitals do not allow smoking in the facility. There may be designated smoking areas outside the building. Inform clients and visitors about the hospital's smoking regulations. Do not allow confused, sedated, or severely incapacitated clients to smoke without direct supervision.
6. Store all combustible materials securely to prevent spontaneous combustion. Appropriate storage and handling are directed by facility safety officers and individuals identified to address Life Safety and Environment of Care.
7. Make sure that all staff and employees participate in and understand fire safety measures, such as extinguishing fires and plan for evacuating clients.

(continued)

Skill 7.1.2 | Preventing Thermal/Electrical Injuries *(continued)*

8. Report and do not use any apparatus that produces a shock, has a broken plug or ground pin, or has a frayed cord. Broken or damaged equipment should be labeled to prevent use.

9. Turn equipment off before unplugging it. ➤ *Rationale:* This prevents sparks that can cause a fire.

10. Use only three-pronged grounded plugs.

Skill 7.1.3 | Providing Safety for Clients During a Fire

Equipment

Appropriate extinguisher for fire:
Water type
Soda-acid type
Foam type
Dry chemical type
ABC extinguisher

Procedure

1. Follow hospital policy and procedure for type of fire safety program (Box 7-9 ■).

Box 7-9 PRIORITIES FOR FIRE SAFETY

R   Rescue and remove all clients in immediate danger
A   Activate fire alarm
C   Confine the fire; close doors, windows; turn off oxygen supplies and electrical equipment
E   Extinguish fire when possible

---

2. Remove all clients from the immediate area to a safe place. Be familiar with fire exits and agency evacuation plan.

3. To remove a client safely from the fire, use carrying method that is most comfortable for you and safe for client.

   a. If moving the bed or equipment that the client is occupying is not feasible, place blanket (or bedspread) on floor. Lower the client onto the blanket. Lift up the head end of the blanket and drag the client out of danger.

   b. Use two-person swing method. Place the client in a sitting position. Form a seat by having two people clasp forearms or shoulders. Lift the client into the "seat" and carry out of danger.

   c. Carry the client using "back-strap" carry method. Step in front of the client. Place the client's arms around your neck. Grasp the client's wrists and hold tight against your chest. Pull the client onto your back and carry to safety.

4. Activate fire alarm.

5. Secure the burning area by closing all doors and windows.

6. Shut off all possible oxygen sources and electrical appliances in the fire area.

7. If possible, employ the appropriate extinguishing method without endangering yourself. Fire extinguishers should not be used directly on an individual.

8. Be familiar with the different types of fire extinguishers and their location. ❶

   Class A
   a. Water-under-pressure type or soda-acid type
   b. Used on cloth, wood, paper, plastic, rubber, or leather
   c. Never used on electrical or chemical fires due to danger of shock

   Class B
   a. Foam, dry chemical, carbon dioxide types
   b. Used on fires such as gasoline, alcohol, acetone, oil, grease, or paint thinner and remover
   c. Class A extinguisher never used on class B fires

❶ Become familiar with the location and use of fire extinguishers in the hospital.

Class C

a. Dry chemical or carbon dioxide types

b. Used on electrical wiring, electrical equipment, or motors

c. Class A or class B extinguishers never used on class C fires

Class ABC combination

a. Contains graphite

b. Used on any type of fire

c. Most common extinguisher in use

9. Keep fire exits clear at all times.

Skill 7.1.4 | Providing Safety for Clients Receiving Radioactive Materials

Equipment

Protective shields for x-ray

Lead-shielded container if required

Film badge if required for dosimetry

Sign for client's door: "Caution, Radioactive Material"

Personal Protection Equipment (PPE)

Procedure

1. Review guidelines (see Box 7-10 ■):

   a. Determine type and amount of radiation used and its side effects and hazards.

   b. Rotate care providers because increased time in the presence of a radioactive source increases exposure to radiation.

   c. Use shields, such as lead walls or lead aprons, to protect from radioactive source. Eye and thyroid shields may be needed.

   d. Inform staff that exposure is greater the closer the individual and longer the exposure to the radioactive source.

   e. Store radioactive material in lead-shielded containers when not in use. Container should be labeled.

   f. Issue monitoring badge to all who enter room to record exposure. ❶

Box 7-10 GENERAL GUIDELINES FOR RADIATION PRECAUTIONS*

Radioactive Implant

- Care time is not to exceed 15 minutes per employee per day.
- No pregnant woman or anyone under age 18 should enter room.
- Visitors are limited to 1–2 hours per day, keeping distance from client.
- There is no special handling of excreta other than standard precautions.
- Bath is usually omitted and client movement is restricted.
- Cleaning of room is often limited.
- All linens, gloves, trash, and dressings are kept in room until cleared by radiation safety officer.

Radiopharmaceuticals

- No lab specimens should be taken without consent of radiation safety officer.
- Use disposable dietary tray.
    - Handle all excreta and secretions with gloves. Wear all necessary PPE to protect clothes.
    - Shoe covers should be used in the client room and removed prior to exit.
- Have client use toilet—flushing twice. Male and female clients should sit to avoid splatter.
- Shielding is not needed.
- Visitors require special instructions—avoid physical contact with client.
- Keep gloves, dressings, linens, and trash in contaminated container.

*Note: See Institutional Policy for Specifics.

CLINICAL ALERT

Pregnant nurses should check hospital policy regarding working with clients receiving radioactive materials.

---

❶ Badge worn when working with clients receiving radioactive material.

(continued)

Skill 7.1.4 | Providing Safety for Clients Receiving Radioactive Materials *(continued)*

2. If nurse or family members are assisting with a radioactive procedure, they must put on a shield.

3. If a radioactive implant is used in a client, all nurses and visitors must be protected with a shield. Limit exposure with the client.

4. Keep track of how much time is spent in the presence of radioactive material. Check film badge frequently.

5. Constantly assess and support clients who are undergoing radiation therapy. Bed rest, isolation, and unpleasant side effects are sometimes common.

6. Follow guidelines for working with clients with unsealed sources of iodine-131.

   a. Wear rubber gloves at all times when providing care.

   b. Wash gloves before removing, and place in designated waste container.

   c. Wash hands with soap and water after removing gloves.

   d. Dispose of all bed linen in contaminated linen bag.

   e. Wrap all nondisposable items that have come in contact with client's blood, saliva, or gastric juices in plastic bag. Send to appropriate hospital department for decontamination (usually nuclear medicine department).

   f. Notify radiation safety officer (usually in radiology department) if clothes or shoes have been contaminated.

   g. Instruct visitors and family member of no visitations for 24 hours.

7. If client is discharged immediately after radioactive iodine, provide client instructions.

   a. Minimize contact (less than 3 feet or 0.6 meter for more than 1 hour each day) with everyone for the first 5 days, and with small children or pregnant women for 8 days.

   b. Do not sit next to someone in an automobile for more than 1 hour.

   c. Sleep in a separate room and use separate bath linen and launder these and underclothing separately for 1 week.

   d. Wash hands with soap and water every time the toilet is used.

   e. Rinse the sink and tub thoroughly after using them.

   f. Use separate eating utensils or disposable eating utensils. Wash eating utensils separately for 1 week. Do not prepare food for others.

   g. Flush toilet two to three times after use for 2 weeks after discharge.

   h. Males should sit when urinating to avoid splashing for 1 week.

> **CLINICAL ALERT**
> **Client Education after Receiving Radioactive Iodine**
> - Check with physician regarding guidelines.
> - Follow the guidelines, if approved by physician.

Skill 7.1.5 | Providing Safety for Clients with Seizure Activity

Equipment
Oral airway
Padding material for side rails
Suction equipment and catheters
Clean gloves

Preparation
1. Identify client at risk for seizure activity (e.g., clients with closed head injury, neurosurgical clients, meningitis, and history of seizures).
2. Place suction equipment and catheters on bedside stand.
3. Tape oral airway to head of bed or place on wall.
4. Pad side rails with blankets or other heavy material.

Procedure
1. Determine type of seizure activity, if client has a previous history of seizures. ➤ *Rationale:* This knowledge assists in determining potential type of seizure activity, client response, and presence of an aura.
2. Place client in side-lying position, with pillow at head of bed and side rails in raised position, if seizure activity is anticipated. ➤ *Rationale:* This protects client from injury.

3. When seizure activity begins, provide privacy; ensure bed is in low position and side rails are raised.

> **CLINICAL ALERT**
> If client is at risk for respiratory arrest, activate the Rapid Response Team or call 911.

4. Maintain client in side-lying position with head flexed slightly forward. Do not restrain client or place anything in client's mouth. ➤ *Rationale:* This prevents injury to jaw or teeth. Flexed head will prevent tongue from occluding airway.
5. Remain with client during seizure to ensure airway is not occluded and client does not require suctioning.
6. Explain that client had a seizure when he or she is alert.
7. Remain with client after seizure to ensure he or she has an uneventful postictal period. Client usually sleeps for a period of time after seizure.
8. Document findings and notify physician of the client's seizure.

Skill 7.1.6 | Assessing Home for Safe Environment

Equipment
Home Assessment Checklist
Outcome and Assessment Information Act (OASIS-B1)

Procedure
1. Identify type of dwelling (i.e., client-owned, boarding home, rental, mobile home).
2. Identify water source.
3. Identify sewer source.
4. Identify type of plumbing available.
5. Determine if any pollutants are present in the environment.
6. Assess exterior of the home for the following:

   a. Condition of sidewalks and steps
   b. Presence of railings on steps
   c. Barriers that prevent easy access to the home
   d. Adequacy of lighting
   e. Adequacy of roof and windows

7. Assess interior of the home for the following:

   a. Presence of scatter rugs or worn carpeting
   b. Uncluttered pathways throughout the house
   c. Adequacy of lighting
   d. Doorways wide enough to permit assistive devices
   e. Cleanliness of house
   f. Presence of insects, rodents, or infective agents
   g. Presence of functioning smoke detectors
   h. Adequate heating and cooling systems
   i. Presence of running water

8. Determine whether hazardous materials are safely stored.
9. Assess for presence of lead-based paint.
10. Determine whether medications can be adequately stored out of reach of children and impaired individuals.

11. Assess stairway and halls for the following:

    a. Adequacy of light
    b. Handrails that are securely fastened to wall
    c. Flooring in good repair
    d. Rugs or carpeting in good repair
    e. Light switches in easy reach and accessible at both ends of stairs or hallway

12. Assess kitchen for the following:

    a. Properly functioning stove
    b. Adequacy of light surrounding stove and sink
    c. Condition of small appliances
    d. Accessibility of appliances to clients in wheelchairs
    e. Adequacy of sewage disposal

13. Assess bathroom for the following:

    a. Skidproof strips or mat in tub or shower
    b. Handrails around toilet and tub or shower
    c. Accessibility of medicine cabinet
    d. Adequate space if wheelchairs, shower or tub chairs, or walkers are used
    e. Temperature of hot water from faucets in sink, tub, or shower

14. Assess bedroom for the following:

    a. Accessibility of closets and cabinets
    b. Ease in getting into and out of bed
    c. Adequate space, if commode or wheelchair is required
    d. Night light availability
    e. Accessibility of medications, water on night stand
    f. Calling system to alert healthcare provider
    g. Flooring in good repair and nonslippery surface

Unit 7.1 Documentation and Evaluation

DOCUMENTATION for Providing a Safe Environment

- Assessment notes
- Actual incidents involving mechanical, chemical, or thermal trauma
- Client education provided
- Safety devices used

- Behaviors occurring before, during, and after seizure activity
- Safety issues instituted for client receiving radioactive iodine
- Completion of home environment forms

(continued)

EVALUATION/Critical Thinking

Expected Outcomes

- Client's environment is safe from potential mechanical, chemical, and fire or electrical hazards.
- All personal articles and call light are within easy reach of the client.
- All electrical equipment is intact and operated safely.
- If oxygen is used, appropriate safety measures are in effect.
- All clients and personnel are protected from radioactive material.
- Client is free of injury after seizure.
- Client does not experience sequelae from seizure activity.

Unexpected Outcomes

- The client, nurse, or visitor experiences an accident or injury related to mechanical, chemical, or thermal trauma.

Alternative Actions

- Provide immediate first aid or care.
- Assess vital signs and notify physician.
- Report the incident according to hospital procedure. Unusual occurrence forms are used to protect the injured individual, the nurse, and the hospital.
- Review safety procedures to ensure a safe environment.
- Report all malfunctioning equipment immediately to the proper department.

- Unfamiliarity with hospital fire and disaster protocol results in poor performance.

- Review protocols frequently to update knowledge base.
- Participate in fire and disaster drills to become familiar with protocols.

- Radium implant becomes dislodged and falls out.

- Put on lead gloves, pick up radium with forceps, and place in lead-shielded container in client's room.
- Notify physician and hospital radiation safety officer immediately.
- Never touch radioactive source directly.

- Spillage of excreta from client with systemic radioactive therapy occurs.

- Cover spillage with absorbent material and notify radiation safety officer.
- Wash with soap and water if skin is contaminated.

Restraints

Nursing Process Data

ASSESSMENT Database

- Assess client's risk for falls on an ongoing basis.
- Assess need for fall prevention measures.
- Assess area under and surrounding a restraint to ensure it is not restrictive.
- Evaluate client's response to restraint use.

PLANNING Objectives

- To identify clients who are at risk for injury
- To prevent a client from injuring himself or herself or others
- To employ fall prevention measures
- To obtain physician's order for restraints if deemed absolutely necessary
- To apply restraints safely and effectively, including applying restraints during procedures
- To restrain a child's elbow to prevent the child from reaching an incision or intravenous site or equipment
- To promote client safety when ambulating or sitting in a chair

IMPLEMENTATION Procedures

DOCUMENTATION AND EVALUATION

Expected Outcomes

- Client is prevented from injuring himself or herself or others.
- Restraints are applied appropriately.
- Client does not develop complications due to restraint use or restraint placement (e.g., agitation, pressure ulcers, circulatory disturbance).
- Child is prevented from reaching the incision site, IVs, or tubes.
- Client remains in restraints for a limited amount of time.
- Client does not endure undue psychological stress while being placed in restraints.

Unexpected Outcomes/Alternative Actions

Pearson Nursing Student Resources

Find additional review materials at **nursing.pearsonhighered.com**.
Prepare for success with NCLEX®-style practice questions and Skill Checklists.

Skill 7.2.1 | Managing Clients in Restraints

Equipment
Appropriate restraint (Box 7-11 ■).

Preparation
1. Identify and evaluate if less restrictive measures have been explored before the client is placed in restraints (Table 7-6 ■).
2. Call physician or licensed independent practitioners (LIP) for restraint order before applying restraints. If restraints must be placed before the order is obtained, ensure the order is obtained within 1 hour for either a nonbehavioral health client or a behavioral health client. ➤ *Rationale:* Physician's order is required to apply restraints.

Note: Follow guidelines for obtaining restraint orders and updating orders according to hospital policy.

CLINICAL ALERT

Restraints are indicated only if there is no other viable option available to protect the client, and then they are implemented only when the client is assessed and evaluated by an appropriate licensed independent practitioner (LIP).

Box 7-11 TYPES OF RESTRAINTS

There are three types of restraints used in clinical practice:

- *Chemical:* Sedating psychotropic drugs to manage or control behavior. Psychoactive medication used in this manner is an inappropriate use of medication.
- *Physical:* Direct application of physical force to a client, without the client's permission, is used to restrict his or her freedom of movement.
- *Seclusion:* Involuntary confinement of a client in a locked room. Physical force may be applied by individuals, mechanical devices, or a combination of any of them.

Source: The Joint Commission (2000)

---

3. According to policy, ensure that a face-to-face assessment is completed on the nonbehavioral health client (may be within 4 hours) and on the behavioral (psychiatric) health client (within 1 hour). ➤ *Rationale:* Frequent assessments prevent complications.
4. Ensure that restraint orders are renewed every 24 hours or sooner according to facility policy for nonbehavioral health clients or every 1 to 4 hours for behavioral health clients. For example, children from 12 to 17 must have orders renewed every 2 hours, for a maximum of 24 hours. ➤ *Rationale:* Restraints should be discontinued as soon as possible.
5. Establish and implement a plan of care for the client to eliminate the need for restraints.
6. Discuss the use of restraints with the client and family members. If possible, elicit the support of the family or use one-to-one supervision to stay with the client rather than place the client in restraints.

CLINICAL ALERT

In acute medical and postsurgical care, a restraint may be necessary to ensure that an IV or tube feeding is not removed, or the client cannot be allowed out of bed after surgery. This type of medical restraint may be used temporarily to limit mobility or prevent injury to the client.

Additional types of activities that may constitute a restraint include the following:

- Tucking a client's sheet so tight that he or she cannot move
- Using a side rail to prevent a client from voluntarily getting out of bed
- Placing the client in a geri-chair with a table
- Placing a wheelchair-bound client so close to the wall that it prevents him or her from moving

---

Table 7-6 Methods to Decrease Use of Physical or Chemical Restraints

Environmental Alterations	Physiologic Approaches
• Use alternatives such as wedge or roll cushions for positional support. • Adjust lighting at night to decrease fear of unknown and facilitate vision of where bed is in room. • Use rolled edge mattresses. • Use low-level beds (7 to 13 in. from floor). • Place mats on floor in case of client fall. • Use special beds. • Place in special unit or locate close to nurses' station where client can be watched more carefully. • Use sitters or family members. • Use upper side rails only for aid in turning and moving. • Use alarms.	• Potential complication assessment (i.e., increased temperature or hypoxia) • Pain relief • Comfort measures • Physical therapy/exercises **Psychosocial Interventions** • Identify and alter factors that are causing client anxiety, if possible. • Talk with client. • Involve client in activities that take his or her mind off what is happening. • Encourage interaction with family members by phone if necessary. • Establish guidelines and expectations for behaviors. • Reorient to expectations as needed. • Adapt interventions to mental status and developmental level.

Procedure

1. Gather appropriate restraint and perform hand hygiene. Many facilities require use of gloves.
2. Identify client using two identifiers and seek client's cooperation with restraint procedure, if possible.
3. Apply restraint according to manufacturer's specific directions.
4. Monitor and assess the client every 15 minutes, or according to facility policy. In some instances, continuous monitoring may be required.
5. Release restraint at least every 2 hours or sooner (The Joint Commission). ➤ *Rationale:* Releasing restraints allows the client to be provided with the following:
   a. Toileting
   b. Fluids and food
   c. Hygiene care such as brushing teeth or washing face and hands
   d. Circulation checked; skin care provided
   e. Body alignment checked
   f. Range of motion to all joints, particularly those in restraints
6. Avoid application of force on long bone joints and pad bony prominences beneath restraint. ➤ *Rationale:* This reduces pressure on skin and joints.
7. Take vital signs every 4–8 hours unless indicated more frequently. (Refer to facility policies.)
8. Bathe client every 24 hours or more often as needed. A warm face cloth may be soothing.
9. Do not interrupt the client's sleep unless indicated by his or her medical condition. Restraints are often removed when client falls asleep. Monitor closely as client awakens.
10. Ensure that a new order and the physician or LIP completes a medical assessment every 24 hours.
11. Obtain a physician's order and discontinue restraints as soon as it is clinically indicated.
12. Document all assessments and findings on appropriate forms.

Skill 7.2.2 | Applying Torso/Belt Restraint

Equipment

Safety belt restraint (usually 2-in. soft webbing material) with waist and side belts (for bed)

Procedure

1. Check physician's order and client care plan for torso/belt restraint. Perform hand hygiene.
2. Obtain belt. Belts may have a key-locked buckle.
   ➤ *Rationale:* This prevents slipping and provides a snug fit. ❶
3. Introduce self and identify client using two identifiers; explain necessity for safety belt to client and family.
4. Apply torso restraint as follows:
   a. Slip waist belt through flat buckle, adjusting to client's size.
   b. Snap hinged plate shut by hooking plain end of key over cross bar and lifting upward.
   c. Attach side belts to bed frame in similar manner.
   d. Release restraint by hooking green end of key over cross bar from below and pulling downward.
5. Document time, rationale, and type of safety belt used in nurses' notes, along with client monitoring, client response, frequency of care measures, and time and rationale for discontinuing restraint. Documentation must be done every 15 minutes.
6. Remove restraint when clinically indicated. Staff convenience is not an appropriate rationale for continued use.

❶ Some belts have a key-locked buckle to prevent slipping and to provide a snug fit.

(continued)

Skill 7.2.2 | Applying Torso/Belt Restraint *(continued)*

EVIDENCE-BASED PRACTICE
Deaths Due to Use of Physical Restraint or Seclusion
A 50-state survey by the *Hartford Courant* in 1998 identified at least 142 deaths related to the use of physical restraint or seclusion since 1988. The true number of deaths is much higher since data regarding this type of information are not public information. According to statistical projections commissioned by the *Courant* and conducted by the *Harvard Center* for Risk Analysis, between 50 and 150 deaths occur every year across the country due to improper restraint procedures. Based on this data, it was felt there is a critical need for mandated monitoring of the use of restraints and seclusion.

In 2012, the ANA reconfirmed its support for reducing client restraint and seclusion in healthcare settings. The ANA also noted that nurses often must work hard to find a balance between protecting the client's rights and needing to prevent harm to clients and staff. This responsibility makes it essential that nurses possess the knowledge and skills to assess clients and determine that restraints and seclusion are used only when clinically appropriate and adequately justified and when no other option is viable.

Source: American Nurses Association (2012)

Skill 7.2.3 | Using Wrist Restraints

Equipment
Commercial cloth restraints with flannel padding
Ace bandages of appropriate size for area to be immobilized
Call bell for communication

Procedure
1. Attempt all other methods of client protection or less restrictive measures before applying restraints.
2. Check physician's order for wrist or ankle soft restraint. If necessary, place restraint on client, then phone physician or LIP for orders within 1 hour of application of restraint.
3. Obtain soft restraints. Check correct size of restraints.
4. When applying restraint, place padded section over the wrist or ankle. ❶ Ensure restraint will not interfere with IVs or tubes. Allow as much movement of extremity as possible while still achieving the desired outcome. It is unusual for only one extremity to be restrained. Assess for fall risk and safety.
5. Secure restraint by pinching long-pronged adapter and inserting into buckle end of restraint, or follow manufacturer's directions. ❷
6. Slip two fingers under restraint (Box 7-12 ■). ➤ *Rationale:* This ensures it is not too tight and will not constrict blood flow.
7. Attach other end of the restraint to the bed frame by using a half-bow knot. Do not attach to the movable part of bed. ❸ ➤ *Rationale:* The half-bow is a quick-release knot and will untie quickly in an emergency.

CLINICAL ALERT
Always keep scissors in easy access to facilitate cutting restraints in case of an emergency.

❶ First, apply padded portion of restraint around wrist or ankle.

❷ Secure restraint by pinching long-pronged adapter and inserting into buckle end of restraint.

8. Release restraints every 2 hours. ➤ *Rationale:* Release is necessary to allow nursing actions:
   a. Check limb circulation and skin condition.
   b. Provide extremity range of motion.
   c. Change client's position.
   d. Attend to elimination, fluid, or other needs.

❸ Secure restraint to bed frame; do not secure to movable bed parts.

9. Document use of and rationale for wrist restraints in nurses' notes. Identify all less restrictive actions tried before restraints.
10. Monitor client every 15 minutes. In some cases, continuous monitoring may be required. ➤ *Rationale:* Frequent monitoring prevents complications.

Box 7-12 ALTERNATE TYPE OF SOFT RESTRAINT

- Slide strap through slit in restraint.
- Tighten strap, leaving fingerbreadth space between restraint and client's limb.

Skill 7.2.4 | Using Mitt Restraints

Equipment
Mitt restraint
Gauze padding
Call bell for communication

Procedure
1. Check physician's order, or after placing mitt restraint, phone physician or LIP for orders.
2. Determine whether less restrictive actions could be used.
3. Perform hand hygiene.
4. Obtain appropriate size mitt restraint and gauze padding, if needed. ❶
5. Identify the client by checking two forms of identification.
6. Explain steps and purpose of procedure to family and client (to gain his or her cooperation) if client is able to understand.
7. Raise bed to high position.
8. Lower side rail as needed.
9. Check condition of skin and circulation in involved extremity.
10. Wrap fingers with gauze to absorb moisture and prevent abrasion, if necessary.
11. Apply mitt; secure wrist ties snugly, but maintain circulation by ensuring that two fingers can be slipped under the restraint.

12. For hand control, use the slip knot to tie restraints to the immovable part of bed frame, not to the side rail. In some cases, mitts without arm movement **limitation** will provide enough of a restraint.
13. Place call bell within access and monitor client every 15 minutes.

❶ Mitt restraint.

(continued)

Skill 7.2.4 | Using Mitt Restraints (continued)

> **CLINICAL ALERT**
>
> Restraints are never used as a substitute for surveillance.
>
> **Note:** In confused ambulatory clients, restraint use has been associated with increased falls.

14. Remove mitt every 2 hours. ➤ *Rationale:* This is necessary to allow nursing actions:

    a. Check adequacy of circulation and skin condition.
    b. Provide extremity range of motion.

    c. Change client's position.
    d. Provide for fluid.
15. Reapply mitt.
16. Raise bed rail and lower bed, according to facility policy.
17. Perform hand hygiene.
18. Chart on nurses' notes: client behavior necessitating restraint, all less restrictive actions taken, condition of skin, adequacy of circulation of involved extremity, time of mitt application, times of release and observed responses, and care needs met. Documentation must be done every 15 minutes.

Skill 7.2.5 | Using Elbow/Pediatric Arm Restraints

Equipment
Elbow/Arm restraint
Soft padding

Procedure

1. Check physician's order. This type of restraint, if used for medical procedures or to protect IVs, does not require specific restraint orders.
2. Obtain elbow restraints (many types are available). **1**
3. Explain necessity of restraints to child's parents.
4. Place restraints over elbow of both arms. Follow manufacturer and facility policies and procedures. **2**
5. Wrap restraints snugly around the arm. Secure by tying the restraints at the top. Many restraints have ties long enough to cross under the child's back and tie under the opposite arm.
6. Release the restraints every 2 hours. Remove restraints more often to monitor IV site. ➤ *Rationale:* This allows for joint mobility. Intravenous infiltration in a small child can lead to complications rapidly.
7. Assess position of restraints, circulation, skin condition, and sensation every hour.
8. Provide diversionary activity for small child.
9. Encourage parents or hospital personnel to hold child to promote a feeling of security.
10. Document use of restraints in nurses' notes. Document release of restraints, skin, and circulatory condition. Documentation must be done every 15 minutes.

1 Elbow restraints prevent children from reaching equipment.

2 Elbow restraints may be used to prevent child from reaching his or her face or head.

Skill 7.2.6 | Applying a Vest Restraint

Equipment
Safety vest
Call bell for communication

Procedure

For Client in Bed

1. Check the physician's order or apply vest and call physician or LIP within 1 hour for order.

2. Determine whether less restrictive actions could be used.

> **CLINICAL ALERT**
>
> The use of vest restraints has been associated with serious injury, including client suffocation. If your facility still uses this restraint, exercise extreme caution in applying restraint and monitor frequently. Many organizations no longer allow use of this type of restraint.

3. Introduce self, identify client, and explain necessity for jacket or vest restraint to client and family.
4. Place vest over gown. Have scissors at bedside if needed. Place safety vest on client so that closed side of vest is in back and front side of vest crosses over chest or according to manufacturer's directions. ➤ *Rationale:* This prevents choking if client slumps forward. ❶
5. Bring strap through slit in front of the vest. ➤ *Rationale:* Criss-crossing vest in the back may cause serious injury.
6. Tie straps to nonmovable upper section of bed frame using slipknot. ➤ *Rationale:* This position minimizes risk of inadvertent release, which may cause subsequent injury.
7. Observe client every 15 minutes to ensure proper fit of jacket.
8. Release vest restraint every 2 hours. Follow interventions for releasing restraints of all types.
9. Document use and rationale for restraint in nurses' notes every 15 minutes.
10. Document client assessment and attendance to fluid and elimination needs regularly.
11. Remove as soon as clinically viable.

For Client in Wheelchair

1. Place client in wheelchair with buttocks against chair back.
2. Place vest on client (zipper vest is best); place zipper to back of client. Zip vest from bottom to top. ❷ Ensure that there is adequate space between vest and client.
➤ *Rationale:* This prevents constriction from vest that is too tight.
3. Pull straps at 45-degree angle to rear of seat and pull vest tails under armrests and cross tails in back of chair.
➤ *Rationale:* Tying vest tails in back of chair prevents client from reaching the tails and untying the vest. ❸
4. Wrap tails around immovable kickspur. ➤ *Rationale:* This anchors the tails and prevents client from slipping out of restraints.
5. Tie each tail to kickspur using half-bow knot. ❹
➤ *Rationale:* This type of knot is used because it can be quickly released if necessary (Box 7-13 ■).
6. Check client every 15 minutes to ensure vest is on correctly and client is not in compromising situation. ❺ Have scissors available in the immediate vicinity of the chair.
7. Document every 15 minutes according to policy. ❻

❶ Vest restraint can be used for client on bed rest.

❷ Zip vest from bottom to top at client's back.

(continued)

Skill 7.2.6 | Applying a Vest Restraint (continued)

3 Pull vest tails under armrests and cross tails in back of chair. Wrap tails around immovable kickspur.

5 Check client every 15 minutes while in restraint.

4 Tie each tail to kickspur using half-bow knot.

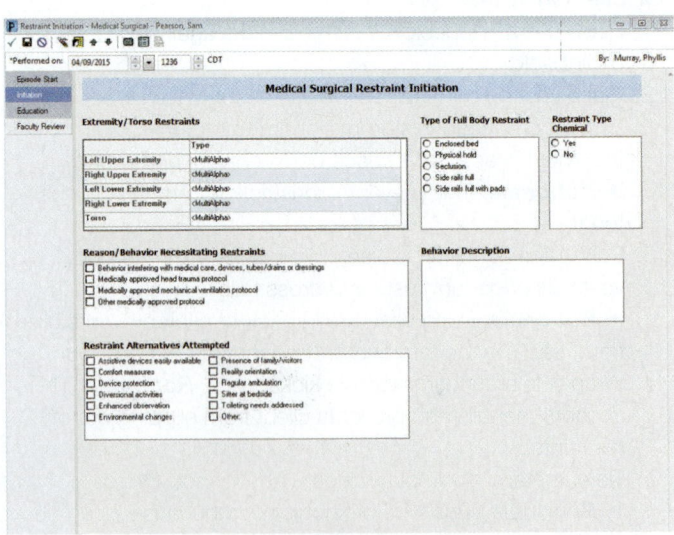

6 Document on Restraint/Seclusion flow sheet.

Source: From Cerner Electronic Health Record. © Cerner Corporation. Pearson has restricted permission to reproduce and distribute this copyrighted work. Further reproduction or distribution is strictly prohibited without written consent of Cerner Corporation.

Box 7-13 **TYING A HALF-BOW KNOT**

Place restraint tie around wheelchair kickspur. Bring free end up, around, under, and over attached end of tie and pull tight.

Tighten free end of tie and bow until knot is secure.

Take free end over and under attached end of tie, but this time make half-bow loop.

Pull end of tie and loosen first crossover tie in an emergency.

LEGAL CONSIDERATIONS FOR ALL RESTRAINTS

Restraints: *Swann v. Len-Care Rest Home Inc.* **(1997)**

Family members requested the confused grandmother be restrained when they were not in attendance. The physician ordered the restraints and wrote a letter indicating he wanted the restraints placed when the client was alone. The client was left unattended and unrestrained, fell, and sustained a head injury. The family brought suit against the facility. During the trial, it was noted this was the client's third fall while she was unrestrained. The court found for the plaintiff. To avoid liability, always follow hospital policies related to use of restraints.

Skill 7.2.7 | Applying Mummy Restraints

Equipment

Blanket large enough to fit child, or sheet, if blanket not large enough for infant.

Procedure

1. Perform hand hygiene.
2. Place the blanket on a secure surface and fold down one corner until tip reaches the middle of the blanket. ❶
3. Place the baby in a diagonal position with the head halfway off the folded edge of the blanket (Box 7-14 ■).
4. Bring one side of the blanket over the infant's arm and trunk, and tuck it under the other arm and around the back. Keep arms in natural position to the side.

❶ A mummy restraint is used when certain procedures are to be done.

(continued)

Skill 7.2.7 | Applying Mummy Restraints *(continued)*

5. Tuck the bottom part of the blanket up onto the infant's abdomen.
6. Fold the second side over the infant, and tuck it snugly around the body.
7. Use the restraint only until procedure is completed.

CLINICAL ALERT

Generally, restraint policies do not apply to the following situations:

- Restriction for security purposes
- Procedure-related immobilization (e.g., for medical, surgical, or diagnostic procedure)
- Use of adaptive support devices (e.g., brace, orthopedic appliances)
- Use of medical protective devices (e.g., tabletop chairs, bed rails)
- Voluntary restraint (client consent)

Box 7-14 MUMMY BOARDS AND PAPOOSE RESTRAINTS

Mummy boards with Velcro straps are used more often in the hospital setting. A diaper or Chux is placed on the board, and the infant is placed on the board and secured with the Velcro straps. Papoose restraints are also used during procedures. Often, pre-procedure sedation can reduce the need for restraints.

Papoose restraint board.

Unit 7.2 Documentation and Evaluation

DOCUMENTATION for Applying Restraints

- Description of specific behaviors leading to restraint
- List of all less restrictive techniques used, or rationale for not using them
- Extent to which client is able to cooperate with restraint procedure
- Any injury to client or others
- All observation data for entire time restraint is applied, including skin integrity, neurovascular changes, and such

- Client's behavior after and during time restraint is applied
- Justification and reassessment for continued use of restraints
- Documentation of review of care plan for effectiveness or rationale for ineffectiveness of care plan

EVALUATION/Critical Thinking

Expected Outcomes

- Client is prevented from injuring himself or herself or others.
- Restraints are applied appropriately.
- Client does not develop complications due to restraint use (e.g., agitation, pressure ulcers, circulatory disturbance).

(continued)

- Child is prevented from reaching the incision site, IVs, or tubes.
- Client remains in restraints for a limited amount of time.
- Client does not experience complications as a result of restraint placement.
- Client does not endure undue psychological stress while being placed in restraints.

Unexpected Outcomes	Alternative Actions
• Skin abrasion, maceration, or rash occurs after application of restraints.	• Reassess absolute need for restraint. • Reassess application method. • Increase padding of soft restraints before application. • Keep restraints off as much as possible and have staff or family member stay with client.
• Impaired circulation or edema evidenced by change in color, sensation, movement, and blanching of nail beds.	• On observation of signs of neurovascular changes, immediately release restraints. Have colleagues present or nearby. • Massage area gently to increase circulation. Inform client about actions prior to implementing. • If extremity is edematous, elevate extremity above level of heart. Encourage range of motion. • Request order for different type of restraint if restraints are still necessary.
• Client unties restraints.	• Camouflage restraint to decrease client's awareness. • Reassess need for restraint. • Exhaust alternative measures to promote safety. • Anticipate and attend to client's needs.
• Client with history of falling has developed acute cognitive changes.	• Alert all personnel that client is high risk for fall. • Review medication regimen (e.g., many medications including psychoactive drugs can cause acute confusion). • Assess for physiologic causes (e.g., hypoxemia, infection, pain, delirium) and address alterations. • Place bedside commode away from bed and remove all obstacles; provide good lighting as well as night light. • Reduce environmental stimuli (e.g., television). • Reorient client with each encounter. • Move client for better surveillance. • Employ monitoring alarm/device or engage family attendance. • Request floor mattress or recliner chair.
• Child is able to reach incision site even with elbow restraints in place.	• Make sure the elbow restraints are tight enough and extend over the elbow. • Check that the restraint is large enough to completely immobilize the elbow. If not, obtain a larger size. • Consider an alternative type of restraint.

Chapter Wrap-Up

GERONTOLOGIC Considerations

Safety Precautions for the Older Adult

- Ensure sensory adaptive devices are used (glasses, hearing aid).
- Use one-half to three-quarter rails rather than full rails.
- Provide adequate lighting.
- Provide and encourage use of call bell or summons device.
- Assess fluid and elimination needs regularly.
- Promote activities of daily living and exercise to maintain muscle strength and flexibility.
- Assist client in **ambulation** if client is unsteady on feet.
- Heed client's summons promptly.
- Put necessary articles for personal hygiene and activities of daily living within easy reach.
- Provide nonslip mats and grab bars in bathtubs, showers, and near toilets.
- Use shower chair.
- Mop up spills promptly.
- Keep hallways clear of obstacles.
- Lock all equipment when not moving client.
- Provide handrails in hallways.
- Apply nonslip footwear and correct size hospital gown or pants.

- Instruct in use of assistive devices when in use.
- Maintain a consistent environment: Keep furniture in established places.

Preventing Thermal Injury

- Skin is fragile and prone to injury as client's age increases. Use thermal treatments with caution. Do not apply *direct* heat to areas with ischemic tissue.
- Check skin frequently when any type of heat therapy (e.g., Aqua K pad) is used.
- Check water temperature before placing client in bathtub (95°F [35°C] for the older adult and those with peripheral circulation impairment).

Wandering-Client Management Plan

- Clients who are identified as potential wanderers from a facility or at risk for falls should wear a monitor device.
- Monitors come in various models, each one designed to identify clients who move away from a designated monitor zone.
- Clients need to be checked regularly to ensure the monitor is appropriately positioned and the alarm functions properly.

MANAGEMENT Guidelines

Each state legislates a Nurse Practice Act for RNs and LVN/LPNs. Healthcare facilities are responsible for establishing and implementing policies and procedures that conform to their state's regulations. Verify the regulations and role parameters for each healthcare worker in your facility.

Delegation

- Before nursing staff is assigned to care for clients requiring restraints, the team leader and/or charge nurse must ensure they have been properly educated in the legal requirements as well as in the application of restraints.
- All personnel must be aware of environmental and client risks for injury. Remind staff to notify RN of risks.
- Nurses must help identify clients at high risk for injury and must be familiar with agency plan/protocol for the prevention of injury.
- Nurses must individualize restraint implementation.

Interprofessional Communication

- Clients at high risk for injury: Report client risk behaviors, attempts to determine underlying cause, attempted alternative protective measures, and rationale for choice of restraint.
- Document type and time restraint initiated, regular monitoring, and client response. According to the FDA, approximately 20 clients die every year from protective restraints. It is critical to instruct all personnel (including CNAs and UAPs who may not administer the restraints, but give client care and therefore, observe restraint use) in the proper use of restraints.

CASE STUDY Applications

Scenario 1

As you enter Mrs. Lake's room, you find her with one leg over the side rail, making attempts to get out of bed unassisted. Mrs. Lake is an 82-year-old client with a history of heart failure (HF). When you question what she is doing, she tells you, "I need to go to the bathroom." She also tells you she is sure her dog needs to be let out because she hasn't been able to get out of the bed all morning. This is your second day caring for Mrs. Lake. Your initial assessment on admission 2 days ago included her being oriented to person, place, time, and situation. The night shift reported off saying she was disoriented all night.

1. What is your first nursing action? Provide rationale for your response.
2. What additional priority nursing actions are justified for Mrs. Lake?
3. What additional information do you need to gather to determine the next step in her plan of care?
4. If, in the assessment completed by the RN, it is determined she needs to be closely monitored for possible falls, what interventions, by priority, will you implement?
5. Identify the legal requirements that must be implemented when a client is placed in restraints.
6. Identify other least restrictive measures that can be utilized before restraints are applied.

Scenario 2

A 75-year-old female was admitted to the hospital after sustaining a fractured hip after a fall on the sidewalk in front of her house. The admission nurse calls the unit to apprise them of the new admission. The nurse explains that the client is not sure what day it is nor where she is at the moment. She did sustain a cut on her forehead in the fall requiring five stitches. You have been assigned to admit the client when she arrives on the unit.

1. Identify the priority assessment you will complete at the time of admission.
2. Describe the environmental alterations that can be initiated to prevent injury to the client.
3. Considering the fall, determine what assessment findings you will evaluate in the initial assessment.
4. Describe two priority nursing interventions that will be included in the client-care plan for this client.
5. The client has surgery the next day and returns to the nursing unit. The client comes back with two IVs, hip dressings with a drain, and O_2 per nasal cannula. The client responds to painful stimuli but is not fully awake. Determine the appropriate safety interventions that will be employed to prevent injury to the client as she awakens.

NCLEX® Review Questions

Unless otherwise specified, choose only one (1) answer.

1. Which one of the following factors is not considered a characteristic that promotes adaptation to the environment?
   A. Environmental influences
   B. Age
   C. Mental status
   D. State of illness

2. What is the primary root cause of a sentinel event?
   A. Poor staffing ratio
   B. Errors in procedure
   C. Inaccurate client assessment
   D. Communication

3. A client has an order for application of wrist restraints as a result of attempting to pull out a peripherally inserted central catheter. How often, in hours, must a renewal order be written?
   A. 2
   B. 4
   C. 8
   D. 24

4. Restraint guidelines include which of the following?
   A. Client must be observed every 2 hours while in restraints.
   B. Wrist restraints must be the first type of restraints used before proceeding to other types of restraints.
   C. Slip knots are used for securing restraints to the bed frame.
   D. Use of restraints is encouraged to replace sitters for clients at risk for falls.

5. When you are preparing to care for a client with a radioactive implant, what is the most important client-care principle?
   A. Keep soiled dressings, gloves, and linens in contaminated container in the room.
   B. Assist client to sit at edge of bed to participate in bathing.
   C. Increase time available for client care; provide care by standing at head or foot of bed.
   D. Instruct visitors to limit visits to no more than 4 hours each day.

6. What is the priority nursing intervention when a client has a seizure?

   A. Turn client on abdomen to prevent tongue from occluding airway.

   B. Insert tongue blade to side of mouth to prevent tongue from falling back.

   C. Place vest restraint on client after initial seizure activity to prevent client from falling out of bed.

   D. Stay with client during postictal state to ensure client has an uneventful recovery.

7. In case of fire in the nursing unit, what is the priority intervention?

   A. Extinguish fire, if possible.

   B. Close doors and windows of clients' rooms.

   C. Remove clients from immediate danger.

   D. Activate the fire alarm.

8. Which one of the following safety precautions is not part of the client teaching plan for an 88-year-old female client who is being discharged to home?

   A. Explain to client that he or she needs to be on bed rest until lower extremity strength and flexibility returns.

   B. Place essential articles for personal hygiene near the bed.

   C. Install grab bars in tubs and near the toilet.

   D. Use a shower chair when bathing the client in the shower.

9. When assessing a client for potential falls, what environmental alteration could be used to prevent the need for restraints?

   A. Placing a rolled-edge mattress on the bed

   B. Placing client in a room near nurses' desk for easy observation

   C. Using a geri-chair and placing client near the nurses' desk

   D. Placing bed in low position, with two upper side rails in the "up" position

10. The client is being positioned in a wheelchair with an order for a Posey vest to prevent him from falling out of the chair. Which actions should be taken by the nurses to secure the vest on the client?

    Select all that apply.

    A. Place vest on client with the zipper in front.

    B. Place vest tails under armrests and cross tails in back of chair.

    C. Tie vest tails using a daisy chain and anchoring on kickspur of the wheelchair.

    D. Tie each tail to the kickspur using half-bow knot.

    E. Tie each tail to the kickspur using a square knot.

QSEN Activity

Domain: Quality Improvement and Client-Centered Care

KSA: Knowledge

Activity:

Staff development meeting to discuss issues around an increased number of clients requiring restraints. Case scenario is used for staff participation and planning.

Background information: The incidence of restraints in a facility had been 4.3 hr/month for 6 months for all clients admitted to the unit. The average number of clients restrained each month was 2. During month 7, the incidence increased to 12 hours for the first 2 weeks of the month with five clients being restrained.

1. Staff were asked to identify three questions they would ask to further their understanding of what led to the increased incidence of restraint use. They stated they wanted to know the

   a. time of day, day of the week when incidents occurred

   b. staffing numbers and changes in staff

   c. medically related problems

Bibliography

The Advisory Board Company. (2012, Nov. 28). Are hospital bed rails safe for patients? Regulators investigate. Retrieved from https://www.advisory.com/daily-briefing/2012/11/28/regulators-investigate-hospital-bed-rail-deaths

American Geriatrics Society. (2015). Guideline for the prevention of falls in older persons. Retrieved from http://www.americangeriatrics.org/health_care_professionals/clinical_practice/clinical_guidelines_recommendations/prevention_of_falls_summary_of_recommendations

American Nurses Association. (2012). Position statements: Reduction of patient restraint and seclusion in health care settings. Retrieved from http://www.nursingworld.org/MainMenuCategories/EthicsStandards/Ethics-Position-Statements/Reduction-of-Patient-Restraint-and-Seclusion-in-Health-Care-Settings.pdf

Centers for Disease Control and Prevention. (2012). Data and statistics. HAI prevalence survey. National and state healthcare-associated infections progress report 2012. Retrieved from http://www.cdc.gov/hai/surveillance/

Center for Medicare & Medicaid Services. (2008). CMS Manual System Pub. 100-07 State Operations Provider Certification §482.13(e) Standard, p 90: Restraint or seclusion. Retrieved from http://www.cms.gov/Regulations-and-Guidance/Regulations-and-Guidance.html

Clugston, D. (2007, Apr.). Falls by older adults. *Advance for Nurse Practitioners 2007, 15*(4), 61–64.

Food and Drug Administration. (2014). A guide to bed safety bed rails in hospitals, nursing homes and home health care: The facts. Retrieved from http://www.fda.gov/MedicalDevices /ProductsandMedicalProcedures/GeneralHospitalDevicesand Supplies/HospitalBeds/ucm123676.htm

Hellwig, K. (2000). Alternatives to restraints: What patients and caregivers should use. *Home Healthcare Nurse, 18*(6), 395.

Jagger, J., & Perry, J. (2002). Realistic expectations for safety devices. *Nursing, 32*(3), 72.

Johnston, J., & Davis, M. (2008, Apr.). When sequential-compression devices cause falls. *American Journal of Nursing, 108*(4), 37–38.

Magill, S. S., Edwards, J. R., Bamberg, W., Beldav, Z. G., Dumyati, G., Kainer, M. A., . . . & Fridkin, S. K. (2014, Mar.). Multistate point-prevalence survey of health care–associated infections. *New England Journal of Medicine, 370*(3), 1198–1208. doi: 10.1056/NEJMoa1306801

National Institutes of Health. (2014). Use of restraints. Retrieved from http://www.nlm.nih.gov/medlineplus/ency/patientinstructions/000450.htm

Peason, K. & Coburn, A. (2011, Dec.) Evidence-based falls prevention in critical access hospitals. www.flexmonitoring.org

Registered Nurses' Association of Ontario. (2005, Oct.). *Prevention of falls and fall injuries in the older adult.* (Revised). Toronto, Canada: Author.

Swann v. Len Care Rest Home, Inc. (1997, Oct. 7). Retrieved from http://caselaw.findlaw.com/nc-court-of-appeals/1242298.html

The Joint Commission. (2015, Apr. 6). Sentinel event data general information 1995–2013. Retrieved from http://www.jointcommission.org/sentinel_event_data_general/

The Joint Commission. (n.d.). Sentinel event data root causes by event type 2004–2014. Retrieved from http://www.jointcommission.org/assets/1/18/Root_Causes_by_Event_Type_2004-2014.pdf

The Joint Commission. (2012). Home care national patient safety goals. Retrieved from http:www.jointcommission.org/HomeCareNationaPatientSafetyGoals

The Joint Commission. (2013). Revised restraint requirement for hospitals and critical access hospitals. Retrieved from http://www.jointcommission.org/issues/article.aspx?Article=A60ZwhfjVk0WTltMZRr4UySBYvozp5CV1Wo47LkIw%2B8%3D

The Joint Commission. (2014). National patient safety goals for 2015. Retrieved from http://www.jointcommission.org/assets/1/6/2015_NPSG_HAP.pdf

United States Department of Labor. (n. d.) Hazard communication safety data sheets. Retrieved from https://www.osha.gov/Publications/HazComm_QuickCard_SafetyData.html

Williams v. Covenant Medical Center, 2000. In Guido, G. W. (2006). *Legal and Ethical Issues in Nursing,* 4th ed. Upper Saddle River, NJ: Prentice Hall, p. 395.

Chapter 8
Bathing, Bedmaking, and Maintaining Skin Integrity

 ## Learning Objectives

8.1 Compare and contrast the steps in making an occupied and unoccupied bed.

8.2 Demonstrate the skill of folding a mitered corner.

8.3 Outline the steps in bathing a bedridden adult client.

8.4 Differentiate between bathing a bedridden client and a critically ill client.

8.5 Compare and contrast the differences in bathing an infant, a child, and an adult client.

8.6 State the advantages of using a commercial bathing system.

8.7 Describe the assessment modalities completed while bathing a client.

8.8 Outline the steps in providing morning care.

8.9 Describe the skin assessment steps that must be completed on a daily basis.

8.10 Outline the steps in providing foot care.

8.11 Describe the changes in skin that occur with aging and appropriate nursing interventions to prevent a skin tear.

8.12 Describe briefly the components of evening care.

8.13 Define the three back care strokes and their use in back care.

8.14 Complete client charting for morning and evening care on nurses' notes.

8.15 Write three nursing diagnoses appropriate for providing basic hygienic care to clients.

Chapter Outline

Terminology

Acne skin condition due to irritation and infection of the sebaceous glands.

Athlete's foot irritation characterized by itching, burning skin; caused by an easily transmitted fungus.

Blanching a whitish hue to an area of the skin when pressure is applied.

Calluses thickened epidermis over area of pressure.

Closed bed a bed not being used by a client; the linens are left to cover the bed.

Complete care the client requires total assistance from the nurse and/or CNA because he or she is not able to care for himself or herself. Complete bathing, skin care, oral care, nail and hair care, care of the feet, eyes, ears, and nose, and a total bed linen change are usually provided.

Corns high calluses caused by pressure on toes, joints, or bony prominences.

Cyanosis blueness of the skin related to decreased oxygenation of the blood.

Drawsheets fabric or waterproof material placed across the shoulder-to-knee area of the bed and tucked in on the sides.

Early morning care or **a.m. care** assistance provided by the night shift or day shift nurse and/or CNA; may include bathing the hands and face; use of the bedpan, urinal, or bedside commode; oral care; and other preparations before breakfast.

Ecchymosis collection of blood underneath skin surface; bruise.

Effleurage long stroking motions of the hands up and down the back in a back rub. Hands do not leave the skin surface. Pressure is light.

Emollient soothing, softening agent applied to body surfaces.

Epidermis superficial, or top, layer of skin.

Erythema redness of skin associated with rashes, inflammation, infections, allergic responses, or congestion of the capillaries.

Evening care (H.S. care, hour of sleep care) evening care usually provided to prepare the client for a relaxing, uninterrupted period of sleep. Activities may include oral care, partial bathing, skin care, a soothing back massage, straightening or changing the bed linen, and offering the bedpan or urinal. The client should also be assessed for the need of food, drink, or medication before sleep.

Flush redness of the face and neck due to dilation of the capillaries.

Footboard usually a solid support placed on the bed where the soles of the feet touch and secured to the mattress or bed frame. Footboards are used to prevent permanent plantar flexion (footdrop) and to exercise leg muscles. The footboard may also have side supports to maintain proper foot alignment.

Hyperemia influx of blood into an area causing redness to the skin.

Incontinent pads large cloth or disposable pads that can be placed under the buttocks area, head, drains, or any place where excess moisture or fluid may collect on the bed.

Independent care the client is able to complete his or her own care. The nurse provides the client with any needed equipment.

Inflammation swelling, pain, heat, and redness of tissue.

Jaundice yellowish appearance caused by deposition of bile pigment in the skin.

Ischemia decreased, insufficient blood supply to body area.

Lesion an area of broken skin as a result of trauma or a pathologic interruption of tissue.

Mucosa mucous membrane lining passages and cavities communicating with the air.

Necrosis cellular death resulting from decreased blood flow to tissue.

Occupied bed the client remains in the bed while it is being made.

Open bed a bed being used by a client; the linens are fanfolded down.

Pallor paleness; absence of skin coloration.

Partial bath cleaning of certain parts of the body such as the face, hands, underarms, back, and perineal area, or areas the client cannot reach.

Partial care the client performs as much of his or her own care as possible. The nurse or CNA completes the remaining care.

Petechiae pinpoint reddish spots.

Petrissage pinching of the skin, subcutaneous tissue, and muscle as you move up and down the client's back with a back rub.

Pigmentation normal or abnormal coloring of the skin.

Plantar warts virus manifested as a deep, often painful, wart on the soles of the feet.

Preoperative care care of clients who will be undergoing surgery or diagnostic tests. It includes removal of dentures, hairpins, makeup, nail polish, contact lenses, and jewelry; locking up valuables; and encouraging to void before leaving for the operating room.

Pressure points areas of skin that can become injured with pressure, especially over bony prominences; areas for exerting pressure to control bleeding.

Pressure ulcer an area of cellular necrosis due to decreased circulation.

Pull sheets sheets placed across the shoulder-to-knee area of the bed that are used to lift the client in the bed. The sides are not tucked under the mattress.

Purpura reddish purple area.

Sensory overload too much stimulation for the senses to adjust to at once.

Shearing force layers of skin moving on each other, which can lead to pressure ulcer or skin damage.

Skin tear traumatic wound resulting from separation of the epidermis from the dermis.

Tapotement alternate striking of fleshy part of hands on client's back as you move up and down the back with a back rub.

Therapeutic bath bath requiring a physician's order; used for specific conditions.

Turgor the degree of elasticity of the skin.

Ulcer an open sore or lesion of the skin or mucous membrane of the body.

Basic Health Care

Clients enter the hospital environment for a variety of reasons requiring immediate care, or for recommended diagnostic procedures or surgery (commonly referred to as an *elective admission*). Whatever the reason, the client must rapidly alter everyday routines and activities of daily living. The client may be concerned about his or her health and well-being and may experience varying degrees of anxiety as a reaction to unfamiliar procedures, hospital personnel, or the hospital environment itself.

After the client has been admitted to the healthcare unit, many **independent care** actions, such as bathing, personal hygiene, and general care may be curtailed by the nature of the illness and confinement. The client may require assistance with even the simplest of actions. Without therapeutic intervention, the total adaptation process may be put in jeopardy as additional physical problems occur. Knowing when and how to intervene and performing such skills as bedmaking, bathing, and personal hygiene facilitate the client's process of adapting to the healthcare environment.

When the client is confined to bed even for a short time, comfort is essential in order to promote rest and sleep. To prevent skin irritation and breakdown, beds must be kept clean and free of debris and wrinkles. The bed needs to be straightened frequently throughout the day to accomplish this. If the client is to remain in bed for an extended time, all care and daily routines are directed from bed. It becomes the center of activity.

Types of Beds

There are many different types of beds and related equipment available to meet the special healthcare needs of individual clients.

The hospital bed is a standard twin-size bed in a frame that allows for different positions to facilitate care and comfort for the client. The height, head, and foot positions in most beds are electrically operated to assist both the client and the nursing staff. The nurse instructs the client in the proper use of bed controls and in bed positions that could be helpful or dangerous for the client.

Support Surfaces

Support surfaces such as mattress overlays filled with foam, gel, or water are commonly used as the first line of defense against skin breakdown. These surfaces prevent pressure on bony prominences, thus reducing **pressure ulcer** incidence. They are cost-effective surfaces that prevent pressure ulcers in clients who are classified as low risk. These surfaces can also be used to treat those clients who already have pressure ulcers. (Pressure ulcers are addressed under wound care.)

Foam overlay support surfaces are used for prevention in low-risk clients. The foam pads are ventilated for moisture control and have an antishearing surface. Foam mattresses and continuous airflow systems can be placed on top of existing mattresses. Alternating pressure mattresses are used as replacements for standard mattresses. A third type of support system keeps skin dry with a continuous airflow and moisture control feature. It also reduces friction and shear. This system is portable and easily transported and is placed on the existing mattress.

Specialty Beds

New types of specialty beds are used to provide care to clients at risk for developing skin breakdown and pressure ulcers. Clients most susceptible to these conditions (where a specialty bed is critical) include spinal cord injury clients or those who need frequent turning and are difficult to move, such as clients who have had a stroke or brain attack.

Specialty beds replace the entire hospital bed and are classified as air fluidized, low air-loss, kinetic therapy, and critical care therapy. High air-loss beds are used for clients with stage III and IV pressure ulcers. These beds have anti-friction/shear surfaces and built-in scales. Low air-loss beds are used for clients who are difficult to reposition or when moving is contraindicated. Air-filled beds are used for clients who require minimal movement. It makes turning easy and facilitates drainage.

There are two additional types of specialty beds used as preventative or treatment measures for clients having special needs. The first type, the kinetic bed, is used to provide continuous passive motion or oscillation for clients with unstable spines. The second type of bed, the bariatric bed, is used for clients who are obese. These beds have a special feature that allows clients to be weighed in the bed, and it can also be converted into a chair.

Bathing

Routine bathing is an essential component of daily care. It is essential to prevent body odor, because excessive perspiration interacts with bacteria to cause odor. Dead skin cells can lead to infection if impaired skin integrity occurs. Excessive bathing, on the other hand, can increase the risk for impaired skin integrity in older adult clients. In older adults, skin may become dry and cracked due to a natural decrease in the production of moisturizing oils, which can lead to infection.

Bathing promotes a feeling of self-worth by improving the individual's appearance. Relaxation and improved circulation are benefits of bathing and play a therapeutic role in the care of clients on bed rest. The apocrine glands, found in the axillae and pubic areas, produce sweat, which leads to odor. Therefore, thorough bathing should be provided to these areas.

In addition to the therapeutic effects, the **therapeutic bath** affords the nurse time to communicate with and assess the client. Assessment of skin conditions, mobility, and self-care deficits can be detected while bathing the client. If the bath is delegated to the CNA, the nurse needs to assess the client's skin and self-care deficits.

In addition to the basin, wash cloth, and soap bathing procedure, there are several types of commercial body cleansing systems currently used in hospitals and other healthcare facilities. The systems are a body bath, shampoo, and a perineal care package. The bath system uses disposable washcloths to cleanse the client. This type of system cleans, moisturizes, conditions, and protects the skin; therefore, it is a good alternative for older adult clients or clients with sensitive skin. The system contains ingredients that are hypoallergenic and bactericidal.

Bathing is accomplished in a variety of ways, according to the client's needs, condition, and personal habits. Bathing is necessary to cleanse the skin and to promote circulation.

Baths may also be used as a treatment to promote healing for a client with burns. Various types of bathing include:

- **Complete bath:** The client, who is usually totally dependent, is bathed in bed by the nurse or CNA due to physical or mental incapacity. The client is encouraged to complete as much of his or her bath as possible.
- **Partial bath:** Face, axilla, hands, back, and genital area are bathed; or the areas the client cannot reach. **Partial bath** may be completed by client, CNA, or nurse.
- **Therapeutic bath:** This bath is used as part of a treatment regimen for specific conditions, such as skin disorders, burns, high body temperature, and muscular injuries. Therapeutic baths require physician's orders, including type of bath, water temperature, solution to be used, and frequency. Medicinal substances, such as oatmeal, Aveeno, and cornstarch, may be included in the bathwater.
- **Shower:** Preferred method of bathing if client is ambulatory or can be transported to use a shower chair.
- **Tub bath:** Used by ambulatory clients as well as those who must be assisted by a device such as the Hoyer lift.
- **Cooling bath:** The client is placed in a tub of tepid water to reduce body temperature.

Skin Conditions

The skin is the largest organ of the body. Skin is exposed to environmental risks as well as physical and mechanical injury. Skin is composed of the **epidermis** (outer layer) and the dermis (inner layer). The skin provides protection, thermoregulation, excretion, metabolism, sensation, and communication for the body.

Skin types, colors, textures, and condition are as different and unique as each individual. The condition of a client's skin is determined by his or her health status, age, activity level, and environmental exposure. For example, the skin of an infant is often more sensitive and delicate than that of an adult because it has not been exposed to many environmental elements. Most infants cannot tolerate strong soaps and lotions and must be handled gently to avoid trauma. Adolescents are often affected by **acne** and have areas of increased oil secretion. Adults may have drier skin, especially as they age. Older adults cannot always tolerate harsh soaps because their skin is more delicate. They require less frequent bathing and more lubrication with oil-rich creams and lotions.

Skin tears are a traumatic wound, usually occurring on the extremities of older adult clients. They are a result of friction, or shearing and friction forces, that cause separation of the epidermis from the dermis. Older adult clients are more susceptible to skin tears because of changes in their skin with aging. The epidermis gradually thins and loses its elasticity. This leads to a less effective barrier against fluid loss, bruising, and infection. Impaired thermoregulation leads to decreased tactile sensitivity and pain perception. Blood vessels become thin and fragile, which presents as **purpura** or the appearance of little hemorrhages under the skin. Skin tears often occur at the site where purpura is present. Skin tears are more prevalent on the arms and hands, but can occur anywhere on the body. A skin tear on the back or buttocks is often mistaken for a pressure ulcer, but its etiology is not the same.

Maintaining skin integrity is an integral part of providing nursing care; being aware of the client's skin condition and alterations in skin integrity is a critical aspect of providing total client care. The feet are especially susceptible to discomfort, trauma, and infection due to the amount of stress they must endure as well as to their distance from main blood supplies. Many conditions can be avoided if proper foot care is taken.

Cultural Awareness

When providing hygienic care for clients, the nurse needs to assess the client's usual pattern of bathing, hygienic products usually used, and cultural rituals and beliefs.

Modesty and bathing rituals and beliefs must be considered in caring for clients. For example, some cultures and religions do not allow members of the opposite gender to see them unclothed (Muslim culture, Southeast Asian cultures). Many Hispanic women have a strong sense of modesty and do not want healthcare workers to see them unclothed.

Nursing Diagnoses

The following nursing diagnoses may be appropriate to include in a client care plan when the components are related to basic care of the client.

NURSING DIAGNOSIS	RELATED TO . . .
Activity Intolerance	Prolonged bed rest, surgery, pain, treatment schedule, weakness, fatigue
Ineffective Health Maintenance	Ineffective coping, lack of motivation, motor impairment, lack of financial resources
Impaired Bed Mobility	Unable to ambulate, difficulty moving into or out of bed, lack of coordination, motor impairment, visual disorders, surgery, muscle weakness, pain
Impaired Skin Integrity	Surgery, immobility, prolonged bed rest, mechanical factors (**shearing force**, pressure)

Source: Herdman, T. H. & Kamitsuru, S. (Eds.) *Nursing Diagnoses – Definitions and Classification* 2015-2017. Copyright © 2014, 1994–2014 by NANDA International. Used by arrangement with John Wiley & Sons Limited. Companion website: www.wiley.com/go/nursingdiagnoses. In order to make safe and effective judgments using NANDA-I nursing diagnosis it is essential that nurses refer to the definitions and defining characteristics of the diagnoses listed in this work.

Unit 8.1
Bedmaking

Nursing Process Data

ASSESSMENT Database

- Assess the client's need to have linen changed.
- Determine whether the client's present condition permits a change of bed linen.
- Determine how many and what type of linens are required.
- Check client's unit for available linens.
- Determine client's prescribed level of activity and any special precautions in movement.
- Assess client's ability to get out of bed during linen change.

PLANNING Objectives

- To provide a clean, comfortable sleeping and resting environment for the client
- To eliminate irritants to skin by providing wrinkle-free sheets and blankets
- To avoid client exertion, do not move client more than necessary when making an occupied bed
- To enhance client's self-image by providing a clean, neat, and comfortable bed
- To properly dispose of soiled linens and prevent cross-contamination
- To correctly align clients to assist in promoting a physically and emotionally safe and comfortable position
- To prevent stress to the nurse's back or limbs during procedure

IMPLEMENTATION Procedures

DOCUMENTATION AND EVALUATION

Expected Outcomes

- Bed remains clean, dry, and free of wrinkles.
- Client's skin is intact and free of irritation.
- Nurse does not experience stress on back or joints during bathing and bedmaking.

Unexpected Outcomes/Alternative Actions

Pearson Nursing Student Resources

Find additional review materials at **nursing.pearsonhighered.com**.
Prepare for success with NCLEX®-style practice questions and Skill Checklists.

Skill 8.1.1 | Folding a Mitered Corner

Equipment
Linens

Procedure
1. Perform hand hygiene.
2. Identify client using two descriptors.
3. Introduce self and explain the procedure that will be done.
4. Tuck sheet tightly and smoothly under mattress at top or bottom of the bed depending on where mitered corner is needed.
5. Grasp edge of sheet with hand and bring sheet onto mattress so that edge forms a right angle.
6. Tuck lower edge of sheet under mattress.
7. Place finger on sheet where it meets mattress and lower top of sheet over finger. ➤ *Rationale:* This action makes the mitered corner neat, tight, and secure.
8. Remove finger without disturbing folds. ❶
9. Tuck sheet securely under mattress.

❶ Mitered corners keep bed linens tight and wrinkle-free.

Skill 8.1.2 | Changing a Pillowcase

Equipment
Clean pillowcase

Procedure
1. Perform hand hygiene.
2. Pick up center of closed end of pillowcase.
3. Continue to firmly grip end of pillowcase; then with other hand, gather pillowcase from open end and fold back (inside-out) over closed end.
4. Pick up center of one end of pillow with the hand holding the gathered pillowcase. ❶
5. Invert pillow so that pillowcase drapes down over pillow.
6. Pull pillowcase over pillow with other hand. Do not place pillow or case under arm, chin, or in teeth. ➤ *Rationale:* Contamination occurs from using these methods.
7. Adjust pillow corners in pillowcase by placing hand between case and pillow. Do not shake the pillow to position it in its case.

❶ Pick up center of one end of pillow with the hand holding the gathered pillowcase and pull case over pillow with the other hand.

Skill 8.1.3 | Making an Unoccupied/Surgical Bed

Equipment
Chair or table
Linen hamper
Linens (in order of use):
Top sheet (used as barrier on chair or table to protect clean linens)
Mattress pad, optional
Bottom sheet
Drawsheet
Incontinent pad, if needed

Top sheet
Blanket
Bedspread
Pillowcase
Clean gloves, as needed

Note: Whenever possible, make an unoccupied bed rather than an **occupied bed**. This is physically less stressful for both the client and the nurse.

Preparation

1. Gather clean linen and hamper and bring to room.
2. Explain need for client to be out of bed during procedure.
3. Perform hand hygiene. Don gloves if needed. ➤ *Rationale:* Linens may be contaminated from urine, stool, or drainage.
4. Assist client out of bed and into chair.
5. Arrange second chair and hamper conveniently for use.
6. Place linen on chair; ensure chair is clean. ➤ *Rationale:* This action provides a clean surface and promotes infection control.
7. Place clean linen on chair in order of use; pillowcase at bottom.
8. Detach call signal from bed linen.
9. Adjust bed to a comfortable working height and use body mechanics principles.

Procedure

1. Lower both side rails and place bed in flat position.
2. Remove spread and blanket. If they are to be reused, fold them and place on the chair.
3. Loosen linen on all sides, including head and foot of the bed.
4. Remove top, draw, and bottom sheet, and place in soiled linen hamper. ➤ *Rationale:* Cross-contamination occurs if dirty linen is placed on the floor.
5. Push mattress to head of bed. Center the mattress if necessary.
6. If mattress pad is not changed, smooth out wrinkles and recenter pad on the bed surface. ➤ *Rationale:* Wrinkles can cause skin abrasions if skin is compromised by age, disease, or malnutrition.
7. Make up one side of the bed, then move to the other side of bed and make it. ➤ *Rationale:* This step saves time and expenditure of nurse's energy.
8. If using a fitted bottom sheet, place sheet on mattress, and continue making bed at Step 13. ❶ If using a flat bottom sheet, place the center fold of the sheet in the middle of the mattress with the end of the sheet even with the end of the mattress, and perform Steps 9–12.
9. Unfold the bottom sheet, and cover the mattress.
10. Tuck the top of the sheet under the head of the bed.
11. Miter the corner of the bottom sheet at the head of the bed. (Procedure for mitered corner appears below.) ➤ *Rationale:* A mitered corner is tighter and less likely to come apart.
12. Tuck the remaining side of the bottom sheet well under the mattress.
13. If the client needs a **drawsheet**, ❷ place the drawsheet on the bed and open drawsheet. Tuck the sheet under the mattress. Smooth out wrinkles.

    a. If a **pull sheet** is needed, fold drawsheet in half or quarters. Position sheet in middle of bed. ➤ *Rationale:* Pull sheets are used with heavy or difficult-to-move clients.

    b. If absorbent pad is needed, center it on bed over draw- or pull sheet.

14. Move to the other side of the bed. Pull linen toward you and straighten out linen.
15. Tuck the top of the sheet under the head of the bed if using a flat sheet.
16. Miter the corner of the bottom sheet at the head of the bed if not using a fitted sheet. See steps for creating a mitered corner. ❸
17. Tuck remaining bottom sheet well under the mattress. Gather sheet into your hand, lean away from the bed, and pull sheet downward. Tuck sheet under mattress.
18. If drawsheet is used, tighten and tuck the same as bottom sheet.
19. Straighten out absorbent pad and pull sheet if used.
20. Place top sheet, blanket, and spread full length on top of bed.
21. Leave a cuff of top sheet and spread at the head of the bed. Fold back top sheet and spread to form a 6-inch (15-cm) cuff. ❹ ➤ *Rationale:* This prevents client's face from rubbing against blanket.
22. Tuck sheet, spread, and blanket well under foot of mattress, one side at a time.
23. Miter corners at the foot of the bed, one side at a time.
24. Make a small pleat or slightly loosen linen to allow room for client's feet. ❺ ➤ *Rationale:* This prevents friction and pressure on feet and toes.
25. Fanfold linen to foot of bed. ➤ *Rationale:* This facilitates client getting into bed.
26. Change pillowcase. See Skill 8.1.2, Changing a Pillowcase.
27. Return bed to lowest position. Reattach call signal to linens.
28. Pull side rail up on side farthest from client. ➤ *Rationale:* This allows client to position self in bed.
29. If the bed is unassigned, leave top linen pulled up, covering the bed.
30. Dispose of soiled linen in dirty utility room or hamper (Box 8-1 ■). ❻
31. Perform hand hygiene.

Note: Some facilities use individualized plastic bags to transfer linens to dirty utility room.

Box 8-1 PRINCIPLES OF MEDICAL ASEPSIS WITH LINENS

- Place dirty linen in hamper.
- Do not place dirty linen on floor.
- Discard all unused linen from client area.
- Do not transfer linen from one client area to another.
- Do not allow dirty linen to touch uniform.
- Perform hand hygiene.

(continued)

Skill 8.1.3 | Making an Unoccupied/Surgical Bed (continued)

❶ Lay the bottom sheet on one side of the mattress. Making up one side of the bed at a time saves time and energy.

❷ Tuck drawsheet in tightly over bottom sheet.

A

C

B

D

❸ Mitering corners: **A.** Smooth linen before mitering corners. **B.** Form triangle. **C.** Tuck in linen. **D.** The mitered linens are tucked under the mattress.

④ Fold cuff of sheet over spread.

A

B

⑤ **A.** Pleat top linen to allow space for feet. **B.** Fanfold linen to foot of bed.

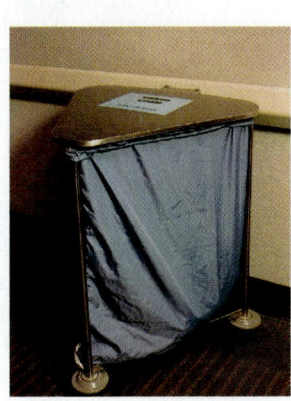

⑥ Keep linen hamper covered to prevent spread of microorganisms. Position hamper outside client's room for easy access.

Skill 8.1.4 | Changing an Occupied Bed

Equipment

Chair or table
Soiled linen hamper
Linens (in order of use):
   Bath blanket or top sheet
   Mattress pad, optional
   Bottom sheet
   Cloth drawsheet
   Incontinent pad, if needed
   Top sheet
   Blanket
   Bedspread
   Pillowcase
Clean gloves, if indicated

Preparation

1. Introduce self, identify the client and explain how he or she can be involved in the procedure.
2. Explain the sequence for the procedure.
3. Arrange furniture and equipment (e.g., soiled linen hamper and chair) for convenience of use.
4. Perform hand hygiene and then collect the clean linen.
5. Place linen on chair; ensure that chair is clean.
6. Detach call signal from linens.
7. Provide for privacy for the client.
8. Adjust the bed to a comfortable working height with side rails up. Help client into a supine position.
9. Don gloves if bed linen is soiled with body fluids.

Procedure

1. Lower side rail on your side of the bed, but make sure side rail on opposite side is in UP position. ➤ *Rationale:* This ensures client safety as client rolls to edge of bed.
2. Loosen top linens.
3. Remove spread, sheet, and blanket at the same time the bath blanket is pulled over the client. Top sheet may be used in place of bath blankets in some facilities.

(continued)

Skill 8.1.4 | Changing an Occupied Bed *(continued)*

➤ *Rationale:* Blanket keeps client warm during bed change. If they are to be reused, fold them and place on the chair.

4. Place top sheet in soiled linen hamper, unless being used to cover client during bedmaking.

5. Push mattress to head of bed. Center the mattress if necessary.

6. Assist client to the side of the bed, place in side-lying position facing away from you as near the far side rail as possible. ❶

7. Loosen bottom linens on your side of the bed. ❷

8. Fold or roll dirty linen under client and remove it. ❸
   ➤ *Rationale:* This keeps soiled linen contained and away from client's skin.

9. Smooth out wrinkles and recenter pad on the bed surface if mattress pad is used but not changed. ➤ *Rationale:* Wrinkles may cause skin irritation.

10. Place clean bottom sheet on mattress with client on the opposite side of the bed. Place the center fold of the sheet in the middle of the mattress with the end of the sheet even with the end of the mattress. ❹

11. Unfold the bottom sheet and cover the mattress. Make sure the clean bottom sheet is underneath any used linen.
    ➤ *Rationale:* This keeps the clean linen uncontaminated.

12. Tuck the top of the sheet under the head of the bed, or position fitted sheet around corner of mattress.

13. Miter the corner of the bottom sheet at the head of the bed if flat sheet is used.

14. Tuck the remaining bottom sheet well under the mattress from head to foot.

15. Center drawsheet on the bed, if the client requires one, and fanfold half of the sheet under the client. Tuck side of the sheet under the mattress. Smooth out wrinkles.

    a. Fold drawsheet in half or quarters if a pull sheet is needed. Position sheet in middle of bed. Fanfold half of the pull sheet under client from client's shoulders to knees.

    b. Fanfold absorbent pad and center it on bed under client's buttocks. Place the pad, absorbent side up and plastic side down, close to the client. ➤ *Rationale:* This position makes it easy to pull through to the other side of the bed.

16. Help the client roll over to the other side of the bed. ❺

17. Tell the client why there is a hump of linen in the center of the bed. Ensure client comfort (i.e., reposition pillows).

18. Raise the side rail. Move to other side of bed.

19. Move linens to the other side of the bed by gently pulling linens toward you.

20. Lower side rail, and loosen bottom sheets.

21. Pull dirty linen to side of bed and roll into a bundle at the foot of the bed or place linen in linen hamper. ➤ *Rationale:* This reduces the spread of microorganisms.

22. Never place dirty linen on the floor. ➤ *Rationale:* Cross-contamination occurs from this action.

23. Pull clean linen across mattress and straighten under client. ❻ ❼

24. Miter the top corner of the flat bottom sheet or tuck fitted sheet over mattress edge.

25. Gather bottom sheet into your hand, lean away from the bed, and pull linens downward at an angle. Tuck remaining bottom sheet well under the mattress. If drawsheet is used, tighten and tuck it in the same way.

26. Help the client into a supine position and adjust the pillow. ❽

27. Place top sheet, blanket, and spread over the client. Leave at least a 6-inch (15-cm) cuff of top sheet at the head of the bed.

28. Remove bath blanket, and straighten top sheet and blanket.

29. Miter corners at foot of bed.

30. Pull up all layers of linen at client's toes. Make a small pleat.
    ➤ *Rationale:* This allows room for client's feet and prevents sheets from rubbing on client's toes.

31. Raise side rail.

32. Remove pillow from bed, and change pillowcase.

33. Return bed to lowest position. Reattach call signal to linens.

34. Position client for comfort.

35. Dispose of soiled laundry.

36. Remove gloves, if used, and perform hand hygiene.

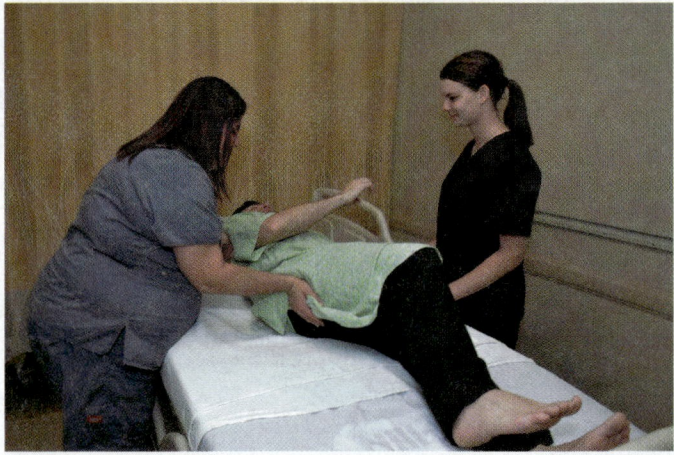

❶ Roll the client to one side of the bed.

❷ Loosen soiled linens and move them to the center of the bed.

3 Roll the client past the dirty linens and remove them from the bed.

6 Center drawsheet in middle of bed.

4 Place and tighten the bottom sheet under mattress, and place drawsheet in the middle of the bed.

7 Smooth and tighten the linens and the drawsheet.

5 Roll the client onto the clean linens.

8 Position the client supine and check for comfort.

EVIDENCE-BASED PRACTICE

To reduce or eliminate the risk for pressure ulcers, research recommends limiting the layers of linen on which a client lies. Use only the minimum amount of bed linens needed for the specific client's needs or condition.

Source: Stotts, Brown, Donaldson, Aydin, & Fridman (2013)

Unit 8.1 Documentation and Evaluation

DOCUMENTATION for Bedmaking

- Specific linens or equipment that cause discomfort for the client
- Special requirements for linens (e.g., certain detergents or elimination of starch)
- Use of pull sheets, incontinent pads, or specified ways to keep bed dry
- Addition or removal of linen to adjust for accurate client weight, if using bed scale

EVALUATION/Critical Thinking

Expected Outcomes
- Bed remains clean, dry, and free of wrinkles.
- Client's skin is intact and free of irritation.
- Nurse does not experience stress on back during bathing and bedmaking.

Unexpected Outcomes	Alternative Actions
Client refuses to have bed made.	• Assess reason for refusal. Client may be in pain or does not want to be disturbed. • Offer to make the bed at a later time. • Change only the pillowcase and drawsheet, if client allows. • Beds do not need to be changed unless soiled or damp, so allow client's independence if possible.
Cross-contamination occurs from improper linen disposal.	• Provide adequate linen hampers for the nursing personnel. • Attend in-service education programs on infection control.
Client's skin becomes irritated from linen or begins to break down.	• Obtain hypoallergenic linen. • Place therapeutic mattress under client. • Provide skin care with appropriate lotion.
The nurse feels stress on back during bedmaking.	• Make sure bed is positioned for comfort of the nurse. High position is generally used. • If client is heavy, ask for assistance with bedmaking, especially in moving side to side. • Use full sheet or Booster Lift for turning. • Attend in-service classes on preventing back strain. • Use body mechanics principles during bedmaking procedure. • Use assistive devices for large clients, as available.

Nursing Process Data

ASSESSMENT Database

- Assess client's need for bathing and other personal hygiene activities.
- Check client's activity order. Note special precautions related to movement or exercise.
- Assess client's ability to perform his or her own care and determine how much assistance he or she needs.
- Discuss client's preferences for the bathing procedure, bath, and personal articles.
- Check client's room for availability of bathing articles and linens.
- Assess client's skin.

PLANNING Objectives

- To decrease the possibility of infection by removing transient bacteria, excessive debris, secretions, and perspiration from the skin
- To eliminate odors and rid body of microorganisms
- To promote circulation
- To maintain muscle tone through active or passive movement during bathing
- To alternate points of pressure on the body by changing client's position during the bath
- To provide comfort for the client
- To assess the client's overall status, skin condition, level of mobility, and comfort

IMPLEMENTATION Procedures

DOCUMENTATION AND EVALUATION

Expected Outcomes

- Client's skin is free of excessive perspiration, secretions, and offensive odors.
- Client feels comfortable and does not experience itching or irritation.
- Client's skin is moist and free of itching sensation.
- Client is able to take bath or shower without excessive fatigue or anxiety.
- Client is able to bathe self using disposable cleansing system.

Unexpected Outcomes/Alternative Actions

Pearson Nursing Student Resources

Find additional review materials at
nursing.pearsonhighered.com.
Prepare for success with NCLEX®-style practice questions and Skill Checklists.

Skill 8.2.1 | Providing Morning Care

Equipment
Basin of warm water
Soap
Towel and washcloth
Emesis basin
Toothbrush and paste
Bedpan or urinal
Toilet tissue
Clean gloves

Preparation
1. Introduce self to client. Determine whether client wishes morning care. ➤ *Rationale:* Morning care is provided to "freshen" the client in preparation for breakfast, physicians' visits, and procedures occurring before bathing. Morning care may be delegated to the CNA.
2. Perform hand hygiene. ➤ *Rationale:* When providing morning care to several clients, it is important to perform hand hygiene between clients so that microorganisms are not transmitted from one client to another.
3. Gather equipment and take it to client's room.
4. Identify client using two indicators.
5. Explain that **early morning care** or **a.m. care** is available while client remains in bed. If client is able, assist him or her to the bathroom.
6. Provide privacy.

Procedure
1. Perform hand hygiene.
2. Offer bedpan or urinal and assist client as needed. Don gloves when giving client bedpan or urinal.
3. Move bed to comfortable working height and lower side rail.
4. Put equipment on overbed table within reach. Place towel under client's chin. ➤ *Rationale:* This keeps gown and linens dry.
5. Wash client's face and hands or assist as needed. Dry face and hands.
6. Offer oral hygiene. Assist as needed. Gloves should be worn if client needs assistance with oral hygiene.
7. Hold emesis basin so client can rinse after brushing teeth.
8. Assist client to comfortable position.
9. Reposition bed, and replace side rails.
10. Remove equipment and draw curtains.
11. Remove gloves, if used.
12. Perform hand hygiene.
13. Document morning care provided.

Skill 8.2.2 | Bathing an Adult Client

Equipment
Basin or sink with warm water 110°–115°F (43.3°–46.1°C)
Soap and soap dish
Personal articles (i.e., deodorant, powder, lotions)
Laundry hamper
Two to three towels and several washcloths
Gloves if appropriate
Bath blanket
Pajamas or hospital gown
Table for bathing equipment (**Note:** For shaving a client, see Chapter 9, Skill 9.2.3, Shaving a Client.)

Note: Use a new cloth for each section of the body to prevent cross-contamination. Clients confined to bed may have increased perspiration and bacterial growth, leading to infections.

Preparation
1. Provide a comfortable room environment (i.e., comfortable temperature, lighting).
2. Identify client; and introduce self talk with client about plan for bathing to meet personal care needs.
3. Encourage client to bathe himself or herself. ➤ *Rationale:* This increases independence and promotes exercise and a sense of self-worth. Bathing activities may be delegated to the CNA.
4. Explain any unfamiliar methods or procedures regarding bathing.
5. Perform hand hygiene.
6. Collect necessary equipment, and place articles within reach on overbed table.
7. Ask the client if he or she needs to void or defecate before starting the bath. ➤ *Rationale:* Warm water of the bath and movement can stimulate the client to void.
8. Position the bed at a comfortable working height.
9. Ensure privacy.

Procedure
1. Place bath blanket over client and over top linen. ❶ Loosen top linen at edges and foot of bed.
   a. Ask client to grasp and hold top edge of bath blanket to keep it in place while you pull linen to foot of bed.
   b. Remove dirty top linen from under bath blanket, starting at client's shoulders and rolling linen down toward the client's feet. If bath blanket is not available, use top sheet.
   c. Place dirty linen in laundry hamper.
2. Help client to the side of the bed closest to you. Keep the side rail on the far side of the bed in the UP position.
3. Remove client's gown. ❷ Most gowns have snaps and can be taken off without disturbing IVs or other tubes. Place gown in laundry bag. Keep client covered with bath blanket. ➤ *Rationale:* This protects client's modesty and keeps the client warm during bathing.

4. Remove pillow if client can tolerate.

5. Place towel under client's head.

6. Don clean gloves if there is risk of exposure to body fluids when bathing client. ➤ *Rationale:* This maintains Standard Precautions.

7. Make a mitt with a washcloth. Fold washcloth around your hand as illustrated. ❸ ➤ *Rationale:* This prevents wet ends of cloth from annoying the client.

❶ Remove top linen and replace with bath blanket.

❷ Remove gown while covering client with bath blanket.

8. Bathe client's face. ➤ *Rationale:* Begin bath at cleanest area and work downward toward feet.

   a. Wash around client's eyes, using clear water. With one edge of washcloth, wipe from the inner canthus toward the outer canthus. ❹ ➤ *Rationale:* This prevents secretions from entering the lacrimal duct. Using a different section of the washcloth, repeat procedure on other eye. Dry thoroughly.

   b. Wash, rinse, and dry client's forehead, cheeks, nose, and area around lips. Use soap with client's permission.

   c. Wash, rinse, and dry area behind and around the client's ears.

   d. Wash, rinse, and dry client's neck.

Note: For shampooing and shaving clients, see Skill 9.2.2, Shampooing Hair, and Skill 9.2.3, Shaving a Client.

A

B

C

❸ **A.** Wrap one edge of cloth around palm and fingers. **B.** Wrap cloth around hand and anchor with thumb. **C.** Tuck far edge of cloth under edge in palm of hand.

9. Remove towel from under client's head.

10. Use a clean washcloth for each section of the body. Bathe client's upper body and extremities. Place towel under area to be bathed.

    a. Wash both arms by elevating client's arm and holding client's elbow area. ❺ Use long, firm strokes from the wrist toward the shoulder, including the axillary area. ➤ *Rationale:* Movement from distal to proximal increases venous return and promotes circulation.

    b. Wash, rinse, and dry client's axillae. Apply deodorant and powder if desired.

    c. Wash client's hands by soaking them in the basin or with a washcloth. ❻ Nails can be cleaned now or after the bath.

(continued)

Skill 8.2.2 | Bathing an Adult Client *(continued)*

    d. Keeping chest covered with the towel, wash, rinse, and thoroughly dry client's chest, especially under breasts. (Apply powder or cornstarch under breasts if desired. ➤ *Rationale:* Using powder or cornstarch under breasts helps prevent the skin under the breasts from becoming damp, which can lead to rashes or infections.)

11. Bathe client's abdomen. Using a towel over chest area and bath blanket, cover areas you are not bathing. Wash, rinse, and dry both abdomen and umbilicus. Replace bath blanket over client's upper body and abdomen. **7**

12. Bathe client's legs and feet. Place towel under leg to be bathed. **8** Drape other leg, hip, and genital area with the bath blanket.

    a. Carefully place bath basin on the towel near the client's foot with knee bent. **9**

    b. With one arm under the client's leg, grasp the client's foot and bend knee. Place foot in basin of water.

    c. Bathe client's leg, moving toward hip with long, firm strokes. Rinse and dry client's leg. ➤ *Rationale:* This promotes circulation.

    d. Wash client's foot with washcloth. Rinse and dry foot and area between toes thoroughly.

    e. Carefully move basin to other side of bed, and repeat procedure for client's other leg and foot.

CLINICAL ALERT

Bathe lower extremities gently if client is at high risk for deep vein thrombosis. DO NOT rub legs. This action could dislodge a clot.

---

6 Wash hands by soaking them in a basin.

7 Keep client covered with towel during bath.

8 Wash client's legs and feet for a total bed bath.

4 Wash eyes first; direction of stroke is from inner to outer canthus.

5 Support elbow area when washing client's arm.

9 Place client's feet in basin while bathing.

13. Change bathwater. Raise side rails when refilling basin.
    ➤ *Rationale:* This ensures client safety. Check the water temperature before continuing with the bath.
14. During the bath, continuously assess the client's skin and musculoskeletal system. Careful attention should be paid to the verbal statements and nonverbal expressions.
    ➤ *Rationale:* This yields information about client's overall condition.
15. Help client turn to a side-lying or prone position. Place towel under area to be bathed. Cover client with a bath blanket.
16. Wash, rinse, and dry client's back, moving from the shoulders to the buttocks. ➤ *Rationale:* Moving from clean to dirty areas of the body helps to prevent transfer of microorganisms.
17. Provide back massage now or after completion of bath. (For procedure, see Skill 8.4.2, Providing Back Care.)
18. Bathe client's genital area if client is unable to do this by self. Cover all body parts except area to be bathed. Place towel under client's hips.

Female Client

a. Bathe perineum from pubis to rectum. ➤ *Rationale:* This prevents contamination from the rectal area to the urethra.
b. Use separate areas of the washcloth for each stroke.
c. Discard soiled washcloths as needed.
d. Clean the labia majora by separating the labia and clean between the majora and labia minora.
e. Wash, rinse, and dry the clitoris, urethral meatus, and vaginal orifice.
f. Ensure all folds of skin are thoroughly dry.

Male Client

a. Place a towel under the penis.
b. Hold the penis by the shaft. If the client is uncircumcised, retract the foreskin before washing if it retracts easily.
   ➤ *Rationale:* This will allow removal of smegma that may have collected, thus decreasing chance of infection.
c. Using a circular motion, wash, rinse, and dry the meatus of the penis and glans in an outward direction.
d. Gently replace foreskin to its original position.
   ➤ *Rationale:* This action minimizes the risk of paraphimosis (venous and lymphatic congestion which can lead to decreased blood flow to the penis).
e. Cleanse the shaft of the penis moving from the tip to the base of the penis.
f. Wash, rinse, and pat the scrotum dry, especially the posterior rugae.

19. Remove gloves and place in receptacle.
20. Assist client to dress in a clean hospital gown or pajamas.
21. Clean and store bath equipment. Dispose of dirty linen.
22. Proceed with any other personal hygiene activities as needed, such as applying deodorant.
23. Replace call light, lower bed, and place side rails in UP position before leaving client.
24. Remove gloves, if used, and perform hand hygiene.

Skill 8.2.3 | Providing Foot Care

Equipment
Basin of warm water
Soap or emollient agent
Washcloth
Two towels
Nail file, emery board, pick, or orangewood stick
Skin care lotion or lanolin
Clean gloves (use if there is risk of contacting body fluids)

Preparation
1. Determine foot care needs based on client's condition and assessment data.
2. Check physician's orders and client care plan. ➤ *Rationale:* Clients with diabetes require specialized foot care.
3. Collect necessary equipment.
4. Introduce self and identify client. Help client into a chair in a comfortable sitting position if possible.
5. Discuss procedure with client.
6. Perform hand hygiene.

Procedure
1. Place towel or bath mat on floor in front of client.
2. Place basin of warm water on towel.
3. Help client place feet in basin. ❶

4. Add **emollient** agent to water, if desired.
5. Assist client with other personal hygiene activities while feet are soaking. Let feet soak for 10 minutes.
6. Using a washcloth, gently wash client's feet with soap and water.
7. Dry each foot thoroughly with a second towel. Dry between each toe.

❶ Place towel on floor in front of client and place feet in basin for soaking.

(continued)

Skill 8.2.3 | Providing Foot Care (continued)

8. If there are no contraindications, use nail clippers to cut straight across the nails. ➤ *Rationale:* This prevents trauma to surrounding tissue.

9. Clean underneath and on sides of nails using a file or orangewood stick.

10. If necessary, push back cuticles using an orangewood stick. Smooth rough edges with an emery board.

11. Apply lotion to entire foot, focusing on **calluses** or dry areas. If client's feet are cracking or excessively dry, instruct client to use a deep-penetrating moisturizer like shea butter.

12. Assist client in putting on clean socks and shoes or slippers.

13. Replace equipment.

14. Assist client to bed or position for comfort in chair.

15. Perform hand hygiene.

Skill 8.2.4 | Bathing a Client in Tub or Shower

Equipment
Two towels and washcloth
Soap
Clean gown, robe, and slippers

Preparation

1. Introduce self and identify client; perform hand hygiene.

2. Assess client's ability to tolerate tub or shower.

3. Cover all tubings and dressings with plastic covering and instruct client to minimize getting these areas wet.

4. Ensure that tub or shower and equipment are cleansed per agency policy. ➤ *Rationale:* This prevents spread of microorganisms.

5. Place a rubber mat or towel on floor. Use shower chair if indicated. ➤ *Rationale:* This prevents client slipping and ensures safety.

6. Fill tub or adjust shower with warm water (temperature if tested 105°F [40.6°C]).

Procedure

1. Assist client into tub or shower. Use hydraulic bathtub chair if necessary (see Skill 8.2.7, Bathing in a Hydraulic Bathtub Chair).

2. Show client how to call for help when needed.

3. Provide client privacy. Assist client with washing back, lower legs, or feet, as needed.

4. Assist client with putting on clean gown, robe, and transporting back to room.

5. Clean shower or tub area and dispose of dirty linen.

6. Perform hand hygiene.

Skill 8.2.5 | Bathing Using Disposable System

Equipment
Commercial cleansing system
Bath blanket
Clean gown
Disposable bag
Clean gloves, if appropriate

Note: Use of disposable cleaning systems is the preferred method in many facilities.

Preparation

1. Obtain package with cleansing cloths. ❶ Cloths are premoistened with an aloe and vitamin E formula.
   ➤ *Rationale:* The cleansing cloths are less drying; they maintain the skin at pH of 4.7–4.9.

2. Heat package in microwave for no more than 45 seconds. Check temperature before applying to skin. ➤ *Rationale:* Increased time could lead to excessive heat and burning of the skin. The commercial system can be used at room temperature.

3. Explain procedure to client. ➤ *Rationale:* This procedure may be new to the client, and an explanation is needed to ensure client understands the difference between a bed bath and a bath using a cleansing system. The client may not think he or she has had a complete bath but only "a sponge bath."

4. Perform hand hygiene.

5. Don gloves if there is a risk of contact with body secretions.

6. Replace top linen and gown with bath blanket or top sheet if bath blanket not available.

❶ Place package containing cleansing cloths in microwave to warm according to directions (usually no more than 45 seconds).

Procedure

1. Open package and remove one cloth at a time. **②**
2. Remove bath blanket at each site when cleansing with cloth.
3. Replace bath blanket when cloth removed. ➤ *Rationale:* This prevents the client from becoming chilled.
4. Use a new cloth for each section of the body as follows:

   a. Face, neck, and chest **③ ④**
   b. Right arm and axilla
   c. Left arm and axilla **⑤ ⑥**
   d. Perineum
   e. Right leg
   f. Left leg
   g. Back
   h. Buttocks

5. Discard cloth after cleansing each area. Do not flush down toilet as it could clog the drains. Rinsing is not required with this system. Replace bath blanket or sheet over each part of the body after it has been cleaned. ➤ *Rationale:* This prevents the client from becoming chilled.
6. Place clean gown on client.
7. Place client in comfortable position.
8. Discard cloths in appropriate receptacle. **⑦**
9. Perform hand hygiene.
10. Document bath on flow sheet or nurses' notes.

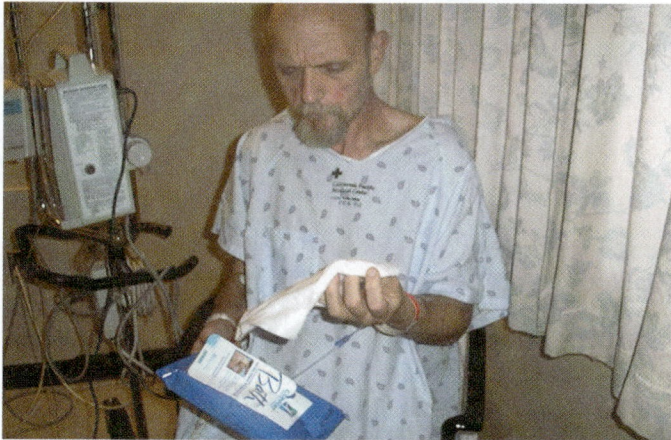

② Each towel is used once and discarded.

③ Disposal bathing—face.

④ Disposal bathing—neck.

⑤ Disposal bathing—arm.

⑥ Disposal bathing—underneath arm.

⑦ Disposing cloth.

(continued)

Skill 8.2.5 | Bathing Using Disposable System *(continued)*

EVIDENCE-BASED PRACTICE
Bath Basins as Potential Sources of Infection

A study (2009) conducted at three acute care hospitals examined 92 bath basins from three intensive care units. Sterile culture sponges were used to obtain samples from the basins. Some form of bacteria grew in 98% of the samples. The organisms with the highest positive rates of growth were enterococci (54%), gram-negative organisms (32%), *Staphylococcus aureus* (23%), vancomycin-resistant enterococci (13%), and methicillin-resistant

Staphylococcus aureus (8%). The conclusion of the study indicated that bath basins are a reservoir for bacteria and may be a source of transmission of hospital-acquired infections.

When a prepackaged bath was used, microbial counts were significantly lower than with basin baths. The study concluded that using a disposable bath is more efficacious for bathing, particularly for high-risk clients.

Source: Johnson, Lineweaver, & Maze (2009)

Skill 8.2.6 | Bathing an Infant

Equipment

Tub or basin filled with warm water (100°F [37.7°C])
Two towels
Washcloth
Suction bulb
Mild soap
Cotton balls
Blanket
Clean clothing
Clean gloves, if indicated

Preparation

1. Provide a comfortable room environment (i.e., warm temperature, soft lighting).
2. Check client ID.
3. Perform hand hygiene.
4. Collect necessary equipment, and place articles within reach.
5. Position the bed at a comfortable working height.
6. Place towel, laid out in diamond fashion, on bed next to basin.
7. Don gloves if there is a risk of exposure to body secretions.

Procedure

1. Test water temperature with your wrist or elbow.
2. Lift infant using football hold.

Note: Some facilities use disposable cleansing systems to bathe neonates and infants. There are four infant-sized washcloths for infants up to 25 pounds. The bathing procedure is the same for infants and adults.

3. Remove all clothing except shirt and diaper.
4. Cover infant with towel or blanket. Never let go of the infant during the bath. ➤ *Rationale:* This is a safety intervention to prevent falls or other injury.

5. Clean infant's eyes using a cotton ball moistened with water. Wipe from inner to outer canthus, using a new cotton ball for each eye. ➤ *Rationale:* This procedure prevents water and particles from entering the lacrimal duct.
6. Make a mitt with the washcloth.

CLINICAL ALERT
Discharge from the eyes may be present for 2–3 days due to prophylactic eyedrops administered at birth.

7. Wash infant's face with water.
8. Suction nose, if necessary, by compressing suction bulb before placing it in nostril. ➤ *Rationale:* This prevents aspiration of moisture. Gently release bulb after it is placed in nostril.
9. Wash infant's ears and neck, paying attention to folds; dry all areas thoroughly. Use mild soap and rinse.
10. Remove shirt or gown.
11. Remove diaper by picking up infant's ankles in your hand.
12. Pick up infant and place feet first into basin or tub. Immerse infant in tub of water only after umbilical cord has healed. Pick up infant by placing your hand and arm around infant, cradling the infant's head and neck in your elbow. Grasp the infant's thigh with your hand. ➤ *Rationale:* The umbilical cord is kept dry to prevent infection.
13. Wash and rinse the infant's body, especially the skin folds.
14. Wash infant's genitalia.

    a. For a female infant: Separate labia and with a cotton ball moistened with soap and water, cleanse downward once on each side. Use a new piece of cotton on each side.
    b. For an uncircumcised male infant: Do not force foreskin back. Gently cleanse the exposed surface with a cotton ball moistened with soap and water.
    c. For a circumcised male infant: Gently cleanse with plain water.

15. Wrap the infant in a towel and use a football hold when washing an infant's head. Soap your own hands and wash infant's hair and scalp, paying attention to the nape of the neck and using a circular motion. Rinse hair and scalp thoroughly. ➤ *Rationale:* Football hold is the most secure for active infants.
16. Place infant on a clean, dry towel with head facing the top corner and wrap infant.

17. Use the corner of the towel to dry infant's head with gentle, yet firm, circular movements.
18. Replace infant's diaper and redress in a new gown or shirt.
19. Provide comfort by holding the infant for a time after the bath procedure.
20. Perform hand hygiene.

Skill 8.2.7 | Bathing in a Hydraulic Bathtub Chair

Equipment
Two towels and washcloth
Soap
Clean gown, robe, and slippers

Procedure
1. Check client's ID using two identifiers; introduce self; perform hand hygiene.
2. Bring client to tub room in wheelchair.
3. Fill tub with water and check temperature. ❶ ➤ *Rationale:* Temperature must not be more than 105°F (40.6°C) or client may burn skin.
4. Release chair to lowest point beside tub ❷. Place towel on floor under chair.
5. Move client into bathtub chair, and attach seat belt.
6. Swing chair into position over tub.
7. Direct client to move legs down, and then lower chair into tub filled with water.
8. Provide assistance. ❸ (May raise chair to prevent back strain.) When client is finished bathing, reverse chair out of tub.
9. Assist client to towel dry.
10. Put clean gown, robe, and slippers on client.
11. Transfer client to wheelchair and transport to room.
12. Assist client to settle comfortably in bed.
13. Perform hand hygiene.

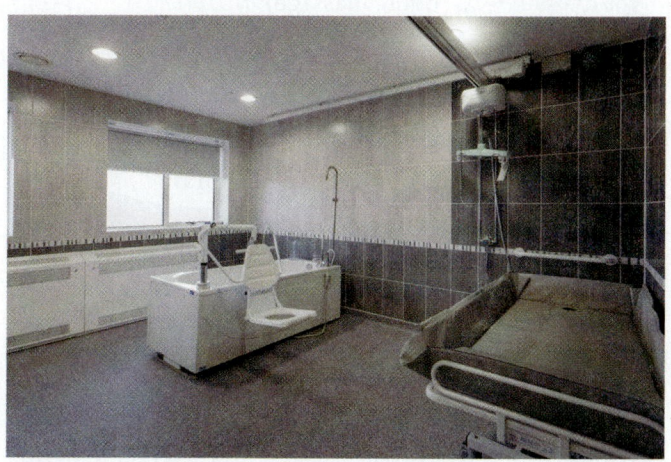

❷ Have seat in low position by the tub.
Source: © Peter Noyce PLB / Alamy

❶ Check that water temperature is not above 105°F (40.6°C).

❸ Secure belt and monitor client safety while assisting with the bath.
Source: © Andréa Aubert / Science Source

Unit 8.2 Documentation and Evaluation

DOCUMENTATION for Bath Care

- Client's overall ability to participate in own care
- Type of bath given (i.e., complete or partial) and by whom (e.g., client, nurse, family member)
- Condition of client's skin and any interventions provided for the skin (e.g., lotion, massage)
- Client's educational needs regarding hygienic care
- Information shared with client or family
- Infant bath demonstration to parents with return demonstration

EVALUATION/Critical Thinking

Expected Outcomes

- Client's skin is free of excessive perspiration, secretions, and offensive odors.
- Client feels comfortable and does not experience itching or irritation.
- Client's skin is moist and free of itching sensation.
- Client is able to take bath or shower without excessive fatigue or anxiety.
- Client is able to bathe self using disposable cleansing system.

Unexpected Outcomes	Alternative Actions
• Client is unwilling to accept a complete bed bath.	• Respect client's wishes and take other opportunities for assessment. • Have client wash hands, face, and genitals. You should wash back and give back care. Reexplain the purpose of the bath to the client and request client participation.
• Client is too shy to allow bath.	• Respect client's privacy and only wash areas client wishes you to do. • Give assistance so client can bathe himself or herself. • Allow spouse or parent to give bath if this is more acceptable to client.
• Client complains of dry, itching skin after the bath.	• Assess for cause of itching. • Ask physician for an order for special lotion. • Do not use soap for the bath.

Skin Integrity

Nursing Process Data

ASSESSMENT Database

- Assess for signs of skin breakdown or the eruption of lesions.
- Assess color of skin.
- Assess color of **mucosa**.
- Check for alterations in skin turgor.
- Assess for complaints of itching, tingling, or numbness.
- Assess texture of skin.
- Assess general hygienic state.
- Observe skin for increased or decreased pigmentation and discoloration.
- Assess client's condition to determine appropriate support surface or specialty bed.

PLANNING Objectives

- To maintain intact skin
- To recognize a break in skin integrity
- To avoid introduction of pathogens through break in skin
- To prevent skin breakdown from **pressure points** or strain
- To prevent excessive dryness, flaking, itching, or burning
- To use support surface or specialty bed to prevent or treat altered skin integrity

IMPLEMENTATION Procedures

DOCUMENTATION AND EVALUATION

Expected Outcomes

- Client's skin is intact.
- Client's skin does not show evidence of dryness, flaking, itching, or burning.
- Client is comfortable with no complaints of pain or discomfort.

Unexpected Outcomes/Alternative Actions

Pearson Nursing Student Resources

Find additional review materials at
nursing.pearsonhighered.com.
Prepare for success with NCLEX®-style practice questions and Skill Checklists.

Skill 8.3.1 | Monitoring Skin Condition

Equipment

Artificial light for observation if natural light is not available

Bath blanket

Gown

Clean gloves, if indicated

Procedure

1. Perform hand hygiene. Introduce self.
2. Check two client identifiers and explain monitoring process to client.
3. Provide privacy for client.
4. Remove linens and gown if necessary. Cover client with bath blanket.
5. Compare color of client's skin with normal range of color within the individual's race. Observe for **pallor** (white color), **flush** (red color), **jaundice** (yellow color), ashen appearance (gray color), or **cyanosis** (blue color). ❶
6. Place the back of your fingers or hand on client's skin to check temperature. ❷ Consider the temperature of the room and of your hands. ➤ *Rationale:* The back of the hand is more sensitive to changes in temperature than the palm.
7. Correlate abnormalities in skin color with changes in skin temperature. ➤ *Rationale:* Skin temperature reflects blood circulation in the dermis layer.
8. Observe for areas of excessive dryness, moisture, wrinkling, flaking, and general texture of skin (Table 8-1 ■).
9. Gently pick up a small section of the skin with your thumb and finger. Observe for ease of movement and speed of return to original position to check for skin **turgor**. ❸
   ➤ *Rationale:* Degree of hydration is reflected in the skin turgor or elasticity of the skin.
10. Press your finger firmly against client's skin for several seconds (especially ankle area). After removing your finger, observe for lasting impression or indentation. ❹
    ➤ *Rationale:* This identifies the severity of pitting edema. It is based on a 4-point scale: +1 (slight) to +4 (very marked).

11. When checking skin temperature and texture, note the client's response to heat, cold, gentle touch, and pressure.
12. Observe the amount of oil, moisture, and dirt on the skin surface. ➤ *Rationale:* Degree of moisture or dryness may indicate disease states or hydration status.
13. Note presence of strong body odor or odor in the skin folds.
14. Observe for areas of broken skin (**lesions**) or **ulcers** (Box 8-2 ■). If present, wear gloves. Check if lesions are present over entire body or if they are localized to a specific area.

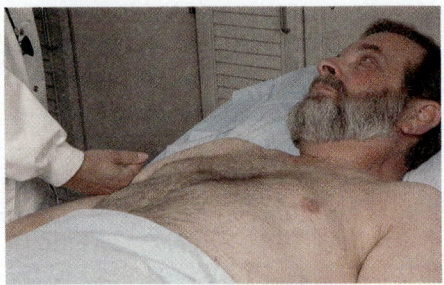

❷ Place back of your fingers or hand on client's skin to check temperature.

❸ Gently pick up a small section of skin with your thumb and finger to check for skin turgor.

❶ Compare color of client's skin with normal range of color within the individual's race.

Box 8-2 RISK FACTORS FOR SKIN TEARS

- Age and gender
- History of previous skin tears
- Dry, fragile skin
- Medications that thin the skin (steroids)
- Bruising and discoloration of skin due to blood leaking into subcutaneous tissue
- Impaired mobility or vision
- Poor nutrition and hydration
- Cognitive or sensory impairment
- Compromised vascularity and skin status due to chronic heart disease, renal failure, and cerebral vascular injuries

Source: Stephen-Haynes & Carville (2011)

Table 8-1 Potential Skin Problems

Skin Condition	Problem	Nursing Responsibility
Xeroderma or dry skin	If skin is extremely dry, it could crack and become infected. May cause pruritus.	Maintain skin integrity. Bathe less frequently. Relieve discomfort. Use emollient or moisturizing lotion after bathing. Encourage nutritious diet. Increase fluid intake. Maintain cool, humid environment.
Skin rash or contact dermatitis. May be allergic or nonallergic reaction; may have exudate.	Erythema, flat or raised eruptions, and **inflammation**. Could cause pruritus, discomfort, and infection if scratched.	Avoid soap and heat, and rubbing area. Bathe area: may use antiseptic soap with orders. Apply ordered lotion or spray (steroids) to prevent itching. Use cool, wet dressing. If exudate present, check bed linens and client's gown, change if moist.
Abrasions	Break in skin integrity could result in infection. Healing may be prolonged due to age (poor circulation, etc.).	Wash abrasions with soap and water. Apply lotion as ordered.
Fungal skin infection	Fungal skin infection: common in diabetics, those on antibiotics or immunosuppressive therapy, and those who are incontinent.	Apply topical antifungal medication as ordered. Dry skin folds well before applying antifungal medication. Apply medication sparingly to prevent skin from becoming too moist. Keep incontinent clients dry and provide good perineal care. Avoid using plastic pants or liners next to client's skin. Use nonocclusive dressings if needed.
Yeast skin infection	Seen with prolonged antibiotic use and in skin folds.	Cleanse and dry skin folds. Apply medicated lotion or cream as ordered.

4 Press your finger firmly against client's skin for several seconds to check for pitting edema.

15. Check for skin discolorations (e.g., **ecchymosis**, **petechiae**, purpura, **erythema**, and altered **pigmentation**). ➤ *Rationale:* These signs may indicate generalized disease states, such as leukemia, vitamin deficiency, or hemophilia.
16. Ensure client is resettled comfortably.
17. Assess client's psychosocial needs while checking skin condition. ➤ *Rationale:* Nonverbal comments can explain as much about how a client is feeling as assessing color and temperature.
18. Perform hand hygiene.
19. Document findings in chart.

Skill 8.3.2 | Preventing Skin Breakdown

Equipment
Skin lotion
Pressure-relieving mattress, support surface, or specialty bed (Box 8-3 ■)
Clean gloves if open lesions are present

Procedure
1. Perform hand hygiene.
2. Check two client identifiers.
3. Provide for client privacy.
4. Inspect skin daily; observe the client's most vulnerable body surfaces for **ischemia**, **hyperemia**, or broken areas. **1**
5. Change the client's body position at least once every 2 hours to rotate weight-bearing areas. **2** Use turning techniques. ➤ *Rationale:* This helps minimize skin injury caused by friction and shear forces. Observe all vulnerable areas at this time. Include right and left lateral, prone, supine, and swimming-type positioning if possible.

1 Observe client's most vulnerable body surfaces for ischemia, hyperemia, or broken skin.

(continued)

Skill 8.3.2 | Preventing Skin Breakdown *(continued)*

 Lubricate dry, unbroken skin to prevent breakdown.

 High-risk, obese clients should be placed on a bariatric bed such as the BariMaxx II or Magnum.

6. If skin is not reddened, massage client's skin and pressure-prone areas (not bony prominences) when client changes position. ➤ *Rationale:* Massage increases risk of breakdown in clients with reddened areas over bony prominences.

CLINICAL ALERT

Current guidelines from the U.S. Department of Health and Human Services advocate no skin massage on reddened skin or skin that has a potential for breakdown because massage causes friction and shearing.

---

7. Lubricate dry, unbroken skin to prevent breakdown.

Note: Products used to prevent skin breakdown and treat impaired skin integrity are selected based on client's skin type, product application, cost, and desired outcome (Table 8-2 ■).

8. Apply lotion to bedridden client's sacrum, elbows, and heels several times during the day.
9. Cleanse skin with warm water and a mild pH-balanced cleansing agent, and then apply moisturizers and a barrier cream as ordered.
10. Protect healthy skin from drainage secretions.
11. Use protective padding on heels and elbows if needed.
12. Keep linens clean, dry, and wrinkle-free.
13. Minimize the layers between the client and mattress.
    ➤ *Rationale:* This allows for proper functioning of pressure relief mattresses.
14. Encourage active exercise or range-of-motion exercise.
15. Encourage client to eat a well-balanced diet with protein-rich foods and adequate fluids.
16. Teach client and family how to prevent pressure areas and pressure ulcer formation.
17. Perform hand hygiene.
18. Document findings in chart.

Table 8-2 Therapeutic Beds

Type of Bed	Client Recommendations
Air fluidized and low air-loss	High risk for skin breakdown
KinAir IV (KCI)	Obese clients
Clinitron Rite Hite (Hill-Rom)	Skin grafts, flaps All four stages of pressure ulcers Wound healing
Air-fluidized	Severe skin disorders
Clinitron II (Hill-Rom)	Pressure ulcers
Fluid Air Elite (KCI)	Burns
Low air-loss	Massive edema
KinAir Med Surg (KCI)	Critical care
Flexicair Eclipse (Hill-Rom)	Pneumonia or other pulmonary problems with compromised skin integrity
Kinetic therapy	Obese: 850–1,000 lbs
Bariatric Client Care Systems	Difficult to move out of bed
MAGNUM II (Hill Rom)	Assistance to place in a sitting position
BariAir (KCI)	Difficult to move due to obesity
BariMaxx II (KCI)	Difficult to move due to obesity
Critical care therapy	Pulmonary condition related to immobility (pneumonia), COPD
TriaDyne Proventa (KCI)	Skin complications related to bed rest
SpO2RT (Hill Rom)	Spinal cord–injured, requiring skeletal traction
RotoRest Delta (KCI) Kinetic	Spinal cord–injured, at risk for respiratory complications

Box 8-3 **SUPPORT SURFACES AND SPECIALTY BEDS**

First Step Plus, an overlay mattress from KCI.

FluidAir Elite, air-fluidized therapy from KCI.

KinAir IV, a low air-pressure bed from KCI.

RotoRest Delta Kinetic, a kinetic bed from KCI.

BariMaxx II, a bariatric pressure bed from KCI.

Skill 8.3.3 | Preventing Skin Tears

Equipment

Lift or turning sheet or booster lift device
Padding for bed rails, or other equipment
Pillows and blankets
Paper tape
Moisturizing agent for skin
Clean gloves as needed

Preparation

1. Identify clients at risk for developing skin tears.
   ➤ *Rationale:* This helps determine appropriate preventative measures. Clients at risk include those on bed rest; those with purpura, ecchymosis, or paper-thin skin such as geriatric clients; those on long-term steroid use; or those with poor vision who may accidentally bump into objects.
2. Identify the category of skin tear, if present (Box 8-4 ■).
   ➤ *Rationale:* This determines correct nursing actions to be completed.
3. Perform hand hygiene before providing client care.

Procedure

1. Check two client identifiers. Introduce self and describe the procedure that will be completed.
2. Use lift sheet or a lift device when moving clients at risk for developing skin tears. ➤ *Rationale:* This will help prevent tears resulting from friction or shearing.

> **CLINICAL ALERT**
> Ensure that all healthcare workers are aware of proper handling of older adult clients with fragile skin. Slight friction and shearing can create a skin tear when turning or lifting these clients.

3. Remove tape from dressings carefully; use only paper or nonadherent dressing for at-risk clients, if possible.
4. Assist clients with ambulation if unsteady gait. Remove objects in pathway. ➤ *Rationale:* This prevents the client from falling or bumping into objects, causing bruises, cuts or skin tears.
5. Ensure clients use glasses, if necessary, when ambulating or transferring into chair. ➤ *Rationale:* This prevents falling or unsteady gait due to impaired vision leading to potential skin tears from falls.
6. Place padding on beds, wheelchairs, or equipment.
   ➤ *Rationale:* This prevents client from rubbing on hard surfaces and causing bruising.
7. Keep head of bed elevated less than 30 degrees unless contraindicated.
8. Support feet and legs when head of bed is elevated.
9. Use lifting devices such as drawsheets, transport boards, and gait belts when moving client.
10. Ensure client is receiving adequate hydration and nutrition.
11. Don gloves and apply moisturizing agent to dry skin to keep moist.
12. Remove gloves and place in appropriate receptacle.
13. Perform hand hygiene.
14. Document findings in chart.

Box 8-4 PAYNE–MARTIN CLASSIFICATION SYSTEM FOR SKIN TEARS

Category I: skin tears without tissue loss
Linear type: epidermis and dermis pulled apart
Flap type: epidermal flap completely covers dermis to within 1 mm of the wound margin

Category II: skin tears with partial tissue loss
Scant tissue loss type: 25% or less of epidermal flap lost
Moderate to large tissue loss type: more than 25% epidermal flap lost

Category III: skin tears with complete tissue loss, no epidermal flap

Category III skin tear.

Source: LeBlanc & Baranoski (2011)

Photo source: © Stefan Sollfors / Alamy

Skill 8.3.4 | Managing Skin Tears

Equipment
Saline
Nontoxic wound cleanser
Moist wound dressing (e.g., Hydrogel, foam)
Nonadherent dressings
Soft silicone dressing
Transparent film
Gauze or Kerlix bandage
Clean gloves

Procedure
1. Perform hand hygiene.
2. Introduce self and check two client identifiers.
3. Don clean gloves.
4. Remove old dressing, being careful to not cause additional skin damage. Moisten dressing with saline before removing if dressing sticks to skin.
5. Assess for signs of infection.
6. Cleanse skin tear with saline or nontoxic wound cleanser. Be careful not to put pressure on skin as you are cleaning.
   ➤ *Rationale:* This prevents additional pain and trauma to skin.
7. If there is tissue that is still attached but not viable, remove it according to physician's orders.
8. Reapproximate viable skin flap when present. Gently cleanse the flap and reposition the flap into place utilizing a moistened applicator. Do not disturb for 5–7 days to allow skin flap to readhere to underlying structure.
9. Choose a dressing appropriate for the wound condition. Most skin tears with minimal drainage on the extremities and where the skin is friable should use a wafer Hydrogel or Hydrogel disk to add moisture to the wound and then be secured with Kerlix bandage roll.
10. When the skin tear is without drainage and has relatively good skin integrity, apply transparent film dressing. ❶ The film ensures that the damaged skin has a moist environment in which to heal.
11. Apply a nonocclusive dressing and wrap the site in a gauze bandage roll when the tear has moderate drainage and is red or warm, or if there is a history of infected skin tears.
12. Apply a foam dressing to absorb the drainage and cushion the wound when there is heavy drainage and the skin surrounding the wound is extremely fragile. Apply a gauze bandage roll to hold it in place.
13. Change dressings according to hospital policy.
14. Remove gloves and place in appropriate receptacle.
15. Perform hand hygiene.
16. Document findings in chart.

❶ If skin tear has no drainage and has relatively good skin integrity, a transparent film dressing can be applied.

Unit 8.3 Documentation and Evaluation

DOCUMENTATION for Skin Integrity

- Client's skin condition: odor, temperature, turgor, sensation, cleanliness, integrity
- Client's mobility
- Turning frequency and client positioning
- Type of care given (e.g., massage, bathing)
- Client's complaints about skin or pressure ulcer
- Time and method used to obtain wound specimen
- Type of lesion, rashes and bruises; state location, size, shape, color
- Alterations in sensation in skin lesion area
- Skin or body odor
- Presence of skin tear and assessment findings
- Treatment given for skin tear including description of drainage and type of dressing applied to wound tear

EVALUATION/Critical Thinking

Expected Outcomes

- Client's skin is intact.
- Client's skin does not show evidence of dryness, flaking, itching, or burning.
- Client is comfortable with no complaints of pain or discomfort.

Unexpected Outcomes	Alternative Actions
• Skin is erythematous but remains intact.	• Monitor fluid balance and nutritional status. • Obtain pressure-relieving mattress. • Turn client every 2 hours. • Ambulate if able.
• Client cannot be positioned in a manner to avoid erythematous areas entirely.	• Turn at least every hour. • Do not turn on erythematous site. • Use protocol for stage 1 ulcer treatment on affected area. • Place support mattress on bed.
• Skin integrity is interrupted, even with skin care.	• Use aseptic technique in treating area to prevent spread of bacteria and promote wound healing. • Use appropriate skin care products. • Place support mattress on bed.
• Skin tear occurs.	• If skin is sensitive and breakdown occurs over large area, the use of a Clinitron unit or air-fluidized bed might be indicated (see Table 8-2).

Nursing Process Data

ASSESSMENT Database

- Review client's usual routines before sleep.
  - Usual time of sleep and length of sleeping period
  - Personal hygiene routines
  - Temperature of room and number of blankets
  - Anticipated elimination needs
  - Religious or meditation needs
- Assess client's understanding and acceptance of safety precautions, such as use of side rails.
- Assess client's needs for comfort and security.
  - Dressings
  - Medication
  - Linen change or adjustment
  - Positioning
  - Television, radio, light
  - Communication needs
- Assess physical and emotional status during evening care.
- Assess condition of back, especially bony prominences.

PLANNING Objectives

- To encourage a period of comfortable, uninterrupted rest
- To evaluate the client's present health status
- To make observations about the client's physical and emotional status
- To provide time for the client and nurse to review the day's events
- To provide time for the client to communicate needs and questions regarding health care
- To provide the client with a clean, secure environment in which to sleep

IMPLEMENTATION Procedures

- **Skill 8.4.1** Providing Evening Care 212
- **Skill 8.4.2** Providing Back Care 212

DOCUMENTATION AND EVALUATION

Expected Outcomes

- Client states he or she is comfortable and ready for sleep after **evening care (H.S. care or hour of sleep care)**.
- Client states that back care has decreased muscle tension and improved comfort level.

Unexpected Outcomes/Alternative Actions

Pearson Nursing Student Resources

Find additional review materials at
nursing.pearsonhighered.com.
Prepare for success with NCLEX®-style practice questions and Skill Checklists.

Skill 8.4.1 | Providing Evening Care

Equipment
Disposable cleansing cloth system or towels, washcloth, and basin with water and soap

Clean linens if needed

Dental care items (i.e., toothbrush, dentifrice, denture cup)

Emesis basin, cup

Fresh drinking water if allowed

Skin care lotion, if desired

Personal care items (e.g., deodorant, skin moisturizers)

Bedpan, urinal, toilet paper

Miscellaneous supplies as needed (e.g., dressing, special equipment)

Clean gloves, if indicated

Preparation
1. Perform hand hygiene.
2. Check two client identifiers. Introduce self.
3. Explain the needs and benefits of evening care; discuss how the client can be involved.
4. Collect and arrange equipment.
5. Adjust the bed to a comfortable working height, and assist the client into a comfortable position.
6. Ensure privacy.
7. Don gloves if indicated.

Procedure
1. Assess for pain. Medicate as necessary.
2. Offer bedpan or urinal if client is unable to use bathroom. Assist with hand washing. Evening care may be delegated to the CNA or unlicensed assistive personnel (UAP).
3. If client needs or requests a bath, provide assistance as needed.
4. Assist with mouth and dental care as needed.
5. Remove equipment, extra linens, and pillows if possible. Remove sequential compression devices, ace wraps, and binders.
6. Change dressings, if necessary. Perform any required procedural techniques. The nurse is responsible for this activity.
7. Wash face, hands, and back. Provide back massage.
8. Assist with combing or brushing hair if desired.
9. Replace sequential compression devices, stockings, and binders.
10. Replace soiled linen, or straighten and tuck remaining linen. Fluff pillow and turn cool side next to client.
11. Straighten top linens. Provide additional blankets if desired.
12. Remove any unnecessary equipment. Place call signal and water (if allowed) within client's reach.
13. Administer sleeping medication if ordered and client requests. This is the nurse's responsibility.
14. Assist client into a comfortable position.
15. Ensure that the client's environment is safe and comfortable.
16. Remove gloves, if used.
17. Raise upper side rails, place bed in LOW position, and turn lighting to low.

Note: Side rails are now considered restraints by the Centers for Medicare and Medicaid Services and the Food and Drug Administration. Check with your facility about agency policies on use of side rails.

18. Perform hand hygiene.
19. Document evening care provided.

Skill 8.4.2 | Providing Back Care

Equipment
Disposable cleansing cloth system or basin of warm water, washcloth, towel, and soap

Skin care lotion

Clean gloves if indicated

Procedure
1. Perform hand hygiene.
2. Check two client identifiers. Introduce self.
3. Explain the purpose of a back rub, and ask client if he or she would like one.
4. Provide privacy. Back care may be delegated to the CNA or UAP.
5. Assess for pain. This is the nurse's responsibility.
6. Warm lotion by holding bottle under water.
7. Raise bed to comfortable height for you, and assist the client into a comfortable prone or semiprone position. Keep farthest side rail in UP position. Placing pillow below breasts may increase comfort for female clients.
8. Don gloves if necessary.
9. Drape bed clothes for warmth, and untie the client's gown. Cleanse back with disposable cleansing cloth or washcloth with soap. ❶
10. Place lotion on your hands and rub hands together to warm lotion.
11. Once you place your hands on a client's back to begin a back rub, your hands should remain in constant skin contact with the client until back rub is complete. ❷ ➤ *Rationale:* This prevents a "tickling" sensation.
12. Repeatedly move your hands up on either side of the client's spine, across shoulders, and down the lateral aspects of the back using the **effleurage** stroke, applying firm and steady pressure.
13. Move your hands down the center of the client's back to sacral area.
14. Massage with a figure-eight motion from the sacrum out over each buttock. ❸
15. Finally, rub lightly up and down the back a few strokes before lifting hands from client's back.

❶ Cleanse back using a disposable cleansing cloth before beginning a back rub.

❷ Without lifting hands from skin surface, massage in continuous motion.

❸ Maintain constant skin contact during care by moving hands in figure-eight motion from shoulder to buttocks and back.

16. Throughout back rub, assess skin for color, turgor, and breakdown.
17. When percussion is desired, the back and buttocks can be lightly struck with the fleshy sides of your hands, called **tapotement**. ❹ Using an alternating rhythm, move up and down the back several times, avoiding the kidney area. In addition, kneading can be accomplished by picking up the skin between the thumb and fingers as you move up the back. This movement is called **petrissage**. ❺
18. Close client's gown, pull up bedcovers, and assist client to change position if desired. Place top half of side rails in UP position. (See Chapter 7 regarding use of side rails.) Place bed in LOW position.
19. Remove gloves, if used.
20. Return lotion to the proper area.
21. Perform hand hygiene.
22. Document care provided.

❹ The *tapotement* stroke stimulates the skin as the hands move up and down the back. The kidney area should be avoided.

❺ The *petrissage*, or kneading stroke, is issued over the shoulders and along back.

Unit 8.4 Documentation and Evaluation

DOCUMENTATION for Evening Care

- Client's level of comfort or discomfort
- Type of care given (i.e., back care, evening care)
- Any significant complaints

- Nature of client teaching if done
- Medication required for discomfort or sleep
- Client's physical and emotional status after evening care completed

EVALUATION/Critical Thinking

Expected Outcomes

- Client states he or she is comfortable and ready for sleep after evening care.

- Client states that back care has decreased muscle tension, improved comfort level, and increased feelings of relaxation.

Unexpected Outcomes

- Client refuses back care because he or she does not want to be touched.

- Client refuses back care because he or she thinks you are too busy or disinterested.

- Client is unable to sleep even after evening care is given.

Alternative Actions

- Tell client that if he or she cannot accept back care as part of the therapeutic regimen, you will stop.

- Make sure you offer the back care in an unhurried and meaningful manner. Do not allow the client to misinterpret your offer for care.
- Return to client and offer back care later in the evening.

- Encourage verbalization of feelings, fears, etc.
- Check to see if sleeping medication can be given.
- Provide additional back care.

Chapter Wrap-Up

GERONTOLOGIC Considerations

Factors That Can Increase Risk of Skin Breakdown and Delay Wound Healing

- Inadequate nutritional intake
- Compromised immune system
- Compromised circulatory and respiratory systems
- Poor hydration
- Decreased mobility and activity

Skin Changes With Age

- There is delayed cellular migration and proliferation.
- Skin is less effective as barrier and slow to heal.
- There is increased vulnerability to trauma.
- There is less ability to retain water.
- Geriatric skin is dry (osteotosis) due to decreased endocrine secretion and loss of elastin. This can cause pruritus, which could lead to skin ulceration.

- Increased skin susceptibility to shearing stress can lead to blister formation and skin tears.
- There is increased vascular fragility.

Skin Assessment Data for Older Adults

- Decreased temperature, degree of moisture, dryness resulting from decreased dermal vascularity
- Skin not intact, open lesions, tears, pressure ulcers as a result of increased skin fragility
- Decreased turgor, dehydration as a result of decreased oil and sweat glands

- Pigmentation alterations, potential cancer
- Pruritus—dry skin most common cause because of decreased oil and sweat glands
- Bruises, tears, scars from increased skin fragility

Bathing Adaptations to Minimize Dryness

- Have client take complete bath only twice a week.
- Use superfatted or mild soap or lotions to aid in moisturizing.
- Use tepid, not hot, water.
- Apply emollient (lanolin) to skin after bathing.

MANAGEMENT Guidelines

Each state legislates a Nurse Practice Act for RNs and LVN/LPNs. Healthcare facilities are responsible for establishing and implementing policies and procedures that conform to their state's regulations. Verify the regulations and role parameters for each healthcare worker in your facility.

Delegation

- All personnel interacting with clients must report any client risk behaviors or signs or symptoms that are unusual or new. Since activities of bathing or bedmaking have predictable outcomes and do not require nursing judgment, they are usually delegated to CNAs or UAPs. When these activities of daily living are delegated to a CNA or unlicensed personnel, the professional nurse remains responsible for total client care and should receive a complete report from the staff member assigned to the client.

- Even though unlicensed personnel are qualified to complete many tasks that involve activities of daily living, if the client is critically ill or unstable, the RN or LVN/LPN should be assigned to such a client. The professional nurse is responsible for assessing the client's total condition, thereby avoiding complications caused by missed assessment parameters.

Interprofessional Communication

- CNAs and UAPs must report any unusual or unanticipated signs or symptoms or risk behaviors to the RN or LVN/LPN responsible for the client's care. This report should include mental status as well as previously unreported physical signs and symptoms observed during the interaction period.
- Clients with alterations in skin integrity may be referred to the wound care specialist if the facility has one on staff.

CASE STUDY Applications

Scenario 1

An 89-year-old male was admitted earlier today, and you were assigned to admit him and provide nursing care for the remainder of the shift (4 hours). His admitting diagnosis is dehydration due to prolonged nausea and vomiting. He lives with his 88-year-old wife. They have some home health care twice a week, and a nursing assistant assists them with bathing and personal hygienic care. He is usually very active, walking, gardening, and attending church every week.

Your nursing history indicates he has not been out of bed for 3 days. He was unable to get to the bathroom and used a urinal, which proved to be difficult for him to manage and he spilled some urine each time he used it. He has not had a bath for 4 days and has also not brushed or cleaned his dentures.

1. Considering the client's issues related to bathing and bedmaking, what is your priority assessment after completing the initial assessment? Provide the rationale for your answer.

2. What information would you place on his plan of care to prevent skin breakdown? List the risk factors the client most likely exhibited.
3. Outline the nursing interventions that will be incorporated in his plan of care for the pressure ulcer.
4. What would you consider priority for his bathing needs? Provide the rationale for your answer.
5. Identify the major preventative measures to prevent skin breakdown or tears that will need to be discussed with the nursing assistant who will continue to care for him when he returns home.

Scenario 2

The client develops a skin tear on the greater trochanter the second day after admission. Refer to Scenario 1 for data.

1. In addition to risk factors identified in Scenario 1, describe additional risk factors that can cause skin tears.
2. Describe nursing interventions that can be used to treat the skin tear.

3. Describe nursing actions you will use when applying a dressing for the skin tear.

4. Explain how skin changes with age and how that leads to skin tears.

5. Are there any bathing changes that will need to be carried out during the time the treatment for the skin tear is being carried out?

NCLEX® Review Questions

Unless otherwise specified, choose only one (1) answer.

1. Which one of the following statements is correct relative to making an occupied bed?
   A. The bed is made by tucking the sheet under the mattress starting at the head of the bed, then pulling the sheet down to the foot of the bed.
   B. One side of the bed is completed first, then the client is moved to that side of the bed while the second side is completed.
   C. Making a bed with the client in the bed consists of changing the drawsheet and pillowcase.
   D. Unoccupied bed changes are completed only when the bed is soiled; then the bed is changed by rolling up the soiled part of the sheet and having the client move to the opposite side of the bed.

2. You are preparing to complete a bed bath for an older adult client who is experiencing difficulty when moving in and out of bed. Place in order the sequence you will use for bathing the client.
   A. Legs
   B. Arms
   C. Abdomen
   D. Back
   E. Face

3. While assessing the skin of an older adult client, you notice the skin is very dry. What is the most appropriate intervention?
   A. Use any fragrant soap when washing the skin.
   B. Bathe the client daily using only lukewarm water and mild soap.
   C. Apply generous amounts of oil-rich cream to the skin.
   D. Have the client only take showers to prevent build-up of soap on the skin.

4. A physician's order must be obtained before you perform which one of the following nursing interventions?
   A. Cooling bath using tepid water
   B. Tub bath requiring the use of a hydraulic bathtub chair
   C. Bath using Aveeno or cornstarch
   D. Partial bath including washing the genitalia

5. A client's diagnosis is heart failure. He has difficulty breathing when he experiences too much activity. Which of the following is the most appropriate intervention for bathing this client?
   A. Give him a bed bath.
   B. Place him in a shower chair, wheel him to the shower, and shower him.
   C. Assist him to the side of the bed and instruct him to complete a partial bath.
   D. Assist him with washing his face and hands if he is able to tolerate the activity.

6. The protocol for client care on the unit where you are gaining clinical practice includes providing morning care to all bedridden clients. What does this activity include?
   Select all that apply.
   A. Offering oral hygiene
   B. Providing a wash cloth and assisting the client with washing his or her face and hands
   C. Changing the drawsheet and pillowcase
   D. Providing back care
   E. Administer zolpidem if ordered

7. Which of the following is a major advantage of using a disposable bathing system for bathing a client?
   A. It is less expensive than using regular linen.
   B. It is warmed to provide a soothing effect for the skin.
   C. It maintains a pH of 4.7–4.9 and is less drying than soap.
   D. It prevents the spread of infection among clients.

8. What is the first step in bathing an infant?
   A. Wash the infant's hair and scalp.
   B. Place the baby into the bathtub and wash the face, neck, and ears.
   C. Cleanse the eyes using a moist cotton ball.
   D. Lower the baby into the bathtub and wash the abdomen, arms, and legs before washing the genitalia.

9. As part of your morning assessment, you are going to check the client's skin condition for signs of hydration. What is the most appropriate method to check for hydration?
   A. Place the back of your fingers or hand on the client's skin to check for resilience.
   B. Gently pick up a small section of the skin with your thumb and forefinger, release, and observe for speed of return to original position.

C. Firmly press your finger against the client's skin for several seconds and observe for **blanching** of skin.

D. Observe for color change in skin of hands.

10. You are working the afternoon shift and the day nurse asks you to carefully assess an older adult client because she thinks she may have the beginning of a skin tear. You complete the assessment as soon as you are out of report.

Your findings are a Category I flap type skin tear on the right arm. What is the most appropriate nursing action?

A. Cleanse the tear with a Betadine swab, and press the tear back onto the skin.

B. Place Tegaderm or adherent dressing over the tear.

C. Place a dry 4×4 dressing over the tear and tape securely.

D. Apply a moist dressing over the tear and immobilize the arm to prevent excess movement.

QSEN Activity

Domain: Safety

KSA Category: Skill

Activity:

As a nurse teaching a new CNA how to safely provide client care for a client using a hydraulic bathtub chair, what safety measures will you explain to the CNA? Provide rationales for the answers.

1. Ensure water temperature is not more than what temperature (°F)?

2. Before taking client to the tub room, what safety action would you complete?

3. Explain how you will place the client in the tub.

4. Once the client is in the tub chair, what safety feature is essential to prevent client from injuring himself or herself?

5. What instructions will you give the client to safely lower himself or herself into a tub?

Bibliography

Johnson, D., Lineweaver, L., & Maze, L. M. (2009). Patient's bath basins as potential sources of infection: A multicenter sampling study. *American Journal of Critical Care, 18(1), 31–40.*

LeBlanc, K. and Baranoski, S. (2011). Skin tears: State of the science: Consensus for the prevention, predictions, assessment, treatment of skin tears. *Advances in Skin and Wound Care, 24(9Suppl 1), 2–15.*

Stephen-Haynes J., & Carville K. (2011, Nov.). Skin tears made easy. *Wounds International, 2(4).* Retrieved from http://www.woundsinternational.com/other-resources/view/skin-tears-made-easy

Stotts, N., Brown D. S., Donaldson N. E., Aydin C., & Fridman, M. (2013, Jan.). Eliminating hospital-acquired pressure ulcers: Within our reach. *Advances in Skin & Wound Care 26(1), 13–18.*

Tyco Healthcare. (n.d.). Wound care/dressing protocol-skin tear. Retrieved from http://www.dhphomedelivery.com/wound-care-skin-tear.pdf

Wounds International. (2014) International best practices guidelines: effective skin and wound management of non-complex wounds. London, England: Author. Retrieved from http://www.woundsinternational.com/Pdf/-ontent_11308.pdf

Chapter 9
Personal Hygiene

Learning Objectives

9.1 Discuss oral hygiene needs of clients.

9.2 Outline the procedure for flossing teeth.

9.3 Compare and contrast oral hygiene for clients with natural teeth and dentures.

9.4 Demonstrate safety awareness when providing oral care for unconscious clients.

9.5 Identify the appropriate method of hair care according to client's condition.

9.6 Outline the steps for shaving a male client.

9.7 Describe procedure for removing lice and nits from hair and other body areas.

9.8 State some of the cautions that apply when using solutions that treat pediculosis.

9.9 Demonstrate proper draping technique for female clients.

9.10 Demonstrate the skill of placing a bedpan for a bedridden client.

9.11 Describe the steps in providing perineal care for male and female clients.

9.12 Describe nursing actions necessary to care for clients with contact lenses.

9.13 State two suggested solutions when hearing is not improved after cleaning a hearing aid.

9.14 State at least two nursing diagnoses pertinent to clients requiring assistance with personal hygiene.

Chapter Outline

Terminology

Abrasion the scraping away of a portion of skin or of a mucous membrane as a result of injury.

Adaptation an alteration or adjustment by which an individual can improve his or her relationship to the environment.

Anticoagulant any substance that suppresses or counteracts coagulation of blood.

Aspiration to inhale GI fluid into the lungs; to withdraw fluid that has collected in an area to obtain a specimen.

Canthus the angle at either end of the slit between the eyelids.

Cornea the clear, transparent anterior portion of the fibrous coat of the eye.

Debilitated feeble; tired; lack of strength.

Dental plaque a thin film on the teeth made up of mucin and colloidal material found in saliva.

Edema a local or generalized condition in which there is excess fluid in the tissues.

Emesis vomiting.

Excoriation an injury to a surface of the body cavity caused by trauma.

Floss a waxed or unwaxed tape or thread used to clean between teeth.

Holistic the philosophy that an individual must be looked at as a whole rather than a sum of the parts.

Hygiene the study and observance of health rules.

Impetigo inflammatory skin disease marked by isolated pustules that rupture and become crusted.

Incontinent inability to retain urine or feces through loss of sphincter control.

Intervention the act of coming between, so as to hinder or modify.

Irritation a source of annoyance; incipient inflammation, soreness, roughness, or irritability of a body part.

Labia the lips of the vulva.

Lesion an injury or wound; a single infected patch in a skin disease.

Louse singular form of the word *lice*.

Microbiome the 100 trillion microorganisms that live in the gut, mouth, skin, and elsewhere in the human body.

Microorganism a minute living body such as a bacterium or protozoan not perceptible to the naked eye.

Mucosa mucous membrane lining passages and cavities communicating with the air.

Nasolacrimal pertaining to the nose and lacrimal apparatus.

Nits lice eggs.

Ophthalmic solution solution designed especially for the eyes.

Oral concerning the mouth.

Palate the roof of the mouth.

Parotid gland either of the largest of the paired salivary glands, located below and in front of each ear.

Pediculosis infestation with lice.

Periodontal disease chronic bacterial infection of the tissues surrounding the teeth.

Perineum the external region between the vulva and anus in a female or between the scrotum and anus in a male.

Sclera the tough, white, fibrous outer envelope of tissue covering all of the eyeball except the cornea.

Semi-Fowler's position semisitting position.

Systemic pertaining to the whole body rather than to one of its parts.

Thrush fungal infection of mouth or throat, especially in infants and young children and in clients with AIDS.

Ulcer an open sore or lesion of the skin or mucous membrane of the body.

Urethra canal for the discharge of urine extending from the bladder to the outside of the body.

Vascular pertinent to or composed of blood vessels.

Hygiene Care

Unfamiliar or life-threatening conditions affect the client's **adaptation** to the healthcare system. A **holistic** approach on the part of the nurse provides individualized care and assists the client to adapt. Basic **hygiene** care is an integral part of the total treatment program. Together with its role in enhancing the client's adaptation to the hospital environment and sense of self-worth, it provides an opportunity for the nurse to do a total assessment and evaluation. This time also allows for establishing a working relationship with the client and offers an opportunity to reduce stress by discussing fears and concerns about being in the hospital or the care the client is receiving.

The manner in which hygiene care is provided by nursing staff influences the client's perception of the staff. If care is administered in a professional and efficient manner, the client's confidence in the healthcare system is increased. The need to provide personal hygiene depends on each client's physical state and ability to care effectively for himself or herself. The nurse's first responsibility is to assess the client's level of ability, and then to assist the client as necessary, providing any assistance or teaching he or she may require.

Oral Hygiene

The condition of the **oral** cavity has a direct influence on an individual's overall state of health. Dental diseases require a "host" (the tooth and gum), an "agent" (plaque), and an "environment" (e.g., the presence of saliva and food). When plaque comes in contact with bacterial enzymes, carbohydrates, and acids, cavitation begins as the enamel of the tooth is decalcified. As long as food and plaque remain in the oral cavity, the possibility of dental decay increases. In the hospital setting, the incidence of caries (cavities) can be decreased by using a dentifrice containing fluoride, proper brushing and flossing, and adequate nutrition. Clients at risk for poor oral hygiene include those who are NPO, mouth breathers, and those with oral surgery.

Oral hygiene is a challenge for clients in long-term care settings. It is one of the most important **interventions** that nurses need to provide for these clients. Evidence links poor oral hygiene to serious **systemic** illnesses, including diabetes, stroke, hypertension, myocardial infarction, and **aspiration** pneumonia.

Hair Care

The appearance and condition of a client's hair may reflect his or her general physical and emotional status, individuality and feelings of worth, and the ability to care for himself or herself. When complex medical care is required during illness or trauma, hair care is often neglected.

Hair care is an important aspect of regular hygiene. To prevent damage to the hair, scalp, and surrounding skin, and to promote the client's sense of well-being, the nurse assesses the condition of a client's hair. Based on the assessment, hair and scalp care, shampooing, and shaving may be provided and interventions done to correct special problems.

Pediculosis

Pediculosis is one of the major health problems in school-age children and easily spreads to family members and friends. The use of terminology varies related to the life cycle of the **louse**. According to biologists, the life cycle of the head louse includes:

Adult Louse: wingless, flat insect about the size of a sesame seed, parasitic on warm blood.

Eggs: head louse eggs are also called **nits**: cemented firmly to hair shaft and take 6–9 days to hatch; nit shells remain on hair shaft.

Nymph: immature louse released when egg hatches; looks like an adult head louse, but the size of a pinhead; takes 7–8 days to become an adult.

Perineal and Genital Care

The **perineum** consists of the area between the thighs and from the anterior pelvis to the anus. This area contains organs and structures related to sexual functioning, reproduction, and elimination.

Hygienic care involves cleaning the perineum and genitalia to prevent bacterial growth, which can rapidly increase in this warm, dark, moist environment. Perineal care is often provided as a routine part of bathing but may be required more frequently to prevent skin **irritation**, infection, discomfort, or odor.

All clients are susceptible to perineal irritation or infection. Clients who are especially vulnerable are those who are immobilized, **incontinent**, **debilitated**, postsurgical, or comatose; those who have indwelling catheters; those who have metabolic and fluid balance disorders; or those who require systemic medications.

Eye Care

The usual eye care provided for hospitalized clients is for the comatose client and the client with contact lenses. There are several types of contact lenses used by clients. The older, hard lenses were the first on the market and were made of solid plastic. They were easy to keep clean because they did not absorb proteins from the eye. They did inhibit oxygenation of the **cornea**; therefore, they could not be worn for long periods of time.

Gas permeable contacts were introduced in the late 1970s. Most gas permeable lenses incorporate silicone, which makes them more flexible than hard contacts. Silicone is oxygen permeable, so oxygen can pass through these lenses, resulting in greater comfort and better eye health. Gas permeable contacts generally transmit more oxygen to the eye than soft contact lenses, although some hydrogen soft lenses are comparable to gas permeable lenses in oxygen transmission. Gas permeable lenses provide better vision, durability, and deposit resistance than soft contact lenses. They last longer than soft lenses and are less expensive.

Soft lenses, the most popular of the lenses, allow more oxygenation of the cornea than hard lenses, but they are less durable and carry a risk of contamination from collection of bacteria, dirt, and chemicals. Extended-wear lenses, a type of soft contact lenses, can be worn up to 7 days and 6 nights without being removed. The Food and Drug Administration (FDA) has also approved the use of continuous 30-day lenses. It is recommended that the lenses be removed every 30 days, cleaned, disinfected, and replaced or discarded. Lenses should not be replaced for 24 hours to allow the eye to rest. Reported side effects with these lenses include conjunctivitis, dry eyes, and mild burning or stinging. Some clients use disposable extended-wear lenses. These are considered one-time-only contacts and are discarded, not cleaned, after they are removed.

Individuals who wear contact lenses must be aware of environmental contaminants such as dust, smoke, and sprays because they can irritate the eyes. Certain drugs cause a decrease in the eye fluid on which the contact lens floats and can lead to irritation of the eye. Common drugs that can lead to this problem include antihistamines, birth control pills, and alcohol. Clients who use eye cosmetics must apply the makeup before they insert the contact lenses so that makeup will not adhere to the lenses.

Cultural Awareness

- Cultures define cleanliness in different ways. Western cultures, because of the abundance of detergents and washing machines, value clean clothes. Some underdeveloped countries have limited access to freshwater and therefore may not wash clothes as frequently.
- Anglo-Americans tend to be fastidious about body cleanliness and the absence of body odor. The use of perfumes, deodorants, and aftershave lotions is a major part of their hygienic care. In some cultures, natural body odor is thought to have sex appeal.
- Some cultures incorporate the participation of family members to provide personal care, particularly assistance with using a bedpan or bedside commode, to maintain modesty. Puerto Ricans, African Americans, and clients of Arab descent should be asked to inform the staff of their preferences for assistance with personal care.

Nursing Diagnoses

The following nursing diagnoses may be appropriate to include in a client care plan when a client is admitted and requires basic hygiene care.

NURSING DIAGNOSIS	RELATED TO . . .
Deficient Knowledge	Misinformation or lack of information, impaired cognitive function, lack of motivation
Noncompliance	Inability to perform tasks, disability, impaired memory
Impaired Oral Mucous Membrane	Inadequate oral hygiene, chemotherapy, malnutrition, dehydration, infection, mechanical trauma
Bathing Self-Care Deficit	Impaired motor or cognitive function, pain, disease condition, surgery
Situational Low Self-Esteem	Impaired motor or cognitive function, chronic illness, chronic pain

Source: Herdman, T. H. & Kamitsuru, S. (Eds.) *Nursing Diagnoses – Definitions and Classification 2015-2017*. Copyright © 2014, 1994–2014 by NANDA International. Used by arrangement with John Wiley & Sons Limited. Companion website: www.wiley.com/go/nursingdiagnoses. In order to make safe and effective judgments using NANDA-I nursing diagnosis it is essential that nurses refer to the definitions and defining characteristics of the diagnoses listed in this work.

Nursing Process Data

ASSESSMENT Database

- Assess whether client wears dentures.
- Evaluate client's knowledge of oral hygiene techniques.
- Assess condition of client's oral cavity, teeth, gums, and mouth.
- Assess for color, lesions, tenderness, inflammation, intactness of teeth, and degree of moisture or dryness of the oral cavity.
- Observe external and internal lips.
- Assess palate (roof and floor of mouth), and inspect under tongue.
- Assess entire oral mucosa, noting inside of the cheek.
- Observe tongue. Note tip, sides, back position, and underside.
- Evaluate condition of gums and teeth.
- Assess condition of throat as client says "Ah."
- If dentures or orthodontic appliances are used, observe relationship of the appliances to client's oral cavity (i.e., fit, irritation, condition of dentures).

PLANNING Objectives

- To remove plaque and bacteria-producing agents from oral cavity
- To allow nurse to assess client's oral health status, knowledge, and routines of oral care
- To decrease possibility of irritation or infection of oral cavity
- To remove unpleasant tastes and odors from oral cavity
- To provide comfort for client
- To provide client teaching when appropriate
- To assess hydration status

IMPLEMENTATION Procedures

DOCUMENTATION AND EVALUATION

Expected Outcomes

- The oral health status of client has been assessed and documented by nurse.
- Oral hygiene care is provided without complications.
- Plaque and bacteria-producing agents are removed.

Unexpected Outcomes/Alternative Actions

Pearson Nursing Student Resources

Find additional review materials at
nursing.pearsonhighered.com.
Prepare for success with NCLEX®-style practice questions and Skill Checklists.

Skill 9.1.1 | Providing Oral Hygiene

Equipment

Toothbrush: small enough to reach back teeth; soft and rounded with nonfrayed rows of nylon bristles

Dentifrice: client's choice, preferably one containing fluoride; special paste for dentures

Cup of water

Emesis basin or sink

Dental **floss**: regular or fine, waxed or unwaxed, depending on client's needs

Tissues or towel

Mouthwash if desired

Clean gloves

Preparation

1. Perform hand hygiene.
2. Collect necessary equipment.
3. Check two forms of client ID and introduce yourself.
4. Assist client to sink or provide privacy if care is to be given in bed.
5. Help client into a comfortable **semi-Fowler's position** or a sitting position. Assist client with the arrangement of equipment if necessary.
6. Don clean gloves.
7. Inspect surface of mouth for any abnormalities.

    a. Inspect surface of mouth, especially buccal **mucosa** (it should be pink, smooth, and moist), for any abnormalities. ❶ ➤ *Rationale:* Alterations from normal may indicate presence of disease states such as measles, mumps, or Addison disease.

    b. Examine condition of teeth and gums. Be alert to changes in gums. ➤ *Rationale:* Gingival hypertrophy, crevices between teeth and gums, pockets of debris, and bleeding with slight pressure are indications of gingivitis.

    c. Ask client about usual oral care routines.

8. Elicit any concerns, comments, or questions client may have about his or her oral health status.
9. Determine oral hygiene needs based on findings.
10. Assess client's need for teaching. Consider educational level; physical, emotional, and mental state; previous experiences; and cultural differences.
11. Assess client's physical condition. Consider diagnoses, lab reports, treatments, fluid status, drugs, diet, and level of comfort or pain.
12. Assess client's ability to care for himself or herself.

Procedure

1. Perform hand hygiene and don clean gloves.
2. Assist client to wash hands if client is performing his or her own oral care.
3. Request that client open mouth wide and hold **emesis** basin under chin.
4. Instruct client to complete following steps or provide the care yourself (Box 9-1 ■). Direct the bristles of the

EVIDENCE-BASED PRACTICE

According to a report by the Harvard Heart Letter, treatment for periodontitis (gum disease) may reduce the physical burden of heart disease, type 2 diabetes, cerebrovascular disease, and pregnancy. In a study of insurance records of more than 300,000 people with **periodontal disease** and one of five conditions—cardiovascular disease, cerebrovascular disease (typically a stroke), type 2 diabetes, rheumatoid arthritis, or pregnancy—researchers discovered that periodontal disease treatment generally correlated with lower medical costs and fewer hospitalizations. Healthcare costs for clients with diabetes and cardiovascular disease who received periodontal treatment were 20%–40% lower than in clients who had no treatments. Reduction in costs for pregnant women who received treatment was a remarkable 74%. Of the five conditions, only rheumatoid arthritis did not show a reduction in healthcare costs after periodontal treatment.

Source: Corlis (2014)

toothbrush toward the gumline for all areas to be brushed. ❷ ➤ *Rationale:* Action removes food particles from gumline (Box 9-2 ■) and stimulates the gums.

❶ Inspect the surface of the mouth for abnormalities.

❷ Providing oral hygiene is an essential component of client care.

(continued)

Skill 9.1.1 | Providing Oral Hygiene *(continued)*

5. Keep the brush positioned over only two or three teeth at a time. Use small rotating movements to cover the outside surfaces of all teeth. If using a sonic toothbrush, see suggestions in Box 9-3 ■.
6. Clean the inner surfaces of all back teeth, using the brushing method described above.
7. Use a firm back-and-forth motion to clean the flat chewing surfaces.
8. Use the bristles on the end of the toothbrush and rotate the brush back and forth across the teeth to clean the inner surfaces of the front teeth.
9. Lightly brush all areas of the tongue, being careful not to stimulate gag reflex. ➤ *Rationale:* This improves the breath.
10. Rinse the client's mouth thoroughly with water. ❸
11. Inspect oral cavity, and repeat brushing if necessary.

Box 9-1 **CLIENT TEACHING ABOUT ORAL CARE**

Begin teaching client about oral care during your initial assessment. Focus teaching on oral health needs and care. This is particularly helpful for clients in home care or prior to discharge from the hospital. You may want to incorporate the following techniques:

- A demonstration and return demonstration to illustrate correct dental care techniques
- If ordered, teach client that disclosure tablets or solutions temporarily stain **dental plaque** pink. This technique helps the client to see where plaque appears on the teeth. After applying tablets or solution, the client brushes and flosses until plaque is removed.

Box 9-2 **GUM DISEASE**

The American Academy of Periodontology estimates that at least half of noninstitutional individuals aged 55 and older have periodontitis and that almost 25% aged 65 and older have lost all of their teeth. Periodontal disease affects glycemic controls in diabetic clients. There is also a significantly higher incidence of cardiovascular complications as a result of periodontal disease.

❸ Assist client to rinse the mouth with water.

12. Floss thoroughly or instruct the client how to floss properly. ➤ *Rationale:* Flossing removes plaque from between teeth. If the client is on blood thinners or aspirin, check with the healthcare provider to determine if flossing is appropriate. ❹

Box 9-3 **SONIC TOOTHBRUSH**

Many dentists and dental hygienists recommend the use of a sonic toothbrush, especially for clients with plaque formation, stains, and periodontal pockets. The usual recommended time for brushing is 2 minutes twice a day. The toothbrush is charged by plugging the charger into the electrical outlet; therefore, electrical safety procedures must be followed. Do not store or place the charger where it can come in contact with water. Client instructions for using the toothbrush are printed in the owner's manual and must be clearly understood before attempting to use the toothbrush.

Note: If the client brings the toothbrush to the hospital, it is not necessary to charge it if hospitalization is less than 2 weeks. If hospitalization is beyond 2 weeks or the toothbrush needs charging, instruct the client's relatives to take the brush home and charge it or have the hospital engineering department charge the battery. It is required by most hospitals that any electrical appliance brought into the hospital must be checked for safety by the hospital engineering department.

A

B

❹ **A.** Instruct the client to floss to prevent build-up of plaque and food particles between the teeth. **B.** Flossing teeth of client.

a. Wrap one length of floss loosely around index fingers of both hands.

b. Hold floss taut between two hands, and gently pull back and forth between each tooth.

c. Move floss up and down sides of teeth to clean plaque. Go as near to gumline as possible without injury to gum. Pull floss back and forth gently, working back toward the biting surface of each tooth. Repeat on other edge of each tooth, using a new section of floss. ➤ *Rationale:* Overly vigorous flossing can damage gums.

d. Floss each tooth several times until all particles of food are removed.

13. Assist client to rinse mouth and expectorate into emesis basin.

14. Wipe off client's mouth and chin.

15. Wash client's toothbrush, rinse, and put the toothbrush and paste away and return additional equipment to the appropriate area.

16. Remove gloves and place in appropriate receptacle.

17. Perform hand hygiene.

18. Check to see that client is comfortable.

EVIDENCE-BASED PRACTICE
Evidence to Support Toothbrushing in Critically Ill Patients
Attention has been focused on oral care as the evidence accumulates to support an association between the bacteria in the oral **microbiome** and respiratory pathogens that cause pneumonia. It is assumed that those respiratory pathogens originating in the oral cavity are aspirated into the lungs, causing infection.

Evidence is accumulating from studies obtained from oral specimens that there are genetically matched bacteria obtained from oral specimens and from organisms in blood specimens.

Eight studies were reviewed to determine whether there was a positive outcome from toothbrushing and oral care as an intervention for clients with ventilator-associated pneumonia (VAP). The results showed no difference between clients who had toothbrushing and clients in the control groups. Several additional study groups evaluated the outcomes of toothbrushing clients and nontoothbrushing clients. It was proven that no significant changes in the incidence of pneumonia occurred with toothbrushing.

Source: Ames (2011)

Skill 9.1.2 | Providing Denture Care

Equipment
Denture toothbrush
Dentifrice (e.g., Polident)
Denture cup, labeled with client's name
Emesis basin
Cleanser or effervescent tablets for dentures
Clean gloves
Mouthwash, if desired
Adhesive dental liner, optional

Procedure

1. Encourage client to use dentures. ➤ *Rationale:* Dentures improve speech, make eating easier, and improve the shape of the mouth, appearance, and self-image.

2. Perform hand hygiene and don gloves.

3. Help client remove dentures. If client is unable to do this, carefully place your finger on the edge of the upper denture. ➤ *Rationale:* This action breaks the seal at the roof of the mouth and allows the denture to easily slide out. Lower denture generally lifts out easily.

4. If client is unable to clean own dentures, place them in an unbreakable container. Either wash dentures over a basin or carry them to the sink. ❶ Place a towel or washcloth on the bottom of the sink. ➤ *Rationale:* This cushions the surface in case you accidentally drop a denture.

5. Hold one denture in your hand. With your other hand, use a toothbrush or special denture brush and a cleaning agent, such as a commercially prepared paste or solution, to brush the denture. Use the same brushing motion as with natural teeth.

6. Rinse denture thoroughly in cold water. ➤ *Rationale:* Hot water can damage dentures. ❷

7. If dentures are to remain out of the mouth for a period of time, as at night, store them in a clearly labeled, unbreakable container of cold water with denture fixative.

8. If dentures are to be worn immediately, help client to rinse oral cavity with warm water or mouthwash.

9. Gently brush client's gums and tongue, if client requests. ➤ *Rationale:* This removes bacteria and freshens breath.

10. Apply adhesive dental liner if client requests. ➤ *Rationale:* This holds dentures in place and provides cushion for more security and comfort.

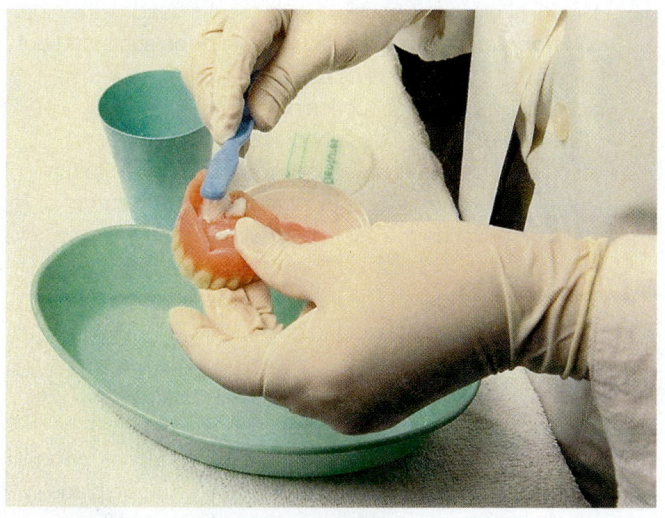

❶ Hold dentures securely while brushing.

(continued)

Skill 9.1.2 | Providing Denture Care (continued)

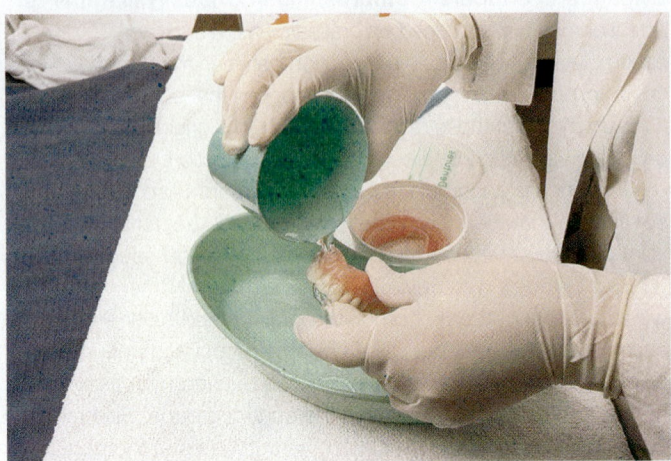

11. Moisten dentures according to client's desire.
12. Help client replace dentures.
13. Clean denture cup and emesis basin and replace in client's bedside stand.
14. Remove gloves, and place in appropriate receptacle.
15. Perform hand hygiene.

② Rinse dentures in cold water.

Skill 9.1.3 | Providing Oral Care for Unconscious Clients

Equipment

Foam toothette oral swabs or toothbrush
Lubricant for lips such as lip balm
Waterpik devices or floss
Bulb syringe or suction equipment
Tongue blades or bite block
Hydrogen peroxide (optional)
Mouthwash (antiseptic or alcohol free)
Gauze pad
Towels
Clean gloves

Procedure

1. Gather equipment. Identify client.
2. Perform hand hygiene and don gloves.
3. If possible, position client on side in a semi-Fowler's position. If this is not possible, turn client's head to the side.
   ➤ *Rationale:* This allows fluid to drain or be suctioned out of mouth and thus prevents aspiration.
4. Place a bulb syringe or suctioning equipment nearby.
   ➤ *Rationale:* This is a safety precaution to use for suctioning oral cavity as needed. You may choose to turn the suction on and place the catheter under the corner of the pillow, covering the suction tip with a clean towel or washcloth.
5. Place a towel under the client's head and an emesis basin under the client's chin and mouth.
6. Insert bite block if necessary to keep mouth open while brushing.
7. Place a small amount of toothpaste on brush. Brush the external surfaces of the teeth in the routine manner, using less water on the brush. **❶** You may use a tongue blade to move the cheeks and lips. Do not put your fingers in the client's mouth. ➤ *Rationale:* This prevents accidental closing down on toothbrush and biting your finger.

❶ Use a padded tongue blade when brushing the teeth.

Toothettes can be used in place of the toothbrush. Floss the client's teeth if appropriate, using the same technique as for a conscious clients.
8. To clean the inner surfaces of the teeth, use a padded tongue blade to separate the upper and lower sets of teeth, if bite block is not used. Brush the teeth and tongue in the usual manner.
9. Clean the interior of the cheeks, roof of the mouth, teeth, and tongue using mouthwash or water and a gauze pad wrapped around an index finger. Rinse the client's mouth carefully, using very small amounts of fluid that can be easily suctioned. **②**
10. Remove bite block. Wipe client's face with a towel.
11. Lubricate client's lips with lip balm or products comprising beeswax, olive oil, shea butter, or cocoa butter.
    ➤ *Rationale:* These products are water soluble, not water repellent like petroleum jelly.
12. Remove gloves and place in appropriate receptacle.
13. Perform hand hygiene.

❷ Rinse the mouth using water-filled syringe and suction.

14. Perform oral care frequently, as often as every 4 hours if necessary. ➤ *Rationale:* Oral care maintains adequate oral health.

Note: Foam toothettes can be moistened with water and used as a toothbrush (Box 9-4 ■).

Box 9-4 **TOOTHETTE SWABS**

Toothette swabs are indicated for the following client conditions: radiation therapy, chemotherapy, bone marrow transplant, immunosuppressed, on a ventilator, nutritionally depleted, or older clients. Toothettes improve the appearance of oral tissue (tongue, **palate**, lips). Toothbrushes are more effective in stimulating gingival tissue and removing debris from the teeth. ➤ *Rationale:* The use of toothette swabs will prevent bleeding in the gums of clients with potential bleeding disorders.

Unit 9.1 Documentation and Evaluation

DOCUMENTATION for Oral Hygiene

- Findings from assessment of mouth; condition of gums, mucous membranes, and teeth
- Assessment of client's oral hygiene needs
- Planning steps taken to meet client's oral hygiene needs
- Oral care provided or observed

- Effectiveness of oral care on client's teeth, gums, and mucosa
- Client's reaction and level of comfort
- Client's level of participation in oral care
- Client's participation in nurse–client teaching

EVALUATION/Critical Thinking

Expected Outcomes
- The oral health status of client has been assessed and documented by nurse.

- Oral hygiene care is provided without complications.
- Plaque and bacteria-producing agents are removed.

Unexpected Outcomes
- Even with increased oral hygiene, client still has odorous breath.

Alternative Actions
- Use antiseptic mouthwash between oral hygiene care.
- Notify the healthcare provider, as this could be a symptom of systemic disease.
- Obtain dental consultation to check for presence of dental caries or gum disease.
- Examine client's nutritional intake. Absent nutrients or imbalanced intake of fats, protein, or carbohydrates can result in bad breath.

(continued)

Unexpected Outcomes	Alternative Actions
• Client complains of extreme oral mucosal irritation or sensitivity.	• Request healthcare provider's order for one of the following solutions: 　Saline solutions for soothing, cleansing rinses 　Anesthetic solutions to dull extreme pain in the oral cavity 　Effervescent solutions (e.g., hydrogen peroxide or ginger ale) to loosen and remove debris from the mouth 　Coating solutions (e.g., Maalox) to protect irritated surfaces 　Antibacterial—antifungal rinses (e.g., nystatin [Mycostatin]) to prevent the spread of organisms that cause **thrush**
• Vigorous flossing results in bleeding and sore gums.	• Give client warm antiseptic mouthwash to relieve soreness. • Investigate gum condition and refer for consultation.
• Client needs care after oral surgery or oral trauma.	• Oral care after surgery or trauma is always ordered by the healthcare provider. No oral hygiene care should be attempted until the healthcare provider has clearly defined the specific care. • Suctioning equipment should always be present. • Assessment of client's head, face, neck, and general status is critical at this time.
• Normal stimulation and cleaning are not sufficient to remove debris and plaque for the unconscious client.	• Try flossing teeth to dislodge debris. • Provide mouth care with toothbrush and dentifrice at least twice daily. • Check with healthcare provider and order sonic toothbrush.
• **Parotid gland** inflammation can occur with improper oral hygiene.	• Rinse mouth with mouthwash. • Use swab to reach back in oral cavity along mandible to temporomandibular area. • Floss teeth at least daily.

Hair Care

Nursing Process Data

ASSESSMENT Database

- Review general physical assessment findings.
- Elicit information regarding loss of hair, tenderness of scalp, or itching.
- Determine client's ability to perform own hair care.
- If unable to care for own hair, find out who usually assists client.
- Observe client's hair and scalp, noting the following:
  Texture
  Color
  Degree of thickness and hair distribution
  Degree of gloss or shine
  Dryness or oiliness
  Areas of irritation, rash, or scaliness on the scalp or surrounding skin
  Matting or snarls
  Pediculosis (lice)
- Assess usual hair care routines, products, and appliances.
- Assess method for providing hair care (e.g., in bed, on gurney, in wheelchair).
- Determine client teaching needs regarding hair care.
- Assess need for frequency of shaving facial hair for male clients.

PLANNING Objectives

- To prevent irritation to the scalp and damage to the hair
- To help maintain or improve client's existing condition of hair and scalp
- To promote circulation to the hair follicle and growth of new hair
- To distribute oils along the hair shaft
- To remove facial hair for client comfort and self-esteem
- To promote self-esteem

IMPLEMENTATION Procedures

DOCUMENTATION AND EVALUATION

Expected Outcomes

- Hair and scalp assessment are performed without complications.
- Appropriate method of hair care provided for client.
- Client's hair and scalp are clean, comfortable, and styled according to client's preference.
- Client is comfortable and resting after shampooing.
- Shaving is accomplished without skin nicks or discomfort.

Unexpected Outcomes/Alternative Actions

Pearson Nursing Student Resources

Find additional review materials at
nursing.pearsonhighered.com.
Prepare for success with NCLEX®-style practice questions and Skill Checklists.

Skill 9.2.1 | Providing Hair Care

Equipment
Blunt-ended comb or pick
Brush
Towel
Mirror
Hair care products and ornaments

Preparation
1. Identify client using two identifiers.
2. Introduce yourself and explain the procedure for hair care.
3. Determine client's hair care needs.
4. Perform hand hygiene.
5. Help client into a comfortable position to perform hair care.
6. Collect and assemble equipment.

Procedure
Routine Hair Care
1. Place all hair care items within reach.
2. Place towel over client's shoulders.
3. Brush or comb client's hair from scalp to hair ends, using gentle, even strokes.
   a. Tangled hair: Use short gentle strokes. Work from end of hair shaft toward scalp. Conditioner may make combing easier.
   b. Curly hair: Use wet comb on wet hair (water or oil) for ease of combing.
4. Style hair in a manner suitable to client.
5. Replace hair care items in appropriate place and clean items as needed.
6. Perform hand hygiene.

Skill 9.2.2 | Shampooing Hair

Equipment
Two bath towels
Gloves
Washcloth
Large container for water
Shampoo
Conditioner, if desired
Hair dryer, if allowed by hospital*
For Disposable System
　　Package containing shampoo cap
　　Face or bath towel
　　Hair care products, as requested by client
Comb and/or brush

Note: Ensure that electrical equipment is checked by maintenance department before using. ➤ *Rationale:* This confirms that equipment is grounded and mechanically safe.

Preparation
1. Identify client. Determine client's hair care needs.
2. Perform hand hygiene. Apply gloves if scalp has **lesions**, cuts, or infestation, or if blood is present.
3. Collect and assemble equipment.
4. Help client into a comfortable position to perform hair care.
5. Shampooing the hair can be accomplished in a variety of ways depending on the client's usual routine and physical condition. In many institutions, a physician's order is necessary before shampooing a client's hair.
6. If possible, the easiest way to shampoo is to assist the client while he or she is in the shower. Caution should be taken to prevent the client from becoming overly tired or weak while in the shower. (Use shower chair if necessary.)

Procedure
Client on a Gurney
1. Have shampoo items readily available.
2. Position gurney with head end at sink.
3. Lock wheels on gurney. ➤ *Rationale:* This prevents the gurney from moving away from the sink.
4. Pad the edge of the sink with a towel or bath blanket.
5. Move the client's head just beyond the edge of the gurney.
   ➤ *Rationale:* This allows water to run off more easily.

> **CLINICAL ALERT**
> If the client is an older adult, do not press the neck down on the edge of the sink—this position can diminish circulation to the brain and has been reported to be a possible cause of strokes.

6. Put a pillow or a rolled blanket under the client's shoulders.
   ➤ *Rationale:* This helps elevate and extend the head.
7. Drape one towel over client's shoulders and around neck. Place another towel within reach.
8. Use a washcloth to protect client's eyes. Wet hair and gently make a lather with shampoo.
9. Rinse thoroughly and repeat if necessary.
10. Towel dry, add conditioner if desired, and rinse again.
11. Using a dry towel, pat hair dry, and wrap turban style to transport back to room.
12. Use hair dryer if available.
13. Style as desired.
14. Replace equipment.
15. Perform hand hygiene.

Note: This procedure is not the first choice for shampooing hair. It should be used for clients who cannot get out of bed. The disposable system for shampooing hair is the most common method today.

Client Using Disposable System

1. Heat shampoo package in microwave for no more than 30 seconds. Follow package directions. ❶
2. Perform hand hygiene.
3. Open package and check temperature. ➤ ***Rationale:*** Clients react to heat at different temperatures; therefore, check the cap temperature with client before placing on client's head.
4. Place cap on head. Ensure that all hair is contained within the cap. For longer hair, place cap on top of head and then tuck all hair up inside cap. ❷
5. Gently massage cap with hands, 1–2 minutes for short hair and 2–3 minutes for longer hair. ➤ ***Rationale:*** This helps saturate the hair with the solution. There is no need to rinse hair after using solution.

Note: If hair is tangled, the cap may need to stay on for longer period of time in order to saturate hair. If blood or other secretions are present on hair, they may need to be removed using washcloths from the disposable bath system before attempting to shampoo the hair.

6. Remove cap and place in appropriate receptacle.
7. Towel dry hair.
8. Complete hair care according to client's needs and desires.
9. Perform hand hygiene.

Note: Disposable hair care systems provide a quick and easy way to freshen client's hair with minimal client movement.

❶ Shampoo system activated by microwave.

❷ Disposable cap can be used for clients on bed rest.

Skill 9.2.3 | Shaving a Client

Equipment
Safety or electric razor, specific to client's needs or wishes
Shaving cream
Aftershave lotion (optional)
Two towels
Basin of warm water
Gloves

Preparation
1. Identify client using two identifiers.
2. Introduce yourself and explain the procedure.
3. Place client in sitting position.
4. Perform hand hygiene.
5. Place towel over chest and under chin.
6. Put up mirror on overbed table.

7. Determine how the client usually shaves (i.e., use of safety edge or electric razor; special products).

> **CLINICAL ALERT**
> Only electric razors can be used to shave clients with excessive bleeding tendencies.
>   According to hospital policy, be sure to have the electric razor checked for safety aspects. Some hospitals do not allow clients to use their own electric razors.

8. Check to see if the client has excessive bleeding tendencies due to pathologic conditions (hemophilia) or the use of specific medications (**anticoagulants** or large doses of aspirin). ➤ ***Rationale:*** If client is accidentally cut, it could lead to some loss of blood.

(continued)

Skill 9.2.3 | Shaving a Client *(continued)*

Procedure

1. If using a safety edge razor:
   a. Don gloves and apply a warm, moist towel to soften the hair.
   b. Apply a thick layer of soap or shaving cream to the shaving area.
   c. Holding skin taut, use firm but small strokes in the direction of hair growth.
   d. Gently remove soap or lather with a warm, damp towel. Inspect for areas you may have missed.

2. If using electric razor:
   a. Use rotating motion of razor and start from lateral aspect of face and move toward chin and upper lip area.
   b. Clean razor with brush or remove razor head and clean facial hair from head of razor.

3. Apply aftershave lotion or powder as desired.
4. Reposition client for comfort if needed.
5. Remove gloves and replace equipment.
6. Perform hand hygiene.

Unit 9.2 Documentation and Evaluation

DOCUMENTATION for Hair Care

- Documentation of hair care assessment and needs
- Shampooing method, outcomes, problems encountered
- Client's tolerance to hair care
- Shaving completed; note specific type of razor
- Unusual bleeding from shaving

EVALUATION/Critical Thinking

Expected Outcomes

- Hair and scalp assessment performed without complications.
- Appropriate method of hair care was provided for client.
- Client's hair and scalp are clean, comfortable, and styled according to client's preference.
- Client is comfortable and rested after shampooing.
- Shaving is accomplished without skin nicks or discomfort.

Unexpected Outcomes

- Extreme matting, snarling, blood, or nonremovable substances appear in client's hair.

Alternative Actions

- Never cut a client's hair unless it is absolutely necessary.
- Check hospital policy regarding haircutting. It may not be allowed in some facilities.
- Apply alcohol to tangled hair or blood-soaked hair. Keep in place for 5 minutes. Wash hair with shampoo to remove alcohol and blood.
- Secure permission of family or physician (if order required).

- Client is cut during shaving procedure.

- Assess extent of cut, and place a clean towel on the area with pressure to stop bleeding.
- If cut appears to be more than a nick, report to the physician and fill out unusual occurrence report.

- Shaving is difficult and painful for the client.

- Place warm towels on area to be shaved for 15 minutes.
- Apply more shaving cream.
- Ensure that razor is sharp.

Pediculosis

Nursing Process Data

ASSESSMENT Database

- Observe head (scalp), body (nape of neck, behind ears, beard, eyebrows, arms, legs), and pubic areas for the following signs:

    Small, hemorrhagic areas on the skin

    Scratches on the skin

    Habitual itching and scratching, feeling like something crawling in hair

    Insect-type bites or pustular eruptions behind the ears or hairline

    Small, white dandruff-like particles

    Gritty feel when running fingers through hair

- Assess client's personal hygiene, living conditions, contact or exposure to others with lice (e.g., school-aged children, sexual partners, siblings).

PLANNING Objectives

- To remove lice from client's hair and prevent further skin problems such as **impetigo** or infection
- To remove cause of itching and intense need to scratch scalp
- To control spread of lice to others

IMPLEMENTATION Procedures

DOCUMENTATION AND EVALUATION

Expected Outcomes

- Lice removed after treatment.
- Client verbalizes cause of problem and preventive measures.
- Client repeats back to nurse instructions for preventing lice infestation and indicates understanding of process.
- Client and family members remain free of lice infestation.

Unexpected Outcomes/Alternative Actions

Pearson Nursing Student Resources

Find additional review materials at
nursing.pearsonhighered.com.
Prepare for success with NCLEX®-style practice questions and Skill Checklists.

Skill 9.3.1 | Identifying the Presence of Lice and Nits (Lice Eggs)

Equipment
Bright lamp/light
Magnifying glass
Clean gloves
Water-resistant gown to protect clothes
Isolation bag
Nit combs or tongue blades (2)

Procedure
Note: Louse becomes adult in 7–8 days. Each louse lays 4–8 eggs/day for the next 18 days, then dies (each louse lays 100–400 eggs). The nits or eggs hatch in 8 days. Adult lice can survive up to 55 hours without a host.

1. Check order and identify client using two forms of ID.
2. Introduce yourself and explain the procedure.
3. Gather supplies. Perform hand hygiene.
4. Don clean gloves and water-resistant gown to protect clothes.
5. Position client so that head or affected body area is well lighted by lamp.
6. Use fine-tooth louse comb after removing tangles and comb from roots to end. After each stroke, examine comb for live louse or a viable egg. Use magnifying glass to observe scalp and hair. ❶

   a. For live lice:
      Gray-white to reddish brown in color
      2–4 mm long; 1 mm wide
      Flat body with six clawed legs
      Live lice crawl, but do not fly, jump, or hop.
      Feed on blood 3–4 times/day
   b. For viable eggs or nymph:
      Tiny and hard
      Yellow to white oval, teardrop-shaped capsules ❷
      Attached firmly to base of hair shaft (Dandruff will fall from hair shaft when touched.)
      Nits hatch after 7–10 days.
      Nits within 6 mm of scalp are usually viable and indicate an active infestation.
      Easiest to detect close behind the ears or at the nape of the neck

7. Identify lice or nits:

   a. Fine-toothed louse comb: After removing tangles, comb from roots to end with the nit comb. After each stroke, examine comb carefully for signs of lice.
   b. Nits present without lice do not indicate that there is an active infestation. Assess further: previous treatment, timing, and distance from scalp.
   c. Put hair strands between two tongue blades and scrape white specks. Determine whether they come off the shaft easily. Observe base of scalp carefully for tiny lice.

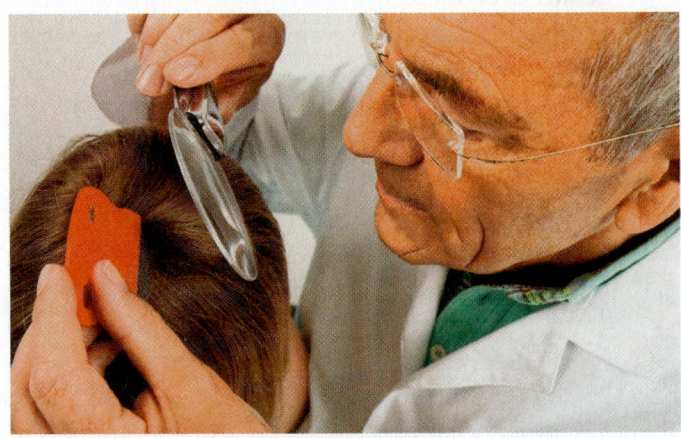

❶ Use magnifying glass when inspecting for head lice.

❷ Examine hair closely for white nits on hair shafts.

Skill 9.3.2 | Removing Lice and Nits

Equipment
Isolation bags (optional)
Topical insecticides/pediculicides:
   Permethrin (Nix, RID)
   Dimeticone 4% liquid gel
   Pyrethrin (A-200, Pronto, Tisit)
   Malathion (Ovice, by prescription)
   ClearLice

Clean linen
Fine-tooth "nit" comb
Disinfectant for comb
Clean gloves
Towels

Procedure

1. Identify client using two forms of identification. Introduce yourself and determine whether client is allergic to ragweed or chrysanthemums. ➤ *Rationale:* Pyrethrin is obtained from these plants and cannot be used to treat lice if client is allergic to them.

> **CLINICAL ALERT**
>
> When using any of the lice treatment products, the nurse needs to check for allergies to ragweed or chrysanthemum flowers. Allergies to ragweed can cause breathing difficulties or an asthmatic attack. Allergies to chrysanthemums can cause pneumonia, muscle paralysis, or death due to respiratory failure.

2. Check order; gather supplies; perform hand hygiene.
3. Don clean gloves. Gloves are used even when completing treatment at home.
4. Remove and bag client's clothing and linens. Client's clothes do not need to be bagged separately and placed in isolation bags if standard precautions are used.
5. Notify physician and other healthcare providers of lice infestation. Begin treatment as ordered by physician (Box 9-5 ■).
6. Follow manufacturer's directions for product ordered.
7. Give the client a towel to protect eyes and face while applying product and rinsing hair. Apply lotion, mousse, or gel to scalp and dry hair, beginning at the roots, and extend to the end of the hair shaft. If using shampoo before treatment, be sure to towel dry hair.

Box 9-5 GUIDELINES FOR DIAGNOSIS AND TREATMENT OF PEDICULOSIS CAPITIS IN CHILDREN AND ADULTS

Diagnosis:
- A live louse or nymph on the scalp or a viable egg is usually found within 1 cm of the scalp.
- Using a fine-tooth louse comb is four times more efficient and two times faster than direct visualization.

Treatment:
- ClearLice is the newest and most efficient method to destroy lice. It only needs to be used once.
- Permethrin has been the treatment of choice because of efficacy and lack of toxicity.
- Pyrethrin and Piperonyl butoxide are not ovicidal and application should be repeated in 7 days.
- Malathion lotion is used for children over 6 years of age.
- Combing wet hair using a conditioner of choice and a louse comb is an alternative regimen and the treatment of choice for children younger than 2 years of age. When using this method, repeat combing needs to be done for the next 2 weeks on days 1, 5, 9, and 13 to break the life cycle.
- A combination of Permethrin and Bactrim should be reserved for cases not responsive to traditional pediculicides and those suspected of having lice-related resistance.

> **CLINICAL ALERT**
> **Cautions for Lice Treatment**
> - Do not use near eyes, eyebrows, eyelids, inside nose, mouth, or vagina.
> - If product gets into eyes, immediately flush eyes with water. If child swallows product, immediately contact a Poison Control Center for directions on care.
> - Stop treatment immediately if client complains of breathing difficulties, eye irritation, or skin or scalp irritation.
> - Adverse reactions and side effects may be more frequent and severe in younger clients. Consult with healthcare provider about treatment dose. Pediculicides are not effective on some resistant strains of lice.

8. Leave product on hair for 10 minutes (leave Malathion longer, according to directions).
9. Rinse hair thoroughly.
10. Comb out nits using a fine-tooth or lice/nit comb for 20 minutes. Hair should remain slightly damp while removing nits. If hair dries during combing, dampen slightly with water. ➤ *Rationale:* Combing is the most important step in the process of lice removal, as eggs can be left behind and hatch at a later time (Box 9-6 ■).
11. Disinfect combs and brushes with the shampoo.
12. Remove gloves.
13. Perform hand hygiene.
14. Instruct client, parent, or significant other to check hair and use "nit comb" every 2–3 days until lice are gone and to check skin for removal of scabies. (Pruritus may last for 2 weeks after treatment.)
15. Wash clothes and linens that the individual has used within 48 hours before treatment. ➤ *Rationale:* Head lice rarely survive more than 48 hours off the body.
16. Place stuffed toys in hot dryer or place in a plastic bag and seal for 2–4 weeks.
17. Instruct client or family to vacuum furniture and floors to rid house of lice. ➤ *Rationale:* One of the biggest causes of reinfestation is not getting the lice out of the environment

---

Box 9-6 REMOVING NITS FROM HAIR

- Part hair into sections; start at top of head and do one section at a time.
- Lift a 1- to 2-inch–wide strand of hair. Place comb as close to scalp as possible and comb with a firm, even motion away from scalp.
- Pin back each strand of hair after combing.
- Clean comb often. Wipe nits away with tissue and discard into a plastic bag. Seal bag and discard to prevent lice from spreading.
- After combing, thoroughly recheck for lice and nits. Recomb as needed.
- Check every 1–3 days for missed lice.

(continued)

Skill 9.3.2 | Removing Lice and Nits (continued)

completely. Lice will live up to 48 hours on the scalp. Nits will survive up to 10 days on a sofa, car seat, or bedding.

18. Administer Bactrim if ordered (usually used with resistant cases). ➤ *Rationale:* This is used if multiple treatments have been tried to rid hair of lice.

19. Inspect all family members using wet louse comb or magnifying glass in bright light for lice and nits (eggs). Look for tiny nits near scalp, beginning at back of neck and behind ears. Examine small sections of hair one at a time. Treat each member infested with lice using the same treatment plan.

20. Discuss the cause, treatment, and preventive measures regarding lice infestation with client and family.

21. Reinspect hair every 1–3 days for signs of reinfestation.

22. Apply second treatment within 7–10 days to kill any newly hatched lice.

Note: ClearLice eliminates lice and nits from the head and home in 1 day. Once the exoskeletons of the lice and nits begin to dissolve, lice and nits cannot survive when exposed to ClearLice.

CLINICAL ALERT
- Do not use more than three applications in 2 weeks.
- Do not use cream rinse, conditioner, or conditioning shampoo before applying pediculicide treatment as it will interfere with the medication.

Unit 9.3 Documentation and Evaluation

DOCUMENTATION for Removing Lice

- Location of lice infestation
- Notification of physician and healthcare providers
- Medicated shampoo applied

- Side effects of medicated shampoo, if any
- Nursing interventions and the results obtained
- Client teaching activities

EVALUATION/Critical Thinking

Expected Outcomes
- Lice were removed after treatment.
- Client verbalizes cause of problem and preventive measures.

- Client repeats back to nurse instructions for preventing lice infestation and indicates understanding of process.
- Client and family members remain free of lice infestation.

Unexpected Outcomes
- Special shampoo is left on hair or scalp too long.

Alternative Actions
- Observe for irritation or burning after rinsing out the shampoo.
- If scalp is burned, notify physician for a medication order.
- Do not repeat treatment unless specifically ordered by physician.

- Other clients or staff become infested with lice.

- Isolate the client's linen and personal hair grooming equipment to prevent spread of lice.
- Instruct client or staff on use of medicated lotion, shampoo, or combination therapy.

- Lice are not eliminated with treatment.

- Repeat treatment using combination therapy as ordered by physician.
- Do not repeat treatment for 7 days.
- Utilize another type of insecticide or wet-combing method.

Bedpan, Urinal, and Commode

Nursing Process Data

ASSESSMENT Database

- Determine client's usual voiding pattern.
- Assess client's ability to assist with the procedure.

PLANNING Objectives

- To assist the client to void when on bed rest or unable to urinate
- To help client void 200–500 mL of urine without discomfort or difficulty

IMPLEMENTATION Procedures

DOCUMENTATION AND EVALUATION

Expected Outcomes

- Client voids 200–500 mL of urine without discomfort or difficulty.
- Bladder does not become distended.
- Genitourinary system is free of infection.
- Client transferred to commode for voiding.

Unexpected Outcomes/Alternative Actions

Pearson Nursing Student Resources

Find additional review materials at **nursing.pearsonhighered.com.**
Prepare for success with NCLEX®-style practice questions and Skill Checklists.

Skill 9.4.1 | Using a Bedpan and Urinal

Equipment
Bedpan or urinal ❶
Toilet tissue
Absorbent pad, if needed
Clean gloves

Procedure
1. Identify client using two identifiers.
2. Introduce yourself and explain the procedure.
3. Perform hand hygiene and don gloves.
4. Obtain bedpan or urinal and warm pan or urinal by running warm water around the edges of the receptacle if cold. Fracture pan is used for clients in traction, body cast, or with casted extremities.

❶ Urinal, bedpan, and fracture pan used for clients on bed rest.

5. Provide privacy.
6. Place client in a supine position, if possible, or position on edge of bed or in a chair.
7. Instruct the client to sit on bedpan or place penis into urinal. If the client needs assistance, follow these steps:

Using a Bedpan
a. Place absorbent pad under hips, if needed.
b. Raise the client's hips and slip your arm under the client or turn the client on his or her side. Roll the client onto the pan. ❷
c. Place a rolled towel or blanket under the client's sacrum.
   ➤ *Rationale:* This provides comfort by padding the bony area.
d. Elevate the head of the bed.

Using a Urinal
a. Place the base of the urinal flat on the bed between the client's thighs.
b. Position the client's penis into opening of the urinal.

Note: It may be easier for clients to use a urinal if they sit on the edge of the bed.

8. Place the signal light or call bell and toilet tissue within easy reach.

❷ **A.** Turn client to side to position on bedpan. **B.** Roll client onto pan and make comfortable.

9. When the client has voided, remove the bedpan or urinal and assist with wiping as necessary.

   a. Remove bedpan by placing hand under small of back.

   b. Assist client to lift buttocks off pan.

   c. Remove pan by pulling toward edge of bed. Keep bedpan flat when moving. ➤ *Rationale:* This prevents spilling urine out of bedpan.

10. Provide an opportunity for the client to perform hand hygiene.

11. Reposition the client for comfort, pull back curtains.

12. Measure and record intake and output if required.

13. Empty bedpan or urinal, clean equipment, and return to proper area in client's room.

14. Remove gloves and perform hand hygiene.

Skill 9.4.2 | Assisting Client to Commode

Equipment
Commode with locking wheels or rubber-tipped legs
Toilet tissue
Nurse's call bell
Slippers
Bath blanket

Procedure
1. Identify client using two identifiers.
2. Introduce yourself and explain the process for assisting client to commode.
3. Place commode at foot of bed. Be sure to lock wheels on commode if needed.
4. Place slippers on client.
5. Raise head of bed to facilitate moving client to edge of bed.
6. Move client to edge of bed and assist to a sitting position at edge of bed. Instruct client to place feet flat on floor.
7. Stand directly in front of client, blocking client's toes with your feet and client's knees with your knees. ➤ *Rationale:* This prevents client from buckling knees.
8. Flex your knees.
9. Place your arms securely around client's waist.
   ➤ *Rationale:* This stabilizes the client for transfer.
10. When starting to transfer, avoid bending at the waist.
    ➤ *Rationale:* This prevents back strain.
11. Instruct client to push self off bed and support his or her own weight.
12. Straighten your knees and hips as you raise client to standing position. ❶
13. Pivot client in front of commode. Instruct client to grasp arm rest on farthest side.
14. Lower client onto commode, using correct body mechanics (flexing your hip and knees but not your back) to ensure client is securely positioned on commode.
15. Place toilet tissue within easy reach.
16. Cover client with bath blanket for warmth and privacy.
17. Place call bell within easy access of client.
18. Provide privacy by closing curtains and shutting door.
19. Assist client to wipe self as necessary.
20. Assist client back to bed.
21. Empty and clean commode.
22. Perform hand hygiene.

❶ Pivot with client and bend knees when seating client.

Unit 9.4 Documentation and Evaluation

DOCUMENTATION for Bedpan, Urinal, and Commode

- Amount, color, appearance, and odor of urine and feces
- Techniques effective in stimulating voiding
- Equipment used (e.g., commode, bedpan)
- Type of support needed for transfer to commode

EVALUATION/Critical Thinking

Expected Outcomes

- Client voids 200–500 mL of urine without discomfort or difficulty.
- Bladder does not become distended.
- Genitourinary system is free of infection.
- Client transferred to commode for voiding as soon as able.

Unexpected Outcomes

- Client unable to turn and has difficulty raising hips

Critical Thinking Options

- Use a fracture pan rather than a bedpan. Powder the fracture pan if approved by the facility.
- Insert the fracture pan with the flat side toward the head, under the client's thighs.
- Assess reason for difficulty.
- Maintain complete privacy.

- Unable to void on bedpan

- Run water in sink.
- Massage the lower abdomen.
- Place a hot washcloth on the abdomen.
- Pour warm water over the perineum with client positioned on toilet or bedpan.

Perineal and Genital Care

Nursing Process Data

ASSESSMENT Database

- Review client's general assessment data.
- Observe for signs of perineal itching, burning on urination, or skin irritation. Ask client if he or she experiences any of these problems.
- Assess client's ability to bathe himself or herself and to perform perineal care.
- While providing privacy, observe the perineal–genital area for abnormal secretions, ulcerations, skin **excoriations** and sensitivity, drainage (amount, consistency, odor, color), swelling, enlarged lymph glands, catheter patency, and comfort.
- Assess client's learning needs related to perineal and genital care.

PLANNING Objectives

- To decrease the growth of bacteria
- To remove excessive secretions
- To promote healing after surgery and vaginal deliveries
- To prevent the spread of microorganisms for clients with indwelling catheters
- To increase client comfort

IMPLEMENTATION Procedures

DOCUMENTATION AND EVALUATION

Expected Outcomes

- Perineal care has been comfortably and effectively provided.
- Perineal area is clean, odor-free, and without irritation or discharge.
- Skin remains intact after perineal care.

Unexpected Outcomes/Alternative Actions

Pearson Nursing Student Resources

Find additional review materials at
nursing.pearsonhighered.com.
Prepare for success with NCLEX®-style practice questions and Skill Checklists.

| Skill 9.5.1 | Draping a Female Client |

Equipment
Bath blanket
Clean gloves

Procedure
1. Bring bath blanket to bedside.
2. Introduce self, identify client using two forms of identification, and explain procedure.
3. Provide privacy.
4. Perform hand hygiene and don gloves.
5. Assess bladder for distention. ➤ *Rationale:* Offer bedpan before providing perineal care to prevent urge to urinate during perineal care.

6. Place bed in HIGH position, and lower side rail nearest you.
7. Place bath blanket over client's top linen so that one corner of the blanket is pointed toward the client's head to form a diamond shape over the client.
8. Instruct client to hold on to bath blanket. Fanfold linen to foot of bed.
9. Request that client flex knees and keep them apart with feet firmly on bed.
10. Wrap lateral corners of bath blanket around feet in a spiral fashion until they are completely covered.
11. The corner of the blanket between knees and extending over perineum can later be folded back over the abdomen.

Skill 9.5.2 | Providing Female Perineal Care

Equipment
Bath blanket or sheet
Basin of warm water
Two to three bath towels or perineal cloths
Protective pad
Three washcloths or disposable cloth package
Clean gloves

Preparation
1. Check to see if specific physician orders are to be followed.
2. Introduce self; identify client using two forms of identification.
3. Talk with client about how she can perform care or assist with procedure. ➤ *Rationale:* This provides a sense of control.
4. Collect and arrange necessary equipment. Warm disposable cloth package if using disposable system. ➤ *Rationale:* Warm cloth is more comfortable for client.
5. Provide privacy by closing door and pulling drapes.
6. Perform hand hygiene.
7. Position client in a comfortable position in bed. Head of bed can be elevated to low-Fowler's position. Drape according to procedure described above. ❶
8. If possible, encourage the client to bend her knees and separate her legs. ➤ *Rationale:* The perineal area can be cleansed more efficiently in this position.

Procedure
1. Place a protective pad or towel under the client's hips. ➤ *Rationale:* This keeps the linen clean and dry.
2. Don gloves.
3. Lift corner of drape away from perineal area.
4. Place first washcloth into basin. Rub cloth with soap, wring out excess water or open disposable cloth package.

❶ Draping protects client's privacy when performing perineal care.

5. Fold washcloth or disposable cloth into mitt or gather into palm of hand.
6. Separate **labia** with one hand to expose **urethra** and vaginal openings. ❷
7. Wash labia minora, from front to back, in a downward motion on one side. ➤ *Rationale:* This promotes the principle of washing from a clean to a dirty area to prevent a urinary tract infection.
8. Take opposite end of washcloth or disposable cloth and wash other side from top to bottom.
9. Do not replace washcloth in basin.
10. Place a second washcloth in water and put soap on it, or take a new disposable cloth; wash the labia majora from top to bottom. ➤ *Rationale:* This prevents contamination from previously cleaned area.

❷ Separate labia and expose urethral and vaginal areas.

11. Take opposite side of washcloth or disposable cloth and clean external labia (labia majora) and perineal area from front to back. ❸
12. Wring out new washcloth or take new disposable cloth and rinse perineum.
13. Thoroughly pat dry perineal area. ➤ *Rationale:* Prevents moisture accumulation and potential fungal infections. ❹
14. Use washcloth or disposable cloth used for rinsing and clean around anal area. ➤ *Rationale:* Anal area is last to be washed to prevent cross-contamination.
15. Discard washcloths in appropriate receptacle.
16. Remove gloves.
17. Position client for comfort.
18. Perform hand hygiene.

3 Use different section of washcloth or disposable cloth for each area of perineum.

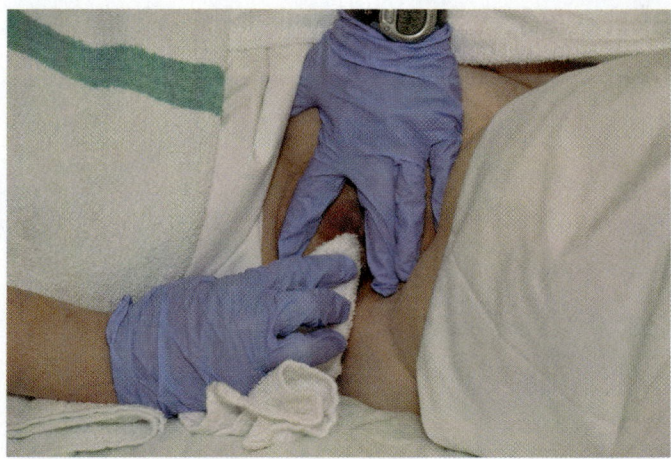

4 Thoroughly pat dry perineal area.

Skill 9.5.3 | Providing Male Perineal Care

Equipment

Bath blanket or sheet
Two bath towels
Protective pad or plastic sheet
Disposable cloths or three washcloths
Basin of warm water
Clean gloves

Preparation

1. Identify client using two forms of identification.
2. Introduce yourself.
3. Collect and arrange necessary equipment.
4. Explain the procedure and discuss with client about how he can perform care or assist with procedure.
5. Ask client to attempt to empty bladder.
6. Provide privacy by closing door and pulling drapes.
7. Perform hand hygiene and don gloves.
8. Cover client with bath blanket or towel over abdomen and cover client's legs with sheet or towel, exposing genital area as little as possible. ➤ *Rationale:* This contributes to client's comfort and privacy.

1 Hold shaft of penis in one hand.

Procedure

1. Place washcloth in basin or open disposable cloth package. Apply soap to washcloth.
2. Wring washcloth out to remove excess water.
   ➤ *Rationale:* This will prevent the protective pad from getting too wet.
3. If the client has not been circumcised, retract his foreskin carefully to expose the glans penis.
4. Gently but securely hold the shaft of the penis in one hand. **1**
5. Using a circular motion, start at the tip of the penis and wash downward toward the shaft with soap and water. Do not repeat washing over an area without using a new washcloth or disposable cloth. **2** ➤ *Rationale:* This procedure prevents cross-contamination.

2 Use circular motion, starting at tip of penis and wash toward shaft.

6. Replace the foreskin over the glans penis and cleanse area.
7. Obtain new washcloth and wash around the scrotum. **3**

(continued)

Skill 9.5.3 | Providing Male Perineal Care *(continued)*

8. Wash the anus last.
9. Use new washcloth and rinse the perineal area.
10. Dry all areas.
11. Remove articles and cover client.
12. Reposition client for comfort.
13. Place disposable cloth in garbage or washcloth in linen hamper.
14. Remove gloves, and place in appropriate receptacle.
15. Perform hand hygiene.

❸ Wash around scrotum using new washcloth.

Skill 9.5.4 | Providing Incontinence Care

Equipment
Commercially prepared package with premoistened perineal washcloths
Cleansing agent if needed
Clean linen, gown as needed
Clean gloves

Preparation
1. Identify client using two forms of identification.
2. Introduce yourself and explain the procedure.
3. Provide privacy for client and explain what you will be doing.
4. Obtain package of three washcloths premoistened with 3% dimethicone, a transparent barrier that remains on the skin to protect it. ➤ *Rationale:* This protective barrier is less messy than zinc oxide or other petroleum-based barriers, and it seals out wetness on the perineum.
5. Place in microwave for 12 seconds. ➤ *Rationale:* Warming for a longer time can potentially burn the client's perineum. Washcloths may be used at room temperature.

6. Take warmed package to room.
7. Don clean gloves.

Procedure
1. Remove client's soiled gown and place in linen hamper. (Change gloves if they become contaminated.)
2. Open package.
3. Clean soiled area by cleansing from front to back for females and tip of penis down shaft for males. ➤ *Rationale:* This prevents contamination. The cloths provide moisturizing, deodorizing, and a barrier protection.
4. Use a different cloth for each area of the perineum.
5. Discard soiled washcloths and package in appropriate receptacle.
6. Place new gown on client and change linen as needed.
7. Place client in position of comfort.
8. Remove gloves and place in appropriate receptacle.
9. Perform hand hygiene.

Unit 9.5 Documentation and Evaluation

DOCUMENTATION for Perineal and Genital Care

- Assessment and care needs for perineal hygiene
- Client's level of understanding and teaching needs
- Perineal care provided and outcomes of care
- Type, amount, and consistency of discharge from perineal area

- Presence of lesions, ulcerations, or other skin lesions
- Response of client to procedure
- Incontinence, number of times, and interventions attempted to control incontinence

EVALUATION/Critical Thinking

Expected Outcomes

- Perineal care has been comfortably and effectively provided.
- Perineal area is clean and odor-free, and without irritation or discharge.
- Skin remains intact after perineal care.

Unexpected Outcomes	Alternative Actions
• Client has foul odor even after perineal care.	• Obtain order for sitz bath. • Request order for medicated solution. • Request culture of discharge so the appropriate treatment can be instituted.
• Client develops urinary tract infection.	• Instruct client on proper technique for perineal care. • Instruct female clients to wash from anterior to posterior aspects of perineum, using different sections of cloth for each wipe. • Instruct male clients to wash from urethral opening down the shaft of the penis.

Eye and Ear Care

Nursing Process Data

ASSESSMENT Database

- Assess whether client is using eyeglasses or contact lenses or is experiencing any eye problems.
- Observe client's eyes for symmetry and clarity.
- Assess skin surrounding client's eyes for excessive dryness, scaling, and irritation.
- Assess eyes for discomfort, irritation, **edema**, crustation, sties, and lesions.
- Assess client's knowledge related to care of contact lenses.
- Observe client's tear duct areas and **sclera** for inflammation and excessive tearing.
- Assess client's pupils for response to light.
- Observe client's eye movements or muscle action.
- Evaluate ability to hear and effectiveness of hearing aid.

PLANNING Objectives

- To ensure that eyes and surrounding skin areas are clear, comfortable, and free of crustation
- To improve or maintain the client's vision
- To prevent irritation and infection
- To maintain or improve the client's appearance and self-esteem
- To increase ability to hear

IMPLEMENTATION Procedures

DOCUMENTATION AND EVALUATION

Expected Outcomes

- Eyes and surrounding area are clear and free of encrustation.
- Vision is maintained or improved.
- Contact lenses are cleaned and replaced without difficulty.
- Hearing is improved after cleaning hearing aid.

Unexpected Outcomes / Alternative Actions

Pearson Nursing Student Resources

Find additional review materials at
nursing.pearsonhighered.com.
Prepare for success with NCLEX®-style practice questions and Skill Checklists.

Skill 9.6.1 | Providing Routine Eye Care

Equipment

Small basin
Water or normal saline solution
Washcloth or cotton balls
Clean gloves

Preparation

1. Determine client's eye care needs, and obtain healthcare provider's order if needed.
2. Identify client using two forms of identification.
3. Introduce yourself.
4. Explain necessity for and method of eye care to client. Discuss how client can assist you.
5. Collect necessary equipment.
6. Perform hand hygiene and don gloves.

Procedure

1. Use water or saline solution at room temperature.
2. Using the washcloth or cotton balls moistened in water or saline, gently wipe each eye from the inner to outer **canthus**. Use separate cotton ball or corner of washcloth for each eye. ▶ *Rationale:* This prevents cross-contamination from one eye to the other.
3. If crusting is present, gently place a warm, wet compress over eye(s) until crusting is loosened.
4. Dispose of used supplies and return basin to appropriate area.
5. Remove and discard gloves.
6. Perform hand hygiene.

Skill 9.6.2   Providing Eye Care for Comatose Client

Equipment
Water or normal saline solution
Washcloth, cotton balls, tissues
Sterile lubricant or eye preparations if ordered by the
   physician
Eye dropper or Asepto bulb syringe
Eye pads or patches
Clean gloves

Procedure
1. Perform hand hygiene and don clean gloves.
2. Cleanse the eyes using a moistened washcloth or cotton
   balls moistened in water or saline. **❶** Gently wipe each
   eye from inner to outer canthus. Use separate cotton ball
   or corner of washcloth for each eye. ➤ *Rationale:* Wiping
   from inner canthus to outer prevents particles and fluid from
   entering **nasolacrimal** duct.
3. Use a dropper to instill a sterile **ophthalmic solution** (liquid
   tears, saline, methylcellulose) every 3–4 hours as ordered by
   healthcare provider. (See Skill 18.2.4, *Instilling Ophthalmic
   Drops* in Chapter 18, Medication Administration.)
   ➤ *Rationale:* Use of ophthalmic solution prevents corneal
   drying and ulceration.

❶ Wash the eye carefully, moving from the center to the
outside corner of the lid.

4. Keep client's eyes closed if blink reflex is absent. If eye pads
   or patches are used, explain their purpose to client's family.
   Do not tape eyes shut. ➤ *Rationale:* Corneal **abrasions**
   and drying occur when eyes lose blink reflex.
5. Remove gloves and perform hand hygiene.
6. Remove patch and evaluate condition of eye every 4 hours.

Skill 9.6.3   Removing and Cleaning Contact Lenses

Equipment
Towel
Contact lens container
Eye wetting solution
Commercially prepared cleaning solution
Commercially prepared disinfecting solution
Commercially prepared rinsing and storing solution
Enzymatic agent (protein remover)
Clean gloves

Procedure
1. Place client in semi-Fowler's position and place a towel
   under the client's chin.
2. Perform hand hygiene and don gloves. Place a drop
   of wetting solution or sterile saline into the eyes.
   ➤ *Rationale:* This moistens the contact surface.
3. Place the tip of your thumb across the lower lid below its margin.
4. Place the tip of the forefinger of the same hand on the upper
   lid above its margin.
5. Spread eyelids apart as wide as possible and locate outer
   edges of soft lens that should appear as a rim around outer
   edge of iris.
6. Place thumb and forefinger directly on soft lens.
7. Ask the client to look up, then pull down the lower eyelid.
   Touch the lower edge of the lens with the index finger and
   slide the contact lens down to the white part of the eye.

Using the thumb and index finger, squeeze the lens gently
and remove it. ➤ *Rationale:* Cornea is not **vascular**, and
use of contact lenses interrupts flow of oxygen into the
cornea. Removing lenses for a period of time allows oxygen
to reach cornea and prevent corneal complications.
8. Release eyelids.
9. Place lens in palm of hand or place disposable lenses in
   trash. Some types of disposable lenses are cleaned and
   reused. Follow eye care specialist directions.
10. Place 2–3 drops of cleaning solution on lens.
11. Clean lens thoroughly by rubbing between fingertip and
    palm of hand for 20–30 seconds.
12. Rinse lens thoroughly with sterile saline solution or rinsing
    solution. Use only lens cleaning system recommended
    by ophthalmologist. Do not interchange cleaning solution
    systems.
13. Place lens in disinfecting solution according to physician
    directions. Time varies from hours to 1 full day.
    ➤ *Rationale:* This destroys **microorganisms** on lenses.
14. Rinse lens thoroughly with rinsing solution.
15. Repeat procedure on second lens. As appropriate, teach
    client about lens care (Box 9-7 ■).
16. Use enzyme tablet or solution according to physician orders,
    usually weekly. ➤ *Rationale:* This removes stubborn protein
    and lipids.

(continued)

Skill 9.6.3 | Removing and Cleaning Contact Lenses (continued)

CLINICAL ALERT

- Extended-wear (overnight) contacts, rigid or soft, increase the risk of corneal **ulcers**—infection-caused eruptions on the cornea that can lead to blindness. Symptoms include visual changes, eye redness, eye discomfort or pain, and excessive tearing.
- Clean, rinse, and disinfect reusable lenses each time they are removed regardless of number of times each day. Always store lenses in storage solution, not water. Microorganisms from water can feed on corneal tissue.

17. Clean lens container daily and leave open to dry. Replace as directed by physician, either weekly or monthly.
18. Remove gloves and perform hand hygiene.

Note: A suction cup can be placed gently against lens for easy removal of lens. Squeeze suction cup with dominant hand, place on lens, open finger slightly to create suction between lens and cup. Rock lens gently to remove it.

Box 9-7 CLIENT TEACHING FOR CONTACT LENS CARE

Instruct the client in the following safety issues:

- Notify physician immediately if eyes are red, not comfortable, or you can't see clearly.
- Use only rinsing solution, not saliva, to wet lenses.
- Use only commercially prepared saline solution or rinsing solution to cleanse lenses.
- Do not interchange types of lens cleaning systems.
- Maintain lens-care regimen prescribed by physician.
- Put on makeup before inserting lenses.
- Use appropriate type of lenses for their intended use. Do not use daily-wear lenses at night or disposable lenses more than once.
- Do not allow soft lenses to dry out.
- Contact lens wearers should be instructed to carry appropriate identification on type and care for specific lens he or she wears.

Skill 9.6.4 | Cleaning and Checking a Hearing Aid

Equipment

Soap
Water
Cotton-tipped applicator
Hearing aid batteries (Box 9-8 ■)
Clean gloves

Procedure

1. Determine ability of client to perform all or part of cleaning procedure, and teach procedure when necessary (Box 9-9 ■). Have client remove hearing aid if able to do so.
2. Perform hand hygiene and don gloves.
3. Wipe casing with dry cloth.

4. Check batteries if hearing aid has not been functioning. Insert new batteries, matching positive (+) and negative (−) signs.
5. Before inserting ear mold, cleanse the outer ear gently with a cotton-tipped applicator. Instruct the client not to insert cotton-tipped applicators into the ear canal.
6. Turn receiver switch to ON. Assist client to adjust volume control to desired level. If whistling or feedback noises occur, check for tightness of fit as ear mold probably has not been inserted properly or there is a buildup of ear wax.
7. Place hearing aid in labeled container when not in use and place in bedside stand.
8. Remove gloves.
9. Perform hand hygiene.

Box 9-8 TYPES OF HEARING AIDS

- **Analog:** Two types, conventional and programmed. Programmed aids adjust amplifier more precisely to match hearing loss and provide greater fitting flexibility.
- **Digital:** Continuous sound waves are broken into small, discrete bits of information, digitizing the signal. Computer programs are written for each client's hearing loss.

Note: 75% of all hearing aids sold are digital.

Box 9-9 CLIENT TEACHING FOR HEARING AIDS

- Replace batteries when needed.
- Turn hearing aid off when not in use.
- Clean hearing aids according to manufacturer's directions.
- Refrain from using hair spray or other hair products.
- Keep hearing aids away from moisture and heat.

Source: National Institute on Deafness and Other Communication Disorders (NIDCD) (2014)

Unit 9.6 Documentation and Evaluation

DOCUMENTATION for Eye and Ear Care

- Documentation of eye assessment and eye care needs
- Method and outcome of eye care provided
- Condition of eye and surrounding structure
- Client's response to client teaching regarding contact lenses
- Response to using hearing aid
- Improved hearing after cleaning hearing aid
- Client's ability to insert, remove, and clean hearing aid

EVALUATION/Critical Thinking

Expected Outcomes

- Eyes and surrounding area are clear and free of crustation.
- Vision is maintained or improved.
- Contact lenses are cleaned and replaced without difficulty.
- Hearing is improved after cleaning hearing aid.

Unexpected Outcomes	Alternative Actions
• Eyelids become crusted from exudate.	• Place warm, moist washcloth across eyes and leave in place for several minutes. • Moisten cotton applicator stick with sterile saline and gently twist the applicator stick over crusted surface to assist in removing crust.
• Wrong solution used on contact lens causes excessive tearing and burning sensation when lens is placed in eye.	• Immediately remove lens from eye and place in proper storage container. • Immediately rinse client's eye with copious amounts of sterile water. • Have client checked immediately by ophthalmologist for emergency care of potentially burned cornea.
• Hearing did not improve with cleaning of hearing aid.	• Check if receiver switch is ON. • Check if batteries are properly in place and that the poles match: positive (+) and negative (−). • Recheck hearing aid with expert.

Chapter Wrap-Up

GERONTOLOGIC Considerations

Clients With Dentures Require Special Nursing Care.

- Check for proper fit when replacing dentures. Ill-fitting dentures interfere with chewing and can lead to altered nutrition. Loss of teeth may limit meal planning and the nurse should assist the client to choose a balanced diet taking into account tooth loss.
- Monitor denture cleaning to ensure client has fresh-tasting mouth to encourage eating. Older adult clients have decreased sensitivity to sweet, sour, salty, and bitter tastes; thus they may compensate by using extra salt. The nurse can counsel the client on alternative seasonings and request dietary consultation.

Fear of the Unknown

- Any treatment or activity may be unfamiliar and frightening to the older adult.

- Explain each procedure before attempting it. Ask client to help when appropriate.

Self-Perception and Self-Concept

- Poor self-concept, depression, and negative feelings are common among older adults.
- Encourage personal hygiene activities to promote a more positive self-image.
- A positive body image is enhanced with good personal hygiene. Nursing care should focus on assisting the client to maintain good personal hygiene.
- Encourage older adult clients to have hair and nail care done frequently to increase self-esteem.

MANAGEMENT Guidelines

Each state legislates a Nurse Practice Act for RNs and LVN/LPNs. Healthcare facilities are responsible for establishing and implementing policies and procedures that conform to their state's regulations. Verify the regulations and role parameters for each healthcare worker in your facility.

Delegation

- The staffing patterns today often require that Certified Nursing Assistants (CNAs) or Unlicensed Assistive Personnel (UAPs) complete personal hygiene activities for most clients because these activities have a predictable outcome and do not require nursing judgment. However, performing these tasks for the client provides an excellent forum for client assessment. When the tasks are delegated to other personnel, the RN and LPN/LVNs responsible for client care must receive specific reports of the client's condition and any unexpected findings. The CNAs and UAPs should receive specific instructions regarding the condition of each client and what to observe for.

- The RN is responsible for assessing all clients because assessment responsibilities cannot be delegated.
- The team member delegating staff assignments should try to implement a staffing pattern that allows professional nurses to be assigned to complete general care, including personal hygiene activities, at least every other day so that important assessment parameters are not missed.
- Check facility's procedure manual for appropriate healthcare worker to remove and replace contact lenses.

Interprofessional Communication

CNAs and UAPs should be educated, encouraged, and rewarded with positive feedback when they give excellent reports on the client for whom they have performed the tasks of personal hygiene. When the unit is extremely busy, this may be the major source of information the professional nurse receives about the client for whom he or she is legally responsible.

CASE STUDY Applications

Scenario 1

You have been assigned to two clients for the 7 a.m. to 12 noon clinical experience.

Client 1:

A 68-year-old female with a total hip replacement 2 days ago. Her past history indicates she had a cataract removed 2 months ago and had a lens fitted a week ago. She has developed a very uncomfortable incision site. It is red and tender to touch. Her dressings are somewhat moist without observable drainage on the dressings. Her vital signs indicate a temperature of 101°F, P 90, R 28 and unlabored. She tells you she doesn't feel like doing anything today.

Client 2:

An 80-year-old female with a fractured hip, unrepaired, admitted this morning from a local long-term care facility. She is in severe pain and requires pain medications every 4 hours. She is unable to use the patient-controlled analgesia (PCA) because she forgets how it works. Her physical assessment indicates her skin is reddened around the coccyx and very dry. She appears to be unkempt, and her hair is matted.

1. Based on the scenario, what is your first action after you hear report? Provide a rationale for your answer.
2. Identify the assessment you will complete on each client. What information will you be gathering in order to make a decision on nursing care for the shift?
3. List, in priority order, the nursing care you will provide for each client and provide rationales for your decision.
4. Which client will you assess first and why?

5. Which of the personal hygiene skills will you provide or can be delegated for each client? Will any adjustments need to be made in the skill in order to provide care for the client? Please state the changes that will need to be made.

Scenario 2

You are working in a pediatric clinic when a mother brings her two preschool children into the clinic. She tells you she is not sure why her children keep scratching their scalps and have something that looks like dandruff. After examining the children's hair you determine they have lice. When the mother receives this information she starts crying and states, "I just knew that preschool was dirty. I should not have sent the children there."

1. What response will be appropriate to this statement?
2. After calming the mother down, how will you approach her to explain the treatment for lice?
3. You begin the explanation with a discussion of potential side effects. What will you tell her about the side effects?
4. Describe the skill of applying a treatment for lice.
5. While shampooing the hair, if the child starts crying and says her eyes are burning, what will you tell the mother to do?
6. Explain the most effective method for removing nits from the child's hair after the treatment.
7. The mother asks you if she needs to do the treatment once and then the lice will be gone. What is your response to her?
8. The mother wants to know if she and her husband can get the lice also. What is your response to her?
9. What is your best response to the mother's question about whether she needs to burn the sheets and children's clothes?

NCLEX® Review Questions

Unless otherwise specified, choose only one (1) answer.

1. You are assigned to provide hygienic care to an unconscious client. Your assessment indicates she needs good oral hygiene. What is the major safety action for this procedure?
   A. Turn the client's head to the side.
   B. Keep a suction bulb or equipment at bedside.
   C. Use a tongue blade to keep the mouth open.
   D. Don clean gloves to prevent spread of bacteria.

2. A client has severely tangled hair. What is the best description of how to provide hair care for this client?
   A. Brush or comb her hair from the scalp to hair ends.
   B. Apply small amount of oil to tangled areas of scalp before combing.
   C. Use a hair pick to untangle hair and then brush hair.
   D. Use short gentle strokes with a wide-toothed comb, starting at the end of hair shaft.

3. Which of the following statements is true regarding lice eggs?
   A. Lice eggs are light brown, crawl, and feed on blood.
   B. Lice eggs are yellow to white and attach to hair shaft.
   C. Lice eggs hatch 17 days after a louse lays eggs.
   D. Lice eggs have clawed legs that assist in jumping and hopping.

4. What identifies a live louse or nymph on the scalp, which is evidenced by nits (eggs) located on the hair shaft?
   A. Less than 1 cm from the scalp they are usually not viable.
   B. Within 10 mm from the scalp they are usually not viable.
   C. Within 6 mm they are usually viable.
   D. Those easily seen on the hair shaft are viable.

5. What is the primary intervention to prevent spread of lice or nits?

   A. Discard all clothing and bedding used by client.

   B. Use one of the products to prevent lice on all family members at the same time client is being treated.

   C. Launder all clothing and bedding in hot water, followed by drying using hot cycle of dryer.

   D. Observe family members for signs of nits near scalp; if present, use same treatment plan as client.

6. The client requires denture care but is unable to remove his or her dentures. When removing the dentures, where will the nurse place his or her finger?

   A. To the side of the lower denture and move it sideways to remove it.

   B. On the middle of the upper denture and ask the client to move it with his or her tongue.

   C. On the edge of the upper denture and gently break the suction.

   D. In the middle of the teeth on the lower denture and gently pull the denture upward to remove it.

7. When moving a client from the bed to the commode, what is the most appropriate movement to prevent client or nurse injury?

   A. Instruct client to place hands around nurse's neck to stabilize stance when standing.

   B. Ensure the nurse bends back and squats when moving client out of bed.

   C. Stand in front of client, block client's toes with your feet and client's knees with your knees before starting to transfer.

   D. Maintain your hips and knees flexed when pivoting client to commode.

8. When providing male perineal care, what step is important to remember?

   A. If the client is not circumcised, wash the penis carefully to prevent retraction of the foreskin.

   B. To wash the penis using a circular motion, start at the base of the shaft and move toward the tip.

   C. When washing the penis, do not wash over the same area without using a new cloth.

   D. Always wash the scrotum first before washing the perineum.

9. What explanation should be included as client teaching for individuals who wear contact lenses?

   A. Daily wear lenses can be worn overnight; however, they need to be disposed of once they are removed.

   B. You can use tap water or rinsing solution to wet reusable contact lenses.

   C. You can use interchangeable types of lens cleaning solutions regardless of type of contact lenses.

   D. Soft contact lenses should not be allowed to dry out.

10. A client asks you about caring for a hearing aid. Which of the following would your response include?
    Select all that apply.

    A. You need to turn off the hearing aids when not in use.

    B. Keep hearing aids away from moisture and heat.

    C. Newer hearing aids do not have batteries that require changing.

    D. Hair spray should not be used when wearing hearing aids.

    E. If whistling sound is heard when turning switch ON, turn off immediately, take out, and clean it again.

QSEN Activity

Domain: Safety

KSA: Skills

Activity: Role Play: Nurse providing oral care for unconscious client

1. Nurse does not identify the client using two forms of identification. She calls the client by name but client is comatose. She gathers the equipment but does not obtain lubricant for lips and tongue blade. She brings in a toothbrush, not toothette oral swabs. The client is on ASA therapy and has a history of bleeding from the gums.

2. When the nurse approaches the bed, she has not washed her hands but does apply gloves. She sets up the bulb suction. She positions the client in a lateral position and takes the pillow away from the client.

3. The nurse proceeds to place a large amount of toothpaste on the toothette, inserts it into the mouth, and begins scrubbing the external surface of the teeth. She then rinses the mouth using a large amount of water and when the client begins to choke, she takes the bulb syringe and suctions the mouth. She sits the client up in Fowler's position and, using her hand and a paper towel, proceeds to wipe out the client's mouth.

Questions:

1. What actions were unsafe for client care?

2. Was there any missing equipment or actions that should have been taken to promote safety for the client?

3. What changes would you make to ensure a safe environment for this client?

Bibliography

Ames, N. J. (2011, May). Evidence to support tooth brushing in critically ill patients. *American Journal of Critical Care, 120*(3), 242–250.

Corlis, J. (2014, Jul.). Treating gum disease may lessen the burden of heart disease, diabetes, other conditions. *Harvard Heart Letter*, July 13, 2014. Retrieved from http://www.health.harvard.edu/blog/treating-gum-disease-may-lessen-burden-heart-disease-diabetes-conditions-201407237293

Feider, L., Mitchell, P., & Bridges, E. (2010). Oral care practices for orally intubated critically ill adults. *American Journal of Critical Care, 19*(2), 175–182.

National Institute on Deafness and Other Communication Disorders (NIDCD). (2014). Hearing aids. Retrieved from http://www.nidcd.nih.gov/health/hearingaid.asp

Schwartz, A., & Powell, S. (2009, Mar.). Brush up on oral assessment and care. *Nursing, 39*(3), 31–32.

Stein, P., & Henry, R. (2009). Poor oral hygiene in long term care. *American Journal of Nursing, 109*(6), 44–49.

Stoessel, K. (2009, Nov.). Hand hygiene: Challenges and strategies. *Infection Control Today, 13*(11), 26–28.

Chapter 10
Vital Signs

 ## Learning Objectives

10.1 Identify the cardinal signs that reflect the body's physiologic status.

10.2 List three mechanisms that increase heat production.

10.3 Explain how disease alters the "set point" of the temperature-regulating center.

10.4 Define hypothermia and list the symptoms of this condition.

10.5 Differentiate between the oral, rectal, axillary, and tympanic methods of taking temperature.

10.6 Describe two nursing actions that can be performed when temperature is not within normal range.

10.7 Describe at least three different types of pulse characteristics.

10.8 Discuss the pulse, and indicate how it is an index of heart rate and rhythm.

10.9 Compare normal heart rate range for adults and children.

10.10 Identify the characteristics of peripheral pulses.

10.11 Explain why the blood pressure cuff should be the appropriate size for the client.

10.12 Define Korotkoff sounds in terms of phases.

10.13 Identify four of the seven factors that affect blood pressure.

10.14 Demonstrate the method of palpating systolic arterial blood pressure.

10.15 Discuss conditions when vital signs may be delegated and when they would not be delegated.

10.16 Demonstrate the proper techniques for obtaining peripheral pulses.

10.17 Describe the most effective method of obtaining a respiratory rate.

10.18 Discuss conditions when respiratory rate would be elevated or decreased.

10.19 Compare normal respiratory rates for adults and children.

Chapter Outline

Terminology

Antipyretic an agent that reduces febrile temperatures.

Apex the pointed end of a cone-shaped part or organ (e.g., lower heart, upper lung).

Arteriosclerosis an arterial disease characterized by inelasticity and thickening of the vessel walls with lessened blood flow.

Atherosclerosis a form of arteriosclerosis in which there are localized accumulations of lipid-containing material within the internal surfaces of blood vessels.

Atrial pertaining to the atrium, the upper cardiac chamber that receives blood from the lungs and systemic circulation.

Atrial fibrillation atrial arrhythmia characterized by rapid, random contractions of the atrial myocardium causing a rapid, irregular ventricular rate.

Autoregulation the intrinsic ability of an organ or tissue to maintain blood flow despite changes in arterial pressure.

Axilla armpit.

Bigeminal pulse a regularly irregular pulse where every second beat has a decreased amplitude.

Bounding pulse increased pulse pressure, felt as a slapping against the fingers because of the rapid upstroke and quick downstroke. It is seen in conditions of increased cardiac output, such as exercise, anxiety, alcohol intake, and pregnancy. It is also noted in pathology with fever, anemia, hyperthyroidism, liver failure, complete heart block with bradycardia, and hypertension.

Bradycardia a pulse rate below 60 beats per minute (beats/min).

Cardiac output the amount of blood ejected by the heart or the stroke volume (SV) times the heart rate (CO = SV × HR).

Cardiogenic originating in the heart itself.

Chemoreceptor a sense organ or sensory nerve ending that is stimulated by and reacts to chemical stimuli.

Contractility having the ability to contract or shorten muscle tissue or cells.

Core temperature the body's interior deep tissue temperature (e.g., the abdominal cavity).

Diastole the period in which the heart dilates and fills with blood; the period of relaxation.

Doppler a type of ultrasound stethoscope or probe that uses an ultrasound beam to detect blood flow.

Febrile feverish, increased body temperature.

Fibrillation quivering, involuntary contraction of individual muscle fibers.

Hypertension blood pressure that is considered to be higher than the normal range.

Hyperthermia unusually high body temperature.

Hypotension blood pressure that is lower than the normal range.

Hypothalamus the part of the brain that lies below the thalamus; it maintains or regulates body temperature, certain metabolic processes, and other autonomic activities.

Hypothermia a body temperature below the average normal range.

Hypovolemia diminished blood volume.

Infarction an area of tissue in an organ or part that undergoes necrosis after cessation of blood supply.

Infrared scanner thermometer a noncontact digital thermometer that measures a client's temperature without physical contact by using infrared technology.

Ischemia local and temporary hypoxia due to obstruction of the circulation to a part.

Korotkoff sounds low-frequency sounds that are regarded by the American Heart Association as the best index of blood pressure in an adult—sounds are produced as a result of changes in blood flow through a compressed artery.

mm Hg millimeters of mercury, used for measuring blood pressure.

Myocardium the middle muscle layer of the walls of the heart.

Normal pulse pulse is smooth and rounded and is felt as a sharp upstroke and gradual downstroke. Provides information about cardiac status and blood volume. Correlates with cardiac contraction.

Normotensive a normal tone, tension or pressure, as in normal blood pressure.

Palpate to examine by touch; feel.

Peripheral pertinent to the periphery, away from the central structure.

Peripheral vascular disease indicates diseases of the arteries and veins of the extremities, especially those conditions that interfere with adequate flow of blood.

Piloerection hair standing on end when heat production is stimulated through vasoconstriction.

Point of maximum impulse (PMI) or apical pulse; palpated at fifth intercostal space, left midclavicular line. Pulse occurs with contraction of left ventricle.

Premature ventricular beats a pacemaker outside the sinus node fires earlier than the sinus node, the normal pacemaker of the heart. Since the beat is early, the stroke volume is less because the ventricles do not have time to fill. This condition causes a pause in rhythm, which may result in a pulse deficit.

Pulse deficit occurs when the heart rate counted at the apex by auscultation is greater than the heart rate counted by palpation of the radial pulse. The pulse wave is not transmitted to the periphery to produce a palpable radial pulse.

Pulse pressure the difference between systolic and diastolic pressure (about 30–40 points).

Pulsus alternans rhythm is regular but the amplitude alternates from beat to beat. May be related to left ventricular failure.

Pulsus paradoxus disappearance of Korotkoff sounds during inspiration phase of breathing, with sounds appearing throughout the respiratory cycle (during inspiration and exhalation) at a pressure 10 mm Hg lower than heard during exhalation alone; detected by blood pressure measurement. This phenomenon occurs in chronic obstructive pulmonary disease (COPD) and with cardiac tamponade and should be further evaluated.

Pyrogen any substance that produces fever.

Set point the constant temperature that the hypothalamus (the body's thermostat) strives to maintain.

Shock state of inadequate tissue perfusion resulting from circulatory failure, precipitated by many factors and identified by various signs and symptoms.

Sinus arrhythmia heart rate change that is common in children and young adults. The rate accelerates with inspiration and slows with expiration.

Sonorous loud (describes breathing).

Sphygmomanometer instrument for indirectly determining arterial blood pressure.

Stertorous loud, noisy (describes breathing).

Tachycardia heart rate greater than 100 beats per minute (beats/min).

Thermoregulation the body's physiologic function of heat regulation to maintain a constant internal body temperature.

Valsalva maneuver attempt to forcibly exhale with the glottis, nose, and mouth closed, producing an increased intrathoracic pressure.

Vasoconstriction constriction of the blood vessels and stimulation of heat production, which is a function of the hypothalamus.

Vasodilation dilation of blood vessels.

Weak or **thready pulse** pulse pressure is diminished. It is smooth and rounded but is felt as a gradual upstroke and prolonged downstroke. It is commonly seen in conditions resulting in decreased cardiac output, such as heart failure and shock, and with obstruction to left ventricular ejection, such as aortic stenosis.

Vital Signs

Vital signs, also termed cardinal signs, reflect the body's physiologic status and provide information critical to evaluating homeostatic balance. Vital signs include four critical assessment areas: temperature, pulse, respiration, and blood pressure. The term *vital* is used because the information gathered is the clearest indicator of overall health status. These four signs form baseline assessment data necessary for ongoing evaluation of a client's condition. If the nurse has established the normal range for a client, deviations can be more easily recognized. Although not a cardinal sign, pain is considered the fifth vital sign and must be assessed at the same time as all other vital signs.

Routine vital signs (including pain assessment) are important to assess on every client. Vital signs should be taken at regular intervals, and comparison of readings is important when assessing overall health status. In fact, trends yield more information than singular readings. The more critical the client's condition, the more often these assessments need to be taken and evaluated. Hospital policy and good nursing judgment typically dictate the frequency of assessment on the basis of the client's medical diagnosis, comorbid conditions, and hospital course. Vital signs are not only indicators of a client's present condition, but are also cues to a positive or negative change in status.

Obtaining the total picture of a client's health status is a major objective of client care. Although vital signs yield important information, they gain even more relevance when compared with the client's diagnosis, laboratory tests, history, and records. The five vital signs are as follows:

1. *Temperature* represents the balance between heat gain and heat loss and is regulated in the **hypothalamus** of the brain. Variations in temperature indicate the health status of the body; thermostatic function may be altered by **pyrogens**, nervous system disease, or injury.

2. The *pulse* is an index of the heart's action; by evaluating its rate, rhythm, and volume, one can gain an overall impression of the heart's action. Pulse points can be found throughout the body and are a good indicator of perfusion. A diminished pulse can be an indication of limited perfusion to the affected extremity.

3. *Respiration*, the act of bringing oxygen into the body and removing carbon dioxide, yields data on the client's entire breathing process. When the pattern of respiration is altered, ongoing evaluation yields important clues to a client's changing condition.

4. *Blood pressure* readings provide information about the condition of the heart, the arteries and arterioles, vessel resistance, and the **cardiac output**. Serial readings provide the best indication of a client's cardiovascular status.

5. *Pain assessment* that is ongoing and constant is essential to maintain the client's homeostasis and quality of life. Pain assessment provides information on location, quality, and intensity, as well as outcomes of relief measures. (See Figure 10-1 ■, Vital Sign Assessment Record.)

Factors Influencing Vital Signs

Factors that cause alterations in vital signs include age, gender, race, heredity, medications, lifestyle, environment, pain, exercise, anxiety, stress, metabolism, circadian rhythms, and hormones. The normal variations in vital signs may be caused by age, disease, trauma, and so on. The most common alterations are listed below.

Age Age influences body temperature. It varies from 96.0° to 99.5°F (35.6–37.4°C) in newborns and 96.8° to 98.3°F (36–36.8°C) in older clients due to **thermoregulation** deficiencies in both age groups. Newborns have an immature thermoregulation mechanism that causes temperature fluctuations in response to the environment. Older adult clients have an ineffective thermoregulating system due to physiologic changes of aging. These changes are related to loss of subcutaneous fat, decreased number of sweat glands, reduced metabolism, and poor vasomotor control. Environmental conditions may also play a role in an older adult's ability to effectively adapt body heat and cooling to changes in external temperature. Respirations vary according to age as well. Newborns have a respiratory range of 30–80 breaths/min with an average rate of 32 breaths/min. As age increases, respirations decrease; adults average 16 breaths/min. The pulse rate also decreases with age. Newborns average 140 beats/min and adults average 80 beats/min. On the other hand, blood pressure may increase with age. The newborn's mean blood pressure is 65/42, while the normal adult client's blood pressure ranges from 120/80 to 100/60.

Gender Women experience greater temperature fluctuations than men, probably due to hormonal changes. Temperature variations occur during the menstrual cycle. During menopause, the instability of the vasomotor controls leads to periods of intense body heat and sweating.

Race and Heredity Studies have been mostly inconclusive as to race and heredity being related factors in vital signs alteration. Blood pressure alterations appear to be the main difference in vital signs, usually as a result of particular groups

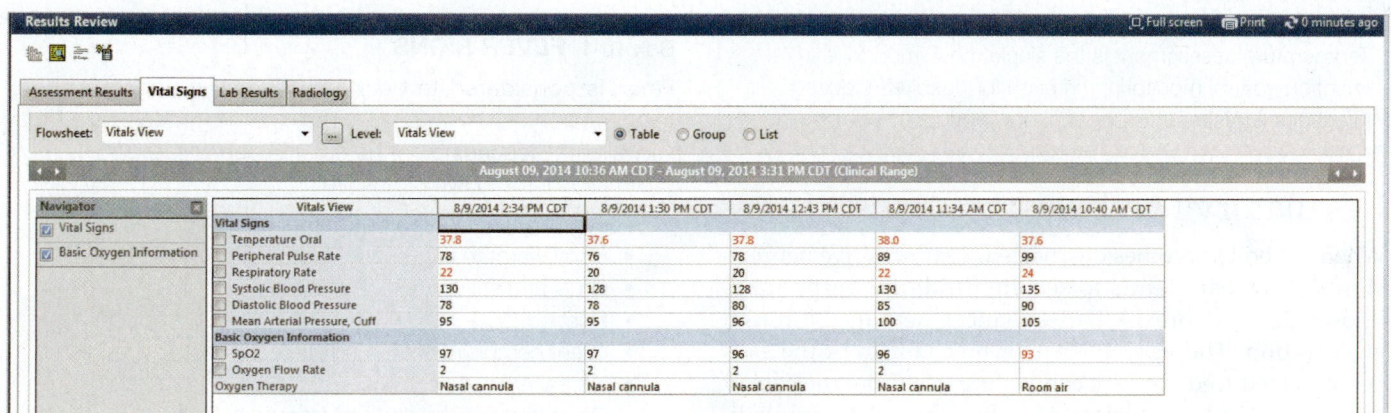

FIGURE 10-1 Vital signs assessment record. Measurements outside normal range appear in red. *Source:* From Cerner Electronic Health Record.
© Cerner Corporation. Pearson has restricted permission to reproduce and distribute this copyrighted work. Further reproduction or distribution is strictly prohibited without written consent of Cerner Corporation.

being more susceptible to hemodynamic alterations. African Americans are more prone to high blood pressure resulting from a combination of genetic and environmental factors.

Medications   Some medications can directly or indirectly alter temperature, pulse, respirations, and blood pressure. For example, narcotic analgesics can depress the rate and depth of respirations and lower blood pressure, while some cold medications can increase the heart rate.

Pain   Acute pain leads to sympathetic stimulation, which in turn increases the heart rate, respiratory rate, and blood pressure. Chronic pain decreases the pulse rate as a response to parasympathetic stimulation and may decrease heart rate and respirations.

Circadian Rhythms   Biological rhythms, or biorhythms, control certain physiologic patterns in conjunction with environmental factors. The most familiar biorhythm is the circadian rhythm that controls sleep patterns. These rhythms influence blood pressure (pressure is lowest in the morning and peaks in late afternoon and evening) and temperature (highest in the evening—8 p.m. to 12 midnight—and lowest in the early morning—4 to 6 a.m.).

Temperature

Temperature control of the body is a homeostatic function, regulated by a complex mechanism involving the hypothalamus. The temperature of the body's interior (**core temperature**) is maintained within 1°F except in the case of **febrile** illness. The surface temperature of the skin and tissues immediately underlying the skin rises and falls with a change in temperature of the surrounding environment. Core temperature is maintained when heat production equals heat loss. The temperature regulating center in the hypothalamus keeps the core temperature constant. Temperature receptors, which determine whether the body is too hot or too cold, relay signals to the hypothalamus.

> **CLINICAL ALERT**
> Temperature assessment is the single most important infection control monitoring criterion for hospital-acquired infections (HAIs) and fever of unknown origin.

Regulatory Mechanisms

When the body becomes overheated, heat-sensitive neurons stimulate sweat glands to secrete fluid; this response is known as diaphoresis. This enhances heat loss through evaporation. The vasoconstrictor mechanism of the skin vessels is reduced, thereby conducting heat from the core of the body to the body surface. Heat loss occurs through radiation, evaporation, and conduction.

When the body core is cooled below 98.6°F (37°C), heat conservation is affected. Intense **vasoconstriction** of the skin vessels results. There is also **piloerection** and a decrease in sweating to conserve heat. Heat production is stimulated by shivering and increased cellular metabolism.

The **set point** is the critical temperature level at which the regulatory mechanisms attempt to maintain the body's core temperature. Above the set point, heat-losing mechanisms are brought into play, and below that level, heat-conserving and heat-producing mechanisms are set into motion.

Disease can alter the set point of the temperature-regulating center to cause fever, a body temperature above normal. Inflammation, brain lesions, pyrogens from bacteria or viruses, or degenerating tissue (i.e., gangrenous areas or myocardial **infarction**) also increase the set point. Dehydration can cause fever due to lack of available fluid for perspiration and by increasing the set point, which brings more heat-conserving and heat-producing mechanisms into play. When the "thermostat" is suddenly set higher, the client complains of feeling cold, has cool extremities, shivers, and has piloerection (Box 10-1 ■). Hypoxia can occur due to increased oxygen use with the increased metabolism of heat production. When the thermostat returns to normal, heat-losing mechanisms again are activated.

When the body temperature falls below the normal range, the client experiences **hypothermia** and complains of being cold, shivers, and has cool extremities. Hypothermia may be caused by accidental cold exposure, frostbite, or hemorrhage. Medically induced hypothermia is used for some cardiovascular and neurosurgical interventions. The ability of the hypothalamus to regulate body temperature is greatly impaired when the body temperature falls below 94°F (34.4°C) and is lost below 85°F (29.4°C). Cellular metabolism and heat production are also depressed by a low temperature.

Measuring Body Temperature

Oral or rectal temperatures reflect the body's core temperature. Tympanic and *axillary* temperatures are somewhat variable but are clinically acceptable for tracking important changes. The normal range of an oral temperature is

---

Box 10-1 **FEVER SIGNS**

Fever is considered to be any abnormal elevation of body temperature (≥100.4°F [38°C]). The cut-off point for "fever" may vary slightly depending on the organization or facility. The most common signs and symptoms are:

- Perspiration over the body surface
- Body warm to the touch
- Chills and shivers
- Flushed face
- Client complaints of feeling alternately cold and hot
- Increased pulse and respirations
- Complaints of malaise and fatigue
- Parched lips and dry skin
- Convulsions, especially in children

97°–99.5°F, or 36°–37.5°C. Rectal temperatures are approximately 1°F higher, ear canal 0.5°F higher, and axillary temperatures are 1°F lower than oral readings. Body temperature may vary according to age (lower for the aged), time of day (lower in the morning and higher in the afternoon and evening), amount of exercise, or extremes in the environmental temperature.

> **CLINICAL ALERT**
> Temperature varies with time of day: It is highest between 5 and 7 p.m. and lowest between 2 and 6 a.m. This variation is termed *circadian thermal rhythm*. A consistent method of body temperature measurement should be used so that readings are comparable.

The thermometer is the instrument used to measure body temperature. In most hospitals, you will find a variety of digital, disposable, and electronic thermometers that can be used to measure oral, rectal, and tympanic temperatures.

The temporal artery thermometer (Exergen) is a relatively new device. Clinicians and nurses should all be trained on how to use these devices properly. Failure to use the recommended technique may result in inaccurate readings. The temporal artery scanner has been found to be accurate for children less than 4 years of age (Reynolds et al., 2014)

Pulse

The pulse is an index of the heart's rate and rhythm. The apical pulse rate is the number of beats per minute (beats/min). With each beat, the heart's left ventricle contracts and forces blood into the aorta. Closure of the heart valves creates the sounds heard. The forceful ejection of blood by the left ventricle produces a wave that is transmitted through the arteries to the periphery of the body. The pulse is a transient expansion of **peripheral** arteries resulting from internal pressure changes. If cardiac output is reduced (such as with a premature or irregular heartbeat), the peripheral pulse is weak; if the radial pulse rate is less than the apical rate, the difference is called a **pulse deficit**. The pulse wave is influenced by the elasticity of the larger vessels, blood volume, blood viscosity, and arteriolar and capillary resistance.

Circulatory System Control

The circulatory system is under the dual control of the autonomic nervous system and **autoregulation** (at the microcirculation level). This dual control allows the circulatory system to vary blood flow to meet the body's requirements. Local control of blood flow is called autoregulation. Blood flow is adjusted according to oxygen need based on changing metabolic activity of different tissues.

The autonomic nervous system regulates circulation through the vasomotor center in the medulla oblongata.

Stimulation of the sympathetic nervous system causes vasoconstriction, increased heart rate and cardiac **contractility**, and a resulting increase in blood pressure. On the other hand, sympathetic inhibition causes **vasodilation**, reduced heart rate, and a reduction in blood pressure.

Pressure receptors, called baroreceptors, located in the walls of the carotid sinus and arch of the aorta, also influence the vasomotor center. Decreased circulating volume (as in hemorrhage) stimulates these receptors, which then transmit signals to the vasomotor center to stimulate the sympathetic nervous system. Resulting cardiovascular responses divert blood flow to vital organs.

Heart Rate and Rhythm

A normal adult heart rate is from 60 to 100 beats/min; the average rate is 72 beats/min. Rates are slightly faster in women and more rapid in children and infants (90–140 beats/min; Table 10-1 ■). The resting heart rate usually does not change with age. **Tachycardia** is a pulse rate over 100 beats/min. **Bradycardia** is a pulse rate below 60 beats/min.

When taking a client's pulse, be aware that many pathologic conditions produce bradycardia. Among the most common causes are decreased thyroid activity, hyperkalemia, cardiac conduction blocks, and increased intracranial pressure.

Tachycardia is associated with stressful conditions, hypoxia, exercise, and fever. Client conditions, such as congestive heart failure, hemorrhage, **shock**, dehydration, and anemia produce tachycardia as a compensatory response to poor tissue oxygenation.

Heart rhythm is the time interval between each heartbeat. Normally, the heart rhythm is regular, although slight irregularities do not necessarily indicate cardiac malfunction. An irregular cardiac rhythm, especially if sustained, requires cardiac evaluation because it may be indicative of cardiac disease.

Variance in heart rate, either increased or decreased, may be attributed to many factors, such as drug intake, lack of oxygen, loss of blood, exercise, and body temperature. When evaluating a pulse rate, it is important to ascertain the normal baseline for each client and then to determine variances from the normal for that particular client. The heart normally pumps about 5 L of blood through the body each minute. This **cardiac output** is calculated by multiplying the heart rate per minute by the stroke volume, the amount of blood ejected with one contraction. Increasing the heart rate is one of the first compensatory mechanisms the body employs to maintain cardiac output.

Evaluating Pulse Quality

The quality of the pulse is determined by the amount of blood pumped through the peripheral arteries. Normally, the amount of pumped blood remains fairly constant; when it varies, it is also indicative of cardiac malfunction. A so-called **bounding pulse** occurs when the nurse is able to feel the pulse by exerting only a slight pressure over

Table 10-1 Normal Vital Sign Ranges Across the Lifespan

	Pulse (per minute)	Respirations (per minute)	Temperature (°C)	Blood Pressure (mm Hg)	
				Systolic	Diastolic
Newborn	100–205 (awake) 90–160 (asleep)	30–80	Normal range: 36.5–37.5	At birth: 50–70[a] At day 10: 90	At birth: 30–45[a] At day 10: 50
Infant	100–180 (awake) 80–160 (asleep)	30–60	Normal range (axillary): 36.5–37.5	Age 1 Boys: 80–89 Girls: 83–90	Age 1 Boys: 34–39 Girls: 38–42
Toddler	98–140 (awake) 80–120 (asleep)	20–40	Normal range: 36–38.5 Extreme range: 35–40	Age 2 Boys: 84–92 Girls: 85–91	Age 2 Boys: 39–44 Girls: 43–47
Preschooler	98–140 (awake) 80–120 (asleep)	22–34	Normal range: 36–38.5 Extreme range: 35–40	Age 4 Boys: 88–97 Girls: 88–94	Age 4 Boys: 47–52 Girls: 50–54
School age	70–120 (awake) 50–90 (asleep)	15–25	Normal range: 36–38.5 Extreme range: 35–40	Age 9 Boys: 95–104 Girls: 96–103	Age 9 Boys: 57–62 Girls: 58–61
Adolescent	50–90	12–20	Normal range: 36–38.5 Extreme range: 35–40	Age 15 Boys: 109–117 Girls: 107–113	Age 15 Boys: 61–66 Girls: 64–67
Adult	60–100	12–20	Normal range: 36–38.5 Extreme range: 35–40	Less than 120	Less than 80
Older adult	60–100	15–20	Normal range: 36–38.5 Extreme range: 35–40	Less than 120	Less than 80

[a]Blood pressure is usually monitored before age 3 only if the client has cardiac issues.

the artery. If, by exerting pressure, the nurse cannot clearly determine the flow, this is called **weak** or **thready pulse**.

The arterial pulse can be felt over arteries that lie close to the body surface and over a bone or firm surface that can support the artery when pressure is applied. In adults and children older than age 3, the radial artery is **palpated** most frequently because it is the most accessible. The femoral and carotid arteries are used in cases of cardiac arrest to determine the adequacy of perfusion.

Peripheral pulses may be absent or weak. The amplitude of a pulse depends on the degree of filling in the artery during systole (ventricular contraction) and emptying during **diastole** (ventricular relaxation). It is important to note characteristics of peripheral pulses: 0 = absent; 1+ = weak; 2+ = diminished; 3+ = strong; and 4+ = full and bounding (refer to your agency procedure manual for additional information).

When peripheral pulses cannot be palpated, a **Doppler** ultrasound stethoscope is used by the nurse to confirm the presence or absence of the pulse. Even though the peripheral pulse is an indicator of cardiac function, it is not always an accurate indication of the force of cardiac contractions. If cardiac contractions are weak or ventricular filling is incomplete, the pulse is weak; however, in the case of aortic stenosis, the pulse may be weak in spite of forceful cardiac contraction.

The pulse should be taken frequently on an acutely ill hospitalized client and less frequently on more stable hospitalized clients. Once a week or even once a month is adequate for clients in long-term care facilities. Do not wait until the next routinely scheduled time if the client develops unexpected symptoms or has experienced trauma.

Respiration

Respiration is the process of bringing oxygen to body tissues and removing carbon dioxide. The lungs play a major role in this process. Another respiratory function is to maintain arterial blood homeostasis by maintaining the pH of the blood. The lungs accomplish this by the process of breathing.

Breathing consists of two phases, inspiration and expiration. Inspiration is an active process in which the diaphragm descends, the external intercostal muscles contract, and the chest expands to allow air to move into the tracheobronchial tree. Expiration is a passive process in which air flows out of the respiratory tree.

The respiratory center in the medulla of the brain and the level of carbon dioxide in the blood both control the rate and depth of breathing. Peripheral receptors in the carotid body and the aortic arch also respond to the level of oxygen in the blood. To some extent, respiration can be voluntarily controlled by holding the breath and hyperventilation. Talking, laughing, and crying also affect respiration.

The diaphragm and the intercostal muscles are the main muscles used for breathing. Other accessory muscles, such as the abdominal muscles, the sternocleidomastoid, the trapezius, and the scalene, can be used to assist with respiration if necessary.

Evaluating Respirations

The respiratory rate is the most overlooked and least recorded vital sign. The quality of breathing is important baseline information and can give early indications of respiratory deterioration. Normal breathing, termed *eupnea*, is almost invisible, effortless, quiet, automatic, and regular. When the breathing pattern varies from normal, it needs to be evaluated thoroughly. For example, bronchial sounds heard over the large airways are fairly loud. There is normally a pause between inspiration and expiration. Softer sounds are heard over peripheral lung areas, and there are no pauses between inspiration, which is a long sound, and expiration, which is a short sound. If breathing is noisy, labored, or strained, an obstruction may be affecting the breathing pattern that could lead to major alterations in homeostasis.

In addition to evaluating the breathing pattern, it is also necessary to evaluate the rate and depth of breathing. The normal rate for a resting adult is 12–18 breaths/min. A rate of 24 or above is considered tachypnea, and a rate of 10 or less is considered bradypnea. The rate for infants ranges from 20 to 30 breaths/min and is often irregular. Older children average about 20–26. The ratio of pulse to breathing is usually 5:1 and remains fairly constant.

The depth of an individual's breathing (tidal volume) is the amount of air that moves in and out with each breath, and it is oftentimes documented as "shallow," "normal," or "deep." The tidal volume is 500 mL in the healthy adult. Alveolar air is only partially replenished by atmospheric air with each inspiratory phase. Approximately 350 mL (tidal volume minus dead space) of new air is exchanged with the functional residual capacity volume during each respiratory cycle. Accurate tidal volume can be measured by a spirometer, but an experienced nurse can judge the approximate depth by placing the back of the hand next to the client's nose and mouth and feeling the expired air. Another method of estimating volume capacity is to observe chest expansion and to check both sides of the thorax for symmetrical movement.

After assessing the pattern, rate, and depth of breathing, it is important to observe the physical characteristics of chest expansion. The chest normally expands symmetrically without rib flaring or retractions. In addition, observation of chest deformities should also be made, as all of these signs yield information about the respiratory process and overall health status of the client. See Chapter 11, Physical Assessment.

Blood Pressure

The heart generates pressure during the cardiac cycle to perfuse the organs of the body with blood. Blood flows from the heart to the arteries, into the capillaries and veins, and then flows back to the heart. Blood pressure in the arterial system varies with the cardiac cycle, reaching the highest level at the peak of systole and the lowest level at the end of diastole. The difference between the systolic and diastolic blood pressure is the pulse pressure, which is normally 30–50 points (**mm Hg**).

There are seven major factors that affect blood pressure:

Cardiac Output The force of heart contractions (the amount of blood ejected by the heart) influences blood pressure, especially systolic pressure.

Peripheral Vascular Resistance (PVR) Resistance to the flow of blood is due to resistant vessels under the influence of the autonomic nervous system. Peripheral vascular resistance is the most important determinant of diastolic pressure.

Elasticity and Distensibility of Arteries Elasticity refers to the action of the blood vessel walls to spring back after blood is ejected into them. When blood is ejected into the aorta and large arteries, the arterial vessel walls distend. Recoil during diastole propels blood through the arterial tree and maintains diastolic pressure. Both elasticity and distensibility decrease with age, resulting in increased systolic pressure and slightly increased diastolic pressure.

Blood Volume Increased blood volume causes an increase in both systolic and diastolic blood pressure, whereas decreased blood volume causes the reverse effect. Hemorrhage decreases blood pressure, whereas overhydration from excessive blood transfusions may cause an increase in blood pressure.

Blood Viscosity Blood viscosity (thickness) influences blood flow velocity through the arterial tree. For example, increased viscosity, which occurs with polycythemia, increases resistance to blood flow, whereas decreased viscosity, resulting from anemia, decreases resistance.

Hormones and Enzymes These substances have an important influence on blood pressure. For example, epinephrine and norepinephrine produce a profound vasoconstrictor effect on peripheral blood vessels (mediators of the sympathetic nervous system). Aldosterone (released by the adrenal cortex), renin (released by the juxtaglomerular apparatus of the kidney), and angiotensin (activated by the renin response) also produce effects that raise blood pressure. Histamine and acetylcholine (a parasympathetic mediator) cause vasodilation, therefore lowering blood pressure.

Chemoreceptors **Chemoreceptors** in the aortic arch and carotid sinus also exert control over the blood pressure. They are sensitive to changes in PaO_2, $PaCO_2$, and pH. Decreased PaO_2 stimulates the chemoreceptors, which stimulate the vasomotor center. Increased $PaCO_2$ and decreased pH directly stimulate the vasomotor center, causing increased peripheral vascular resistance.

Measuring Blood Pressure

Measuring arterial blood pressure provides important information about the overall health status of the client. For example, the systolic pressure provides data about the condition of the heart and great arteries. The diastolic pressure indicates arteriolar or peripheral vascular resistance. The **pulse pressure**, or difference between the systolic and diastolic pressure, provides information about cardiac function and blood volume. A single blood pressure reading, however, does not provide adequate data from which conclusions can be drawn about all of these factors. Rather, a series of blood pressure readings should be taken to establish a baseline for further evaluation.

The *indirect method* (noninvasive blood pressure [NIBP]) of taking a blood pressure using a recently calibrated aneroid manometer and a stethoscope is accurate for most clients. Electronic blood pressure devices can monitor systolic, diastolic, and mean readings constantly or at preset time intervals and are helpful to measure blood pressure trends in clients who are at risk for **hyper-** or **hypotension**. These devices can also be synchronized to transmit findings directly to the electronic health record (EHR). If a stethoscope is unavailable or the brachial artery amplitude is decreased, the brachial or radial artery can be palpated as the blood pressure cuff is inflated to determine the systolic blood pressure (palpated pulse disappears at this point). Alternatively, an inflated blood pressure cuff may be slowly deflated; the point at which distal pulsation is first palpated reflects systolic blood pressure. Those who are severely *hypotensive* or *hypertensive* (hemodynamically unstable), have low blood volume, or are on vasoactive drugs should have blood pressure measured by direct (intra-arterial) method. The *direct method* is continuous and measures mean arterial pressures. With this method, a needle or catheter is inserted into the brachial, radial, or femoral artery. An oscilloscope displays arterial pressure waveforms.

Normal blood pressure in an adult varies between 100 and 120 systolic and 60 and 80 diastolic. (See the table on Blood Pressure Classification in Skill 10.4.1.) As blood moves toward smaller arteries and into arterioles, where it enters the capillaries, pressure falls to 35. It continues to fall as blood goes through the capillaries, where the flow is steady and not pulsatile. As blood moves into the venous system, pressure falls until it is the lowest in the venae cavae.

Blood pressures vary widely and are influenced by age, gender, health, race, and ethnicity as well as socioeconomic status, occupation, personal factors, and environmental factors. A blood pressure of 100/60 may be normal for one individual but may be hypotensive for another. Hypotension (90–100 systolic) in a healthy adult without other clinical symptoms is little reason for concern.

Blood pressure readings are recorded in association with **Korotkoff sounds**. These sounds are described as "K" phases. The systolic, or first, pressure reading occurs with the advent of the first Korotkoff sound. The systolic reading represents the maximal pressure in the aorta after contraction of the left ventricle and is heard as a faint tapping sound.

According to The American Heart Association standards, the diastolic, or second, reading should be taken at the time of the last Korotkoff sound (phase V) for adults. The diastolic reading represents the minimal pressure

---

Box 10-2 HYPERTENSION: FREQUENCY AND SUGGESTED LIFESTYLE MODIFICATIONS

Hypertension is a modifiable risk factor for cardiovascular disease. Hypertension affects one in three adults nationwide. Approximately 68 million adults have hypertension and only half of these people have their hypertension under control.

Currently, there are five methods of lifestyle modification suggested for management of hypertension:

1. Weight reduction
2. Diet modification (one rich in fruits and vegetables, with a reduced amount of saturated and total fat)
3. Sodium reduction
4. Physical activity—regular aerobic exercise
5. Moderate alcohol intake

The other important method of reducing blood pressure is prescriptive medications, monitored by a healthcare provider.

---

exerted against the arterial walls at all times. In children under age 13, pregnant women, and clients with high cardiac output or peripheral vasodilation, sounds are often heard to a level far below muffling and sometimes to levels near 0. In these individuals, muffling (phase IV) should be used to indicate diastolic pressure, but both muffling (phase IV) and disappearance (phase V) should be recorded (e.g., 110/80/20).

Frequency of blood pressure assessment should be individualized or as ordered. Blood pressure for an acutely ill client should be taken every 15 minutes to 1–2 hours and the blood pressure of more stabilized clients should be taken every 4–8 hours to once a day. Clients with severe hypotension or **hypertension**, with low blood volume, or those on vasoactive drugs require checking every 5–15 minutes.

> **CLINICAL ALERT**
> When a client moves from recumbent to standing position, orthostatic hypotension can occur. Systolic pressure can fall 10–15 mm Hg and diastolic may rise by 5 mm Hg. This may result in dizziness and falls.

Hypertension is a significant health concern in the United States (Box 10-2 ■).

Pain

According to The Joint Commission, pain should be considered the fifth vital sign. Pain must be evaluated every time vital signs are taken, and it should be documented on the vital sign record. Refer to Chapter 16, Pain Management, for a more in-depth explanation of pain and the options available for pain management.

Cultural Awareness

Many cultures believe that certain substances protect one's health. For example, many Italians, Greeks, and Native Americans believe that garlic or onions eaten raw or worn on the body will prevent an illness such as high blood pressure. If a client wishes to include these items in his or her diet or wear them, the nursing staff should respect this practice, since it is an important cultural tradition for many groups.

Nursing Diagnoses

The following nursing diagnoses are appropriate to use on client care plans when the components are related to vital signs.

NURSING DIAGNOSIS	RELATED TO . . .
Ineffective Airway Clearance	Obstruction of airway, increased secretions, fatigue
Ineffective Breathing Pattern	Change in rate, depth, or pattern of breathing that alters normal gas exchange
Decreased Cardiac Output	Hypovolemia, rapid pulse, changes in breathing patterns, alteration in heart rhythm or rate, or vascular tone
Deficient Fluid Volume	Excessive urinary output, abnormal fluid loss, infection, fever, diarrhea
Excess Fluid Volume	Decreased cardiac output, fluid retention, inflammatory process, low protein diet, increased fluid intake
Chronic Pain	Chronic disease conditions, tissue trauma, injury
Ineffective Thermoregulation	Disease, infection, drug reactions, damage to the hypothalamic temperature regulating center, possibly dehydration
Ineffective Peripheral Tissue Perfusion	Vascular disorders, hypovolemia, medications, hypoxemia
Impaired Spontaneous Ventilation	Metabolic factors, respiratory muscle fatigue

Source: Herdman, T. H. & Kamitsuru, S. (Eds.) *Nursing Diagnoses – Definitions and Classification 2015-2017.* Copyright © 2014, 1994–2014 by NANDA International. Used by arrangement with John Wiley & Sons Limited. Companion website: www.wiley.com/go/nursingdiagnoses. In order to make safe and effective judgments using NANDA-I nursing diagnosis it is essential that nurses refer to the definitions and defining characteristics of the diagnoses listed in this work.

Temperature

Nursing Process Data

ASSESSMENT Database

- Determine number of times temperature needs to be taken daily.
- Assess temperature in relationship to time of day and age of client.
- Compare temperature with other vital signs to establish baseline data.
- Determine the method most appropriate for obtaining temperature.

Oral Method

- Accurate method of determining body temperature
- Used only for alert and cooperative clients; not recommended for unconscious clients
- Not appropriate for use with tachypneic or mouth-breathing clients
- Not appropriate for clients with oral inflammatory processes or oral surgery
- Delivery of oxygen by nasal cannula does not affect oral temperature readings.
- Determine client has not ingested hot or cold liquids or smoked for 15–30 minutes before taking temperature orally.

Rectal Method

- Appropriate for tachypneic, uncooperative, confused, or comatose clients or for clients on seizure precautions
- Used for clients with open-mouth breathing, such as those with nasal or oral intubation
- Appropriate for clients with wired jaws, facial fractures, or other abnormalities, or for clients with nasogastric tubes who cannot breathe easily with mouth closed
- Contraindicated for infants or clients who have had surgery involving the rectum

Axillary Method

- Less accurate, but safe
- Often used for infants and young children
- Used in recovery rooms to avoid turning clients
- Time-consuming

Electronic Thermometer

- Accurate for oral or rectal temperature measurement, but inaccurate for axillary temperature measurement
- Time-efficient and easy to read

Infrared Ear Thermometer

- Measures body heat radiating from the tympanic membrane
- Noninvasive, safe, efficient
- Important to use proper technique for accurate reading
- Less sensitive in detecting fever in the very young child and infant

Temporal Artery Scanner Thermometer

- Measures temperature using a touch or no-touch technique via infrared technology
- Used for children or unconscious clients

Heat Sensitive Tape

- Disposable and nonbreakable
- Appropriate for children when proper cleaning of thermometer is difficult

PLANNING Objectives

- To determine whether the body temperature is within normal range
- To provide baseline data for further evaluation
- To determine alterations in disease conditions

IMPLEMENTATION Procedures

DOCUMENTATION AND EVALUATION

Expected Outcomes

- Temperature is within normal range.
- Temperature readings are compared with age, time of day, and previous readings.
- Alterations in temperature are detected early and treatment initiated.
- Appropriate method of temperature taking is determined for each client.
- Correct length of time is used for thermometer insertion to obtain an accurate reading.

Unexpected Outcomes/Alternative Actions

Pearson Nursing Student Resources

Find additional review materials at
nursing.pearsonhighered.com.
Prepare for success with NCLEX®-style practice questions and Skill Checklists.

Skill 10.1.1 | Using a Digital Thermometer

Note: The process for taking temperature via the oral, axillary, or rectal route is consistent regardless of type of thermometer.

Equipment
Client's individual digital thermometer
Disposable sheaths, if multiple client use
Gloves, if necessary

Procedure
1. Perform hand hygiene.
2. Don gloves if risk of contact with saliva.
3. Introduce self; identify client with two forms of ID.

Oral Temperature
a. Wait 20–30 minutes to take oral temperature if client has been eating, drinking, chewing gum, smoking, or exercising. ➤ **Rationale:** These activities may alter the temperature.
b. Place thermometer in client's mouth under front of tongue and along gumline. ❶ ➤ **Rationale:** Location ensures contact with large vessels under tongue.
c. Have client hold lips closed and leave thermometer in place for 45–90 seconds. ❷ The alert sound will indicate time. ➤ **Rationale:** Open-mouth breathing produces abnormally low readings.
d. Remove thermometer and read temperature displayed in digital window.

Axillary Temperature
a. Perform hand hygiene.
b. Don gloves if risk of contact with body fluids possible.
c. Identify client with two forms of ID.
d. Assist client to comfortable position and expose **axilla** area.

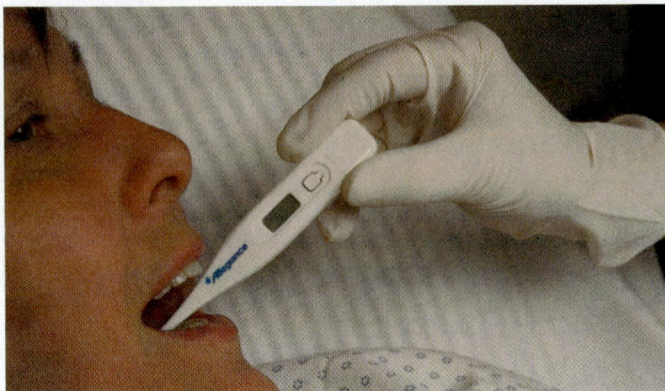

❶ Place individual digital thermometer in client's mouth under tongue.

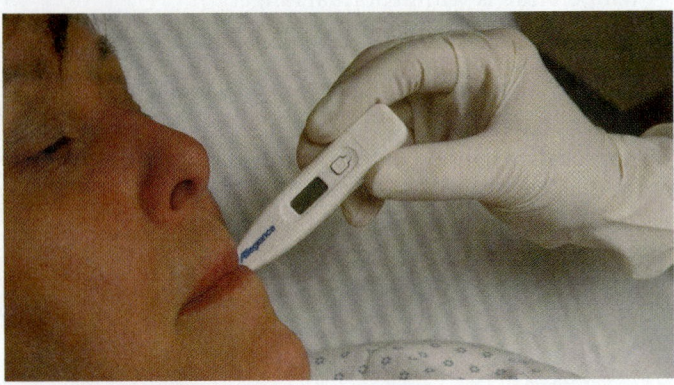

❷ Ask client to hold lips closed and leave individual digital thermometer in place for 45–90 seconds.

e. Dry axilla if necessary. ➤ **Rationale:** A false low reading may result if axilla is moist.
f. Place thermometer in center of axilla and lower arm down across the chest. ➤ **Rationale:** This position allows thermometer to be in contact with large vessels.
g. Leave in place for 1–2 minutes. ➤ **Rationale:** Axillary temperature recordings take a longer time to register.
4. Record temperature, noting route. Be sure to document per facility policy (Centigrade or Fahrenheit); see Table 10-2 ■.
5. Perform hand hygiene.

Table 10-2 Comparing Centigrade and Fahrenheit Temperatures

Degrees Centigrade (°C)	Degrees Fahrenheit (°F)
36.0	96.8
36.5	97.7
37.0	**98.6**
37.5	99.5
38.0	100.4
38.3	101.0
39.0	102.2
39.5	103.1
40.0	104.0

To convert degrees F to degrees C, subtract 32, then divide by 1.8. To convert degrees C to degrees F, multiply by 1.8, then add 32.

Skill 10.1.2 | Using an Electronic Thermometer

Equipment

Electronic thermometer unit with digital readout and probe ❶
Disposable cover for thermometer
Lubricant on tissue (for rectal temperature)
Clean gloves

Procedure

1. Perform hand hygiene; don gloves if necessary.
2. Place disposable sheath over probe. ❷
3. Introduce self.
4. Provide privacy for rectal temperature.

Oral Temperature

a. Perform hand hygiene.
b. Don gloves if risk of contact with saliva.
c. Identify client with two forms of ID.
d. Instruct client to open mouth. Slide probe under front of client's tongue and along the gumline in the sublingual pocket. ❸ ➤ *Rationale:* The larger blood vessels in the pocket more accurately reflect the core temperature.

5. Instruct client to close lips (not teeth). Lips should close at the ridge on the probe cover.

❶ Electronic thermometer unit with digital probe.

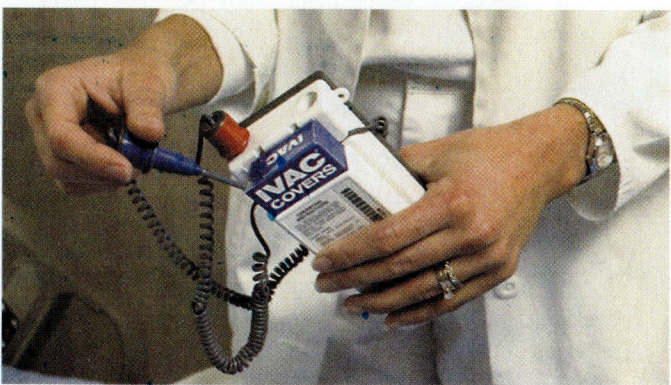

❷ Cover probe of thermometer before taking temperature.

❸ Slide probe under front of tongue to sublingual pocket.

> **SAFETY ALERT**
> The temperature of an unconscious client is never taken by mouth. The rectal, tympanic, or scanner method is preferred.

Rectal Temperature

a. Perform hand hygiene.
b. Identify client with two forms of ID.
c. Don clean gloves. ➤ *Rationale:* This prevents exposure to feces.
d. Position client on side facing away from you, separate buttocks, instruct client to take in a deep breath, and insert covered and lubricated probe ¼–1½ in. (0.5–3.75 cm), depending on the client's age, through anal sphincter. ➤ *Rationale:* Taking in a deep breath relaxes the sphincter, and the lubrication prevents tissue trauma.
e. Position probe to side of rectum to ensure contact with tissue wall. ➤ *Rationale:* This ensures probe is in contact with large vessels of rectal wall.
f. Remove probe when audible signal occurs. Client's temperature is now registered on the screen.
g. Discard probe cover into trash.
h. Wipe anal area with tissues to remove lubricant and stool.
i. Discard tissue and gloves. ➤ *Rationale:* Proper disposal prevents transmission of microorganisms.

6. Assist client to comfortable position.
7. Perform hand hygiene.
8. Record temperature.

> **CLINICAL ALERT**
> Only use client's own dedicated electronic thermometer (including rectal and oral) if diagnosis includes *Clostridium difficile*-associated diarrhea because of the potential for spreading the bacteria and increasing the risk of transmitting an HAI to other clients.

Skill 10.1.3 | Measuring an Infant or Child's Temperature

Equipment
Digital or electronic thermometer with disposable probe
    cover
Water-soluble lubricant
Gloves, if necessary

Procedure
1. Determine appropriate thermometer and route for child.
   ➤ *Rationale:* Oral route is appropriate only for child over 3 years of age. Electronic, nonbreakable thermometer or scanner is preferred.
2. Perform hand hygiene and identify client with two forms of ID.
3. Introduce self. Explain procedure so child can understand.
4. Remove probe from cover or attach probe tip to electronic thermometer.

Oral Route (only for child 3 years or older)
a. Place probe under child's tongue, one side or the other.
b. Have child close mouth and either hold thermometer in place or monitor while taking temperature.
c. Leave digital thermometer in place for 45–90 seconds, or remove electronic thermometer when audible signal occurs.

Rectal Route
Rectal temperature is contraindicated in newborns and clients with recent rectal surgery, rectal disease, diarrhea, neurologic disease (spinal cord injury), and/or neutropenia (low white blood cell count) as it increases the risk of infection.
a. Place infant or child in prone or side-lying position.
b. Lubricate probe.
c. Insert thermometer ¼–½ in. (0.5–1.25 cm) into rectum for infant or ½–1 in. (1.25–2.5 cm) for child and hold in place.
d. Remove probe when tone or beep is heard.
5. Discard probe cover into trash.
6. Wipe anal area with tissues to remove lubricant and stool.
7. Discard tissue and gloves. ➤ *Rationale:* Proper disposal prevents transmission of microorganisms.

8. Assist client to comfortable position.
9. Perform hand hygiene.
10. Record temperature.

Axillary Route
a. Perform hand hygiene.
b. Don gloves if there is risk of contact with bodily fluids.
c. Identify client with two forms of ID.
d. Assist infant or child to a comfortable position and expose axilla.
e. Dry axilla if necessary. ➤ *Rationale:* A moist axillary area can produce a false low reading.
f. Place thermometer in center of axilla. ❶ Lower child's arm down and across the chest. ➤ *Rationale:* This position ensures that thermometer remains in contact with large vessels of axilla.
g. Leave in place 1–2 minutes or until tone is heard.
   ➤ *Rationale:* Axillary temperature recordings take longer to register than oral or rectal readings.
h. Read and record temperature; indicate method.
i. Discard probe cover into trash by pushing ejection button, or return digital thermometer into its case.

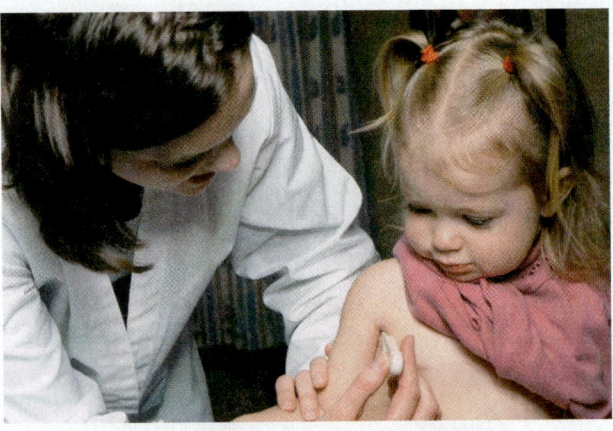

❶ Axillary temperature reading in a young child.

Skill 10.1.4 | Obtaining a Tympanic Temperature

Equipment
Infrared thermometer unit
Disposable probe cover

Note: A tympanic thermometer measures the infrared energy that naturally radiates from the tympanic membrane and surrounding tissues.

Procedure
1. Perform hand hygiene and identify client with two forms of ID.
2. Attach disposable cover centering probe on film and press firmly until backing frame of probe cover engages base of probe. ➤ *Rationale:* Cover protects client from transmission of microorganisms.
3. Turn the client's head to one side and stabilize the client's head.
4. Pull pinna upward and backward for an adult or down and backward for a child. ❶ ➤ *Rationale:* This procedure provides better access to the ear canal.
5. Center probe and gently advance into ear canal to make a firm seal, directing probe toward tympanic membrane. ❷ ➤ *Rationale:* Pressure close to the tympanic membrane seals ear canal and allows for accurate reading.

❶ Position client so ear canal is easily seen and pull pinna back and up.

❷ Place probe in client's ear and advance into ear canal to make a firm seal.

6. Press and hold temperature switch until temperature reading displays (approximately 3 seconds). ➤ *Rationale:* Method records core body temperature.
7. Remove thermometer. Discard probe cover.
8. Return thermometer to home base or storage unit for recharge.
9. Keep lens clean using lint-free wipe or alcohol swab, then wipe dry. Do not use povidone-iodine (Betadine).
10. Perform hand hygiene and record temperature.
11. May be used for clients over 3 months of age.

CLINICAL ALERT

Do not use ear thermometer in infected or draining ear or if adjacent lesion or incision exists.

EVIDENCE-BASED PRACTICE

Correct Technique for Taking a Tympanic Temperature

Studies on the correct technique for taking a tympanic temperature indicate that the ear tug (pulling the pinna upward and backward for an adult and down and backward for a child) is essential for an accurate reading. Eliminating this step will not allow the thermometer to be aimed directly at the tympanic membrane.

Skill 10.1.5 | Using a Temporal Thermometer (Infrared)

Equipment

Temporal artery scanner thermometer (temporal infrared thermometer or scanner)

Procedure

Note: This method is not recommended for diaphoretic clients; alternate sites may be used.

1. Perform hand hygiene.
2. Introduce self and identify client with two forms of ID.
3. Check orders for scanner device.
4. Follow manufacturer's directions for scanning device:
   a. No-touch thermometer is placed up to 2 in (5 cm). from center of the forehead.
   b. Touch thermometer requires a gentle stroke across forehead and a tap behind the ear. ❶
5. Press power button to turn device on.
6. Press and hold scan button in appropriate location(s).
7. Release scan button and note reading that is displayed. ❷

8. Clean device with antiseptic wipe.
9. Document temperature.

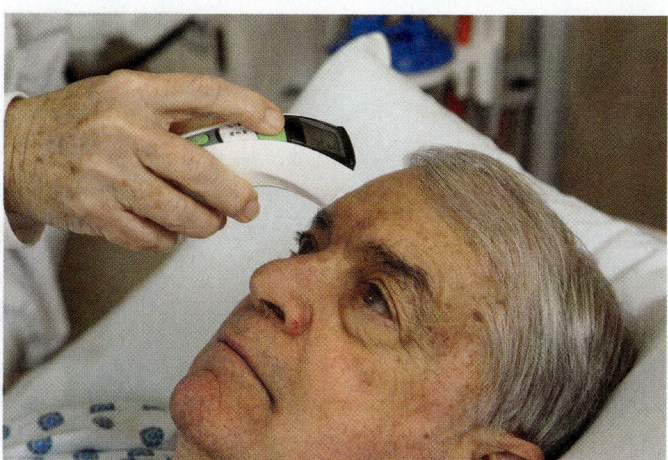

❶ Follow manufacturer's directions for scanner device.

(continued)

Skill 10.1.5 | Using a Temporal Thermometer (Infrared) *(continued)*

❷ After releasing scan button, note the reading in the window.

EVIDENCE-BASED PRACTICE
Accuracy of Temporal Artery Thermometers
A recent study by Emergency Nurses Association (ENA) on temporal artery thermometer accuracy found that among the pediatric participants ($N = 52$), temporal artery temperatures were within the acceptable range set by the experts to use as a noninvasive substitute for core body temperatures (Reynolds et al., 2014).

Skill 10.1.6 | Using a Heat-Sensitive Wearable Thermometer

Equipment
Wearable thermometer, chemical strip tape, or liquid crystal thermometer

Procedure
1. Check orders for continuous-reading thermometer and identify client with two forms of ID. Introduce self.
2. Dry forehead or axilla area, if necessary.
3. Place strip on forehead ❶ or deep in client's axilla ❷—may stay in place for 2 days.
4. Read correct temperature by checking color changes or dots that turn from green to black.
5. Record temperature on appropriate form or record.

LEGAL ALERT
Nurses' Negligence
The client had transthoracic vagotomy. The doctor ordered vital signs q 15 minutes × 1 hour and q hour for 10 hours. Vital signs were recorded four times for 1 day. The next day the client's temperature was 102°F (38.9°C) and it remained there until the day after, when it was 105°F (40.6°C). The nurse administered aspirin when it rose to 106°F (41°C). The nurse then contacted the doctor who found signs of serious wound infection. The client suffered organic brain syndrome as a direct result of the continued high temperature. The court found that the nurses breached standard of care when they failed to notify the doctor of the client's high temperature.

❶ Liquid crystal thermometer is placed against lower forehead for 15 seconds.

❷ Place a continuous-reading, wearable thermometer deep in the client's axilla.

Unit 10.1 Documentation and Evaluation

DOCUMENTATION for Temperature

- Site designated: "O" (oral), "R" (rectal), "A" (axillary), "T" (tympanic), or "TA" (temporal artery)
- Temperature documented on vital sign sheet and graph
- Nursing interventions used for alterations in temperature
- Condition of skin related to alterations from normothermia (e.g., diaphoresis)
- Signs and symptoms associated with alterations in temperature (e.g., shivering, dehydration)

EVALUATION/Critical Thinking

Expected Outcomes

- Temperature is within normal range.
- Temperature readings are compared with age, time of day, and previous readings.
- Alterations in temperature are detected early and treatment begun.
- Appropriate method of temperature taking is determined for each client.
- Correct length of time is used for thermometer insertion to obtain an accurate reading.

Unexpected Outcomes

Alternative Actions

- Fever develops.

- Check possible sources of infection and take preventative measures.
- Notify healthcare provider.
- Employ cooling methods if temperature is dangerously high, such as tepid sponge bath, cool oral fluids, ice packs, or **antipyretic** drugs.
- Assess all vital signs.

- Despite initial cooling measure, temperature remains elevated due to hypothalamus damage from brain disease or injury.

- Check possible sources of infection and take preventative measures.
- Notify healthcare provider and request cooling blanket.
- Monitor temperature every 15–30 minutes and record.
- Continue to administer antipyretic drugs as ordered.

- Temperature remains elevated because of bacteria-produced pyrogens.

- Check for order to obtain culture of possible sources of infection.
- Give antipyretic drugs as ordered.
- Decrease room temperature and remove excess covers.
- Give tepid sponge bath.

- Temperature remains subnormal.

- Extreme low temperature can cause vasoconstriction; assess for blood clots.
- Institute measures to promote vasodilation (application of warmth).
- If extremity is ischemic, monitor that heat source does not exceed body temperature.

- Using a tympanic thermometer, client's temperature reading seems too low.

- Be sure client has been indoors for at least 10 minutes.
- Replace probe cover and retake temperature.
- Check that probe cover and lens are clean and intact.
- Reposition client so ear canal is easily seen.

Nursing Process Data

ASSESSMENT Database

- Assess appropriate site to obtain pulse.
- Check pulse with health status changes, as ordered by healthcare provider, or before administering certain medications.
- Assess for rate, rhythm, volume, and quality.
- Assess an apical pulse on clients with irregular rhythms or those on cardiac medications.
- Obtain baseline peripheral pulses with initial assessment or in any client undergoing cardiac or vascular surgery. Also obtain pulse for medical clients with diabetes, arterial occlusive diseases, **atherosclerosis**, or aneurysm, or any color or temperature changes in the periphery.
- Obtain an apical–radial pulse when deficits occur between apical and radial measurements.
- Assess the need to monitor pulses with an ultrasound or electronic device.

PLANNING Objectives

- To determine whether the pulse rate is within normal range and if the rhythm is regular
- To evaluate the quality (amount of blood pumped through peripheral arteries) of arterial pulses
- To determine whether peripheral pulses are equal in amplitude when compared with corresponding pulses
- To determine presence of peripheral pulses with ultrasound device when palpation is ineffective
- To monitor and evaluate changes in the client's health status
- To determine apical pulse rate before heart medications are administered

IMPLEMENTATION Procedures

Note: See also Skill 30.3.2, Using Pulse Oximetry, page 1187

DOCUMENTATION AND EVALUATION

Expected Outcomes

- Pulse is palpated without difficulty.
- Pulse rate is within normal range and rhythm is regular.
- All peripheral pulses are equal in amplitude when compared bilaterally and when compared with the next proximal site.
- Apical pulse is easily detected and counted.

Unexpected Outcomes/Alternative Actions

Pearson Nursing Student Resources

Find additional review materials at **nursing.pearsonhighered.com.**
Prepare for success with NCLEX®-style practice questions and Skill Checklists.

Skill 10.2.1 | Palpating a Radial Pulse

Equipment

Watch with sweeping second hand or digital watch that indicates seconds.

Note: To assess a pulse correctly, the nurse's watch must have second-measuring capability.

Procedure

1. Perform hand hygiene.
2. Introduce self. Check client identity with two forms of ID and place client in comfortable position.
3. Ask about activity level within last 15 minutes. ➤ **Rationale:** Pulse rate increases with activity, then returns to preactivity rate.
4. Palpate arteries by using pads of the middle three fingers of your hand. ➤ **Rationale:** The nurse may mistakenly feel own pulse if palpating with the thumb.

   a. Radial artery is usually used ❶ because it lies close to the skin surface and is easily accessible at the wrist.

   b. Press the artery against the bone or underlying firm surface to occlude vessel and then gradually release pressure. ➤ **Rationale:** Too much pressure obliterates the pulse.

   c. Note pulse characteristics, that is, quality (strength) of pulse (Box 10-3 ■). ➤ **Rationale:** Strength of the pulse is an indication of stroke volume or amplitude.

   d. If pulse is difficult to palpate, try exerting more pressure on the most distal palpating finger. ➤ **Rationale:** This amplifies the pulse wave against the two more proximal palpating fingers.

5. Count pulse for 30 seconds, and multiply by 2 to obtain pulse rate. ❷ ➤ **Rationale:** This is sufficient time for rate determination if pulse rhythm is regular.

Note: When other sites are inaccessible or in emergency situations, the carotid pulse can be used. ❸

6. Count radial pulse for at least 1 minute if rhythm is irregular or difficult to count. ➤ **Rationale:** It may take a minute or so

---

Box 10-3 PULSE CHARACTERISTICS

When counting the pulse rate, pay attention to:

- Rate: Average is 72 beats/min. The normal adult heart rate range is 60–100 beats/min. If pulse rate is below 60 or above 100 beats/min (outside the normal parameters), notify the healthcare provider.
- Rhythm: The pattern of beats, either regular or irregular.
- Volume or amplitude: The force of blood with each beat; can range from absent to bounding.
- Symmetry: Bilateral uniformity of pulse.

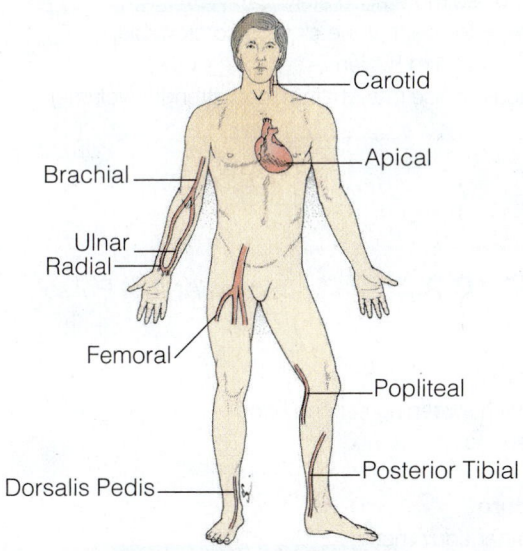

❶ Radial artery is the most commonly used site for determining pulse rate. Use the pads of middle three fingers, not the thumb, for accurate results.

❷ Count pulse for at least 30 seconds and multiply by 2 to obtain pulse rate.

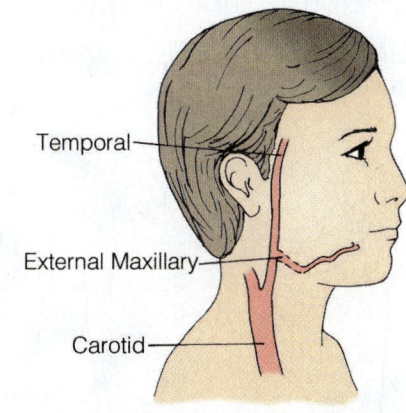

❸ Carotid artery is used when other sites are inaccessible or when there is a cardiac arrest to determine the adequacy of perfusion during CPR.

(continued)

Skill 10.2.1 | Palpating a Radial Pulse *(continued)*

to detect the irregularity. This method assists you to count the pulse more accurately.

7. Check to see that the client is comfortable.
8. Perform hand hygiene.
9. Record pulse rate, rhythm, and strength (volume).

EVIDENCE-BASED PRACTICE
Pulse Rate Measurement

It is recommended to count the pulse for 30 seconds and multiply by 2 if it is regular. If it is irregular, count the pulse for a full 60 seconds to ensure accuracy.

Skill 10.2.2 | Taking an Apical Pulse

Equipment

Watch with sweeping second hand
Stethoscope

Procedure

1. Gather equipment.
2. Perform hand hygiene.
3. Clean stethoscope bell and diaphragm with alcohol swab or equivalent.
4. Check two forms of client ID. Introduce self.
5. Provide privacy.
6. Explain procedure to client.
7. Place client in a supine position and expose chest area. If possible, stand at client's right side. ➤ **Rationale:** Auscultation of heart sounds is often enhanced when examiner is at client's right side.
8. Locate the apical impulse, termed *the point of maximal impulse* (PMI), by palpating the angle of Louis just below the suprasternal notch. ❶ This is the angle between the manubrium, top of the sternum, and the body of the sternum.

   a. Place your index finger just to the left of the client's sternum and palpate the second intercostal space.
   b. Place your middle finger in the third intercostal space and continue palpating downward until you locate the apical impulse or **PMI** at the fifth intercostal space. ❷
   c. Move your index finger laterally along the fifth intercostal space to the midclavicular line (MCL). ❸

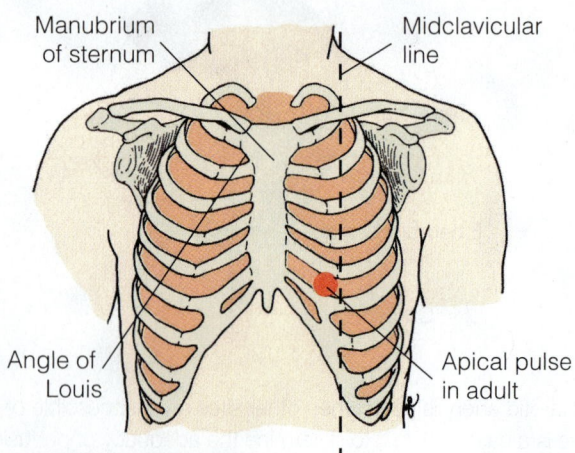

❶ Apical pulse site in adult.

Manubrium of sternum
Midclavicular line
Angle of Louis
Apical pulse in adult

❷ Place one finger in third intercostal space and continue to move downward to the fifth intercostal space.

❸ Move index finger along fifth intercostal space to midclavicular line.

9. Warm the stethoscope in the palm of your hand for 5–10 seconds. ➤ **Rationale:** Warming the stethoscope prevents startling the client.
10. Count client's apical pulse.

    a. Place diaphragm of stethoscope firmly over apical impulse site. ❹ ➤ **Rationale:** Heart sounds are high-pitched and most clearly heard with diaphragm of stethoscope.
    b. Count the rate for 1 minute when taking an apical pulse. Count *lub-dub* sound as one beat. ➤ **Rationale:** More

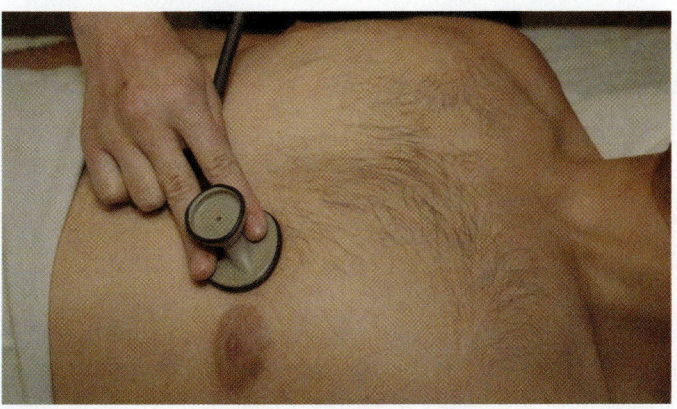

4 Accurate apical pulse is found in fifth intercostal space, left of sternum at midclavicular line or mitral area.

accurate readings are obtained over 1 minute, especially if pulse is irregular.

c. Determine if pattern is regular, regularly irregular, or chaotic. ➤ **Rationale:** This finding helps describe the rhythm disturbance.

11. Check to see that client is comfortable.
12. Perform hand hygiene and clean stethoscope.
13. Document apical pulse rate, rhythm, and intensity.

> **CLINICAL ALERT**
> The best practice for taking a pulse for infants or children is to listen to the heart itself, rather than palpating the pulse. Too much pressure may obliterate it, and inadequate pressure may not detect it.

EVIDENCE-BASED PRACTICE
Effect of Music on Vital Signs
One hundred and fifteen clients who were scheduled to undergo ophthalmic procedures and who were exposed to live classical piano music showed a statistically significant decrease ($P < 0.0001$) in blood pressure, heart rate, and respiratory rate.

Source: Camara, Ruskowskis, & Worak, (2008)

Skill 10.2.3 | Taking an Apical–Radial Pulse

Equipment
Watch with sweeping second hand
Stethoscope
Another nurse to assist with procedure (optional)

Procedure
1. Gather equipment.
2. Perform hand hygiene.
3. Clean stethoscope bell and diaphragm with alcohol swab or equivalent.
4. Check two forms of client ID. Introduce self.
5. Provide privacy.
6. Explain procedure to client, especially if two nurses are taking the pulse. ➤ **Rationale:** Clients may be apprehensive when two nurses are at the bedside, so a full explanation helps allay fears.
7. Assist client to a supine position and expose chest area.
8. Place watch where clearly visible to both nurses.
   ➤ **Rationale:** Both nurses count pulse rates within the same time span, preferably using one watch.
9. Warm stethoscope in palm of your hand. ➤ **Rationale:** This prevents startling the client with cold stethoscope.
10. Locate radial pulse. The second nurse locates apical pulse at the fifth intercostal space left of sternum at the midclavicular line and firmly places diaphragm of stethoscope on the site. **1** ➤ **Rationale:** Firm application helps transmit high-pitched heart sounds.

1 A. Auscultate apical pulse and palpate radial pulse simultaneously. **B.** This can also be done by two nurses.

(continued)

Skill 10.2.3 | Taking an Apical–Radial Pulse *(continued)*

11. With assistant, select number on watch to start counting pulse (e.g., 12:00).
12. Signal to the other nurse with your hand when to start taking the pulse and when to stop. Both nurses simultaneously count pulse for 1 full minute.
13. Auscultate the apical pulse and palpate the radial pulse simultaneously (preferably using two nurses, one at each site).

    a. Note a pulse deficit between apical and radial pulses when rhythm is irregular. ➤ *Rationale:* Atrial dysrhythmias and premature ventricular beats generally produce pulse deficits (apical greater than radial rate). A pulse deficit results from the ejection of a volume of blood that is too small to initiate a peripheral pulse wave.

    b. If a significant pulse deficit is found, assess for other abnormal signs (BP).

    c. Assess pulse volume by feeling the pressure of the beat. The quality is described as normal, weak, strong, or bounding.

14. Subtract radial rate from apical rate to obtain pulse deficit. ➤ *Rationale:* The pulse deficit represents the number of ineffective or nonperfused heartbeats.
15. Position client for comfort.
16. Perform hand hygiene.
17. Chart apical and radial rate and pulse deficit.

Skill 10.2.4 | Palpating a Peripheral Pulse

Equipment
Felt-tipped pen
Watch with second hand

Procedure
1. Gather equipment.
2. Perform hand hygiene.
3. Check two forms of client ID. Introduce self.
4. Provide privacy. Explain procedure.
5. Place client in a supine position with relaxed legs.
6. Palpate peripheral pulses: radial, carotid (when other sites are inaccessible), brachial, femoral, popliteal, dorsalis pedis, posterior tibial. (For special cases, after carotid surgery, palpate temporal pulse also.)
7. Compare pulse sites bilaterally by palpating with pads of the middle three fingers of your hand.
8. Press artery against the bone or underlying firm structure to occlude vessel and then gradually release pressure. ❶
9. Palpate weak pulses gently. ➤ *Rationale:* Too much pressure obliterates a weak pulse.
10. Assess if bilateral pulses are equal in amplitude (strength).

    a. If pulse is not immediately palpable, examine proximal area. ➤ *Rationale:* This action identifies where interruption or alteration in circulation occurs in an extremity.

    b. Since pulse locations differ, mark pulse locations with felt-tipped pen, especially when they are difficult to palpate. ➤ *Rationale:* Marking site allows the next nurse to find location without spending extra time.

    c. Compare presence and characteristic of peripheral pulses with previous findings. ➤ *Rationale:* This action allows early identification of alterations in peripheral circulation.

11. Check to see that client is comfortable.
12. Perform hand hygiene.
13. Record pulse rate, rhythm, pattern, and volume (Box 10-4 ■).

> **CLINICAL ALERT**
> If palpating the carotid pulse, avoid pressing on the carotid sinus in the upper neck area near the jaw. *Do not* palpate both carotids simultaneously because this decreases blood flow to the brain.

Box 10-4 **CHARACTERISTICS OF PERIPHERAL PULSES**

Peripheral pulses may be absent or weak. The size (amplitude) of a pulse depends on the degree of filling of the artery during systole (ventricular contraction) and emptying during diastole (ventricular relaxation). The amplitude of a pulse is described as being large or small and determines the pulse pressure (the difference between systolic and diastolic pressure).

    0 = Absent
    1+ = Weak
    2+ = Diminished
    3+ = Strong
    4+ = Full and bounding

❶ Apply firm pressure against underlying structure, then release to find the peripheral pulse.

Skill 10.2.5 | Monitoring Peripheral Pulses With a Doppler Ultrasound Stethoscope

Equipment

Doppler ultrasound stethoscope or probe
Conductive jelly (not K-Y)

Procedure

1. Gather equipment.
2. Perform hand hygiene. Introduce self.
3. Check two forms of client ID; explain procedure.
4. Provide privacy.
5. Uncover extremity to be assessed.
6. Place extremity in a comfortable position.
7. Locate anatomical region of pulse point.
8. Apply conductive gel to client's skin. ➤ *Rationale:* The ultrasound beam travels best through gel and requires an airtight seal between the probe and the skin.
9. Hold probe (at tapered end of plastic core) against skin at a 90-degree angle to the blood vessel being examined. ❶
10. Turn on Doppler.
11. Move probe over site if pulse is not detected. Keep it in direct contact with skin, and adjust volume to detect blood flow. ➤ *Rationale:* This action should facilitate detection of whooshing pulse sounds.
12. Reapply new gel if pulse is still not detected and, with light pressure, place probe over site and turn switch ON. Increase volume control, or check if batteries are weak.

❶ Hold probe against skin at a 90-degree angle.

13. Mark site where pulsations were heard. ➤ *Rationale:* This facilitates future assessments.
14. Clean gel from skin and Doppler probe. Replace cover over extremity.
15. Position client for comfort.
16. Replace Doppler equipment to appropriate location.
17. Perform hand hygiene.

Note: For pulse oximetry measurement, see Skill 30.3.2, Using Pulse Oximetry, page 1187.

Unit 10.2 Documentation and Evaluation

DOCUMENTATION for Taking a Pulse

- Type of pulse taken
- Rate, rhythm, intensity, and quality of pulse
- Pulse deficit, if any, present

- Characteristics of all peripheral pulses—use rating scale
- Use of Doppler stethoscope, if needed
- Effects of nursing interventions or medical treatments on abnormal pulse rates or rhythms

(continued)

Unit 10.2 Documentation and Evaluation *(continued)*

EVALUATION/Critical Thinking

Expected Outcomes

- Pulse is palpated without difficulty.
- Pulse rate is within normal range and rhythm is regular.
- All peripheral pulses are equal in amplitude when compared with the corresponding pulse on the other side and when compared with the next proximal site.
- Apical pulse is easily detected and counted.

Unexpected Outcomes	Alternative Actions
• Apical, femoral, and carotid pulses are absent.	• *Note:* For all unexpected outcomes, assess all vital signs and status of the client. • Activate emergency response system. • Initiate CPR immediately, and continue to assess the femoral or carotid pulse during resuscitation. • For absent femoral pulse, assess for systemic circulation and presence of disorders affecting circulation to extremities. • Use Doppler stethoscope to assess for presence of pulse.
• Abnormal heartbeats are present.	• Relieve anxiety, fear, or stress through communication and pertinent information. • If client has pain, relieve with change of position, back rub, and analgesic. • If new onset, notify healthcare provider.
• Tachycardia (pulse rate over 100 beats/min in adults or 140 in children)	• Decrease heart rate by reducing an elevated temperature to normal. • Take vital signs every 15 minutes to 2 hours until condition stabilizes and pulse rate is within normal limits. • Determine significance of pulse rate as it affects blood pressure, sensorium, and client comfort. • Reassess client for shock because a rise in pulse rate is one of the earliest signs of shock. • Notify healthcare provider if persistent tachycardia continues or if there is a change in blood pressure. • Determine whether tachycardia is normal for this client.
• Bradycardia (pulse rate less than 60 in adults or less than 70 in children)	• Compare to baseline; many clients who are in excellent physical condition have a resting pulse rate of <60 beats/min. • Notify healthcare provider for electrocardiogram request to determine if heart block is present. • If client is on digitalis, hold the drug, or on beta-blockers or other medications, notify healthcare provider. • Have atropine and temporary pacemaker available for healthcare provider if pulse is consistently slow (less than 50) and client is not an athlete (who may well have a pulse less than 50). • Continue monitoring pulse rate every 15 minutes to 2 hours until pulse is within normal limits.

Unexpected Outcomes	Alternative Actions
• Ectopic beats (premature ventricular or atrial contractions)	• Relieve pain if irregularity is due to **premature beats** associated with pain. • Administer oxygen if client has an order to do so. • If associated with stimuli from noise, visitors, caffeinated beverages, or smoking, eliminate the cause of the stimulation. • Notify healthcare provider to request a medical order for an electrocardiogram since premature beats in a client with myocardial infarction may be potentially harmful. • Obtain order from healthcare provider to draw serum electrolytes, especially magnesium or potassium. Low levels can cause ectopic beats. • Continue monitoring pulse rate every 15 minutes to 2 hours until irregularity is controlled.
• Peripheral pulse is absent.	• Report immediately. • Assess for other signs and symptoms of circulatory impairment such as pallor and cool temperature.
• Loss of peripheral pulse.	• Use a Doppler ultrasound and stethoscope to find pulse and report to healthcare provider.
• Doppler stethoscope is unable to detect sounds.	• Check that conductive jelly is used because salt from lubricants such as K-Y Jelly can damage the probe. • Check that batteries are less than 6 months old. The date should be indicated on all batteries. • Check that abnormal pressure is not applied, as this obliterates pulse.
• Client is in isolation and requires vascular assessment.	• After assessment, immediately clean according to manufacturer's recommendations.

Respirations

Nursing Process Data

ASSESSMENT Database

- Assess client's respiratory rate, depth, and rhythm.
- Note any abnormalities found during inspection and palpation or by percussion and auscultation.
- Assess presence of dyspnea or cyanosis.
- Assess for presence of abnormal sounds, such as **stertorous** or **sonorous** breathing.
- Assess if accessory muscles are used for breathing.

PLANNING Objectives

- To note respiratory rate, rhythm, and depth
- To establish baseline information on admission to the unit
- To note labored, difficult, or noisy respirations or cyanosis
- To identify alterations in respiratory pattern resulting from disease condition
- To determine whether respiratory rate is within normal range compared with pulse and blood pressure readings

IMPLEMENTATION Procedures

DOCUMENTATION AND EVALUATION

Expected Outcomes

- Respiratory rate, rhythm, and depth are within normal limits.
- Baseline information upon admission is documented.
- Labored, difficult, or noisy respirations are evaluated.
- Alterations in respiratory patterns resulting from disease conditions are identified.

Unexpected Outcomes/Alternative Actions

Pearson Nursing Student Resources

Find additional review materials at
nursing.pearsonhighered.com.
Prepare for success with NCLEX®-style practice questions and Skill Checklists.

Skill 10.3.1 | Obtaining the Respiratory Rate

Equipment
Watch with a second hand

Procedure
1. Perform hand hygiene. Introduce self.
2. Check two forms of client ID and explain procedure to client.
3. Check lighting to ensure it is adequate for procedure.
4. Maintain client's privacy.
5. Place hand on chest or observe chest rise and fall and count respirations. ❶
6. Note relationship of inspiration to expiration. Note also depth and effort of breathing.
7. Count respirations for preferably 1 minute, or for 30 seconds, and multiply by 2. ➤ *Rationale:* One full minute is more accurate for abnormal breathing patterns.
8. Perform hand hygiene.
9. Compare respiratory rate with previous recordings.
10. Document respiratory rate. Record if rhythm or depth deviates from normal (Box 10-5 ■ and Table 10-3 ■).

Box 10-5 **NORMAL RESPIRATORY RATE**

Adults: 12–20 per minute
Young children: 20–25 per minute
Infants: Up to 40 per minute

Note: Counting respirations for 15 seconds versus a full minute produced a significant difference in the rate; the safest approach is to count respirations for a full minute.

❶ Place hand on chest when respirations are difficult to count.

Table 10-3 Abnormal Breathing Patterns

Pattern	Description	
Apnea	Absence of breathing.	——————
Biot's respirations	Abrupt interruptions between a faster, deeper respiratory rate.	
Bradypnea	Slow, regular respirations. Rate is below 10 per minute.	
Cheyne–Stokes	Periods of apnea appear throughout cycle. Respirations become deeper and faster than normal followed by a slower rate and progressing to periods of apnea lasting from 15 to 60 seconds.	
Hyperpnea	Abnormal increase in depth and rate.	
Kussmaul's respirations	Deep, gasping breathing. Attempt to blow off carbon dioxide as respiratory compensation for metabolic acidosis (e.g., diabetic ketoacidosis).	
Tachypnea	Respiratory rate increased above 24 breaths per minute. Rate remains regular but shallow in pattern.	

LEGAL ALERT

Failure to Assess and Monitor Vital Signs

A client entered the hospital with pain from a kidney stone. From 4:35 p.m. to 10:30 p.m., he received three 5-mg doses of morphine, 1 mg of Dilaudid, and an additional 15 mg of morphine with 50 mg of Phenergan IV. At 1:05 a.m., the night shift found the client in respiratory and cardiac arrest. He died shortly thereafter. After having been transferred from the emergency department to a unit at 8:15 p.m., the client had not had his vital signs taken, even though hospital policy stated that after IV narcotic administration, the client must be monitored every hour for respiratory depression for 24 hours. The court found a breach of standard of care by the nurse's failure to assess, monitor, and document care of a client receiving narcotics.

Source: McMinn v. Mount Carmel Health, 1998

Unit 10.3 Documentation and Evaluation

DOCUMENTATION for Respiration

- Rate, depth, and rhythm of respirations
- Abnormal sounds associated with breathing
- Effectiveness of therapy if needed to correct respiratory problems
- Ratio of inspiration and expiration
- Alterations from baseline respiratory patterns

EVALUATION/Critical Thinking

Expected Outcomes

- Respiratory rate, rhythm, and depth are within normal limits.
- Baseline information upon admission is documented.
- Labored, difficult, or noisy respirations are evaluated.
- Alterations in respiratory patterns resulting from disease conditions are identified.

Unexpected Outcomes	Alternative Actions
• Apnea (absence of breathing) occurs, may be intermittent.	• *Note:* For all unexpected outcomes, assess client for all vital signs and comfort/condition. • Begin rescue breathing. • Summon help immediately; activate emergency response system.
• Tachypnea (rate faster than normal and more shallow >24) occurs.	• Identify cause. • Relieve anxiety, fear, and stress through communication and pertinent information. • Correct respiratory insufficiency with low-flow oxygen administration, good pulmonary toilet, and deep breathing and coughing exercises.
• Bradypnea (rate slower than normal <10) occurs.	• A sleeping adult's respirations can be less than 10 per minute; if so, use other vital signs to check condition. • If due to respiratory depressant drugs, such as opiates, barbiturates, and tranquilizers, be prepared to assist respirations or administer mouth-to-mask resuscitation. • Administer oxygen at 4–6 L/min via nasal cannulae as ordered. • Stimulate client to take breaths at least 10 times per minute.
• Hyperpnea (increased depth of respiration) occurs.	• Rest after period of exertion. • Relieve fear, anxiety, or stress. • May be indicative of respiratory compensation for metabolic acidotic state (Kussmaul pattern).

Unexpected Outcomes

- Cheyne–Stokes respirations (respiratory cycle in which respirations increase in rate and depth, then decrease, followed by a period of apnea) occur.

Alternative Actions

- Follow healthcare provider's orders to treat underlying disease state (e.g., heart failure, increased intracranial pressure).
- Monitor respirations every 15 minutes to hourly, depending on client's status.
- Evaluate cause—one of the indicators that death is approaching.

- Biot (irregular pattern—slow and deep or rapid and shallow, followed by apnea) respirations occur.

- Assess for central nervous system (CNS) abnormalities (increased intracranial pressure, meningitis).

- Kussmaul (deep and gasping breaths—more than 20 breaths/min) respirations occur.

- Follow orders to treat for renal failure, septic shock, or diabetic ketoacidosis.

Nursing Process Data

ASSESSMENT Database

- Assess blood pressure initially and whenever there is a change in client's status.
- Assess size of cuff needed for accurate reading.
- Assess the beginning and disappearance of Korotkoff sounds during a blood pressure reading.
- Assess presence of factors that can alter blood pressure readings.
- Note any changes from prior assessments.

PLANNING Objectives

- To determine whether arterial blood pressure reading is within normal range for the individual client
- To assess condition of heart, arteries, blood vessel resistance, and stroke volume
- To establish a baseline for further evaluation
- To identify alterations in blood pressure resulting from a change in disease condition
- To correlate blood pressure readings with pulse and respirations

IMPLEMENTATION Procedures

DOCUMENTATION AND EVALUATION

Expected Outcomes

- Blood pressure readings provide information regarding the overall health status of client.
- Major changes from prior assessments are documented.
- Accurate readings are taken by using correct cuff size and procedure.
- Beginning and disappearance of Korotkoff sounds during a blood pressure reading are evaluated and documented.
- The presence of factors that can alter blood pressure readings is identified.

Unexpected Outcomes/Alternative Actions

Pearson Nursing Student Resources

Find additional review materials at
nursing.pearsonhighered.com.
Prepare for success with NCLEX®-style practice questions and Skill Checklists.

| **Skill 10.4.1** | Measuring a Blood Pressure |

Equipment

Sphygmomanometer with proper size cuff
Stethoscope
Alcohol wipe

Procedure

1. Gather equipment. Clean stethoscope before use. Be sure the cuff is an appropriate size (Box 10-6 ■) for the client. ❶
   ➤ *Rationale:* A cuff that is too narrow results in erroneously high readings; a cuff too large may result in false low readings.
2. Provide quiet environment.
3. Perform hand hygiene.
4. Clean stethoscope with alcohol swab or equivalent.
5. Check two forms of client ID. Introduce self.
6. Explain procedure to client. If client is a child, take blood pressure after the other vital signs. ➤ *Rationale:* This intervention may upset the child and affect pulse and respirations.
7. Place client in relaxed reclining or sitting position. ❷ (Sitting position with feet on the floor is the preferred position.)
   ➤ *Rationale:* Blood pressure can vary by position in certain individuals.
8. Prepare client for blood pressure reading.

   a. Assess whether client has smoked or exercised within last 15 minutes.
   b. Allow client to rest several minutes before beginning a reading.
   c. Client should be instructed not to cross legs or talk during the procedure. ➤ *Rationale:* Client activities and a slouched position yield false high readings.

CLINICAL ALERT
- Avoid measuring blood pressure in an arm with extensive axillary node dissection (e.g., radical mastectomy) or an arteriovenous fistula (e.g., for dialysis).
- Ultrasound techniques such as using a Doppler stethoscope can be used to measure systolic blood pressure when auscultatory sounds are too faint to be heard.

Box 10-6 **BLOOD PRESSURE CUFF SIZES**
- Standard (12–14 cm wide) for the average adult arm
- Narrower cuff for infant, child, or adult with thin arms
- For children (younger than 13 years), bladder large enough to encircle the arm completely (100%)
- Wider cuff (18–22 cm) for client with obese arms or for thigh pressure readings

The cuff's inflatable bladder width should be 40% of the circumference of the limb on which it is used. The length of the bladder should be twice its width.

❶ Blood pressure cuffs come in various sizes.

❷ Before starting procedure, explain steps and position the client in a relaxed position.

EVIDENCE-BASED PRACTICE

Body Positioning Affects Blood Pressure

A study in an ambulatory cardiac clinic found that clients seated in proper position (in a chair with back support, feet on the floor, and arms at heart level) had readings 12%–14% lower than those who were seated on exam tables (Turner, 2008).

Blood Pressure Measurement in Obese Clients
- Be cautious when using a thigh cuff on the upper arm. It may approximate the correct diameter but often it is too long, extending into the axilla and beyond the antecubital fossa.
- Extra-long cuffs are not suitable alternatives and do not meet AHA standards.
- Use sensitivity when taking blood pressure of an obese client (McFarlane, 2012).

(continued)

Skill 10.4.1 | Measuring a Blood Pressure (continued)

9. Expose upper part of client's arm and position it with palm upward, arm slightly flexed with the whole arm supported at heart level. ➤ *Rationale:* If arm is below level of heart, the blood pressure reading is higher than normal, and if above the heart, it is lower than normal. ❶ Blood pressure cuffs come in various sizes. ❷ Before starting procedure, explain steps and position the client in a relaxed position.

10. Choose appropriate size cuff and wrap totally deflated cuff snugly and smoothly around upper part of arm (lower border of cuff 1 in. [2.5 cm] above antecubital space) with center of cuff bladder over brachial artery (pressure dial at zero). ❸

11. Locate and palpate brachial artery with fingertips (medial aspect of antecubital fossa).

12. Position stethoscope ear pieces in ears. The ear pieces should tilt slightly forward. ➤ *Rationale:* With a forward tilt, sounds are heard more clearly.

13. Ensure stethoscope hangs freely from ears. ➤ *Rationale:* Rubbing of stethoscope against an object can cause artifacts and inaccurate readings.

14. Close valve on sphygmomanometer pump.

15. Inflate cuff rapidly (while palpating radial artery) to a level 30 mm Hg above level at which radial pulsations are no longer felt. ➤ *Rationale:* This level ensures that cuff is inflated to a pressure exceeding the client's systolic pressure. Slow inflation can yield gaps in pressure readings.

16. Note level and rapidly deflate, waiting 60 seconds. ➤ *Rationale:* This is enough time for venous congestion to decrease.

17. Place bell (or diaphragm) of stethoscope lightly on the medial antecubital fossa where brachial artery pulsations are located and rapidly inflate cuff to 30 mm Hg above point where radial pulse disappeared.

Note: Bell and diaphragm of stethoscope yield similar results.
❹–❻ ➤ *Rationale:* This pressure ensures that cuff is inflated to exceed client's systolic pressure. ❹ **A.** Bell of stethoscope. **B.** Diaphragm of stethoscope. ❺ Place stethoscope on medial antecubital fossa. ❻ Palpate brachial artery on medial antecubital fossa.

18. Deflate cuff gradually at a constant rate by opening valve on pump (2–4 mm Hg/sec) until the first Korotkoff sound is heard. This is the systolic pressure, or phase I, of Korotkoff sounds. ➤ *Rationale:* Slower or faster deflation yields false readings.

19. Read pressure on manometer at eye level. ❼ ➤ *Rationale:* This ensures accurate reading.

❹ **A.** Bell of stethoscope. **B.** Diaphragm of stethoscope.

❺ Place stethoscope on medial antecubital fossa.

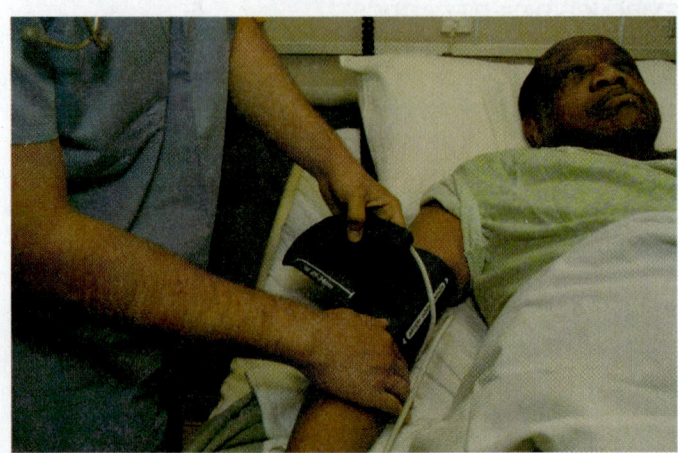

❸ Wrap blood pressure cuff snugly around upper arm.

❻ Palpate brachial artery on medial antecubital fossa.

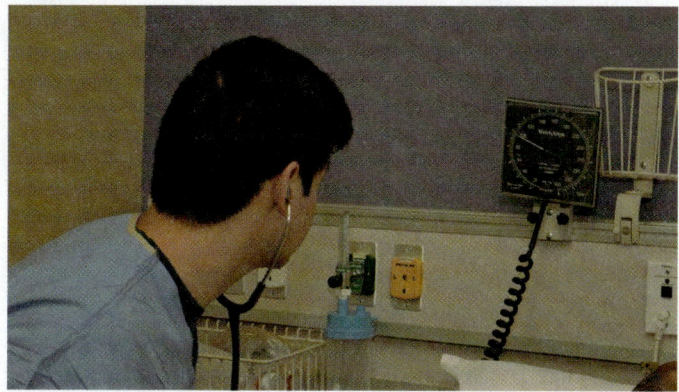

7 Read manometer at eye level.

20. Continue to deflate cuff at a rate of 2–4 mm Hg/sec until the last Korotkoff sound is heard. This will prevent missing an auscultatory gap. Do not reinflate without letting cuff totally deflate. ➤ *Rationale:* Reinflating cuff results in erroneously high readings. **7** Read manometer at eye level.

21. Note point at which Korotkoff sounds begin (phase I) and when they disappear completely (phase V). Disappearance of sounds (phase V) is regarded by the American Heart Association as the best index of diastolic blood pressure in individuals over age 13. If the child is younger than 12 years, the best indication of diastolic pressure is the distinct muffling of sounds at phase IV (Box 10-7 ■).

Note: Some facilities require that all five phases be recorded.

22. Do not leave cuff inflated for a prolonged period. ➤ *Rationale:* Leaving cuff inflated produces client discomfort.

23. Deflate cuff completely and wait at least 1–2 minutes before rechecking the blood pressure. ➤ *Rationale:* This allows time for blood vessels to return to normal.

Note: Check level of comfort of client and level of consciousness (as well as other vital signs) when evaluating blood pressure reading. If all signs and symptoms do not correlate, reevaluate blood pressure.

Box 10-7 KOROTKOFF SOUND PHASES

Phase I: The pressure level at which the first faint, rhythmic tapping sounds are heard. The sounds gradually increase in intensity as the cuff is deflated. This phase coincides with the reappearance of a palpable pulse (systolic sound).

Phase II: That time during cuff deflation when a murmur or "whooshing" sounds are heard.

Phase III: The period during which sounds are crisper "knocking" sound and increase in intensity.

Phase IV: That time when a distinct, abrupt, muffling of sound (usually of a soft, blowing quality) is heard (diastolic sound in children or physically active adults).

Phase V: That pressure level when the last sound is heard and after which all sound disappears (second diastolic sound).

In some clients, there is no distinct V sound; in this instance, you will document the pressure when you hear the IV sound.

24. Remove cuff from client's arm.

25. Clean the diaphragm/bell and cuff with an approved antiseptic. If possible, each client should have a disposable blood pressure cuff. ➤ *Rationale:* Studies have shown that cuffs (as well as stethoscopes) can become contaminated.

EVIDENCE-BASED PRACTICE

Stethoscopes—Carriers of Bacterial Infection

Researchers investigated the incidence of contamination level of physician hands and stethoscopes and found the level of contaminant of a stethoscope after a single examination was comparable to the dominant hand of the provider. The leading contaminant identified was methicillin-resistant *Staphylococcus aureus* (MRSA). Stethoscopes need to be cleaned in-between clients, similar to hand hygiene protocols.

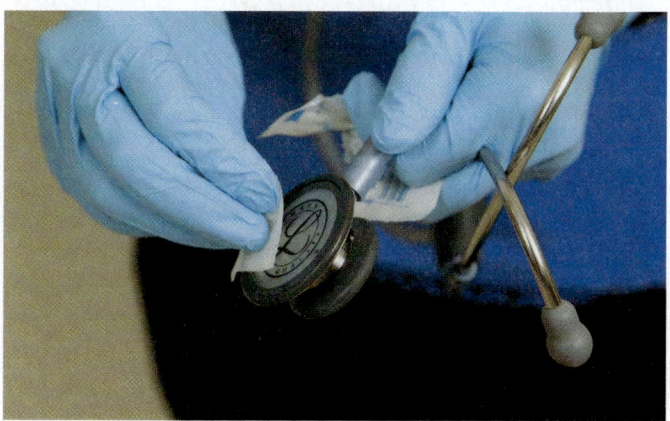

Clean the bell/diaphragm of the stethoscope after taking client's blood pressure.

Source: Longtin et al. (2014)

26. Check that client is comfortable.

27. Compare blood pressure reading with previous recordings.

28. Perform hand hygiene.

29. Record blood pressure readings using two phases: 120/80 where 120 is the systolic (phase I) and 80 is the diastolic (phase V) pressure; or three phases: 130/110/80 where 130 is the systolic (phase I), 110 is the first diastolic (phase IV), and 80 is the second diastolic (phase V) pressure. See Table 10-4 ■ for blood pressure classifications.

Table 10-4 Blood Pressure Classification

Blood Pressure	Systolic	Diastolic
Normal	<120	<80
Prehypertension	120–139	80–89
Stage I high blood pressure	140–159	90–99
Stage II high blood pressure	160 and higher	100 and higher

Source: National Center for Health Statistics. (2011)

(continued)

Skill 10.4.1 | Measuring a Blood Pressure *(continued)*

30. Repeat this procedure on the opposite arm if this is an initial reading. ➤ *Rationale:* Clients may have a difference of 10 points between the two arms. For ongoing monitoring, note that BP should be taken on the arm with the higher blood pressure.

Note: If there is more than a 20-point difference, report to healthcare provider.

Skill 10.4.2 | Palpating Systolic Arterial Blood Pressure

Equipment
Sphygmomanometer with proper size cuff

Procedure
1. Gather equipment. Check that cuff is appropriate size for client. ➤ *Rationale:* A cuff that is too narrow results in erroneously high readings.
2. Perform hand hygiene.
3. Clean stethoscope with alcohol swab or equivalent.
4. Check two forms of client ID. Introduce self.
5. Explain procedure to client.
6. Place client in relaxed position and support arm at heart level.
7. Wrap cuff snugly and smoothly around the upper part of the arm (1 in. above antecubital space) with center of bladder over brachial artery.
8. Keep pressure level in cuff at zero.
9. Locate radial artery pulsations on cuffed arm.
10. Inflate cuff rapidly (while palpating radial artery) ❶, to a level 30 mm Hg above level at which radial artery pulsations are no longer felt. ➤ *Rationale:* This level ensures that cuff is inflated to a pressure exceeding client's systolic pressure.
11. Continue to palpate artery and release pressure from cuff slowly (2–3 mm Hg/sec). The first palpated beat is the systolic pressure. This should be the same point at which the last pulsation was felt during inflation of cuff.
12. Remove cuff and return equipment.
13. Perform hand hygiene.
14. Record systolic blood pressure reading as "palpated systolic pressure."

❶ Palpate the radial artery while inflating cuff and releasing pressure.

> **CLINICAL ALERT**
> Children as young as 3 should have their blood pressure checked to identify possible heart disease. Children under age 3 can have their BP checked by palpation method. The normal systolic BP can be determined by using the formula $80 + 2 \times$ the child's age. A newborn's systolic BP ranges between 50 and 80 mm Hg and diastolic between 25 and 55 mm Hg.

Skill 10.4.3 | Measuring Lower-Extremity Blood Pressure

Equipment
Stethoscope
Sphygmomanometer with standard or large-size cuff

Procedure
1. Gather equipment.
2. Perform hand hygiene.
3. Clean stethoscope with alcohol swab or equivalent.

4. Check two forms of client ID. Introduce self.
5. Explain procedure to client.
6. Wrap cuff snugly and smoothly around lower leg with cuff's distal edge at the malleolus. **1**
7. Locate either the dorsalis pedis or posterior tibial artery pulsations.
8. Inflate cuff rapidly while palpating foot artery, to a level 30 mm Hg above level at which artery pulsations are no longer felt.
9. Place bell (or diaphragm) of stethoscope quickly on pulse site.
10. Deflate cuff slowly (2–4 mm Hg/sec) while auscultating sounds over the selected artery.
11. Remove cuff and return equipment.
12. Check to see that client is comfortable.

1 Wrap cuff snugly around lower leg and locate dorsalis pedis.

13. Record readings for first (systolic) and last (diastolic) sounds, noting site and client position.

Alternative Methods

14. Measure blood pressure in thigh by using a large cuff with bladder placed over posterior mid-thigh and bottom edge above knee. ➤ *Rationale:* The cuff bladder must be directly over the posterior popliteal artery for accurate reading. Listen with stethoscope at popliteal fossa with client in prone position, or supine with knee flexed enough for stethoscope placement.

Note: The systolic pressure is 20–30 mm Hg higher than in the brachial artery. The diastolic pressure is the same.

15. Measure blood pressure in forearm by placing appropriate size cuff around forearm 13 cm from elbow; listen for Korotkoff sounds over radial artery at wrist.
16. Compare blood pressures measured indirectly in the arm, leg, and thigh to reveal similar values. Measurements may be difficult to obtain in clients with **peripheral vascular disease**.

> **CLINICAL ALERT**
>
> Traditionally, vital signs provided the basis for assessing the need for and adequacy of sedation in clients who are critically ill. If the client is on drug therapy, vital signs may not always be a reliable indicator of sedation, because they do not directly reflect the level of consciousness.

Skill 10.4.4 | Measuring Blood Pressure by Flush Method in a Small Infant

Equipment
Sphygmomanometer with appropriate cuff
Elastic bandage
Assistant for observing flush
Well-lighted room

Procedure
1. Gather equipment.
2. Perform hand hygiene.
3. Check two forms of client ID. Introduce self.
4. Wrap blood pressure cuff snugly and smoothly just above wrist or ankle.
5. Elevate extremity above heart level.
6. Wrap elastic bandage firmly around exposed hand or foot.
   ➤ *Rationale:* Bandage compression empties the veins.

7. Lower extremity to heart level when compression is complete.
8. Inflate cuff rapidly to 200 mm Hg.
9. Remove elastic bandage.
10. Deflate cuff slowly (not exceeding 5 mm Hg/sec).
11. Instruct assistant to watch for appearance of flush in the extremity distal to cuff. ➤ *Rationale:* An assistant is necessary so that pressure at which flush appears can be precisely noted. This reading more clearly reflects the *mean* blood pressure than the systolic pressure.
12. Document that blood pressure was taken by flush method.

> **CLINICAL ALERT**
>
> Flush pressures are taken on small infants or on adults when unable to auscultate or palpate blood pressure readings.

Skill 10.4.5 | Using a Continuous Noninvasive Monitoring Device

Equipment
Blood pressure cuff
Display monitor

Procedure
1. Check two forms of client ID; introduce self; wash hands.
2. Gather equipment. Select proper size blood pressure cuff. (Size should be two-thirds the size of upper arm.) **Note:** In most institutions, the cuffs are one-time use to ensure infection-control practices. Attach the cuff to the air hose by firmly pushing the valve from the cuff into the air hose and twisting to secure fit. ❶
3. Squeeze the air from the cuff.
4. Wrap the cuff securely around the extremity (usually the arm).
   a. Place cuff over brachial artery with lower edge 1 in. above antecubital fossa.
   b. If skin is fragile, place single layer of cotton under cuff.
5. Turn power switch ON.
6. Position the extremity at the level of the heart. ➤ **Rationale:** If arm is below heart level, reading will be higher than normal.
7. Set arterial pressure alarm limits for both HIGH and LOW parameters. ➤ **Rationale:** The alarm parameters provide a safety factor by alerting the nurse when the readings exceed the parameters.
8. Set time frames for continuous monitoring depending on client's condition. **Note:** Many continuous noninvasive

devices communicate directly with EHRs to provide ongoing documentation. An example can be seen in Box 10-8 ∎.
9. Press START button.
10. Alternate extremities if device is used for a prolonged period of time.
11. Check position of cuff and skin under cuff frequently.
    ➤ **Rationale:** It is important to note bruises or skin trauma and to check if position of cuff has changed.
12. Perform hand hygiene.
13. Always plug in continuous monitoring blood pressure device to avoid draining batteries.

EVIDENCE-BASED PRACTICE
Trendelenburg Position and Blood Pressure
The use of Trendelenburg position has not been found to lead to beneficial changes in blood pressure or cardiac output or cardiac index. As a result, this position is probably not useful in rescue efforts (Halm, M., 2012).

Box 10-8 **NEW TRENDS: ELECTRONIC STETHOSCOPE**

A new electronic stethoscope is now available. It measures a client's blood pressure via Bluetooth-enabled Cardioscan and sends the results directly into the client's computer record for immediate evaluation.

❶ Continuous monitoring of blood pressure is done by attaching the cuff to the display monitor.

Unit 10.4 Documentation and Evaluation

DOCUMENTATION for Blood Pressure

- Two phases of Korotkoff sounds (e.g., 120/80) and site
- Three phases of Korotkoff sounds (e.g., 130/110/80) and site
- Response to alternative nursing actions
- Response to position changes
- Document vital signs in chart, in addition to attaching digital readouts

EVALUATION/Critical Thinking

Expected Outcomes

- Blood pressure readings provide information regarding the overall health status of the client.
- Major changes from prior assessments are documented.
- Accurate readings are taken by using the correct cuff size and procedure.
- Beginning and disappearance of Korotkoff sounds during a blood pressure reading are evaluated and documented.
- The presence of factors that can alter blood pressure readings is identified.

Unexpected Outcomes

- Blood pressure reading is abnormally high without apparent physiologic cause.

Alternative Actions

- Check if arm was unsupported.
- Check if cuff was not snug.
- Check if cuff was deflated too slowly or reinflated during deflation, causing venous engorgement and abnormally high diastolic readings.
- Ask if client has pain, was anxious (white coat syndrome), or had just exercised, eaten, or smoked. Recheck pressure as indicated.
- Check blood pressure on both arms. The normal difference from arm to arm is usually no more than 5 mmHg.
- Check if insufficient rest before assessment.

- Blood pressure reading is very low and there are no significant clinical indicators.

- Assess if cuff is too wide.
- Check if client's arm was above heart level.
- Check if inflation was too slow. This reduces intensity of Korotkoff sounds.
- Assess if Korotkoff sounds were barely audible. Raise client's arm, and then recheck. Sounds should be louder.
- Identify if stethoscope was misplaced and was not on brachial artery.
- Take blood pressure 3 minutes after client rises from supine to standing if postural hypotension is suspected.

- Blood pressure cannot be measured on upper extremity due to casts or other causes of inaccessibility.

- Use lower extremity to obtain blood pressures.

(continued)

Unit 10.4 Documentation and Evaluation (continued)

Unexpected Outcomes	Alternative Actions
• Continuous BP monitoring system displays 00 instead of blood reading. (00 indicates the unit is unable to determine parameters.)	• Check cuff placement and size to determine if appropriately placed. • Ensure cuff is attached to monitor and not loose. • Recalibrate if needed.
• Hypotension (systolic pressure less than 90 mm Hg) develops.	• Take all vital signs more frequently (every 15 minutes to 2 hours) until condition has stabilized. • Assess cause of hypotension, and notify healthcare provider. • Increase or administer fluids as ordered by healthcare provider. • Observe postoperative clients for signs of bleeding. • Administer oxygen.
• Hypertension (blood pressure consistently over 140/90 mm Hg)	• For clients with severe, acute hypertension, take vital signs more frequently (every 15 minutes to 2 hours) until condition has stabilized. • Notify healthcare provider. • If client is anxious or excited, institute relaxation techniques to lower blood pressure. • Allow client to rest after strenuous exercise. • Relieve pain with reassurance, change of position, and analgesia as ordered by healthcare provider. • For clients with essential hypertension, administer antihypertensive and diuretic drugs as ordered by the healthcare provider. Evaluate response by checking blood pressure in reclining and standing position.

• Client's blood pressure continues to be high with a diagnosis of hypertension.	• Evaluate any medication client is taking, including antihypertensive agents.
	• Teach client about lifestyle modifications as a cornerstone for managing hypertension:
	  1. Lose excess weight.
	  2. Maintain a low-fat diet with many fruits and vegetables.
	  3. Limit alcohol intake.
	  4. Stop smoking.
	  5. Exercise regularly.
	  6. Include extra minerals in diet: potassium, calcium, and magnesium.
	  7. Reduce sodium intake and switch to sea salt.
	  8. Practice stress-reducing exercises such as meditation, yoga, and t'ai chi.

Chapter Wrap-Up

GERONTOLOGIC Considerations

Cardiac Status—Changes

- Changes in cardiovascular status with aging are often insidious and may become apparent when system is stressed and there is increased demand for cardiac output (which may occur with illness and hospitalization). Nursing care assessment should focus on client's cardiovascular status, even when diagnosis does not include a cardiac condition.
- Blood pressure measurement should take age into account. If client has severe joint stiffness, pseudohypertension may be present. If this is suspected, raise the cuff pressure above the systolic blood pressure and, if the radial pulse remains palpable, the reading may show 10–15 mm Hg in error.
- Postural hypotension is common in the older adult (positional drop of less than 20 mm Hg); nurses should take note when helping a client out of bed. Hypertension is also common in this age group.
- A rise in blood pressure may be associated with reduced cardiac output, vasoconstriction, increased blood volume, or fluid overload.
- Pulse changes, particularly an irregular pulse, can be related to hypoxia, airway obstruction, or electrolyte imbalance.
- The arteries in older adult clients may feel stiff and knotty due to decreased elasticity. Excessive pressure to site when taking pulse may obliterate it. The normal rate is 60–90 beats/min.
- If pulses are not palpated, a Doppler may need to be used.

Respiratory Status—Changes

- Changes in the respiratory system may be subtle and gradual with the older adult: Oxygen saturation is decreased to 93%–94%; there is often poor cough response and incomplete lung expansion—all of which leads to increased risk of pulmonary infection when the older adult client is hospitalized.
- Slightly irregular breathing patterns are not unusual in the older adult.

Temperature—Changes

- With the older adult, temperature may be as low as 95°F (35°C). Because they may be easily dehydrated with increased temperature, nursing assessment should include baseline temperature at admission and continued monitoring during hospitalization.
- Older adults with acute infections may have a subnormal temperature.
- Increased temperatures can lead to increased metabolism, thus increasing the body's demand for oxygen. This causes the heart to work harder.
- Oral temperatures are the preferred method for obtaining the older adult client's temperature.

MANAGEMENT Guidelines

Each state legislates a Nurse Practice Act for RNs and LPN/LVNs. Healthcare facilities are responsible for establishing and implementing policies and procedures that conform to their state's regulations. Verify the regulations and role parameters for each healthcare worker in your facility.

Delegation

- Taking vital signs for clients may be assigned to any healthcare worker provided they have been assessed for competency in the procedure. This includes LPN/LVN, unlicensed assistive personnel (UAP), and EMT.
- The registered nurse must identify parameters for which the healthcare worker is to notify the nurse (i.e., blood pressure above or below a certain reading, pulse rate, or irregular pulse).

- The nurse must provide detailed explanations and/or demonstrate alterations in the procedure or specific methods of obtaining the vital signs to UAP, or EMTs.
- Obtaining peripheral pulses by use of the Doppler is the responsibility of the RN or LPN/LVN. A UAP is not responsible for using the Doppler.
- The UAP may monitor blood pressure using the noninvasive monitoring device; however, the UAP is not responsible for initiating the procedure or setting the alarms.

Interprofessional Communication

- Directions must be given to healthcare workers on documentation procedures. Do they complete the graphic record, enter data into the EHR, write the findings on a vital sign sheet at the nurses' desk, or give the results to the nurse?

- The registered nurse must evaluate all abnormal or changed vital signs identified by the healthcare workers. The nurse maintains total responsibility for client care even though someone else performs the task of taking the vital signs.

- The registered nurse must ensure that the healthcare workers know the parameters for reporting unusual vital signs. Periodic checks with the workers may be necessary.

CASE STUDY Applications

Scenario 1

Mr. Trager (age 92) has been admitted to your unit with a temperature of 103°F (39.4°C), BP 140/90, P 114, and R 30 and labored. He reports a history of 3 days of diarrhea and fever and asks you for something to drink.

1. From your analysis of the admission data, determine the following:
   a. Appropriate nursing diagnosis in order of priority for this client.
   b. The metabolic effects of fever on pulse and respiration.
   c. Age factors that contribute to the existing problem.
2. What are the other assessment findings indicative of the diagnosis established from primary admitting data?
3. Develop a plan of care for this client.
4. Describe the evaluative outcomes for problem resolution.

Scenario 2

Mr. Sondheim is admitted to the hospital with unstable hypertension for evaluation. He has a family history of hypertension and heart disease. The nurse will complete a physical exam and a history.

1. What information is missing in the family history that the nurse will want to elicit from the client?
2. Which questions regarding lifestyle would be appropriate to ask?
3. Which aspects of client teaching would the nurse want to cover before Mr. Sondheim is discharged?

Scenario 3

You are caring for a client, and when checking his vital signs, you are unable to palpate his radial pulse.

1. What would be your follow-up intervention?
2. When you still cannot find a pulse clear enough to document, what would be your next intervention?
3. What parameters of the pulse will you pay attention to when assessing and recording a client's pulse?

NCLEX® Review Questions

Unless otherwise specified, choose only one (1) answer.

1. During a shift assessment, the nurse notes that the client's peripheral pulses are absent. What would the next intervention be?
   A. Palpate the peripheral pulse.
   B. Use a Doppler to assess peripheral pulse.
   C. Notify the healthcare provider.
   D. Administer O_2 as ordered.

2. When a pulse deficit is detected in a client, what would the nurse expect the client is experiencing?
   A. Premature ventricular beats
   B. Bradycardia
   C. Tachycardia
   D. Heart block

3. A client's temperature remains elevated despite the administration of antipyretic drugs. What would be the first intervention after determining this condition?
   A. Administer a cool bath.
   B. Assess all remaining signs.

C. Request orders for a cooling blanket.
D. Obtain an order for a blood culture.

4. When taking a client's blood pressure that has been within normal limits, the nurse gets a reading that is very low without any significant clinical indicators. Which intervention would be appropriate?
   A. Assess if the BP cuff is too narrow.
   B. Assess if the BP cuff is too wide.
   C. Assess if the client's arm was positioned below heart level.
   D. Notify the healthcare provider.

5. When taking a client's blood pressure, the nurse finds the reading very different from previous readings recorded on the chart. What is the first intervention?
   A. Recheck the blood pressure with different equipment.
   B. Notify the healthcare provider.
   C. Validate the reading with another nurse.
   D. Check the client's circulatory status.

6. Which of the following breathing patterns of adults are abnormal?

   Select all that apply.

   A. Apnea

   B. Rate of 12–20 per minute

   C. Hyperpnea

   D. Biot

   E. Bradypnea

7. When assessing a client newly admitted to the ED, which of the following would be recognized as an early sign of shock?

   A. Pulse rate of 120

   B. Blood pressure of 110/70

   C. Respiratory rate of 24

   D. Fever of 101°F (38.3°C)

8. When using the tympanic route for taking a temperature, what is the rationale for directing the probe toward the tympanic membrane?

   A. Pressure seals the ear canal.

   B. The probe will not record unless it is near the tympanic membrane.

C. This method records the core temperature.

D. This method provides better access to the ear canal.

9. The RN is in charge of the team assigned to care for six clients for morning shift. The staffing includes the RN, an LPN/LVN, and two UAPs. All clients need to have vital signs taken as part of their shift assessment. How will the RN best assign these duties?

   A. The LPN/LVN should do all of the vital signs.

   B. The RN and LPN/LVN should split the vital signs.

   C. The RN should assign vital signs to the two UAPs.

   D. The RN should do all of the vital signs.

10. When you observe a UAP assessing the blood pressure of an obese client with a thigh cuff, what would you do next?

    A. Do nothing, as this is an acceptable practice.

    B. Inform the UAP that a thigh cuff is not appropriate and that a properly fitting cuff is required.

    C. Find an extra-long cuff as a replacement.

    D. Recommend the UAP adjust the systolic and diastolic reading by adding 20 mm Hg to the reading.

QSEN Activity

Domain: Communication

KSA: Skill

Activity: Have the learner create an SBAR that he or she will have to give to the oncoming shift based on the following scenario:

A 59-year-old male admitted this morning for infection of left great toe secondary to poorly managed type 2 diabetes mellitus. Vital signs on arrival: T 100.1 (37.8°C), P 92, R 16, BP 114/96. Mid-day vital signs: T 100.7 (38.2°C), P 108, R 19, BP 107/88. End-of-shift vital signs: T 101.5 (38.6°C), P 118, R 23, BP 98/76.

Bibliography

Camara, G. G., Ruskowskis, J. M., & Worak, S. R. (2008). The effect of live classical music on the vital signs of patients undergoing ophthalmic surgery. *Medscape Journal of Medicine, 10*(6), 149.

Centers for Disease Control and Prevention. (n.d.). *High blood pressure.* Retrieved from http://www.cdc.gov/bloodpressure/

Halm, M. (2012). Trendelenburg position: "Put to bed": Or angled toward use in your unit. *American Journal of Critical Care, 6* (21), 449–452.

LeMone, P., & Burke, K. M. (2012). *Medical–surgical nursing: Critical thinking in clinical care* (5th ed.). Upper Saddle River, NJ: Prentice Hall Health.

Longtin, Y., Schneider, A., Tschopp, C., Renzi, G., Gayete-Ageron, A., Schrenzel, J., & Pittet, D. (2014). Contamination of stethoscopes and physicians' hands after a physical examination. *Mayo Foundation for Medical Education and Research, 89*(3), 291–299.

McFarlane, J. (2012). Blood pressure measurement in obese patients. *Critical Care Nursing, 32,* 70–73.

National Center for Health Statistics. (2007–2010). *National Health and Nutrition Examination Survey;* Centers for Disease Control and Prevention. (2011). Retrieved from http://www.nhlbi.nih.gov/health/health-topics/topics/hbp/

Reynolds, M., Bonham L., Gueck M., Hammond K., Lowery J., Redel C., Rodriguez C., Smith S., Stanton A., Sukosd S., & Craft M. (2014, Jan.). Are temporal artery temperatures accurate enough to replace rectal temperatures measurement in the pediatric ED patients? *Journal of Emergency Nursing, 40*(1), 46–50.

Turner, M. (2008). University of Virginia Health System reported by the Academy of Medical-Surgical Nurses.

Chapter 11
Physical Assessment

Learning Objectives

11.1 Outline the essential elements obtained from a health history.

11.2 List the four techniques of physical assessment.

11.3 Demonstrate six steps of the focus assessment.

11.4 Describe the abnormal manifestations associated with each specific body system for one client with whom you are familiar.

11.5 List four normal responses that determine the client's level of consciousness.

11.6 Describe four abnormal responses in pupil assessment.

11.7 State three assessment components of the skin.

11.8 Describe normal and abnormal lung sounds.

11.9 Describe the assessment techniques used in an abdominal assessment in sequential order.

11.10 Outline the steps of breast assessment.

11.11 Identify the four areas for heart sound auscultation.

11.12 List at least five essential elements included in a mental status assessment.

11.13 Compare and contrast three elements of the antepartum obstetrical assessment.

11.14 Relate the elements of a "9" score on the Apgar test as part of a newborn assessment.

11.15 Describe basic components of a pediatric physical assessment.

Chapter Outline

Assessment

Basic assessment discussed in this chapter can be performed in less than 10 minutes using a stethoscope, penlight, reflex hammer, your hands, and observational skills. Although you may not be able to perform assessment rapidly at first, you will have many opportunities to practice your skills, because every client should be assessed at least once a shift.

While interviewing the client, note such characteristics as hair, skin, posture, facial expression, and body language—in other words, the general appearance of the client. Then proceed with a head-to-toe systems assessment using the four techniques of assessment: inspection, palpation, percussion, and auscultation (IPPA). This IPPA sequence is used for all systems except for the abdominal assessment, which requires auscultation *before* palpation and percussion in order not to alter bowel motility and affect data obtained for bowel sounds. These methods are described in the following pages. Observe the client's response as each system is assessed.

Equipment

The stethoscope is the primary instrument used for assessment. Remember that any movement of the tubing or chest piece by clothing or hands can cause extraneous noise that obliterates the sounds you want to hear. The diaphragm piece should be applied firmly to the skin. The diaphragm enhances high-pitched sounds (breath sounds, normal heart sounds, bowel sounds). The bell piece should be placed very lightly to pick up low-pitched sounds, such as vascular sounds and abnormal heart sounds. Note that if the bell is pressed firmly, it stretches the skin and acts as a diaphragm.

Other equipment includes the penlight, reflex hammer, ophthalmoscope, otoscope, and tuning fork.

Health History

A total client assessment begins with a nursing health history. Using open-ended questions such as "Tell me about...," the nurse collects data about past health conditions, current problems, and present needs. The information is obtained through objective (observed) and subjective (stated-by-client) data collection.

Information obtained from the interview and the physical assessment constitutes the basis for identifying nursing diagnoses and establishing the individualized client care plan. A complete health history includes the following elements:

- *Biographic information:* age, gender, ethnicity, educational level, marital status, living arrangements.
- *Chief complaint:* condition that brought client to healthcare facility; reason for visit; any recent changes.
- *Present health status or illness:* onset of the problem; clinical manifestations, including severity of symptoms; pain characteristics if present.
- *Health history:* general state of health, past illnesses, surgeries, hospitalizations, allergies, over-the-counter (OTC) medications, herbal supplements, current medications, and general habits such as smoking, alcohol consumption, or recreational drug use.
- *Family history:* age and health status of parents, siblings, and children; cause of death for immediate family members.
- *Psychosocial factors, lifestyles:* cultural beliefs that influence health management; religious or spiritual beliefs.
- *Nutrition:* dietary habits, preferences, or restrictions.
- *Domestic violence:* physical and behavioral indicators.

Nurse's Role

The nurse's role in obtaining a health history and completing a physical assessment has expanded dramatically over the last 40 years. Today, nurses must be adequately instructed to perform a total assessment, as well as a focus assessment, including the use of equipment that was formerly the domain of physicians only. The skill of performing a physical assessment must be practiced repeatedly to acquire expertise.

Examination Techniques

Inspection

Observe the client while facing him or her in the bed or chair (Figure 11-1 ■). Observe the client's skin color and texture; check for lesions and hair distribution. Look at overall body structure. If the client can be out of bed, observe gait and stance. Note all parts of the body as the examination proceeds. Inspection also evaluates verbal and behavioral responses and mental status.

Auscultation

Note: *Always* auscultate before palpating the abdomen to avoid distorting sounds.

Auscultation is accomplished by using a stethoscope to listen to breath, heart, and bowel sounds. Place the

FIGURE 11-1 Inspection.

FIGURE 11-2 Auscultation.

stethoscope on the client's bare skin to listen for the presence and characteristics of sound waves (Figure 11-2 ■). The bell of the stethoscope is held lightly against the skin to detect low-pitched sounds; the diaphragm is placed firmly on the skin to detect high-pitched sounds. Note variations in intensity, pitch, duration, and quality.

Palpation

Palpation is performed using fingers and hands to assess for organ size, organ displacement, and chest expansion.

It is also useful when assessing for masses and crepitus. Obtain information by pressing the hands and fingers to palpate. A light or deep palpation depends on the area being palpated. The palmar surface of fingers and finger pads are used to determine position of the organs, size, and consistency, fluid accumulation, pain, and masses (Figure 11-3 ■). The ulnar surface of the hand is used to distinguish temperature. The moisture and warmth of the skin can also be determined during palpation.

Percussion

Percussion is performed using fingers and a tapping motion to assess abnormalities of sound within the body. Sound waves are produced by using the fingers as a hammer. The interphalangeal joint of the middle finger is placed on the skin surface of the nondominant hand (Figure 11-4 ■). The tip of the middle finger of the dominant hand strikes the placed finger. Vibration is produced by the impact of the fingers striking against underlying tissue. Sound or tone of the vibration is determined by body area or organ percussed. Normal lung areas produce a resonance sound; liver sounds are dull, and a flat sound is heard over muscle. Ascites produces tympanic sounds near the umbilicus and dullness over the flanks. Percussion sounds can be distorted in clients who are obese.

FIGURE 11-3 Palpation.

FIGURE 11-4 Percussion.

Assessment: Focus (Shift)

A full, comprehensive physical assessment is completed upon admission. A focus assessment, also called a bedside or shift assessment, is performed at the beginning and ending of the shift and concentrates on vital assessment parameters. It tracks changes or problem-oriented assessments from shift-to-shift and should take no more than 5 minutes to complete. Several activities in the assessment can be completed at the same time. Usually, it is individualized to fit the client's condition, diagnosis, and level of acuity.

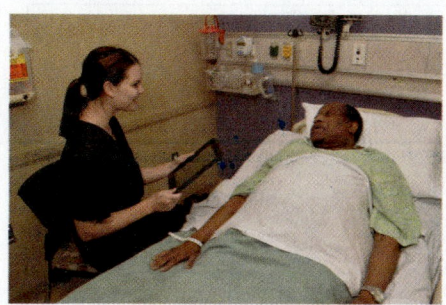

FIGURE 11-5 Step 1.

Step 1

Evaluate the client's level of consciousness, eye contact and responsiveness, color and texture of the skin, and any IVs, dressings, or visible drainage tubes (Figure 11-5 ■). Ask appropriate questions to determine orientation to time and place. Establish the nurse–client relationship at this time.

FIGURE 11-6 Step 2.

Step 2

Assess vital signs. While taking the client's pulse (Figure 11-6 ■), feel skin temperature and moisture. Check bilateral radial pulses. Observe for overall edema. Individualize the assessment; for example, with a neurologic condition, check the pupils.

FIGURE 11-7 Step 3.

Step 3

Remove client's gown or raise the gown. Be sure to provide for privacy. Use stethoscope to listen to heart sounds, apical pulse, and breath sounds bilaterally (Figure 11-7 ■). Observe breathing patterns, symmetry of chest movement, shape of chest, and depth of respirations. Check for skin turgor.

FIGURE 11-8 Step 4.

Step 4

Auscultate abdomen for bowel sounds (Figure 11-8 ■). Use palpation and percussion techniques only if appropriate to diagnosis. Palpate bladder if necessary (based on output). If catheter is in place, observe urinary output for color, odor, consistency, and amount.

FIGURE 11-9 Step 5.

Step 5

Assess lower extremities for warmth, color, moisture, and presence of pedal or popliteal pulses, muscle tone, and sensation (Figure 11-9 ■). Assess for pedal edema or general edema in the lower extremities. Check traction or casted areas for skin breakdown, alignment, and placement.

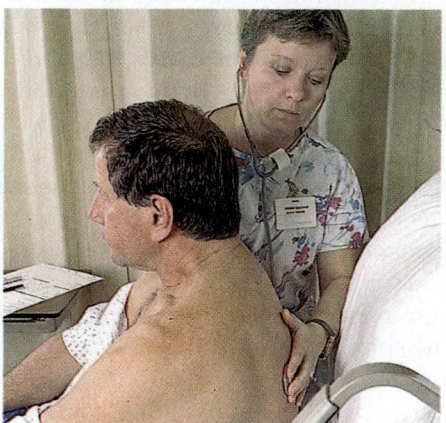

FIGURE 11-10 Step 6.

Step 6

Have client turn onto side or sit at edge of bed. Assess posterior lung fields and symmetry of chest movement with inspiration (Figure 11-10 ■). Assess skin for pressure areas, particularly coccyx and heels when client returns to side-lying position. Evaluate client's ability to move in bed.

Assessment of the Nervous System

Assessment of the nervous system includes the following:

- Level of Consciousness
  - Glasgow Coma Scale
  - Respiratory Assessment
  - Cranial Nerves
  - Spinal Nerves
- Pupil Assessment
- Motor Function Assessment
- Coordination Assessment
- Reflex Assessment
- Sensory Function
- Vital Signs

An understanding of the function of each lobe of the brain allows the nurse to be able to identify potential client problems when an injury occurs to that portion of the brain (Figure 11-11 ■).

The brain comprises three segments: the brainstem, cerebrum, and the cerebellum. There are 12 cranial nerves (Figure 11-12 ■), which are discussed later in this chapter, and 31 pairs of spinal nerves with dorsal and ventral roots.

The brainstem is divided into four sections: The *diencephalon* comprises the thalamus, which screens and relays sensory impulses to the cortex, and the hypothalamus, which regulates the autonomic nervous system, stress response, sleep, appetite, body temperature, water balance, and emotions. The *midbrain* is responsible for motor coordination and conjugate eye movements. The *pons* controls involuntary respiratory reflexes and contains projection tracts between the spinal cord, medulla, and brain. The *medulla* contains cardiac, respiratory, vomiting, and vasomotor centers. In addition, all afferent and efferent nerve tracts must pass between the spinal cord and brain through the medulla.

The cerebral hemispheres have an outer layer formed by cellular gray matter, called the cerebral cortex. The two

FIGURE 11-11 Lobes of the brain.

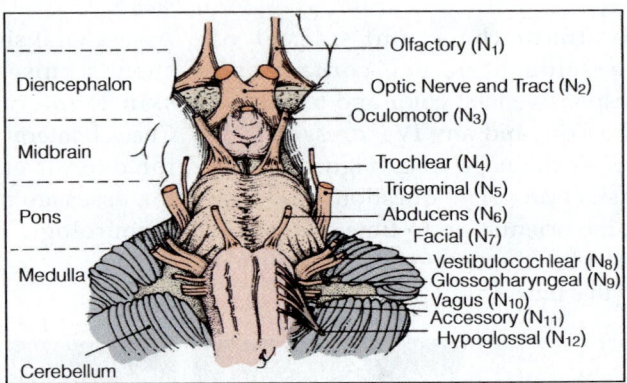

FIGURE 11-12 Brain segments and cranial nerves.

cerebral hemispheres are divided into four major lobes. The frontal lobe controls emotions, judgments, motor function, and the motor speech area. The parietal lobe integrates general sensations; interprets pain, touch, and temperature; and governs discrimination. The temporal lobe contains the auditory center and sensory speech center. The occipital lobe controls the visual area. The cerebellum coordinates muscle movement, posture, equilibrium, and muscle tone.

The 12 cranial nerves are summarized in Table 11-1 ■. The 2nd through 12th nerves arise from the brainstem. The cranial nerves are 12 pairs of parasympathetic nerves with their nuclei along the brainstem.

Table 11-1 Cranial Nerves and Their Function

Cranial Nerve	Function	Testing Cranial Nerves
I Olfactory	Sensory nerve	Recognizes odor in each nostril separately (e.g., coffee)
II Optic	Sensory nerve: conducts sensory information from the retina	Demonstrates visual acuity: can read newsprint
III Oculomotor	Motor nerve: controls four of the six extraocular muscles; raises eyelid and controls the constrictor pupillae and ciliary muscles of the eyeball	Responds to light: pupils constrict; moves eyes medially; elevates upper eyelid
IV Trochlear	Motor nerve: controls the superior oblique eye muscle	Move eyes to the right, up then down, and to the left
V Trigeminal	Mixed nerve with three sensory branches and one motor branch: the ophthalmic branch supplies the corneal reflex	Demonstrates normal facial sensation; clenches teeth with no lateral jaw deviation; blinks as wisp is touched to cornea
VI Abducens	Motor nerve: controls the lateral rectus muscle of the eye	Moves eyes laterally

Table 11-1 Cranial Nerves and Their Function *(continued)*

Cranial Nerve	Function	Testing Cranial Nerves
VII Facial	Mixed nerve: sensory supply to anterior tongue, motor supply to glands of nose, palate lacrimal submaxillary, and sublingual; motor branch supplies hyoid elevators and muscles of expression and closes eyelid	Elevates eyebrows; puffs cheeks; recognizes tastes (sugar, salt)
VIII Acoustic	Sensory nerve with two divisions: hearing and semicircular canals	Hears whisper separately with each ear
IX Glossopharyngeal	Mixed nerve: motor innervates parotid gland; sensory innervates auditory tube and posterior portion of taste buds	Demonstrates gag reflex to tongue blade when touched to back of tongue
X Vagus	Mixed nerve: motor branches to the pharyngeal and laryngeal muscles and to the viscera of the thorax and abdomen; sensory portion supplies the pinna of the ear, thoracic, and abdominal viscera	Same as IX
XI Accessory	Motor nerve: innervates the sternocleidomastoid and trapezius muscles	Shrugs shoulders
XII Hypoglossal	Motor nerve: controls tongue muscles	Sticks tongue out in midline without deviation

The neurologic examination begins with the initial contact with the client. Evaluation of movement, verbal responses, and sensation is carried out throughout the examination. In addition, functions of the cerebrum, cerebellum, cranial nerves, spinal cord, and peripheral nerves are assessed. The level of consciousness is the most sensitive and reliable index of cerebral function (Table 11-2 ■).

Table 11-2 Glasgow Coma Scale

A. Motor response	Points
1. Obeys a simple command	6
2. Localizes painful stimuli; attempts to remove offending stimulus; lack of obedience	5
3. Withdrawn—moves purposelessly in response to pain	4
4. Abnormal flexion—decorticate posturing	3
5. Extensor response—decerebrate posturing	2
6. No motor response to pain	1
B. Verbal response	**Points**
1. Oriented—to time, place, and person	5
2. Confused conversation; disorientation in *one* or more spheres	4
3. Inappropriate or disorganized use of words (cursing); lack of sustained conversation	3
4. Responds with incomprehensible sounds	2
5. No verbal response (record T if an endotracheal or tracheostomy tube is in place)	1
C. Eye opening	**Points**
1. Spontaneous when an individual approaches	4
2. In response to speech	3
3. Only in response to pain	2
4. Eyes do not open, even to painful stimuli	1

Note: This scale is a tool for assessing a client's response to stimuli. Scores range from 3 (deep coma) to 15 (normal). Add numbers to get a total score.

Assessment: Neurologic

Assessment	Normal Responses	Abnormal Responses
Level of Consciousness		
Apply **Glasgow Coma Scale** (see Table 11-2)	A score of 15 is evaluated as normal	A score under 15 is not normal; a comatose client is 7 or less
Evaluate **verbal responses and orientation**	Alert	Drowsy
If client seems awake and alert but does not respond properly, check to see if client is blind, deaf, or speaks another language	Mood appropriate to situation	Difficult to awaken
	Responds to verbal command	Unable to give date, month, place
	Answers questions appropriately	Irritable
	Speaks clearly	Memory defect
	Oriented to time, person, place, and purpose	Difficulty finding words
	Recent and remote memory intact	Does not recognize family
		Does not respond to own name
Observe and test symmetry of **motor responses** on both sides of body	Eyes open	Eyes closed
	Follows command to stick out tongue, squeeze fingers, move extremities	Does not follow directions to stick out tongue, squeeze fingers, or move extremities
Exert pressure on nailbed with pen	Responds to painful stimuli by reaching out or trying to stop pressure	Does not localize or withdraw from painful stimuli or withdraws abnormally
Apply pressure to supraorbital ridge		Assumes *decorticate posturing* (Figure 11-13 ■ top) (legs extended; feet extended with plantar flexion; arms internally rotated and flexed on chest): may be due to lesion of corticospinal tract near cerebral hemisphere
Pinch Achilles tendon		Assumes *decerebrate posturing* (see Figure 11-13 bottom) (arms stiffly extended and hands turned outward and flexed; legs extended with plantar flexion): may be due to lesion in diencephalon, pons, or midbrain
Test each side independently		Assumes *flaccid posturing* (no motor response): may be due to extreme brain injury to motor area of brain
		Involuntary movements Choreiform (jerky and quick): present in Sydenham chorea
		Athetoid (twisting and slow): present in cerebral palsy
		Tremors: hyperthyroidism, cerebellar ataxia, parkinsonism
		Spasms: cord-injured clients
		Seizures: brain injury, heat stroke, electrolyte imbalance
		Asterixis: metabolic encephalopathy due to liver or kidney failure

Decorticate posturing—abnormal flexor posturing

Decerebrate posturing–abnormal extensor posturing

FIGURE 11-13 Decorticate posturing–abnormal flexor posturing. Decerebrate posturing–abnormal extensor posturing.

Note: In the charts throughout this chapter, the information in the third column provides abnormal responses or variations from normal.

Assessment	Normal Responses	Abnormal Responses

Respiratory Assessment

Clients with neurologic damage are at risk for respiratory complications

Respirations are normal
Oxygen levels are normal

Respiratory complications may include traumatic or spinal cord injury

Cranial Nerves

See Table 11-1 for specific functions and testing.
Spinal Nerves (Figure 11-14 ■)
Thirty-one pairs of peripheral nerves that originate on the spinal cord from anterior roots. Each pair of spinal nerves is related to a specific region of the body.

Cervical nerves C_1 - C_8

Thoracic nerves T_1 - T_{12}

Lumbar nerves L_1 - L_5

Sacral nerves S_1 - S_5

FIGURE 11-14 Spinal nerves.

Pupil Assessment

Observe **pupils** using penlight and pupil gauge or an automated pupillometer
Size of pupils

Diameter: 1.5–6 mm

Unilateral dilation: sign of third cranial nerve involvement
Bilateral dilation: sign of upper brainstem damage
Unilateral dilation and nonreactive: sign of increased intracranial pressure (ICP) or ipsilateral oculomotor nerve (III) compression from tumor or injury

Shape of pupils

Round and midposition

Midposition and fixed: sign of midbrain involvement
Pinpoint and fixed: sign of pontine involvement or opiate effect

Equality of pupils

Equal

Unequal: sign that parasympathetic and sympathetic nervous systems are not in synchronization

(continued)

Assessment: Neurologic *(continued)*

Assessment	Normal Responses	Abnormal Responses
Observe **reaction to light** by using penlight in darkened room (Figure 11-15 ■)	Pupil constricts promptly	Sluggish reaction or failure to react to light: early warning of deteriorating condition or elevated ICP

FIGURE 11-15 Move light toward client's eye from side position.

Assessment	Normal Responses	Abnormal Responses
Open eyelid being tested; cover opposite eye		Light reflex is the most important sign differentiating structural (cranial involvement) from metabolic coma due to extracranial cause (e.g., diabetic coma), which does not alter light reflex
Observe consensual **light reflex** Hold both eyelids open Shine light into one eye only Observe opposite eye	Both pupils constrict	Pupil does not constrict: sign that connection between brainstem and pupils is not intact
Check **accommodation** (ability of lens to adjust to objects at varying distances)	Lens can adjust	When the lens thickens (often in the fifth decade of life) accommodation can be limited

Motor Function Assessment

Assessment	Normal Responses	Abnormal Responses
Assess bilateral **muscle strength** Test hand grip by asking client to squeeze your fingers (Figure11-16 ■) Rate muscle strength from 0 to 5, with 0 indicating no muscle contraction and 5 (normal) indicating full range of motion against gravity with full resistance	Muscle strength is equal bilaterally	Absent or weak muscle function on one side may be sign of hemiplegia (paralysis of one side of the body); or hemiparesis (weakness on one side); paraplegia (paralysis of the legs or lower part of the body); tetraplegia or quadriplegia (paralysis of arms and legs)
Test arm strength by asking client to close eyes and hold arms out in front with palms up	Maintains position for 20–30 seconds	Cannot maintain position—downdrifts one extremity

FIGURE 11-16 Test client's hand grip.

Assessment	Normal Responses	Abnormal Responses
Muscle Grading Scale		
Muscle Graduations	**Description**	
5—Normal	Complete range of motion against gravity with full resistance	
4—Good	Complete range of motion against gravity with some resistance	
3—Fair	Complete range of motion against gravity	
2—Poor	Complete range of motion with gravity eliminated	
1—Trace	Evidence of slight contractility, no joint motion	
0—Zero	No evidence of contractility	
Assess **flexion** and **extension** strength in extremities Stand in front of client, place your hand in front of client, and ask client to push your hand away Place your hand on client's forearm and ask client to pull arm upward	Equal response in both arms	Unequal response in arms Asymmetrical response Inability to perform movements
Position client's leg with knee flexed and foot resting on bed; as you try to extend leg, ask client to keep foot down Place one hand on client's knee and one hand on client's ankle; ask client to straighten leg as you apply resistant force to knee and ankle	Equal response in both legs	Unequal response in legs
Assess **muscle tone** Flex and extend client's upper extremities to assess how well client resists your movements Flex and extend client's lower extremities to assess resistance	Client resistance is apparent	Increased resistance: sign of increased muscle tone from muscle rigidity or spasticity in upper motor neuron (UMN) lesions; for example, as with cerebrovascular accident (CVA) and parkinsonism Decreased resistance to leg extension and arm flexion in UMN lesion (CVA) Weakness in lower motor neuron (LMN) and cerebellar lesion
Coordination Assessment		
Hand coordination		
Ask client to pat both thighs as rapidly as possible Ask client to turn hands over and back in quick succession Ask client to touch thumb with each finger in rapid succession—repeat with other hand	Client able to perform coordinated movements on request: hand, foot, hand and leg positioning	Uncoordinated movements: may be due to cerebellum or basal ganglia involvement Clumsy movement with cerebellar involvement

(continued)

Assessment: Neurologic *(continued)*

Assessment	Normal Responses	Abnormal Responses
Foot coordination Place your hands close to client's feet Ask client to tap your hands alternately with the balls of feet		
Hand positioning coordination With client's eyes open, extend your hand in front of client's face Ask client to touch nose with index finger several times in rapid succession Repeat test with client's eyes closed		Tremor as nose is approached indicates cerebellar involvement Inability to perform task with eyes closed: may be due to loss of positioning sense
Leg positioning coordination Ask client to put heel on opposite knee and to slide heel down leg to foot		

Reflex Assessment

Blink reflex Hold client's eyelid open Approach client's eye unexpectedly from side of head with a wisp of sterile cotton Complete corneal touch	Eyes close immediately	Absence of blink response; eyelid continuously in open position: due to fifth or seventh cranial nerve (pons) involvement; blindness
Gag and swallow reflex Open client's mouth and hold tongue down with tongue blade Touch back of pharynx on each side with applicator stick	Gag and swallow reflex present	Absence of gag and swallow reflex; inability to swallow food or liquid: due to 9th or 10th cranial nerve (medulla) involvement
Plantar reflex (Figure 11-17 ■) Run top of pen along outer lateral aspect from heel to little toe of client's foot Continue tracing a line across ball of foot toward great toe	Toes are pointed down (Figure 11-18 ■)	Babinski response: great toe dorsiflexes; other toes fan on foot of paralyzed side in CVA, and bilaterally in spinal cord injury (SCI) (Figure 11-19 ■)

FIGURE 11-17 Testing plantar reflex.

FIGURE 11-18 Normal plantar reflex.

FIGURE 11-19 Babinski response (abnormal).

Deep tendon reflex Ask client to relax Position limb to be assessed so that muscle is somewhat stretched Using reflex hammer, strike tendon quickly Assess according to scale	Biceps reflex: flexion at elbow and contracting of biceps muscle Triceps reflex: extension at elbow and contraction of triceps muscle Patellar reflex: extension of knee and contraction of quadriceps	Absent or diminished: sign of cervical cord (C–5 or C–6) involvement Absent or diminished: C–7 or C–8 cord involvement Absent or diminished: L2–3 or L3–4 cord involvement

Assessment	Normal Responses	Abnormal Responses
Grading Scale 4+ Hyperactive or exaggerated 3+ More brisk than usual but not indicative of disease state 2+ Average or normal 1+ Slightly diminished, low normal 0 No response		Indicates upper motor neuron (UMN) lesion or SCI Seen with lower motor neuron (LMN) lesion
Sensory Function Assess **superficial sensations**		
Pain Ask client to close eyes Stroke or touch skin with cotton-tipped applicator, alternating cotton tip with wooden end Ask client to distinguish sharp and dull pain	Ability to distinguish between sharp and dull sensations	Alterations in pain or temperature sensations: indicate lesion in posterior horn of spinal cord or spinothalamic tract of cord
Temperature Fill two test tubes with water, one hot, one cold Ask client to close eyes and touch client's skin with test tubes	Ability to distinguish between hot and cold	
Touch Ask client to close eyes Stroke cotton wisp over client's skin	Ability to identify light touch—equal bilaterally	Anesthesia = loss of light touch Analgesia = absence of sense of pain Hypoalgesia = decreased pain sensation Hyperalgesia = exaggerated sensitivity to pin prick (pain)
Positioning Ask client to close eyes Grasp client's finger with your thumb and index finger Move client's finger up and down Ask client to identify direction finger is moving. Repeat with great toe.	Ability to identify position or mimic position with other hand	Inability to determine direction of movement: may be due to posterior column or peripheral nerve disease
Vital Signs Temperature Apical/radial pulses Respiration Blood pressure		
Assess **temperature** If client is semiresponsive or nonresponsive, take rectal, axillary, or tympanic temperature If rectal temperature is contraindicated or there are signs of increased ICP, use alternate method.	Ability to maintain normal body temperature (approximately 98.6°F, or 37°C)	Inability to maintain normal temperature: may be due to damage to hypothalamus No sweating below level of injury; due to spinal cord injury Hypothermia

(continued)

Assessment: Neurologic (continued)

Assessment	Normal Responses	Abnormal Responses
Assess **apical** and **radial pulses** (Figure 11-20 ■) Note character of pulses Count heart rate Count radial pulse rate **FIGURE 11-20** Assess client's radial and apical pulse.	Regular rhythm Rate 60–100 beats/min Apical and radial rates are equal	Fast heart rate due to decreased blood volume, arrhythmia, heart failure, fever, medulla dysfunction Irregular rhythm with premature beats due to hypoxia, cardiac irritability, or electrolyte imbalance Pulse deficit due to premature beats or ineffectual cardiac contraction.
Assess **respiration** Assess rate and pattern of breathing	Regular rate: 12–20 breaths per minute	Cheyne-Stokes (rhythmic increase in depth of breathing followed by period of apnea) may be due to deep cerebral or cerebellar lesion or condition altering cerebral perfusion Central neurogenic (sustained) hyperventilation due to upper brainstem involvement Ataxic (Biot) breathing unpredictably irregular, due to lower brainstem involvement
Monitor arterial blood gases if signs of respiratory imbalances occur	pH: 7.35–7.45 PCO_2: 35–45 mm Hg HCO_3^-: 22–26 mEq/L	Alterations in pH and PCO_2 values indicate respiratory imbalances: pH below 7.35 and PCO_2 above 45: sign of respiratory acidosis (hypoventilation) pH above 7.45 and PCO_2 below 35: sign of respiratory alkalosis (hyperventilation) HCO_3^- above 26 indicates metabolic compensation for chronic respiratory acidosis (hypoventilation)
Assess **blood pressure** Position neurologic clients in low to semi-Fowler position	Normal pressure (range 120/80); see Box 11-1 ■ for Korotkoff sounds and Box 11-2 ■ for blood pressure classification	Systolic blood pressure rises with diastolic pressure remaining the same (widening pulse pressure): sign of increased intracranial pressure Blood pressure over 140/90 is a sign of stage 1 hypertension Blood pressure below 90/60 is a sign of hypotension

Box 11-1 KOROTKOFF SOUND PHASES FOR BLOOD PRESSURE

Note: See also Chapter 10, Vital Signs.

Phase I: The pressure level at which the first faint, clear tapping sounds are heard. The sounds gradually increase in intensity as the cuff is deflated. This phase coincides with the reappearance of a palpable pulse (systolic sound).

Phase II: That time during cuff deflation when a murmur or swishing sounds are heard.

Phase III: The period during which sounds are crisper and increase in intensity.

Phase IV: That time when a distinct, abrupt, muffling of sound (usually of a soft, blowing quality) is heard (diastolic sound in children or physically active adults).

Phase V: That pressure level when the last sound is heard and after which all sound disappears (second diastolic sound).

Box 11-2 BLOOD PRESSURE CLASSIFICATION

Blood Pressure	Systolic	Diastolic
Normal	<120	<80
Pre high blood pressure	120–139	80–89
Stage I high blood pressure	140–159	90–99
Stage II high blood pressure	160 and higher	100 and higher

Source: National Center for Health Statistics (2011)

Assessment of the Head and Neck

Assessment of the head and neck often referred to as HEENT, includes examining the head for gross abnormalities; in addition to an eye, ear, and nose assessment. The mouth assessment includes lips, buccal cavity, and throat. Lastly, the neck is examined to include range of motion, tenderness, lymphadenopathy, and thyroid assessment.

The names of the regions of the head are derived from the bones that form the skull (Figure 11-21 ■). Knowing the names of the bones and regions of the skull can help when describing the location of physical findings.

The size and shape of the head should be noted, as well as the placement of the eyes and facial structures. Note any lesions or discharge from the ears. If there are any lesions of the lips or mouth, assess further.

When palpating the neck, note the head position and neck muscles. Using your fingers, palpate the lymph nodes in the neck to determine swelling. Check the thyroid gland in the front of the neck, and if enlarged, note that this condition requires further assessment.

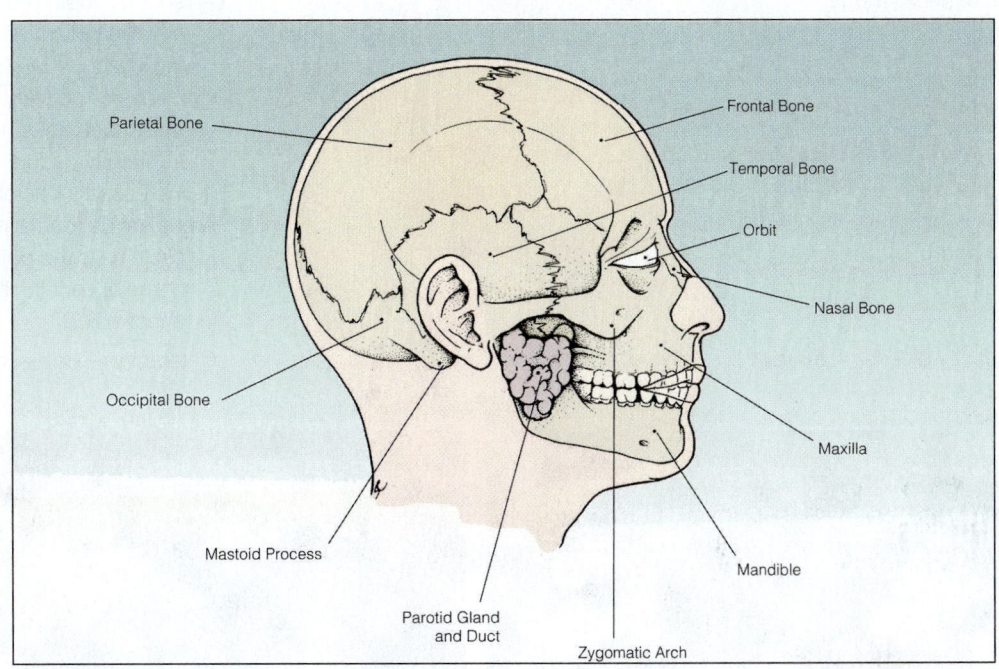

FIGURE 11-21 Bones that form the skull.

Assessment: Head and Neck

Assessment	Normal Responses	Abnormal Responses
Eye Assessment		
Note **visual acuity** by observing client performance of activities of daily living	Adequate performance of activities of daily living	Age-related macular degeneration (AMD)
Factors influencing visual acuity include client's previous status and age	Appropriate responses to environment	Hyperopia (farsightedness)
Note exact location, size, and color of any **external lesions** (Figure 11-22 ■)	No external lesions	Myopia (nearsightedness)
Palpate for mobility and firmness		Cataract (opacification of the lens)
		Enucleation (loss of an eye): may have prosthesis in place
		Circumocular ecchymosis: may be sign of basal skull fracture
		Xanthelasma (small, yellowish, well-circumscribed plaques): may appear on eyelids of clients with lipid disorders. *Example*: atherosclerosis

FIGURE 11-22 Anatomy of the eye.

Assessment	Normal Responses	Abnormal Responses
Note **equality of eyelid movement**	Eyelids are equal in movement	Ptosis (paralytic drooping of the upper eyelid)
Note color, consistency, amount, and origin of **discharge** from eyes	No discharge	Sty or hordeolum
Note **internal lesions**	No internal lesions	Thick white discharge; may be due to conjunctivitis
Assess differences between **pupil size and reaction** (Figure 11-23 ■)	Both pupils are the same size	Conjunctival or ciliary injection (dilatation of the blood vessels)
Note presence of hemorrhage		Anisocoria (indicates unequal pupil size): may be indicative of neurologic trauma or deficit
		Corneal edema (very soft, movable mass that looks like raw egg white): frequently occurs in clients who have increased intracranial pressure
		Arcus senilis (partial or complete whitish circle near the outer edge of the cornea); usually due to aging; does not affect vision
Observe for opacity of lens—**cataract** (Figure11-24 ■)	No opacity noted	Cataract present—one or both eyes

FIGURE 11-23 Assess pupil size and reaction.

FIGURE 11-24 Cataract: Opacity of the crystalline lens.

Assessment	Normal Responses	Abnormal Responses
Ear Assessment		

Note **auditory acuity** (Figure 11-25 ■) by asking client to indicate if he or she hears normal sounds as you make them

Adequate responses to normal sounds
Auditory changes due to aging

Deafness or impaired hearing; excess cerumen in auditory canal
Abnormal sounds in the ears (ringing or buzzing) may be caused by ototoxic drugs

FIGURE 11-25 Anatomy of the tympanic membrane (ear drum).

Note exact size, color, and location of any **external** lesions
Palpate lesions for mobility and firmness

No external lesions

Battle sign (ecchymosis behind the ear): may be sign of basilar skull fracture

Examine tympanic membrane using an otoscope (Figure 11-26 ■)

Membrane intact, flat, gray, with no scarring

White patches show prior infections: yellow or red patches may be infection of middle ear
Bulging membrane may indicate increased pressure in middle ear
Depressed membrane may indicate vacuum due to blocked eustachian tube.

FIGURE 11-26 Technique for positioning and inserting an otoscope into ear before viewing.

Note color, quantity, and consistency of any **discharge** from the ears
Test clear fluid for glucose using a Labstix

No discharge
Wax buildup
Glucose test negative

Redness, swelling, and pain may be signs of otitis externa
Cerebrospinal fluid (CSF) leak: may be due to head injury. If drainage is blood and CSF, it will develop a "halo" (Figure 11-27 ■) with a reddish area in the center surrounded by a whitish circle if placed on white material
Perforation of tympanic membrane: serosanguineous or purulent drainage
Glucose test of clear drainage is positive if CSF

Red blood

Cerebrospinal fluid

FIGURE 11-27 "Halo" sign.

(continued)

Assessment: Head and Neck (continued)

Assessment	Normal Responses	Abnormal Responses
Nose Assessment		
Note any **structural changes** in the nose by observing client breathing Gently occlude one nostril at a time; ask client to breathe through the nonoccluded nostril	Regular breathing with mouth closed Breathing through nonoccluded nostril	Breathing through the mouth only: furuncles may occlude breathing Obstruction in the nose due to deviated nasal septum, swelling of the nasal turbinates, or excessive mucus secretions
Note color, quantity, and consistency of any **discharge** from the nose	Minimal discharge	Cerebrospinal fluid leak (fluid tests positive for glucose with test strip) Copious, watery-to-thick, mucopurulent discharge: may be due to acute rhinitis Excessive buildup of mucous secretions
Mouth and Lip Assessment		
Note size, color, and location of any **external lesions** Palpate for mobility and firmness	No external lesions	Dehydrated mouth or lips Fissures Pressure sores Necrosis
Note size, color, and location of any **internal lesions** Palpate for mobility and firmness	No internal lesions	Candidiasis (a fungal infection indicated by adherent, white patches)
Neck Assessment		
Note any **lesion or swelling** in the neck (Figure 11-28 ■) Ask client to relax and flex neck slightly Palpate the neck, using the pads of your fingers to move the skin and underlying tissues	Occasional small, mobile, discrete, nontender lymph nodes	Enlarged tender immobile nodes

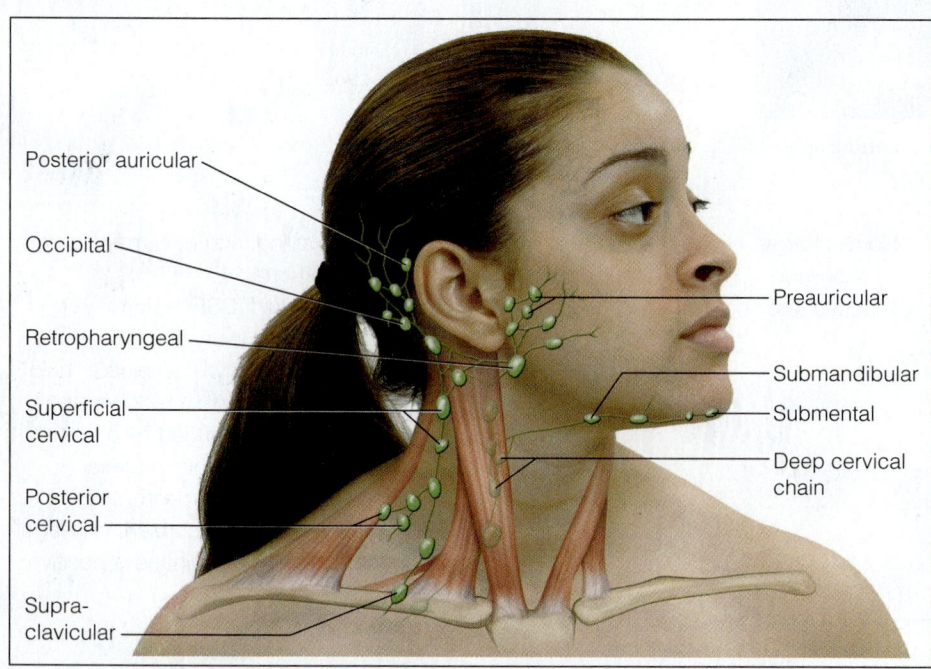

Posterior auricular
Occipital
Retropharyngeal
Superficial cervical
Posterior cervical
Supra-clavicular
Preauricular
Submandibular
Submental
Deep cervical chain

FIGURE 11-28 Lymph nodes in the head and neck.

Assessment of the Skin and Nails

The skin is the body's first line of defense against disease and injury. It is made up of three layers: the epidermis, the dermis, and the subcutaneous tissues (Figure 11-29 ■).

The epidermis is divided into two avascular, or bloodless, layers: an outer layer that consists of dead keratinized cells and an inner layer that consists of live cells where keratin and melanin are formed. The dermis contains blood vessels, connective tissue, sebaceous glands, and some of the hair follicles. The subcutaneous tissues contain the remainder of the hair follicles, fat, and the sweat glands.

Hair, nails, sweat glands, and sebaceous glands are appendages of the skin. There are two types of sweat glands: eccrine and apocrine. Eccrine glands are distributed over most of the body except for the palms and soles. These glands help control body temperature through their sweat production. The apocrine glands are found mainly in the axillary and genital areas and are stimulated by

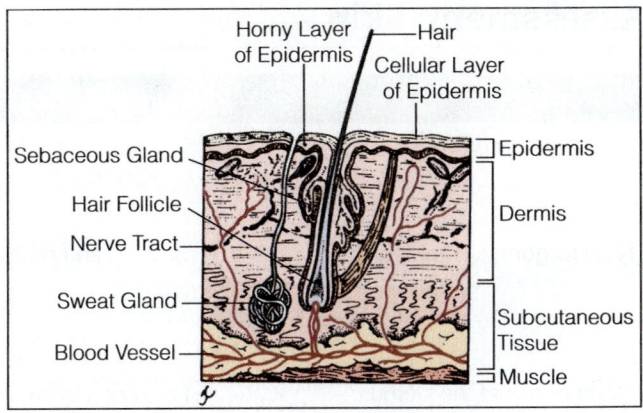

FIGURE 11-29 Anatomy of the skin.

emotional stress. Bacterial decomposition by apocrine sweat glands causes adult body odor.

The nail body is made up of dead keratinized cells. Nail production occurs at the nail root. Underlying vessels give the nail its pink color.

Assessment: Skin

Assessment	Normal Responses	Abnormal Responses
Skin Assessment		
Note **color** of the skin by assessing the oral mucous membranes, the conjunctiva, and the nailbeds	Pink, tan, or brown, depending on the client's basic skin color (Figure 11-30 ■) Oral mucous membrane: moist, pink Conjunctiva: moist, pink Nailbeds: pink	Pallor (decrease in color) *Example*: anemia from acute blood loss (hemorrhage), renal failure, dietary deficiencies, or arterial insufficiency Jaundice (icterus): due to the presence of conjugated or unconjugated bilirubin in the blood and tissues; appears most frequently in the face and sclerae; seen best under natural light *Example*: liver disease Cyanosis (blue, blue-gray, or purple discoloration of the skin and mucous membranes): caused by hypoxia, a result of an increased amount of reduced hemoglobin Peripheral: seen in nailbeds and earlobes *Example*: vasoconstriction, venous insufficiency Central: seen in nailbeds, lips (circumoral), and oral mucosa Erythema (redness of the skin): caused by capillary congestion; occurs with inflammation or infection; usually a local finding

FIGURE 11-30 Check quality of the skin.

(continued)

Assessment: Skin *(continued)*

Assessment	Normal Responses	Abnormal Responses
Note **pigmentation**	Discolored spots may be due to normal aging	Hyperpigmentation (especially in skin creases) *Example:* use of oral contraceptives, pregnancy, Addison disease, and hyperthyroidism
Note **turgor** and **mobility**	Smooth and elastic	Tight or stretched and difficult to move: due to local or generalized edema Wrinkled: due to dehydration or caused by rapid weight loss
Pinch skin over the sternum If the fold persists, skin turgor is poor	Resilient and supple	Thin and translucent (parchment) *Example:* chronic steroid use Thin, shiny, and smooth with alopecia on lower extremities *Example:* chronic arterial insufficiency
Assess for **edema** (Figure 11-31 ■) Press finger firmly for 5 seconds into skin on top of foot or inner ankle bone	Resilient and no depression remains after pressure released	Pitting edema: excess interstitial fluid (Figure 11-32 ■) *Example:* congestive heart failure, renal failure, cirrhosis of the liver, venous stasis

FIGURE 11-31 Check client for edema.

FIGURE 11-32 Grading pitting edema.

Note **moistness** and **temperature** of the skin	Warm and dry	Warm (hot) and moist due to temperature elevation Cool and moist (cold and clammy): may be due to shock states Abnormally dry: may be due to dehydration, decreased sebaceous gland secretions, or the excessive use of soap
Assess for **sensation**—response to external stimuli	Feels touch, sensitive to heat and cold and pressure	Absence of touch or pain sensation *Example:* spinal cord injury or nerve damage Diminished heat and cold sensation *Example:* peripheral vascular disease Itching and tingling *Example:* peripheral vascular disease, peripheral neuropathy, allergy
Note **lesions** on the skin Physical characteristics include color, elevation, shape, mobility, and contents	No lesions present	Macules (flat localized changes in color) *Example:* petechiae, first-degree burns, purpura Papules, plaques, nodules (solid, elevated, varying in size) *Example:* psoriasis, xanthomas Cancerous lesions *Examples:* Basal cell epithelioma— small, smooth papule with atrophic center Melanoma—pigmented tumor; may arise from a blue-black mole

Assessment	Normal Responses	Abnormal Responses
		Squamous cell—macules with indistinct margins; surface may be crusted
		Wheals (elevated, circumscribed, transient)
		Example: urticaria, insect bites
		Vesicles and bullae (clear, fluid-filled pockets between skin layers)
		Example: second-degree burns
		Pustules (vesicles or bullae filled with purulent exudate)
		Example: furuncles, acne
		In the obese client it is essential to examine skin folds; under the breast, panniculus and perineal areas.
Nail Assessment		
Note condition of the nails	Smooth transparent layer with white crescent called a lunula	Clubbing occurs with hypoxia or decreased tissue perfusion, cirrhosis, and other conditions such as fungal infections.
		Spoon-shaped nails may indicate iron deficiency.
		Thickened nails may relate to circulatory disorder.
		Cracked, split, or broken nails may result from nutrient deficiencies.

Assessment of the Chest, Lungs, and Heart

The chest, or thorax area, extends from the base of the neck to the diaphragm. The overall shape of the thorax should be elliptical, although deformities such as barrel chest, pigeon chest, or funnel chest do occur. Total assessment includes the external aspect: The nurse should observe for movement, posture, shape, and symmetry, especially of the breast and axilla area, and the internal components of the lungs and the heart.

The lungs anteriorly extend from 2 to 4 cm above the inner third of the clavicle to the eighth rib at the midaxillary line and the sixth rib at the midclavicular line (Figure 11-33 ■).

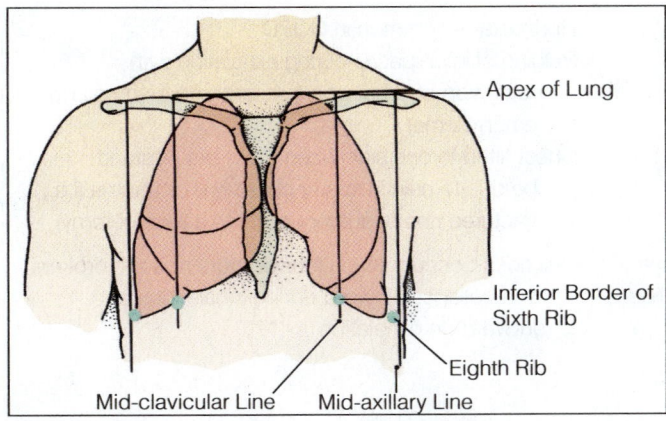

FIGURE 11-33 Anterior anatomical relationship of lungs to skeletal structure.

Apex of Lung

Inferior Border of Sixth Rib

Eighth Rib

Mid-clavicular Line   Mid-axillary Line

Posteriorly the lungs extend from the third thoracic spinous process and descend to the 10th process or, on deep inspiration, to the 12th process.

Chest assessment begins with inspection, proceeds to palpation, and then to auscultation. Breath sounds of clients differ due to the depth of breathing, underlying disease, or obesity. Because of these differences, it is difficult to compare the breath sounds of one client with another. The basic principle to remember when auscultating the lungs is to do a comparison between the right and left lung. To make these comparisons, begin auscultating at the apices of one lung, alternating sides as you work down through both lungs. By comparing similar areas in both lungs, you can note changes and determine causes for these changes more easily.

Examination of the chest usually proceeds from posterior to anterior. For posterior assessment of the lungs, place the client in an upright sitting position with shoulders pulled forward. For anterior assessment, the client can be sitting or supine (especially if female). If the client is lying on his or her side, the lung closest to the bed is mechanically compressed, and true lung sounds cannot be heard.

Ask the client to breathe a little deeper than usual through the mouth. Breathing through the nose produces extra sounds that mask true lung sounds.

The heart is located directly behind the sternum, with the left ventricle projecting into the left chest. The heart is usually thought to be in the left chest for two reasons: the left ventricle produces the most movement (ventricular contraction), and three of the valve sound areas are located to the left of the sternum.

The action of the heart should be assessed both proximally and distally. Proximal assessment involves evaluating heart sounds, heart rate, and rhythm to obtain information about the mechanical activity of the heart. Distal assessment involves evaluating the peripheral pulses to obtain information about the effectiveness of the heart's pumping action.

One method for assessing heart sounds is to start at the aortic area, moving slowly across to the pulmonic area, down to Erb point and the tricuspid area, and over to the mitral area. This same general progression can also be used in reverse, starting at the mitral area and progressing up to the aortic area. Most clinicians begin the assessment at the mitral area, which is the point of maximum impulse where the apical pulse is the loudest. When assessing heart sounds in the morbidly obese client, adipose tissue makes auscultation difficult. Steps that can be taken are minimizing extraneous noises and having the client lie on his or her left side, which brings the heart closer to the chest wall.

The most important point to remember in heart assessment is to use the same method every time, repeating the same steps in the same sequence. By using one systematic approach, you learn how to compare the different sounds more easily and not neglect any areas of the chest.

Breast assessment should include observing for lumps, drainage, dimpling of breast tissue, and presence of asymmetry. The client should also be asked if she has noted any recent changes.

Assessment: Chest, Lungs, and Heart

Assessment	Normal Responses	Abnormal Responses
Chest Assessment		
Note respiratory rate—increase may be due to fever, pain, anxiety	A normal or increased rate does not assume a normal tidal volume	Clients may have an increased rate to compensate for decreased tidal volume, but the resultant minute volume is still not sufficient. (Normal minute volume is 6–8 L/min.) Increased depth: due to neurologic disease, intracranial pressure (ICP) from trauma, drug overdose, exertion, fear, or anxiety Decreased depth: due to neurologic disease, ICP from trauma, drug overdose, respiratory disease, pneumothorax, or pain Other abnormal breathing patterns (Table 11-3 ■)
Note the **general appearance** of the chest and movement when client breathes	Straight spine, level shoulders	Breathes sitting forward with arms on pillows or overbed table (present with emphysema)
	Relaxed breathing; rib cage moves symmetrically with respirations	Uses accessory muscles (i.e., scalene, trapezius, sternocleidomastoid, pectoralis, or intercostal)
Note **shape of chest**	Anterior–posterior dimension is half of transverse dimension	Anterior–posterior dimension increased in emphysema (barrel chest) Deformities such as scoliosis (lateral curvature), kyphosis (forward curvature), or kyphoscoliosis
Note **position of ribs**	Ribs slant downward	Horizontal is common in COPD Bulging of interspaces during exhalation with retraction on inhalation (present with asthma and emphysema) Chest tilted to one side when client sits or stands: may be due to pain in ribs or chest wall or trauma (i.e., fractured ribs or surgery such as a thoracotomy)
Measure **chest excursion** for range and symmetry: place hands parallel to 10th rib (under scapulae) with thumbs beside spine. (Figure 11-34 ■) Bunch up fold of skin pushing thumbs medially. Ask client to inhale.	On inhalation, the thumbs move equidistant away from midline indicating equal expansion	Flail chest: occurs when four or more ribs are broken; area collapses inward during inhalations and outward on exhalation

Assessment	Normal Responses	Abnormal Responses
For anterior assessment, place hands over lower thorax, push medially, then have client inhale. Note equidistant lateral movement of hands.	 **FIGURE 11-34** Measure chest excursion while client takes deep breath.	Asymmetrical (unequal) chest expansion occurs with pneumothorax, fractured ribs, atelectasis, or when client's chest splints due to pain

Tactile and Vocal Fremitus

Tactile fremitus (vibrations felt on surface of chest as sound passes through tissue) Palpate upper thorax and ask client to say "ninety-nine"; vibrations detected as hands move down thorax (Figure 11-35 ■)	Varied because it depends on thickness of chest wall **FIGURE 11-35** Palpation for tactile fremitus.	Decreased sounds: obesity, emphysema, pneumothorax, and possible Increased sounds: heard when lung is filled with fluid-consolidation (pneumonia) or tumors Absent sounds: atelectasis or pleural effusion Asymmetric sounds: abnormal Normal sounds: found with bronchitis or pulmonary edema

Lung/Respiratory Assessment

Complete a **general assessment** of the lungs		
Respiratory rate *Respiratory depth or volume*	12–20 respirations/minute Normal depth is equal to about 500 mL	Increased respiratory rate: may be due to increased metabolic needs (fever), mechanical injury, surgery, or trauma to chest wall
Auscultation: note location and quality of **lung sounds** (Figure 11-36 ■)		In the morbidly obese individual, move skins folds to the side and place the diaphragm firmly over the area.
Note presence of *adventitious (extra) sounds*, such as rales/crackles, wheezes, and rhonchi, or pleural friction rub	No extra sounds heard—symmetrical areas should be the same in quality and intensity	*Discontinuous Sounds*: *Crackles* (rales) are due to sudden opening of closed airways, indicating hypoventilation; usually heard as soft, high-pitched scratching sounds, like hair strands rubbing together at end of inspiration Heard in dependent areas of bedridden clients or in early congestive heart failure. May be collapsed or fluid-filled alveoli. Simulate by rubbing hair together in front of your ear *Continuous Sounds*: *Wheezes* are produced by air passing through airways narrowed by edema, spasm or mucus; may be heard on inspiration but more often louder on expiration; high-pitched and musical *Rhonchi* are low-pitched rumbling, coarse; sounds heard on inhalation and exhalation. Fluid-blocked airways—may be cleared with coughing.

FIGURE 11-36 Stethoscope placement sites for posterior (left) and anterior (right) auscultation of breath sounds. Follow arrows for sequence of examination.

(continued)

Assessment: Chest, Lungs, and Heart (continued)

Assessment	Normal Responses	Abnormal Responses

Sibilant wheezes are high-pitched, musical sounds; may be caused by asthma, increased secretions, or edema

Pleural friction rub is produced when inflamed pleurae rub together in the absence of normal pleural fluid; localized, high-pitched, harsh, and scratchy; frequently transient; may be heard on inspiration and expiration

Stridor is an inspiratory wheeze heard in the neck due to partial obstruction at upper airway—tracheal or laryngeal level

In the morbidly obese client, the weight of the chest and fatty deposits may result in diminished breath sounds.

FIGURE 11-37 Listen to posterior breath sounds.

Evaluate **breath sounds**

Bronchovesicular breath sounds
Heard over the mainstem bronchi below the clavicles and adjacent to the sternum, between scapulae

Moderate to high pitch, with moderate amplitude
Hollow, muffled quality
Inspiration and expiration equal in duration

Bronchial or bronchovesicular sounds heard in the perimeter where vesicular sounds are expected indicate consolidation such as pneumonia. The client's spoken and whispered words are also clearly heard by the examiner over consolidated lung areas

Vesicular (normal) breath sounds
Heard over lung parenchyma (heart will mask breath sounds on the left side)

Low to medium pitch, with low amplitude
Soft, whooshing quality

Breath sounds may be absent over areas of atelectasis, pneumothorax, or pleural effusion

Lungs extend anteriorly to the sixth intercostal space

Inspiration two to three times longer than expiration

Bronchial breath sounds

Heard over the trachea above the sternal notch

High pitch and amplitude
Harsh, loud, tubular quality
Expiration longer than inspiration

Lungs extend posteriorly to T10v on expiration, to T12 on deep inspiration (Figure 11-37 ■)

Breath sounds are decreased (faint) with hypoventilation, early atelectasis, and COPD

Table 11-3 Abnormal Breathing Patterns

Apnea	Absence of breathing.	————————	**Hyperpnea**	Abnormal increase in depth and rate.	∿∿∿
Biot's respirations	Abrupt interruptions between a faster, deeper respiratory rate.	⋀⋀⋁⋀⋀	**Kussmaul's respirations**	Deep, gasping breathing. Attempt to blow off carbon dioxide as respiratory compensation for metabolic acidosis (e.g., diabetic ketoacidosis).	∿∿∿∿∿
Bradypnea	Slow, regular respirations. Rate is below 10 per minute.	⌒ ⌒ ⌒	**Tachypnea**	Respiratory rate increased above 24 breaths per minute. Rate remains regular but shallow in pattern.	∿∿∿∿∿∿∿
Cheyne–Stokes	Periods of apnea appear throughout cycle. Respirations become deeper and faster than normal followed by a slower rate and progressing to periods of apnea lasting from 15 to 60 seconds.	⋀⋁⋀⋀⋀ ⋀⋁⋀			

Assessment	Normal Responses	Abnormal Responses

Heart Assessment (Figure 11-38 ■)

Evaluate **atrioventricular heart sounds** (S_1 heart sound). Use diaphragm of stethoscope—best for picking up high-pitched sounds

S_1 (the first heart sound, a combination of the mitral and tricuspid closure) heard best over the mitral and tricuspid areas. S_1 louder than S_2 in this area (Figure 11-39 ■)

Heart sounds not heard in the area prescribed (e.g., with left ventricular hypertrophy, mitral sound moves laterally)

Mitral value sounds

Heard best at left, fifth intercostal space at, or medial to, the midclavicular line

Tricuspid valve sounds

Heard best at fifth intercostal space, left sternal border

S_1 also heard at this area and is louder than S_2

Evaluate **semilunar heart sounds** (S_2 heart sounds)

S_2 (the second heart sound, a combination of the aortic and pulmonic closure): heard best over the aortic and pulmonic areas

Sounds altered with aortic stenosis (thrill) and hypertension (accentuated sound)

FIGURE 11-38 Auscultate heart sounds.

FIGURE 11-39 S_1 is heard best over mitral and tricuspid areas. S_2 is heard best over aortic and pulmonic areas.

Aortic area, *Pulmonic area*, *Tricuspid area*, *Mitral area*

Aortic valve sounds

Heard best at second intercostal space, right sternal border

Pulmonic valve sounds

Heard best at second intercostal space, left sternal border

Part of S_2 is louder than S_1 in this area. May be heard separately from aortic closure if client inhales deeply

Accentuated with pulmonary hypertension

Evaluate presence of **diastolic heart sounds**

Use bell of stethoscope—best for picking up low-pitched sounds and gallops. Place lightly on chest with client in left side lying position.

Quiet and low-pitched

Murmurs originating from stenotic valves

S_3 (ventricular gallop)

Heard just after S_2, at the apex or at lower, left sternal border

May be a physiologic finding in children and young adults

Abnormal finding in older clients

Almost always signifies heart failure in client over age 40

(continued)

Assessment: Chest, Lungs, and Heart (continued)

Assessment	Normal Responses	Abnormal Responses
S_4 (atrial gallop)		
Heard just before S_1, at the apex or at lower, left sternal border; occurs when blood flow from atrial contraction meets increased resistance in ventricle	Normal finding in older adult	Heard in older individual with hypertension
Assess for **heart murmurs**, heard between heart sounds (Box 11-3 ■) Produced by atypical flow of blood through the heart (e.g., irregularity or partial obstruction, increased flow in normal area, flow into dilated chamber, flow through abnormal passage); regurgitant flow Occurs during systole (between S_1 and S_2) or during diastole (between S_2 and S_1)	Faint sound More common during systole Often found in children and young adults	Faint or loud enough to be heard without a stethoscope Occurs during systole or diastole (diastolic murmurs are almost always pathologic)—found in older clients with heart disease or infants and children with congenital heart defects
Evaluate the **apical pulse** when assessing for general heart rate and rhythm of contractions	Regular rhythm Heart rate: 60–100 beats/min	Irregular rhythm (dysrhythmia) may be regularly irregular or irregularly irregular (i.e., atrial fibrillation)
Auscultate at the apex of the heart (left, fifth intercostal space at the midclavicular line)	Moderate bradycardia common in well-trained athletes	Bradycardia (less than 60 beats/min)
Palpate and view pulse on chest wall if client's chest wall is thin enough Assess for **irregular apical pulse**	Mild tachycardia possible with stress, infection, or fever	Tachycardia (more than 100 beats/min)
With another nurse, take apical and radial pulses *simultaneously* Compare beats per minute for both pulses	Equal apical and radial pulses × no pulse deficit	Fewer beats at the radial area may indicate an irregular apical pulse, producing ineffective pumping
Auscultate apical pulse and compare to carotid pulse (Figure 11-40 ■)	Two pulses are synchronous	Apical pulse greater than carotid pulse indicates a pulse deficit

Box 11-3 DESCRIBING A MURMUR

Murmurs are classified by timing and are heard between heart sounds:

Timing—When does it occur? Between systolic (S_1 and S_2) sounds or between diastolic (S_2 and S_1) sounds.

Location—Point where murmur is loudest.

Radiation—Where murmur starts (point of maximum intensity) and moves to surrounding areas.

Quality—Blowing, harsh, musical, or rumbling.

Pitch—High, low, medium.

Intensity—Grade 1, barely audible; to grade 6, audible with stethoscope just off client's skin.

Pattern—Intensity over time; soft to loud/loud to soft.

Source: Smith (2016)

FIGURE 11-40 Compare apical and carotid pulses to identify pulse deficit.

Assessment	Normal Responses	Abnormal Responses
Palpate **peripheral pulses:** radial, brachial, femoral, popliteal, dorsalis pedis (Figure 11-41 ■), posterior tibial. (For special cases, after carotid surgery, palpate temporal pulse also)	Easily palpated Equally strong on both sides Posterior tibial pulse usually weaker than femoral	Difficult to palpate Unequal pulses Weak pulse Absent pulses

Guidelines for palpating peripheral pulses:

If pulse is not immediately palpable, examine adjacent area—pulse locations differ with clients. Palpate proximal pulse point.

Palpate weak pulses gently so that you do not obliterate pulse with too much pressure

If you cannot differentiate your pulse from client's pulse, check your radial or carotid pulse, or observe monitor pattern

When peripheral pulses cannot be palpated, use a Doppler ultrasound stethoscope and grade according to scale

FIGURE 11-41 Palpate peripheral pulse, dorsalis pedis.

Note: See Skill 10.2.4, Palpating a Peripheral Pulse.

Assessment of the Abdomen, Spleen, Kidney, Liver, and Genitourinary Tract

The abdomen extends from the diaphragm to the pelvis. Generally speaking, there are two body systems present in this area: the gastrointestinal system and the genitourinary system (Figure 11-42 ■).

The gastrointestinal system begins at the mouth and ends at the anus. It consists of the esophagus, stomach, the small and large intestines, and associated organs that include the liver, pancreas, and spleen.

The urinary tract consists of the kidneys, ureters, bladder, and the urethra. The urinary tract should be assessed frequently and accurately because changes in urine production reflect changes in other body systems.

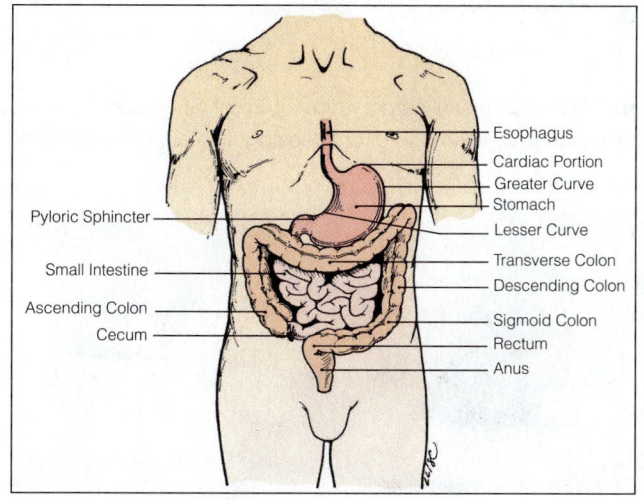

FIGURE 11-42 Assessment requires knowledge of abdominal organ anatomy.

The most common way to assess the urinary tract is to note the quantity and quality of the urinary output. Some medications or foods produce unusual odors and colors in urine (e.g., sulfasalazine [Azulfidine] turns urine a yellow-orange color; asparagus gives urine a musty odor).

External male genitalia include the penis, the scrotum, and the testicles. External female genitalia include the vulva, the urethral orifice, and the vagina.

Assessment: Abdomen, Liver, Spleen, Kidney, and Genitourinary Tract

Assessment	Normal Responses	Abnormal Responses
Abdominal Assessment		
Have client lie flat in bed At the client's abdominal level, inspect the **general contour** of the abdomen	Abdomen flat from chest to pubis with concave indentation at umbilicus	Scaphoid (concave) abdominal contour: due to inadequate nutritional intake to meet caloric need or inadequate food absorption Distended abdomen: caused by gas and fluid accumulation due to lack of peristalsis, hemorrhage, or intestinal leakage after trauma (e.g., motor vehicle crash or surgery), or ascitic fluid (e.g., liver or cardiac failure)
Inspect for bruising around umbilicus and over flanks	No change of skin color around umbilicus or flanks	Acute abdomen
Observe for scars, stretch marks, dilated veins, presence of hernia	Correlate with health history	Dilated veins caused by liver disease Bulge seen with defect in abdominal wall
Assess **circumference** for intraabdominal hemorrhage or ascites by placing a tape measure around the largest circumference of the abdomen. Draw two lines around client's entire abdomen, one line at the top of the tape measure, one line at the bottom of the tape measure; perform measurement when client exhales Auscultate abdomen to assess presence and quality of **bowel sounds** (Figure 11-43 ■)	No increase in abdominal circumference	Abdominal circumference increases steadily within 1–2 hours Bowel sounds may be difficult to auscultate because of the amount of adipose tissue in the morbidly obese client.
Place diaphragm of stethoscope firmly on right lower quadrant and count sounds for 1 minute	Bowel sounds gurgle, about 5–30 per minute	Hyperactive bowel sounds due to blood in GI tract, diarrhea, or to partial bowel obstruction (sounds become high-pitched and tinkling or come in "rushes," followed by silence as obstruction progresses)

Note: After abdominal surgery, the return of GI function is determined by the (1) return of flatus, (2) bowel movement, (3) hunger, (4) no nausea or tolerance of oral feeding, (5) flat abdomen/nondistension, rather than the return of bowel sounds.

FIGURE 11-43 Auscultate abdomen for bowel sounds.

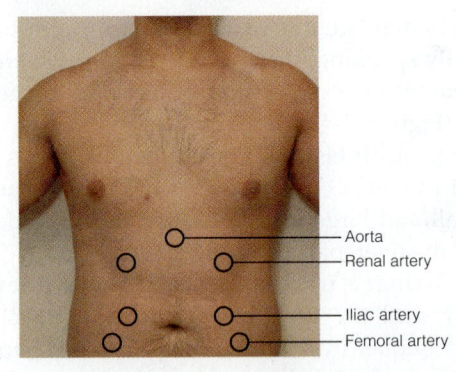

Aorta
Renal artery
Iliac artery
Femoral artery

Assessment	Normal Responses	Abnormal Responses
Listen at all quadrants, near the center, for several minutes if sounds not heard initially	Varying frequency of sounds with clients and time of day (i.e., more sounds right before and after eating)	
	Decreased or absent bowel sounds after surgery	Bowel sounds hypoactive, quiet, and infrequent: may be due to peritonitis, paralytic ileus, or no obvious cause
	After general anesthesia, normal sounds in 1–2 days	
	After abdominal surgery, normal sounds in 3–5 days	Absent bowel sounds: may be due to complete bowel obstruction or systemic illness
Palpate abdomen lightly to determine area of tenderness (Figure 11-44 ■). Palpate deeper to check **abdominal muscles** and organs beneath muscles. Assist client to relax, lie flat in bed, and flex knees. Have client mouth-breathe.	No tenderness, abdomen is relaxed.	Tenderness is present—hypersensitivity.

FIGURE 11-44 Palpate client's abdomen.

Assessment	Normal Responses	Abnormal Responses
Place your hand flat on client's abdomen, holding your four fingers together and depress 1/2 in. or 1 cm.	Soft, pliant musculature when relaxed	Rigid, tender muscles/pain produced with cough: may be due to presence of muscle spasm, inflammation, or infection (peritonitis)
Have client cough to determine any areas of abdominal tenderness	Cough does not produce pain in abdomen	
Begin palpation at the pubis, moving upward. Palpate any problem areas last to minimize effects of discomfort.	No bulges felt	Pain or tenderness with quick release of pressure indicates rebound tenderness suggesting peritoneal inflammation
	No masses felt	
Palpate all quadrants of abdomen to assess organs contained in each quadrant		If hernia is suspected, have client raise head and shoulders and observe for abdominal bulge
Light or superficial palpation: use slight pressure only with your fingers extended		
Deep palpation: indent the abdominal wall 4–5 cm—may use one hand over the other to apply pressure	No masses felt	Masses felt with colon disease, vascular aneurysm, dilated bowel, distended bladder, or cancer

Liver Assessment

Assessment	Normal Responses	Abnormal Responses
Palpate **liver** by placing left hand behind 11th and 12th ribs with right hand on right abdomen lateral to rectus muscle (Figure 11-45 ■)	Normal liver (difficult to palpate) may feel like sharp ridge with smooth surface	Tenderness may be due to inflammation (hepatitis)
		Enlarged liver with nontender edge may be due to cirrhosis

(continued)

Assessment: Abdomen, Liver, Spleen, Kidney, and Genitourinary Tract (continued)

Assessment	Normal Responses	Abnormal Responses

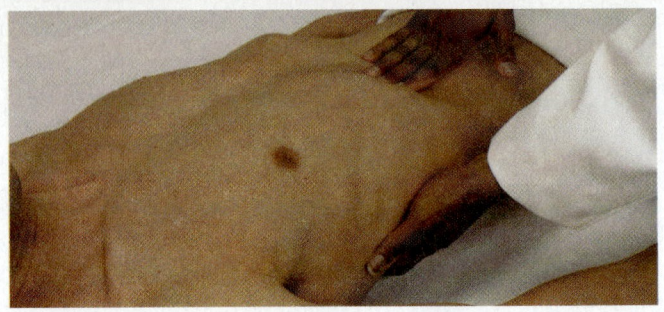

FIGURE 11-45 Palpation of the liver.

Spleen Assessment

Standing on client's right side, palpate spleen. Place left hand under rib cage on left side and elevate rib cage. Press fingers of right hand into left costal margin area and ask client to take a deep breath (Figure 11-46 ■). You should feel spleen move forward toward right hand.

A normal spleen is usually not palpable

Enlarged spleen (which can be palpated) occurs in acute infections such as mononucleosis

FIGURE 11-46 Palpation of the spleen.

Urinary Tract Assessment (Figure 11-47 ■ and Figure 11-48 ■)

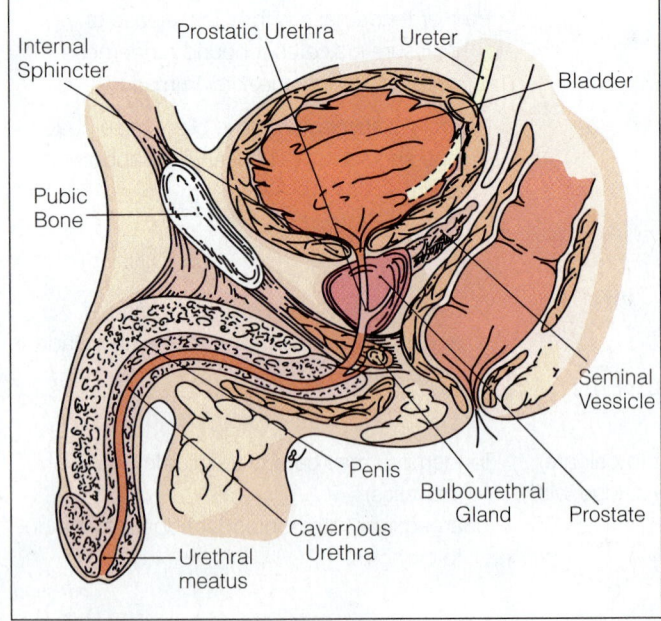

FIGURE 11-47 Male genitourinary system.

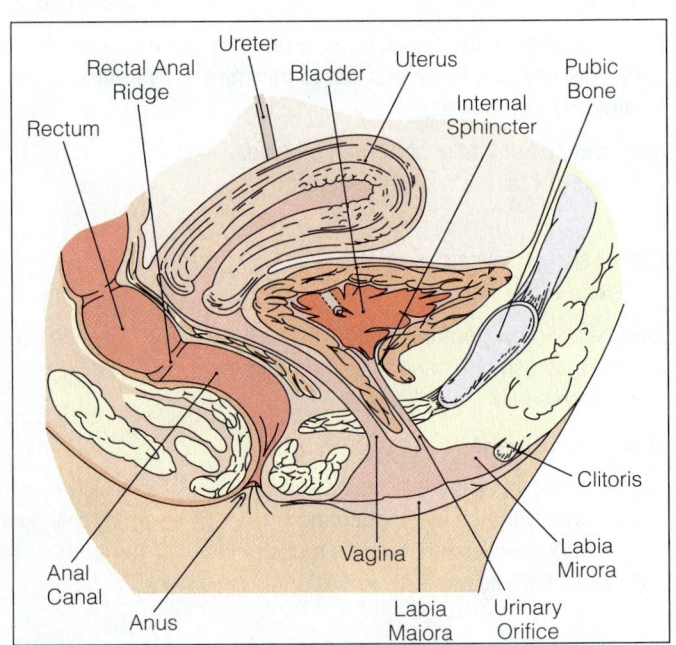

FIGURE 11-48 Female genitourinary system.

Assessment	Normal Responses	Abnormal Responses
Assess the **external urethra**	Orifice is pink and moist; clear, minimal discharge	Burning or pain at urethral orifice: may indicate urinary infection
Assess the quantity, color, odor, specific gravity, and pH of **urine output**	Output: average 1,200–1,500 mL/24 hours, or 30–50 mL/hour—should equal oral and IV intake	Increased output: may indicate increased intake, diuresis, potential diabetes mellitus, or inappropriate antidiuretic hormone (ADH) response (e.g., diabetes insipidus) Frequent small amounts of urine output indicate urinary retention or urinary tract infection Decreased output: may indicate dehydration, acute nephritis, cardiac disease, renal failure, or excess ADH response (e.g., head injury)
	Clear, yellow-amber color (vegetarians may have slightly cloudy urine)	Cloudy (turbid): may indicate possible urinary tract infection Dark amber: may indicate very concentrated urine due to dehydration Dark amber to green: may indicate hepatitis or obstructive jaundice
	Slight odor (ammonia-like odor indicates that specimen has been sitting for some time)	Foul-smelling: may indicate urinary tract infection, drug or specific food ingestion (e.g., asparagus) Sweet odor: may indicate acetone from ketoacidosis (i.e., diabetes mellitus)
	Specific gravity: 1.003–1.030	Specific gravity of more than 1.030: indicates dehydration Constant specific gravity of 1.010, regardless of fluid intake: indicates renal failure
	pH range from 4.5–7.5; average is 6–7	Acidic pH—when below 6.0 may indicate starvation or acidosis Alkaline pH greater than 7.0: indicates metabolic alkalosis or alkaline ash diet (e.g., vegetarian)
Assess for **blood** in urine using Hemastix or Labstix	No blood present	Smoky to mildly pink-tinged to grossly red-colored urine: indicates blood in urine
Palpate for **bladder distention**	Not normally palpated	Distended bladder (firm, round mass) accompanied by discomfort and urge to void: indicates urine retention (common following surgery, where catheter is not used)

Kidney Assessment

Assess (palpate) for kidney pain on either side of vertebrae column between last thoracic and third lumbar vertebrae Use indirect percussion to further assess the kidneys (Figure11-49 ■)	When palpated, client feels no pain 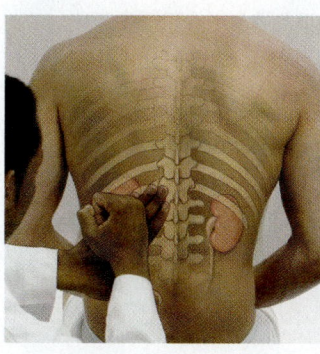	Severe pain, discomfort, or tenderness in the flank region (below rib cage posteriorly and lateral to spine), costovertebral angle (CVA) indicates inflammation, kidney infection, stones, or kidney disease. Kidney enlargement may indicate neoplasm or polycystic disease.

FIGURE 11-49 Use of indirect percussion will identify pain.

(continued)

Assessment: Abdomen, Liver, Spleen, Kidney, and Genitourinary Tract (continued)

Assessment	Normal Responses	Abnormal Responses
Genital Assessment Male		
Visually examine the **male genitalia**	Clean	Unclean
Retract the foreskin of the uncircumcised penis to note cleanliness, any **lesions**, and **discharge**	No odor	Odor
	No lesions	Lesions and discharge may indicate venereal disease or cancer
Lift scrotum to inspect for rash	No discharge	Oval and round, dark erosion: may indicate syphilitic chancre
	Size of penis and scrotum vary	
Noting groin area, ask client to strain down	Urethra opens midline of the tip of the glans	Hypospadias: due to congenital displacement of the urethral meatus
	No bulges in groin area	Bulge on straining seen with hernias
		Indurated nodule or ulcer: may indicate carcinoma
Testicular Examination		
Palpate scrotum, testes, and observe shape and contour.	Should be pear-shaped with left side lower than right; no masses; testes nontender, smooth, and solid	Swelling may indicate orchitis or scrotal edema; scrotal hernia or testicular torsion; varicocele
Observe for swelling, redness, and distended veins or lesions in inguinal area.	Flat, no evidence of masses	Mass may be related to inguinal hernia or cancer
Using thumb and first two fingers, gently palpate each testicle for size, shape, and consistency	Two testicles in the scrotum	Mass in scrotum: indicates possible hernia, hydrocele, testicular tumor, or cyst
	No nodules felt, no swelling or tenderness	Pain indicates inflammatory disease
Female		
Document last menstrual period (LMP)	Clean	Unclean
Visually examine **female genitalia**	No odor	Odor (musty with bacterial infection)
Assess for signs of sexual abuse	No signs	Bruises, welts, burns, unusual swelling
Assess for **lesions** or **discharge** or complaints of itching	Minimal, clear discharge	Thick; thin, white, yellowish, or green discharge: may indicate trichomoniasis
	Menstrual flow	Thick, white, and curdy discharge with pruritus may indicate candidiasis
	Lochia (normal discharge after delivery)	Lesions: could indicate syphilitic chancre, herpes infection, venereal wart, or carcinoma of vulva
	No lesions	
	No pruritus	
Breast Assessment		
Inspect **size, symmetry,** and **contour** of breasts, comparing one side with the other	Size varies with each client	Masses, skin thickening, dimpling, or flattened areas: indicate possible cancer
Place client in sitting position	Breasts should be fairly equal in size and contour and symmetric in position	
Have client remove clothing from waist up		
Have client raise arms over her head		
Color, edema, and **venous pattern of skin**	Normal skin color with darker area surrounding nipples	Erythema: indicates infection or inflammatory carcinoma
	No edema or prominent vessels	Edema or increased venous prominence: indicates carcinoma
Inspect **size and shape of nipples.** Note direction in which they point, and any **rashes or discharge**	Simple inversion of nipples is common	Flattening, nipple retraction, or axis deviation of nipple points: may be due to fibrosis associated with cancer
To palpate breasts, position client supine or on side		Ulcerations of nipples and areola: may be due to Paget disease
Place a pillow under the shoulder of the side being examined		Discharge: may not be malignant but should be observed closely

Assessment	Normal Responses	Abnormal Responses
Using three fingers in a circular motion, compress breast tissue gently against chest wall (Figure11-50 ■)		Mobile nodules may indicate cystic disease
Systematically examine entire breast, top to bottom, moving medially to laterally into the axilla	Soft, elastic tissue with mobile nodules	Hard nodules fixed to skin or underlying tissue may indicate cancer
Examination of women with breast implants proceeds in a similar fashion; palpate the breast to identify the edge of the implant. Be careful not to palpate too aggressively as this can cause the implant to rupture or leak.		When nodules are present: Describe location and quadrant of breast where found Note size in centimeters Describe consistency and shape Note tenderness and mobility of nodule in relationship to underlying tissue

FIGURE 11-50 Examine breast tissue in circular movement.

Palpate nipples		
Compress nipple and areola between thumb and index finger to inspect for discharge	No discharge or small amount of milky discharge in previously nursing mother	Bloody discharge: may indicate papilloma
Note **elasticity** Observe for erection of nipple with palpation	Elastic, no retraction of nipple	Loss of elasticity: indicates possible cancer Inversion, flattening, or retraction: may indicate cancer

Mental Health Assessment

The mental assessment is completed throughout the physical assessment during the history taking. It is not generally considered a separate entity. Mood, memory, orientation, and thought processes can be evaluated while obtaining the health history. Nutritional preferences and restrictions can be determined as a part of a client care plan and may or may not be included in the general client assessment.

A spiritual assessment can be obtained as a part of the health history, although specific sociocultural beliefs may need to be ascertained separately. The purpose of a spiritual assessment is to facilitate the client adapting to the hospital environment and to help the staff understand stressors the client may be experiencing as a result of belief systems.

The purpose of a mental status assessment is to evaluate the present state of psychological functioning and to monitor safety needs of the client. It is not designed to make a diagnosis. Rather, it should yield data that contribute to the total picture of the client as he or she is functioning at the time the assessment is made.

The specific rationale for completing a mental status assessment is:

- To collect baseline data to aid in establishing the cause, diagnosis, and prognosis
- To evaluate the present state of psychological functioning

- To evaluate changes in the individual's emotional, intellectual, motor, and perceptual responses
- To determine the client's ability to cope with the present situation
- To assess the need and availability of support systems
- To ascertain if some seemingly psychopathologic response is, in fact, a disorder of a sensory organ (i.e., a deaf individual appearing hostile, depressed, or suspicious)
- To determine the guidelines of the treatment plan
- To document altered mental status for legal records

The initial factors that the nurse must consider in completing a mental status assessment are to correctly identify the client, the reason for admission, record of previous mental illness, present complaint, any personal history that is relevant (living arrangements, role in family, interactional experience, history of alcoholism, domestic violence), family history if appropriate, significant others and available support systems, assets, and interests.

The actual assessment process begins with an initial evaluation of the appropriateness of the client's behavior and orientation to reality. The assessment continues by noting any abnormal behavior and ascertaining the client's chief verbalized complaint. Finally, the evaluation determines if the client is in contact with reality enough to answer particular questions that further assess the client's condition.

Note: For more information on a spiritual–religious assessment, see Chapter 4.

Assessment: Mental Status

Assessment	Normal Responses	Abnormal Responses
General Appearance, Manner, and Attitude		
Assess **physical appearance**	General body characteristics, energy level	Inappropriate physical appearance, high or low extremes of energy
Note **grooming**, mode of dress, and **personal hygiene**	Grooming and dress appropriate to situation, client's age, and social circumstance	Poor grooming
		Inappropriate or bizarre dress or combination of clothes
	Clean	Unclean
Note **posture**	Upright, straight, and appropriate	Slumped, tipped, or stooped
Note speed, pressure, pace, quantity, volume, and diction of **speech**	Moderated speed, volume, and quantity	Tremors
		Accelerated or retarded speech and high quantity
	Appropriate diction	Poor or inappropriate diction
Note relevance, content, and organization of **responses**	Questions answered directly, accurately, and with relevance	Inappropriate responses, unorganized pattern of speech
		Tangential, circumstantial, or out-of-context replies
Expressive Aspects of Behavior		
Note **general motor activity**	Calm, ordered movement appropriate to situation	Overactive (e.g., restless, agitated, impulsive)
		Underactive (e.g., slow to initiate or execute actions)
Assess **purposeful movements and gestures**	Reasonably responsive with purposeful movements, appropriate gestures	Repetitious activities (e.g., rituals or compulsions)
Assess style of **gait**		Command automation
		Parkinsonian movements
		Ataxic, shuffling, off-balance gait
Consciousness	Alert, attentive, and responsive	Disordered attention; distracted, cloudy consciousness
Assess **level of consciousness**	Knowledgeable about time, place, and person	Delirious
		Stuporous
Thought Processes and Perception		
Assess **coherency, logic**, and **relevance** of thought processes by asking questions about personal history (e.g., "Where were you born?" "What kind of work do you do?")	Clear, understandable responses to questions	Disoriented in time, place, person
	Attentiveness	Disordered thought forms
		Autistic or dereistic (absorbed with self and withdrawn); abstract (absent-mindedness); concrete thinking (dogmatic, preaching)
Assess **reality orientation**: time, place, and person awareness	Orderly progression of thoughts based in reality	Disorders of progression of thought; looseness, circumstantial, incoherent, irrelevant conversation, blocking
	Awareness of time, place, and person	Delusions of grandeur or persecution: neologisms, use of words whose meaning is known only to the client
		Echolalia (automatic repeating of questions)
		No awareness of day, time, place, or person
Assess **perceptions** and reactions to personal experiences by asking questions, such as "How do you see yourself now that you are in the hospital?" "What do you think about when you're in a situation like this?"	Thoughtful, clear responses expressed with understanding of self	Altered, narrowed, or expanded perception illusions
		Depersonalization

Assessment	Normal Responses	Abnormal Responses
Thought Content and Mental Trend		
Assess degree of anxiety Ask questions to determine general themes that identify **degree of anxiety** (e.g., "How are you feeling right now?" "What kinds of things make you afraid?")	Mild or 1+ level of anxiety in which individual is alert, motivated, and attentive	Moderate to severe (2+ to 4+) levels of anxiety
Assess **ideation** and **concentration**	Ideas based in reality Able to concentrate	Ideas of reference Hypochondria (abnormal concerns about health) Obsessional Phobias (irrational fears) Poor or shortened concentration
Mood or Affect		
Assess prevailing or **variability in mood** by observing behavior and asking questions, such as "How are you feeling right now?" Check for presence of abnormal **euphoria**	Appropriate, even mood without wide variations high to low	Cyclothymic mood swings; euphoria, elation, ecstasy, depressed, withdrawn
If you suspect **depression**, continue questioning to determine depth and significance of mood (e.g., "How badly do you feel?" "Have you ever thought of suicide?")	May be sad or grieving but mood does not persist indefinitely	Flat or dampened responses Inappropriate responses Ambivalence
Memory		
Assess **past and present memory** and **retention** (ability to listen and respond with understanding or knowledge); ask client to repeat a phrase (e.g., an address)	Alert, accurate responses Able to complete digit span Past and present memory appropriate	Hyperamnesia (excessive loss of memory); amnesia; paramnesia (belief in events that never occurred) Preoccupied Unable to follow directions
Assess **recall** (recent and remote) by asking questions, such as "When is your birthday?" "What year were you born?" "How old are you?" "Who is the president of the United States now?"	Good recall of immediate and past events	Poor recall of immediate or past events
Judgment		
Assess **judgment, decision-making ability**, and **interpretations** by asking questions, such as "What should you do if you hear a siren while you're driving?" "If you lost a library book, what would you do?"	Ability to make accurate decisions Realistic interpretation of events	Poor judgment, poor decision-making ability, poor choice Inappropriate interpretation of events or situations
Awareness		
Assess **insight**, the ability to understand the inner nature of events or problems, by asking questions, such as "If you saw someone dressed in a fur coat on a hot day, what would you think?"	Thoughtful responses indicating an understanding of the inner nature of an event or problem	Lack of insight or understanding of problems or situations Distorted view of situation
Intelligence		
Assess **intelligence** by asking client to define or use words in sentences (e.g., recede, join, plural)	Correct responses to majority of questions	Incorrect responses to majority of questions indicate possible severe psychiatric disorders

(continued)

Assessment: Mental Status *(continued)*

Assessment	Normal Responses	Abnormal Responses
Assess **fund of information** by asking questions, such as "Who is the president of the United States?" "Who was the president before him?" "When is Memorial Day?" "What is a thermometer?" (Consider client's cultural and educational background and his or her grasp of English)	Correct responses to majority of questions	Deteriorated or impaired cognitive processes
Sensory Ability Assess the **five senses** (i.e., vision, hearing, taste, feeling, and smell)	Able to perceive, hear, taste, feel, touch, smell appropriate to stimulus	Lack of response Suspicious, hostile, depressed Kinesthetic imbalance
Developmental Level Assess **developmental level** compared with normal	Behavior and thought processes appropriate to age level	Wide span between chronologic and developmental age Intellectually and developmentally delayed (I/DD)
Lifestyle Patterns Identify **addictive patterns** and effect on individual's overall health	Normal amount of alcohol ingested Smoking habits, number of years Prescriptive medications Adequate food intake for physical characteristics	High quantity of alcohol taken frequently Heavy smoker Addicted to illegal drugs Habituative medication; user of over-the-counter or legal medications Anorexic eating patterns Obesity or food overindulgence
Coping Devices Identify **defense-coping mechanisms** and their effect on individual	Conscious coping mechanisms used appropriately, such as compensation, fantasy, rationalization, suppression, sublimation, or displacement Mechanisms effective, appropriate, and useful	Unconscious mechanisms used frequently, such as repression, regression, projection, reaction formation, insulation, or denial Mechanisms inappropriate, ineffective, and not useful

Obstetrical Assessment

Assessment: Obstetrical

Assessment	Normal Responses	Abnormal Responses
Baseline Data Assess **breasts** and **nipples: to include implants, reductions, nipple piercings** Contour and size		
Presence of lumps Secretions	No lumps Colostrum secretions in late first trimester or early second trimester	Lumps Secretions, other than colostrum

Assessment	Normal Responses	Abnormal Responses
Assess **abdomen**		
Contour and size Changes in skin color	*Linea nigra* (black line of pregnancy along midline of abdomen) Primiparas: coincidentally with growth of fundus Multiparas: after 13–15 weeks' gestation	
Striae (reddish-purple lines)	On breasts, hips, and thighs during pregnancy After pregnancy, faint silvery-gray	
Scar, rashes, or other skin disturbances	Usually none present	
Fundal height in centimeters (fingerbreadths less accurate): measure from symphysis pubis to top of fundus	Fundus palpable just above symphysis at 8–10 weeks Halfway between symphysis and umbilicus at 16 weeks Umbilicus at 20–22 weeks	Large measurements: Expected date of confinement, or delivery (EDC) is incorrect; tumor; ascites; multiple pregnancy; polyhydramnios, hydatidiform mole Less than normal enlargement: fetal abnormality, oligohydramnios, placental dysmaturity, missed abortion, fetal death
Perineum: assess for scars, lesions, or discharge	None present	Rash, warts, discharge
Evaluate **weight**		
Take **vital signs, blood pressure** (BP), **temperature, pulse,** and **respiration** (TPR)	Vital signs normal	
Evaluate **lab findings** Urine: sugar, protein, albumin	Negative for sugar, protein, and albumin throughout pregnancy	Positive for sugar, protein, and/or albumin
Hematocrit (HCT) Hemoglobin (Hgb) Blood type and Rh factor	38%–47% 12–16 g/dL	If Rh negative, father's blood should be typed If Rh positive, titers should be followed; possible RhoGAM at termination of pregnancy
Pap smear Venereal disease, cervical dysplasia, human papilloma virus (HPV)	Negative	
Antepartum Assessment		
During the prenatal visit ask about drug use (illicit, OTC, and herbal remedies), smoking, and alcohol consumption Ask client if she is in a "safe environment" and explore potential for intimate partner violence (IPV)	Denies	Alcohol consumption during pregnancy has been associated with fetal alcohol syndrome Have available resources if safety is an issue Pregnant women are especially vulnerable to IPV
Evaluate **weight** to assess maternal health and nutritional status and growth of fetus	Minimum weight gain during pregnancy: 24 lb If underweight: gain 28–42 lb If obese: gain 15 lb or more Normal weight gain: 25–35 lb	Inadequate weight gain; possible maternal malnutrition Excessive weight gain: if sudden at onset, may indicate preeclampsia; if gradual and continual, may indicate overeating
Evaluate **blood pressure**	Fairly constant with baseline data throughout pregnancy	Increased: possible anxiety (client should rest 20 to 30 minutes before you take BP again) Rise of 30/15 above baseline data: sign of preeclampsia Decreased: sign of supine hypotensive syndrome. If lying on back, turn client on left side and take BP again

(continued)

Assessment: Obstetrical (continued)

Assessment	Normal Responses	Abnormal Responses
Evaluate **fundal height**	Drop around 38th week: sign of fetus engaging in birth canal Primipara: sudden drop Multipara: slower, sometimes not until onset of labor	Large fundal growth: may indicate wrong dates, multiple pregnancy, hydatidiform mole, polyhydramnios, tumors Small fundal growth: may indicate fetal demise, fetal anomaly, retarded fetal growth, abnormal presentation or lie, decreased amniotic fluid
Determine **fetal position, using Leopold maneuvers** (Figure 11-51 ■). Complete external palpations of the abdomen to determine fetal position, lie, presentation, and engagement		

FIGURE 11-51 Steps of Leopold maneuvers.

First maneuver: to determine part of fetus presenting into pelvis *Second maneuver:* to locate the back, arms, and legs: fetal heart heard best over fetal back *Third maneuver:* to determine part of fetus in fundus *Fourth maneuver:* to determine degree of cephalic flexion and engagement	Vertex presentation	Breech presentation or transverse lie
Evaluate **fetal heart rate** by quadrant, location, and rate	120–160 beats/min	>160 or <120: may indicate fetal distress. *Notify healthcare provider*
Check for presence of **edema**	In lower extremities toward end of pregnancy	In upper extremities and face: may indicate preeclampsia
Evaluate **urine** (clean catch midstream)	Negative for sugar, protein, and albumin	Positive for sugar: may indicate subclinical or gestational diabetes Positive for protein and/or albumin: may indicate preeclampsia
Evaluate **levels of discomfort**		
Intrapartum Assessment Assess for **lightening** and **dropping** (the descent of the presenting part into the pelvis)	Several days to 2 weeks before onset of labor Multipara: may not occur until onset of labor Relief of shortness of breath and increase in urinary frequency	No lightening or dropping: may indicate disproportion between fetal presenting part and maternal pelvis

Assessment	Normal Responses	Abnormal Responses
Check if **mucus plug** has been expelled from cervix	Usually expelled from cervix before onset of labor	Frank bleeding, placenta previa
Assess for "**bloody show**"	Clear, pinkish, or blood-tinged vaginal discharge that occurs as cervix begins to dilate and efface	
Assess for **ruptured membranes** Time water breaks	Before, during, or after onset of labor	Breech presentation: frank meconium or meconium staining
Color of **amniotic fluid**	Clear, straw color	Greenish-brown: indicates meconium has passed from fetus, possible fetal distress Yellow-stained: fetal hypoxia 36 hours or more before rupture of membrane or hemolytic disease Bloody
Quantity of amniotic fluid	Normal is 500–1,000 mL of amniotic fluid, rarely expelled at one time	**Polyhydramnios**—excessive amniotic fluid over 2,000 mL Observe newborn for congenital anomalies: craniospinal malformation, orogastrointestinal anomalies. Down syndrome, and congenital heart defects **Oligohydramnios**—minimal amniotic fluid, less than 500 mL Observe newborn for malformation of ear, genitourinary tract anomalies, and renal agenesis
Odor of fluid	No odor	Odor may indicate infection; deliver within 24 hours
Fetal heart rate (tested at every stage of labor)	110–160 beats/min	Decreased: indicates fetal distress with possible cord prolapse or cord compression
	Regular rhythm	Accelerated: initial sign of fetal hypoxia Absent: may indicate fetal demise
Labor and Delivery Assessment **Evaluate Contractions**		
Frequency: from start of one contraction to start of next	3–5 minutes between contractions; if client is on oxyocin (Pitocin), check contractions every 2–3 min	Irregular contractions with long intervals between: indicates false labor
Duration: from beginning of contraction to time uterus begins to relax	50–90 seconds	>90 seconds: uterine tetany; stop oxytocin if running
Intensity (strength of contraction): measured with monitoring device	Peak 25 mm Hg End of labor may reach 50–75 mm Hg	>75 mm Hg: uterine tetany or uterine rupture
First-Stage		
Latent phase (0–4 cm dilation)	0–3 to 4 cm; average 6.4 hours	Prolonged time in any phase: may indicate poor fetal position, incomplete fetal flexion, cephalopelvic disproportion, or poor uterine contractions
Active phase (4–8 cm) *Transitional phase* (8–10 cm)	Length of time varies—may be 1–2 hours	If total labor 63 hours: indicates precipitous labor, increasing risk of fetal complications, or maternal lacerations and tears

(continued)

Assessment: Obstetrical (continued)

Assessment	Normal Responses	Abnormal Responses
Assess for **bloody show** Observe for presence of **nausea or vomiting** Assess **perineum** Evaluate **urge to bear down**	Beginning to bulge	Often uncontrolled Multipara: can cause precipitous delivery "panting" (can be controlled until safe delivery area established)
Second stage (10 cm to delivery)	Primipara: up to 2 hours Multipara: several min to 2 hours	>2 hours: increased risk of fetal brain damage and maternal exhaustion
Assess for **presenting part**	Vertex with ROA or LOA presentation	Occiput posterior, breech, face, or transverse lie
Assess **caput** (infant head) Multipara: move to delivery room when caput size of a dime Primipara: move to delivery room when caput size of a half-dollar	Visible when bearing down during contraction	If client "crowns" in room other than delivery room, do not move client. Delivery is imminent
At every stage of labor, assess **fetal heart rate (FHR)** Bradycardia, drop of 20 beats/min below baseline (<120 beats/min) Tachycardia, increase in FHR over 160 beats/min for 10 min	110–160/min	Decreased: may indicate supine hypotensive syndrome (turn client on side and take again) Hemorrhage (check for other signs of bleeding: notify healthcare provider) Increased or decreased: may indicate fetal distress secondary to cord progression or compression (place client in Trendelenburg or knee–chest position; give oxygen if necessary. Other conditions that cause altered FHR include smoking, drugs, infection and alcohol use. Inform healthcare provider)
Evaluate **fetal heart rate tracing**	Short-term variability is present Long-term variability ranges from 3–5 cycles/min	Absence of variability (no short term or long term present) Severe variable decelerations (fetal heart rate <70 for longer than 30–45 seconds with decreasing variability)
Deceleration	Early deceleration (10–20 beat drop), usually due to head compression Recovery when acme contraction passes—often not serious	Monitor closely—distinguish from decrease with hypertonic contraction; leads to fetal distress
Variable deceleration; decrease in FHR, below 120/min	Mild; may be within normal parameters—continue to monitor	Cord compression—may result in fetal difficulty
Loss of beat-to-beat variation	If continues less than 15 minutes, no problem apparent	Late deceleration pattern occurs—monitor for hypertonic contraction; leads to total distress.
Evaluate **breathing**	Controlled with contractions	Heavy or excessive: may lead to hyperventilation and/or dehydration
Evaluate **pain** and **anxiety**	Medication required after dilated 4–5 cm unless using natural childbirth methods. In some instances, the client may require pain meds or an epidural during the initial stages of dilation	Severe pain early in first stage of labor: inadequate prenatal teaching, backache due to position in bed, uterine tetany, low pain threshold

Assessment	Normal Responses	Abnormal Responses
Third stage (from delivery of baby to delivery of placenta)	Placental separation occurs within 30 minutes (usually 3–5 min)	Failure of placental separation Abnormality of uterus or cervix, weak, ineffectual uterine contraction, tetanic contractions causing closure of cervix >3 hours: indicates retained placenta
Fourth stage (first hour postpartum)		Mother in unstable condition (hemorrhage usual cause) Highest risk of hemorrhage in first postpartum hour
Temperature	97.7°F–99.5°F (36.5°C–37.5°C)	>99.5°F (37.5°C): may indicate infection Slight elevation: due to dehydration from mouth breathing and NPO
Pulse	Pulse: 60–100	Increased: may indicate pain or hemorrhage
Respiration	Respirations: 12–22	
Blood pressure	Blood pressure: 120–140/80	Increased: may indicate anxiety, pain, or posteclamptic condition Decreased: hemorrhage

Postpartum Assessment
Cardiovascular

Assess **vital signs** every 15 minutes for 1 hour, every 30 minutes for 1 hour, every hour for 4 hours, every 8 hours, and as needed	Pulse may be 45–60/min in stage 4 Pulse to normal range about third day	Decreased BP and increased pulse: probably postpartum hemorrhage Elevated temperature <100.4°F (38°C) indicates possible infection Temperature elevates when lactation occurs
Additional assessment includes: Thromboembolism assessment, level of consciousness	No evidence of DVT Alert and oriented	Postpartum clients are at risk for pulmonary embolism
Assess **fundus** every 15 minutes for 1 hour, every 8 hours for 48 hours, then daily	Firm (like a grapefruit) in midline and at or slightly above umbilicus Return to prepregnant size in 6 weeks: descending at rate of 1 fingerbreadth/day	Boggy fundus: immediately massage gently until firm; report to healthcare provider and observe closely; empty bladder; medicate with oxytocin if ordered Fundus misplaced 1–2 fingerbreadths from midline: indicates full bladder (client must void or be catheterized)
Assess incision if postcesarean birth	Incision dry and intact	Evidence of dehiscence, notify healthcare provider
Assess **lochia** every 15 minutes for 1 hour, every 8 hours for 48 hours, then daily	3 days postpartum: dark red (rubra) 4–10 days postpartum: clear pink (serosa)	Continued dark red
Color	10–21 days postpartum: white, yellow brown (alba)	Red
Quantity	Moderate amount, steadily decreases	Heavy, bright-red: indicates hemorrhage (massage fundus, give medication on order, notify healthcare provider) Spurts: may indicate cervical tear No lochia: may indicate clot occluding cervical opening (support fundus; express clot)
Odor	Minimal	Foul: may indicate infection
Assess **breasts** and **nipples** daily	Days 1–2: soft, intact, secreting colostrum Days 2–3: engorged, tender, full, tight, painful	Sore or cracked (clean and dry nipples; decrease breastfeeding time; apply breast shell between feeding)

(continued)

Assessment: Obstetrical *(continued)*

Assessment	Normal Responses	Abnormal Responses
	Day 3+: secreting milk Increased pains as baby sucks: common in multiparas	Milk does not "let down": help client relax and decrease anxiety; give glass of wine or beer if not culturally, religiously, or otherwise contraindicated
Assess **genitourinary system**		
Assess **perineum** daily	Episiotomy intact, no swelling, no discoloration	Swelling or bruising: may indicate hematoma
Assess **bladder** every 4 hours If urinary catheter in place, assess. Assess **kidneys**	Voiding regularly with no pain Remove as soon as possible No costovertebral angle (CVA) tenderness	Not voiding: bladder may be full and displaced to one side, leading to increased lochia (catheterization may be necessary) Distension, dark yellow urine, burning on urination, CVA tenderness
Assess **gastrointestinal system** Nausea and vomiting, emesis Bowel sounds	Spontaneous bowel movement 2–3 days after delivery Denies emesis Spontaneous return of bowel sounds	Fear associated with pain from hemorrhoids, episiotomy, and perineal trauma
Assess mother–infant **bonding**	Touching infant, talking to infant, talking about infant	Refuses to touch or hold infant
Evaluate **Rh-negative status**	Client does not require RhoGAM	RhoGAM administered
Maternal History: Definition of Terms		
Abortion: pregnancy loss before fetus is viable (typically <500 g)	*Multigravida:* refers to second or any subsequent pregnancy	*Nullipara:* refers to female who has never carried pregnancy to viable age for fetus
Gravida: any pregnancy, including present one	*Para:* past pregnancies that continued to viable age (20 weeks); infants may be alive or dead at birth	*Multipara:* refers to female who has given birth to two or more viable infants; either alive or dead
Primigravida: refers to first-time pregnancy	*Primipara:* refers to female who has delivered first viable infant; born either alive or dead	

Newborn Assessment

Assessment: Newborn

Assessment	Normal Responses	Abnormal Responses
Apgar Score		
Obtain Apgar score at birth and at 5 minutes (Table 11-4 ■)	Score of 7–10	Score of 0–6
Assess head	Head at birth: about 2 cm greater than chest	
Skin Assessment		
Note skin **color, pigmentation, lesions,** and **turgor**	Pink Mongolian spots	Cyanosis, pallor, beefy red Petechiae, ecchymoses, or purpuric spots: signs of possible hematologic disorder

Assessment	Normal Responses	Abnormal Responses
	Capillary hemangiomas on face or neck	Café-au-lait spots (patches of brown discoloration): possible sign of congenital neurologic disorder Raised capillary hemangiomas on areas other than face or neck
	Localized edema in presenting part	Edema of peritoneal wall Poor skin turgor: indicates dehydration
	Milia (small white pustules over nose and chin) Jaundice after 24 hours; gone by second week	Impetigo neonatorum (small pustules with surrounding red areas) Jaundice at birth or within 12 hours Dermal sinuses (opening to brain) Holes along spinal column Low hairline posteriorly: possible chromosomal abnormality Sparse or spotty hair: congenital goiter or chromosomal abnormality
Note color of **nails**	Pink	Yellowing of nail beds (meconium stained)
Note **muscle strength/tone**	Strong, tremulous	Flaccid, convulsions Muscular twitching, hypertonicity
Head and Neck Assessment		
Note **shape of head**	Fontanels: anterior open until 18 months; posterior closed shortly after birth	Depressed fontanels indicate dehydration; closed or bulging indicate congenital anomalies; full or bulging indicate edema or increased ICP Cephalohematoma that crosses the midline Microcephaly and macrocephaly
Assess **eyes**	Slight edema of lids	Purulent discharge Lateral upward slope of eye with an inner epicanthal fold in infants not of Asian descent Exophthalmos (bulging of eyeball): may be congenital anomaly, sign of congenital glaucoma or thyroid abnormality Enophthalmos (recession of eyeball): may indicate damage to brain or cervical spine
	Pupils equal and reactive to light by 3 weeks of age Intermittent strabismus (occasional crossing of eyes)	Constricted pupil, unilateral dilated fixed pupil, nystagmus (rhythmic nonpurposeful movement of eyeball): continuous strabismus

Table 11-4 Apgar Scoring

Sign	0	1	2
Heart rate	Absent	Slow (less than 100)	Over 100
Respiratory effort	Absent	Slow, irregular	Good, crying
Muscle tone	Flaccid	Some flexion of extremities	Active motion
Reflex irritability	No response	Cry	Vigorous cry
Color	Blue, pale	Body pink, extremities blue	Completely pink

APGAR scoring system is a method of evaluating a newborn's condition at 1 and 5 minutes after birth.

- Newborns who score 7–10 are considered free of immediate danger.
- Newborns who score 4–6 are moderately depressed.
- Newborns who score 0–3 are severely depressed.

Scores less than 7 at 5 minutes, repeat every 5 minutes for 20 minutes. Infant may be intubated unless 2 successive scores of 7 or more occur.

(continued)

Assessment: Newborn *(continued)*

Assessment	Normal Responses	Abnormal Responses
	Conjunctival or scleral hemorrhages	Haziness of cornea
	Symmetrical light reflex (light reflects off each eye in the same quadrant): sign of conjugate gaze	Absence of red reflex; asymmetrical light reflex
Note **placement of ears,** shape and position	The top of the ear should be on an imaginary line from the edge of the eye; cartilage should be well formed	Low-set ears: may indicate chromosomal or renal system abnormality
Assess **nose**	Discharge, sneezing	Thick, bloody nasal discharge
Assess **mouth**	Sucking, rooting reflexes	Cleft lip, palate
	Retention cysts	Flat, white nonremovable spots (thrush)
	Occasional vomiting	Frequent vomiting: may indicate pyloric stenosis
		Vomitus with bile: fecal vomiting
		Profuse salivation: may indicate tracheoesophageal fistula
Assess feedings, whether bottle or breast, amount mL per feeding with bottle, sucking quality.	Bottle every 3–4 hours, breast every 2–3 hours	Poor sucking quality, poor latch on, impaired feeding

EVIDENCE-BASED PRACTICE
Weight Loss in Breastfed Neonates
During the first hours of life, exclusively breastfed neonates will predictably lose up to 10% of their body weight. Neonates delivered by cesarean demonstrate an even greater loss. By 72 hours of life, neonates will begin to regain weight.

Source: Flaherman, Schaefer, Kuzniewicz, Li, Walsh, & Paul (2015)

Assessment	Normal Responses	Abnormal Responses
Assess **neck**	Tonic neck reflex (Fencer position); should have full range of motion	Distended neck veins
		Fractured clavicle
		Unusually short neck
		Excess posterior cervical skin
		Resistance to neck flexion
Assess **cry**	Lusty cry	Weak, groaning cry: possible neurologic abnormality
		High-pitched cry: newborn drug withdrawal (may occur 6–12 months after birth); hoarse or crowing inspirations; catlike cry: possible neurologic or chromosomal abnormality
Chest and Lung Assessment		
Assess **chest**	Circular; head at birth about 2 cm greater than chest	Chest larger than head or much smaller than head
	Enlargement of breasts	Depressed sternum
	Milky discharge from breasts	Broken clavicle (from shoulder dystocia)
		Head smaller than chest or much larger than chest
		Retractions, asymmetry of chest movements: indicates respiratory distress and possible pneumothorax
Assess **respirations and lungs**	Respiratory rate: 30–50	Thoracic breathing, unequal motion of chest, rapid grasping or grunting respirations, flaring nares, retractions
	Respiration movement irregular in rate and depth	Deep sighing respirations
	Resonant chest (hollow sound on percussion)	Grunt on expiration: possible respiratory distress
		Hyper-resonance of chest or decreased resonance

Assessment	Normal Responses	Abnormal Responses
Heart Assessment		
Assess the **rate, rhythm,** and **murmurs** of the heart	Rate: 100–160 at birth; stabilizes at 120–140 Regular rhythm Murmurs: significance cannot usually be determined in newborn	Heart rate >200 or <100 Irregular rhythm Dextrocardia, enlarged heart
Abdomen and Gastrointestinal Tract Assessment		
Assess the **abdomen**	Prominent	Distention of abdominal veins: possible portal vein obstruction
Evaluate condition of cord	Umbilical cord with one vein and two arteries Soft granulation tissue at umbilicus	One artery present in umbilical cord: may indicate other anomalies Wet umbilical stump or fetid odor from stump
Assess abdomen	Firm and rounded, no masses detected	Midline suprapubic mass: may indicate Hirschsprung disease
Assess the **gastrointestinal tract**	Bowel sounds present Liver 2–3 cm below right costal margin Spleen tip palpable	Visible peristaltic waves Increased pitch or frequency: intestinal obstruction Decreased sounds: paralytic ileus Distention of abdomen Enlarged liver or spleen Spleen enlarged or mass
Genitourinary Tract Assessment		
Assess **kidneys and bladder**	May be able to palpate kidneys Bladder percussed 1–4 cm above symphysis pubis	Enlarged kidney Distended bladder; presence of any masses
Assess the **genitalia**	Edema and bruising after delivery Unusually large clitoris in females a short time after birth Vaginal mucoid or bloody discharge may be present in the first week	Ambiguous genitalia (chromosomal abnormality) Vaginal or bloody discharge after first week Inguinal hernia
Urethral orifice	Urethra opens on ventral surface of penile shaft	Hypospadias (urethra opens on the inferior surface of the penis) Epispadias (urethra opens on the dorsal surface of the penis) Ulceration of urethral orifice
Testes	Testes in scrotal sac or inguinal canal	Hydroceles in boys Undescended testes in boys
Spine and Extremities Assessment		
Assess the **spine**	Straight spine	Spina bifida, pilonidal sinus; scoliosis
Assess **extremities**	Soft click with thigh rotation, full ROM, symmetric gluteal folds, feet in normal alignment, 10 digits	Asymmetry of movement Sharp click with thigh rotation: indicates possible congenital hip Uneven major gluteal folds: indicates possible congenital hip Polydactyly (extra digits on a hand or foot); syndactyly (webbing or fusion of fingers or toes)
Neuromuscular	Tone, cry, activity normal Reflexes normal	Tone, cry, activity outside normal limits Reflexes weak or absent
Pain	No evidence of pain Neonatal Infant Pain Scale (NIPS) score less than 3 (Figure 11-52 ■).	Score greater than 3 on NIPS
Assess **anus and rectum**	Patent anus	Closed (imperforate) anus: no meconium

Characteristic	Scoring Criteria
Facial Expression 0 = Relaxed muscles 1 = Grimace	■ Restful face with neutral expression ■ Tight facial muscles; furrowed brow, chin, and jaw (Note: At low gestational ages, infants may have no facial expression.)
Cry 0 = No cry 1 = Whimper 2 = Vigorous cry	■ Quiet, not crying ■ Mild moaning, intermittent cry ■ Loud screaming, rising, shrill, and continuous (Note: Silent cry may be scored if infant is intubated, as indicated by obvious facial movements.)
Breathing Patterns 0 = Relaxed 1 = Change in breathing	■ Relaxed, usual breathing pattern maintained ■ Change in breathing, irregular, faster than usual, gagging, or holding breath
Arm Movements 0 = Relaxed/restrained 1 = Flexed/extended	■ Relaxed, no muscle rigidity, occasional random (with soft restraints) movements of arms ■ Tense, straight arms; rigid; or rapid extension and flexion
Leg Movements 0 = Relaxed/restrained 1 = Flexed/extended	■ Relaxed, no muscle rigidity, occasional random (with soft restraints) movements of legs ■ Tense, straight legs; rigid; or rapid extension and flexion
State of Arousal 0 = Sleeping/awake 1 = Fussy	■ Quiet, peaceful, sleeping; or alert and settled ■ Alert and restless or thrashing; fussy

FIGURE 11-52 Neonatal Infant Pain Scale (NIPS).
Sources: Lawrence (1993) and Morrow (2010)

Pediatric Assessment

Assessment: Pediatric

Assessment	Normal Responses	Abnormal Responses
Measurements		
Measure **height** and **weight** and plot on a standardized growth chart	Height/weight proportional Sequential measurements: pattern follows normal growth curves	Height/weight below fifth percentile Sudden drop in percentile range of height and/or weight: possible sign of disease process or congenital problem Sudden and persistent increase (above 95th percentile)
Assess **temperature** (axillary or tympanic until 6 years of age)	Axillary: 97.7–99.5°F (36.5°–37.5°C) Elevations after eating or playing not unusual Rectal: 97.8–99°F (36.6°–37.2°C)	Temperature of 104°–105°F (40–40.6°C): comparable to 101°–102°F (38.3–38.9°C) in an adult Large daily temperature variations Hypothermia: usually result of chilling
Measure **circumference of head and chest**		
Examine or check circumferences when child is less than 2 years old	Head at birth: about 2 cm greater than chest During first year: equalization of head and chest	Increase in head circumference greater than 2.5 cm per month: sign of hydrocephalus
Compare measurements with standardized charts	After 2 years: rapid growth of chest; slight increase in size of head	
Assess **pulse** apically	Birth–1 year: 100–170 1 year: 80–130 2 years: 80–120 3 years: 70–120 Over 3 years: 70–120	Pulse over 180 *at rest* after first month of life: cardiac or respiratory condition Inability to palpate or very weak femoral and pedal pulses: possible coarctation of the aorta

Assessment	Normal Responses	Abnormal Responses
Assess **respirations**	Birth: 30–80 6 years: 16–22 Puberty: 12–30 (Young children have abnormally high respiration rate with even slight excitement)	Consistent tachypnea: usually a sign of respiratory distress Respiratory rate over 100; lower respiratory tract obstruction Slow rate: may be sign of CNS depression
Assess **blood pressure**	Birth: 50–70/30–45 1 year: 80–90/34–42 Rise in both pressures: 2–3 points per year of age Adult level reached at puberty	Elevated blood pressure in upper extremities *and* decrease in lower extremities: coarctation of aorta Narrowed pulse pressure (normal or elevated diastolic with lowered systolic; less than 30 points difference between systolic and diastolic readings): possible sign of aortic or subaortic stenosis or hypothyroidism Widened pulse pressure: possible sign of hyperthyroidism
Appearance		
Observe **general appearance**	Alert, well-nourished, comfortable, responsive	Lethargic, uncomfortable, malnourished, gross anomalies, dull
Listen to **voice and cry**	Strong, lusty cry Facial expression animated No indications of pain	Weak cry, low- or high-pitched cry: may indicate neurologic problem or chromosomal abnormality Stridor: possible upper airway edema or obstruction or hoarse cry, unresponsive Doubling over, rubbing a body part, general fretfulness, irritability
Assess presence of **odor**	No odor	Musty odor: sign of phenylketonuria, diphtheria Odor of maple syrup: may be maple syrup urine disease Odor of sweaty feet: one type of acidemia Fishy odor: may be metabolic disorder Acetone odor: acidosis, particularly diabetic ketoacidosis
Skin Assessment		
Assess **pigmentation**	Usually even Pigmented nevi common Large, flat, black and blue areas over sacrum, buttocks (mongolian spots)	Multiple café-au-lait spots: possible neurofibromatosis Cyanosis Jaundice Pallor
Assess **lesions**	Usually none Adolescence: acne	Erythematous lesions Multiple macules, papules, or vesicles Petechiae and ecchymoses: may indicate coagulation disorder
Assess **signs/symptoms of abuse**	None present	Hives (allergy) Subcutaneous nodules: may indicate juvenile rheumatoid arthritis Any unexplained bruises, welts, scars, burn marks, rope marks, failure to thrive, x-ray findings of multiple bone injuries, passive, noncommunicating child
Note **consistency of skin**	Good turgor Smooth and firm Check fontanel in infant	Poor turgor Dryness Edema Lack or excess of subcutaneous fat: sign of malnutrition or excess nutrition (obesity)
Assess **nails**	Nailbeds: normally pigmented Good nail growth	Cyanosis Pallor Capillary pulsations Pitting of the nails: possible sign of fungal disease or psoriasis Broad nailbeds: possible sign of Down syndrome or other chromosomal abnormality

(continued)

Assessment: Pediatric (continued)

Assessment	Normal Responses	Abnormal Responses
Assess **hair** (consistency appropriate to ethnic group)	No excessive breaking Consistent growth pattern	Dry, coarse, brittle hair: possible sign of hypothyroidism Alopecia (loss of hair): may be psychosomatic or due to drug therapy Unusual hairiness in places other than scalp, eyebrows, and lashes: may indicate hypothyroidism, vitamin A poisoning, chronic infections, reaction to Dilantin therapy Tufts of hair over spine or sacrum: may indicate site of spina bifida occulta or spina bifida Absence of the start of pubic hair during adolescence: possible hypothyroidism, hypopituitarism, gonadal deficiency, or Addison disease
Assess **lymph nodes**	Nontender, movable, discrete nodes up to 3 mm in diameter in occipital, postauricular, parotid, submaxillary, sublingual, axillary, and epitrochlear nodes Up to 1 mm in diameter inguinal and cervical nodes	Tender or enlarged nodes: may be sign of systemic infection

Head and Neck Assessment

Assessment	Normal Responses	Abnormal Responses
Assess **scalp**	Usually without lesions	Ringworm, lice Seborrheic dermatitis
Assess frontal and maxillary **sinuses**	Nontender	Tenderness: indicative of inflammatory process
Assess **face**	Symmetrical movement	Asymmetry: signs of facial paralysis Twitching: could be due to psychosomatic causes; vitamin/mineral deficiency

Evaluate the eyes
  Gross screening of vision
  Snellen chart
	With younger child, ability to focus and follow movement and to see objects placed a few feet away	Inability to follow movement or to see objects placed a few feet away

Sclerae	Completely white	Yellow sclera: sign of jaundice Blue sclera: may be normal or indicative of osteogenesis imperfecta
Placement in eye socket	Normally placed	Exophthalmos (protrusion of eyeball) Enophthalmos (deeply placed eyeball)
Iris	At rest: upper and lower margins of iris visible between the lids	Setting sun sign (iris appears to be beneath lower lid): if marked, may be sign of increased intracranial pressure or hydrocephalus
Movement	In newborn, intermittent strabismus or nystagmus	Fixed strabismus or intermittent strabismus continuing after 6 months of age: indication of muscle paralysis or weakness Involuntary, repetitive oscillations of one or both eyes: normal with *extreme* lateral gaze Nystagmus: may be cerebellar dysfunction indicative of use of certain drugs (anticonvulsants, barbiturates, alcohol)
Eyelids	Fully cover eyes Fully raised on opening	Ptosis of eyelid: may be an early sign of a neurologic disorder Sty
Conjunctiva	Clear	Inflammation (conjunctivitis) Hemorrhage Stimson lines (small red transverse lines on conjunctiva)

Assessment	Normal Responses	Abnormal Responses
Cornea	Clear	Opacity: sign of ulceration Inflammation Redness
Discharge	Tears	Purulent discharges: note amount, color, consistency (bacterial conjunctivitis)
Pupils	Round, regular Clear, equal Brisk reaction to light Accommodation reflex (ability of lens to adjust to objects at different distances)	Sluggish or asymmetrical reaction to light: indicates intracranial disease Lack of accommodation reflex
Lens	Clear	Opacities (cataracts)
Evaluate the **ears** Sinuses	No abnormality	Small holes or pits anterior to ear: may be superficial but could indicate presence of a sinus leading into brain
Position	Top of ear above level of eye	Top of ear below level of eye: associated with some congenital defects
Discharge	None	Discharge: note color, odor, consistency, and amount
Hearing	In infant: turning to sound In older child: responds to whispered command	Diminished hearing in one or both ears
Assess the **nose**	No secretions Breathing through nose	Secretions: note characteristics Any unusual shape or flaring of nostrils Breathing through mouth
Assess the **mouth**		Circumoral pallor: possible sign of cyanotic heart disease, scarlet fever, rheumatic fever, hypoglycemia; also seen in other febrile diseases Asymmetry of lips: seen in nerve paralysis
	Intact palate Teeth in good condition In older child presence of permanent teeth	Cleft palate Delayed appearance of deciduous teeth: may indicate cretinism, rickets, congenital syphilis, or Down syndrome; may also be normal Poor tooth formation: may be seen with systemic diseases Green or black teeth: seen after iron ingestion or death of tooth Stained teeth: may be seen after prolonged use of tetracyclines
Assess the **gums**	Retention cysts in newborn	Inflammation, abnormal color, drooling, pus, tenderness Black line along gums: may indicate lead poisoning
Assess the **tongue**	Moves freely Pink, with conical, filiform nontender papillae	Tremors on protrusion: may indicate chorea, hypothyroidism, cerebral palsy Protruding tongue—Down syndrome White spots (thrush) Tongue-tie (frenulum) Strawberry tongue (scarlet fever)
Assess the **throat**	Tonsils normally enlarged in childhood	White membrane over tonsils (diphtheria) White pus on sacs, erythema (bacterial pharyngitis), tender: vitamin deficiencies, anemia
Assess the **larynx**	Normal vocal tones	Hoarseness or stridor: possible upper respiratory tract obstruction
Assess the **neck**	Short in infancy Lengthens at 2–3 years Trachea slightly right of midline	Trachea deviated to left or right: may indicate shift with atelectasis

(continued)

Assessment: Pediatric (continued)

Assessment	Normal Responses	Abnormal Responses
Thyroid	Not enlarged	Enlarged: may be due to hyperactive thyroid, malignancy, goiter
Movement	Full lateral and upward/downward motion	Limited movement with pain: may indicate meningeal irritation, lymph node enlargement, rheumatoid arthritis, or other diseases
Lungs and Thorax Assessment		
Assess the **lungs**	Normally clear and equal breath sounds bilaterally	Presence of rhonchi, crackles, or wheezes
		Diminished breath sounds heard over parts of lung
	No retractions	Mild to severe intercostal or sternal retractions indicative of respiratory distress
	Symmetry of diaphragmatic movement	Asymmetry of movement (phrenic nerve damage)
Assess the **sputum**	None or small amount of clear sputum in morning	Thick, tenacious sputum with foul odor
		Blood-tinged or green sputum
Assess the **breasts**	Slightly enlarged in infancy	Discharge or growth in male
	Generally slightly asymmetrical at puberty	Masses (especially solid, fixed nonmobile) in older adolescent
Heart Assessment		
Assess **heart sounds**	S_1, S_2, S_3	S_4 indicates congestive heart failure
Assess **femoral pulses**	Strong	Weak
Note **edema**	None present	Edema—note location (initially periorbital) and duration, bulging fontanelles
Note **clubbing** of fingers	None present	Clubbing—congenital cyanotic heart defects; note location and duration
Note **murmurs**		Murmur grade 3 or higher is always abnormal
		No change in quality with positional changes
Note **cyanosis**	None normally present	Circumoral or peripheral cyanosis: indicates respiratory or cardiac disease (hypoxemia); congenital heart defects
Abdomen Assessment		
Assess **skin condition**	Soft	Hard, rigid, tender
Assess for **peristaltic motion**	Not visible	Visible peristalsis—may indicate pyloric stenosis (olive-shaped mass, palpable, in area of pylorus)
Assess **shape**	"Pot-bellied" toddlers	Large protruding abdomen: may indicate pancreatic fibrosis, hypokalemia, rickets, hypothyroidism, bowel obstruction, constipation, inguinal hernias, unilateral or bilateral: observe for reducibility
	Slightly protuberant in standing adolescent	
	Umbilical protrusion	Umbilical hernia
Genitourinary Tract Assessment		
Assess **female genitalia**		
Discharge	Mucoid, no odor	Foul or copious discharge; any bleeding before puberty
Signs of abuse	No signs	Bruises, welts, swelling, discharge, bleeding
Assess **male genitalia**	Orifice on distal end of penis	Hypospadias or epispadias (urethral orifice along inferior or dorsal surface)
Presence of urethral orifice		
Urethral opening	Normal size	Stenosis of urethral opening
Foreskin	Covers glans completely	Foreskin incompletely formed ventrally when hypospadias present
Placement of testes	Descended testes	Undescended testes
		Enlarged scrotum
Signs of abuse	No signs	Bruises, welts, swelling, discharge, bleeding
Assess **urine output**	Full, steady stream of urine	Urine with pus, blood, or odor (infection)
		Excessive urination or nocturia: possible sign of diabetes
Check **anus and rectum**	No masses or fissures present	Hemorrhoids, fissures, prolapse, pinworms
		Dark ring around rectal mucosa: may be sign of lead poisoning

Assessment	Normal Responses	Abnormal Responses
Musculoskeletal Assessment		
Assess **extremities**	Coloration of fingers and toes consistent with rest of body	Cyanosis—indicates respiratory or cardiac disease, or hypothermia in newborn
		Clubbing of fingers and toes indicates cardiac or respiratory disease
	Quick capillary refill on blanching	Sluggish blood return on blanching indicates poor circulation
	Temperature same as rest of body	Temperature variation between extremities and rest of body indicates neurologic or vascular anomalies
	Presence of pedal pulses	Absence of pedal pulses indicates circulatory difficulties
	No pain or tenderness	Presence of localized or generalized pain
	Straight legs after 2 years of age	Any bowing after 2 years of age may be hereditary or indicate rickets
	Broad-based gait until 4 years of age; feet straight ahead afterwards	Scissoring gait indicates spastic cerebral palsy
		Persistence of broad-based gait after 4 years of age indicates possible abnormalities of legs and feet or balance disturbance
		Any limp or ataxia
Assess **spine**	No dimples	Presence of dimple or tufts of hair indicates possible spina bifida
	Flexible	Limited flexion indicates central nervous system infections
		Hyperextension (opisthotonos) indicates brainstem irritation, hemorrhage, or intracranial infection
Have child bend forward at waist and check level of scapulae (scoliosis screening)	No lateral curvature or excessive anterior posterior curvature	Presence of lordosis (after age 2 years), kyphosis, or scoliosis
	Scapulae at same height	
Assess **hips**	Symmetrical full range of motion	Asymmetrical thigh folds, clicks on adduction—hip dysplasia
Assess **joints**	Full range of motion without pain, edema, or tenderness	Pain, edema, or tenderness indicates tissue injury
Assess **muscles**	Good tone and purposeful movement	Decreased or increased tone
	Ability to perform motor skills approximate to development level	Spasm or tremors may indicate cerebral palsy
		Atrophy or contractures

Chapter Wrap-Up

GERONTOLOGIC Considerations

Head and Neck and Neurologic System
Physiologic Changes With Age
- Decreased speed of nerve conduction and delay in response and reaction time, especially with stress
- Diminution of sensory faculties; decreased vision, loss of hearing, diminished sense of smell and taste, greater sensitivity to temperature changes with low tolerance to cold

- Tooth loss
- Poor dentition, inadequate chewing, poor swallowing reflex
- Condition of teeth, gums, buccal cavity
- Periodontal disease

Taste sensation decreases.

- Chronic irritation of mucous membranes
- Atrophy of up to 80% of taste buds
- Loss of sensitivity of those on tip of tongue first: sweet and salt
- Loss of sensitivity of those on sides later: salt, sour, bitter

Assessment

- Facial symmetry
- Poor reflex reactions
- Level of alertness—presence of organic brain changes: memory impairment
- Motor function—strength

Skin

Physiologic Changes With Age

Skin less effective as barrier:

- Decreased protection from trauma
- Less ability to retain water
- Decreased temperature regulation

Skin composition changes:

- Dryness (osteotosis) due to decreased endocrine secretion
- Loss of elastin
- Increased vascular fragility
- Thicker and more wrinkled on sun-exposed areas
- Melanocyte cluster pigmentation

Sweat glands:

- Decreased number and size
- Decreased function of sebaceous glands

Hair:

- General hair loss
- Decreased melanin production
- Facial hair increases in women

Nails:

- More brittle and thick

Assessment

Skin:

- Temperature, degree of moisture, dryness
- Intactness, open lesions, tears, decubiti
- Turgor, dehydration
- Pigmentation alterations, potential cancer
- Pruritus—dry skin most common cause
- Bruises, scars

Condition of nails (hard and brittle):

- Presence of fungus
- Overgrown or horny toenails, ingrown

Condition of hair:

Infestations (scabies, lice)

Chest

Physiologic Changes With Age

Respiratory muscles lose strength and become rigid.

Ciliary activity decreases.

Lungs lose elasticity:

- Residual capacity increases.
- Larger on inspiration
- Maximum breathing capacity decreases; depth of respirations decreases.
- Alveoli increase in size, reduce in number.
- Fewer capillaries at alveoli
- Dilated and less elastic alveoli

Gas exchange is reduced:

- Arterial blood oxygen PaO_2 can decrease after age 70.
- Arterial blood carbon dioxide $PaCO_2$ unchanged

Coughing ability reduced—less sensitive mechanism

More dependent on the diaphragm for breathing

System less responsive to hypoxia and hypercardia

Assessment

- Shape of chest excursion
- Lung and breath sounds
- Quality of cough, if present; sputum

Rib cage deformity

Dyspnea, hypoxia, and hypercarbia

Breast—size, symmetry, contour:

- Presence of lumps
- Size and shape of nipples

Heart

Physiologic Changes With Age

Mitral and aortic valves thicken and become rigid.

Cardiac output decreases 1% per year after age 20 due to decreased heart rate and stroke volume.

Vessels lose elasticity:

- Less effective peripheral oxygenation
- Position change from lying-to-sitting or sitting-to-standing can cause blood pressure to drop as much as 65 mm Hg.

Increased peripheral vessel resistance:

- Blood pressure increases: systolic may normally be 170 mm Hg, diastolic may normally be 95 mm Hg.
- Smooth muscle in arteries is less responsive.

Blood clotting increases.

Assessment

Heart sounds—murmurs

Peripheral circulation, color, warmth:

- Apical pulse
- Jugular vein distention

Orthostatic hypotension:

- Dizziness
- Fainting

Edema

Activity intolerance

Dyspnea

Transient ischemic attacks (TIAs)

Abdomen
Physiologic Changes With Age

Esophagus dilates and has decreased motility.

Stomach:

- Hunger sensations decrease.
- Secretion of hydrochloric acid decreases.
- Emptying time decreases.

Peristalsis decreases and constipation is common.

Absorption function is impaired:

- Body absorbs fewer nutrients due to reduced intestinal blood flow and atrophy of cells on absorbing surfaces.
- Decrease in gastric enzymes affects absorption.

Hiatal hernia common (40%–60% of older adults)

Diverticulitis common (40% over age 70)

Liver:

- Fewer cells, with decreased storage capacity
- Decreased blood flow
- Enzymes decreased
- Increased risk for drug toxicity

Impaired pancreatic reserve

Decreased glucose tolerance

Assessment

- Indications of possible hiatal hernia
- Bowel distention
- Bowel sounds

Genitourinary Tract
Physiologic Changes With Age

Kidneys:

- Smaller due to nephron atrophy
- Renal blood flow decreases 50%.
- Glomerular filtration rate decreases 50%.
- Tubular function diminishes: less able to concentrate urine; lower specific gravity; proteinuria 1+ is common; blood urea nitrogen (BUN) increases.
- Renal threshold for glucose increases.

Bladder:

- Muscle weakens.
- Capacity decreases to 200 mL or less, causing frequency.

- Emptying is more difficult, causing increased retention.
- Increased risk of incontinence (*Note:* Incontinence is not a normal age-related occurrence.)

Prostate enlarges to some degree in 75% of men over age 65 (hypertrophy).

Menopause occurs by mean age of 50.

Perineal muscle weakens.

Vulva atrophies.

Vagina:

- Mucous membrane becomes drier due to decreased estrogen.
- Elasticity of tissue decreases, so surface is smooth.
- Secretions become reduced, more alkaline.
- Flora changes.

Sexuality:

- Older people continue to be sexual beings with sexual needs.
- No particular age causes an individual's sexual functioning to cease.
- Frequency of genital sexual behavior (intercourse) may tend to decline gradually in later years, but capacity for expression and enjoyment continues far into old age.

Assessment

- Condition of skin—dehydration
- Urinary output; blood in urine; color; specific gravity; prothrombin time (PT)
- Incontinence
- Bladder distention
- Genital assessment

Musculoskeletal System
Physiologic Changes With Age

Contractures:

- Muscles atrophy, regenerate slowly, strength diminishes.
- Tendons shrink and sclerose.

Range of motion of joints decreases:

- Lack of adequate joint motion, ankylosis
- Slight flexion of joints

Assessment

Mobility level:

- Ambulate with more difficulty
- Limitation to movement
- Muscle strength diminishes and cramps occur.
- Gait becomes unsteady.
- Presence of kyphosis
- Pain in joints

MANAGEMENT Guidelines

Each state legislates a Nurse Practice Act for RNs and LPN/LVNs. Healthcare facilities are responsible for establishing and implementing policies and procedures that conform to their state's regulations. Verify the regulations and role parameters for each healthcare worker in your facility.

Delegation

- RNs must complete the admission assessment and document the findings. They cannot delegate this activity to anyone else on the team.
- LPN/LVNs may complete focus assessments each shift; however, any changes in assessment findings must be reported and verified with the RN.
- Unlicensed assistive personnel may not perform assessments on clients.

Interprofessional Communication

- Changes in assessment data identified in report or in the client's chart must be reported to the appropriate nurse assigned to complete the focus assessment.
- LPN/LVNs delegated the responsibility to complete focus assessments on clients must have clear direction on what is essential information to report back. Remind the LPN/LVNs they must verify with the RN any changes identified in the assessment.
- Remind LPN/LVNs that if there are any questions on the client status as a result of their assessment, they must notify the RN immediately.

CASE STUDY Applications

Scenario 1

Mrs. Smiley has had a history of hypertension for several years. She has recently experienced an inability to use her right arm and leg and has lost ability to express herself. She has been admitted to your unit with the diagnosis of R/O left CVA (stroke) and has been placed on a continuous heparin IV drip.

1. Based on admitting data, make a judgment about what deviations from normal you would find in the physical examination.
2. List appropriate nursing diagnoses based on her physical state and immobility status (this affects virtually all systems).

3. In view of all these existing and potential problems, identify *priority* concerns (all are important concerns) for this client.
4. Develop a plan of care addressing these priority concerns.

Scenario 2

You are caring for a woman in labor and monitoring the fetal heart rate. You note that early deceleration has occurred (a 10- to 20-beat drop in the fetal heart rate).

1. From these symptoms, indicate your priority intervention.
2. What would you conclude about the viability of the fetus?
3. What does this change in condition of the fetus imply?

NCLEX® Review Questions

Unless otherwise specified, choose only one (1) answer.

1. Components of the chest assessment include which of the following? (*Select all that apply.*)
   A. General appearance
   B. Shape of chest
   C. Position of ribs
   D. Costovertebral angle tenderness
   E. Retractions
   F. Curvature of the spine

2. The nurse suspects that a client has appendicitis. When assessing for rebound tenderness, what should the nurse do?
   A. Perform this assessment first.
   B. Have the client take a deep breath.
   C. Palpate deeply with quick release of pressure.
   D. Have the client lie flat with legs extended.

3. A client comes into the clinic for evaluation of a burn injury from hot liquid. The lesions are flat and red. The nurse should document the presence of what type of lesion?
   A. Macules
   B. Wheals
   C. Vesicles
   D. Papules

4. The nurse is assessing a client's deep tendon reflexes. How would the nurse document a normal response?
   A. +1
   B. 0
   C. +2
   D. +4

5. Which cranial nerve is assessed when testing for the "gag reflex"?

   A. XI accessory

   B. VII facial

   C. IX glossopharyngeal

   D. XII hypoglossal

6. During a cardiac assessment, where can S_1 heart sound be heard the loudest?

   A. At the second intercostal space

   B. At the pulmonic valve region

   C. Over the aortic area

   D. At the apex of the heart

7. When assessing the lymph nodes in the neck, what should the nurse instruct the client to do?

   A. Raise the chin.

   B. Lie in a supine position.

   C. Swallow a sip of water.

   D. Flex the neck slightly.

8. When completing a physical assessment, the nurse is unable to palpate a peripheral pulse, the dorsalis pedis. What would the next intervention be?

   A. Notify the healthcare provider.

   B. Examine the adjacent area.

   C. Obtain a new Doppler.

   D. Move on to the next area.

9. The urinary tract assessment includes checking the specific gravity of the client's urine to determine if it is within normal limits. The normal range of specific gravity is ___ to ____.

10. Suspecting that the client you are assessing may be exhibiting cognitive decline or dementia, which of the following questions would be appropriate?

    A. "How do you feel today?"

    B. "What work did you do 20 years ago?"

    C. "Who is the president of the United States?"

    D. "Tell me why you are in the hospital."

QSEN Activity

Domain: Client Centered Care

KSA: Knowledge

Activity:

When collecting data for a physical exam for clients of different ethnic backgrounds, what are some considerations to explore? What are some genetic predispositions to consider:

If your client is Hispanic?

If your client is African American?

If your client is of Jewish descent?

If your client is of Mediterranean descent?

Bibliography

Cowdell, F. & Radley, K. (2014, Mar.). What do we know about skin hygiene care for patients with bariatric needs? Implications for nursing practice. *Journal of Advanced Nursing*, 70 (3), 543–552 doi: 10.1111/jan.12208

Flaherman, V. J. F., Schaefer, E. W., Kuzniewicz, M. W., Li, S., X., Walsh, E. M., & Paul, I. M., (2015, Jan.). Early weight loss nomograms for exclusively breastfed newborns. *Pediatrics*, 135(1), e16–e23.

Koti, A. & Roetzheim, R. (2015, Jan.). Patient factors associated with documented provision of JNC 7: Recommended hypertension care at an academic family medicine office. *Journal of the American Board of Family Medicine*, 28(1), 97–104. Doi:10.3122/jabfm.2015.01.140258

Lawrence, J., Alcock, D., McGrath, P., Kay, J., MacMurray, S. B., & Dulberg, C. (1993, Dec.). The development of a tool to assess neonatal pain. *Neonatal Network, 12*(6), 61.

Morrow, C. (2010, Jun.). Reducing neonatal pain during routine heel lance procedures. *American Journal of Maternal Child Nursing*, 35(6), 346–354.

National Center for Health Statistics. (2007–2010). *National Health and Nutrition Examination Survey*. Centers for Disease Control and Prevention. (2011) retrieved from http://www.nhlbi.nih.gov/health/health-topics/topics/hbp/

Phillips, J. (2013). Care of the bariatric patient in acute care. *Journal of Radiology Nursing, 32*, 21–31.

Smith, S. F. (2016). *Sandra Smith's review for NCLEX-RN*, (13th ed.). Burlington, MA: Jones & Bartlett Learning, LLC.

Chapter 12
Body Mechanics and Positioning

Learning Objectives

12.1 Discuss the primary function of the skeletal muscles, joints, and bones.

12.2 Describe nursing measures that assist in preserving joints, bones, and skeletal muscles.

12.3 Describe the ANA Standards that promote safe handling of clients and prevention of injury to healthcare workers.

12.4 Describe a minimum of two principles of correct body mechanics.

12.5 Explain practice guidelines to prevent injury to clients and healthcare workers as outlined in OSHA guidelines.

12.6 State two expected outcomes of using proper body mechanics.

12.7 Discuss the objectives for moving and turning clients.

12.8 Describe the position of the head of the bed in the four Fowler's positions.

12.9 Explain how the client is positioned in a lateral and prone position.

12.10 Describe the correct placement of the canvas pieces when placing a client on the floor-based client lift.

12.11 Explain the rationale of assisted ambulation for clients.

12.12 Demonstrate the procedures for moving a client to the side of the bed and dangling a client.

12.13 Outline the steps in logrolling a client.

12.14 Describe requirements for lift team members.

12.15 List the pertinent data that should be charted when moving a client from the bed.

12.16 Write a client care plan using at least three nursing diagnoses for a client requiring moving and turning interventions.

Chapter Outline

Terminology

Alignment referring to posture; the relationship of body parts to one another.

Ambulate walking; able to walk.

Assistive equipment used to move clients without placing pressure on back and trunk.

Atrophy a wasting; decrease in size of an organ or tissue.

Balance A result of body alignment that maintains equilibrium, coordination and stability of the body in space.

Base of support surface area on which an object rests (e.g., for a client lying in prone position, the base of support is the entire undersurface of the body).

Body mechanics movement of the body in a coordinated and efficient way so that proper balance, alignment, and conservation of energy is maintained.

Cartilage nonvascular, dense, supporting connective tissue. Found in joints, thorax, larynx, trachea, nose, and ear.

Center of gravity midpoint or center of the body weight. In an adult, it is the midpelvic cavity between the symphysis pubis and umbilicus.

Dangle The position in which a client's feet are placed over the edge of the bed and allowed to hang freely.

Ergonomics applied science concerned with designing and arranging things people use so that the people and things interact most efficiently and safely.

Flexion the act or condition of being bent.

Fowler's position head of bed is at a 45-degree angle; client's knees may or may not be flexed.

Gravity the force that pulls objects toward the earth's surface.

High-Fowler's position head of bed is at a 60-degree angle; often used to achieve maximum chest expansion.

Hoyer lift a mechanical device that enables one individual to safely transfer a client from bed to chair.

Joint the portion of the body where two or more bones join together.

Leverage the use of a lever to apply force.

Ligament a band or sheet of strong fibrous connective tissue connecting the articular ends of bones serving to bind them together and to facilitate or limit motion.

Manual client handling tasks such as lifting, transferring, and repositioning of clients without use of assistive devices.

Mobility state or quality of being mobile; facility of movement.

Musculoskeletal pertaining to the muscles and bones.

Orthosis use of external device or special equipment to stabilize or immobilize a body part, protect against injury, or assist with function.

Paralysis temporary or permanent loss of function, especially loss of sensation or voluntary motion.

Posture attitude or position of body.

Prone lying horizontal with face downward.

Reverse Trendelenburg position mattress remains unbent, but head of bed is raised and foot is lowered.

Semi-Fowler's position head of bed is at a 30-degree angle; often used for clients with cardiac and respiratory problems.

Skeletal system system of separate bones (206) bound together by ligaments and responsible for supporting, moving, and giving shape to the body.

SPHM acronym for Safe Patient Handling and Mobility. Safe patient handling and mobility programs and standards aim to reduce the risk of injury to clients and healthcare workers in all healthcare settings.

Stable when the center of gravity is close to the base of support.

Strain injury caused by excessive force or stretching of muscles or tendons around the joint.

Trendelenburg position mattress remains unbent but the head of the bed is lowered and the foot is raised. "Shock blocks" may be used under the legs of the bed to achieve this position.

Trochanter either of the two bony prominences below the neck of the femur.

Musculoskeletal System

The **musculoskeletal** system protects the body, provides a structural framework, and allows the body to move. The primary structures in this system are muscles, bones, and joints.

Skeletal Muscles

Skeletal muscles move the bones around the joints by contracting and relaxing so that movement can take place. Each muscle consists of a body, or belly, and tendons, which connect the muscle to another muscle or to bone.

When skeletal muscles contract, they cause two bones to move around the joint between them. One of these bones tends to remain stationary while the other bone moves. The end of the muscle that attaches to the stationary bone is called the origin. The end of the muscle that attaches to the movable bone is called the insertion.

Muscles are designated flexors or extensors according to whether they flex the joint (decrease the angle between the bones) or extend the joint (increase the angle between the bones). For example, when the deltoid muscle contracts, it abducts the arm and raises it laterally to the horizontal position. The anterior fibers aid in **flexion** of the arm, and the posterior fibers aid in extension of the arm.

Joints

Joints are the places where bones meet. Their primary function is to provide motion and flexibility. Although the internal structure of joints varies, most joints are composed of **ligaments**, which bind the bones together, and **cartilage**, or tissue, which covers and cushions the ends of the bones.

Bones

Bones provide the major support for all the body organs. Bone is composed of an organic matrix, deposits of calcium salts, and bone cells. The organic matrix provides the framework and tensile strength for the bone. The calcium salts, which are about 75% of the bone, provide compressional strength by filling in the matrix. As a result, it is very difficult to damage a bone by twisting it or by applying direct pressure.

Bone cells include osteoblasts, osteocytes, and osteoclasts. Osteoblasts deposit the organic matrix; osteocytes and osteoclasts reabsorb this matrix. Because this process is usually in equilibrium, bone is deposited where it is needed in the **skeletal system**. If increased stress is placed on a bone, such as the stress of continued athletic activity, more bone is deposited. If there is no stress on a bone, as is often the case with clients on prolonged bed rest, part of the bone mass is reabsorbed, or lost.

System Alterations

Alterations in **mobility** can result from problems in the musculoskeletal system, the nervous system, and the skin. A primary cause for alterations in muscles is inactivity. With forceful activity, muscles increase in size. With inactivity, muscles decrease in size and strength. When clients are in casts, in traction, on prolonged bed rest, or unable to exercise, their muscles become weak and atrophied.

Alterations in joints result when mobility is limited by changes in the adjacent tissues. When muscle movement decreases, the connective tissue in the joints, tendons, and ligaments becomes thickened and fibrotic.

Chronic flexion and hyperextension can also cause alterations in the joints. Chronic flexion can cause joints to become contracted in one position so that they are unmovable. Hyperextension occurs when joints are extended beyond their normal limits, which is usually 180 degrees. The results of hyperextension are pain and discomfort to the client and abnormal stress on the ligaments and tendons of the joints.

Alterations in bone are caused by disease processes, decalcification, and breaks caused by trauma or twisting. Encouraging clients to stand and to walk is important because the body functions best when it is in a vertical position. Physical activity forces muscles to move and increases blood flow, which improves metabolism and facilitates such body functions as gastrointestinal peristalsis.

Many body systems are affected by immobility (Table 12-1 ■). Even a few days of immobility can lead to alterations in many body systems. The following chart indicates a few of the systems affected and what occurs with immobility.

In addition to the system alterations, mental health can be affected. Alterations in mental health can range from depending upon others for care and loss of independence to isolation and depression.

Nursing Measures

Nursing care measures to preserve the joints, bones, and skeletal muscles should be carried out for all clients who require bed rest. Positions in which clients are placed and methods of moving and turning should all be based on the principles of maintaining the musculoskeletal system in proper **alignment**. The nurse must also use good **body mechanics** when moving and turning clients to preserve her or his own musculoskeletal system from injury. These nursing measures are also performed by the home care providers.

In addition to paying attention to the body positioning and moving and turning, it is essential to:

- Avoid using the Valsalva maneuver when turning or moving a client.
- Perform range-of-motion exercises—maintain blood circulation and muscular activity, as well as promote oxygenation to the cells and tissues.
- Provide frequent turning, proper positioning, and repositioning—essential to prevent skin breakdown (also described as pressure ulcer prevention). Protect areas of bony prominence, which are especially vulnerable to skin breakdown.
- Increase fluids to maintain blood flow, unless contraindicated by the client's condition. Consider time of day of fluid ingestion to decrease frequency of getting out of bed during the night.

Table 12-1 Pathophysiologic Effects of Immobility

System Affected	Result
Cardiovascular Heart effects	• Veins become engorged, which may contribute to valve damage due to lack of muscular activity (peripheral edema). • Increased risk of clot formation is due to slowing of blood flow and inadequate circulation of blood to cells and tissues (deep vein thrombosis and pulmonary embolism). • Valsalva maneuver, caused by holding the breath when trying to raise up in bed or when having a bowel movement, leads to increased workload on the heart. • Blood pressure may decrease, causing orthostatic hypotension when standing and potentially leading to falls.
Respiratory	• Thick secretions accumulate, pooling in the lower respiratory structures. • Immobility prevents lung expansion, decreases movement of secretions in the airways, and decreases expectoration of secretions • Risk increases for reduced oxygenation and perfusion, and development of pneumonia.
Gastrointestinal	• An indirect effect of immobility on the GI system occurs during the intake of nutrients, both food and water. • Decreased metabolic needs can cause anorexia. • Decreases in food intake may lead to protein deficiency. • Constipation or diarrhea may occur due to fecal impaction, weakened muscle tone, and not feeling the urge to defecate.
Urinary	• Immobility causes the kidneys to force urine against **gravity**. • Sluggish flow leads to pooling of urine in the kidney and increases the risk of renal calculi and infection. • Loss of sphincter muscle tone can lead to urinary incontinence, resulting in losing the urge to void and increased urine dribbling.
Musculoskeletal	• Loss of muscle tone and deterioration of bone leads to weakness and stiffness. • Loss of elasticity and demineralization of bones leads to osteoporosis.

- Instruct the client in coughing and deep-breathing exercises to prevent and remove secretions from the airways and promote oxygenation. Position to promote oxygenation.
- Provide nutritious meals, especially high calcium for bone health and protein to protect skin integrity.

Safe Patient Handling and Mobility

Knowledge of a client's body and how it moves is important. Knowledge of your own body and what happens to it when you care for clients with altered mobility is also important. Before you lift or move a client, determine the causes and consequences of the client's illness and use Safe Patient Handling and Mobility Algorithms, if available, to determine the appropriate client moving or lifting and transfer protocols. These guidelines also indicate the equipment needed for safe client transfer or moving or the need for the lift team. This knowledge enables you to move the client safely.

In the past, the most common client handling approaches used in the United States included manual client lifting, education related to body mechanics, education in safe lifting techniques, and the use of back belts. However, there is strong evidence that each of these approaches is not effective in reducing caregiver injuries. Evidence-based practice indicates that reduced injury to both clients and staff is associated with use of client handling equipment and devices, client care ergonomic assessment protocols, "No Lift" policies, education in proper use of client handling equipment and devices, and client lift teams. Other benefits include improved quality of care and client outcomes, increased

client and staff satisfaction, reduced workforce turnover, and reduced costs due to development of complications and workman compensation. A system-wide, sustained commitment to emphasize a culture of safety is at the core of safe patient handling and mobility programs and actions.

The physical environment of the healthcare setting and the aging of the nursing workforce also contribute to work-related injuries. The "tight quarters" and configuration of client rooms, nurses' work areas, and equipment can affect use of appropriate body mechanics as well as equipment for moving clients. The most common tasks leading to injury are lifting, transferring, and repositioning. Musculoskeletal disorders (MSDs) account for 33% of all injuries (Figure 12-1 ■).

A well-designed client care environment and access to equipment assist the staff in using ergonomically sound procedures that improve client handling. Trying to lift or move too much weight forces you to use your body incorrectly and frequently causes injuries. The National Institute for Occupational Safety and Health (NIOSH) states that

Nonfatal Occupational Injuries and Illnesses by Private Industry Sector (2011)

- 387,820 MSD cases (33% of all cases)
- Occupations with most MSDs:
  - o Nursing assistants
  - o Laborers
  - o Janitors and cleaners
  - o Truck drivers
  - o Registered nurses
  - o Stock clerks

FIGURE 12-1 Nonfatal occupational injuries and illnesses.
Source: Bureau of Labor Statistics.

the average worker should not manually lift more than 35 lb under controlled and limited circumstances. However, even with lighter weights, cumulative microinjuries of the spine can result in debilitating injury. Incorrect lifting may put pressure on the muscles of the lower back or other vulnerable parts of the body. If you do not follow guidelines for promoting proper body mechanics or using equipment, you are putting your own health and safety in jeopardy. For this reason, many organizations have developed policies stating that healthcare workers must use lifts to move clients, and the U.S. Department of Labor Occupational Safety and Health Administration (OSHA) recommends minimizing manual lifting and eliminating lifting whenever possible (Box 12-1 ■). To prevent injury, it is advisable that healthcare workers do simple exercises to strengthen and stretch the abdominal muscles and muscles that support the back (ANA, 2013).

Proper use of body mechanics helps prevent injuries to clients and all members of the health team. The following guidelines underlie the implementation of body mechanics:

- Request assistance from others or use client-handling equipment or devices when working with heavy clients to avoid **strain**.
- Assume a proper stance before moving or turning clients.
- Distribute workload evenly before moving or turning clients.
- Establish a comfortable height when working with clients. Keep the client as close to your body as possible when moving.
- Push when moving an individual or object; do not pull.
- Use large muscles for lifting and moving, not back muscles. Move the hips and shoulders as one unit.
- Avoid leaning and stretching.
- Avoid twisting your body.
- Keep the low back in neutral position.

In addition to proper use of body mechanics, ergonomic protection and education programs must be implemented in all healthcare facilities to decrease risk factors related to back injuries. The use of body mechanics, equipment, and devices alone does not prevent back injuries and musculoskeletal disorders among nurses. However, appropriate use of body mechanics combined with a safe client handling or client care **ergonomics** program can decrease both the number and severity of injuries.

LEGAL ALERT
Back Injuries From Lifting and Transferring

A suit was filed against a large nursing home chain by nursing assistants at five Pennsylvania nursing homes. The complaint with OSHA alleged they had sustained back injuries from lifting and transferring clients. After a 15-month investigation, OSHA issued citations against the nursing home for ergonomics violations under the "general duty" clause of the Occupational Safety and Health Act. The clause states that an employer must provide employees with a workplace free of recognized hazards that are causing or likely to cause death or physical harm. OSHA argued that transferring clients exposed CNAs to serious injury to the upper back and upper extremities. OSHA settled with the nursing home chain. Under the terms of the settlement, the nursing home chain agreed to purchase mechanical lifting equipment at all facilities, nationwide, and to train all workers in the use of the equipment.

Source: Mellinger (2002)

ANA Promotes Safe Patient Handling and Mobility

Safe patient handling and mobility has been a priority for the ANA for many years. In 2003, ANA launched the Handle with Care Program in an effort to prevent injuries and MSDs. In June 2013, new Safe Patient Handling and Mobility Interprofessional National Standards were released (Harrington & Brigham, 2013). Nurses and other healthcare workers face many hazards in their work environments. Every day nurses sustain debilitating and often career-ending MSDs. The current statistics (ANA, 2011) indicate that 62% of nurses fear they will develop a disabling MSD, 56% of nurses state they have experienced MSD pain that was made worse by their job, and 80% of nurses report pain from MSDs but continue to work.

Home Care

Knowledge of body mechanics and how to use these principles when giving care is important to both the healthcare provider and the client. Correct use of body mechanics decreases the caregiver's potential for injury and provides safety for the client. Recently, there has been an increase in the number of back injury incident claims among home healthcare providers. One reason for the increase is the improper use of body mechanics while performing skills in

---

Box 12-1 **PRACTICE GUIDELINES**

Preventing Injury to Clients and Healthcare Workers

OSHA has developed the following lifting guidelines for healthcare workers to prevent injury to the client and the worker.

- Never transfer clients/residents when off **balance**.
- Never lift clients alone, particularly those who have fallen. Use team lifts or use mechanical assistance.
- Lift loads close to the body.
- Limit number of allowed lifts per worker per day.
- Avoid heavy lifting, especially with spine rotation.
- Complete training in when and how to use mechanical assistive devices.

Source: Occupational Safety and Health Administration (n.d.)

the home setting. Also, there may be no one to assist the care provider when lifting and turning clients in the home. The nurse may need to improvise, as the equipment may not be adequate or adjustable. More home care agencies assist clients in obtaining assistive devices.

The purpose of this unit is to consider adaptations necessary for providing safe care to the client while using proper body mechanics. In the home setting, much of the care is given by the family; therefore, it is essential that they also be taught good body mechanics.

Cultural Awareness

Different cultures may have cultural variances regarding distance and space. When clients are being moved or transferred to a bed or gurney, the client is brought close to the nurse's body. It is important to explain the transfer process to clients, particularly American, Canadian, and British clients. They may be threatened by invasion of personal space and touch. Asians, Middle East clients, and Hispanics may not be as concerned about personal space.

Nursing Diagnoses

The following nursing diagnoses are appropriate to use on client care plans when the components are related to body mechanics.

NURSING DIAGNOSIS	RELATED TO . . .
Activity Intolerance	Impaired motor function, weakness, paralysis, or pain
Risk for Injury	Altered mobility, impaired sensory function, prolonged bed rest
Impaired Physical Mobility	Trauma or musculoskeletal impairment, surgical procedure, muscle weakness, pain, decreased strength
Impaired Transfer Ability	Weakness, flaccidity, amputation, decreased strength
Impaired Walking	Muscle weakness, impaired motor function, orthopedic surgery, or dysfunction
Ineffective Breathing Patterns	Musculoskeletal dysfunction; decreased energy
Ineffective Peripheral Tissue Perfusion	Mechanical reduction of venous and/or arterial blood flow

Nursing Process Data

ASSESSMENT Database

- Evaluate personnel's knowledge of the principles of body mechanics.
- Evaluate personnel's knowledge of how to use correct muscle groups for specific activities.
- Assess knowledge and correct any misinformation about body alignment and how to maintain it with each position.
- Assess knowledge of physical science and application to balance and body alignment.
- Assess the competency of spinal cord and associated musculature.
- Assess the muscle mass of the long, thick, and strong muscles of the shoulders and thighs.

PLANNING Objectives

- To promote proper body mechanics while caring for clients
- To maintain good posture, thereby promoting optimum musculoskeletal balance
- To provide knowledge of the musculoskeletal system, body alignment, and balance in order to assist the nurse in caring for clients
- To correct body mechanics, promote health, enhance appearance, and assist body function

IMPLEMENTATION Procedures

DOCUMENTATION AND EVALUATION

Expected Outcomes

- Correct body mechanics are used when preparing for and providing client care.
- Injuries are prevented to both the nurse and the client.
- Proper body mechanics facilitate client care.
- Clients and nurses are not injured when nursing care is provided.
- Center of gravity is maintained when lifting objects.
- Back care exercises promote back health.

Unexpected Outcomes/Alternative Actions

Pearson Nursing Student Resources

Find additional review materials at
nursing.pearsonhighered.com.
Prepare for success with NCLEX®-style practice
questions and Skill Checklists.

Equipment
Small pillow

Note: This skill is for nurses to prevent back strain.

Preparation
1. Check the physician's orders or client's chart to determine the types of exercises to be carried out.
2. Gather any equipment needed for the exercises.
3. Identify the client using two identifiers.
4. Introduce yourself and explain the procedure.
5. Perform hand hygiene and provide privacy.

Procedure
1. Complete the four exercises in order, and repeat 10 cycles.
   ➤ **Rationale:** These exercises assist in strengthening stomach, buttocks, and thigh muscles and stretching lower back muscles to prevent back injuries (see Box 12-2 ■).
2. Complete posterior pelvic tilt exercises.
   a. Lie flat on your back with head on a small pillow or stand against a wall.
   b. Bend knees and hips so that feet are flat on the hard surface.
   c. Push lower back onto floor or against wall (back needs to be flat).
   d. Tighten abdominal muscles, and then exhale.
   e. Tighten gluteal muscles, and then exhale.
   f. Lift hips from floor, or away from wall, and tilt whole pelvis forward while maintaining back flat against hard surface. Hold position for count of 10.
   g. Slowly relax.
3. Complete 10 lumbar stretches to keep natural curves of spine in shape.
   a. Lie flat on floor with head on pillow.
   b. Bend knees and slowly bring them toward your chest. Place hand behind thigh to assist in bending knees.
   c. Keep head on pillow, and elevate buttocks as high as possible off the floor. Keep knees as close to chest as possible.
   d. Hold position, holding on to thighs and keeping knees to chest for count of 10.
4. Complete hamstring stretches for 10 cycles to promote easy bending.
   a. Lie on a hard surface with knees close to the chest in a relaxed position.
   b. Slowly extend one leg toward ceiling; flex foot and push heel upward to feel hamstring muscles stretch. Hold position and count to 10. Bend leg and bring knee back toward chest.
   c. Extend second leg while lowering first leg and complete step b.
   d. Repeat exercise 10 times and then bring both knees toward chest, roll to one side, and take a standing position.
5. Complete reverse sit-ups to strengthen abdominal muscles.
   a. Sit on floor in upright position with knees bent.
   b. Lock hands together behind head and hold arms out to side.
   c. Slowly lean back 15 degrees while tightening stomach muscles. Hold position for count of at least 5.
   d. Slowly lean back about 20 degrees, hold the position, and count to 10.
   e. Slowly return to an upright position; repeat exercises 10 cycles.

Box 12-2 GUIDELINES ON PREVENTION OF LOW BACK PAIN FOR WORKERS

- Physical exercise is recommended for prevention of low back pain. There is insufficient evidence to recommend for or against any specific type or intensity of exercises.
- Lumbar supports or back belts are not recommended.
- Shoe inserts/**orthoses** are not recommended. There is insufficient evidence to recommend for or against insoles, soft shoes, soft flooring, or antifatigue mats.
- Temporary modified work and ergonomic workplace adaptations can be recommended to facilitate early return to work for individuals with low back pain.
- There is insufficient consistent evidence to recommend physical ergonomic interventions alone for prevention of low back pain.
- Further research is necessary to determine appropriate prevention of low back pain. Future studies need to be high quality, using randomized, controlled trials.

CLINICAL ALERT
Stop exercises if you experience pain or if it gets more difficult with repetitions. Check with your physician before attempting exercises.

Skill 12.1.2 | Applying Body Mechanics

Procedure

1. Determine need for assistance in moving or turning a client following OSHA Lifting Guidelines. ➤ *Rationale:* Half of all back pain is associated with lifting or turning clients. (See Box 12-2 for prevention of low back pain.) ❶–❹ The most common back injury is strain on the lumbar muscle group.

❶ Gait belts are routinely used to assist in manual transfer in most facilities.

❷ Manual transfers from bed to chair should be done only if client is able to stand.

❸ Use proper body mechanics whenever moving clients or objects.

❹ Ensure that height of bed allows you to work without causing injury.

2. Place bed at the correct height for staff: waist level when providing care; hip level when moving a client.
3. Establish a wide, **stable** base with your feet by placing both feet flat on the floor. Distribute the weight evenly on both feet.

CLINICAL ALERT

According to the ANA, smaller, lighter healthcare recipients do not warrant use of **SPHM** technology. **Reality:** All manual lifting should be eliminated.

4. Try to keep the work directly in front of you to avoid rotating the spine.
5. Slightly bend both knees. ➤ *Rationale:* This allows strong muscles of legs to do the lifting.
6. Hold abdomen firm and tuck buttocks in so that spine is in alignment. ➤ *Rationale:* This position protects the back.
7. Hold head erect and assume firm stance.
8. Use this stance as the basis for all actions in moving, turning, and lifting clients.

9. Maintain weight to be lifted as close to your body as possible. ➤ *Rationale:* This position maintains the **center of gravity** and provides **leverage** that reduces lower back strain.
10. Align the three natural curves in your back (cervical, thoracic, and lumbar). ➤ *Rationale:* Weight of client is evenly distributed throughout spine, lowering risk of back injury.
11. Prevent twisting your body when moving the client. ➤ *Rationale:* This prevents injury to the back.

EVIDENCE-BASED PRACTICE
Back Brace to Prevent Back Injury?

Two early studies on prevention of low back pain using a back support differed in their conclusions. One study, Linton and van Tulder (2001), researched the literature and found 27 investigations that were consistently negative about the use of back braces to prevent low back pain. They found strong evidence not only that lumbar supports or back belts are ineffective in prevention, but that they are no more beneficial than either no intervention or preventative interventions and might be detrimental. In contrast, the study indicated that exercises showed positive results in the randomized controlled trials, providing consistent evidence of their function in prevention.

Another study (Kraus, 1996) found the opposite results. The UCLA study "found compelling evidence that back support can play an important role in helping reduce back injuries among workers who do a lot of lifting." The study indicated that low back injuries are reduced by one-third when workers wear a back support. This study recommends worker training and proper workplace ergonomics design and indicates that back supports should be part of an overall back injury prevention program.

NIOSH reviewed the scientific findings in the UCLA study and issued a report that concluded the benefit of back supports remained unproven and not recommending their use. A number of preventive measures have been introduced to prevent work-related back injuries. Training, job screening, and ergonomic modification are recommended by NIOSH, but objective evidence of their effectiveness alone or in combination has been elusive and subject to many issues and problems.

There have been numerous studies done on the benefit, or nonbenefit, of utilizing the back belt as a form of injury prevention (Patee, 2015). Several studies were completed with the same conclusion, that back belts are not helpful in preventing back injuries. It has been determined that the best injury prevention for low back pain is proper engineering and ergonomics.

Best current practice is implementation of Illness and Injury Prevention Programs (IIPPs) geared towards identification and elimination of hazards before injuries, illnesses, or deaths occur (OSHA, n.d.). Six core elements of IIPPs are: management leadership, worker participation, hazard identification and assessment, hazard prevention and control, education and training, and program evaluation and improvement.

Skill 12.1.3 | Maintaining Proper Body Alignment

Procedure

1. Begin with the proper stance established in the previous intervention.
2. Evaluate working height necessary to achieve objective.
   a. Test parameters of possible heights (i.e., bed moves within an approximate range of 18 in. [46 cm] from floor).
   b. Establish a comfortable height at which to work; usual height is between waist and lower level of hip joint.

3. Test that this level minimizes muscle strain by extending your arms and checking that your body maintains proper alignment.
4. If you need to work at a lower level, flex your knees. ➤ *Rationale:* Bending over at the waist results in back strain.
5. Make accommodations for working at high surface levels. ❶ ➤ *Rationale:* Reaching up may result in injury to the back through hyperextension of muscles.

(continued)

Skill 12.1.3 | Maintaining Proper Body Alignment *(continued)*

A   B

❶ A. *Correct:* Keep body in correct alignment when turning and reaching for objects to prevent muscle strain or back injury.
B. *Incorrect:* Do not use stretching or twisting movements when you reach for objects out of close proximity to your body.

6. Work close to your body so that your center of gravity is not misaligned and your muscles are not hyperextended. **❷**
   ➤ *Rationale:* This prevents back strain.

7. Use your longest and strongest muscles (biceps, quadriceps, and gluteal) when moving and turning clients.
8. Whenever possible, roll and push objects instead of lifting.

A   B

❷ A. *Correct:* Work close to the body so that center of gravity is not misaligned. **B.** *Incorrect:* Bending over incorrectly can injure back muscles and cause undue strain.

Skill 12.1.4 | Using Coordinated Movements

Procedure

1. Plan muscle movements to distribute workload before you actually begin turning, moving, or lifting clients.

   a. Establish a clear plan of action before you begin to move.
   b. Take a deep breath so oxygen is available for energy expenditure.
   c. Tense antagonistic muscles (abdomen) to those you will be using (diaphragm) in preparation for the movement.
   d. Release breath and mobilize major muscle groups (abdominal and gluteal) to do the work.

2. Move muscles in a smooth, coordinated manner. **❶**
   ➤ *Rationale:* This avoids putting strain on one muscle and is more efficient.
3. Do not make jerky, uncoordinated movements.
   ➤ *Rationale:* This may cause injury or frighten the client.
4. When you are working with another staff member, coordinate plans and movements before implementing them.

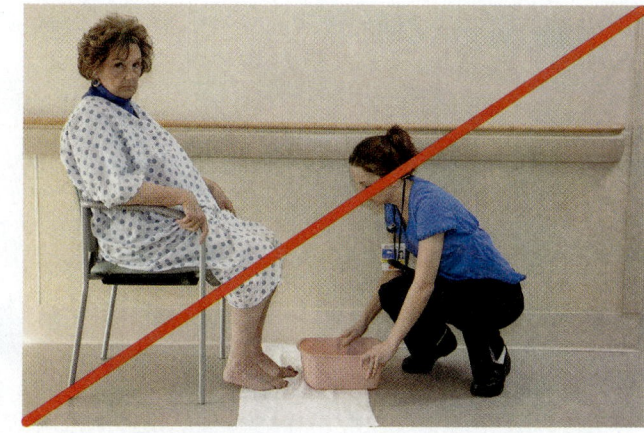

❶ A. *Correct:* Move muscles as a unit and in alignment rather than twisting. **B.** *Incorrect:* Do not twist or rotate upper body when working at lower surface levels.

Skill 12.1.5 | Using Basic Principles

1. Move an object by pushing to expend minimal energy.
   a. Stand close to the object. ❶
   b. Place yourself in proper body alignment stance.
   c. Tense muscles, and prepare for movement.

   d. Avoid pulling.
   e. Push away from you by leaning toward object, using body weight to add force and letting arms, hips, and thighs (*not back*) do the work.

❶ A. *Correct:* When pushing an object, place yourself in proper body alignment. **B.** *Incorrect:* Standing away from object puts the body out of proper alignment.

2. When changing direction, use pivotal movement—moving muscles as a unit and in alignment, rather than rotating or twisting upper part of body.
3. When working at lower surface levels, do not stoop by bending over. Flex body at knees and, keeping back straight, use thigh and gluteal muscles to accomplish task. ❷
4. Use muscles of arms and upper torso in an extended, coordinated movement parallel to body stance when reaching to prevent twisting or hyperextension of muscles.
5. Lift clients or objects with the maximum use of these body alignment principles:

   a. Determine that the movement is within your capability to perform without injury.
   b. Place yourself in proper body alignment stance.
   c. Stand close to and grasp the object or individual near the center of gravity. ❸
   d. Prepare muscles by taking a deep breath, and set muscles.
   e. Lift object with arms or by stooping and using leg and thigh muscles.
   f. Carry object close to your body to prevent strain on your back.
   g. Take frequent rest periods to prevent additional strain.

(continued)

Skill 12.1.5 | Using Basic Principles *(continued)*

② **A.** *Correct:* Keep body in proper alignment by bending knees and keeping back straight when lifting objects. **B.** *Incorrect:* Leaning forward while lifting puts more strain on back muscles; for proper alignment, bend at knees and use leg muscles.

 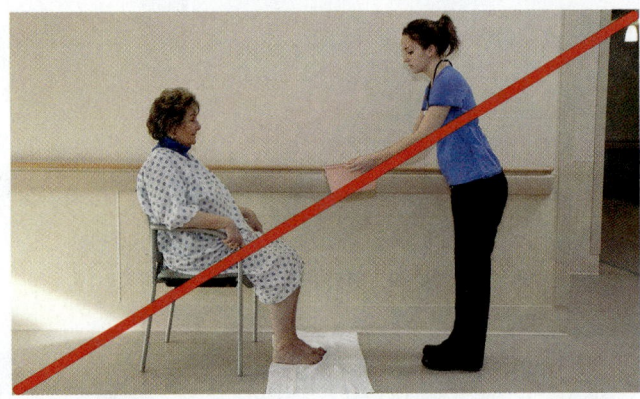

③ **A.** *Correct:* Hold objects close to the body to prevent muscle strain and possible back injury. **B.** *Incorrect:* Holding objects away from the body may cause back strain or injury.

Unit 12.1 Documentation and Evaluation

DOCUMENTATION for Body Mechanics

- Devices needed for turning and moving
- Number of personnel required for turning and moving
- Ways in which client assists in moving
- Special requirements of client for proper body alignment, such as support pillows

- Complete an unusual occurrence report for client or nurse injury during transfer or moving of client. (Some facilities refer to this as a Safety Report or Incident Report.)

EVALUATION/Critical Thinking

Expected Outcomes
- Correct body mechanics are used when preparing for and providing client care.
- Injuries are prevented to both the nurse and the client.

- Proper body mechanics facilitate client care.
- Clients and nurses are not injured when nursing care is provided.
- Center of gravity is maintained when lifting objects.

Unexpected Outcomes	Alternative Actions
• Incorrect body mechanics are used while giving client care.	• Identify areas of your body where you feel stress and strain. • Evaluate the way you use body mechanics. • Attend an in-service program on using body mechanics appropriately. • Concentrate on how you are using your body when moving and turning clients. • Position bed and equipment at a comfortable height and proximity to working area. • Use your longest and strongest muscles to prevent injury.
• Nurse injures self while giving client care.	• Report any back strain immediately to supervisor. • Complete unusual occurrence form. • Go to health service or emergency room for evaluation and immediate care. • Evaluate any activities that led to injury to determine contributing factors. • Prevent additional injury by obtaining assistance when needed. Seek accommodations. • Avoid manual lifting; use assistive devices.
• Nurse uses poor body mechanics and injures client.	• Assess the extent of client's injury. • Notify client's physician. • Complete unusual occurrence form. • Carry out physician's orders for follow-up treatment. • Document client condition. • Notify family per organization policy. • Provide support to client.
• Nurse is unable to obtain sufficient assistance with turning and moving clients.	• Place turning sheets on bed for all clients who are difficult to move. Take steps to prevent skin breakdown. • Use principles of leverage in moving clients. • Until adequate staff is available, turn and position client from side to side at least every 2 hr. • Use Hoyer lift.
• Number of client/healthcare worker injuries increases in nursing unit.	• Determine cause of injury and nursing units involved. • Based on causes, compile a survey and walking rounds on all shifts and units to gather data regarding injury status. Look for trends and personnel behaviors. • Request that safety committee evaluate data and review IIPP plan or develop plan related to issues associated with injuries. • If indicated, determine appropriate equipment based on level of injury and dependency. Bring in vendors to demonstrate equipment based on findings. • Complete in-service staff development program on proper use of equipment and safety principles before implementing program. • Continue to keep detailed notes on client and/or staff injury reports after implementation of new protocols. Analyze data and compare with prior injury rates and types.

Moving and Turning Clients

Nursing Process Data

ASSESSMENT Database

- Observe the client and identify ways to improve the client's position and alignment.
- Determine the client's physical ability to assist with positioning.
- Assess appropriate mechanical device for moving clients requiring assistance.
- Note the presence of tubes and incisions that alter the positioning and alignment procedures.
- Assess joint mobility.
- Assess skin condition with each turn.

PLANNING Objectives

- To provide increased comfort
- To provide optimal lung excursion and ventilation
- To prevent contractures due to constant joint flexion
- To promote optimal joint movement
- To help maintain intact skin
- To prevent injury due to improper movement
- To move and transfer clients using mechanical devices

IMPLEMENTATION Procedures

DOCUMENTATION AND EVALUATION

Expected Outcomes

- Client's comfort is increased.
- Skin remains intact without evidence of breakdown as a result of moving and turning.
- Breathing is adequate and unlabored.
- Joint movement is maintained.
- Footdrop is prevented.
- Body alignment is maintained.
- Mechanical equipment and devices are used in client transfers and repositioning as needed.
- Client is moved safely using appropriate device.

Unexpected Outcomes/Alternative Actions

Pearson Nursing Student Resources

Find additional review materials at
nursing.pearsonhighered.com.
Prepare for success with NCLEX®-style practice questions and Skill Checklists.

Skill 12.2.1	Assessing Clients for Safe Moving and Handling

Equipment

Mechanical equipment or devices based on assessment of functional level.

Procedure

1. Perform hand hygiene.
2. Check if physician orders need to be obtained for client transfers or moving (joint replacement, spinal cord injury, or surgical procedure).

3. Use two indicators to identify client and introduce yourself.
4. Explain use of assessment criteria in preparation for safe moving and handling. ❶ ❷ See Table 12-2 ■ for positions.
5. Complete checklist or document findings in nurses' notes.

    a. Identify client's level of assistance.

    (1) Independent: able to perform task safely with or without staff assistance or assistive devices

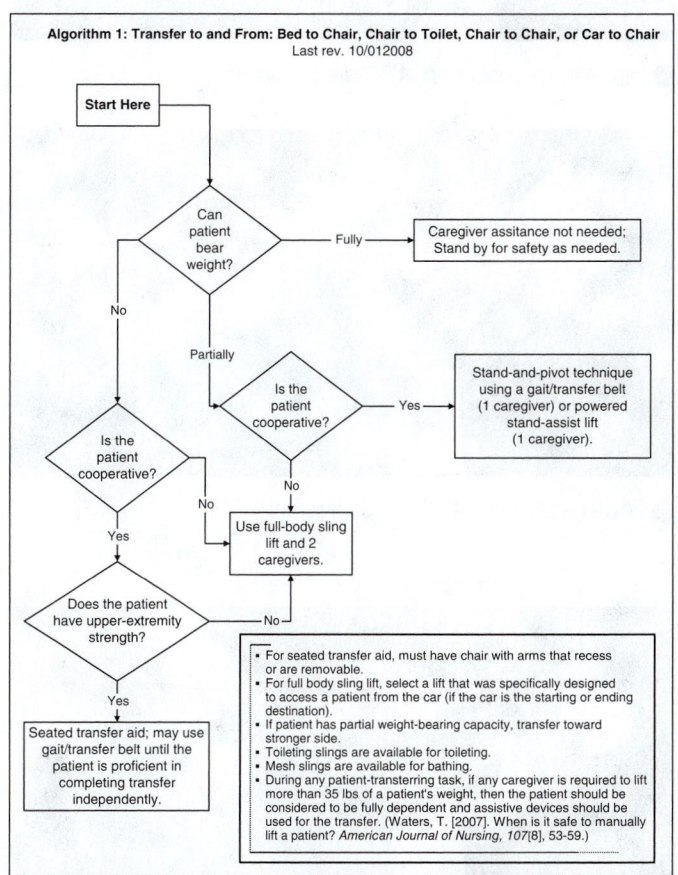

❶ Assessment criteria and care plan for Safe Patient Handling and Movement.

❷ Sample algorithm for client transfer.

Source for both images on this page: Waters, Nelson, Hughes, & Menzel (2009)

Table 12-2 Bed Positions for Client Care

Positions	Placement	Use
High-Fowler's (Image ❶) (See images below table.)	Head of bed 60-degree angle	Thoracic surgery, severe respiratory conditions
Fowler's (❸)	Head of bed 45–60-degree angle; hips may or may not be flexed	Postoperative, gastrointestinal conditions, promote lung expansion
Semi-Fowler's (❻)	Head of bed 30-degree angle	Cardiac, respiratory, neurosurgical conditions
Low-Fowler's (❿)	Head of bed 15-degree angle	Necessary degree elevation for ease of breathing, promotes skin integrity, client comfort
Knee-gatch (❸)	Lower section of bed (under knees) slightly bent	For client comfort; contraindicated for vascular disorders
Trendelenburg (❺)	Head of bed lowered and foot raised	Percussion, vibration, and drainage (PVD) procedure; promotes venous return
Reverse Trendelenburg (❺)	Bed frame is tilted up with foot of bed down	Gastric conditions, prevents esophageal reflux

(continued)

Skill 12.2.1 | Assessing Clients for Safe Moving and Handling *(continued)*

Ⓐ High-Fowler's position at 60-degree angle.

Ⓔ Elevated knee gatch.

Ⓑ Fowler's position at 45–60-degree angle.

Ⓕ Trendelenburg position.

Ⓒ Semi-Fowler's position at 30-degree angle.

Ⓖ Reverse Trendelenburg position.

Ⓓ Low-Fowler's position at 15-degree angle.

(2) Partial assist: requires stand-by assistance cueing or lifting no more than 35 lb of client's weight by staff

(3) Dependent: requires staff to lift more than 35 lb of client weight or is unpredictable in amount of assistance needed; assistive devices need to be utilized.

b. Weight-bearing capacity

(1) Full

(2) Partial

(3) None

c. Bilateral upper extremity strength

d. Client's ability to transfer weight, assist with repositioning of body before contractures occur

e. Client's level of cooperation and comprehension

(1) Cooperative: may need prompting; able to follow simple commands

(2) Unpredictable or varies: Client's behavior changes frequently; client is not cooperative or is unable to follow simple commands.

f. Record client's:

(1) Height

(2) Weight

(3) Client more than 300 lb must use bariatric algorithms for assistance.

g. Identify client's physical condition, which will likely affect transfer and repositioning techniques (i.e., pin sites, surgical incision, fragile skin, fractures, presence of IVs and tubes, and the like).

Note: See Tampa Research and Education Foundation (2015) for more on safe patient handling.

6. Determine appropriate procedure for safe transfer: assistive devices, lift team, number of workers required for procedure for safe transfer.

7. Review algorithms or appropriate use of equipment and devices to determine equipment necessary to meet the client's needs (Boxes 12-3 ■ and 12-4 ■).

8. Complete care plan, identifying type of client transfers and specifics to be carried out during transfers.

9. Ensure all staff are properly instructed in techniques and equipment utilized as assistant devices. ➤ *Rationale:* This promotes safe handling of clients during transfer.

Box 12-3   BARIATRIC CONSIDERATIONS

Lifting and transferring bariatric clients has become a concern for healthcare providers. When the body mass index (BMI) is greater than 30, special bariatric equipment may be required. If the BMI is 40 or higher, the client is considered to be severely or morbidly obese.

Equipment may need to be ordered if not available in the facility. To ensure that appropriate equipment is available, the needs assessment should be part of the hospital admission assessment.

Frequently required equipment includes:

- Wider wheelchairs
- Wider beds
- Walkers
- Shower/commode chairs

Box 12-4   KINETIC BED THERAPY

Kinetic bed therapy reduces the odds of developing healthcare-associated (nosocomial) pneumonia in mechanically ventilated clients. It has not shown a significant reduction in mortality, duration of mechanical ventilation, or length of ICU or hospital stays.

Skill 12.2.2 | Placing a Trochanter Roll

Equipment

Bath blanket

Procedure

1. Perform hand hygiene, use two identifiers to identify client, and place client in supine or **prone** position.

2. Place folded bath blanket on bed next to client. (See also Box 12-5 ■ for a handroll.)

3. Extend blanket from greater trochanter to thigh or knee. ❶

Box 12-5   HANDROLL POSITIONING

When positioning clients who are on long-term bed rest, all areas of the body must be considered. Handrolls made from folded washcloths rolled into a cone shape (or commercially available) may be used to position and maintain wrist and fingers in a functional position. The purpose is to prevent deformity and contractures.

❶ Use trochanter rolls made from bath blankets to align the client's hips.

(continued)

Skill 12.2.2 | Placing a Trochanter Roll *(continued)*

4. Place blanket edge under leg and buttocks to anchor.
5. Roll bath blanket toward client by rolling it under.
6. Rotate affected leg to slight internal hip rotation.
   ➤ *Rationale:* The purpose is to prevent external rotation of the head of the femur in the acetabulum.
7. Tighten the roll by tucking the roll under the hip joint.

8. Allow affected leg to rest against trochanter roll. Hip should be in normal alignment, not internally or externally rotated. Patella should be facing upward if client in supine position. ➤ *Rationale:* This is used most commonly for clients who have a muscle weakness or **paralysis** of that side of the body.

Skill 12.2.3 | Turning to Lateral Position

Equipment
Pillows for positioning
Lateral-assist device or friction-reducing sheet
Drawsheet for trochanter roll

Procedure
1. Introduce self. Use two identifiers to identify client and perform hand hygiene.
2. Explain rationale for procedure to client.
3. Lower head of the bed completely or to a position as low as client can tolerate.

4. Elevate bed to a comfortable working height.
5. Move client to your side of bed. Put side rails up, and move to other side of bed. Use lateral-assist device or friction-reducing sheet if necessary.
6. Flex client's knees.
7. Place one hand on client's hip and one hand on client's shoulder; roll onto side.
8. Position pillow to maintain proper alignment. ❶
9. Be sure to position client's arms so they are not under the body. ❷
10. Perform hand hygiene.

❶ Use pillows to support proper alignment.

❷ Lateral (side-lying) position.

Skill 12.2.4 | Turning to a Prone Position

***Note**: Prone positioning is contraindicated for many conditions.*

Equipment
Pillows for positioning ❶ ❷
Lateral-assist device or friction-reducing sheet

Procedure
1. Use two identifiers to identify client, and perform hand hygiene.
2. Introduce self and explain rationale for procedure to client.
3. Lower head of bed completely or to a position that is as low as client can tolerate.

4. Elevate bed to a comfortable working height.
5. Move client to side of bed away from side where he or she will finally be positioned. Use lateral-assist device or friction-reducing sheet if necessary.
6. Position pillows on side of bed for client's head, thorax, and feet.
7. Roll client onto pillows, making sure that client's arms are not under his or her body.
8. Reposition pillows as necessary for client's comfort.
9. Perform hand hygiene.

❶ Supine position.

❷ Prone position.

Skill 12.2.5 | Moving Client Up in Bed

Note: Manual lifting should be avoided if possible.

Equipment
Trapeze (optional) ❶
Friction-reducing sheet

Procedure
1. Introduce self. Use two identifiers to identify client and perform hand hygiene.
2. Explain rationale for procedure to client.
3. Lower head of bed so that it is flat or as low as client can tolerate.
4. Raise bed to a comfortable working height. ➤ *Rationale:* This allows nurse's center of gravity to assist in turning.
5. Remove pillow and place it at head of bed. ➤ *Rationale:* This prevents striking client's head against bed.
6. Place one arm under client's shoulders and other arm under client's thighs. ❷ Use this method of moving only if the client can assist with move.
7. Flex your knees and hips. Move feet close to bed. ❸
8. Place your weight on your back foot.

❷ Place one arm under shoulders and other under thighs.

❸ Maintain proper body alignment when moving client up in bed.

9. Instruct client to put arms across chest, bend legs, and put feet flat on the bed.
10. Shift your weight from back to front foot as you lift client up in bed. ➤ *Rationale:* Shifting weight reduces the force needed to move client up in bed.
11. Ask client to push with feet as you move him or her.
12. Position client comfortably, replacing pillow and arranging bedding as necessary.
13. Perform hand hygiene.

Note: There are several other methods of moving a client up in bed—including using assist devices such as friction-reducing sheet or total lift devices for clients who are unable to assist with moving and turning.

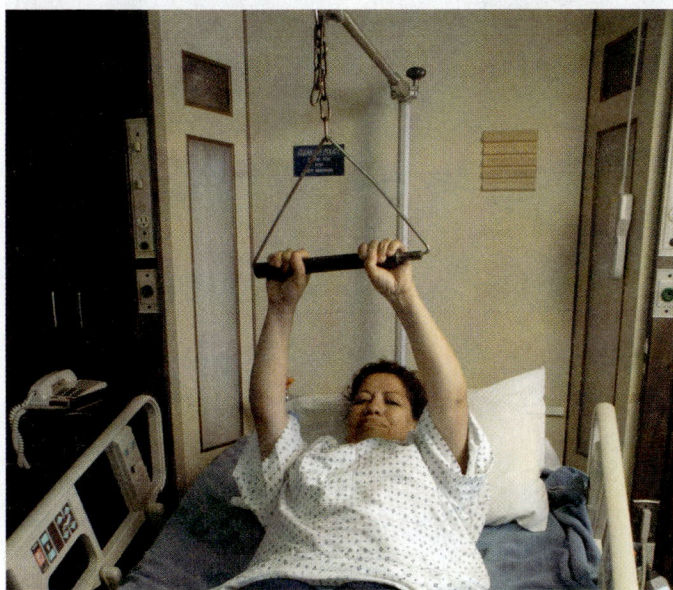

❶ Encourage client to help when repositioning.

(continued)

Skill 12.2.5 | Moving Client Up in Bed (continued)

EVIDENCE-BASED PRACTICE
Recommendations for Positioning
- Client experiences consolidated pneumonia in one lung: Position good lung down to increase oxygenation.
- Progressive mobilization to dangling legs, standing, and walking are safe positions for intubated clients.
- Clients increase their oxygenation with head of bed elevated.

- Turning every 2 hr is not sufficient to prevent healthcare-associated pneumonia.
- Using kinetic and continuous lateral rotation therapy decreases risk of ventilator-acquired pneumonia (VAP) in clients on ventilators. Eighteen hours of rotation per day and early placement in kinetic bed are necessary to prevent VAP.

Source: Rauen, Chulay, Bridges, Vollman, & Arbour (2008)

Skill 12.2.6 | Moving Client With Assistance

Equipment
Friction-reducing sheet

Procedure
1. Use two identifiers to identify client and perform hand hygiene; bring sheet to bedside.
2. Introduce yourself and explain rationale for procedure to client.
3. Lower head of bed so that it is flat or as low as client can tolerate.
4. Raise bed to a comfortable working height.
5. Remove pillow, and place it at head of bed. ➤ *Rationale:* This prevents head being bumped when moved.
6. Coordinate the movements of all nurses. ➤ *Rationale:* One nurse is responsible for stating when to move client, "on count of three."
7. Position client with two nurses or staff members.
   a. Position one nurse on each side of client. Assume broad **base of support**; position front foot facing head of bed, and body slightly turned toward head of bed.
   b. Assist client to flex knees, if possible.
   c. Each nurse firmly grasps sheet at level of client's upper back with one hand and at level of buttocks with other hand.
   d. Each nurse places weight on back foot.
   e. Then with one firm, coordinated, rocking movement (shifting weight from back to front foot), lift client toward head of bed. ❶
   f. Place client in a comfortable position.
8. Perform hand hygiene.

> **CLINICAL ALERT**
> OSHA states that healthcare workers should lift no more than 35 lb. It is advisable to use lifting and transferring devices.

❶ Use friction-reducing sheet and shift weight from back to front leg when moving client up.

Skill 12.2.7 | Logrolling the Client

Equipment
Pillows, towels, blankets for positioning
Turning sheet

Procedure
Note: It is recommended that a friction-reducing sheet be used instead of manual turning. However, sometimes the logrolling technique is necessary.

1. Check order for logrolling client and client care plan as to exactly why client needs to be logrolled.
2. Identify the client using two identifiers. Perform hand hygiene.
3. Obtain sufficient assistance to complete procedure with ease (Box 12-6 ■). Three nurses are preferable.
4. Place a pillow between the client's knees before moving the client. ➤ *Rationale:* This prevents adduction of hip. This will prevent spinal torque.

5. Position two nurses on side of bed to which client will be turned. ❶ Position third nurse on opposite side of bed.
6. Designate individual at head of bed to be in charge of coordinating move.
7. Assume correct position for client move:
   a. Nurse at head: one arm supports client's head, second arm supports shoulders and neck.
   b. Second nurse: one hand grasps client's other shoulder, the other hand and arm around knee.
   c. Third nurse: on the opposite side of the bed, nurse holds drawsheet firmly to support torso. ➤ *Rationale:* This maintains the body in alignment. ❷
8. Instruct client to place arms across chest to keep body straight.
9. Assume broad stance with one foot ahead of the other and knees flexed.
10. Rock onto back foot, and use leg and arm muscles to push client in one coordinated movement when nurse at head of bed signals to move client. ➤ *Rationale:* To maintain

❸ Maintain client's position with pillow support under client's back.

proper alignment, all of the body parts must be moved at the same time. If not, injury to client's neck and spinal column may occur.

11. Maintain client's position in alignment with pillows, towels, or folded blankets. ❸
12. Change client's position frequently (minimum every 2 hr) according to physician's orders.

❶ Position nurses on each side of client.

Box 12-6 **CLIENT LIFT TEAMS**

A lift team consists of two physically fit individuals competent in lifting techniques who work together to perform high-risk client transfers. The individuals on the team must have no prior history of a musculoskeletal injury and must depend on their physical strength and capabilities. They must have had a physical examination and an x-ray of their spine, in addition to having no history of back injury. They are trained in the use of mechanical lifting devices.

Several clinical trials have been conducted on the use of client lift teams. The outcomes indicated that this intervention was effective in decreasing the loss of work days and compensable injury costs.

❷ Maintain proper alignment while turning client.

Skill 12.2.8 | Transferring Client From Bed to Gurney

Equipment

Transfer board: polyethylene board, about 18–22 in. wide by 72 in. long (Table 12-3 ■)

Sheets to cover board, gurney, and client

Bath blanket (optional)

Gurney, bed, or CT table

Procedure

1. Use two identifiers to identify the client and perform hand hygiene.
2. Introduce self and explain procedure to client and show client transfer board. ➤ *Rationale:* Seek to allay client's fears of being dropped from board.
3. Cover client with sheet or bath blanket and cover board and gurney with sheets.
4. Position client on side of bed away from gurney in lateral position. ❶
5. First nurse supports client while second nurse places board as close to client as possible. (If manual lifting is necessary, as many healthcare providers as possible should participate to decrease stress on each worker.) ➤ *Rationale:* This allows client to be positioned entirely on the board after the turn.
6. Instruct client to turn onto back, directly onto board. Client may need assistance to turn.
7. Place both nurses on side of gurney or bed toward which client will be turned. ❷
8. Assume appropriate body mechanics (broad base of support, one foot in front of the other, knees and hips flexed). Place weight on front foot.
9. Transfer weight on count of three from front to back foot as you lift board and pull it toward you.
10. Center client on gurney or bed and remove board by pulling board out and up using handholds along edge of board and using good body mechanics. ❸ ❹
11. Place side rails in UP position, or according to facility policy.

Note: Lateral-assist devices can be used to transfer clients from bed to gurney.

❶ Move client to side of bed in lateral position and position transfer board.

❸ Use handholds on board to move client to gurney; maintain proper body mechanics.

❷ Two nurses move to transfer board side of gurney before moving client.

❹ Remove transfer board after centering client on gurney.

Table 12-3 Assistive Devices for Moving and Turning Clients

Equipment/Device	Use for Client Moving or Handling
Gait belt	Assists client to walk when he or she has leg strength, can cooperate, and requires minimal assistance.
Lateral-assist devices (roller boards, side boards, friction-reducing lateral-assist devices)	Assists clients in lateral transfers, bed-to-gurney, and reduces client-surface friction during transfers, thus preventing skin breakdown and client discomfort. Friction-reducing sheets are used to position clients in bed and in lateral transfers.
Electric beds	Assists clients in lateral transfers. Position the bed so transfer surface (gurney) is slightly lower than bed to allow client to move onto new surface. Beds can be placed in high-Fowler's position to assist client into sitting position for easier transfer out of bed.
Nonmechanical sit-to-stand aids	Assists clients with some arm strength and weight-bearing ability and who can follow simple directions to move out of bed. Once client stands, pulling self up by holding on to bars, a seat flap is lowered, and the client can rest on the seat. Transfers to commodes, toilets, and showers can be accomplished using this device.
Powered stand-assist device	Assists clients who can bear weight on at least one leg and can follow simple instructions. Client is instructed to place feet on footrest while a sling is placed under arms and around back. Legs are positioned against padded shin rest and client's hands are placed on handles. Machine will lift client to a standing position, once electronic hand control is pushed by nurse. Device can be used to transport client to bathroom or chair.
Powered full-body lifts	Assists clients who are unable to bear any weight. These lifts can also be used to pick up clients off the floor after falls. Sling is placed under client, then attached to a positioning bar. Client is then lifted from bed or floor. These lifts are portable or ceiling mounted.

Skill 12.2.9 | Dangling at the Bedside

Procedure

1. Use two identifiers to identify client and perform hand hygiene.
2. Introduce self and explain procedure to client.
3. Lower bed to lowest position.
4. Move client to edge of bed and instruct client to bend knees. ❶ ➤ *Rationale:* This allows client to easily move legs and feet over side of bed onto floor.
5. Turn client onto side, keeping knees flexed, or place bed in Fowler's position (head elevated at 45-degree angle). ❷ ➤ *Rationale:* This position is sometimes preferred; it may be easier for nurse to pivot client to sitting position.
6. Stand at client's hip level. Assume broad base of support with forward foot closest to client. Flex your knees, hips, and ankles. ❸

❷ Turn client onto side, maintaining knees in flexed position.

❶ Move client to side of bed and instruct to flex knees.

❸ Maintain broad base of support as you pivot client to sitting position.

(continued)

Skill 12.2.9 | Dangling at the Bedside *(continued)*

7. Place one of your arms under client's shoulders and other arm beneath client's thighs near knees. Instruct client to use arms to push shoulders up from bed. ➤ *Rationale:* This prevents client falling backward onto bed.

8. Lift client's thighs slightly and pivot on balls of your feet as you move client into sitting position. Use gluteal, abdominal, leg, and arm muscles to move client.

9. Stand in front of client until client is stable in upright position. ➤ *Rationale:* Client may experience orthostatic hypotension if he or she has been on bed rest for a period of time.

10. Take vital signs, especially if this is first time client is dangled. ➤ *Rationale:* You need to determine if orthostatic hypotension is present.

11. **Dangle** client with feet down for a few minutes before transferring to chair or ambulating. ④ ➤ *Rationale:* When feet are on floor, it helps to prevent clot formation.

④ Dangle client with feet down for several minutes before transferring to chair or ambulating.

Skill 12.2.10 | Moving From Bed to Chair

Equipment
Chair
Gait belt

Procedure

1. Introduce self. Use two identifiers to identify the client and perform hand hygiene.
2. Lock bed in place.
3. Place chair at head of bed. If using wheelchair, remove arm and foot closest to bed to facilitate transfer. ①

4. Lock chair wheels or have someone hold chair as you move client.
5. Follow steps in Skill 12.2.9, *Dangling at the Bedside*. ②
6. Dangle client until he or she is stable.
7. Give client nonskid shoes or slippers.
8. Place gait belt around client's waist and move client to side of bed using gait belt for support (Box 12-7 ■). ③ ➤ *Rationale:* This helps stabilize client to prevent falls during transfer to chair.

① When using wheelchair, remove arm and foot closest to bed for ease of transfer.

② Pivot client to dangling position before placing feet on floor.

③ Move client to side of bed using gait belt for support.

④ Stand with your foot between client's feet; assist client to standing position.

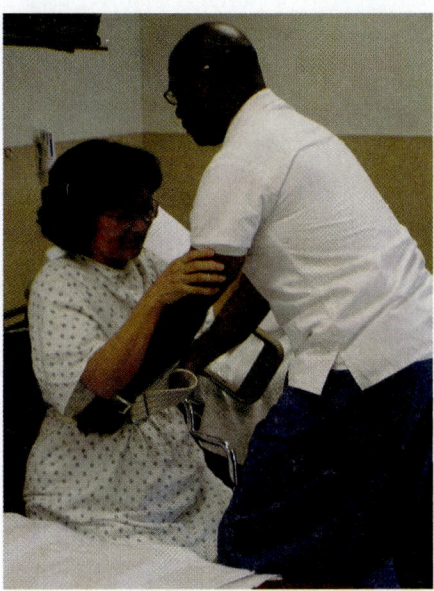

⑤ Grasping gait belt for safe transfer, use leg muscles to pivot client into chair.

⑥ Slowly lower client into chair while holding gait belt securely.

9. Stand as close to client as possible; place your foot closest to chair between client's feet. ④
10. Bend your hips and knees, keeping back straight.
11. Rock client and, on count of three, assist client to standing position.
12. Grasp gait belt firmly for safe transfer while using leg muscles to pivot client to chair. ⑤ Move your body in direction in which transfer is taking place.

13. Slowly lower client into chair. ⑥
14. Position client in chair to prevent pressure areas. If client has circulatory impairment, elevate legs while out of bed. ➤ *Rationale:* This promotes venous return.

Note: It is preferable to use the nonmechanical sit-to-stand aid for transferring clients out of bed unless they require minimal assistance.

Box 12-7 EFFECTIVENESS OF SAFE CLIENT HANDLING USING ASSISTIVE EQUIPMENT AND DEVICES

Healthcare Staff Benefits

- Use of assistive client handling equipment and devices has made **manual client handling** unnecessary.
- New assistive devices control the ergonomic hazard associated with lifting and transferring clients, preventing injuries to staff.
- Injuries to nursing staff have decreased with use of the new devices and equipment, leading to cost savings for facilities for workers' compensation benefits.

Client Benefits in Use of Assistive Devices and Equipment

- Reduction in client falls and skin tears as a result of the new equipment and devices.
- Clients feel more secure with transfer and ambulation with new equipment and devices.
- Client is more comfortable in moving and turning using the new devices and equipment.
- Client's dignity is protected by using **assistive equipment** and devices.
- Assistive devices and equipment are selected to match the client's ability to assist in own movement, allowing client more autonomy.

| **Skill 12.2.11** | Using a Floor-Based (Sling) Lift |

Equipment

Floor-based lift (such as a Hoyer); assistive devices shown in Table 12-4 ■
2 canvas pieces: 1 large, 1 small
2 sets of canvas straps

Procedure

1. Check orders and client care plan. Determine that lift can safely move the weight of the client (Box 12-8 ■).
2. Introduce self. Use two identifiers to identify client and explain procedure to client. ➤ *Rationale:* Clients may be frightened by use of a mechanical device.

(continued)

Box 12-8 CRITERIA FOR SELECTION OF LIFTING AND TRANSFER DEVICES

- Appropriate for task to be accomplished
- Safe and stable for client's caregiver
- Comfortable for client
- Can be managed with relative ease
- Maneuverable in confined work space
- Efficient use of time
- Minimal maintenance required
- Equipment storage requirements reasonable
- Adequate numbers of device available
- Cost effectiveness

3. Perform hand hygiene.
4. Bring floor-based frame to bedside.
5. Provide privacy for client.
6. Lock wheels of bed.
7. Place client's chair by the bed. Allow adequate space to maneuver the lift.
8. Raise bed to HIGH position and adjust head and knee gatch so that mattress is flat.
9. Keep side rail on opposite side in UP position.
10. Roll client away from you.
11. Place lower edge of wide canvas piece under client's knees. ❶

12. Place upper edge of narrow canvas piece under client's shoulders.
13. Raise side rail on your side of bed.
14. Move to opposite side of bed and lower side rail.
15. Roll client away from you to opposite side and straighten out canvas pieces. Turn client to supine position.
16. Place U base of frame under bed on side where chair is positioned.
17. Lock wheels of frame. Lower side rail.
18. Attach canvas straps from swivel bar to each canvas piece using hooks.
19. Place straps evenly on canvas pieces. Sling extends from shoulders to knees. ➤ *Rationale:* This supports client's weight equally.
20. Elevate head of bed.
21. Raise client by turning release knob clockwise to close pressure valve. ❷
22. Pump lift handle until client is lifted clear of the bed.
23. Maneuver client over the chair.
24. Lower client by turning release knob *slowly* counterclockwise.
25. Guide client into chair. ❸
26. Align client into chair.
27. Remove straps from bar and move lift out of the way.
28. Check for client's comfort in chair; place call bell close at hand.
29. Perform hand hygiene.
30. Return client to bed using reverse method.

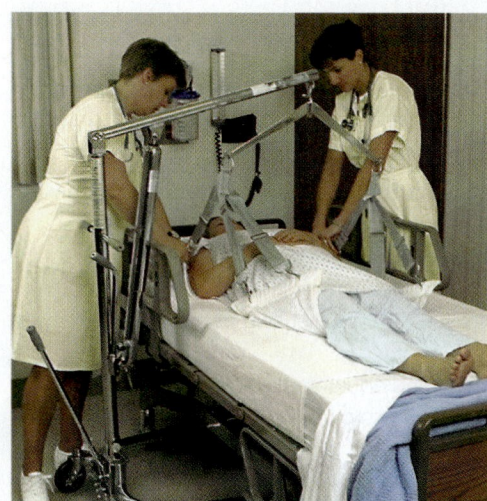

❶ Place canvas piece under client from knees to shoulders.

❷ Raise client off bed by turning release knob clockwise.

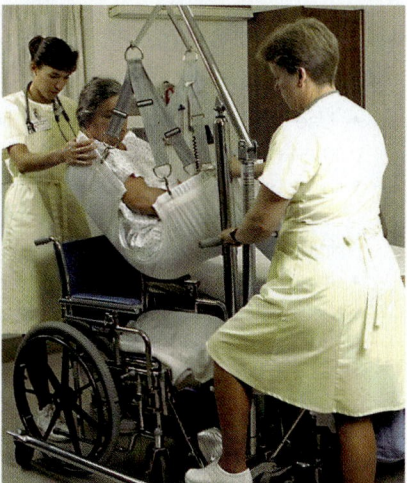

❸ Use one nurse to stabilize client as second nurse guides client into chair.

Skill 12.2.11 | Using a Floor-Based (Sling) Lift *(continued)*

Table 12-4 Safe Client Handling Devices

	Device	Use
	Gait belt	Assist client in walking if he or she has leg strength, can cooperate, and requires minimal assistance.
	Lateral-assist device	Slide boards can be used to transfer clients from bed to gurney.
	Nonmechanical sit-to-stand aid	Use to assist clients who have some arm strength and some weight-bearing ability out of bed. Client pulls self up by holding on to bar. Unfold a seat flap and have client sit on seat.
	Friction-reducing sheet	Use to position clients in bed without causing shearing of the skin.
	Powered full-body lift	Use for clients unable to bear weight. Clients can be moved out of bed or lifted off the floor after a fall. Ceiling-mounted lifts are also available.

Note: Follow manufacturer's directions for use of these assist devices.

Skill 12.2.12 | Using a Hydraulic Lift

Equipment
Sling
Mechanical lift device ❶
Wheelchair

Preparation
1. Check physician's orders for type of assistive device ordered for client (check policy and procedure guide for available types of devices in facility).

(continued)

Skill 12.2.12 | Using a Hydraulic Lift (continued)

1 Ceiling mounted lift device for client transfer.

2 Turn client to side and pull sling under client.

3 Position client in center of sling.

4 Secure leg straps.

2. Check equipment to ensure lift sling is intact (no frayed material or weak stitching; straps, hooks, and chains are intact), and mechanical lift device is functioning appropriately (Box 12-9 ■). Check manufacturer's instructions and safety precautions.

3. Use two forms of identifiers to identify client; introduce yourself to client and explain how the hydraulic lift will transfer the client to the chair or wheelchair.

4. Complete an assessment to determine client's willingness and ability to assist with transfer.

5. Check client's weight. ▶ **Rationale:** Some lifts state a weight restriction. If over weight level, a bariatric hydraulic device will need to be ordered.

6. Bring equipment to room.

7. Perform hand hygiene.

8. Provide privacy.

Procedure

1. Place wheelchair close to head of bed, leaving space to maneuver lift between bed and wheelchair.

2. Ensure bed wheels are locked, flat, and in HIGH position.

3. Roll client on side, and with client holding side rail, place sling under client. **2**

4. Roll client to other side and pull sling through and straighten sling flat.

5. Place client in supine position and place leg loops over thighs. Follow manufacturer's instructions to place loops correctly. **3** **4**

Box 12-9 NURSING CONSIDERATIONS TO MINIMIZE RISKS WHEN USING LIFTS

Learn to use client lifts properly to prevent head trauma, fractures, and deaths.

Receive training and understand how to operate lifts.

Match sling to specific lift and weight of client.

Do not exceed weight for lift and sling.

Make sure sling is not stressed at seams or frayed. Do not use if damaged.

Prior to transferring, make sure client is not agitated or restless.

Keep base of lift (legs) at maximum open position.

Keep client's arms inside sling.

Keep all latches, clips, and hanger bars securely fastened during operation.

Lock wheels of wheelchair, bed, and so on.

Follow instructions for washing and maintaining sling.

Create and follow a maintenance safety inspection checklist.

Source: Food and Drug Administration (2014)

5 Ensure that sling is securely attached to assist device.

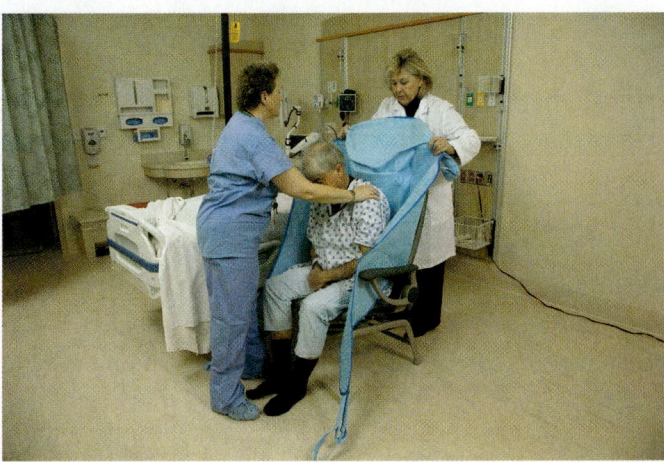

7 Remove sling from the shoulders for client comfort.

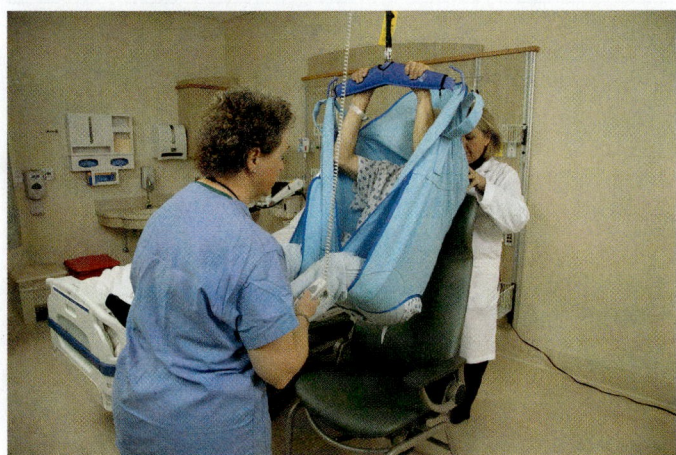

6 Move client directly over chair.

6. Roll lift under bed as far as possible. The lift arm should be over client if appropriately placed. Ensure lift base is wide open. ➤ *Rationale:* This provides stability for lift.
7. Attach sling straps to lift arm. If using hooks, they should be pointed away from client. **5**
8. Elevate head of bed to place client in sitting position. Check manufacturer's instruction for client's hand placement.

9. Ensure wheelchair wheels are locked and client is instructed to remain very still during transfer. ➤ *Rationale:* This maintains the lift's stability.
10. Slowly raise sling until buttocks are just above mattress. ➤ *Rationale:* Self-leveling lift maintains client in sitting position.
11. Turn client to face second nurse who operates the lift. During turning, the client's legs are dangled off bed. Do not pull on client or the lift arm during this step of procedure.
12. Move lift away from bed by grasping steering bar and position client over wheelchair seat. **6**
13. Slowly lower client onto wheelchair until he or she reaches a comfortable position.
14. Unhook sling from lift arm or remove chains or straps from sling. Keep sling in place under client. **7** ➤ *Rationale:* Sling will be reattached to lift device to transfer back to bed.
15. Ensure client is positioned maintaining good body alignment.
16. Evaluate client's response to transfer and document findings.
17. Place overbed table near client. Place fluids, tissues, and personal items in easy reach.
18. Perform hand hygiene.

Skill 12.2.13 | Using a Footboard

Equipment
Footboard

Procedure
1. Provide a footboard if client is unable to place feet in dorsal flexion or plantar flexion.
2. Cover footboard with a bath blanket to protect feet from rough surfaces.
3. Place footboard on bed in a place where client's feet can firmly rest on it without sliding down in bed.
4. Observe legs to ensure that they are not in a flexed position when feet are against the board.

5. Tuck top linen under mattress at foot of bed, and bring linen up over the footboard to the top of the bed. Do not drape top linen over footboard as it can easily be pulled off the bed.
6. Put feet and ankles through range-of-motion exercises every 4 hr for clients on prolonged bed rest.
7. Observe heels, bottom of feet, and ankles frequently for signs of skin breakdown.
8. Place pillow under client's calves (not under heels), allowing heels to be off mattress if skin breakdown is assessed.

Unit 12.2 Documentation and Evaluation

DOCUMENTATION for Moving and Turning Clients

- How often client is turned or moved
- Condition of skin and joint movement
- Unexpected problems with moving or positioning client and solutions to problems
- Client's acceptance of and feelings about the procedure

- Number of staff needed to complete the procedure
- Type of assistive devices needed from bed to chair, if appropriate
- Time client was in chair or dangling at bedside
- Use of a footboard or trochanter roll

EVALUATION/Critical Thinking

Expected Outcomes
- Client's comfort is increased.
- Skin remains intact without evidence of breakdown as a result of moving and turning.
- Breathing is adequate and unlabored.
- Joint movement is maintained.

- Footdrop is prevented.
- Body alignment is maintained.
- Mechanical equipment and devices are used in client transfers and repositioning as needed.
- Client is moved safely using appropriate device.

Unexpected Outcomes	Alternative Actions
• Client unwilling to move due to fear of pain or discomfort.	• Explain rationale and need for the procedure more thoroughly. • If possible, check if client can be medicated before the procedure. • Obtain additional assistance to decrease client's apprehension.
• Client unable to assist with movement.	• Use a friction-reducing sheet to provide more support for client. • Obtain additional assistance to help with moving "dead" weight.
• Client unable to maintain any type of position without assistance.	• Use trochanter roll to prevent external rotation of client's hip. • Use foam bolsters to maintain side-lying positions. • Use folded towels, blankets, or small pillows to position client's hands and arms to prevent dependent edema.
• Skin begins to break down.	• Change client position every 2 hr. • Request physician's order for therapeutic mattress or dressings for pressure ulcer(s) care.
• Client frightened to use assistive device.	• Explain use of equipment (i.e., comfort and safety in transferring). • Demonstrate equipment before using.

Adaptations for Home Care

Nursing Process Data

ASSESSMENT Database

- Assess safety factors in home.
- Check equipment for safety features.
- Determine client's safety in home.
- Determine caretaker's ability to provide client care and safety.
- Determine need for additional client equipment to promote client and caregiver safety.

PLANNING Objectives

- To provide a comfortable and safe client environment
- To ensure caregiver's safety while providing client care
- To provide necessary home care treatments utilizing appropriate safety equipment

IMPLEMENTATION Procedures

DOCUMENTATION AND EVALUATION

Expected Outcomes

- Safe environment is provided for client.
- Healthcare worker's safety is maintained during home visit.

Unexpected Outcomes/Alternative Actions

Pearson Nursing Student Resources

Find additional review materials at
nursing.pearsonhighered.com.
Prepare for success with NCLEX®-style practice
questions and Skill Checklists.

Skill 12.3.1 | Evaluating Client's Safety

Preparation

1. Identify client using two identifiers and introduce yourself.
2. Explain the purpose of asking the following questions.
3. Provide privacy.

Procedure

1. Evaluate client's cognitive abilities: level of consciousness, orientation, ability to make appropriate judgments, and ability to follow commands and directions.

   a. Knowledge of how to operate appliances (e.g., stoves and heaters)
   b. History of alcohol or drug abuse
   c. Knowledge of medication times and doses to be taken
   d. Knowledge of how to call for help: physician, nurse, fire, police

2. Evaluate client's sensory and motor function.

   a. Hearing and vision acuity
   b. Ability to **ambulate** with assistance
   c. Need for assistive devices or support in ambulation

3. Determine client's ability to manage self-care.

   a. Bathing, grooming, and dressing
   b. Preparing food and feeding
   c. Toileting
   d. Housekeeping, shopping, and transportation to physician and pharmacy

4. Assess if client needs alternatives to physical restraints.

   a. Determine if environment needs to be modified by removing unsafe objects or barriers.
   b. Remove wheels from chairs or bed.
   c. Install bed check system or alarm device.
   d. Decrease auditory and visual stimuli.
   e. Place supplies close to bed or chair (e.g., tissues, water).
   f. Develop routine for client.

5. Evaluate most effective type of restraint, if one is absolutely necessary.

   a. Determine that less restrictive methods have been attempted.
   b. Assess purpose of restraint to determine most appropriate type.
   c. Obtain physician's order for restraint. Order must include reason, type, and time of restraints.
   d. Obtain informed consent from client or guardian before applying.
   e. Explain purpose of restraints to client and family members.
   f. Ensure caregiver is instructed on use of restraints.
   g. Evaluate effectiveness and continued need for restraints.

6. Determine client's financial support.

   a. Determine healthcare insurance plan, workers' compensation, Medicare, and Medicaid.
   b. Determine need for social service intervention.

Note: The safety issues in the home are similar to the safety issues of hospitalized clients.

Skill 12.3.2 | Assessing Caregiver's Safety

Procedure

1. Determine caregiver's cognitive function.

   a. Ability to understand and carry out interventions
   b. Ability to make safe decisions and judgments
   c. Willingness to care for client

2. Determine caregiver's sensory and motor function.

   a. Ability to hear client's needs
   b. Visual acuity to read directions, medication labels
   c. Ability to feel temperature changes (e.g., water for bathing)

3. Determine caregiver's motor function and strength.

   a. Ability to assist client in transfer, moving, turning, and activities of daily living (ADLs)
   b. Ability to provide treatments and care for client
   c. Ability to prepare food and do housekeeping chores
   d. Ability to do shopping and provide transportation for physician visits

4. Determine need for client care assistance with ADLs.

   a. Type of wheelchair, with or without removable arms
   b. Over-the-toilet commode or shower chair
   c. Raised toilet seat

5. Determine need for type of transfer-assist devices for safe client handling.

   a. Gait belts: provide secure grip without holding on to client's clothes or limbs ➤ *Rationale:* These prevent caregiver strain, as client weight is closer to caregiver and he or she can assume upright position.

b. Slide board/transfer board: used for seated lateral transfers, such as between bed and wheelchair or commode ➤ *Rationale:* Caregiver does not need to manually lift client.

c. Turning discs: These are used to pivot seated clients who can bear weight and stand. The client is guided to a standing position without adjusting his or her feet. The client must be able to stand or the caregiver will have to exert excessive force in an awkward position.

d. Mechanical lift devices such as the Lean–Stand Assist Lift and Sling–Type Full Lift are used for clients who cannot support their own weight.

e. Repositioning devices: These mechanically pull client up in bed without need for caregiver to assist client.

f. Trapeze lifts: This is a bar device suspended above the bed that allows clients to reposition. Client must have upper-body muscle strength in order to reposition in bed.

Unit 12.3 Documentation and Evaluation

DOCUMENTATION for Home Care

- Client's assessment findings determining ability to care for self and transfer from bed to wheelchair/chair
- Type of assistive devices used in moving and/or transferring client
- Client's ability to assist with transfer and repositioning
- Client's response to moving and repositioning

EVALUATION/Critical Thinking

Expected Outcomes

- Client is safely repositioned or transferred without injury to client or caregiver.
- Appropriate assistive devices are utilized to transfer client.
- Caregiver is able to manage turning, repositioning, and using assistive devices.
- Appropriate body mechanisms are utilized by caregiver.

Unexpected Outcomes	Alternative Actions
• Caregiver is unable to transfer client from bed to wheelchair due to excess weight.	• Determine if wheelchair without arms or transfer board can aid in transfer. • Contact social services to obtain bariatric assist devices. • Determine if other family members can assist with transfer. • May need home health aide services to assist with transfer.
• Injury occurs to client when caregiver attempts transfer to wheelchair.	• Do not continue to reposition client, place in bed. • Complete sensory, motor, and pain assessment. • Notify physician. • Document findings.

Chapter Wrap-Up

GERONTOLOGIC Considerations

Physiologic Age Changes in the Musculoskeletal System That Affect Nursing Care of the Older Adult

- Contractures—muscles atrophy, regenerate slowly; tendons shrink and sclerose.
- Range of motion of joints decreases—lack of adequate joint motion, ankylosis.
- Mobility level is limited—muscle strength lessens and gait may be unsteady.
- Kyphosis occurs—cervical vertebrae may be flexed; intervertebral discs narrow.
- Bodies of thoracic vertebrae compress slowly with aging, leading to the hunchback appearance—loss of overall height results from disk shrinkage and kyphosis.
- Bone changes occur—loss of trabecular bones and bones become brittle.
- Osteoporosis occurs as a result of calcium loss from the bone and insufficient replacement.
- Osteoarthritis increases with age, equally affecting men and women. This condition results in physical stress on joints as a consequence of long-term mechanical, horizontal, chemical, and genetic factors.

Psychosocial and Physiologic Changes in Older Adults Who Are Immobilized

- Older adults are at risk for confusion, depression, and disorientation—keep clock and calendar in room to help reorient to time and place.

- Older adults are also more susceptible to hazards of immobility—maintain own ADLs as much as possible and change position every 2 hr.

Aging and Changes in Ability to Maintain Activity Levels

- As aging occurs, there is a decrease in the rate or speed of activity.
- Loss of muscle mass interferes with activities that require strength, such as bending down, dressing, and reaching for objects.
- Dexterity decreases, leading to a change in performing manipulative skills.

Nursing Care for Positioning Older Adult Clients

- Ambulate within limitations of age.
- Alter position every 2 hr; align correctly.
- Prevent osteoporosis of long bones by providing exercises against resistance as ordered.
- Provide active and passive exercises—rest periods necessary and exercise paced throughout the day for the older adult.
- Provide range-of-motion exercises to all joints three times a day.
- Educate family that allowing the client to be sedentary is not helpful.
- Encourage walking, which is the best single exercise for the older adult.

MANAGEMENT Guidelines

Each state legislates a Nurse Practice Act for RNs and LVN/LPNs. Healthcare facilities are responsible for establishing and implementing policies and procedures that conform to their state's regulations. Verify the regulations and role parameters for each healthcare worker in your facility.

Delegation

- All levels of healthcare workers can be assigned to move and turn clients and provide assistance with transfers.
- Positioning clients in bed can be assigned to all levels of healthcare workers.
- Frequently, the physical therapist is assigned to work with postoperative clients or clients requiring special

transfer techniques or ambulation until clients are released to nursing.

- Before assigning staff to logroll a client or use assistive devices for moving a client out of bed, ensure they have been properly instructed in the procedures and safety issues associated with these activities.

Interprofessional Communication

- The RN must give specific directions to the healthcare workers on appropriate positions for clients on bed rest or specifics on how to transfer clients to a chair or gurney.
- Before physical therapy releases clients to nursing for transfer or ambulation activities, the RN must obtain

explicit information on the procedures to be used. This information must be written on the Kardex, SBAR, or computer record, as well as reviewed with all staff assigned to the client.

- A team conference may be necessary if special equipment or specific activities are required by a client. This conference ensures all staff will be given a demonstration and provided information necessary for safe client care.

- The RN must ensure that all new personnel are proficient in transfers, logrolling, and use of the assistive devices before assigning them to care for clients requiring these skills.

- It is crucial for safe client care that the RN monitors healthcare workers when they perform logrolling or use mechanical devices for transfer after the initial demonstration.

CASE STUDY Applications

Scenario 1

You are assigned to a medical unit where many of the clients require assistance moving in and out of bed. The following clients are assigned to you for care on the day shift.

- Onica Jones, 89-year-old (CVA) client who has weakness on the right side and is unable to communicate but seems to understand directions. She has been in the hospital for 4 days and will be transferred to an SNF this afternoon.

- James Metcalf, 60-year-old (MI) client who is about to be discharged. However, you notice he still has not been able to ambulate by himself.

- Madeline Oscar, 70-year-old client with Parkinson's disease and hospitalized for pneumonia. She was admitted last night. She has orders to be up in the chair BID.

- Joseph Nichols, 40-year-old client, hospitalized for possible kidney stones. He is in severe pain and the MD has ordered that he remain on bed rest until further orders.

1. Which client will you assess first? Provide rationale for your answer.

2. How will you determine the client's ability to assist with his or her own care and movement in bed?

3. For each client, identify the type of assistance he or she might need; provide rationale for your answer.

4. Describe the body mechanics you will use when moving clients; this will be based on the type of moving that will need to be performed for each of the four clients.

Scenario 2

You are assigned to care for a client who weighs 300 lb. The client was out of bed for lunch and now insists on getting back into bed. There are insufficient staff members available to help you. The client is able to bear weight but needs maximal assistance to stand.

1. Suggest creative resolutions to this problem.

2. Describe the procedure you will use to transfer the client from chair to bed.

3. If mechanical devices are not available, what action will you take?

NCLEX® Review Questions

Unless otherwise specified choose only one (1) answer.

1. What is the most effective method for teaching student nurses principles of moving clients?
   A. Using a back brace when lifting clients
   B. Instructions on safe lifting techniques using two to three nurses for heavy clients
   C. Education related to body mechanics
   D. Proper use of lift teams and equipment for moving clients

2. According to the National Institute for Occupational Safety and Health (NIOSH), what is the average client weight that should be lifted by healthcare workers?
   A. 35 lb
   B. 51 lb
   C. 75 lb
   D. 100 lb

3. Applying body mechanics includes which of the following principles?
   Select all that apply.
   A. Establish a base of support by placing the feet close together.
   B. Hold abdomen firm and bend at the waist when lifting a client.
   C. Keep weight to be lifted as close to your body as possible when moving clients.
   D. Align three natural curves in your back when moving clients.
   E. Do not flex your knees when moving clients.

4. Maintaining proper body alignment is critical for nurses to prevent injuries when providing client care. Which of the following steps would not be included in teaching appropriate body alignment?

   Select all that apply.

   A. The most comfortable height at which to provide client care is above the nurse's waist.

   B. Flex your knees if you need to work at lower than waist level.

   C. Triceps, quadriceps, and gluteal muscles are used when moving and turning clients.

   D. Push, pull, or roll objects instead of lifting whenever possible.

   E. Avoid twisting your body when moving clients.

5. If you are injured while providing client care, what is important for you to do immediately?

   A. Complete an unusual occurrence (or incident report) form.

   B. Inform the charge nurse you need to go home to rest and apply ice.

   C. Report the injury to your supervisor.

   D. Ask for a change in your assignment to prevent reinjury.

6. There is an order for a client to be placed in a low-Fowler's position. You will place the bed in a _____ -degree position.

   A. 60

   B. 45

   C. 30

   D. 15

7. During report the team leader stated, "The client needs to be turned to a lateral position every two hours." What is the best way to turn the client?

   A. Ask a second nurse to assist you in turning the client to his or her side.

   B. Ask the lift team to come every 2 hr to turn the client.

   C. Place a friction-reducing sheet under the client to assist in turning.

   D. Explain to the client that he or she needs to move up in bed before you can assist in turning the client to a lateral position.

8. A client is being moved from the bed to a gurney using a transfer board. Which of the following directions are given to the client?

   A. "You need to move toward the side of the bed nearest to the gurney before being placed on the slide board."

   B. "Roll directly onto the transfer board and position yourself on your side."

   C. "The nurse will place the board close to you and you need to roll over the edge of the board onto the gurney while staying in a side-lying position."

   D. "Turn onto your back, directly onto the transfer board."

9. A client assessment indicates the client has some arm strength and weight-bearing ability and can follow simple directions to move out of bed. What is the most appropriate assistive device to move this client out of bed?

   A. Powered full-body lift

   B. Powered stand assist device

   C. Nonmechanical sit-to-stand aid

   D. Lateral-assist device

10. As part of a home care admission assessment, what assessment criteria would you include to determine a client's ability to participate in ambulation?

    Select all that apply.

    A. Weight-bearing capability

    B. Client's level of cooperation and comprehension

    C. Client's decision that he or she is ready to ambulate

    D. Need for assistive device

    E. Visual acuity

QSEN Activity

Domain: Client Centered Care

KSA: Knowledge

Activity:

Engage clients and family in active partnerships that promote health and safety and self-care.

A client requires assistance to transfer from bed to chair and back. Describe teaching points that the nurse should share with the client and spouse during and after the transfer.

Bibliography

American Nurses Association (ANA). (2013). *National standards for safe patient handling and mobility.* Silver Spring, MD: Author.

American Nurses Association. (2014). *Safe patient handling and mobility: Interprofessional national standards.* Washington, DC: ANA.

Demoulin, C., Marty, M., Genevay, S., Vanderthommen, M., Mahieu, G., & Henrotin, Y. (2012). Effectiveness of preventive back educational interventions for low back pain: A critical review of randomized controlled clinical trials. *European Spine Journal, 21*(12), 2520–2530. doi: 10.1007/s00586-012-2445-2OK

Food and Drug Administration. (2014). Patient lifts. Retrieved from http://www.fda.gov/medicaldevices/productsandmedical procedures/generalhospitaldevicesandsupplies/ucm308622.htm

Harrington, S., & Brigham C. J. (2013). Navigate new safe patient handling and mobility interprofessional national standards. ANA NURSECE. Retrieved from https://ananursece. healthstream.com/Pages/Product.aspx?ID=8c29ae61-b3ce-e211-ae19-001517135351&DisplayName=Navigating%20the%20 New%20Safe%20Patient%20Handling%20and%20Mobility%20 Interprofessional%20National%20Standards

Kraus, J.F. Brown, K.A., McArthur, D.L., Peek-Asa C., Samaniego L., & Kraus, C. (1996, Oct.). Reduction of acute low back injuries by use of back supports. *International Journal of Occupational Environmental Health.* (2)4, 264–273.

Krill, C., Raven, C., & Staffileno, B. A. (2012). Moving from a clinical question to research: The implementation of a safe patient handling program. *Medsurg Nursing, 21*(2), 104–106, 116. Retrieved from http://search.proquest.com/docview/1008665093?accountid=3588

Linton, S. J., & van Tulder, M. W. (2001). Preventive interventions for back and neck problems: What is the evidence? *Spine, 26*(7), 778–787.

McIntyre, D.R., Bolte, K.M., & Pope, M.H. (1996, Dec.). Study provides new evidence of back belts' effectiveness. *Occupational Health & Safety.* 65(12), 39–41.

Mellinger, R. (2002, January). Nursing home company settles case. *OSHA Archive Report.* Retrieved from https://www.osha.gov/pls/ oshaweb/owadisp.show_document?p_table=news_releases &p_id=1264

National Institute for Occupational Safety and Health (NIOSH) (June 2014, pages last reviewed). Back Belts-Do They Prevent Injury? www.cdc.gov/niosh/docs/94-1271/94–127/

Occupational Safety and Health Administration. (n.d.). Healthcare wide hazards: Ergonomics. Retrieved from https://www.osha. gov/SLTC/etools/hospital/hazards/ergo/ergo.html

Occupational Safety and Health Administration. (n.d.). Illness and injury prevention programs. Retrieved September 16, 2014 from https://www.osha.gov/dsg/topics/safetyhealth/

Ogg, M. J. (2011). Introduction to the safe patient handling and movement series. *AORN Journal, 93*(3), 331–333. doi:10.1016/j. aorn.2010.12.004

Pain research; studies from Washington University describe new findings in back pain. (2013). *Health & Medicine Week,* 3976. Retrieved from https://books.google.com/ books?id=_5fqLrsR1zIC&pg=PA1&lpg=PA1&dq=back+pain,+ Washington+University,+2013,+health+%26+medicine+week &source=bl&ots=BYT6U1cZhU&sig=s2EnkoPpVpXy30Uzp rFf3_Kva68&hl=en&sa=X&ved=0CB4Q6AEwAGoVChMI8_ izxf_YxgIVAjI-Ch2hIQBE#v=onepage&q=back%20pain%2C%20 Washington%20University%2C%202013%2C%20health%20%26%20 medicine%20week&f=false

Patee, N. (April 27, 2015.) Back Belts in the Workforce-What Does the Research Say? Retrieved from www.workrightnw.com/ back-in-the-workforce-whatdoes.

Pullin, R. (2008, Mar.). Using a hydraulic lift for patient transfer. *Nursing, 38*(3), 54–56.

Rasmussen, C. D. N., Holtermann, A., Mortensen, O. S., Søgaard, K., & Jørgensen, M. B. (2013). Prevention of low back pain and its consequences among nurses' aides in elderly care: A stepped-wedge multi-faceted cluster-randomized controlled trial. *BMC Public Health, 13,* 1088. doi:10.1186/1471-2458-13-1088

Rauen, C. A., Chulay, M., Bridges, E., Vollman, K. M., & Arbour, R. (2008). Seven evidence-based practice habits: Putting some sacred cows out to pasture. *Critical Care Nurse, 28*(2), 98–124.

Tampa Research and Education Foundation. (2015). Safe patient handling, p. 54ff. Retrieved from http://www.tampavaref.org/ safe-patient-handling/UPLUnitSPHBinder.pdf

van Tulder, M. W. & Waddell, C. (2005) Evidence-based medicine for non-specific low back pain. B*est Practice and Research Clinical Rheumatology. 19*(4), vii–ix. doi:10.1016/j. berh.2005.03.009

van Tulder, M. W., Kaes, B. W., Baulter., J.M. (1995). A Cost-Illness Study of Back Pain in the Netherlands. Pain,. *62*(2). 233–40.

Waters, T. R., Nelson, A., Hughes, N., & Menzel, N. (2009). Safe patient handling for schools of nursing: Curricular materials. Washington, DC: National Institute for Occupational Safety and Health, 16, 38. Retrieved from http://www.cdc.gov/niosh/docs/2009-127/ pdfs/2009-127.pdf

Chapter 13
Exercise and Ambulation

Learning Objectives

13.1 Define rehabilitative nursing.

13.2 Compare and contrast preservative and restorative methods of care.

13.3 Identify the joints and the type of movement they accommodate.

13.4 Compare and contrast passive and active range-of-motion exercises.

13.5 Demonstrate passive range-of-motion exercises using all muscle groups.

13.6 Explain the rationale of assisted ambulation for clients.

13.7 Describe the procedure the nurse will carry out when the ambulating client appears to be falling.

13.8 Complete a client teaching guide for clients requiring muscle-strengthening exercises.

13.9 Demonstrate the proper method for measuring crutches.

13.10 Compare and contrast the four crutch-walking gaits.

13.11 Demonstrate the four crutch-walking gaits.

13.12 List the components of crutch walking that require documentation.

13.13 Identify the steps in measuring a client for a cane.

13.14 Describe client instructions for using a cane.

13.15 Describe client instructions for using a walker.

13.16 Write three nursing diagnoses that are appropriate for clients requiring exercise and ambulation activities.

13.17 Describe safety steps necessary when home care client requests use of assistive devices.

Chapter Outline

Terminology

Abduction movement of a bone away from the midline of the body or body part, as in raising the arm or spreading the fingers.

Adduction movement of a bone toward the midline of the body or part, as in lowering the arm from a raised position.

Alignment arranged in a straight line; position of body parts in relation to each other.

Ambulate to walk.

Antagonists anything that exerts an action opposing that of prime mover.

Atrophy a wasting or decrease in size of any organ or body part due to lack of nutrients or oxygen, causing death and reabsorption of cells.

Base of support foundation on which an individual's body weight is supported.

Balance a result of body alignment that maintains equilibrium, coordination, and stability of the body in space.

Circumduction to revolve around an axis in such a way that the proximal end of a limb is fixed and the distal end traces a circle.

Contractility ability of muscle to shorten, tighten, and contract.

Dorsiflexion flexion of the foot at the ankle joint; the act of turning the foot and toes upward, as in standing on the heel.

Elasticity ability of strained muscle to regain original size and shape when applied force is removed.

Eversion turning outward; movement of the foot at the ankle joint so that the sole faces outward.

Excitability capacity of muscle to respond to stimulus without intervention of motor nerves.

Extensibility ability of muscle to stretch in response to applied force.

Extension a movement that increases the angle between two bones, straightening a joint.

Fibrous consisting mainly of fibers or fiber-containing materials, such as fibrous connective tissue.

Flaccid having decreased muscle tone.

Flexion a movement that decreases the angle between two bones; the act of bending a joint.

Hyperextension continuation of extension beyond the anatomic position, as in bending the head backward.

Inversion turning inward; movement of the foot at the ankle joint so that the sole faces inward.

Ligament a band or sheet of strong fibrous connective tissue connecting the articular ends of bones serving to bind them together and to facilitate or limit motion.

Mobility state or quality of being mobile; facility of movement.

Musculoskeletal pertaining to the muscles and bones.

Orthostatic hypotension a decrease in systolic blood pressure of 20 mm Hg or a decrease in diastolic blood pressure of 10 mm Hg within 3 min of standing when compared with blood pressure from the sitting or supine position.

Paralysis temporary or permanent loss of function, especially loss of sensation or voluntary motion.

Plantar flexion extension of the foot at the ankle joint; the foot and toes are turned downward toward the sole of the foot, as in standing on tiptoe.

Posture attitude or position of body.

Prime movers muscles responsible for the essential movement of contraction.

Pronation rotation of the forearm so that the palm faces backward or downward; movement of the whole body so that the face and abdomen are downward.

Prone lying horizontal with face downward.

Protraction movement of the clavicle (collar bone) or mandible (lower jaw) forward on a plane parallel to the ground.

Proximal nearest the point of attachment or reference point.

Range of motion extent to which a joint can move through active or passive exercises.

Retraction movement of the clavicle or mandible backward on a plane parallel to the ground.

Rotation movement of a bone around its own axis, as in moving the head to indicate "no" or turning the palm of the hand up and then down.

Spasticity increase in muscle tension.

Sprain injury caused by wrenching or twisting of a joint that results in tearing or stretching of the associated ligaments.

Strain injury caused by excessive force or stretching of muscles or tendons around the joint.

Supination rotation of forearm so that the palm faces forward or upward; movement of the whole body so that the face and abdomen are upward.

Synergists muscles that enhance action of prime mover.

Tendons fibrous connective tissue serving for the attachment of muscles to bones and other parts.

Tonicity ability of muscle to maintain steady contraction, which determines its firmness.

Ulcer a lesion of the skin marked by inflammation, necrosis, and sloughing of damaged tissue.

Rehabilitation Concepts

Rehabilitation nursing is a specialty area involved in diagnosis and treatment of individuals and groups with actual or potential health problems resulting from altered functional ability and altered lifestyle. The specialty includes prevention and correction of alterations in the **musculoskeletal** system. In fact, the definition of rehabilitative nursing is the process of restoring an individual's ability to live and work in as normal a manner as possible. To assist clients to achieve and maintain optimal **mobility**, both preservative and restorative methods are used.

Preservative methods, such as exercises and assisted ambulation, include those interventions that are needed to help clients maintain their normal mobility. Because the changes that occur in the human body when an individual is hospitalized are varied and subtle, preservative methods are used with every client. *Restorative methods*, such as crutch walking and splinting, are used with clients who have decreased mobility caused by such factors as debilitating illness or major surgery. The purpose of applying restorative methods is to assist the client in achieving the level of mobility he or she enjoyed before becoming ill.

The general goals for using these methods are to assist the client to strive for optimal function, to prevent further injury, and to restore the client's mobility to as close to normal function as possible. To achieve these goals of care, it is important for the nurse to accept the philosophy underlying rehabilitative nursing: that every illness is accompanied by the intrinsic threat of disability and that this part of total client care must begin with the initial client contact. Finally, it is important to accept that the principles of rehabilitation are basic to the care of all clients and that rehabilitation must begin early in the client's hospitalization.

Being hospitalized and immobile seriously affects an individual's body image, behavior, and overall adaptation and adjustment. The greater the disability, the more aspects of an individual's life are affected. The nurse's responsibility in providing total client care is to be aware of these responses and to take them into account when developing a client care plan.

Musculoskeletal System

The musculoskeletal system is composed of bones, muscles, joints, cartilage, bursa, **tendons**, and **ligaments**. The bones form the infrastructure of the system. The ability of bones to provide weight bearing and mobility is in direct relationship to the size and shape of the bones.

Joints, in conjunction with muscles, provide motion and flexibility. Skeletal muscles are under voluntary control as a result of being innervated by somatic nerves. Muscles, through their ability to contract, convert energy into mechanical work, maintain body **alignment**, and cause movement.

The muscular system is a system of more than 600 fibers that are attached to bones. The system allows for body movement under the control of the voluntary nervous system. Muscles provide for body movement or locomotion, support the body, and perform several body functions, such as the partial production of heat. The fibers of the voluntary muscles are grouped together in a sheath of connective tissue. Each bundled group of muscle fibers is surrounded by a connective tissue sheath. The sheath tissue may be continuous with fibrous tissue that extends from the muscle as a tendon.

There are several properties of muscle fibers. The first is **excitability**, or the capacity of a muscle to respond to stimulus without intervention of the motor nerves. Another property is **contractility**, the ability of a muscle to shorten, tighten, or contract. Muscles are also able to maintain steady contraction (**tonicity**), stretch in response to applied force (**extensibility**), and regain their original size and shape when applied force is removed (**elasticity**).

Muscle Function

Skeletal muscles produce body movements by pulling on the bones. Bones serve as levers, and joints serve as fulcrums of these levers. Each muscle has a point of origin and a point of insertion that are usually attached to the bone. Muscles that move a body part usually do not extend over that part. These muscles usually perform with group action; some contract, and others relax. **Prime movers** are muscles responsible for the primary movement of contraction. **Antagonists** are muscles that exert an action opposing that of the prime movers. **Synergists** are muscles that enhance action of the prime mover. The accessory parts to muscles are the ligaments and the tendons.

Joints

A joint of the body is the point at which two or more bones join together. The function of a joint is skeletal flexibility and motion. Joints are classified according to structural variations that allow for different kinds of movements. There are three main types of classification: synarthrotic, amphiarthrotic, and diarthrotic joints.

Synarthrotic joints are immovable and include those areas where tissue grows between articulating surfaces, such as the suture lines of the skull. Amphiarthrotic joints have limited movement. Diarthrotic joints have two freely movable parts. This type of joint is a cavity enclosed by a capsule lined with synovial membrane, which secretes a lubricant. The following types of joint movement allow for structural variations:

- Hinge: allows single directional movement (elbow)
- Ball-and-socket: allows bending (hip)
- Saddle: allows multidirectional shifting (thumb)
- Pivot: allows rotary movement (neck, cervical spine)
- Gliding: allows limited sliding of bones against each other (wrist, ankle, invertebral joints)

Each of these types of joints have specific kinds of movements they can perform. These movements can be described in relationship to the three body planes: sagittal, transverse, and coronal. The sagittal plane divides the body into two portions with a straight vertical line between the two parts. The transverse plane divides the body into upper–lower portions with a horizontal line. The coronal plane divides the body into anterior–posterior portions at right angles to the sagittal plane. The joints accomplish a variety of movements that range from flexion–extension to rotation and circumduction.

Exercise

Muscles that are not used become weak and shortened. During prolonged bed rest, strength and endurance decrease rapidly. Clients can regain muscle strength and mobility by practicing specific groups of exercises daily.

Box 13-1 PHYSICAL ACTIVITY GUIDELINES

The CDC (2014) describes physical activity guidelines for America, including both aerobic and muscle-strengthening exercise. Supporting the 2008 Physical Activity Guidelines for America, it states that regular physical activity reduces the risk of many adverse health outcomes. Adults should avoid inactivity and participate in physical activity to gain some health benefit. There is a greater increase in health benefits as the amount of physical activity increases. Older adult clients need to be encouraged to participate in regular physical activity, including aerobic muscle strengthening and flexibility activities. Aerobic exercise should be vigorous enough to get the individual sweating, but it does not need to be done all at one time. Segments of at least 10 minutes provide benefits. **Balance** training for older adult clients will decrease the risk of falls.

Source: CDC (2014)

Promoting exercise, both passive and active, is one of the most important nursing functions. The purpose of exercises is to promote proper alignment, prevent contractures, stimulate circulation, and prevent thrombophlebitis and pressure **ulcers** (Box 13-1 ■). Exercise reduces joint pain and stiffness and increases flexibility and endurance. Exercise also prevents edema of the extremities and promotes lung expansion.

The nurse both performs and teaches several types of exercises as a component of providing total client care. Passive exercises are carried out by the therapist or nurse without assistance from the client. These exercises enable the client to retain as much joint **range of motion** as possible, as well as stimulating circulation. Active exercises, although supervised by the nurse, are performed by the client. These exercises increase muscle strength when the client is partially immobile.

Resistive exercises, another rehabilitative measure, provide resistance in order to increase muscle power. These active exercises are performed by the individual working against resistance. Isometric or muscle-setting activities are similar to resistive exercises. These exercises maintain strength in a muscle when the joint is immobilized. They are performed by the individual without assistance.

Range-of-motion (ROM) exercises are the most common form of exercises for maintaining joint mobility and increasing maximal motion of a joint when the client is totally or partially immobilized. Passive range-of-motion exercises are completed by the nurse or physical therapist (PT). The therapist puts an extremity through its full range so that the joint is moved through all the appropriate planes. Before beginning these exercises, it is important that the therapist or nurse assess the client's condition and the baseline ROM capabilities, establish the extent of ROM to be carried out, and ensure that the client is comfortable. Be aware that clients might be fearful of this type of exercise and that a full explanation of what you are going to do is helpful to allay fears. Enlist the cooperation of the client for maximum benefit. Discontinue all range-of-motion exercises if the client complains of pain, for it is at this point that the exercises become counterproductive.

Ambulation

Ambulation, or walking, is an important function that most of us accomplish automatically; that is, without thinking or conscious effort. When an individual has been immobilized, confined to bed after surgery or an injury, or unable to **ambulate**, this seemingly simple activity can become a major hurdle to overcome. The longer an individual is immobilized, the more difficult it is to regain ambulatory ability; likewise, the sooner an individual begins to ambulate after being bedridden, the more easily he or she will regain preimmobilization status. Early ambulation decreases hospitalization time and prevents complications, such as paralytic ileus or thrombophlebitis. The client who is weak or has other deficits related to ambulation is often referred for evaluation by a PT. The PT evaluates for strength and need for assistive devices and develops a plan of care specific to PT's scope of practice. Nurses and PTs are true collaborators in the area of client mobility and fall prevention.

The human body functions best when it is frequently placed in a vertical position. Ambulation improves physical and mental well-being. Ambulation increases muscle strength and joint mobility. It also increases gas exchange, gastrointestinal muscle tone and function, and circulation. Without stress on bones, calcium deposits occur anywhere in the body, especially in damaged areas, and renal problems also increase from calcium-based calculi.

Balance, coordination, and good body alignment are aspects important to walking. One must be able to move forward and maintain an upright balance; use muscles, bones, and joints correctly for coordination; and keep the head erect and vertebral column fairly straight with feet and knee caps pointed forward in order to maintain a good body alignment.

The major muscle groups used for walking are the thigh and leg muscles. If these muscles have not been used or exercised because the client has been in bed for a long period of time, ambulation must be accomplished step by step. Weak muscles cannot support a human frame for the mechanics of walking. It is important, then, to begin the process of ambulation by administering muscle-strengthening exercises. It is often at this stage that referrals are made to the PT. Several different types of exercises were described previously; however, the most important preambulatory preparation is quadriceps-setting and gluteal-setting exercises. Carried out several times a day, these exercises restore muscle strength and prepare the legs for weight bearing.

Before actually assisting the client to walk, explain precisely what you are going to do, and prepare the client by completing the ambulatory procedure in stages. For example, begin with the muscle-strengthening exercises. Then assist the client to sit up in bed to determine if he or she is experiencing vertigo. Have the client move to the side of the bed with legs down, and only when he or she is ready and feels comfortable in doing so, assist the client to stand beside the bed. You may decide to take the client's vital signs after dangling to determine if they are stable and if there are orthostatic changes. Allow the client to remain there with the bed as support until he or she feels totally secure. Finally, and with the assistance of one or two nurses (depending on the assessment of the client's ability and readiness to ambulate), have the client walk by taking short steps and walking only as long as he or she can tolerate. It is best to have an assistive device available if needed. Assessing oxygenation by pulse oximetry may aid in understanding the client's physiologic reaction to activity. Throughout this procedure, provide support and encouragement to the client.

Assistive Devices

A variety of assistive devices are available to give the client support when ambulating. Assistive devices are used to relieve the client's body weight to enable the client to ambulate. Walkers and crutches allow for complete non–weight-bearing ambulation. Such devices may give the client confidence (especially important with the older adult), stability, support for a weak limb, or reduced pressure on a limb. Devices may include canes (standard cane, T-handled cane, tripod cane, and quad cane), hemiwalkers (sometimes called a hemicane), and walkers (standard or with wheels). Crutches are another type of assistive device used to lessen or remove weight from one or both legs. Clients may also feel insecure in the initial learning stages when using assistive devices.

Crutches

Crutches are an aid to walking by providing support during ambulating when the lower extremities are unable to support the body weight. Generally crutch use is temporary, but even if it is permanent, crutches do allow independence of movement that otherwise could not occur.

There are three main types of crutches: the axillary (most common for short-term use), the Lofstrand, or Canadian (a forearm crutch with a metal band and handle), and the platform, for clients who are unable to use their wrists to bear weight.

Several safety factors should be taken into account before assisting the client to use crutches. The measurement should be 5 cm (2 in.) from the axillary fold to the crutch bar. The handpiece should be adjusted to allow 20–30-degree elbow flexion, and rubber suction tips should be placed on the bottom of the crutches. Finally, the client should be informed that while using crutches, he or she needs shoes that fit well and have nonslip soles.

The type of crutch used by the client depends on the ability to ambulate, the muscle strength needed for support, and the individual needs of the client.

Walkers

Walkers assist the client with balance and with walking. The client's arms are used to support all or part of the client's body and take weight off the lower limbs as he or she ambulates. Some walkers have seats so that clients are able to sit as needed. This type of walker has hand brakes to prevent client injury. Walkers offer more stability than a cane.

Walkers are a necessary assistive device for postoperative clients requiring help with ambulation. These clients include, for example, those with major spinal cord surgery or hip replacement surgery, or those who were or are weak from major surgery, a medical condition, or prolonged hospitalization and are unsteady with ambulation.

Walkers are constructed with or without wheels or platforms. Wheels may be on the front legs of the walker or on all four legs. All walkers that have rubber tips should be checked frequently to ensure that they are in good repair.

The height of the walker is adjusted by lowering or raising the legs of the extension piece to fit the client's height properly. The handles of the walker should be at the level of the client's greater trochanter.

Canes

Canes are used to provide additional balance during ambulation and to help protect clients from falls. Clients who are unsteady, lose their balance, are weak, or have a leg(s) that cannot hold the client in the upright position are candidates for canes. A PT should evaluate to ensure correct selection of assistive device.

Using a cane may afford the client the confidence to ambulate and maintain his or her independence. Canes, just like crutches, are measured for a proper fit. The cane is turned upside down with the handle on the floor, and the rubber tip is removed. The client is instructed to stand with his or her arms at the sides of the body. The correct measurement is from the floor to the level of the greater trochanter. Most canes are aluminum and can be adjusted to within 1 in. (2.5 cm) of the desired height.

If the cane has a rectangular base with four supports (a quad cane), each should have a rubber platform. Canes with four supports offer more stability than canes with two supports. Canes may have either a "c" (curved) handle or a functional grip (straight handle). Straight handles allow for a better grip by the client.

A hemiwalker, also called a *hemicane* or *side-stepper cane*, is a mobility device sometimes classified as a cane but that also has some characteristics of a walker. It offers more support than a cane but less than a walker, has a larger base than any cane, and may have an additional lower grip to help an individual get up from a sitting to a standing position.

Adaptation to Home Care

Knowledge of body mechanics and how to use these and other principles of safe client mobility and handling is important to both the healthcare provider and the client when care is provided in the home setting. Back injuries can occur among healthcare providers in the home as easily as in other healthcare settings. Contributing factors may be that there is no one to help the care provider when assisting and turning clients in the home, and equipment may not be adequate or adjustable.

The purpose of this unit is to consider adaptations necessary for providing safe care to the client while using proper body mechanics. In the home setting, much of the care is given by the family; therefore, it is essential that they also be taught principles of safety when providing care.

Nursing Diagnoses

The following nursing diagnoses are appropriate to use on client care plans when the components are related to exercise and ambulation needs of clients.

NURSING DIAGNOSIS	RELATED TO . . .
Activity Intolerance	Nutritional disorders, disease states, impaired motor function, pain, inadequate gas exchange
Impaired Home Maintenance	Chronic disease process, lack of knowledge, insufficient funds, lack of support or community resources
Impaired Physical Mobility	Neuromuscular impairment, musculoskeletal impairment, surgical procedure, trauma
Acute Pain	Musculoskeletal disorders, inflammation, immobility
Self-Care Deficit (Bathing, Dressing, Feeding, Toileting)	Neuromuscular impairment, musculoskeletal impairment, visual disorders, external devices, decreased strength and endurance

Source: Herdman, T. H. & Kamitsuru, S. (Eds.) *Nursing Diagnoses – Definitions and Classification 2015-2017.* Copyright © 2014, 1994–2014 by NANDA International. Used by arrangement with John Wiley & Sons Limited. Companion website: www.wiley.com/go/nursingdiagnoses. In order to make safe and effective judgments using NANDA-I nursing diagnosis it is essential that nurses refer to the definitions and defining characteristics of the diagnoses listed in this work.

Range of Motion

Nursing Process Data

ASSESSMENT Database

- Determine client's physical ability to perform exercises (i.e., level of consciousness, presence of casts, traction).
- Ascertain client's baseline level of joint movement and muscle strength.
- Note amount of spontaneous movement shown by the client.
- Assess client's understanding of ROM exercises.

PLANNING Objectives

- To improve or maintain joint function
- To improve or maintain muscle tone and strength
- To enhance or maintain soft tissue integrity
- To counteract effects of prolonged bed rest or immobilization
- To facilitate passive range of motion
- To prevent contractures
- To increase client comfort
- To prepare the client for ambulation

IMPLEMENTATION Procedures

DOCUMENTATION AND EVALUATION

Expected Outcomes

- Client improves range of motion and muscle tone after performing range-of-motion exercises.
- Client is able to progress through range of motion with minimal to no pain.
- Client is able to ambulate without difficulty following a period of bed rest.

Unexpected Outcomes/Alternative Actions

Pearson Nursing Student Resources

Find additional review materials at
nursing.pearsonhighered.com.
Prepare for success with NCLEX®-style practice questions and Skill Checklists.

Skill 13.1.1 | Performing Passive Range of Motion

Equipment
Hospital bed

Procedure

1. Check physician's order to determine if passive range of motion can be performed (according to facility policy).
2. Check two forms of client ID and introduce yourself.
3. Explain procedure to client and caregiver who may be delivering range of motion at home.
4. Perform hand hygiene.
5. Position client on his or her back with bed as flat as possible. Place bed in HIGH position.
6. Expose limb to be exercised.
7. Put all joints through range of motion slowly and gently (Table 13-1 ■ ❶–❿, Table 13-2 ■ ⓫–⓲). Start at head.
8. Protect against gravity and detrimental movement when performing range-of-motion exercises.
9. Provide support above and below joint using a cradling support while performing the exercises.
10. Follow sequence of exercises for upper and lower body according to chart.
11. All joints should be put through five full-range-of-motion exercises to each joint at least twice daily.
12. Encourage client to do active exercises as soon as possible. ➤ *Rationale:* Passive exercises only help prevent contractures but do not maintain muscle.
13. Discontinue exercises if client complains of pain or discomfort. ➤ *Rationale:* Range-of-motion exercises should be performed in pain-free movement.
14. Reassess client's ability to perform ROM exercises and adjust schedule accordingly.

Table 13-1 Range of Motion: Upper Body

	Neck	Shoulder	Elbow	Forearm	Wrist	Finger and Thumb
Flexion	Move head forward 90 degrees with chin on chest.	Raise arm 180 degrees from side to above head.	Bend elbow so arm moves up toward shoulder.		Bend hand 90 degrees toward inner arm.	Make a fist so fingers are all bent inward.
Extension	Move head up from chest 90 degrees to erect position.	Move arm to side of body.	Straighten elbow and return to position.		Move hand straight, pointed out.	Move fingers 90 degrees to straight position.
Abduction		Hold arm away from side 180 degrees to above head.			Bend wrist out, away from arm.	Spread fingers as much as possible.
Adduction		Move arm from side across chest.			Bend wrist inward toward radius.	Move fingers and thumb together.
External rotation		Hold arm out to side with elbow bent 90 degrees; move forward so palm faces forward.				
Internal rotation		Move arm to side at shoulder level with elbow bent 90 degrees. Lower arm so palm faces back.				
Rotation	Move head in side-to-side motion— looking over one shoulder, then the other, but never forcing against any resistance.					
Circumduction		Move arm in full circle.				

(continued)

Skill 13.1.1 | Performing Passive Range of Motion (continued)

Table 13-1 Range of Motion: Upper Body (continued)

	Neck	Shoulder	Elbow	Forearm	Wrist	Finger and Thumb
Supination				Rotate arm so palm faces up (toward ceiling if client is lying in bed).		
Pronation				Rotate arm so palm is down (toward floor if client is lying in bed).		

Table 13-2 Range of Motion: Lower Body

	Trunk	Hip	Knee	Ankle	Toes
Flexion	Bend forward 90 degrees.	Move leg forward and up 90 degrees.	Bend knee 90 degrees; foot moves back and up.		Point down 90 degrees ("curl").
Extension	Stand in straight position.	Move leg in straight alignment with trunk.	Move foot 90 degrees with knee straight and leg in line with body.		Straight out from foot.
Hyperextension	Bend backward 30 degrees.	Move leg backward 50 degrees.			Point up 45 degrees.
Lateral flexion	Bend to both sides 45 degrees.				
Internal rotation		Turn leg and foot inward 90 degrees.			
External rotation		Turn leg and foot outward 90 degrees.			
Abduction		Move leg away from body 45 degrees.			Spread apart 15 degrees.
Adduction		Move leg toward body 45 degrees.			Bring together in normal position.
Plantar flexion				Point toes downward.	
Dorsiflexion				Point toes upward.	
Eversion				Move sole of foot lateral to outside.	
Inversion				Move sole of foot medial to inside.	

Note: ROM exercises should be incorporated into activities of daily living whenever possible.

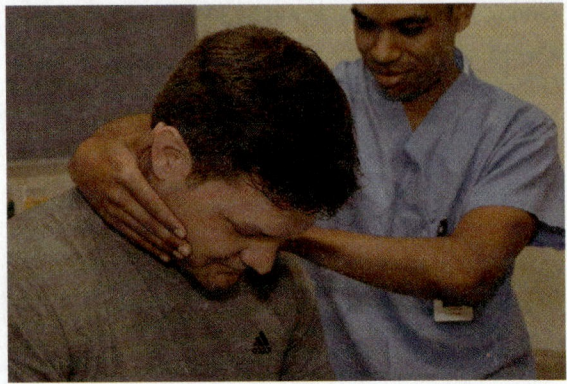

❶ Flexion of neck—move head forward 90 degrees with chin on chest.

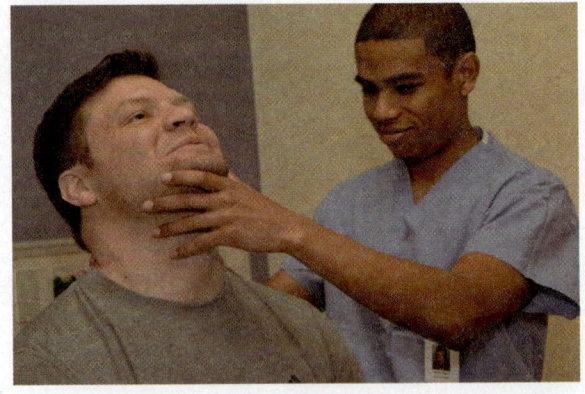

❷ Extension of neck—move head up from chest 90 degrees.

3 Internal rotation of shoulder.

4 External rotation of shoulder.

5 Abduction of shoulder.

6 Adduction of shoulder.

7 Extension of elbow.

8 Rotation of the wrist.

9 Extension of finger joints.

10 Adduction–abduction finger exercises.

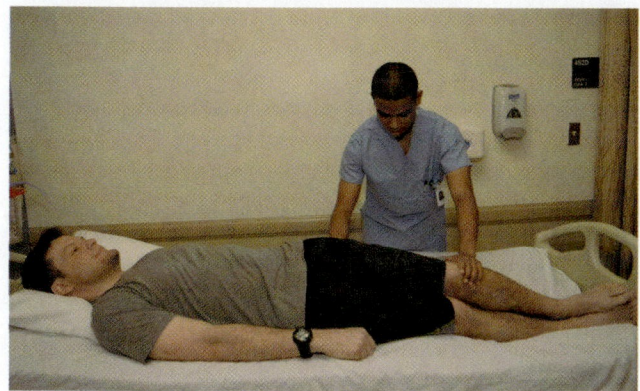
11 Rotate lower trunk outward 90 degrees.

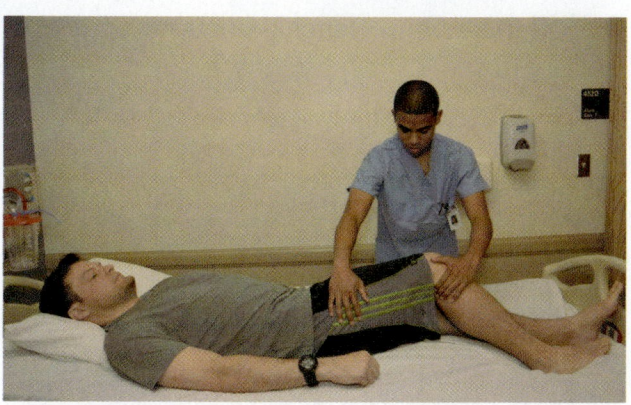
12 Rotate lower trunk to other side 90 degrees.

(continued)

Skill 13.1.1 | Performing Passive Range of Motion *(continued)*

13 Flex hip and knee.

14 Straight leg raise.

15 Abduction—Move leg away from the body.

16 Adduction—Move leg toward midline of body.

17 Plantar flexion—Move foot down and away from leg.

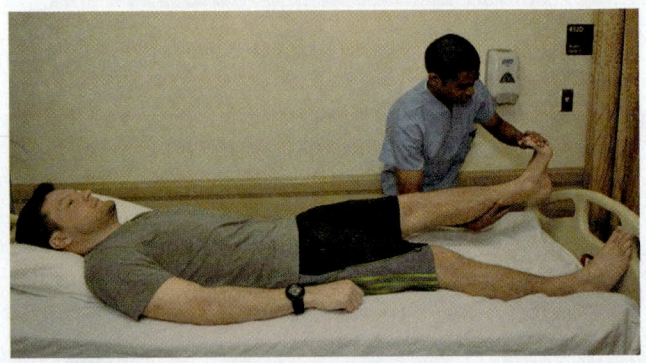

18 Dorsiflexion—Move foot up and toward leg.

Skill 13.1.2 | Teaching Active Range of Motion

Equipment

Hospital bed
Sturdy nonslip shoes or slippers

Procedure

1. Explain the rationale for the procedure to the client.
2. Demonstrate the exercises that the client should perform. (See Skill 13.1.1, *Performing Passive Range of Motion* for specific steps in exercises.)
3. Observe as the client performs the exercises.
4. Assist with the exercises as needed.

5. Verbally redirect the client if you notice any problems with the client's movements.
6. Encourage client to perform as many of the exercises as possible.
7. Instruct client to do range-of-motion exercises every 4 hr, exercising all joints. Dorsiflexion and plantar flexion (ankle pumps) should be done more frequently while awake and in bed or sitting to prevent deep vein thrombosis in lower extremities.
8. Move extremities through range of motion five cycles each procedure.

Unit 13.1 Documentation and Evaluation

DOCUMENTATION for Range of Motion

- Amount of time needed to complete exercises
- Any changes in condition of joint or joint mobility
- Movements that caused unusual pain or discomfort
- Amount of client participation
- Specific joints put through range of motion
- Alterations in usual procedure
- Degree of mobility improvement after exercises

EVALUATION/Critical Thinking

Expected Outcomes

- Client improves range of motion and muscle tone after performing range-of-motion exercises.
- Client is able to progress through the range-of-motion exercises with minimal to no pain.
- Client is able to ambulate without difficulty after a period of bed rest.

Unexpected Outcomes

- Client continues to lose mobility and strength despite nursing intervention.

- Client experiences pain and discomfort during range-of-motion exercises.

Alternative Actions

- Discuss the need for additional measures to improve joint range with the health team.
- Refer client to PT if range of motion is to be performed by nursing staff only.
- Assess client for the need to use splints and braces to maintain the best physiologic position between exercise periods, and discuss your findings with the physician.

- Assess amount and type of pain and report findings to physician.
- Reevaluate your technique to ensure you are performing the exercises correctly.
- Start exercises with less stress on joints. Do exercises for a shorter period of time and gradually increase time and range of joint mobility.

Nursing Process Data

ASSESSMENT Database

- Assess client's previous activity level.
- Check physician's orders for activity.
- Assess vital signs and physical ability to ambulate.
- Assess need for safety belt or assistive devices.
- Assess client for vertigo when moved into an upright sitting position.
- Determine if client feels pain from operative site.
- Observe client's balance.
- Assess any sensory deficits (visual, perceptual).

PLANNING Objectives

- To promote increased feelings of physical and mental well-being
- To develop increased tolerance for exercise
- To decrease hospitalization time
- To regain independence by regaining ability to walk
- To prevent paralytic ileus by increasing abdominal wall and gastrointestinal tract muscle tone
- To prevent thrombophlebitis by increasing circulation in the legs
- To promote healing by increasing circulation and muscle contraction

IMPLEMENTATION Procedures

DOCUMENTATION AND EVALUATION

Expected Outcomes

- Feelings of physical and mental well-being increase.
- Balance and muscle tone improve.
- Client progresses from being dependent with ambulation to becoming independent in ambulation.
- Complications of immobility are prevented with ambulation.
- Client uses assistive devices correctly without supervision.

Unexpected Outcomes/Alternative Actions

Pearson Nursing Student Resources

Find additional review materials at
nursing.pearsonhighered.com.
Prepare for success with NCLEX®-style practice questions and Skill Checklists.

Skill 13.2.1 | Minimizing Orthostatic Hypotension

Equipment

Elastic stockings, if ordered

Robe and slippers

Stethoscope and sphygmomanometer

Procedure

1. Review client's chart before ambulation to check for a history of **orthostatic hypotension** (Box 13-2 ■), medication that contributes to orthostatic hypotension, and intake and output. (Is the client adequately hydrated?) ➤ *Rationale:* This condition may occur in any client, but it is more common in the older adult or with clients who have been immobilized.
2. Perform hand hygiene.
3. Check two forms of client ID, introduce yourself, and review procedure with client.
4. Place compression stockings, if ordered, on client's legs. ➤ *Rationale:* Compression stockings help to reduce blood stasis and promote venous return.
5. Move bed to LOW position. (Always confirm that bed is in locked position.) ➤ *Rationale:* This position enables client to have feet on the floor and is safer if client experiences vertigo.
6. *Slowly* raise head of bed (HOB) to Fowler's position. ➤ *Rationale:* The more slowly the client's position is changed, the less the effect of postural hypotension.
7. Move client to edge of bed by placing one arm behind client's back and one arm under both thighs. Pivot client to a sitting position and assist to dangle legs over side of bed. ➤ *Rationale:* Dangling with feet flat on floor for several minutes with legs in a dependent position will reduce effects of postural hypotension.
8. Take client's blood pressure and pulse and observe for vertigo, fainting, pallor, and so on.

9. *Slowly* assist client to stand. Instruct client to take a deep breath and exhale. If there is no evidence of orthostatic hypotensive symptoms, begin ambulation or transfer to a chair.

Note: If hypotension continues, client should be returned to flat position in bed.

> **CLINICAL ALERT**
>
> If the client has been on prolonged bed rest or has been immobilized, the risk of orthostatic hypotension is increased. Raising and lowering HOB several times to stimulate baroreceptors will help to prevent this condition.

Box 13-2 MEASURING ORTHOSTATIC HYPOTENSION

Postural or orthostatic hypotension is often present after prolonged bed rest or immobilization. It can be also be chronic, symptomatic, or asymptomatic. It is a sudden drop in blood pressure (20 mm Hg systolic or 10 mm Hg diastolic) when the client moves from a horizontal to a vertical position (lying to sitting or standing) at 3 minutes (actual procedures may vary between facilities). An increase in pulse rate of 20 beats or more per minute is considered an abnormal finding. Symptoms include dizziness, lightheadedness, blurred vision, fainting, pallor, or nausea. To measure orthostatic hypotension:

- With client in supine position for 5 minutes, measure pulse and blood pressure. ➤ *Rationale:* This amount of time allows for blood pressure to stabilize.
- Assist client to stand, wait for 3 minutes, and recheck pulse and blood pressure. Evaluate oxygenation by pulse oximetry if vital signs indicate orthostatic hypotension or there are symptoms present. ➤ *Rationale:* This amount of time will allow for compensatory mechanisms to work.
- Notify healthcare provider. Document findings and notification information.

Skill 13.2.2 | Ambulating With Two Assistants

Equipment

Robe or second hospital gown (put on backward so that client is not exposed)

Shoes or slippers that fit well and have nonslip soles

Procedure

1. Perform hand hygiene.
2. Check two forms of client ID, introduce yourself, and explain the rationale for the procedure to the client.
3. Move client to side of bed ❶ and assist client to sit on the edge after placing bed in LOW position. Assist client to sitting position. ❷
4. Assess the client for vertigo or faintness. Keep client in sitting position until he or she is able to stand without

becoming dizzy. ➤ *Rationale:* Orthostatic hypotension can occur with prolonged bed rest (see Skill 13.2.1, Minimizing Orthostatic Hypotension).

5. Position one nurse on each side of the client and have each nurse grasp the client's upper arm with the hand that is closest to the client.
6. Have each nurse grasp the client's hand with the other hand and instruct the client to stand.
7. Encourage the client to maintain erect **posture** and look straight ahead, not down.
8. Ask the client to lift each foot to take a step. The client should not shuffle. ❸ ❹
9. Walk the client only as far as he or she is capable of walking and returning without exhaustion.

(continued)

Skill 13.2.2 | Ambulating With Two Assistants *(continued)*

❶ Move client to side of bed.

❷ Assist client to sit at edge of bed with feet on floor.

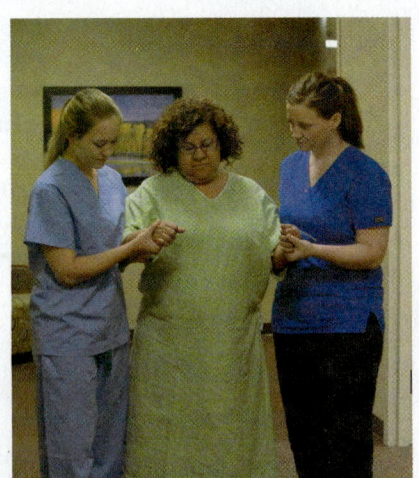

❸ Support is provided by two nurses when client's condition requires.

❹ Grasp client's arms firmly on both sides to provide support.

EVIDENCE-BASED PRACTICE

Progressive Mobility in Critically Ill Clients

Progressive mobility is defined as a series of planned movements done in a sequential manner beginning at a client's current mobility status, with a goal of returning to his or her baseline (Advancing Nursing LLC). It includes elevation of the head of the bed, manual turning, passive and active range-of-motion exercises, continuous lateral rotation therapy (CLRT) and **prone** positioning, movement against gravity, upright leg-down position, chair position, dangling, and ambulation.

A meta-analysis of 39 randomized trials examining the effect of bed rest on 15 different medical conditions and procedures showed that bed rest was not beneficial and may be associated with complications. The short-term outcomes of bed rest for critically ill clients included ventilator-associated pneumonia (VAP) and hospital-acquired pneumonia, delayed weaning off of mechanical ventilation due to muscle weakness, and the development of pressure ulcers. The major long-term complication is the diminished quality of life after discharge due to physical deconditioning that takes place during the client's stay in the ICU. Outcomes from survivors of acute respiratory distress syndrome indicated that they had lost 10% of their body weight at discharge and had significant functional limitations 1 year later due to muscle wasting and fatigue.

Source: Vollman (2010)

Skill 13.2.3 | Ambulating With One Assistant

Equipment

Robe or second hospital gown (put on backward so that client is not exposed)

Shoes or slippers that fit well and have nonslip soles

Safety or gait belt if indicated

Procedure

1. Check client's chart for ambulation problems, orthostatic hypotension, or any specific healthcare provider's orders.
2. Perform hand hygiene.

3. Check two forms of client ID, introduce yourself, and explain rationale for procedure to client.

4. Help client sit on side of bed after placing bed in LOW position.

5. Assess client for vertigo or faintness. ➤ *Rationale:* Keeping client in this position until he or she is able to stand without becoming dizzy will prevent falling.

6. Apply safety belt if client is unsteady. ❶ ➤ *Rationale:* The belt provides support if client is weak and prevents injury. ❷

7. Bend forward facing the client, grasp belt, and gently rock back and forth about three times.

8. Instruct the client to assist with standing while pulling client upward with rocking motion, and on the third rocking motion, pull the client to a standing position. Have client take a deep breath and exhale while standing.

9. Stabilize client in a standing position. Grasp belt firmly at client's back when ambulating. ❸

10. Stand on weaker side, when client is moderately weak; for client with cerebrovascular accident (CVA or stroke), stand on unaffected side. ➤ *Rationale:* **Flaccid** muscles on affected side do not provide sufficient muscle strength for you to grasp and support client.

11. Encourage client to maintain good posture and to look straight ahead. ➤ *Rationale:* Tendency is for client to look down, which may increase vertigo.

12. Instruct client to lift each foot to take a step, not to shuffle.

13. Walk client as far as he or she is capable of walking without becoming exhausted. Remember client must walk back to room, so take this into consideration when walking. A wheelchair or walker can be pushed behind client for use if he or she becomes tired.

14. If client is collapsing, try to break the fall with your body and guide client to the floor. Call for help. If possible, use the wall to support the client. If client is unsteady or appears to be falling, support his or her body, especially the head and trunk, maintaining your body in good alignment with line of gravity within your widened **base of support**. This alignment prevents injury to yourself, while giving the client adequate support. If necessary, guide the client all the way to the floor. ❹

❶ Use gait belt to assist client out of bed.

❷ Gait belt provides for stability when ambulating.

❸ Grasp belt firmly at client's back when ambulating.

❹ **A.** Grasp client under both arms if she begins to fall. **B.** Break client's fall using your body to prevent injury.

Skill 13.2.4 | Ambulating With a Walker

Equipment

Robe or second hospital gown (put on backward so that client is not exposed)

Shoes or slippers that fit well and have nonslip soles

Walker with safety tips and rubber hand grips (nonrolling walker is used for clients beginning ambulation) or hemiwalker

> **CLINICAL ALERT**
>
> The client who has had a total knee or hip joint replacement surgery may need more help with balance and walking than can be provided with crutches or a cane. Four solid prongs on the bottom of the cane may give the most stability.

❶ **A.** Hemiwalker. **B.** Place walker directly in front of client. Instruct client to hold on to hand grips.

Procedure

1. Perform hand hygiene.
2. Check two forms of client ID, introduce yourself, and explain rationale for procedure to client.
3. Move client to edge of bed and seat client so feet touch floor.
4. Place walker directly in front of client at a comfortable distance. ❶ Instruct client to grasp hand grips on walker. ➤ *Rationale:* A walker provides stability when getting up.
5. Ensure legs of walker are level to ground.
6. Instruct client to push self off bed. Client is cautioned to not step completely against front bar of walker. ➤ *Rationale:* Client can lose balance.
7. Have client bend elbows slightly ❷ and move walker forward about one step ahead (6–8 in. [15–20 cm]). Keep all four feet of walker on floor.
8. Instruct client to move weaker side first ❸ by supporting body weight on handles and advancing weaker leg into center of walker.
9. Instruct client to balance self and then move unaffected side by placing that foot even with first foot.
10. Have client move walker forward and continue same pattern of ambulating.

Note: When moving to a chair, instruct client to back all the way to the chair until legs touch the front. Release hands from the walker and grasp the armrests of the chair. Instruct client to slowly lower herself or himself into the chair. Once in the chair, instruct to slide until back touches chair.

> **CLINICAL ALERT**
>
> Adjust walker handles to level of greater trochanter.

❷ Instruct client to bend elbows slightly and move walker forward.

❸ Instruct client to move weaker side first.

Skill 13.2.5 | Ambulating With a Cane

Equipment
Appropriate type of cane with rubber tips
  Straight-legged or standard cane
  Tripod or three-pronged cane
Quad cane
Sturdy shoes with nonskid soles
Safety or gait belt (optional)

Procedure
1. Check physician's orders and client care plan. ➤ **Rationale:** It's important to ensure that the client is ready to use a cane and to ascertain that the cane provides sufficient support for the client.
2. Perform hand hygiene.
3. Check two forms of client ID, introduce yourself, and explain the purpose of using a cane for ambulation, and answer client questions.
4. Demonstrate use of cane if client is unfamiliar with its use.
5. Assist client to put on appropriate shoes and socks for walking.
6. Assist client to standing position with feet firmly on the floor.
7. Instruct client to hold the cane on the stronger side of the body. ❶, ❷ ➤ **Rationale:** This offers the most support.
8. Check that cane extends from greater trochanter to floor with 20–30 degrees for elbow flexion. ➤ **Rationale:** If cane is too long or too short, client may injure back.
9. Place cane about 12 in. (about 30 cm) in front of the foot and slightly to the outside. ➤ **Rationale:** This position provides the best balance, because the client's center of gravity is within the base of support.
10. Determine that client can maintain balance and does not experience vertigo before taking the first step. Hold cane on unaffected side, keeping the cane close to the body. ➤ **Rationale:** This distributes weight away from affected side and prevents the body from leaning forward. Instruct client to grasp handrail, if possible.
11. Have client move cane and affected leg 4 in. (10 cm) forward. ❸
12. Instruct client to shift his or her weight to affected leg and cane. Then move unaffected leg forward, ahead of cane.
13. Have client move cane and affected leg forward simultaneously. Repeat these steps when walking with the cane.
14. Accompany client by walking beside him or her on the unaffected side, or use safety or gait belt if needed. ➤ **Rationale:** If the client loses his or her balance, supporting client on unaffected side is most effective. Simply insert your hand and arm underneath the client's axilla and support his or her arm with your other hand.
15. Evaluate client's ability to use the cane, and instruct about its use as needed.
16. Reinforce the client's achievement to assist him or her to gain confidence in ambulating.

❶ Specially marked cane indicates disability.

❷ Direct client to hold cane on stronger side of body.

(continued)

Skill 13.2.5 | Ambulating With a Cane *(continued)*

❸ Instruct client to move affected leg forward first, even with cane.

LEGAL ALERT

Whenever the nurse is teaching clients how to use assistive devices, ensure that written instructions are also provided. Document what was taught, results of return demonstrations on use of equipment, and client's understanding of use of equipment. The nurse and hospital can be held liable for negligence if the client falls and sustains an injury using an assistive device and there is no documentation of client teaching.

17. Continue to accompany client until the time for walking is completed.
18. Assist client to return to the room and to bed if indicated.
19. Position client for comfort.
20. Assess client's response to ambulation.
21. Perform hand hygiene.
22. Chart client's progress, and evaluate plan for increased periods of ambulation in terms of client's capability.

Box 13-3 MANAGING STEPS USING A CANE

Going upstairs, lead with "good" or unaffected leg; going downstairs, lead with "bad" or affected leg. An easy way to remember this is: Up with the good; down with the bad.

Upstairs

- Take first step up with strong leg. With cane on opposite side of affected leg, grasp handrail.
- Move cane and affected leg to the same step.
- Move unaffected leg to next step.
- Have the client continue this procedure all the way up the stairs.

Downstairs

- Take first step by placing cane and affected leg one step down.
- Lower unaffected leg to same step.
- Have the client continue this procedure all the way down the stairs.

Unit 13.2 Unit Documentation and Evaluation

DOCUMENTATION for Ambulation

- Client's ability to balance
- Client's posture and gait during ambulation
- Time and distance of ambulation
- Strength or weakness of lower extremities
- Use of correct procedure for walker or cane
- Client's perceptions of ambulation

EVALUATION/Critical Thinking

Expected Outcomes

- Client is able to ambulate independently.
- Client is not experiencing complications of immobility.
- Client is able to prevent orthostatic hypotension by following protocol for moving out of bed.
- Client is able to ambulate using assistive devices without assistance.
- Client is able to ambulate safely with assistance.

Unexpected Outcomes	**Alternative Actions**
• Client experiences vertigo or feels faint.	• If in the client's room, help the client return to the chair or bed. • If in the hall, ease the client down the wall to the floor. Do not attempt to hold the client. • Summon help if possible.
• Client is too weak to ambulate.	• Provide active and passive ROM before attempting ambulation. • Begin ambulation protocol as soon as possible using assistive device.
• Client is heavy or has poor balance.	• Ask other nurses or staff to help you ambulate the client until able to walk on his or her own. • If necessary, enlist the aid of a stronger assistant whose presence may give the client additional psychological as well as physical support. • Gradually increase ambulation as muscle tone improves and balance improves. • Request assistance for ambulation from PT. • Obtain walker to assist client with ambulation. The walker will also provide reassurance to client.
• Client feels unsafe to ambulate.	• Ambulate more frequently for shorter periods and with more assistance to increase confidence. • Medicate with mild pain medication at least 1 hour before ambulation to decrease pain. • With abdominal surgery, check with healthcare provider for an order for a binder to decrease fear of dehiscence and pain, if present. • Establish rapport with the client so you can discuss fears about ambulation. • Use assistive devices for client security.

Nursing Process Data

ASSESSMENT Database

- Assess physical ability to use crutches and strength of the client's arm, back, and leg muscles.
- Observe client's ability to balance self.
- Note any unilateral or unusual weakness or vertigo.
- Assess which gait is appropriate for client.
- Assess client's understanding of crutch-walking technique.

PLANNING Objectives

- To improve client's ability to ambulate when he or she has lower extremity injury
- To increase muscle strength, especially in the arms and legs
- To increase feeling of well-being when client can ambulate
- To promote joint mobility
- To resume activities of daily living after injury or surgery

IMPLEMENTATION Procedures

DOCUMENTATION AND EVALUATION

Expected Outcomes

- Client is able to ambulate without assistance.
- Client is able to use crutches to ambulate without fear or anxiety.
- Client is able to move in and out of chair with crutches.
- Crutches are measured appropriately to prevent numbness or tingling in fingers.
- Client is able to resume activities of daily living.

Unexpected Outcomes / Alternative Actions

Pearson Nursing Student Resources

Find additional review materials at
nursing.pearsonhighered.com.
Prepare for success with NCLEX®-style practice questions and Skill Checklists.

Skill 13.3.1 | Teaching Muscle-Strengthening Exercises

Equipment

Books, boards, or other firm surface for each hand

Procedure

1. Check the client care plan for physician's orders.
2. Perform hand hygiene.
3. Check two forms of client ID, introduce yourself, and explain rationale for exercises to client.
4. Demonstrate the exercises that client will practice.

Quadriceps-Setting Exercises

a. Try to hyperextend the client's leg by pushing the popliteal area (the area behind knee) into the bed and lifting heel off the bed.
b. Instruct client to contract muscle for a count of 5, then relax for a count of 5.
c. Have client repeat exercise two to three times, gradually working up to 10–15 times an hour.

Gluteal-Setting Exercises

a. Tell client to pinch his or her buttocks together for a count of 5 and then to relax for a count of 5.
b. Have client repeat exercise 10–15 times an hour.

Push-Ups in Sitting Position

a. Tell client to sit up in bed with arms at sides.
b. Put books, boards, or something firm under the client's hands and have the client push down, raising hips off the bed. (This exercise may also be practiced while sitting in a chair.)
c. Have client repeat exercise until he or she can do 10–15 push-ups an hour.

Push-Ups in Prone Position

a. Tell client to lie prone in bed.
b. Ask client to place hands on the bed, close to the shoulders.
c. Tell client to extend arms and to push the upper part of the body into an upright position.
d. Have client repeat exercise until he or she can do 10–15 push-ups an hour.

5. Monitor as the client performs the exercises and correct any problems that may occur.
6. Assess the client for increasing strength as he or she continues to practice the exercises.
7. Perform hand hygiene.

Skill 13.3.2 | Measuring Client for Crutches

Equipment

Measuring tape
Hard-soled street shoes
Safety or gait belt

Procedure

1. Perform hand hygiene.
2. Check two forms of client ID, introduce yourself, and explain rationale for procedure to client.
3. Ask client to put on the shoes she or he will be wearing when using the crutches, if possible. Shoes should be low heeled and nonskid.
4. Assist client to standing position. Have walker in place for support. Another staff member should be present to provide for safety.
5. Measure distance from client's axilla (armpit) to a point 15–20 cm (6–8 in.) out from heel. ❶
6. Adjust hand bars on the crutches so that client's elbows are always slightly flexed.
7. Instruct client to stand with crutches under arms.
8. Measure the distance between client's axilla and arm pieces on the crutches. You should be able to put two of your fingers in the space between axilla and crutch bar.
   ➤ *Rationale:* Crutches that do not fit client correctly or crutches that are used incorrectly can damage the brachial plexus and cause **paralysis** of the arms.

Note: Use of gait belt can be beneficial when client is beginning to use crutches. ➤ ***Rationale:*** The gait belt provides safety in preventing falls and promotes security for client.

2 Fingers width from axilla to crutch bar

A   B

❶ **A.** Measure from axilla to heel for crutch height, with crutch tip positioned 6–8 in. (15–20 cm) from foot. **B.** Teach tripod crutch stance for balance in crutch walking.

Skill 13.3.3 | Teaching Crutch Walking: Four-Point Gait

Equipment
Properly fitted crutches with rubber tips and axillary pads
 or Lofstrand or Platform crutch.
Regular, hard-soled street shoes
Safety belt, if needed

Procedure
1. Perform hand hygiene.
2. Check two forms of client ID, introduce yourself, and explain
   the rationale for the procedure to the client.

   a. The gait is rather slow but very stable.
   b. The gait can be performed when the client can move and
      bear weight on each leg.

3. Demonstrate the crutch-foot sequence to the client. ❶

   a. Move the right crutch.
   b. Move the left foot.
   c. Move the left crutch.
   d. Move the right foot.

4. Help the client practice the gait. Be ready to help with
   balance if necessary. Use safety belt if necessary.

Step 1   Step 2   Step 3   Step 4

❶ Four-point gait.

5. Assess client's progress and correct mistakes as they occur.
6. Perform hand hygiene.

Skill 13.3.4 | Teaching Crutch Walking: Three-Point Gait

Equipment
Properly fitted crutches with rubber tips and arm pads
Regular, hard-soled street shoes
Safety belt, if needed

Procedure
1. Perform hand hygiene.
2. Check two forms of client ID, introduce yourself, and explain
   the rationale for the procedure to the client.

   a. The gait can be performed when the client can bear
      little or no weight on one leg or when the client has only
      one leg.
   b. This gait is fairly rapid and requires strong upper
      extremities and good balance.

3. Demonstrate the crutch-foot sequence to the client. ❶

   a. Two crutches support the weaker extremity.
   b. Balance weight on the crutches.
   c. Move both crutches and affected leg forward.
   d. Move unaffected leg forward.

4. Assess the client's progress, and correct any mistakes as
   they occur.

5. Remain with client until crutch safety is ensured. Use safety
   belt if necessary.
6. Perform hand hygiene.

Step 1   Step 2   Step 3

❶ Three-point gait.

Skill 13.3.5 | Teaching Crutch Walking: Two-Point Gait

Equipment
Properly fitted crutches with rubber tips and arm pads
Regular, hard-soled street shoes
Safety belt, if needed

Procedure
1. Perform hand hygiene.
2. Check two forms of client ID, introduce yourself, and explain rationale for procedure to client.

    a. Procedure is a rapid version of the four-point gait.
    b. Gait requires more balance than the four-point gait.

3. Demonstrate the crutch-foot sequence to the client. ❶

    a. Advance the right foot and the left crutch simultaneously.
    b. Advance the left foot and the right crutch simultaneously.

4. Help the client practice the gait. Use safety belt if necessary.
5. Assess the client's progress and correct any mistakes as they occur.
6. Perform hand hygiene.

Step 1   Step 2

❶ Two-point gait.

Skill 13.3.6 | Teaching Swing-To Gait and Swing-Through Gait

Equipment
Properly fitted crutches with rubber tips and arm pads
Regular, hard-soled street shoes
Safety belt, if needed

Procedure
1. Perform hand hygiene.
2. Check two forms of client ID, introduce yourself, and explain rationale for procedure to client.

    a. These gaits are usually performed when the client's lower extremities are paralyzed.
    b. The client may require braces.

3. Demonstrate the crutch-foot sequence to the client.

    a. Move both crutches forward.
    b. Swing-to gait: Lift and swing the body to the crutches. ❶
    c. Swing-through gait: Lift and swing the body past the crutches.
    d. Bring crutches in front of the body and repeat.

4. Help the client practice the gaits. Use safety belt if necessary.
5. Assess the client's progress and correct any mistakes as they occur.
6. Perform hand hygiene.

A   Step 1   Step 2   B   Step 1   Step 2

❶ **A.** Swing-to gait. **B.** Swing-through gait.

Equipment

Properly fitted crutches with rubber tips and arm pads
Regular, hard-soled street shoes
Safety belt, if needed

Procedure

1. Perform hand hygiene.
2. Check two forms of client ID, introduce yourself, and explain rationale for the procedure to the client.
3. Apply safety belt if client is unsteady or requires support.
4. Demonstrate procedure using a three-point gait. ❶

Going Downstairs

a. Start with weight on the unaffected leg and crutches on the same level.
b. Use handrail. Place both crutches under opposite arm.
c. Have the client hold affected leg forward and place crutches on lower step.
d. Have the client place affected leg on lower step and move the unaffected leg to the same step. If no handrail is available, keep a crutch on each side, place both crutches on lower step, follow with affected leg, then unaffected leg. Advise caution to avoid forward falls.
e. Have client repeat until he or she understands the procedure.

Going Upstairs

a. Start with the crutches and unaffected extremity on the same level. Use safety belt when client is first learning to navigate stairs.
b. Have the client put weight on the crutch handles and lift the unaffected extremity onto the first step of the stairs.

c. Have the client lift affected extremity to the step.
d. Repeat until client understands the procedure.
5. Help the client practice.
6. Make sure that the client has adequate balance. Be ready to assist if necessary.
7. Assess the client's progress and correct any mistakes as they occur.
8. Perform hand hygiene.

❶ Demonstrate going up or down stairs using a three-point gait.

Equipment

Properly fitted crutches with rubber tips and arm pads
Regular, hard-soled shoes
Safety belt, if needed

Procedure

1. Perform hand hygiene.
2. Check two forms of client ID, introduce yourself, and explain procedure to client.
3. Apply safety belt if client is unsteady with crutches.
4. Instruct client to follow these steps.

Moving Into Chair

a. Stand in front of the chair, facing forward.
b. Place both crutches in hand on affected side.
c. Move backward slowly until back of lower legs touch center of chair.
d. Hold on to chair arm on unaffected side.

e. Lower self into chair by bending knees and hips, keeping back straight.
f. Use crutches and unaffected leg as a support.

Moving out of Chair

a. Move forward in chair by using unaffected side to slide body to edge of chair.
b. Hold on to chair arm on unaffected side.
c. Place both crutches in hand on affected side.
d. Lift self out of chair by grasping the chair arm and supporting self with crutches. Put weight on unaffected leg as you lift body out of chair.
e. Stand with back straight, bearing weight on unaffected leg and crutches.
f. Place crutches in front and slightly to side of body and begin crutch walking.

5. Perform hand hygiene.

Unit 13.3 Documentation and Evaluation

DOCUMENTATION for Crutch Walking

- Time and distance of ambulation on crutches
- Balance
- Reason for safety belt, if used
- Problems noted with technique

- Remedial teaching
- Client's perceptions of ambulation with crutches
- Ability to move in and out of chair
- Fear of using crutches

EVALUATION/Critical Thinking

Expected Outcomes

- Client is able to ambulate without assistance.
- Client is able to use crutches to ambulate without fear or anxiety.

- Client is able to move in and out of chair with crutches.
- Crutches are measured appropriately to prevent numbness or tingling in fingers.

Unexpected Outcomes

- Client states he or she is frightened of the crutches.

Alternative Actions

- Observe as the client practices the procedures to make sure that he or she is completing the steps correctly for each gait.
- Explain that it takes time to become proficient.
- Reassure the client that he or she will improve with continued practice.
- Assess the client's ability to use the crutches and evaluate level of confidence.
- Place safety or gait belt on client until he or she feels confident.
- Check with physician about obtaining an order for a walker until the client feels more confident.

- Client fears falling while dependent on crutches.

- Slow down crutch protocol until client gains confidence at every level of mastery (e.g., four-point gait to two-point gait).
- Remain with client and give verbal reassurance and feedback for improvement.

- Shoulder girdle is too weak to bear client's weight for crutch support.

- Increase exercise of shoulder (biceps and triceps setting) to gain strength.
- Ask physician to write an order for overhead frame with trapeze for shoulder exercise sets.

- Slipping occurs with crutch walking.

- Check crutch tips to ensure they cover all metal or wood.
- Observe the client's stance or gait to determine if it is too broad.
- Be sure that floor surface is dry and free of scatter rugs.

- Client complains of numbness and tingling in fingers when crutch walking.

- Remeasure distance between axilla and crutch bars to determine if two finger breadths can be inserted.
- Observe client's gait to determine if he or she is leaning on crutch inappropriately.

Adaptation for Home Care

Nursing Process Data

ASSESSMENT Database

- Assess family's knowledge of the principles of body mechanics.
- Assess home care provider's knowledge of how to use correct muscle groups for specific activities.
- Assess knowledge of how to improvise for a nonhospital bed.
- Assess knowledge and correct any misinformation about body alignment and ability to move client up in bed without assistance.

PLANNING Objectives

- To promote safe client handling and mobility while caring for clients
- To move clients without assistance, preventing back injury
- To provide knowledge of the musculoskeletal system, body alignment, and balance in order to prevent back injury when providing care for a client in the home
- To provide methods of improvising for a nonhospital bed
- To discuss four safety tips for home care clients requiring assistive devices

IMPLEMENTATION Procedures

DOCUMENTATION AND EVALUATION

Expected Outcomes

- Correct body mechanics are used in caring for clients.
- Injuries are prevented to both nurse and client.
- Client care is facilitated by proper body mechanics.
- Client is able to move without assistance.
- Center of gravity is maintained when lifting objects.
- Nonhospital bed is easily adapted for home care.

Unexpected Outcomes/Alternative Actions

Pearson Nursing Student Resources

Find additional review materials at
nursing.pearsonhighered.com.
Prepare for success with NCLEX®-style practice
questions and Skill Checklists.

Skill 13.4.1 | Positioning Nonhospital Bed for Client Care

Procedure

1. Position foam wedges to simulate change in position when HOB does not move (high-Fowler's, 90 degrees; Fowler's, 60 degrees; semi-Fowler's, 30 degrees).
2. Use correct body mechanics to adjust height (Box 13-4 ■).
   a. Flex body at knees and keep back straight if bed is only slightly low.
   b. Kneel on pillow by bed or sit in chair alongside bed if bed is extremely low.
3. Lock each wheel or leg of bed in position by securing with bricks or blocks of wood.
4. Make footboard of lumber or item such as a TV tray; position legs of tray under mattress so that tray becomes footboard.

Box 13-4 CORRECT BODY MECHANICS

- Place both feet flat on the floor and keep your back straight to prevent back injury.
- Hold objects close to the body to prevent muscle **strain** and possible back injury.
- Keep body in proper alignment by bending your knees and keeping back straight when lifting objects to prevent injury to back muscles. Lifting and moving without assistance place both caregiver and client at risk. Avoid manual lifting. Use mechanical lift devices that are available for home care clients.

Skill 13.4.2 | Moving a Helpless Client up in Bed Without Assistance

Note: Every attempt should be made to avoid moving a client without assistance.

Procedure

1. Lower HOB and place pillow at HOB.
2. Stand at side of client's bed.
   a. Face far corner at foot of bed.
   b. Place one foot behind the other, assume a broad stance, and flex knees.
3. Flex arms so forearms are level with bed. Place one arm under client's head and one under small of back.
4. Rock and shift weight from forward to rear foot; hips will move downward.
5. Guide the client as he or she slides diagonally across bed toward head.
6. Repeat for trunk and leg sections.
7. Move to other side of bed and repeat Steps 2 through 5.
8. Repeat until client is satisfactorily positioned in bed.

Note: Mechanical lift devices are made for home care clients. See Chapter 12.

Skill 13.4.3 | Using Assistive Devices in Home

Note: Consult with PT to ensure appropriate equipment is available and appropriate to the client's level of functioning.

Equipment

Appropriate device for:
Assistance with walking
Cane
Walker
Crutches
Gait belt (optional)

Procedure
Cane

1. Ensure client was measured appropriately for cane (Skill 13.2.5).
2. Review steps in working with a cane. Demonstrate, if necessary.
3. Use gait belt if unsure of client's balance.

4. Assist client to walk stairs as needed.
5. Review safety issues with cane: Observe tips of cane to ensure rubber covers top completely.
6. Instruct caregiver in proper method to walk with cane.

Crutches

1. Ensure client was measured appropriately for crutches (Skill 13.3.2).
2. Review steps in crutch walking according to type of gait: two point, four point, and so on.
3. Demonstrate appropriate gait.
4. Instruct client to demonstrate gait; use gait belt constantly with crutches.
5. Instruct client to walk up and down stairs if needed and have client return demonstration.
6. Instruct client on how to sit down on chair using crutches.
7. Instruct client and caregiver to examine rubber tips and change if they become worn.

(continued)

Skill 13.4.3 | Using Assistive Devices in Home *(continued)*

Walker

1. Ensure client was measured appropriately for walker and appropriate type of walker was selected (with wheels, with seat, and so on.).
2. Review steps in using walker.

3. Demonstrate moving the walker and using the proper foot. After moving the walker, move the weaker side first.
4. Discuss how to grasp handles on walker with both hands.
5. Instruct client and caregiver to examine rubber tips on walker and change if worn.

Skill 13.4.4 | Instructing Caregiver on Safety Issue

Procedure

1. Inspect household for general safety issues. Instruct caregiver and client on change necessary to promote safety for clients using assistive devices.
2. Ensure adequate space to allow client to move throughout the home.

   a. Remove small scatter rugs from pathway.
   b. Keep electrical cords out of pathway.
   c. Wipe up spills that can cause slips.
   d. Position furniture to make space for assistive devices.

   e. Keep frequently used household items in easy access on lower shelves to prevent client from falling.
   f. Install nonslip bath mats and grab bars next to toilet and in shower. Install raised toilet seat and shower or tub seats.
   g. Encourage client to use fanny pack or apron to carry items about the home.
   h. Discuss issues related to house pets and safety.

3. Instruct caregiver to watch for warning signs and to notify physician if any signs appear.

Unit 13.4 Unit Documentation and Evaluation

DOCUMENTATION for Home Care

Using appropriate home care forms, document the following:

- Environmental assessment and safety instruction
- Client's ability to use assistive devices safely

- Support needed for assisting client utilizing assistive devices
- Caregiver's ability to move client up in bed

EVALUATION/Critical Thinking

Expected Outcomes

- Client has safe environment in home for ambulation using assistive devices.
- Client was provided appropriate instruction to ambulate using assistive devices.

Unexpected Outcomes

- Client is not stable ambulating with crutches or cane.

Alternative Actions

- Place safety belt on client and ambulate with walker.
- Increase both upper and lower muscle strength to increase ambulation with cane or crutches.

- Single healthcare worker is unable to lift client up in bed.

- If a second individual is available, utilize him or her to assist in moving.
- Use sliding board if two healthcare workers are available.
- Rent a hydraulic lift or Hoyer lift to assist with moving up in bed or getting out of bed.

- Client is not ambulating.

- Discuss with caregiver and client reasons why client is not ambulating.
- If client is afraid of falling, ensure that a gait belt is worn and the client uses a walker to start with and then moves to a cane, if possible.
- Use two individuals to assist with walking, if available.

Chapter Wrap-Up

GERONTOLOGIC Considerations

The Older Adult Can Sustain Impaired Mobility and Disability Due to Decreased Physical Function or Injuries

- Nearly 23% of older people living in the community have some degree of disability.
- Over 2 million Medicare beneficiaries are living in nursing homes and other residential facilities; 82.5% of them have mobility difficulties ranging from 50.7% for individuals under age 65 to 94.9% over 85.
- Impaired mobility can lead to many subsequent problems, including depression, negative self-image, dependent behavior, and loss of independence.
- Effects of disability can influence the individual's body image, physical appearance, and bodily sensations.
- Posture becomes more flexed and center of gravity shifts.

Special Assessment Parameters Are Important for the Older Adult

- Specific source of disability or impaired mobility
- Presence of accompanying disease state: arthritis, stroke, dementia, diabetes, heart failure, COPD
- Presence of pain
- Condition of skin
- Drug effects: sedation, incontinence, orthostatic hypotension
- Motivation for rehabilitation
- Nutritional status
- Best assistive aid for client
- Be aware of any vision problems your client may have, especially cataracts, glaucoma, or macular degeneration. Note poorly lighted areas in the home or dark areas in the corridors, throw rugs, uneven or uncarpeted areas adjoining carpeted areas, and the like, which may cause the client to stumble or fall.

- Check your client's ability to be mobile—gait, balance, and posture, and whether the client shuffles or is able to pick up his or her feet. Check if the client leans forward and is therefore off balance. Poor or unsteady mobility is often a direct cause of falling.
- Assess the client's degree of muscle strength and flexibility on both sides of body, because as age increases, they may decline, which can result in a fall. Check the degree of range of motion to all joints before ambulating. Even a poor hand grip can be dangerous if the client is walking down stairs. If leg muscles are weak, it may be difficult to get off a bed or up from a chair and the client may lose his or her balance.
- Assess for certain medications the client is taking that may cause vertigo, poor balance, blurred vision, weakness, or even drowsiness. Review the medications for older adult clients, keeping in mind that they may require only half the normal dose due to their age and decreased ability to metabolize drugs. The use of alcohol may contribute to falls in the home environment, so if the client uses alcohol there should be client teaching that focuses on that potential danger.
- Chronic diseases such as osteoarthritis, Parkinson, Alzheimer, and diabetes with peripheral neuropathy can all contribute to falls. Clients who have these diseases may require special assessment and interventions to prevent falls.
- Most older adult clients are aware of the danger of falling and breaking a hip or a leg, so fear is often present when they are moving or walking. Proper intervention and instructions with an assistive device (cane, walker, wheelchair, or the like) will help to allay these fears, which may become so overpowering that they cause immobilization and depression. Even fear itself, with its concomitant caution, may result in a fall. A therapeutic intervention

is for the nurse to work with the client to discuss fears about falling and specific behaviors to prevent falling.

Develop Nursing Care Plan to Meet Older Adult Client's Needs

- Focus on disability or impaired mobility.
- Establish supportive relationship.
- Determine activities that must be accomplished each day for individual to care for own needs and be as independent as possible. Support independence and client decision making and participation.
- Use assistive devices until client is stable and able to ambulate independently.
- Increase activities as individual progresses and is able to resume activity.
- Give positive reinforcement for all effort expended.

MANAGEMENT Guidelines

Each state legislates a Nurse Practice Act for RNs and LVN/LPNs. Healthcare facilities are responsible for establishing and implementing policies and procedures that conform to their state's regulations. Verify the regulations and role parameters for each healthcare worker in your facility.

Delegation

- Range of motion is usually performed for the first time by or under the supervision of a licensed PT or RN. If these team members are not available, the nurse or healthcare worker must understand the principles of the skill before performing it on the client. Range of motion is important for the client who is immobilized or on long-term bed rest, so if the skill is ordered more than once per day, it will probably be delegated to an LVN/LPN, CNA, or unlicensed assistive personnel (UAP). This staff member should be assigned to observe and be checked by personnel who understand the skill.
- Ambulation may be done by any healthcare worker and is often assigned to a CNA or UAP. However, the first time a client is ambulated, an assessment is very important for safety reasons, and this should be performed by an RN or LVN/LPN. In many medical–surgical settings, a PT may ambulate specific high-risk clients for the first time. A licensed nurse performing this task will minimize the possibility of orthostatic hypotension occurring, because assessment and vital signs are an important part of the skill.
- Crutch walking is a skill often performed initially with specialized personnel, such as the PT. However, the nurse should understand the principles of crutch walking so that he or she may reinforce the correct steps of the procedure whether the client is in the hospital or in the home setting.

Interprofessional Communication

- Range-of-motion and muscle-strengthening exercises, ambulation, and crutch walking should all be included in the verbal report at change of shift to all personnel and charted in the client's record.
- Any problems that occur with the exercises or ambulation should also be noted and, if present, the task should be reassigned to licensed personnel. It is especially important to note occurrence of orthostatic hypotension and what actions were effective to minimize the effects on the client.

CASE STUDY Applications

Scenario 1

You are assigned to care for two clients during the day shift.

Client A: A 65-year-old client who is obese had a hysterectomy yesterday. Her orders include ambulation and up-in-chair TID on the first postop day.

Client B: A 70-year-old female client who is to be discharged today after having an inguinal hernia repair yesterday.

1. What is your priority of care of these two clients?
2. What assessment will you focus on for both clients and which assessment will be your priority?
3. Briefly describe the discharge teaching that will be done for Client B.
4. When you approach Client B and tell her you would like to do her discharge teaching, she informs you, "Oh, at my age, I can be a couch potato so I don't need you to tell me anything." What is your best response?
5. Based on the information provided, what generalizations can you make about the general health and projected health of this client?
6. What is the primary danger to the health of this client? Describe how you will explain this to the client.
7. What plan (part of discharge teaching) can you devise to positively affect this situation?
8. You have elicited the help of a nursing assistant to help you ambulate Client A. As you are ambulating the client, she begins to fall. What steps should both you and the nursing assistant take to prevent client injury?
9. After your initial intervention, what other actions should be taken for this client?
10. What preliminary actions should have been taken to prevent this from happening?

Scenario 2

You are a student on an orthopedic unit and are assigned to assist the RN in the care of her clients for the day shift. You obtained the following information during report.

Client A: Client had a right-sided CVA 4 days ago and needs to be instructed on the use of a walker before being discharged to a long-term care facility this morning.

Client B: Client was instructed on the use of a cane yesterday, but no one has seen him practicing with the cane. He had a CVA several years ago and still has some instability when walking. He is 80 years old, wears a hearing aid, and is very independent.

Client C: Client is a 20-year-old who had an arthrotomy last night for injuries from football. He stayed overnight as a result of being nauseated and with low blood pressure. He is to be discharged this morning with crutches.

1. Which client should be assessed first?
2. Provide rationale for your choice.
3. Discuss your priority interventions for each of the clients.
4. Client A: Identify the major nursing action for this client before beginning instruction on the use of a walker.
5. Client B: What hunches do you have regarding why the client may not have been practicing with the cane?

NCLEX® Review Questions

Unless otherwise specified, choose only one (1) answer.

1. What is the movement of a bone away from the midline termed?
   A. Flexion
   B. Eversion
   C. Adduction
   D. Abduction

2. Passive range-of-motion (ROM) exercises were ordered for the client. The nurse has just performed the exercises on the client, who is on strict bed rest. What should documentation for this skill include?
   Select all that apply.
   A. Total time for exercises
   B. Specific joints put through ROM
   C. Specific joints that client was able to exercise independently
   D. Movements that caused unusual pain
   E. Number of times client performed exercises daily

3. During morning report the nurse states that the client assigned to you experienced orthostatic hypotension when getting out of bed. What would your priority intervention be before taking the client to the bathroom?
   A. Move client to side of bed and assist him to transfer to a walker.
   B. Take vital signs before allowing client to stand up.
   C. Raise and lower head of the bed slowly several times before attempting to assist client out of bed.
   D. Obtain assistance from another health team member to assist client to ambulate.

4. Client teaching needs to be completed before the client uses a walker. Which instructions would be included?
   A. "Place the walker approximately 2 feet (60 cm) in front of you and push yourself off the bed, stand erect, and grasp the hand grips on the walker."
   B. "Move the walker by pulling legs of the walker slightly off the floor as you move the unaffected leg forward."
   C. "Move the weaker side of the body first by supporting body weight on handles of the walker and then advancing the weaker leg."
   D. "Grasp the handles of the walker and move the weaker leg first by moving the body toward the center of the walker."

5. What should instructions provided to a client who is using a cane for the first time include?
   A. "You will need to place the cane on the weaker side of your body."
   B. "The cane is placed directly to the side of your weaker leg to help maintain balance."
   C. "The cane and unaffected leg are moved together when walking."
   D. "You need to move the cane forward at the same time as the affected leg."

6. What instructions would you include for the client who is learning to use a cane when walking steps?
   A. "When going downstairs, the unaffected leg is placed on the step, followed by the cane."
   B. "When going downstairs, the unaffected leg and cane are moved to the step before moving the affected leg to the same step."
   C. "When going upstairs, the first step is placing the affected leg and cane on the step, then the unaffected leg."
   D. "When going upstairs, the unaffected leg is placed on the step, followed by the cane and affected leg."

7. What is the correct method for measuring crutches before the client uses them?

   A. Ensure the axilla rests on the top bar of the crutches and that the tip of the crutch is next to the heel.

   B. Measure from the axilla to heel while lying in bed.

   C. Measure from the axilla to the crutch tip at 6–8 in. (15-20 cm) from heel while the client is standing next to the bed.

   D. Measure from the axilla to the heel, keeping the crutch tight to the client's side.

8. A client who can move and bear weight on each leg will be taught which type of gait for crutch walking?

   A. Three-point

   B. Four-point

   C. Two-point

   D. Swing-through

9. How should clients going upstairs with crutches start?

   A. Place weight on the uninjured leg on the step, and place crutches on upper step.

   B. Place weight on the uninjured leg and crutches at same level.

   C. Place crutches on the upper step and then bring the injured leg to the step.

   D. Move injured leg to first step with one crutch, and then move second crutch and uninjured leg to the next step.

10. The client states that when she uses the crutches, she slips. Which of the following critical thinking options should be implemented?
Select all that apply.

   A. Observe client using the crutches to see if she is leaning on them inappropriately.

   B. Reassure the client that this will not occur as she becomes more proficient with the crutches.

   C. Observe the client's stance or gait to check if it is too broad, causing her to slip.

   D. Check the crutch tips to ensure they cover all the metal or wood from the crutches.

   E. Ask the client if she would like to use the gait belt when walking.

QSEN Competency

Domain: Safety

KSA: Knowledge

Activity

A client has been using a cane for support while ambulating for many years. His wife reports that recently he has been unsteady, especially when climbing stairs. What are appropriate nursing actions?

Bibliography

Centers for Disease Control. (2014). How much physical activity do adults need? Retrieved from http://www.cdc.gov/physicalactivity/everyone/guidelines/adults.html

Krill, C., Raven, C., & Staffileno, B. A. (2012, Feb.). Moving from a clinical question to research: The implementation of a safe patient handling program. *Medsurg Nursing, 21*(2), 104–106, 116. Retrieved from http://search.proquest.com/docview/1008665093?accountid=3588

Lanier, J., Mote M. B., & Clay, E. C. (2011, Sep. 1). Evaluation and management of orthostatic hypotension. *American Family Physician, 84*(5), 527–536.

Muscle weakness may persist for months after ICU stay. (2014, Apr. 7). *HealthDay News.* Retrieved from http://news.health.com/2014/04/07/muscle-weakness-may-persist-for-months-after-icu-stay/

Rauen, C. A., Chulay, M., Bridges, E., Vollman, K. M., & Arbour, R. (2008, Feb.). Seven evidence-based practice habits: Putting some sacred cows out to pasture. *Critical Care Nurse, 28*(2), 98–124.

Vollman, K. M. (2010, Apr.). Introduction to progressive mobility. *Critical Care Nurse, 30*(2). Retrieved from www.ccnonline.org

Chapter 14
Infection Control

 Learning Objectives

14.1 Describe the six steps in the chain of infection.

14.2 Explain what is meant by the body's natural defenses.

14.3 Describe eight conditions that predispose clients to infection.

14.4 Define the term *healthcare-associated (nosocomial) infection*.

14.5 List the major organisms responsible for healthcare-associated infections.

14.6 State the main purpose of hand hygiene.

14.7 Demonstrate donning and removing personal protection equipment.

14.8 Define the terms *surgical asepsis* and *medical asepsis*.

14.9 State the isolation procedure for removing specimens and equipment from an isolation room.

14.10 List three precaution principles and explain their main purpose.

14.11 List blood and body fluid protection protocol.

14.12 Describe the difference between the first and second tier of precautions.

14.13 Compare and contrast infection control practices in the home and hospital.

14.14 Differentiate assessment modalities to determine potential for infection in home care and hospitalized clients.

Chapter Outline

Terminology

AIDS acquired immunodeficiency syndrome—a serious condition characterized by a defect in natural immunity against disease. When the immune system is suppressed, the individual is vulnerable to a host of opportunistic infections.

Antibody a protein substance developed by the body to fight disease organisms. Not effective against a virus that is inside the cells.

Antimicrobial an agent that prevents the development or pathogenic action of microbes.

Antiseptics agents that are applied to body tissues, such as skin or mucous membrane, to destroy or retard the growth of microorganisms.

Asepsis the absence of disease-producing microorganisms.

Autoinfections infections that arise from an individual's own body flora.

Bacteriostatic a substance that prevents the growth or multiplication of bacteria.

Barrier nursing any technique that reduces the risk of cross-contamination.

Biohazard waste any solid or liquid waste that may present a threat of infection.

Carrier an individual or animal without signs of illness but who carries pathogens on or within his or her body that can be transferred to others.

Colonization organisms present in body tissue but not multiplying or invading the tissue.

Contagious disease a disease conveyed easily to others.

Contamination introduction of disease, germs, or infectious materials into or on normally clean or sterile objects.

Detergents compounds (surfactants) that possess a cleaning action, often referred to as soaps. They are composed of a hydrophilic and a lipophilic substance.

Disinfectants chemical agents that are used to destroy or reduce microorganisms on inanimate surfaces and objects.

Disinfection a process that employs physical and chemical means to remove, control, or destroy most of the organisms that may be present on equipment or materials.

Endogenous related to organisms natural to an individual's own body.

Enteric precautions isolation practices designed to prevent transmission of pathogens through contact with fecal matter and vomitus.

Epidemic an outbreak of a disease that is widespread or can spread rapidly.

Epidemiology the study of the distribution or patterns and determinants (causes) of health-related events in defined populations.

Exogenous related to organisms external to an individual's own body.

False negative a negative test in someone who in fact has been infected by a microorganism but for some reason has not developed antibodies.

False positive a positive test for an antibody, usually the result of an artifact of the laboratory test, in an individual who has not in fact been exposed to the microorganisms. All individuals who test positive should have the test repeated.

Healthcare-Associated Infection (HAI) (formerly hospital-acquired infection or nosocomial infection) an infection not present and without evidence of incubation at the time of admission to a healthcare setting.

HIV human immunodeficiency virus; a blood-borne retrovirus that has a different life cycle from a normal virus.

Host an animal or individual on which or within which microorganisms live.

Incubation period the time between infection from a microorganism and the onset of symptoms. It seems to range from 6 months to 7 years for AIDS. Not everyone who is exposed to the virus develops the disease.

Infection establishment of a disease process that involves invasion of the body tissue by microorganisms and the reaction of the tissues to their presence and to the toxins generated by them.

Isolation technique practices designed to prevent the transmission of communicable diseases.

MDR-TB multidrug-resistant tuberculosis; an in vitro resistant strain of TB to antituberculosis drugs.

Medical asepsis all practices that limit the number and growth of microorganisms and their transmission.

Microorganism minute living body, such as a bacterium, protozoan, or virus, not perceptible to the naked eye.

Nosocomial infection see HAI.

Outbreak a critical incident in which infections occur above an established level and are caused by the same infective agent.

Pandemic an epidemic of an infectious disease that becomes widespread, affecting a whole region or large area such as a continent.

Pathogen a microorganism that can cause infectious disease in the human body.

PEP postexposure prophylaxis; recommendations from the CDC on how to treat a healthcare worker's exposure to HIV.

Protocol description of steps to be taken in exact order—may be legally binding.

Resident (normal) flora organisms natural to an individual's own body. Organisms multiply in the environment, not merely surviving there.

Retrovirus a virus with a life cycle in which the genetic information is in reverse of that in an ordinary virus: The RNA code is transcribed backward into DNA.

Sepsis a condition resulting from the presence of pathogenic bacteria and their products.

Sterile free from any living microorganisms.

Surgical asepsis practices that will maintain area free from microorganisms, as by a surgical scrub or sterile technique.

Susceptible site an area that is sensitive to or can be invaded by a bacterium or other infectious agent.

Virulence the ability of recognized pathogenic organisms to invade and propagate in normal, intact, and uncompromised individuals. Some organisms that are avirulent for normal individuals become pathogenic when defense mechanisms are impaired.

Virus a minute, parasitic organism that depends on nutrients inside cells for its metabolic and reproductive needs. These organisms cause a variety of infectious diseases and stimulate host antibodies. Unlike bacteria, viruses are unable to survive long on their own and are not affected by antibiotics.

Waterless antiseptic agent an antiseptic agent that does not require use of exogenous water. Agent dries automatically after applying to hands and rubbing hands together.

Chain of Infection

For an **infection** to occur, a chain of events must take place. If the chain is broken through the implementation of infection control measures, the infection is less likely to occur. The chain of infection involves six steps (Figure 14-1 ■).

Infectious Agent (Microorganism) The first step in the chain involves the presence of an infectious agent, or **microorganism**. Whether the microorganism is capable of producing an infection depends on a number of circumstances: the virulence and number of organisms present, the susceptibility of the **host**, the existence of a portal of entry, and the affinity of the host to harbor the microorganism.

Reservoir A reservoir must provide a favorable environment for growth and multiplication of the microorganism. These reservoirs include blood and the respiratory, gastrointestinal, reproductive, and urinary tracts.

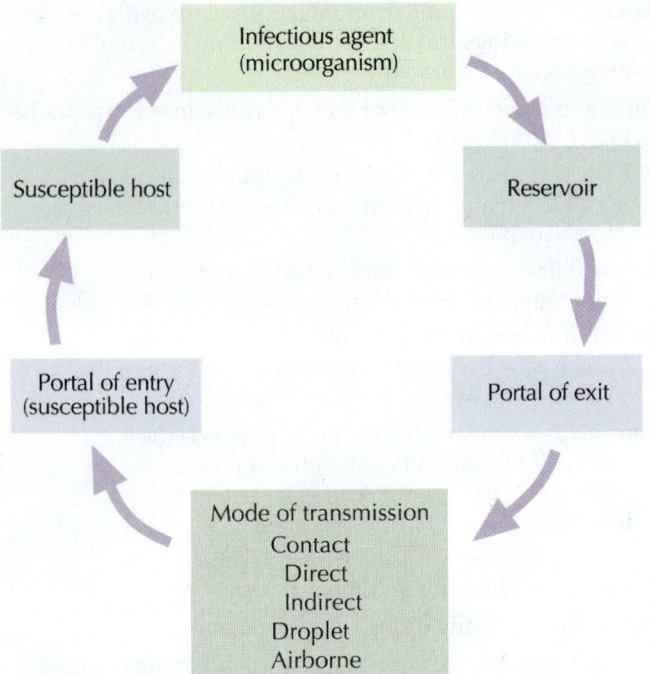

FIGURE 14-1 Six steps in the chain of infection.

Portal of Exit The third link in the chain must be a portal of exit, which allows the microorganism to move from the reservoir to the host. Without a portal of exit, an infection cannot occur. The portal of exit is directly associated with the reservoir. For example, if the reservoir is the respiratory tract, the portal of exit is through sneezing, coughing, breathing, or talking. If the reservoir is blood, the portal of exit is through an open wound, needle puncture site, or nonintact skin surface.

Mode of Transmission The fourth step is transmission of microorganisms. There are five routes of transmission; the three primary routes are contact, droplet, and airborne. Two lesser routes are common vehicle (transmission by contaminated items such as food, water, devices, or equipment) and vector borne (transmission by vectors such as mosquitoes, fleas, or rats). This last mode of transmission is more significant in other parts of the world than in the United States.

Contact transmission, the most frequent source of healthcare-associated infection, is transmitted via two modes—direct and indirect contact. Direct contact involves a direct transmission, body-to-body, and the physical transfer of microorganisms from one infected individual to another; for example, through sexual contact, kissing, or even touch. It also may occur when a healthcare worker touches a client, gives a client a bath, or performs other care activities. Indirect transmission involves contact with a contaminated intermediate object such as a needle, instrument, or dressing. This also occurs when contaminated hands are not washed, gloves are not changed between clients, and whenever there is a break in technique.

Droplet transmission is a form of contact transmission, but the mechanism of **pathogen** transfer is so different that

it is considered a separate route of transmission. It occurs when droplets from the infected source are projected a short distance to the host's nasal mucosa, mouth, or conjunctiva. These droplets are not suspended in the air, so it is not considered airborne transmission.

Airborne transmission occurs by dissemination of either small-particle nuclei of evaporated droplets or dust particles containing the infectious agents. These agents can be dispersed widely by air currents, as with Legionnaire disease, and may be inhaled by a susceptible host. These microorganisms include *Mycobacterium tuberculosis*, rubeola, and varicella **viruses**.

Portal of Entry The most effective barrier to transmission of microorganisms is intact skin. For an infection to occur, it must have a means of entering the body. A disruption in the integrity of the skin provides such a portal of entry for microorganisms. Microorganisms also enter the body the same way they leave the body. The respiratory system provides a viable portal of both exit and entry.

Susceptible Host For an infection to occur, a susceptible host is needed—someone who is "at risk." This includes clients who are immunosuppressed, fatigued, stressed, anemic, not immunized, poorly nourished, or those who have underlying diseases. Hospitalized clients with wounds, catheters, and IVs are at high risk for developing infections. Clients who require invasive procedures, blood specimen collections, and surgery are also in the high-risk category.

Barriers to Infection

An individual's ability to resist infection is determined by the status of the body's defense mechanisms and by the individual's general health. Factors that contribute to susceptibility to infection include altered nutritional status, stress, fatigue, disease, drugs, metabolic functions, and age. Clients with severe underlying diseases are most likely to develop healthcare-associated infections. The body is protected against infection by immunities, by the inflammatory process, and by anatomic barriers that include the skin and mucous membranes.

When the integrity of the skin or mucous membrane is broken, **resident flora** and transient flora, as well as bacteria, have a direct route to the internal tissues of the body. To prevent the spread of infection, the body's internal defense mechanisms mobilize and begin clearing and repairing the damaged site. How quickly a wound heals depends on the degree of vascularization in the injured area, the location and cleanliness of the wound, and the degree of tissue damage.

The second way the body resists infections is through immunity, antitoxins, and vaccines. Natural immunity is inherited. Acquired immunity occurs after an individual has been exposed to a disease or infection or has been vaccinated.

The third way the body resists infection is through the inflammatory process. Inflammation involves use of metabolic energy, increased blood flow to the inflamed area, and, in many cases, drainage of inflammatory debris to the external environment.

When an area becomes inflamed, cells at the site activate the plasmin system, the clotting system, and the kinin system. The result of the activation of these systems is the release of histamine, which creates increased vascular permeability around the injured site, and the release of chemotoxic agents, which summon phagocytes into the vascular and tissue spaces. Phagocytes are white blood cells that combat and prevent infection by ingesting harmful microorganisms.

The Body's Natural Defenses

Any alteration in the body's natural defenses increases the probability that an infection will occur. Almost any organism can be the cause of a significant healthcare-associated infection, given the proper circumstances. Some of the variables that help determine which organism emerges as the pathogen are the **virulence** and number of organisms, the exposure and attachment of the organism to a **susceptible site,** and the duration of the client's exposure to the infectious challenge. The following formula illustrates these variables:

$$\frac{\text{Dose} \times \text{Virulence}}{\text{Host Resistance}} = \text{Infection}$$

Using this formula, the client's risk factors can be evaluated. The inherent health and immunologic status of the client are also major factors in determining whether an infection occurs.

Alterations in the skin barrier include any physiologic break in the integrity of the skin. Intentional breaks are caused by the use of percutaneous catheters and needles and by surgical procedures. Unintentional causes of skin breakdown include the development of pressure ulcers and traumatic wounds.

Healthcare-Associated Infections

Healthcare-associated infections (HAIs; also previously known as nosocomial infections) are infections that are acquired while the client is in the hospital—infections that were not present or incubating at the time of admission. In 2011, it was estimated that there were 722,000 HAIs (about 1 in 25 hospital clients) in U.S. acute care hospitals and 75,000 deaths (Magill, 2014). Over half of the infections occurred outside of intensive care units. HAIs are often caused by poor hand hygiene, as healthcare workers transmit infections between clients. Hand hygiene is the single most important intervention to prevent these infections, yet various studies have shown that there is very poor compliance with hand washing techniques by healthcare workers. Other interventions important to the prevention of HAIs are the use of **sterile** technique when indicated, keeping the environment as free as possible of pathogens, and identifying and protecting at-risk clients.

The five most common HAIs currently are pneumonia, gastrointestinal illness, urinary tract infections, primary bloodstream infections, and surgical site infections. The organisms responsible for the majority of HAIs are *Clostridium difficile* and methicillin-resistant *Staphylococcus aureus* (MRSA).

Clostridium difficile

Clostridium difficile is a gram-positive anaerobic spore-forming bacillus that produces two exotoxins (toxins A and B) and accounts for 15%–25% of all episodes of antibiotic-associated diarrhea (CDAD). This is currently the most common HAI, and rates have been increasing over the past several years. Eighty percent of all infections are associated with health care. Because it is often resistant to **antimicrobial** therapy, *C. difficile* is able to proliferate in the hospital setting. There has also been an increase in more severe strains with increases in mortality.

Clients who are at risk include those who are immune compromised, on antibiotic therapy, have a serious underlying illness, or have a long length of stay in a healthcare setting. *C. difficile* is found in fecal matter and can be transferred to clients by contaminated surfaces such as commodes and through poor healthcare worker hand hygiene. Hand hygiene is essential in preventing the spread of *C. difficile* and requires the use of soap and water. Alcohol-based rubs do not kill the spores and are not an effective means of hand hygiene. The use of gowns, gloves, dedicated equipment, and private rooms or cohorting of clients is also helpful. *Cohorting* refers to placing clients with the same infection in semiprivate rooms together if private rooms are not available (CDC, 2012a).

CLINICAL ALERT

Hand sanitizer does *not* kill *C. difficile*, so soap and water must be used (CDC, 2012a). Gloves and gowns should be worn, even for short treatment visits, with clients who have *C. difficile*. A spore-killing **disinfectant** such as bleach should be used to wipe down equipment after use by a client with *C. difficile*.

EVIDENCE-BASED PRACTICE

Clostridium difficile on the Rise

A study done at 30 community hospitals in the Duke Infection Control Outreach Network showed that *C. difficile* infections are on the rise and have surpassed MRSA. The rate of HAI *C. difficile* was 0.28 cases per 1,000 client days and the rate for MRSA was 0.22 cases per 1,000 client days.

Source: Miller (2010)

Founded in 1991, the IHI offers healthcare facilities information on how to best control hospital infections.

For example, the project JOINTS (Joining Organizations IN tracking SSIs) was an initiative to help spread evidence-based practices to prevent SSIs (surgical site infections) after hip and knee replacement surgery. The IHI provided the tools and resources to support this federally funded initiative. The IHI has many free tools and resources on its website to help nurses and healthcare organizations prevent infections as well as deliver high quality and safe care. For more information, go to the IHI website.

"Superbugs" have become a significant problem in healthcare. However, there is hope on the horizon. A new antibiotic called teixobactin, derived from friendly bacteria that scientists found in a grassy field in Maine, shows the ability to wipe out even drug-resistant bacteria. The drug's effectiveness is attributed to the mechanism by which it works. It destroys the bacterium's lipid or fat molecules, whereas most antibiotics generally attack the proteins. This is an amazing breakthrough on the war on "superbugs" like MRSA, which have become a threat to client safety.

The Centers for Disease Control (CDC) and the Institute for Healthcare Improvement (IHI) have information and best practice bundles on their websites to help healthcare practitioners and clients learn more about preventing and managing HAIs, including the latest data, statistics, and guidelines (Box 14-1 ■). New drugs continue to be sought that will be effective against drug-resistant organisms (Box 14-2 ■).

MRSA

The second most common infection is MRSA. This condition often occurs in clients who have invasive procedures such as intravenous or respiratory therapy treatments or surgical procedures. Healthcare personnel easily transmit MRSA to clients because it frequently colonizes skin, and people who carry MRSA may not have signs of the infection. According to the CDC, about 2 out of every 100 people carry MRSA. Although MRSA is still a major threat, invasive infections declined by 54% between 2005 and 2011 in healthcare settings (CDC, 2013e).

VRE

VRE is vancomycin-resistant enterococci. Enterococci are bacteria normally present in the human body in the intestines and the female genital tract. They can sometimes cause infections. In some cases, the enterococci have become resistant to the drug vancomycin that is used to treat the infection. Most VRE infections occur in hospitals and can cause infections of the urinary tract, bloodstream, or surgical sites. Clients at increased risk for VRE include those previously treated with antibiotics (including vancomycin), clients with weakened immune systems, clients who have had long stays in the intensive care unit, and clients who have urinary or central intravenous catheters.

CRKP

CRKP or carbapenem-resistant *Klebsiella pneumoniae* has emerged as a new and potentially deadly HAI for clients in healthcare facilities and nursing homes. It is resistant to carbapenem antibiotics, one of the last lines of defense. Between 1999 and 2010, bacterial samples that showed resistance to cephalosporins and that could therefore only be treated with carbapenems more than doubled (from 5.3% to 11.6%).

Meanwhile, according to the Center for Disease Dynamics, Economics and Policy (2013), the incidence of CRKP rose from less than 0.1% in 2002 to 4.5% in 2010. These statistics are particularly alarming given the 40% mortality rate associated with the infection (Buki, 2013).

Surgical Site Infections

Surgical site infections are infections that occur within 30 days of the operation and involve the area in which the operation occurred. To prevent surgical site infection, it is important that all healthcare workers follow a set of guidelines and practices recommended by agencies such as the Centers for Disease Control and Prevention (CDC). Many hospitals and ambulatory surgical centers have adopted these guidelines that include:

- Preoperative **antiseptic** showering
- Clipping hair immediately before the operation instead of shaving the client the night before
- Performing skin preparation in the operating room
- Preoperative hand and forearm antisepsis by the surgical team (see Chapter 25, Skill 25.1.1)
- Keeping infected surgical personnel away from clients
- Administration of an antimicrobial agent just before the operation begins

Postoperative incision care includes covering a closed surgical incision with a sterile dressing for the first 24–48 hr. If the incision is left open to heal by secondary intention, then it is packed with sterile moist gauze and covered with a sterile dressing.

Respiratory Tract Infections

Common alterations in the respiratory tract that facilitate the development of an infection include endotracheal intubation, tracheostomy, bronchotracheal suctioning, and stasis due to poor respiratory excursion for clients on bed rest.

The bronchi and trachea are so sensitive to foreign matter that they initiate the cough reflex whenever irritation occurs. Ciliated, mucus-coated epithelium lining the trachea and lungs aids in clearing the respiratory tract of bacteria and mucus by the beating motion of the cilia. Intubation bypasses the cough reflex and compromises the effectiveness of this action. Although the trachea is usually considered sterile, it does not remain sterile after 48–72 hr of intubation. Infections associated with endotracheal intubation include pneumonia, tracheitis, and purulent bronchitis. Pneumonia is one of the leading HAIs occurring in acute care hospitals, according to the CDC in 2011 (Magill, 2014).

Catheters placed directly in the trachea can force pathogenic microorganisms into the respiratory system. In addition, catheters may damage the mucous lining of the respiratory tract, further compromising the effectiveness of its clearing mechanisms.

Urinary Tract Infections

A urinary tract infection (UTI) is an infection involving the urethra, bladder, ureters, and/or kidneys. UTIs are the most common type of infection occurring in healthcare institutions. Seventy-five percent of the UTIs that occur in hospitals are associated with a urinary catheter (a tube inserted into the bladder to drain urine). The risk of developing a catheter-associated UTI (CAUTI) increases the longer a catheter is left in place. Currently, the CDC has guidelines recommending that urinary catheters should only be used for specific indications and they should be removed as soon as they are no longer needed. Healthcare workers must also use sterile technique when inserting urinary catheters and must clean around the catheters on a regular basis to help prevent infections.

Primary Bloodstream Infections

Invasive devices such as centrally inserted catheters are associated with an increased risk of bloodstream infections. The risk is 2–855 times higher with a central line than with a peripheral venous catheter. Therefore, many healthcare institutions have taken steps to reduce the use of central catheters and to create a sterile environment when inserting central catheters. These procedures include full body draping and use of rigorous guidelines for skin preparation and dressing changes. This is part of a bundle of best practice guidelines aimed at reducing central line-associated bloodstream infections (CLABSIs), which can be found on the CDC website.

Standard Precautions

In 1985, universal precautions were instituted as a result of the human immunodeficiency virus (**HIV**) **epidemic** in the United States. Blood and body fluid precautions were practiced on all clients regardless of their potential infectious state. In 1987, body substance isolation (BSI) was proposed. The intent of this isolation system was to isolate all moist and potentially infectious body substances (blood, feces, urine, sputum, saliva, wound drainage, and other body fluids) from all clients, regardless of their infectious status, primarily through the use of gloves.

In the late fall of 1994, the CDC drafted new guidelines. The revised guidelines contain two tiers of precautions: Standard Precautions and Transmission-Based Precautions.

The first tier, *Standard Precautions*, blends the major features of universal precautions (blood and body fluids precautions) and BSI into a single set of precautions to be used in the care of all clients in hospitals, regardless of their diagnosis or presumed infection status. The new Standard Precautions apply to blood; all body fluids, secretions, and excretions, whether or not they contain visible blood; nonintact skin; and mucous membranes. These precautions are designed to reduce the risk of transmission of both recognized and unrecognized sources of infection in hospitals. As a result of the new category of Standard Precautions, clients with diseases or conditions that previously required category-specific or disease-specific precautions are now covered under this category and do not require additional precautions. The precautions include hand hygiene, use of gloves, gown, mask, eye protection, or face shield, and safe injection practices (Figure 14-2 ■).

New elements were added into Standard Precautions in the 2007 guidelines revisions. Two of these areas are Respiratory Hygiene/Cough Etiquette and safe injection practices. Respiratory Hygiene/Cough Etiquette was prompted by the severe acute respiratory syndrome (SARS) **outbreak** and is aimed primarily at educating clients and families about the need to take preventive steps, such as covering their mouth and nose with a tissue when coughing. Elements of Respiratory Hygiene/Cough Etiquette also include hand hygiene, using masks on coughing clients, and proper disposal of used tissues. Safe injection practices aimed at reducing infections include use of single-dose vials when possible and use of a sterile single-use, disposable needle and syringe for each injection.

FIGURE 14-2 The use of personal protective equipment is an important measure in supporting Standard Precautions. Shown is a supply stand that provides convenient access to PPE in the hospital setting.

Transmission-Based Precautions

The second tier, *Transmission-Based Precautions*, is designed only for the care of specified clients. (*Note:* This term and *isolation precautions* are used interchangeably in much of the literature.) This tier reduces the disease-specific precautions into three sets of precautions based on routes of transmission. These categories are designed for clients documented or suspected to be infected or colonized with highly transmissible or epidemiologically important pathogens for which additional precautions must be used to interrupt transmission to others in the hospital (Table 14-1 ■).

The three types of Transmission-Based Precautions include *airborne*, *droplet*, and *contact* precautions. Airborne precautions reduce the risk of airborne transmission of infectious agents, such as measles, varicella, and tuberculosis. Droplet precautions are used to prevent the transmission of diseases such as meningitis, pneumonia, scarlet fever, diphtheria, rubella, and pertussis. Contact precautions are used for clients known to have or suspected of having serious illnesses easily transmitted by direct contact, such as herpes simplex, staphylococcal infections, hepatitis A, respiratory syncytial virus, and wound or skin infections. Contact precautions are subdivided into *direct* and *indirect*. Direct transmission describes transmission from one infected individual to another. Indirect transmission describes transfer of the infectious agent from a contaminated surface such as the hands of a healthcare worker or a client care device (e.g., a stethoscope) to an individual. Table 14-2 ■ outlines specific recommendations for Transmission-Based Precautions.

Transmission-Based Precautions now include educational information to help family members and visitors. They should be taught or informed via fact sheets, pamphlets, and other material about preventing transmission of infections. It is also important to include rationale, risks to household members, and other routine infection prevention strategies, which are a part of respiratory precautions.

All three types of precautions may be used at one time when multiple routes of transmission are suspected in a client. These precautions are always used in conjunction with Standard Precautions.

Fundamental Principles Certain fundamental principles should be applied to all clients (Box 14-3 ■). *The first is hand hygiene.* Hand hygiene is the single most important means of preventing the spread of infection. Many diseases are spread by not washing hands with soap and water to effectively remove germs. *A second fundamental principle involves the use of gloves.* Gloves are worn to provide a protective barrier, prevent gross **contamination** of the hands when touching body substances or blood, and reduce the risk of exposure to blood pathogens. Gloves also prevent the spread of microorganisms to other clients and to healthcare personnel.

The third fundamental principle is the proper placement of clients in the hospital to prevent the spread of microorganisms to others or to the client. Clients may not always be placed in private rooms when they are infected. They can be placed in a room where the second client has the same infectious process.

The fourth fundamental principle is the appropriate use of isolation equipment to prevent the spread of microorganisms to healthcare workers and other clients. The equipment required, often referred to as personal protection equipment (PPE), is based on the specific transmission route of the microorganism. Specific handling of client care items needs to be considered in preventing the spread of infection.

Hand Hygiene Wash hands with nonantimicrobial soap or use **waterless antiseptic agent** for routine hand hygiene and after removing gloves. An antimicrobial or antiseptic agent should be used for control of specific outbreaks of infection (Box 14-4 ■).

Gloves Clean, nonsterile gloves (or latex-free gloves if latex allergy is present) are worn when touching blood, body fluids, secretions, excretions, and contaminated items. Put gloves on just before touching mucous membranes and nonintact skin. Remove gloves immediately after use and wash hands before touching noncontaminated items and environmental surfaces or giving care to another client. Gloves should be discarded immediately and not reused.

Mask, Eye Protection, Face Shield Wear mask and eye protection during procedures in which splashes or sprays could come in contact with eyes and mucous membranes. Face shields protect the mucous membranes of the eyes, nose, and mouth from splashes of blood, body fluids, secretions, and excretions. Suctioning clients and assisting physicians with insertion of hemodynamic monitoring lines are examples of situations in which this type of protection is required.

Table 14-1 Disease Indications for Transmission-Based Precautions*

Modes of Transmission		
Contact (Direct and Indirect)	**Droplet**	**Airborne**
Clostridium difficile	Pertussis	Tuberculosis
E. coli	Streptococcal	Chickenpox
Impetigo	pharyngitis	Herpes zoster
Scabies	Scarlet fever	Measles
Rotavirus infection	Rubella	
Smallpox	Mumps	
Rubella–chickenpox	Meningitis	
	Parvovirus B19	

*Listed above are some common diseases/conditions in which Transmission-Based Precautions are required or advised as a part of the treatment protocol. See Centers for Disease Control website or agency policies for a more complete listing.

Table 14-2 HICPAC* Recommendations for Transmission-Based Precautions

	Contact	Droplet	Airborne
Purpose	• Prevent transmission of known or suspected infected or colonized microorganisms by direct hand or skin-to-skin contact that occurs when providing direct client care. • Prevent transmission through indirect contact with client care devices or shared toys.	• Prevent transmission of large-particle droplets, larger than 5 microns (μm).	• Prevent transmission of small-particle residue of 5 microns (μm) or smaller droplets.
Client Placement	• Private room • Can be placed in room of client with same microorganism	• Private room • Can be placed in room of client with same diagnosis	• Private room • Can be placed in room of client with same diagnosis • Monitor negative air pressure. • Keep door closed. • Keep client in room.
Respiratory Protection	• Mask not necessary • Family, visitors: respiratory hygiene/cough etiquette	• Use mask when entering the room or working within 6–10 feet of client.	• NIOSH certified N95 or higher respirator • Do not enter room of clients with rubeola or varicella if susceptible to these infections.
Gloves and Gown	• Wear gloves and gown when entering room. • Change gloves after contact with infective material, such as wound drainage or fecal material. • Wash hands immediately after removing gloves.	• Follow Standard Precautions.	• Follow Standard Precautions.
Client Transport	• Transport only if essential. • Ensure precautions are maintained to minimize risk of transmission.	• Transport only if essential. • Place mask on client when outside room.	• Transport only if essential. • Place mask on client when outside room.
Client Care Items	• Client care items and environmental surfaces are cleaned daily. • Dedicate equipment to single client use (i.e., stethoscope, thermometer).		

*Hospital Infection Control Practices Advisory Committee
Source: Siegel, Rhinehart, Jackson, & Chiarello (2007)

Box 14-3 **CDC RECOMMENDATIONS FOR HAND HYGIENE, HAND ANTISEPSIS, AND GLOVING**

• Hands must be washed with antiseptic soap and water or alcohol-based hand rub:

1. Before and after client contact and between clients
2. After contact with a source of microorganisms
3. After removing gloves. Before donning gloves
4. After touching equipment or surfaces that may be contaminated
5. Before handling an invasive device (regardless of glove **protocol**)
6. After contact with body fluids, excretions, nonintact skin, and wound dressings
7. Before handling medication and/or preparing food
8. If moving from a contaminated body site to a clean body site during client care

• Gloves should be used as an adjunct to, not a substitute for, hand hygiene:

1. Remove gloves and wash hands after any hand contaminating activity.
2. Change gloves between clients.
3. Change gloves during care of a single client when moving from one procedure to another. (This is critical when moving from a contaminated to a clean body site.)
4. Use disposable gloves only once.
5. Do not touch any body surface that is moist without gloves. (Moisture can be considered potentially contaminated.)
6. Have latex-free gloves available for personnel with an allergy or sensitivity to latex.
7. Decontaminate hands before donning sterile gloves.

See CDC website on hand washing for more information (CDC, 2013c).

Box 14-4 **PRINCIPLES OF HAND HYGIENE**

Wash hands or use alcohol-based gel:

- At the beginning of the shift before providing client care
- Before and after providing client care
- Before and after preparing medications
- After touching client surroundings (i.e., after handling soiled linen, equipment, or supplies)
- Between contact with different clients
- After removing gloves
- After you have sneezed or coughed
- Before and after eating
- After body fluid exposure/risk
- Just before leaving the nursing unit

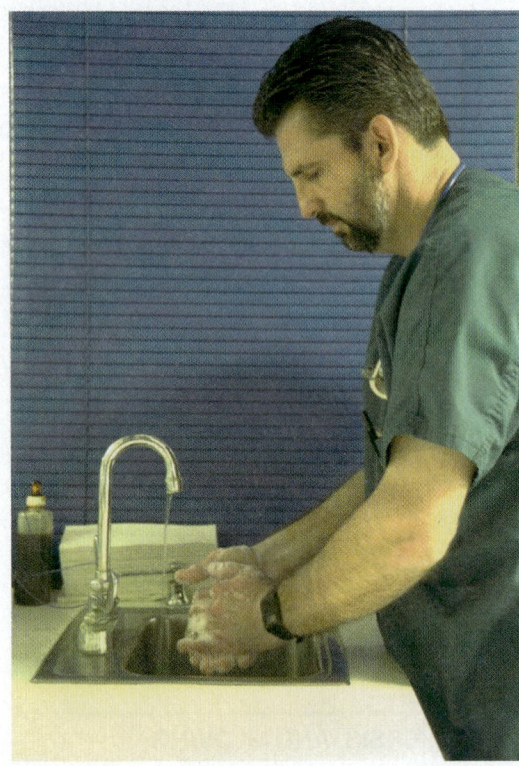

The single most important nursing action to decrease the incidence of healthcare-associated infection is washing your hands.

Gowns Nonsterile disposable gowns are used to protect the skin and clothing from contamination while providing client care. Gowns should be worn whenever there is a risk of contamination from blood, body fluids, secretions, or excretions. Soiled gowns should be removed immediately and hands washed to prevent the spread of microorganisms.

Linen Transport soiled linens in a manner that prevents skin and mucous membrane exposure, contamination of clothing, and transfer of microorganisms to other clients

and environments. This is usually accomplished through double-bagging linen before taking it to the laundry facility.

Occupational Health and Bloodborne Pathogens Take precautions to prevent injuries caused by needles, scalpels, or other sharp instruments or devices. Only use safety needles. The use of needleless systems for IV management has dramatically decreased needlestick injuries.

Never recap used needles, purposely bend or break needles by hand, remove needles from disposable syringes, or otherwise handle needles directly. All such instruments should be placed in puncture-resistant containers for disposal.

Mouth pieces, resuscitation bags, or other ventilation devices should be used as an alternative to mouth-to-mouth resuscitation.

Biohazard waste should be disposed of according to established guidelines (Box 14-5 ■).

Client Placement Clients who are at risk for contaminating the environment or who are unable to maintain appropriate hygiene or environmental control should be placed in a private room. If this is not possible, other arrangements need to be made in consultation with the hospital's infection control department.

In addition to healthcare workers following Standard Precautions, the following guidelines should be considered when providing client care:

- Healthcare workers who have open lesions, upper respiratory infections, or weeping dermatitis should refrain from all direct client contact and from handling client care equipment.
- Because of the risk of transmission of HIV and hepatitis B virus (HBV) from mother to fetus, pregnant healthcare workers should be especially familiar with, and strictly adhere to, precautions to minimize risk of these viruses. Currently, pregnant healthcare workers are not known to be at greater risk of contracting HIV or HBV than other workers.

Needlestick Safety and Prevention Act

In 2000, the OSHA Bloodborne Pathogen standard was modified to provide more protection for healthcare workers from exposure to bloodborne pathogens such as hepatitis and HIV from needlestick injuries. The new guidelines require employers to provide equipment, training, and surveillance to employees with the goal of decreasing exposure and instituting safer work practices, including the use of safer medical devices such as safety needles and needleless systems (Figure 14-3 ■) (Wilburn, 2004).

Box 14-5 PROPER HANDLING OF BIOHAZARD WASTE

What Is Biohazard Waste?

Any solid or liquid waste that may present a threat of infection is considered **biohazard waste**. This could include laboratory waste, blood or blood products, body fluids, absorbent material saturated with blood or body fluids (either wet or dry), discarded sharps, and nonabsorbent disposable devices (such as drains, excretions, gloves, urine specimens, and the like).

Why Separate Biohazard From Other Medical Waste?

It is critical that the biohazard waste be separated at the point of origin or before it leaves the client's room. This reduces the risk of exposure considerably. The principles of separation are:

- Use an impermeable red plastic bag labeled "biohazard"; close bag securely while inside the client's room.
- Use a second red-labeled bag outside the room and place the inside bag in it so that the waste is "double-bagged."
- Do not place red-labeled bag with other waste material, because it could contaminate all waste.
- Sharps should be separated from all other waste and placed in a leak- and puncture-proof container with a biohazard symbol on the outside.
- Scalpels should NOT be placed in fiberboard waste containers.
- Sharps containers should not be overfilled, because items could fall out.

How Should Biohazard Material Be Stored?

Biohazard waste must be appropriately sealed. It may be stored for 30 days; time starts when material is placed in the sharps container or biohazard bag. All biohazard waste must be restricted, locked up, or placed in a separate storage area. Biohazard waste must be in a room with *no* carpeting. Sealed cement is necessary so that a spill can be cleaned up. Biohazard material must be labeled correctly so that there is a tracking method for each bag, container, and such. Labels should say "medical waste" and "biohazard" and be dated when the bag was first placed in the area.

How Should Biohazard Waste Be Transported?

When transporting biohazard waste within the facility, containers must remain intact. Trash chutes must *not* be used. Outdoor containers should be secured against vandalism and marked or labeled. A contingency plan for spilled material:

- Spilled or leaked biohazard material must be cleaned with industrial-strength **detergent** and then disinfected.
- Onsite treatment and disposal of waste must be steamed, incinerated, or cleaned with an alternative method (chemical, dry heat, and the like).
- Each facility must post a "Spill Contingency Plan," which includes which substance should used to disinfect.

If each facility has an administrative code that includes a total plan, policies, and procedures for dealing with biohazard waste, as well as a training program for all employees in how to handle biohazard waste, the incidence of exposure could be dramatically decreased.

FIGURE 14-3 Safety needles.

AIDS

Epidemiology and Modes of Transmission

The CDC estimate of people newly infected with HIV is about 47,500, making it a serious health problem in the United States. This rate has remained stable since the mid-1990s. However, it continues to affect certain groups disproportionately, including African Americans, Latinos, and gay and bisexual men of all races and ethnicities (CDC, 2014b). There are approximately 33,000 new **AIDS** diagnoses each year, and in 2009 there were about 476,000 people living with AIDS. Efforts aimed at HIV testing, prevention, and treatment programs have kept the number of new HIV cases from increasing, in addition to helping people living longer lives with HIV infections.

Definitions

AIDS is the most severe form of a continuum of illnesses associated with HIV infection. AIDS is defined by the CDC as an HIV infection in an individual with a CD4+ T-lymphocyte count of less than 200 cells/microliter (µL) of blood or a CD4+ percentage of less than 14. Twenty-six clinical conditions are listed in the CDC AIDS surveillance case definition in category C (described under HIV). Once clients have a condition listed in category C, they remain in that surveillance category. Among those 26 conditions listed in the category are cytomegalovirus (CMV) retinitis; Kaposi's sarcoma; *Mycobacterium avium* complex (MAC) (which includes the *M. avium* and *M. intracellulare* organisms) or *M. kansasii*; *M. tuberculosis*, any site; *Pneumocystis carinii*; and recurrent pneumonia.

Human Immunodeficiency Virus HIV is a bloodborne infective **retrovirus** that invades the CD4+ T-lymphocyte (immunity) cell, renders it useless, and then duplicates itself by means of that cell. With loss of the client's immune function, the disease becomes clinically manifested. Infection with HIV progresses to AIDS in at least 35% of those infected. Once a client has been diagnosed with HIV, the usual approach to care includes evaluation of the immune system and classification by CDC grouping: (A) asymptomatic, (B) acute symptomatic, and (C) AIDS-indicator conditions. Identification and treatment of infectious and neoplastic complications, initiation of approved antiretroviral therapy, and consideration of experimental measures are also included in the evaluation.

HIV is transmitted through high-risk behaviors or other contact with the virus, including:

- Sexual contact with HIV-infected individuals
- Sharing needles with HIV-infected individuals
- Transfusions of blood or blood products from infected individuals (not common today, but new cases are still reported)
- Transmission from the infected mother to her baby before or during birth, or through breast-feeding
- Contact with contaminated needles, blood, secretions, or excretions from an HIV-infected client

Healthcare Workers' Exposure to HIV

Prospective studies of healthcare workers have estimated that the average risk for HIV transmission after a percutaneous exposure to HIV-infected blood is approximately 0.3%, after a mucous membrane exposure is 0.1%, and after skin exposure is less than 0.1% (CDC, 2013d). Healthcare workers with a potential exposure can take a rapid HIV **antibody** test, which takes about 10–20 minutes. If positive, a follow-up Western blot analysis is done. If a positive result is found, the healthcare worker is immediately referred for postexposure prophylaxis (PEP).

The Public Health Service provides recommendations for management of **PEP** for healthcare workers exposed to HIV. The decision to recommend HIV PEP takes into account the nature of the exposure, needlestick or mucous membrane contact, and the amount of blood or body fluid involved in the exposure. Healthcare facilities should have the protocols available, and prompt reporting and postexposure care should be considered a healthcare emergency and treated as such. This includes access to clinicians who can provide postexposure care during all working hours and immediate availability of the antiretroviral agents for PEP. Healthcare workers must be educated to report occupational exposures immediately after they occur because PEP should be started within 24–36 hours after exposure.

Other Infectious Diseases

Tuberculosis

Tuberculosis is an infectious disease caused by the tubercle bacillus *M. tuberculosis*. The main reservoir for the organism is the human respiratory tract, and transmission occurs between individuals through respiratory contact. The tubercle bacillus enters the respiratory tract on droplets transmitted through productive coughing from the infected individual. Symptoms may occur in 4–12 weeks after exposure or may go unnoticed for many years. Active pulmonary tuberculosis has a slow, insidious onset. The progression of the active disease and symptoms of cough, weight loss, and fever usually occur within the first 2 years after the infection. Latent infections, which are asymptomatic, are not infectious and may last a lifetime. Without treatment, tuberculosis progresses to other body sites. Disseminated tuberculosis occurs in many of the body areas, not just the lungs. The incidence of tuberculosis cases in this country has increased greatly, due in large part to the AIDS epidemic. Immunosuppressed hosts are very vulnerable to the bacillus. In addition to immunosuppressed individuals, others considered at high risk for infection include alcoholics; IV drug abusers; individuals who share a closed environment with the infected individual; residents of institutions such as long-term care and correctional facilities; foreign-born individuals from countries with a high prevalence of tuberculosis, such as Asia, Latin America, Africa, Mexico, and the former Soviet Union; low-income populations who are medically underserved; and clients who are noncompliant and do not complete the appropriate drug therapy. Healthcare workers who come in contact with any of the high-risk populations are at risk for infection.

Multidrug-resistant tuberculosis (**MDR-TB**) is in-vitro resistance of a strain of TBC to antituberculosis drugs. The disease can progress from diagnosis to death in as short a period as 4–16 weeks. According to the CDC (2012b), since 1997 the percentage of U.S.-born clients with MDR TB has remained below 1.0%. However, of the total number of reported primary MDR TB cases, the proportion occurring in foreign-born individuals increased from 25.3% (103 of 407) in 1993 to 86.1% (62 of 72) in 2012. The increasing incidence of MDR-TB can be attributed to delays in treatment, inadequate isolation and infection control practices, and lack of follow-through after hospital discharge. Some clients develop resistance to the standard drug regimen (two first-line therapies, isoniazid and rifampin) as a result of noncompliance and/or inappropriate drug therapy. MDR-TB is also caused by individual-to-individual contact through sneezing or coughing or from an individual with primary drug resistance.

Early recognition and treatment of tuberculosis must be initiated promptly and isolation measures instituted to prevent the spread of the disease. The CDC describes effective tuberculosis control requirements as early identification, isolation, and treatment of individuals with active tuberculosis. The purified protein derivative (PPD) skin test is used to identify the infection quickly in the absence of clinical symptoms. Sputum specimens for acid-fast bacillus (AFB) TB culture and sensitivity and chest x-rays are also ordered to rule out TB. A PPD skin test is read 48–72 hr after the injection. A positive skin test is indicated by an induration of 5–10 mm at the site of the injection.

A two-step method is now being used, particularly with healthcare workers. This procedure involves the first PPD injection to be given and read within 48–72 hr. If the PPD is negative or doubtful, the PPD is repeated in 1 week. If the client has a positive reaction, he or she is started on a prophylaxis regimen. A client who is known to be HIV positive with a 5 mm or larger induration at the site of the PPD injection should be considered positive for tuberculosis.

The CDC recommendation for tuberculosis isolation includes a directional airflow, negative pressure ventilation system in the room of tuberculosis clients. Negative pressure ventilation pulls air away from hallways and exhausts it out of the room to areas away from air intake vents. Six air changes each hour are required to provide microbial dilution within the room. Ultraviolet irradiation lamps can be used to supplement ventilation systems when the risk of tuberculosis transmission is high.

Anyone entering the client's room should wear a mask that forms a tight-fitting seal against particulates 1–5 microns (μm). NIOSH recommends an N-95 mask or respirator be worn for all respiratory isolation rooms and these masks be fit-tested to ensure they properly fit the individual wearing them. All treatments and procedures should be performed in the client's room if at all possible. If the client must leave the room, a valveless particulate respirator must be used.

Viral Hepatitis

There are six forms of hepatitis. Each form differs in regard to **incubation period**, route of transmission, antigenic properties, and progression to chronicity. All forms of hepatitis produce an inflammatory response to the liver, which is characterized by liver cell necrosis, inflammation, and cell regeneration. The three major forms of hepatitis are hepatitis A virus (HAV), HBV, and hepatitis C virus (HCV). Hepatitis D virus (HDV) is not as common, and hepatitis E virus (HEV) is rare in the United States. Hepatitis G virus (HGV) is a recently isolated bloodborne infectious agent transmitted by needlesticks and blood transfusions.

HAV is spread via the fecal–oral route and sexual transmission. Poor sanitation and hand hygiene is a major source of infection. Approximately 152,000 infections occur in the United States each year. Ninety-nine percent of those infected recover without any serious problems. HAVRIX vaccine is available to prevent HAV. If exposed to the infection or as a preventative therapy, immune serum globulin is administered intramuscularly.

HBV is spread through infected blood or body fluids and through two nonparenteral routes: sexual contact and perinatal transmission. Contaminated needles, syringes, and blood products are the most common mode of transmission, although about 30% of the cases are spread through sexual contact. An estimated 140,000 individuals are infected yearly in the United States. Two to 10% of adults become chronically infected with HBV after an infection. HBV is 100 times more infectious than HIV. HBV vaccine provides active

immunity in more than 95% of recipients. The two common vaccines are Engerix-B and Recombivax HB. Hepatitis B immune globulin provides passive immunity to individuals who have had contact with HBV-contaminated material.

HCV is transmitted primarily by contact with contaminated blood and blood products. Eighty-five percent of those infected with HCV will remain chronically infected. Chronic HCV infection is the main causal factor for nearly one-third of all liver transplants. There are three types of interferons used to treat HCV.

The CDC recommends the use of Standard Precautions with clients known to have hepatitis. The precautions should be maintained for 1 week after the onset of symptoms.

Seasonal Flu

Influenza (the flu) is a contagious respiratory illness caused by the influenza virus. It can cause mild to severe illness, sometimes resulting in death. The virus infects the nose, throat, and lungs and is transmitted mainly by droplets when people cough, sneeze, or talk. It can also be transmitted when people touch a surface that has flu virus on it and then touch their own mouth, eyes, or nose. The flu is contagious 1 day before symptoms begin and up to 5–7 days after becoming ill. Symptoms include: fever, cough, sore throat, nasal congestion, muscle aches, headaches, fatigue, and (in some cases) vomiting/diarrhea. Flu is very unpredictable and varies from season to season depending on which viruses are spreading, how much flu vaccine is available, how well the flu vaccine is matched to the influenza virus, and how many people get vaccinated. Certain people are at increased risk for complications from the flu, including older adults, young children, pregnant women, and people with certain health conditions.

The CDC recommends that everyone over the age of 6 months get a flu vaccination every year. This is especially important for those at high risk, which includes healthcare workers. Many healthcare agencies now require their employees to get vaccinated or to wear a mask while at work to protect clients and coworkers during flu season.

> **CLINICAL ALERT**
> During outbreaks of influenza, clients who are suspected of having influenza are placed in droplet precautions. When this occurs, healthcare workers are often encouraged not to reuse isolation or N-95 masks, unless there is a shortage, in order to lessen the chances of contamination and spread of this highly **contagious disease**. Other precautions may include restrictions on visitors under the age of 12 or visitors who are ill (fever, cough, flu-like symptoms).

Emerging Viruses (Possible Pandemic Threats)

Table 14-3 ■ describes **pandemic** influenza preparedness and response.

Table 14-3 Pandemic Influenza Preparedness and Response

Precautions for Staff	Responses (to Infection)
Modify transmission-based infection control strategies to match organism.	Use airborne infection isolation rooms, including HEPA filter.
Use personal protective equipment: gloves, gown, goggles, face shields, and so on.	Use single hospital rooms, or place clients with same organism (H1N1) together.
Modify administrative controls.	Limit number of individuals entering area.
Use safe working practices (i.e., stringent hand hygiene).	Limit client transport.
	Use vigorous hand hygiene measures.
	Employ standard practices for used client care equipment.
	Educate clients on hand hygiene and cough etiquette.

Note: The World Health Organization (WHO) maintains a global surveillance system that monitors presence of an influenza pandemic in progress. Pandemic status evolves and is not always accurately assessed or projected.

Ebola Virus Disease

The 2014 West African Ebola epidemic was the largest in history, affecting multiple countries in that region including Sierra Leone, Liberia, and Guinea. Ebola, previously known as Ebola hemorrhagic fever, is caused by the Ebola virus and is a rare and deadly disease. There are five known strains of the Ebola virus, four of which cause disease in humans. Ebola was first discovered in 1976 near the Ebola River in what is now the Democratic Republic of the Congo. The outbreak hit the United States in September 2014 when the first case of Ebola was diagnosed in Texas in a client who had travelled from Liberia but was not symptomatic until 4 days after arriving in the United States.

Ebola is spread through direct contact with blood and body fluids (e.g., urine, saliva, sweat, feces, vomit, breast milk, semen) of an infected individual. It is not spread through the air or water or generally by food, except in Africa through handling of bushmeat. During outbreaks, Ebola can spread rapidly within healthcare settings, especially if staff are not wearing appropriate personal protective equipment (PPE). Once people recover from the virus they can no longer spread the disease.

Additional PPE training and the use of observers during the donning and removing of PPE are initiated during the care of Ebola clients as recommended by the CDC (2014c), due to the high risk of exposure of healthcare workers who care for these clients. PPE for Ebola clients requires full body coverage with no skin exposure and double gloving.

Severe Acute Respiratory Syndrome

In 2003, there was a multicountry outbreak of a viral respiratory illness caused by a coronavirus (the common cold) called SARS-CoV. SARS-CoV was first reported in Asia in February of 2003 and spread rapidly over the next 2 months before it was contained. According to the World Health Organization (WHO), a total of 8,098 people worldwide became ill and 774 people died. The disease spread primarily through respiratory droplets produced when an individual coughed or sneezed. The droplets were propelled up to 3 feet. The virus also spread through contact with surfaces and may have spread more broadly through airborne transmission. Extensive protocols were put into place during the SARS-CoV outbreak but there have been no cases since 2004.

Middle East Respiratory Syndrome

Middle East Respiratory Syndrome (MERS) is a viral illness caused by a coronavirus. It causes acute respiratory illness that in some cases can be severe. Symptoms include fever, cough, and shortness of breath. It is unknown where the virus originated, but it has been found in animals in the Middle East. Infections can spread through close contact, including contact with healthcare workers. The first case of MERS was reported in Saudi Arabia in 2012 and the first case in the United States was in May 2014 (CDC, 2015). At this time, there are no available treatments other than supportive care.

Avian Influenza

Avian (bird) influenza A (H5N1) usually does not infect humans. However, rare cases of human infections are reported. Since November 2003, there have been 600 cases reported, primarily in Asia, Africa, the Pacific, Europe, and the Near East. On January 8, 2014, a case in the Americas was reported in Canada. The disease carries a high mortality rate, and most cases are thought to occur as a result of close contact with sick or dead infected poultry. Diagnosis is made based on laboratory testing through a throat swab within the first few days of onset of symptoms. It is treated primarily with antiviral drugs. Healthcare personnel caring for clients with suspect infections should wear PPE and use appropriate precautions (CDC, 2013a).

Home Care Adaptations

In the home setting, **medical asepsis**, or clean technique, is often used instead of sterile technique. The major reasons for this protocol change are the nature of the setting and the personnel providing care.

The greatest infection control problem in hospitals is healthcare-associated infections due to the large numbers of antibiotic-resistant organisms present in a hospital setting. When clients are in their own environment, they tend to develop fewer infections because they are subjected to fewer organisms. In the home setting, focus is on protecting home care staff and family, not other clients. While there may be transmission of organisms among individuals in the home, there are minimal data on the incidence of home care–associated infections. Infection-preventing strategies in the home should focus on IV therapy and urinary tract, respiratory, and wound care.

Sterile equipment, such as prepackaged catheter and irrigation kits, parenteral fluid equipment, and dressings, is often purchased for home care. When sterile technique is required, it is the responsibility of the nurse to provide the instruction and evaluate the family's ability to perform the skill accurately. Hospital techniques may need to be modified for the home setting, and ideal environmental working conditions may not be present. Just as in the hospital, effective hand hygiene is the *most* effective means of infection control in the home setting. There is one major difference between hospital and home: Equipment (soap, running water, and paper towels) that is readily available to the nurse in the hospital may not be available in the home. Even if running water is available, there may not be soap or clean towels. Nurses must bring their own hand washing supplies.

A decrease in the duration of hospital stays has dramatically increased the expanded scope of the home care nurse. Unfortunately, infection surveillance, prevention, and control efforts have not kept up. Many home care infection control practices have been based on ritual and acute care practice, rather than scientific principles. Changes in infection control procedures in the home are currently occurring based on a scientific approach.

Home care assessment for potential infections relies on clinical signs and symptoms and tests, such as the urine dipstick, that can be performed in the home. Routine tests used in hospitals to diagnose infections of the urinary tract, respiratory tract, and wound or skin sites are not routinely done, as the current reimbursement system does not support cultures and laboratory tests. Only cultures that confirm and treat bloodstream infections for clients requiring home infusion therapy are obtained.

If the home care client is suspected of or diagnosed as having an infectious disease or the client is infected or colonized with VRE or MSRA, the nurse should use the same PPE and protocol used in the hospital setting. The equipment includes gloves, disposable gown or apron, mask, cap, and goggles. Reusable equipment, such as stethoscopes and blood pressure cuffs, should stay in the home and not be used on other home care clients. If possible, affected clients should be seen at the end of the day.

Cultural Awareness

Many cultures believe that certain substances or practices protect one's health. If a client wishes to include certain food items in his or her diet or engage in certain cultural practices, the nursing staff should respect this as much as possible, since it is an important cultural tradition for many groups.

Nursing Diagnoses

The following nursing diagnoses may be appropriate to use on client care plans when the components are related to clients requiring isolation protocol or sterile procedures.

NURSING DIAGNOSIS	RELATED TO . . .
Ineffective Community Coping	Deficits in social support, disease follow-up protocols, inadequate resources for disease prevention
Deficient Knowledge	Lack of access to healthcare facilities, lack of education, cognitive limitation
Ineffective Health Maintenance	Participation in high-risk activities, substance abuse, infectious states, religious or cultural beliefs detrimental to health
Infection, Risk for	Immunosuppressed hospitalized clients, HIV/AIDS clients, invasive procedures, lack of immunization Inadequate defenses (loss of skin integrity, leukopenia, low hemoglobin)
Latex Allergy Response	Allergies to certain foods, allergy to latex, lack of safety procedures for latex allergy
Noncompliance	Lack of motivation, education, or readiness; information misinterpretation; cultural or religious beliefs Medical condition (communicable disease, HIV-positive), hospitalization, terminal illness
Ineffective Protection	Poor compliance to protocols, lack of knowledge, lack of resources
Ineffective Family Health Management	Choices of daily living precludes maintaining treatment modalities (e.g., drug therapy, hand hygiene).

Source: Herdman, T. H. & Kamitsuru, S. (Eds.) *Nursing Diagnoses – Definitions and Classification 2015-2017.* Copyright © 2014, 1994–2014 by NANDA International. Used by arrangement with John Wiley & Sons Limited. Companion website: www.wiley.com/go/nursingdiagnoses. In order to make safe and effective judgments using NANDA-I nursing diagnosis it is essential that nurses refer to the definitions and defining characteristics of the diagnoses listed in this work.

Nursing Process Data

ASSESSMENT Database

- Assess method of hand hygiene that is most appropriate for assigned task.
- Identify clients at risk for infection.
- Assess availability of equipment for frequent hand hygiene (soap and water or antiseptic cleansing agent).
- Evaluate health status of the nurse.
- Check agency policy for hand hygiene protocol.
- Assess need for use of nonsterile gloves.
- Assess nurses and clients for latex allergies.
- Assess need for latex-free equipment and/or environment.

PLANNING Objectives

- To deliver client care with pathogen-free hands
- To prevent pathogenic microorganisms from spreading client to client, environment to client, or healthcare personnel to client
- To protect clients from cross-contamination
- To protect healthcare workers

IMPLEMENTATION Procedures

DOCUMENTATION AND EVALUATION

Expected Outcomes

- Decreased number of bacteria on hands from client to client
- Delivered care with pathogen-free hands to clients
- Prevented spread of microorganisms from healthcare workers or environment to clients
- Prevented cross-contamination between clients

Unexpected Outcomes/Alternative Actions

Pearson Nursing Student Resources

Find additional review materials at **nursing.pearsonhighered.com.** Prepare for success with NCLEX®-style practice questions and Skill Checklists.

Skill 14.1.1 | Hand Hygiene (Medical Asepsis)

Equipment

Nonantimicrobial soap* for routine hand washing
  (Box 14-6 ■, Box 14-7 ■)
Orangewood stick for cleaning nails
Running warm water
Paper towels
Trash basket

Procedure

1. Stand in front of but away from sink. ➤ **Rationale:** Clothing should not touch sink to avoid contamination.
2. Ensure that paper towel is hanging down from dispenser.
3. Turn on water using foot pedal or faucet so that flow is adequate, but not splashing. ❶
4. Adjust temperature to warm. ➤ **Rationale:** Cold does not facilitate sudsing and cleaning; hot is damaging to skin.
5. Wet hands under clean running water, keeping hands below elbow level. ➤ **Rationale:** Wet hands facilitate distribution of soap over entire skin surface. ❷

According to 2007 HICPAC recommendations.

❶ Use foot pedals when available to prevent contamination of hands.

❷ Wet hands thoroughly before applying soap to facilitate removal of pathogens.

EVIDENCE-BASED PRACTICE

Hand Sanitizer Dispensing Door Handles

Several studies have shown that placement of accessible hand sanitizer dispensers has been associated with increases in hand hygiene compliance. Building on this idea, a pilot project introduced a hand sanitizer-dispensing device that functions as a door knob and is installed on the client's exam room door. Each time the door is opened, the handle dispenses sanitizer into the user's hand. The pilot project demonstrated an increase in compliance with hand hygiene during the trial use of the dispensers from 24.5% at baseline to 77.1%.

Source: Babiarz, Savoie, McGuire, McConnell, & Nagy (2014)

6. Place a small amount, 1–2 teaspoons (3–5 mL), of liquid soap on hands. Thoroughly distribute over hands. Soap should come from a dispenser, not bar soap. ❸ ➤ **Rationale:** This prevents spread of microorganisms.
7. Rub vigorously, using a firm, circular motion, while keeping your fingers pointed down, lower than wrists. Start with each finger, then between fingers, and then palm and back of hand. ➤ **Rationale:** This creates friction on all surfaces. ❹
8. Wash your hands for at least 20 seconds. ➤ **Rationale:** Duration of washing is important to produce mechanical action and to allow antimicrobial products time to achieve desired effect.
9. Clean under your fingernails with an orangewood stick. (This should be done at least at start of day and if hands are heavily contaminated.) Move rings up and down fingers to clean if rings are left on.

CLINICAL ALERT

CDC Alert: The CDC has stated that healthcare workers in contact with clients must remove all artificial fingernails because they serve as a reservoir for microorganisms.

EVIDENCE-BASED PRACTICE

Hand Hygiene Strategies to Prevent HAIs

- Measure hand hygiene compliance.
- Use tracking systems or reminder systems.
- Make sure all surfaces of the hands are covered with the hand hygiene product.
- 20–30 seconds for hand rubbing and 40–60 seconds for hand washing are suggested.
- Keep nails trimmed to less than a quarter inch and do not wear artificial nails.

Source: Ellingson, Haas, Aiello, Kusek, Maragakis, Olmsted, . . . & Yokoe (2014)

(continued)

Skill 14.1.1 | Hand Hygiene (Medical Asepsis) *(continued)*

Box 14-6 **HEALTHCARE INITIATIVE FROM WHO**

An initiative was launched by WHO in 2009 to tackle healthcare-associated infection. Focused on hand hygiene, it introduced a major global effort to follow a detailed action plan to save lives. This plan is based on global evidence that hand hygiene is integrally linked to transmission of infection by healthcare workers. Some international studies indicate that compliance is as low as 8% and even in developed countries, rates range from 5% to 15%. These rates can affect 10%–40% of clients admitted to intensive care units. WHO has an improvement strategy that includes "My 5 Moments for Hand Hygiene," which details when hand hygiene needs to be applied:

1. Before touching a client
2. Before clean or aseptic procedures
3. After body fluid exposure or risk
4. After touching a client
5. After touching client surroundings

Your 5 Moments for Hand Hygiene

1 BEFORE TOUCHING A PATIENT

2 BEFORE CLEAN/ASEPTIC PROCEDURE

3 AFTER BODY FLUID EXPOSURE RISK

4 AFTER TOUCHING A PATIENT

5 AFTER TOUCHING PATIENT SURROUNDINGS

Source: World Health Organization (2009). WHO acknowledges the Hôpitaux Universitaires de Genève (HUG), in particular the members of the Infection Control Programme, for their active participation in developing this material.

Box 14-7 **NEW TRENDS: TECHNOLOGY-ASSISTED HAND HYGIENE MONITORING SYSTEMS**

To support hand hygiene compliance, technology has a new role. Mobile devices and videos are being used to assist in the monitoring and data collection of hand hygiene compliance. Advance technologies or "intelligent" systems are being developed to record hand hygiene opportunities and provide reminders to healthcare personnel. These systems utilize personal wearable electronic monitors that communicate with wifi or radio frequency signals. They establish defined zones around client beds or at the thresholds of client rooms and can capture entry and exit into a client zone.

---

10. Rinse your hands under running water, keeping fingers pointed downward. **5** ➤ *Rationale:* This position prevents contamination of arms.
11. Resoap your hands, rewash, and rerinse if heavily contaminated.
12. Dry hands thoroughly with a paper towel, while keeping hands positioned with fingers pointing up. ➤ *Rationale:*

Moist hands tend to gather more microorganisms from the environment.

Note: Surgical hand antisepsis is found in Chapter 25, Skill 25.1.1.

13. Turn off water faucet with dry paper towel, if not using foot pedal. ➤ *Rationale:* To avoid recontaminating the hands. **6**

3 Use a generous amount of soap and friction during hand washing procedure.

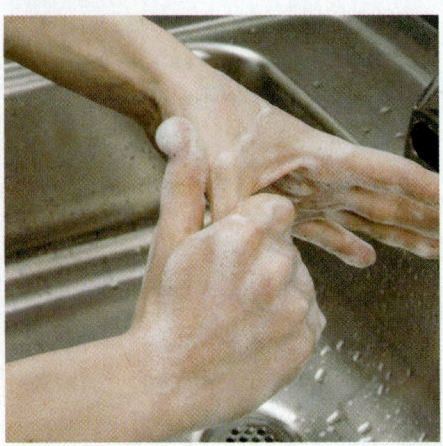

4 Wash your hands for at least 20 seconds.

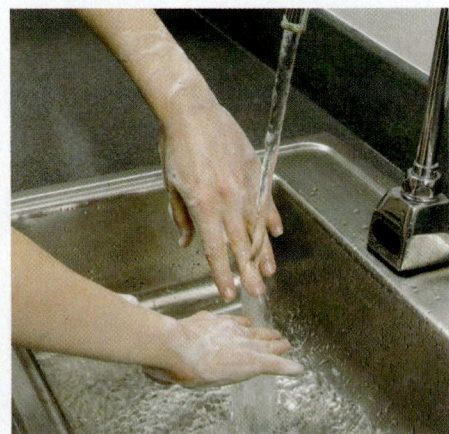

5 Point hands down when rinsing to rinse away contamination.

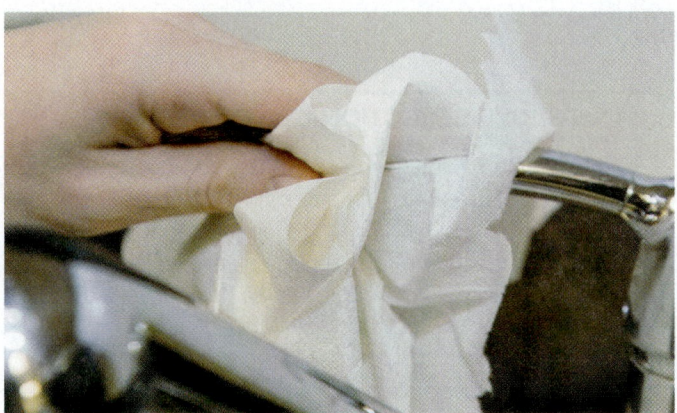

6 If foot pedal is not available, turn water off using a paper towel as a barrier.

7 Waterless hand sanitizer kills 99.9% of the most common germs in 20 seconds.

14. Restart procedure at Step 5 if your hands touch the sink at any time between Steps 5 and 13.

Using Waterless Antiseptic Agents (Foam or Gels)

1. Check dirt on hands and use waterless agent only if hands are clean. ➤ *Rationale:* Hands soiled with dirt or organic matter require soap or detergents that contain antiseptic and water to clean effectively.
2. Apply alcohol-based rub, foam, or gel (3–5 mL) on palm of hand. **7**
3. Rub hands together vigorously, covering all surfaces, sides of hands, and fingers. ➤ *Rationale:* Failure to cover all surfaces can leave contaminated areas on the hands.
4. Rub hands until dry—waterless agent will dry quickly and automatically without using a towel.

Note: Disposable germicidal wipes are available that are effective at killing 99.99% of harmful bacteria. These wipes are also effective at removing soil from hands because of natural friction when wiping.

> **CLINICAL ALERT**
> Antimicrobial soap or waterless agent should be used when there is an identified resistant bacteria, a **colonization** outbreak, or a hyperendemic infection, with the exception of *C. difficile* and *norovirus*, which are not killed by an alcohol-based gel. For these pathogens, soap and water must be used.

Skill 14.1.2 | Cleaning Washable Articles

Equipment
Equipment to be cleaned
Cleaning agent (according to facility policy)
Clean gloves

Procedure
1. Complete hand hygiene and don clean gloves.
2. Remove organic material using recommended cleaning agents per agency protocol.
3. Return item(s) to proper place or prepare for sterilization or **disinfection** if indicated (Siegel, Rhinehart, Jackson, & Chiarello, 2007).
4. Remove gloves; complete hand hygiene.

Skill 14.1.3 | Donning and Removing Clean Gloves

Equipment
Clean gloves
Trash receptacle

Procedure
1. Complete hand hygiene. ➤ *Rationale:* Donning gloves with unclean hands can transfer microorganisms outside gloves. **1**

2. Remove glove from glove receptacle (Box 14-8 ■). **2**
3. Hold glove at wrist edge and slip fingers into openings. Pull glove up to wrist. **3**
4. Place gloved hand under wrist edge of second glove and slip fingers into opening. **4**
5. Remove glove by pulling off, touching only outside of glove at cuff so that glove turns inside out. **5 6**

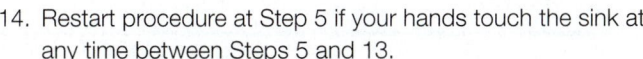

(continued)

Skill 14.1.3 | Donning and Removing Clean Gloves) *(continued)*

6. Place rolled-up glove in palm of second hand. **7**
7. Remove second glove by slipping one finger under glove edge and pulling down and off so that glove turns inside out. Both gloves are removed as a unit. **8** **9**
8. Dispose of gloves in proper container, not at bedside. **10**
9. Complete hand hygiene.

A

B

1 Complete hand hygiene **(A)** by using anti-bacterial gel or **(B)** by washing hands.

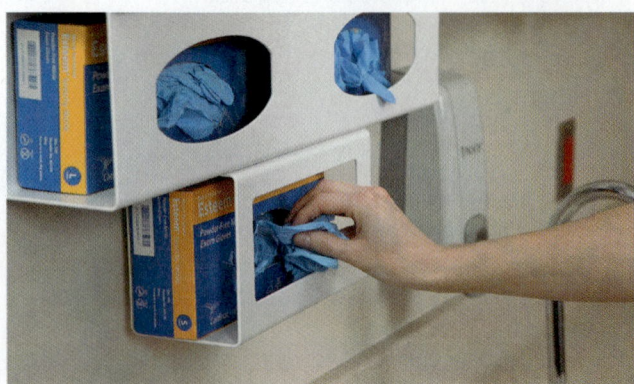

2 Remove glove from dispenser.

Box 14-8 **GLOVE SELECTION**

- Use sterile gloves for procedures involving contact with normally sterile areas of the body.
- Use examination gloves for procedures involving contact with mucous membranes, unless otherwise indicated, and for client care or procedures that do not require use of sterile gloves.
- Change gloves between clients.
- Do not wash, disinfect, or reuse surgical or examination gloves.
- Use general purpose utility gloves (rubber household gloves) for housekeeping tasks that involve potential blood contact and for instrument cleaning and decontamination procedures.

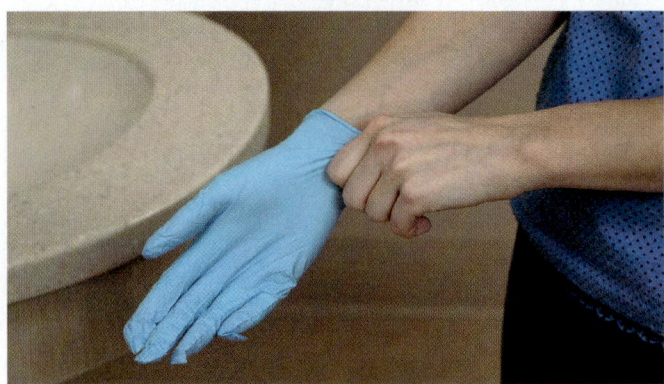

3 Hold glove at wrist edge and slip fingers into openings. Pull glove up to wrist.

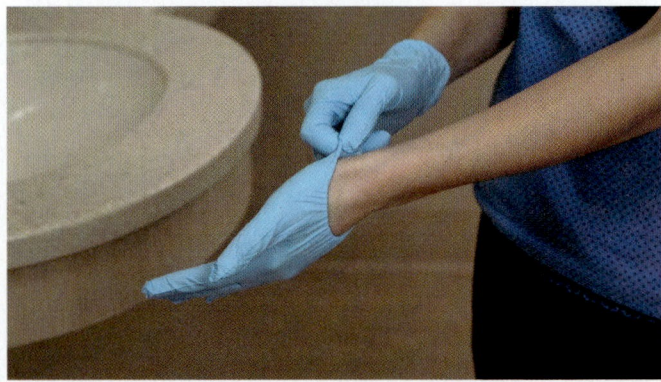

4 Place gloved hand under wrist edge of second glove and slip fingers into the opening.

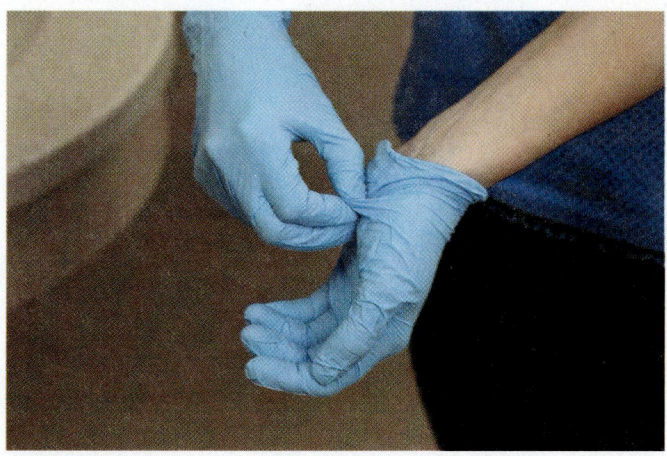

5 Remove glove by pulling it off. Touch only outside of glove at cuff so that glove turns inside out.

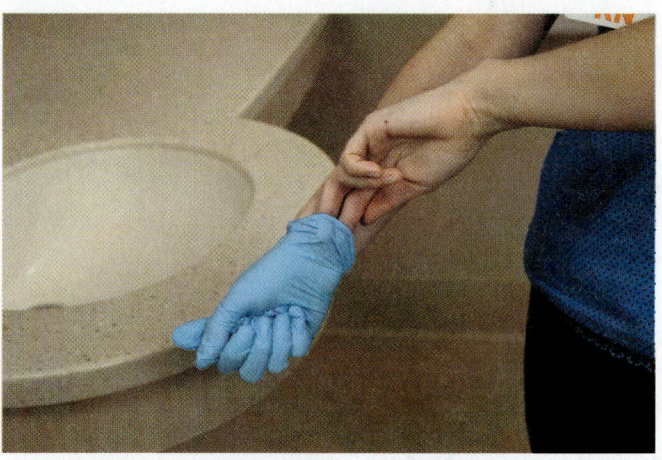

8 Remove second glove by slipping fingers under glove edge.

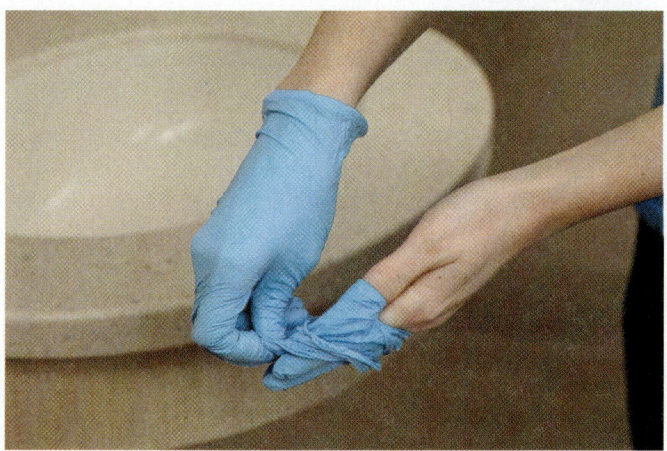

6 Continue pulling off first glove until it is inside out.

9 Pull glove down and off so that glove turns inside out, enclosing other glove.

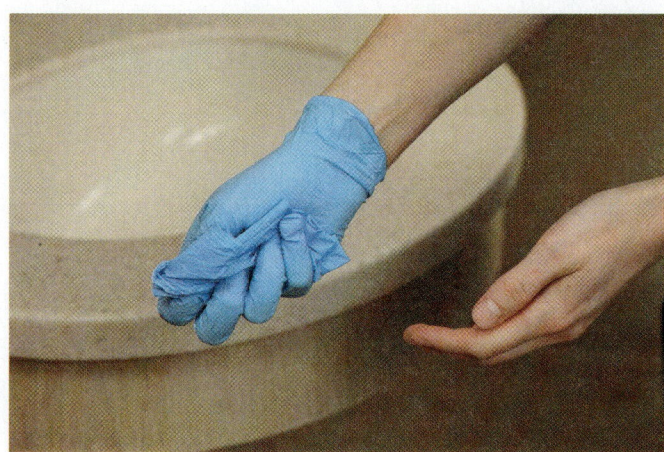

7 Fold rolled-up glove in palm of second hand.

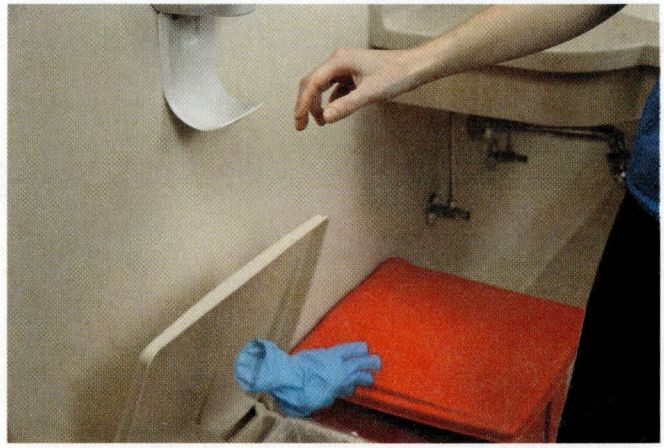

10 Dispose of gloves in proper container, not at bedside. Complete hand hygiene.

Skill 14.1.4 | Managing Latex Allergies

Equipment
Latex-free gloves
Latex-free syringes
Latex-free IV tubing and bags of solution
Latex-free cart with supplies for client with latex allergy ❶

❶ Provide a latex-free cart—supplies for staff and clients with latex allergies.

Procedure
1. Assess clients at high risk or suspected sensitivity to latex (high latex exposure, congenital defects, indwelling catheters, and such).
2. Assess clients and staff with allergies to cherries, apricots, tomatoes, avocados, bananas, papaya, kiwi, or chestnuts.
   ➤ *Rationale:* They may have cross-sensitivity to latex.
3. Recognize symptoms of latex allergy.

   a. Contact dermatitis
   b. Type IV: facial swelling, itching, hives, rhinitis, eye symptoms
   c. Type I: potentially dangerous bronchospasms, generalized edema, difficulty breathing, cardiac arrest

> **CLINICAL ALERT**
> Latex allergy or hypersensitivity can be life threatening, so recognize the primary symptoms in both clients and staff.

4. Replace latex-containing products (especially gloves) with nonlatex alternatives.
5. Obtain a latex-free cart when a client is identified as having a latex allergy.

   a. Place cart inside client's room.
   b. Check that cart is supplied with latex-free gloves, syringes, IV tubes, suction catheters, and such.
6. Ensure that anaphylaxis medication is available for both clients and staff if latex allergy is suspected. ➤ *Rationale:* If there is a severe reaction, this medication may be lifesaving.

Unit 14.1 Documentation and Evaluation

DOCUMENTATION for Basic Medical Asepsis

- Infection control measures used
- Clean gloves used for procedure
- Latex allergy identified
- Use of latex-free gloves

EVALUATION/Critical Thinking

Expected Outcomes
- Decreased number of bacteria on hands from client to client
- Delivered care with pathogen-free hands to clients
- Prevented spread of microorganisms from healthcare workers or environment to clients
- Prevented cross-contamination between clients

Unexpected Outcomes	Alternative Actions
• Infection occurs in clients or healthcare providers.	• Assess mode of transmission of microorganism. • Administer antibiotics specific to microorganism as ordered. • Review hand washing technique. • Attend in-service program on infection control procedures. • Notify nurse manager of allergy.
• Latex allergy is identified in healthcare worker or client.	• Institute latex safety procedures for staff and client (if identified). • Educate staff about latex allergy. • Replace latex-containing objects (particularly gloves) with nonlatex alternatives. • Create a latex-free environment in which those who are allergic can work safely.

Standard Precautions *(Tier 1)*

Nursing Process Data

ASSESSMENT Database

- Assess for skin integrity.
- Assess for presence of drainage from lesions or body cavity.
- Assess for ability to deal with oral secretions.
- Assess for compliance to hygiene measures and respiratory hygiene and cough etiquette (i.e., covering mouth when coughing, ability to control body fluids).
- Assess ability to carry out activities of daily living (ADLs).
- Assess extent of PPE needed (i.e., gloves, gown, mask, protective eyewear).
- Assess need for special equipment (i.e., hazardous waste bags, plastic bags for specimens).

PLANNING Objectives

- To prevent the spread of the microorganism to health professionals
- To reduce potential for the transmission of microorganisms
- To protect hospital personnel and others from contamination
- To provide appropriate equipment and techniques for preventive measures
- To prevent clients (especially compromised clients) from acquiring healthcare-associated infections.

IMPLEMENTATION Procedures

DOCUMENTATION AND EVALUATION

Expected Outcomes

- Prevented spread of microorganisms between clients and/or healthcare workers
- Reduced potential for transmission of microorganisms occurs
- Protected hospital personnel and others from contamination
- Provided appropriate equipment and techniques for preventive measures
- Reduced incidence of healthcare-associated infections

Unexpected Outcomes/Alternative Actions

Pearson Nursing Student Resources

Find additional review materials at **nursing.pearsonhighered.com.**
Prepare for success with NCLEX®-style practice questions and Skill Checklists.

Skill 14.2.1 | Donning Personal Protective Equipment

Equipment
Disposable gloves
Gown
Mask
Protective eyewear

Procedure

1. Use alcohol-based antiseptic or wash hands using nonantimicrobial soap and dry. Follow Standard Precautions guidelines. ❶
2. Put on gown by placing one arm at a time through sleeves. ❷ Wrap gown around body so that it covers clothing completely. ➤ *Rationale:* Gowns are worn when it is likely that personal clothing will come in contact with blood, body fluids, secretions, and excretions (Box 14-9 ■).

3. Don mask or respirator. ❸ ➤ *Rationale:* Masks are worn when there is an anticipated contact with respiratory droplet secretions, the client has a persistent cough and does not cover mouth, or when suction will be performed.
4. Don protective eyewear such as face shield. ➤ *Rationale:* Face shields will protect the nurse from splashing of blood or body fluids while caring for clients.
5. Don disposable gloves. ➤ *Rationale:* Gloves will prevent contamination of hands when there is contact with blood, body fluids, secretions, or excretions.

STANDARD PRECAUTIONS
For all patient care

PROCEDURE	🖐	🧤	👤	👓	😷
Talking to patient					
Adjusting IV fluid rate or non-invasive equipment					
Examining patient *without* touching blood, body fluids, mucous membranes	X				
Examining patient *including* contact with blood, body fluids, mucous membranes	X	X			
Drawing blood	X	X			
Inserting venous access	X	X			
Suctioning	X	X	*Use gown, mask, eyewear if bloody body fluid splattering is likely*		
Inserting body or face catheters	X	X	*Use gown, mask, eyewear if bloody body fluid splattering is likely*		
Handling soiled waste, linen, other materials	X	X	*Use gown, mask, eyewear only if waste or linen are extensively contaminated and splattering is likely*		
Intubation	X	X	X	X	X
Inserting arterial access	X	X	X	X	X
Endoscopy	X	X	X	X	X
Operative and other procedures which produce extensive splattering of blood or body fluids.	X	X	X	X	X

❶ Standard Precautions.

❷ CDC guidelines for donning PPE.

(continued)

Skill 14.2.1 | Donning Personal Protective Equipment *(continued)*

A

B

C

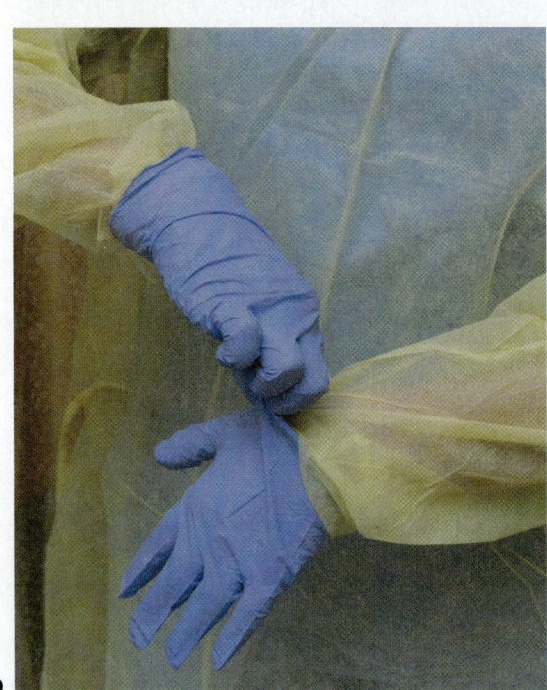

D

❸ **A.** Put on the gown. **B.** Don the mask. **C.** Put on the face shield. **D.** Put on gloves.

Box 14-9 STANDARD PRECAUTION GUIDELINES

The following Standard Precautions are recommended for use with clients to prevent transmission of infectious agents. Please follow these guidelines when caring for clients.

- Wash hands thoroughly or use alcohol-based antiseptic after removing gloves and before and after all client contact.
- Wear gloves when there is direct contact with blood, body fluids, secretions, excretions, and contaminated items. This includes a neonate before first bath. Wash as soon as possible if unanticipated contact with these body substances occurs.
- Protect clothing with gowns or plastic aprons if there is a possibility of being splashed or direct contact with contaminated material.
- Wear masks, goggles, or face shield to avoid being splashed; includes during suctioning, irrigations, and deliveries.
- Do not break or recap needles; discard them intact into puncture-resistant containers.
- Place all contaminated articles and trash in leakproof bags.

- Place clients at risk for contaminating the environment in a private room with separate bathroom facilities, or with another client with same infectious organism.
- Transport infected clients using appropriate barriers, that is, mask and gown.

Place sharps container in area for easy access.

Large sharps containers are available for areas where usage is greater.

Skill 14.2.2 | Removing Personal Protective Equipment

Equipment
Linen hamper
Garbage bag

Procedure

1. Remove gloves grasping the outside of glove with the opposite gloved hand. ➤ *Rationale:* Outside of glove is contaminated. ❶
2. Remove second glove by sliding fingers of ungloved hand under the remaining glove at wrist and peeling off glove (refer to Skill 14.1.3, Donning and Removing Gloves).
3. Remove face shield or goggles by handle, headband, or earpieces and dispose in designated receptacle. ❷
4. Remove gown, unfasten ties, and pull away neck and shoulders touching inside of gown only. Roll up gown and place in designated receptacle. ➤ *Rationale:* Gown front and sleeves are contaminated.
5. Remove mask by grasping bottom, then top ties or elastic, and remove. Discard in designated receptacle. ➤ *Rationale:* The front of the mask is contaminated.
6. Complete hand hygiene.

❶ CDC guidelines for safe removal of PPE.

(continued)

Skill 14.2.2 | Removing Personal Protective Equipment *(continued)*

A

D

B

E

C

❷ **A.** Remove gloves. Remove first glove by pulling it off so glove turns inside out. Place rolled-up glove in palm of second hand and remove second glove. **B.** Remove shield, taking care to hold it by the ties and not to touch the bottom of the shield. **C.** Remove gown by first untying string at waist or neck, and take it off by pulling down from the shoulders. **D.** Turn the gown inside out and pull arms out as you pull the gown off. **E.** Take off mask, holding it by the ties; be careful not to touch the bottom of the mask.

Unit 14.2 Documentation and Evaluation

DOCUMENTATION for Standard Precautions

- Standard Precautions maintained
- Client's response to care and protocol used
- Specimens sent to laboratory if appropriate
- Disposal precautions utilized if appropriate

EVALUATION/Critical Thinking

Expected Outcomes

- Prevented spread of microorganisms between clients and/or healthcare workers
- Reduced potential for transmission of microorganisms
- Protected hospital personnel and others from contamination
- Provided appropriate equipment and techniques for preventive measures
- Reduced incidence of healthcare-associated infections

Unexpected Outcomes

- Contaminated blood or body fluid comes in contact with nurse's skin or mucous membranes.

Alternative Actions

- Report incident and follow agency policy that may include being seen by employee health. (Very important for follow-up legal and medical implications.)
- Follow facility guidelines (they may differ per facility) for PEP.
- Continue to monitor nurse's health status and carry out specific activities to build immune system.
- Eat well-balanced meals with reduced fat intake.
- Exercise frequently.
- Obtain adequate sleep and rest.
- Learn and practice stress reduction activities (stress is known to lessen effectiveness of immune system).

Unit 14.3

Transmission-Based Precautions (*Tier 2*, Isolation)

Nursing Process Data

ASSESSMENT Database

- Identify appropriate times for hand hygiene.
- Identify type of PPE clothing required for **barrier nursing**.
- Identify **epidemiology** of the disease to determine how to prevent infection from spreading.
- Identify equipment needed to prevent spread of organisms.
- Assess method of terminal cleaning and disposing of equipment.

PLANNING Objectives

- To prevent the spread of endogenous and exogenous flora to other clients
- To reduce potential for transferring organisms from the hospital environment to the client
- To protect hospital personnel from becoming infected
- To prevent immunosuppressed clients from acquiring healthcare-associated infections

IMPLEMENTATION Procedures

DOCUMENTATION AND EVALUATION

Expected Outcomes

- Prevented client-to-client spread of endogenous and exogenous flora
- Protected hospital personnel from becoming infected
- Prevented immunosuppressed clients from acquiring healthcare-associated infections
- Reduced transference of organisms from hospital environment to clients

Unexpected Outcomes/Alternative Actions

Pearson Nursing Student Resources

Find additional review materials at **nursing.pearsonhighered.com.**
Prepare for success with NCLEX®-style practice questions and Skill Checklists.

Equipment

Specific equipment depends on isolation precaution system used

   Soap* and running water

Isolation cart containing masks, gowns, gloves, plastic bags, and isolation tape

   Linen hamper and trash can, when needed

Paper towels

Door card indicating precautions

Procedure

1. Check physician's order for isolation.
2. Obtain isolation cart from central supply, if needed.
3. Check that all necessary equipment to carry out the isolation order is available.
4. Place isolation card on the client's door. ❶
5. Ensure that linen hamper and trash cans are available, if needed.
6. Explain purpose of isolation to client and family (Box 14-10 ■).
7. Instruct family in procedures required.
8. Wash hands with antimicrobial soap or use alcohol-based gel before and after entering isolation room. Type of antimicrobial soap or agent depends on infectious agent and client condition.

Note: For donning and removing isolation attire, see Skills 14.2.1 and 14.2.2.

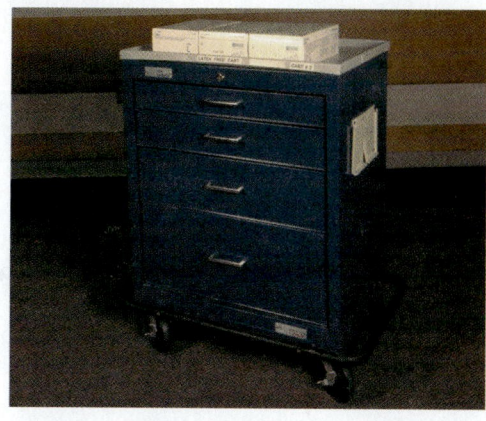

❶ Place isolation cart outside client's door when cart is required.

Box 14-10 **PEDIATRIC CONSIDERATIONS**

Isolation precautions can increase an already stressful situation for a hospitalized child. Younger children have limited cognitive abilities to understand the implications of isolation. Particularly frightening for them is the presence of people in gowns and masks. To help decrease their fears, preparation is important. Letting the children see and play with the equipment lessens some of the anxiety. Healthcare workers should introduce themselves to the child before donning a mask. Frequent visits to the child can also lessen the fear and loneliness associated with isolation.

EVIDENCE-BASED PRACTICE
Airborne Infection Isolation (AII) Rooms

A client with an infection that can be transmitted via airborne route should be admitted to an airborne infection isolation (AII) room. AII rooms have a directional air-flow negative pressure ventilation system with a connected anteroom. The door should be kept closed at all times, and the air should undergo 12 air exchanges per hour to dilute the concentration of airborne contaminants. The exhaust fan should be labeled "Caution: Negative Pressure Isolation Room Exhaust" to ensure that maintenance workers do not accidentally vent it improperly. Air should be filtered through a HEPA filter or discharged directly to the outside toward unoccupied areas and away from openings into the building.

Source: Sabuncuyan (2013)

View from anteroom to client's isolation room with directional air-flow negative pressure ventilation system.

Anteroom connected to isolation room. Staff should use this access to client's room and keep door closed at all times.

Skill 14.3.2 | Using a Mask

Equipment
Clean mask

Procedure
1. Obtain mask from box. ❶
2. Position mask to cover your nose and mouth.
3. Bend nose bar so that it conforms over bridge of your nose.
4. If you are using a mask with string ties, tie top strings on top of your head to prevent slipping. If you are using a cone-shaped mask, tie top strings over your ears.
5. Tie bottom strings around your neck to secure mask over your mouth. There should be no gaps between the mask and your face.
6. *Important:* Change mask every 30 minutes or sooner if it becomes damp. ➤ *Rationale:* Effectiveness is greatly reduced after 30 minutes or if mask is moist.
7. Complete hand hygiene before removing mask.
8. To remove mask, untie lower strings first, or slip elastic band off without touching mask. ➤ *Rationale:* Only strings are considered clean.

9. Discard mask in a trash container.
10. Complete hand hygiene.

> **CLINICAL ALERT**
> Respiratory N95 or HEPA respirators (high-efficiency particulate air) masks are required for infectious diseases transmitted by airborne mode, such as multidrug-resistant tuberculosis.
>
> - Masks are fitted to the worker. Mask should have a good sealing surface with no leakage around the edge, providing a tight seal over the nose and mouth.
> - Refer to agency policy regarding reuse of N95 masks.
> - Discard mask if it becomes contaminated with secretions or bodily fluids.
> - When not in use, store mask in zip-lock bag in safe area.
> - Masks are expensive and can be used repeatedly (up to five times unless otherwise specified) unless it is difficult to breathe through them.

> **CLINICAL ALERT**
> Protective gear such as goggles and face shield are worn when there is a risk of splashes or sprays from blood, secretions, excretions, or body fluids. Eyewear is removed before taking off mask.

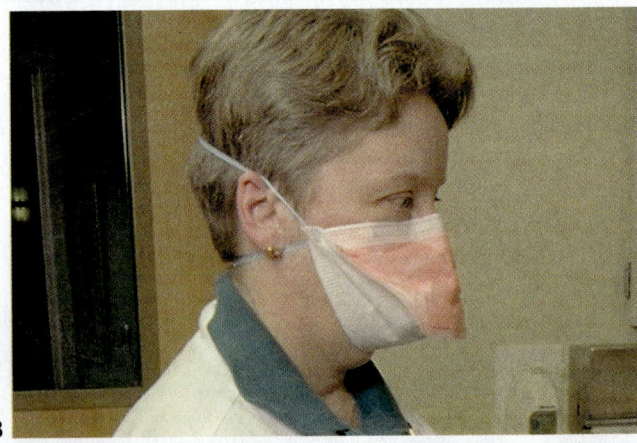

❶ **A.** Sample masks used for isolation protocol. **B.** The particulate filter respirator mask must be airtight.

Skill 14.3.3 | Guidelines When Assessing Vital Signs of Client in Isolation

Equipment
Thermometer
Stethoscope
Blood pressure cuff and sphygmomanometer
Thermometer stand
Watch with sweep second hand
PPE

Procedure
1. Complete hand hygiene and identify client using two forms of client ID.
2. Don PPE as required by type of isolation.
3. Proceed to take vital signs as you would for any client.

4. Place equipment in appropriate area if it is to be left in room. Follow appropriate protocol to remove equipment from isolation room.
5. Remove PPE according to protocol.

6. Complete hand hygiene.
7. Wipe watch if accidentally contaminated. Use appropriate solution.

Skill 14.3.4 | Removing Items From Isolation Room

Equipment
Large red biohazard bags
Specimen container
Plastic bag with biohazard label
Laundry bag
Red plastic container for sharps
Cleaning articles

Procedure
1. Place laboratory specimen in biohazard plastic bag. ❶
2. Dispose of all sharps in appropriate red plastic container in room.
3. Place all linen in linen bag.
4. Use dedicated equipment such as blood pressure cuffs and thermometers for clients in Transmission-Based Precautions and ensure the equipment is cleaned thoroughly before being used on other clients.
5. Dispose of all garbage in plastic bags.

> ### CLINICAL ALERT
> Linen and trash are disposed of in the same manner. Ensure that when placing bags in containers in "dirty" utility room, you place them in the correct container according to bag contents.

6. Replace all bags, such as linen bag and garbage bag, in appropriate container in room. ⬜
7. Clean client's room as necessary, using germicidal solution, according to facility protocol.
8. Prepare to leave the client's room. Place red biohazard bag in appropriate container. ❸ See Skill 14.3.5, Removing a Specimen From Isolation Room.

❷ Set up new biohazard bag for continued use in client's room.

❶ Close biohazard bag securely and label contents, if necessary.

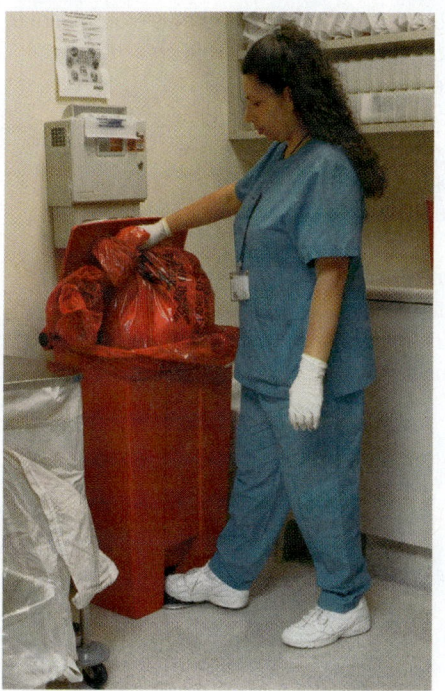

❸ Place red biohazard bag in specified area for disposal.

14.3.5   Removing a Specimen From Isolation Room

Equipment
Specimen container
Clean biohazard bag

Procedure
1. Follow PPE protocol for entering isolation room, or, if you are already in the isolation room, continue with Step 2.
2. Mark a specimen container with the client's name, type of specimen, and the word *isolation* before entering an isolation room.
3. Collect specimen, and place container in a clean plastic biohazard bag outside the room. ➤ *Rationale:* Use clear bags so that laboratory personnel can see the specimen easily. ❶
4. Complete hand hygiene.
5. Send specimen to laboratory with appropriate laboratory request form attached to outside of the bag.

❶ Biohazard bag for transportation of specimens from isolation room.

Skill 14.3.6   Transporting Isolation Client Outside the Room

Equipment
Transport vehicle
Bath blanket
Mask for client if needed

Procedure
1. Explain procedure to client.
2. If a client who is on airborne precautions is being transported, instruct him or her to wear a mask for the entire time out of isolation. ❶ ➤ *Rationale:* This prevents the spread of airborne microbes.
3. Cover the transport vehicle with a bath blanket if there is a chance of soiling when transporting a client who has a draining wound or diarrhea.
4. Help client into transport vehicle. Cover client with a bath blanket.
5. Tell receiving department what type of isolation client needs and what precautions hospital personnel should follow.
6. Remove bath blanket and handle as contaminated linen when client returns to room.

7. Instruct all hospital personnel to complete hand hygiene before they leave the area.
8. Wipe down transportation vehicle with an antimicrobial solution if soiled.

❶ Place surgical mask on a client who needs to be transported outside room.

Skill 14.3.7   Removing Soiled Large Equipment From Isolation Room

Equipment
Antimicrobial agent or appropriate agent and articles needed to wash equipment
Plastic bag

Procedure
1. Don PPE garb as recommended.
2. Remove equipment from the room.

3. Wash equipment per agency protocol. See Box 14-11 ■ for a new type of cleaning device used in ORs.
4. Remove PPE, and complete hand hygiene outside the room.

> **CLINICAL ALERT**
>
> When possible, use dedicated equipment with the client who is on Transmission-Based Precaution to prevent transmission of infections. When this is not possible, equipment should be disinfected after use per manufacturer's recommendations and agency protocols.

Box 14-11 ROBOTS REDUCE RATES OF SURGICAL SITE INFECTIONS IN THE OR

Hospitals have started using specialized robots as an added step in ensuring the operating rooms are thoroughly disinfected. This is especially helpful when clients are infected with particularly virulent organisms or there is an outbreak of a pathogen that can be traced back to a specific operating room. There are two types of technologies available that are used: pulse-xenon UV and HPV.

- Pulse-xenon works by pulsing xenon, an inert gas, twice in a xenon UV flash lamp into the room; this produces UV C radiation.
- HPV delivers heat-generated hydrogen peroxide through a high velocity air stream.

In both systems, the room is first cleaned manually by the environmental cleaning staff; then the robot is brought in and placed in key positions for the disinfection procedure. The UV system works faster than HPV, but both show a reduction in multidrug resistant organisms after the cleaning procedures. Currently, these systems are used primarily in ORs because the rooms need to be closed and clients and cleaning staff cannot be in the room during the procedures.

Source: Adding (2013)

Unit 14.3 Documentation and Evaluation

DOCUMENTATION for Isolation

- Type of isolation protocol being practiced
- Specimens sent to laboratory
- Client's reactions to sensory deprivation
- Vital signs if appropriate

EVALUATION/Critical Thinking

Expected Outcomes

- Prevented client-to-client spread of endogenous and exogenous flora
- Protected hospital personnel from becoming infected
- Prevented immunosuppressed clients from acquiring healthcare-associated infections
- Reduced transference of organisms from hospital environment to clients

Unexpected Outcomes

- Outbreak of disease occurs despite isolation environment.

Alternative Actions

- Identify cause of outbreak, and contact the infection control practitioner for consultation.
- Examine hand washing and infection control practices among staff.
- Attend in-service education program on **isolation techniques** to increase your awareness of appropriate procedures.

Home Care Adaptation

Nursing Process Data

ASSESSMENT Database

- Assess need for hand hygiene.
- Identify clients at risk for infection.
- Assess need for cleaning equipment and decontaminating equipment.
- Identify type of waste material requiring special disposal.
- Assess equipment needed to deliver care in the home.
- Assess need for teaching preventive measures in the home of HIV or AIDS client.

PLANNING Objectives

- To deliver client care with pathogen-free hands
- To clean equipment properly to prevent cross-contamination
- To protect client from cross-contamination
- To protect the nurse from infection
- To properly dispose of contaminated waste material
- To protect client's significant others from contamination of infected material

IMPLEMENTATION Procedures

DOCUMENTATION AND EVALUATION

Expected Outcomes

- Cross-contamination is prevented.
- Nurse is protected from infection.
- Equipment is cleaned appropriately.
- Waste is disposed of in proper manner.

Unexpected Outcomes/Alternative Actions

Pearson Nursing Student Resources

Find additional review materials at
nursing.pearsonhighered.com.
Prepare for success with NCLEX®-style
practice questions and Skill Checklists.

Skill 14.4.1 | Preparing for Client Care in the Home

Equipment

Community health nursing bag
Liquid soap
Antibacterial gel for hand hygiene
Disposable gloves
Disposable apron or gown
Goggles
Masks, air-purifying mask
Thermometers (oral and rectal)
Thermometer sheaths
Vaseline or lubricant
Cotton balls
Alcohol, one small bottle
Antimicrobial wipes
Cotton-tipped applicators
Tongue depressors
Sterile 4×4s
Band-Aids
Bandage scissors
Nonallergenic tape
Plastic bags with ties
Keto-Diastix and Chemstrips
Sphygmomanometer
Stethoscope
Paper cups
Bleach, one small bottle

Procedure

1. Arrange equipment in bag before making home visit so that hand hygiene equipment is accessible. Bring only the supplies needed. ➤ *Rationale:* This procedure decreases the possibility of cross-contamination.
2. Place bag on flat, dry surface to establish a clean work area during visit. Use of disposable barrier under bag is recommended. ➤ *Rationale:* This prevents potential spread of infection between clients' homes. The risk can be high for transmitting undiagnosed infections between home clients.
3. Perform hand hygiene.
   a. Use liquid soap and paper towels from bag and client's water supply. Wash hands with clean running water and apply soap. Rub hands together to make a lather and scrub all surfaces. Rub hands for 15–20 seconds. Rinse

hands well under running water. Dry hands using paper towel from nurse's bag. Turn off faucet using paper towel.
   b. Use antimicrobial gel as alternative for hand washing when soap and water are not available. Squeeze small amount of germicide onto palm of hand and rub all surfaces of hands, fingers, and nails. Rub until hands and fingers are dry. Germicide evaporates into air, making towels unnecessary.
4. Don disposable gloves when appropriate for infection control, especially when handling blood and body fluids.
5. Take other equipment that will be needed during the visit out of the bag and place on clean work surface.
6. Keep bag closed when not in use to promote cleanliness, safety, and security. Care should be taken not to reenter bag wearing soiled gloves. Washing hands between reentering bag is not necessary unless soiled.
7. Wear disposable apron or gown and goggles or mask if necessary. ➤ *Rationale:* This protects the caregiver from blood or body fluid exposure.
8. Cleanse thoroughly any equipment that left clean area and is to be returned to the bag on completing care.
   a. Rinse equipment (such as bandage scissors, forceps) under *cold* water, and wash with soap and water. Use client's personal equipment or disposable equipment whenever possible.
   b. Return stethoscope and blood pressure cuff to nursing bag. ➤ *Rationale:* Clean items can be returned to nursing bag if no visible soiling.

> **CLINICAL ALERT**
> If item is soiled and cannot be returned to the bag, place in separate container for transport to agency. Clean item when it is returned to agency. Most items for home care are disposable.

9. Ensure nursing bag is monitored regularly for safety.
   a. Keep bag out of reach of children.
   b. Keep bag in trunk of car or keep in your home overnight. ➤ *Rationale:* Unattended bags in cars are more often stolen.
   c. Clean bag monthly and PRN.

Skill 14.4.2 | Disposing of Waste Material in the Home Setting

Equipment

Plastic bags, heavy duty
Disposable gloves
Receptacle, rigid and puncture-proof
Bleach
Germicide

Procedure

1. Dispose of wastes contaminated with blood or body fluids.
   a. Place waste products in impenetrable, heavy-duty plastic bag.
   b. Remove plastic gloves by rolling inside out (so contaminated side is on inside) and drop into plastic bag.

(continued)

Skill 14.4.2 | Disposing of Waste Material in the Home Setting (continued)

c. Seal plastic bag with tie.

d. Discard in client's trash.

e. Perform hand hygiene with soap and water or germicide.

2. Dispose of body wastes, such as urine, feces, respiratory secretions, vomitus, and blood by flushing them down the toilet. (This is true whether the toilet empties into a septic tank or a sewage system.)

3. Dispose of needles and sharp objects.

   a. Do *not* remove needle from syringe or bend, break, clip, or recap after use.

   b. Drop entire disposable safety syringe intact into rigid, puncture-proof receptacle provided by agency.

   c. Complete hand hygiene.

4. Discard other trash.

   a. Place in plastic bag.

   b. Discard in client's trash.

Note: Clothing and bedding from clients with potentially transmissible infectious pathogens do not require special handling or laundering. They can be washed with warm water and detergent.

Skill 14.4.3 | Cleansing Equipment in the Home Setting

Equipment
Article to be cleansed
Soap
Running water
Paper towels
Plastic bags
Disposable gloves

Procedure

1. Don gloves when working with equipment contaminated with any body fluid or blood.

2. First rinse article with cold running water. ▶ *Rationale:* Cold water releases organic material from the equipment and warm water may make it adhere to the surface.

3. Second wash with hot, soapy water using friction. Additional steps may be needed for equipment such as urinary drainage bags (Box 14-12 ■).

4. Rinse well with clear water.

5. Dry thoroughly.

6. Disinfect equipment or article as indicated: one part chlorine bleach (Clorox) to nine parts water.

> **CLINICAL ALERT**
> If durable medical equipment cannot be sterilized by ethyl oxide or autoclaved, it should be cleaned with 10% chlorine bleach solution after washing with hot soapy water.

7. Dry thoroughly.

8. Remove disposable gloves.

9. Dispose of gloves (inside out) into plastic bag.

10. Perform hand hygiene.

Box 14-12 DISINFECTING URINARY DRAINAGE BAGS

Urinary drainage bags can be disinfected in the home. Use one part vinegar to three parts water. Soak the bag for 20 minutes, rinse thoroughly with warm water, and hang to dry (Cleveland Clinic, 2013).

Skill 14.4.4 | Teaching Preventive Measures in the Home Setting

Procedure

1. Discuss the inadvisability of allowing any individual who is ill or who has depressed immune function to come in contact with the client.

2. Teach the client these appropriate hygiene principles:

   a. Wash hands after use of toilet or contact with any body fluids.

   b. Do not share thermometers, razors, razor blades, toothbrushes, douche, or enema equipment.

   c. Do not cough without covering mouth.

   d. Be careful to dispose of nasal secretions in tissue, then in plastic bags.

3. Teach these guidelines for sharing kitchens and bathrooms:

   a. Good household cleaning practices prevent spread of infection.

   b. Do not share eating and drinking utensils. After use, they must be cleaned with hot water (hot enough to necessitate use of gloves) and soap. Use of a dishwasher and soap is appropriate.

   c. Kitchen and bathroom surfaces should be cleaned every day with scouring powder or with chlorine bleach solution (10%, one part bleach to nine parts water). Use disposable bathroom cups. Use covered individual toothbrush holders.

   d. Clean refrigerators regularly with soap and water; remove old food to prevent mold.

   e. Mop floors in bathroom and kitchen weekly. Pour dirty water down the toilet and disinfect with bleach solution.

   f. Clean toilet, tub, and shower weekly or as often as necessary with 10% bleach solution. If urine or diarrhea spills on toilet or floor, wipe immediately with the 10% bleach solution.

   g. Sponges used to clean floors or body fluid spills should be soaked for 5 minutes in a 10% bleach solution.

4. Teach the following principles of food preparation:

   a. Wash hands thoroughly before any food preparation.

   b. Do not lick fingers or taste from the mixing spoon while cooking.

   c. Avoid unpasteurized milk (danger of contact with *Salmonella*), do not eat old or moldy food (danger of food poisoning), and cook poultry thoroughly.

   d. Wash all fresh (raw) fruits and vegetables before eating.

5. Teach how to care for linens and laundry.

   a. When clothing or linen is soiled with blood or body fluids, it should be stored separately in a plastic bag. Wash separately with very hot water, detergent, and bleach. Use Clorox II for colored clothing.

   b. Wear disposable gloves when touching soiled clothes or linen.

   c. Do not share used towels or washcloths, and wash separately. (Towels and washcloths are, however, safe to use after washing.)

   d. Change towels and washcloths daily.

6. Inform client and family of measures for disposing of trash.

   a. Flush body wastes down the toilet.

   b. Discard dressings, diapers, Chux, or any materials soiled with secretions in a plastic bag. Discard into the regular trash.

   c. Sharp items (e.g., razors, needles) should be placed in a rigid, puncture-proof container with a solution of 10%

bleach. Incinerate when container is full. Pharmacies collect the used containers in some areas.

7. Discuss procedures for caring for pets.

   a. Clean bird cages wearing gloves. Birds can spread psittacosis (*Chlamydia psittaci*) or *Cryptococcus*.

   b. Clean cat litter boxes wearing gloves to prevent spread of toxoplasmosis.

   c. Tropical fish tanks should not be cleaned by the individual with AIDS to prevent spread of *Mycobacterium*.

8. Teach general principles of preventing cross-infection.

   a. Wear gloves when handling body fluids, linens, or other objects contaminated with body fluids.

   b. Disposable gowns or aprons protect clothing from becoming soiled.

   c. Caregivers should not provide care when ill themselves.

   d. Maintain adequate ventilation in the living quarters.

9. Discuss steps to prevent spread of contagious disease; cold, flu, strep throat.

   a. Clean hands thoroughly before eating or touching food, after using the bathroom, taking out trash, playing with a pet, or being in contact with someone who is ill.

   b. Use tissues when sneezing or coughing, cover mouth and nose, and discard tissue immediately. If tissue is not available, cover mouth and nose with bend in your elbow or your hands. Clean hands immediately.

   c. Avoid contact with others if you are ill.

   d. Maintain up-to-date vaccinations.

10. Medical supplies should be kept in a clean, dry location. If refrigeration is required, place medication in sealed plastic storage bag.

Unit 14.4 Documentation and Evaluation

DOCUMENTATION for Home Care Adaptations

- Document findings on appropriate home care forms.
- Therapies provided and client response
- Follow treatment plan and document goal achievement.
- Client status, physical findings, ability to care for self

- Clinically significant observations stated objectively related to potential infection
- Clinically significant observations related to environmental findings related to potential infections

EVALUATION/Critical Thinking

Expected Outcomes

- Clients do not acquire infections during home care visits.
- Early detection of potential infections is identified through appropriate assessment techniques.

- Infections are treated appropriately and not transmitted to other home care clients or the nurse because effective preventative measures are utilized.

(continued)

Unexpected Outcomes

- There are potential infection sources in the home environment.

Alternative Actions

- Explain the necessity of keeping the environment free of potential organisms by keeping it clean and uncluttered.
- Instruct the client and family members on proper hand hygiene technique.
- Explain and develop a plan for family members to discard soiled dressings, diapers, and the like to prevent potentially infecting other household members.

Chapter Wrap-Up

GERONTOLOGIC Considerations

- Social isolation resulting from infection control requirements is more intense with the older adult. They need frequent contact with healthcare workers. Sometimes being ill is the only attention they receive.
- Older adult clients can become confused in the hospital, and when placed in isolation, there is an even greater risk. Frequent monitoring for safety issues is necessary.

- Frequent explanations of why isolation is necessary are important for the older adult. They may have a lapse of memory and forget earlier discussion about isolation.
- Ensure that call lights are easily accessible and that the client understands how to call for assistance. They may have impaired hearing and sight, which can interfere with communications.

MANAGEMENT Guidelines

Each state legislates a Nurse Practice Act for RNs and LVN/LPNs. Healthcare facilities are responsible for establishing and implementing policies and procedures that conform to their state's regulations. Verify the regulations and role parameters for each healthcare worker in your facility.

Delegation

- LVN/LPNs and CNAs may be assigned to clients requiring infection control precautions and barriers. Ensure that all healthcare workers have been properly educated in infection control procedures before assigning them to clients requiring these measures.
- It is the RN's responsibility to make assignments that take into account the type of isolation precautions and potential cross-contamination of other clients in the care of the healthcare worker. For example, the same healthcare worker should not take care of a client in contact isolation and an immunosuppressed client.

Interprofessional Communication

- Ensure that appropriate designations are posted on the door of the room indicating the type of isolation precautions necessary for the client.
- Indicate the type of isolation precautions on the client's chart.
- During shift report and team report, review the type of isolation precautions being maintained for the client.
- Inform and instruct all visitors on the isolation precautions.
- Monitor that all hospital staff practice good hand hygiene technique. Review appropriate technique with those who do not practice these techniques.
- Review isolation precautions, particularly Standard Precautions, with all new personnel and on a regular basis with all personnel to ensure compliance with hospital policy.
- Monitor healthcare workers for appropriate use of gloves, masks, and gowns when caring for clients in isolation. Instruct healthcare workers in proper use of these items when providing client care.

CASE STUDY Applications

Scenario 1

You are assigned to care for two clients. One client has just returned from surgery for an abdominal resection. The second client is hospitalized with an acute case of tuberculosis.

1. Is this assignment appropriate, considering the two diagnoses? Provide a rationale for the answer.
2. What special precautions will you take when providing care for these two clients?
3. CDC guidelines are specific for clients with tuberculosis. Identify the differences in providing care for this client versus other clients requiring barrier nursing.

4. Describe the procedure for leaving the tuberculosis client's room. Provide a rationale for the prioritized steps.

Scenario 2

You are assigned to take two clients' vital signs, complete a focus assessment, provide hygienic care, monitor IVs, and complete a dressing change for a client with an abdominal resection.

1. What task will have priority with this assignment?
2. Develop a time management plan and provide a rationale for the time frames and activities.

NCLEX® Review Questions

Unless otherwise specified, choose only one (1) answer.

1. When assessing the following client care situations, which situation would require the nurse to wear gloves? **Select all that apply.**
   A. Changing a dressing
   B. Taking blood pressure
   C. Catheterizing the urinary bladder
   D. Emptying a Foley drainage collection bag
   E. Taking a temporal temperature

2. A client is on contact precautions for *Clostridium difficile*. When the nurse performs hand hygiene, what cleansing agent should he or she should use?
   A. Waterless antiseptic
   B. 1:10 bleach solution
   C. Soap and water
   D. Alcohol solution

3. Arrange the steps in priority order for donning personal protection equipment (PPE):
   A. Putting on gown
   B. Putting on gloves
   C. Putting on face shield
   D. Putting on mask

4. When working with infants, what is the most important action for breaking the chain of infection?
   A. Use of sterile technique
   B. Isolation of ill people near the infant
   C. Treatment with antibiotics
   D. Proper hand hygiene

5. When in the home administering insulin to a client with diabetes, what is the best way to dispose of contaminated needles and syringes?
   A. Break the needle from the syringe and dispose of it.
   B. Place them in a puncture-resistant container in the home.

C. Recap them and bring them to an appropriate disposal area.
   D. Soak them in bleach and then dispose of them in the trash.

6. A nurse is giving an emaciated client an injection. While withdrawing the needle from the site, the needle slips and pierces the nurse's finger. What is the most appropriate action?
   A. Recap the needle and save it for laboratory analysis.
   B. Break the needle and discard it in a puncture-proof container.
   C. Obtain an order for the client to receive gamma globulin.
   D. Wash the finger with an antiseptic and water solution.

7. The nurse observes a nursing assistant putting on gloves to deliver lunch trays to clients. What therapeutic intervention would the nurse take?
   A. Commend the nursing assistant for the action.
   B. Explain to the nursing assistant that gloves do not need to be worn if there is no client contact.
   C. Ask the nursing assistant to wear a gown also.
   D. Make sure the nursing assistant does not touch the client.

8. What is the most frequent mode of transmission of healthcare associated or HAI (nosocomial) infections?
   A. Soiled linens
   B. Hands of healthcare workers
   C. Medical equipment
   D. Food trays

9. Place the steps for removing personal protection equipment into correct priority order.
   A. Perform hand hygiene.
   B. Take off your mask.
   C. Remove your gloves.
   D. Remove your gown.

10. What should the home care nurse do to prevent the spread of infection between clients?

   A. Use only disposable supplies and equipment in the home and dispose of them in the home before leaving.

   B. Take out necessary supplies from the bag and bring them into the house, leaving the bag in the car.

   C. Take needed supplies from the bag and place them on a clean work area, then close the bag immediately.

   D. Wear clean gloves throughout the visit, and place them in the garbage as you leave the house.

QSEN Activity

Domain: Quality Improvement

KSA: Practice aligning the aims, measures, and changes involved in improving care.

Activity:

You are a student nurse on a busy surgical unit. You have been asked by your nurse manager to help create awareness around the importance of hand washing and the transmission of infections. You know that it is crucial to educate staff nurses about the importance of hand hygiene. Using resources found on the CDC website, design an educational campaign to raise staff awareness about when they should be washing hands. Create a plan to monitor compliance with hand washing.

Bibliography

Babiarz, L. S., Savoie, B., McGuire, M., McConnell, L., & Nagy, P. (2014). Hand sanitizer-dispensing door handles increase hand hygiene compliance: A pilot study. *American journal of infection control*, 42(4), 443–445.

Buki, A. (2013). Multidrug-resistant CRKP bacteria a growing threat in US hospitals and nursing homes, new study shows. Retrieved from http://www.cddep.org/blog/posts/multidrug_resistant_crkp_bacteria_growing_threat_us_hospitals_and_nursing_homes_new_study

Centers for Disease Control. (2003). Exposure to blood: What health care personnel need to know. DHHS 2003. CDC.org

Centers for Disease Control. (2012a). Life-threatening germ poses threat across medical facilities. Retrieved from http://www.cdc.gov/media/releases/2012/p0306_cdiff.html

Centers for Disease Control. (2012b). Multidrug-Resistant Tuberculosis (MDR TB). Retrieved from http://www.cdc.gov/tb/publications/factsheets/drtb/mdrtb.htm

Centers for Disease Control. (2013a). Avian flu (bird flu). Retrieved from http://wwwnc.cdc.gov/travel/diseases/avian-bird-flu

Centers for Disease Control. (2013b). Blood/body fluid exposure option. Retrieved from http://www.cdc.gov/nhsn/PDFs/HPS-manual/exposure/3-HPS-Exposure-options.pdf

Centers for Disease Control. (2013c). Handwashing: Clean hands save lives. Retrieved from http://www.cdc.gov/hand/hygiene/training.html

Centers for Disease Control. (2013d). Infection control. Retrieved from http://www.cdc.gov/oralhealth/infectioncontrol/faq/bloodborne_exposures.htm

Centers for Disease Control. (2013e). Methicillin-resistant Staphylococcus aureus (MRSA) infections. Retrieved from http://www.cdc.gov/mrsa/healthcare/index.html

Centers for Disease Control. (2014a). Healthcare-associated infections (HAI). Retrieved from http://www.cdc.gov/hai/

Centers for Disease Control. (2014b). HIV/AIDS. Retrieved from http://www.cdc.gov/hiv/

Centers for Disease Control. (2014c). Infection prevention and control recommendations for hospitalized patients with known or suspected Ebola virus disease in U.S. hospitals. Retrieved from http://www.cdc.gov/vhf/ebola/hcp/infection-prevention-and-control-recommendations.html

Centers for Disease Control. (2015). MERS in the Arabian Peninsula. Retrieved from http://wwwnc.cdc.gov/travel/notices/alert/coronavirus-saudi-arabia-qatar

Cleveland Clinic. (2013). Medical devices: Care of the urine drainage bag and leg bag. Retrieved from http://my.clevelandclinic.org/health/medicaldevices/hic-care-of-the-urine-drainage-bag-and-leg-bag

Ellingson, K., Haas, J. P., Aiello, A. E., Kusek, L., Maragakis, L. L., Olmsted, R. N., Perencevich E., ... & Yokoe, D. S. (2014). Strategies to prevent healthcare-associated infections through hand hygiene. *Infection Control*, 35(08), 937–960.

Ling, L. L., Schneider, T., Peoples, A. J., Spoering, A. L., Engels, I., Conlon, B. P., ... & Lewis, K. (2015). A new antibiotic kills pathogens without detectable resistance. *Nature*, 517(7535), 455–459.

Magill, S. S., Edwards, J. R., Bamberg, W., Beldavs, Z. G., Dumyati, G., Kainer, M. A., ... & Fridkin, S. K. (2014). Multistate point-prevalence survey of health care–associated infections. *New England Journal of Medicine*, 370(13), 1198–1208.

Mangram, A. J. (1999). Guidelines for prevention of surgical site infection, *American Journal of Infection Control* 21(2), 97–134

Miller, B. (2010). The impact of hospital-onset healthcare facility associated (HO-HCFA) *Clostridium difficile* infection (CDI) in community hospitals: Surpassing methicillin-resistant Staphylococcus aureus (MRSA) as the new superbug. Paper presented at the Fifth Decennial International Conference on Healthcare–Associated Infections, Society for Healthcare Epidemiology of America, Atlanta, Mar. 18–22, 2010. Retrieved from http://shea.confex.com/shea/2010/webprogram/Paper2801.html

Patterson, P. (2013). Could technology lend a hand in cleaning of ORs? *OR Manager*, 29(3), 12–14.

Sabuncuyan, A. (2013). Air distribution patterns within airborne infectious isolation rooms. *Health Care Design*. Retrieved from http://www.healthcaredesignmagazine.com/article/air-distribution-patterns-within-airborne-infectious-isolation-rooms

Siegel, J. D., Rhinehart, E., Jackson, M., Chiarello, L., and the Healthcare Infection Control Practices Advisory Committee. (2007). Guideline for isolation precautions: Preventing transmission of infectious agents in healthcare settings. Retrieved from http://www.cdc.gov/ncidod/dhqp/pdf/isolation2007.pdf

The Joint Commission. (2009). Measuring hand hygiene adherence: Overcoming the challenges. Retrieved from http://www.jointcommission.org/assets/1/18/hh_monograph.pdf

Wilburn, S. (2004, Sep. 30). Needlestick and sharps injury prevention. *Online Journal of Issues in Nursing*, 9(3), manuscript.

World Health Organization. (2009). WHO guidelines on hand hygiene in health care: Patient safety. Five moments for hand hygiene. Retrieved from http://www.who.int/gpsc/tools/Five_moments/en/

Chapter 15
Disaster Preparedness

 ## Learning Objectives

15.1 Discuss the concept of preparedness for a terrorist attack.

15.2 List the effects on infrastructure that may result from a mass casualty incident.

15.3 State the chain of command and reporting requirements when a mass casualty incident occurs.

15.4 Compare and contrast external and internal communication systems.

15.5 Explain the term *triage* and list the steps of triage.

15.6 Differentiate among biological, chemical, and radiation attacks.

15.7 Describe how to measure external radiation levels.

15.8 Discuss why ethical issues are important during a mass casualty event.

15.9 Discuss diversity considerations when healthcare workers are responding to a terrorist event.

15.10 List components of a home safety plan.

15.11 Discuss safety principles in relation to natural disasters.

15.12 Identify two diarrhea-related diseases.

15.13 List signs and symptoms of various biological agents and describe how to distinguish between them.

15.14 Discuss the clinical features of smallpox.

15.15 Describe the major agents of a chemical attack.

15.16 List the primary interventions necessary to care for the psychological needs of disaster victims.

15.17 Review the equipment included in Standard Precautions.

15.18 List the steps of decontamination via triage.

15.19 Explain the protective equipment necessary for biological exposure (individualize for anthrax, plague, botulism, and smallpox).

15.20 Differentiate methods of decontaminating victims after a biological versus a chemical attack.

15.21 Demonstrate decontamination procedures for victims of a radiological attack.

15.22 Discuss establishing public health parameters for triage.

15.23 Demonstrate the steps for treating life-threatening conditions.

15.24 Discuss posttraumatic stress disorder.

Chapter Outline

Terminology

Aerosol very fine liquid or solid particles suspended in air—small particles in a gaseous medium.

Airborne attack microorganisms spread by droplets dispersed in the air; could be spread by using an aerosol delivery system.

Antidote a substance that neutralizes a poison or the effects of a poison.

Bioterrorism the planned, deliberate use of a chemical or biological agent (bacteria, virus, fungi, or toxin) with the intent to harm or kill people.

Centers for Disease Control and Prevention (CDC) U.S. government agency with the stated purpose of preventing the transmission of communicable diseases. This agency is responsible for identifying and disseminating standards and guidelines for isolation precautions.

Chemical terrorism use of a chemical agent (nerve, blood, blister, volatile) with intent to harm or kill people.

Communicable disease a disease that can be transmitted from individual to individual.

Community disaster plan a document that specifies who is in charge, lines of communication, and agencies and resources that will be involved in responding to a disaster.

Contamination introduction of disease, germs, or infectious materials into or onto normally clean or sterile objects.

Decontamination process of removing contamination from people, equipment, or environment—usually done through a physical (i.e., shower) or chemical process.

Disaster an event of such magnitude that essential services are disrupted and current resources are overwhelmed.

Emergency any event or situation that occurs as an unexpected and sudden incident demanding immediate action.

EMTALA Emergency Medical Treatment and Labor Act—a federal law to stop hospital emergency departments (EDs) from refusing to treat poor or uninsured clients or from transferring clients to other facilities before their medical conditions have stabilized.

Exposure inhalation or contamination by a substance that contains a biological, chemical, or radioactive agent.

FBI (Federal Bureau of Investigation) investigative agency of U.S. Department of Justice; it has authority and responsibility to investigate specific crimes, such as a bioterrorist event.

Federal Emergency Management Agency (FEMA) primary or lead federal agency that responds to a disaster, such as a terrorist incident.

First responder first trained personnel to arrive at an emergency.

Gray a measurement of the absorbed dose of radiation; used more often than RAD—(1 Gy = 100 RADS).

Hazardous material any substance that is potentially toxic to a biological system.

HAZMAT model model for dealing with hazardous materials that is used for situations involving certain toxic or chemical exposures.

Homeland Security the Department of Homeland Security (DHS) coordinates all activities related to a terrorist attack.

Immunization process of rendering an individual immune, usually done through vaccination.

Incident Command System (ICS) local and national command structure that organizes emergency responses.

Incubation period time between infection from a microorganism and onset of symptoms.

Infection establishment of a disease process that involves invasion of body tissue by microorganisms, reaction of tissues to their presence, and to toxins generated by them.

Inhalational related to exposure to a substance through the respiratory tract.

Isolation practices or actions designed to prevent transmission of communicable diseases.

Ionizing radiation radiation that has the energy to cause atoms to lose electrons and become ions—alpha, beta, gamma, and x-rays are examples.

Isotopes elements that have neutrons (they have neither a positive nor negative charge). Not all isotopes are radioactive; those that are radioactive, are called radionuclides. Cobalt-69 is an example of a radioactive isotope.

Mass casualty incident (MCI) an incident or emergency event associated with many casualties (airplane crash, terrorism, chemical spill) that has a negative impact on emergency resources.

Microorganism a minute living body, such as a bacterium, protozoan, or virus, not perceptible to the naked eye.

NBC military acronym for nuclear, biological, and chemical weapons.

Nerve agent a chemical agent that acts on the body by disrupting normal function of the nervous system.

Outbreak critical incident in which infections occur above an established level and are caused by the same infectious agent.

Pandemic a disease that affects the population of a large region, country, or continent.

Pathogen a microorganism that can cause disease; may be bacteria, fungi, parasites, or viruses.

Percutaneous agent a substance that can be absorbed through the skin.

Personal protective equipment (PPE) equipment for protection of emergency personnel; includes gloves, masks, gowns, eye shields, biohazard bags, and in some cases, head and shoe covers.

Poison any substance that enters the body by absorption, ingestion, inhalation, or infection and interferes with normal physiologic functions.

RAD radiation absorbed dose—the unit of measure for radiation exposure.

Radiation energy in the form of waves or particles that is emitted from radioactive material or equipment.

Radiation dose quantity of radiation energy deposited in a material by the radiation to which victim is exposed.

Radioactive contamination radioactive material distributed over some area, equipment, or individual; decontamination is required.

REM roentgen equivalent man—the unit of dose or measure of any ionizing radiation— takes into account type of radiation producing the exposure and its effect on humans.

Sodium hypochlorite 0.5% diluted bleach, the active ingredient used for decontamination.

START acronym that stands for "simple treatment and rapid triage," an initial triage system used for triaging large numbers of victims.

Standard Precautions a system of disease control; assumes that direct contact with body fluids is infectious and recommends a series of procedures to protect the staff.

Terrorism the use of force or violence against people or property in violation of the criminal laws of the United States for purposes of intimidation, coercion, or ransom (FBI).

Threat assessment an evaluation of a community's vulnerability and risk potential.

Toxin poisonous substance produced by a living organism.

Trauma multisystem condition or injury that is potentially life-threatening to the individual.

Vaccine preparation of a killed or weakened microorganism used to induce immunity against disease.

Vesicles blisters on the skin.

Virus an infectious microorganism that normally lives within other living cells and cannot reproduce outside the cell.

Weapons of mass destruction (WMD) nuclear, biological, chemical, incendiary, or conventional explosive agents that pose a threat to health, safety, food supply, property, or the environment.

Overview

It is fair to say that the perspective of the United States changed on September 11, 2001. Since that time, citizens have had to adopt the awareness that we are vulnerable; that biological, chemical, and even nuclear **terrorism** is a possibility; and that we must change our perspective of how to function in the world. Senator Bill Frist stated it clearly: "The United States faces a grave and growing threat from **bioterrorism**." In addition, mass killings such as those at Columbine, CO, Fort Hood, TX, and Sandy Hook, CT, as well as the bombing of the Boston Marathon and other events, have affected our need to make disaster preparedness part of our everyday lives.

A page in history has been turned. The medical community—indeed, the world—must face terrorism and the probability of disasters. We cannot predict, but we can prepare. In order to steer a course toward a viable future, we must be prepared to cope with disasters.

Not all nurses can or should be prepared as **first responders**. All nurses, however, must have sufficient knowledge and skill to recognize the potential for a **mass casualty incident (MCI)** or disaster, identify when such an event may have occurred, know how to protect themselves, know how to provide immediate care for individuals involved, recognize their own role and limitations, and know where to seek additional information and resources (College of Registered Nurses of Nova Scotia, 2007). Preparedness for a terrorist-caused disaster is critical for containment and protection of the population. There must be coordinated **emergency** preparedness plans in place in order for a prompt and effective response to any form of attack.

In the United States, licensed nurses and even student nurses can assist in disaster relief. The American Red Cross responds to approximately 70,000 natural and manmade disasters in the United States, ranging from forest fires to tornadoes, airline crashes, and explosions. The goal of the American Red Cross is to provide relief, shelter, food, health and mental health services in times of catastrophic events. Nurses are encouraged to participate locally and internationally. Competencies required for nurse volunteers in disaster relief include communication skills, flexibility, critical thinking, and the ability to work as part of a team.

EVIDENCE-BASED PRACTICE

Preparedness for Disaster

Hospital-based nurses from rural communities in Texas were surveyed on their perceptions of personal disaster preparedness. Using a 58-item Disaster Readiness Questionnaire, findings revealed that most nurses are not confident in their ability to respond to major disaster events. Based on these findings, the authors suggest nurses should actively seek opportunities to participate in actual disaster events, mock drills, and additional educational opportunities to prepare themselves better for specific events.

Source: Baack & Alfred (2013)

Natural Disasters

Although disasters may be natural or manmade, there are numerous definitions of a disaster. For our purposes, natural disasters will be examined regarding how they affect health and health services. From this standpoint, the type and timing of a disaster event will create the types of injuries and illnesses that occur. Disasters that have a prior warning, such as hurricanes or floods, generally have fewer injuries and deaths than those that occur with little or no warning, such as tsunamis or earthquakes. Disasters tend to have more casualties when individuals have little time to prepare or to evacuate before the disaster strikes, or when there is a combination of disasters, like Hurricane Katrina being followed by severe flooding in New Orleans.

Natural disasters have the potential to affect public health significantly, since access to medical care can be severely limited and resources such as food, water, and medicines become scarce or unavailable.

Common natural disasters include:

- Earthquakes
- Hurricanes
- Floods
- Tornadoes

- Tsunamis
- Volcanic eruptions
- Wildfires
- Landslides and mudslides
- Extreme heat, cold, and/or blizzards

Disaster Defined

Disaster is defined as an event of such magnitude that essential services are disrupted and current resources are overwhelmed (Box 15-1 ■). Disasters may be natural (as listed) or caused by human actions such as civil disturbance, a **hazardous material** incident, or an act of terrorism.

Whatever their type, disasters have several characteristics in common: They are unexpected and there has been little or no warning; lives, public health, and the environment are endangered; and emergency services and personnel must be called to action if not available during the initial stages of the event. The terrorist attacks that occurred in Washington, D.C., New York City, and Shanksville, PA, on September 11, 2001, and the Katrina disaster in 2005 were two such events. They carried an unforeseen and immediate threat to public health and required the intervention of others to provide outside resources.

Critical survival issues that can occur with disasters of any kind include the following:

- Lack of safe shelters
- No safe food or water
- No access to needed medicines (insulin, heart drugs)
- No access to medical care for injuries or diseases
- Chaos in the streets

Public Policy
Mass Casualty Characteristics

- MCIs are community-wide incidents—not confined to individual hospitals.
- Event occurs in local community.
- Local government provides "first responders."
- State and federal government become involved if the incident is large enough.
- Hospitals are the last link in community response to an MCI.
- Hospitals receive the most seriously injured and ill casualties.

Box 15-1 LESSONS FROM NATURAL DISASTERS

The implications of natural disasters for nurses and other healthcare providers are profound. For example, throughout a storm-devastated area, nurses may be called upon to provide hospital care under extreme conditions caused by the lack of electricity, food, water, and medical supplies, as well as the inability to evacuate clients. Other nurses who assist at evacuation centers may be overwhelmed by the surge of sick and injured.

Potential Threats From Natural Disasters

Certain natural disasters, such as earthquakes and tornadoes, are very unpredictable; others, like Hurricane Katrina in 2005, are carefully tracked. As a major storm approaches, the national weather agencies estimate the potential for major damage and disruption (i.e., wind velocity, snow depth, temperature, tidal surges), which are widely publicized by the media. The lesson is to hope for the best, but prepare for the worst. Soon after Katrina, another hurricane threatened the Gulf region. When residents of several Texas cities followed evacuation orders, they experienced traffic delays, gasoline and water shortages, and other obstacles during their disorderly evacuation.

Do Not Assume Government Agencies Will Provide Immediate Relief

The government agencies involved with disaster relief include local police, National Guard, **Federal Emergency Management Agency (FEMA)**, federal troops, the U.S. Coast Guard, and many nongovernmental organizations, such as the Red Cross. The coordination among all these organizations has often failed in a morass of bureaucracy and red tape. Several dire predictions have been made concerning the potential threat to an area from

a disaster, with effective response plans either not in place or that have not been tested.

Learn to Cope Without Electricity and Water

Storms involving strong wind, snow, or ice usually disrupt electrical power. So do earthquakes, wildfires, and floods. A severe hurricane's winds can topple trees into power lines and blow down cell phone towers. A storm surge and flood can disable emergency generators and disrupt water and sewer service. Normal communications are crippled as cell phones and cordless phones do not operate. Television, air conditioning, refrigeration, hospital equipment, and other services that depend upon electricity are disrupted. The ability to communicate with the "outside world" may be extremely limited, leaving hospitals and evacuation centers unable to communicate their emergency needs or to learn when and in what form they could expect assistance.

Disruption of the water service can result in extreme hardship to many thousands of stranded survivors. People may have to endure several days without adequate water, ice, or food until they are either rescued or make their way to an emergency center. The implication of the loss of utilities for the individual nurse is that you must keep an emergency supply of water at home, in your automobile, and at work (in case you are stranded at work or in transit), enough to last for 3 days. Refer to Skill 15.1.1, Creating a Safety Plan for Disasters, for a checklist of emergency supplies.

Another lesson learned from natural disasters is that healthcare professionals who may be called upon to assist with disaster relief should be up to date with tetanus, hepatitis A, and other preventative injections.

Hospitals are the most comprehensive community health resource. As the last link in the community chain of readiness, the hospital is the organization that, by default, will have to make up for inadequacies in community preparedness.

Hospitals must follow federal legislation known as **EMTALA** (the Emergency Medical Treatment and Labor Act), which governs what a hospital must do when clients present themselves. If the emergency department (ED) is closed because of client overload or to protect the health of current clients, by federal law the hospital is not allowed to turn away clients. EMTALA ensures that all individuals who appear at an ED must be screened, evaluated, and stabilized before being transferred. If the State Survey Agency determines that a violation has occurred, it begins the process to terminate the hospital's Medicare provider agreement. Triage is not equivalent to medical screening. A hospital could easily be overwhelmed in a disaster, even when victims are processed in the field via triage.

Bioterrorism Response Act

The Public Health Security and Bioterrorism Response Act of 2002, signed into law in June 2002, authorized $4.3 billion to combat terrorism. As of January 2005, the U.S. Department of **Homeland Security** (DHS) has provided $2.2 billion in counterterrorism grants to the states. The federal government has focused on three components: detection, treatment, and containment.

One aspect of the law is to allocate funds for the training of healthcare workers, including nurses. The American Nurses Association (ANA), together with Health and Human Services (HHS), has established the National Nurses Response Team (NNRT). This team, made up of a large number of nurses, is poised to respond to any major disaster, such as an anthrax or smallpox attack.

In the event of a disaster, NNRT nurses, as well as other healthcare professionals, will be "federalized," thus receiving umbrella coverage for licensure, liability, and expenses. Deployments will be limited to 2 weeks. If a biological assault were to occur, healthcare professionals may well be the first to recognize it. Early detection and response to a threat to public health will make the difference between containment and catastrophe.

To encourage hospitals to be ready to combat bioterrorism, the federal Health Resources and Services Administration has provided millions of dollars in grants, including $800,000 to each of 10 hospitals designated as disaster resource centers that will coordinate emergency training and preparedness. These centers will be required to implement procedures that can deal with a "worst case scenario" or a disaster affecting hundreds of thousands of casualties.

In the aftermath of 9/11, the DHS was created. The DHS coordinates multiple agencies such as FEMA, Transportation Security Administration, Customs and Border Protection, U.S. Coast Guard, and the Secret Service.

Box 15-2 **HOME EMERGENCY KIT***

Prescription medications (to last a minimum of 1 month)
First aid kit and handbook; gloves for work and protection
Bottled water (1 gallon/individual/day; minimum 15 days)
Nonperishable foods that do not have to be prepared; comfort snack foods high in protein and calories; can opener
Extra pet food
Battery or hand-cranked radio, extra batteries
Emergency lighting (flashlights, oil lamps)
Cellular phone or CB radio
Emergency cash in small bills
Emergency phone numbers
Tools and supplies: whistle (to alert rescuers to your location); wrench (to turn off water and gas); duct tape (for broken windows, etc.); buckets and heavy plastic bags for waste
Blankets, sleeping bags, warm clothing, rain gear
Comfort items (games, books, teddy bears, and the like)
Special items for adults (contact lens equipment, glasses) and children (formula, diapers, powdered milk)
Place items in waterproof containers that are easily accessible.
Replace perishable items (water, food, medications, batteries) yearly.

*An emergency planning and preparation guide can be found on the DHS website.

The Disaster Medical Assistance Team (DMAT) is a regional group under the control of Homeland Security. These groups are trained to activate as a unit that can deploy for any type of disaster; they are trained to provide care for any type of casualty. The three major responsibilities of DMAT are triage, staging, and providing medical care.

Nurses are an essential part of the disaster team and must be prepared to function in the event of either a man-made or a natural disaster. To accomplish this effectively, nurses must have a personal and family disaster plan (Box 15-2 ■), for it is difficult to care for others if one's own family is not safe.

Disaster Impact on the Infrastructure

When a disaster occurs, the impact on the infrastructure may be severe. Services and delivery systems, transportation, utilities, fuel, food, water supplies, and communication systems may be affected. Disaster experts point out that when one of the support systems breaks down, it has a domino effect that can impact all elements of the infrastructure. Some of the ways in which the infrastructure can be affected after a disaster are shown in Table 15-1 ■.

Disaster Mitigation

When examining how to mitigate the effects of a disaster, safety precautions and preparation must be considered first, that is,

Table 15-1 Effects of Disasters on Community Services

Service	Effect
Transportation	Inability to get emergency service personnel into the affected area
	Inability to transport victims away from the area
Electrical	Increased risk of fire and electrical shock
	Possible disruption to transportation system if downed lines are across roads
Telephone	Lost contact between victims, service providers, and family members
	System overload due to calls from and to friends or relatives
Water	Disruption of service to homes, businesses, and medical providers
	Inadequate water supply for firefighting
	Increased risk to public health if there is extensive damage to the water supply or if it becomes contaminated
Fuel supplies	Increased risk of fire or explosion from ruptured fuel lines
	Risk of asphyxiation from natural gas leaks in confined areas

FIGURE 15-1 A Community Emergency Response Team (CERT) organizational structure.

personal safety, home preparation, and community preparation. Individual safety and home preparation need to be dealt with on a personal level. Focusing on both natural and manmade disasters, each family or community should develop a Preparedness Plan. In addition, each healthcare facility must have its own Preparedness Plan, developed enough to implement under the chaotic circumstances of a disaster.

The purpose of this chapter is to focus on natural and manmade disasters, such as a terrorist event, and to suggest how the medical community, specifically nurses, could develop their own Preparedness Plan to cope with a mass casualty disaster.

Community Response Plan

Apart from personal safety and home preparation before a disaster, a planned community response is a critical element. A CERT that is trained and prepared to intervene will do more to mitigate disaster outcomes than any other planned approach (Figure 15-1 ■). A CERT organizational structure would look like this:

Strategic Plan for Responding to Biological or Chemical Terrorism

The **Centers for Disease Control and Prevention (CDC)** has formulated a Strategic Planning Workgroup to combat the deliberate dissemination of biological or chemical agents. The plan includes detection and surveillance, laboratory analysis, emergency response, and communication systems. Success of the plan hinges on the relationship between

medical and public health professionals working together for emergency management.

Five focus areas in the CDC's strategic plan are as follows:

- *Preparedness and Prevention:* Emergency coordinated preparedness teams are to be developed in all cities and states in order to respond effectively. The CDC will assist in developing tools and strategies to prevent and mitigate illness and injury.
- *Detection and Surveillance:* Early detection is critical for prompt responding. The CDC will develop disease surveillance systems, as well as mechanisms for detecting, evaluating, and reporting suspicious events. This will be done in partnership with frontline medical–hospital emergency professionals. Reporting of unexplained injuries and illnesses will be part of routine surveillance systems.
- *Diagnosis and Characterization of Biological–Chemical Agents:* The CDC and its partners will create a multilevel laboratory response network to analyze biological agents. Diagnostic technology will be disseminated to state laboratories for diagnostic confirmation and reference support for terrorism response teams.
- *Response:* The CDC will develop a comprehensive public health response to a terrorist event that will encompass investigation, medical treatment, prophylaxis for infected individuals, and disease prevention and **decontamination** measures.
- *Communication Systems:* The ability of the United States to be prepared and intervene effectively when a terrorist event has been identified is dependent on well-trained healthcare and public health professionals having access to emergency information via state-of-the-art communication systems.

Effective communication with the public is also essential. Through this sophisticated communication network, the CDC will disperse information regarding disease **outbreaks**, dissemination of diagnostic results, and emergency health information.

The DHS and federal, state, and local agencies have developed a series of planning scenarios for various types of disasters. These include a general description, timeline dynamics, secondary events, key implications, interventions, and recovery. They were designed to provide the foundation structure for the development of national preparedness standards from which capabilities can be measured. Please check the Homeland Security website for more information about disaster planning for your facility.

The Joint Commission Standards

The Joint Commission has focused on security management to protect those involved in assistance in case of disaster. The plan provides for designation of personnel to report and investigate security incidents, provide identification for participants, and control access and egress to sensitive areas. It was modified to include communication and coordination between healthcare organizations.

To meet The Joint Commission standards, hospital EDs are expected to include four specific phases of disaster management: mitigation, preparedness, response, and recovery. They are also expected to participate in at least one annual drill.

The Joint Commission, together with Homeland Security, has insisted that hospitals strengthen their disaster plans. Hospitals that are renovating or expanding must include new features like decontamination showers, **personal protective equipment (PPE)**, hurricane-resistant glass windows, and reliable power generators. Hospitals must also develop a plan to recover from a disaster and return to predisaster status.

Hospitals Must Be Disaster Ready

A major step in creating a disaster plan is to evaluate the individual hospital's vulnerability in different situations. For example, a hospital on the San Andreas fault in northern California would be vulnerable in different ways than a hospital on the Florida coast. Unique aspects should be taken into account when a **community disaster plan** is formulated. A sample plan for disaster preparation in an earthquake region is shown in Table 15-2 ■. The plan should also be open, up to date, and frequently examined.

Table 15-2 Disaster Preparation—Earthquake

	Focus of Concern-Safety	Preparation and Coping
Power	Electricity—Millions may lose power for days. Gas—Natural gas, the main source of heat for many, will be lost when gas lines rupture. Gas may leak into homes, especially from fallen water heaters. Oil—Damaged oil refineries or oil lines could catch fire, resulting in no oil available.	Have flashlights and batteries or oil lamps on hand. Turn off gas if you smell it. Carefully anchor a gas-powered water heater. Have wood available to burn for heat if you are in a cold climate.
Structures	Homes could become uninhabitable, especially after an earthquake. Inspect any damage before living in a structure. Schools—Many do not yet meet current standards for seismic retrofitting.	Bolt down home to foundation or refit to meet seismic requirements. Have buildings inspected and reinforced. Attach large pieces of furniture to the wall. Plan safe areas in the home (basement) for tornadoes, high winds, or hurricanes. Protect window glass with wood shutters, for example. Keep an ax close in case you have to break out of structure.
Communication	Land lines—Most may survive, but if there is an earthquake or flood, they will be interrupted. Power grid—If down, no calls will go through. Wireless—Cell phone towers could topple, leaving "dead" zones.	Have at least one phone that does not require electricity. Have wind-up radio or extra battery-powered radio to receive information after disaster.
Water	If water comes into the home by pipeline, clean water access could be interrupted or destroyed for weeks or months. Wells could be destroyed by a disaster.	Keep 1 gallon pure water/individual/day for a minimum of 15 days. Have a portable water purifier on hand to make clean drinking water from pools, ponds, creeks, and the like.

Disaster Management

Everyday communication systems are likely to be over-whelmed in a disaster. Preparing for this eventuality by establishing backup and redundant communication systems is essential.

First responders will be local. They will work in conjunction with the state and federal organizations, so there must be an integrated system of in-hospital and out-of-hospital team members with state and federal agencies.

Local systems, both in and out of the hospital, constitute the critical human infrastructure for responding to **weapons of mass destruction (WMD)** incidents. Communication coordination is an essential component in this infrastructure system. One measure is to include a 24-hr wireless radio dedicated communication system to communicate with other healthcare facilities if telephone lines and the internet do not function.

Communication among the triage team establishing victim care priorities out of hospital, the hospital or treatment staff (in-hospital), and state and federal agencies' forensic investigation units must also be established as a cooperative effort. Training drills and scenarios provide practice so that these vital communication functions can be implemented instantly in the event of a WMD incident. To date, states throughout the nation participate in annual countywide disaster drills. It is through these mock events that issues and potential problems are identified.

During a disaster, the local communication system is crucial. There should be one single community-identified individual or small group in command acting as a liaison agent. The state and federal response teams will be integrated into the communication system (Figure 15-2 ■). An example of a local system used nationally might be the **Incident Command System (ICS)**, commonly used

MASS CASUALTY COMMUNITY-WIDE COMMUNICATION NETWORK

FIGURE 15-2 A mass casualty community-wide communication network.

among EMS personnel. This logical management command-and-control structure should be part of hospital planning. In this structure, specific roles carry specific duties and responsibilities. Each position has a prioritized list of tasks that are checked off as they are completed. When an emergency occurs, the "incident commanders" take charge. They can appoint liaison or safety officers or any other position to communicate back to any local or regional ICS, according to the needs created by the emergency. This system organizes emergency responses into five categories: command, planning, operations, logistics, and administration.

A new program introduced by the CDC expands on the ICS model. This program, National Incident Management System (IMS), or NIMS, includes guidelines that all community organizations, including healthcare facilities, are required to follow if they receive grant funds for disaster preparation. All employees involved in disaster response must show evidence of having learned about the NIMS guidelines.

Hospital Evacuation Plans

Evacuation plans must be in place with a designated authority who will order the implementation. There are several types of evacuation:

- *Shelter in Place:* Staying where everyone is may be the safest plan, especially if there is a known contaminant released in the area or it is too dangerous to leave due to a storm, hurricane, etc.
- *Moving Either Up or Down Levels:* Moving all people (clients, staff, and visitors) to another, safer level. Examples are moving up to avoid flood waters or down to the basement to take shelter from a tornado or an **airborne attack**.
- *Total Evacuation:* Removing all people from a building and relocating them to a safe area.

Once the evacuation plan is in place, the staff must be drilled on a regular basis so that the plan may be carried out safely.

The hospital should also have a plan to accommodate special populations if they must evacuate the hospital (Box 15-3 ■). For example, if they must evacuate babies, they should have on hand special aprons that hold several babies in pockets.

Box 15-3 **HOSPITAL EVACUATION**

During superstorm Sandy in 2012, Manhattan evacuated clients from area hospitals. Officials described large-scale power failures in critical areas, including the emergency room, the transplant unit, and obstetrics, where emergency systems did not function. In some instances, clients were connected to battery-operated monitors and pumps. In addition, many of the hospitals appeared to have no emergency or landline phones on some units. Nurses were the front line in assisting with evacuation efforts.

Source: Sifferlin (2012)

Internal (or In-Hospital) Communication

Hospitals will have to expand their sphere of influence to include community-level teams. They must have an ongoing, open channel of communication with emergency response teams who are notified first of an MCI. A community-wide network with a single channel of communication is necessary.

Family and friends, calling to learn about their loved ones after the arrival of casualties, can rapidly overload the system and isolate the hospital. To cope with this problem, a single communication site for obtaining victim and locator information should be established. The Red Cross or comparable organization may serve as this third-party, off-site source of information.

A clear and open information system, using both telecommunications and a position-to-position cascade in the event of the primary system being overloaded, is necessary. This cascade should be designated by position (e.g., emergency room supervisor), not individual, due to turnover, multiple shifts, and personnel reassignment during a disaster. One hospital instituted a text message alert that could be sent to many personnel at one time. In addition to a communication system being established, adequate equipment, such as cell phones, walkie-talkies, even runners, must be available because phone landlines may be totally overwhelmed.

Triage Systems

Triage is from a French word (*trier*) meaning "to sort." It is a medical process of prioritizing treatment urgency. One example of a triage system is **START**, developed in the 1980s in California. An acronym for "simple triage and rapid treatment," this standardized system provides a framework for triage decisions, especially when triaging large numbers of victims at an emergency incident.

ED personnel use triage to quickly assess large numbers of people with multiple problems. Rapid identification in the hospital is important to determine which clients require immediate treatment and which can safely wait.

A three-level triage system has been used for years to differentiate the levels of emergency cases waiting to be seen. A five-level system (discussed later in this section) is preferred by some, because it decreases the ambiguity of the middle level of emergency care (where most casualties fall). There are several methods of categorizing casualties according to the three-level system. One option is as follows:

1. **Emergent** triage refers to a life-threatening or potentially life-threatening condition that requires immediate treatment. These conditions could include multisystem failure, cardiopulmonary arrest, bleeding, airway loss, multiple **trauma**, severe shock, cervical spine injury, and so on.

2. **Immediate** or Urgent triage is not life-threatening or acute, but refers to clients who need treatment as soon as possible (within 2 hr). These clients have stable vital signs and there is no immediate crisis. This category would include fever, minor burns, lacerations, significant pain, and fractures.

3. The third category is **Nonemergent** or Nonurgent, which includes clients who have a condition that would not be affected by a delay in treatment. These are clients with chronic or minor injuries, strains, rash, back pain, and so on.

A second way of implementing the three-level strategy of triage is as follows:

1. **Immediate (I)**—the victim has a life-threatening injury (airway, bleeding, or shock) that demands immediate attention (the same as Emergent).

2. **Delayed (D)**—the victim has an injury that does not jeopardize the victim's life if definitive treatment is delayed.

3. **Dead (DEAD)**—the victim has no respiration after two attempts to open the airway. (CPR is not performed in a disaster environment because it demands extensive resources, including personnel time.)

The I-D-DEAD strategy is often used if there is a mass casualty disaster, because **the goal of triage is to do the greatest good for the greatest number**. Triage must occur as quickly as possible after victims are located.

An example of a five-level system of triage is the Emergency Severity Index (ESI), developed by two physicians in the late 1990s. Table 15-3 ■ shows the five levels of the ESI. The assessment begins with whether the client has a life-threatening condition or if the problem is potentially fatal. Included in this assessment are vital signs and, for the lower acuity casualty, the number of resources required. A level from 1 (most acute) to 5 (least acute) is assigned. Some U.S. hospitals have switched from a three- to a five-level system and have developed their own criteria. A five-level system improves client flow and allows nonacute clients to be screened without taking space in an ED bed. Many hospitals feel that this system is more effective and reliable than the three-level system for handling disaster casualties.

Field Triage

During a disaster, instead of a finite number of victims coming to EDs that are able to utilize all of the hospital's resources, victims may arrive in huge numbers that overwhelm the ED. In these cases, triage must occur in the field, thus the term *field triage*.

Field triage is used in cases of major disaster—either natural (earthquake, tornado, hurricane), or manmade, such as a chemical spill, plane crash, explosion, fire, or a terrorist event. Field triage is done when the numbers of injured exceed the resources of any emergency medical personnel at the scene. Thus, decisions will be triage driven, not treatment driven. Victims are classified according to a color-coding tag system. See Box 15-4 ■ for triage categories used during a disaster.

Box 15-4 TRIAGE CATEGORIES FOR USE DURING A DISASTER

Field Triage

Red	=	Emergent (hyperacute—1st priority)
Yellow	=	Immediate (serious—2nd priority)
Green	=	Urgent (injured—3rd priority)
Blue	=	Nonurgent (first aid and psychological support)
Black	=	Dead or imminently dying

Catastrophic Triage (First Option)

I	=	Immediate (life-threatening)
D	=	Delayed (may delay treatment without death)
Dead	=	Dead

Catastrophic Triage (Second Option)

Red tag = Potential to survive
No other victims tagged.

START Categories

Color Tag			Decontamination Priority
Red	=	Immediate	1. Serious signs/symptoms Known agent **contamination**
Yellow	=	Delayed	2. Moderate-to-minimal signs/symptoms Known agent or **aerosol** contamination Close to point of release
Green	=	Minor	3. Minimal signs/symptoms No known **exposure** to agent
Black	=	Deceased/Dying	4. Very serious signs/symptoms Grossly contaminated Unresponsive

Table 15-3 Emergency Severity Index

Level No.	Level Name	Description
Level 1	Most Acute	Life-threatening—potentially fatal
Level 2	Emergent	Unstable with signs of potential deterioration. Includes vital signs assessment: Is this a high-risk situation? Is the client experiencing new onset confusion, lethargy, or disorientation? Is the client experiencing severe pain or distress?
Level 3	Lower Acuity	Stable—resources required from this level to 5: labs, IV fluids, ECG, x-ray, IV, IM, laceration repair (versus complex laceration repair)
Level 4	Less Urgent	Stable—just one type of resource anticipated (e.g., x-ray)
Level 5	Least Acute	Not life-threatening—minimal resources

Catastrophic Triage

When events are cascading out of control or disaster has wiped out primary treatment resources, the choice of triage system will be limited. Basically, there are two options. One option is to use the first and second steps identified below, and the other is severely limited to those who have the potential to survive—they will be tagged Red. Thus, triage categories may change during a disaster. The primary assessment is one of acuity, but the victim must have the ability to survive. Making these decisions is terribly difficult, but this system is the only realistic method of categorizing thousands of victims from a deadly disaster.

First Step The most direct and expedient method of field triage is to evaluate victims according to these categories:

I	=	Immediate treatment
D	=	Delayed treatment
Dead	=	Dead

Everyone must be tagged.

Second Step Treat victims immediately.

Check airway and breathing rate	►	Initiate airway management
Check circulation	►	Initiate bleeding control
Check mental status	►	Treat for shock

Document Results Documentation is necessary for:

Effective deployment of resources

Information on location of victims

Quick record of number of casualties by degree of severity

Triage Victim Flow

From triage, victims are taken to a designated medical treatment area (Immediate Care, Delayed Care, or Morgue), and from this location they are transported out of the disaster area. There are various methods of implementing triage that include minimal to massive numbers of victims. Whichever triage method or strategy is chosen, the community or identified team must be aware of the specific categories.

Decontamination

Every facility should have a protocol and site for decontamination, both outside and inside. Rooms with negative pressure are especially important for toxic areas and soiled infectious areas. For example, if there is a **pandemic** flu, affected clients should be isolated and the air in those rooms exhausted to the outside to prevent it from contaminating the rest of the facility.

Triage and Decontamination

While triage is an essential component of disaster management, decontamination prioritization is also critical to determine the need for and order of victim decontamination. Both processes may be implemented simultaneously. The same triage rule applies, namely, to provide the greatest benefit to the greatest number.

If there are mass casualty victims inside a "hot zone," the Incident Commander may assign personnel to manage both medical triage and decontamination. The first step may be to group victims into ambulatory and nonambulatory categories. Prioritization of these victims may be done using the medical triage system, START.

The highest priority for Ambulatory decontamination (classified as *Immediate*) casualties includes:

- Victims closest to the point of release
- Those who report exposure to aerosol
- Victims with evidence of liquid deposits on skin or clothing
- Those who are clinically symptomatic (i.e., shortness of breath) but were not as close to point of release
- Victims evidencing conventional injuries, such as open wounds

Nonambulatory casualties include:

- Victims who are unconscious or unresponsive and will remain in place while further prioritization for decontamination occurs
- Those triaged as *Delayed* (casualties who may have serious injuries, but who can wait without compromising their outcome)

Highest priority for overall decontamination includes casualties:

- Who are medically triaged as *Immediate*
- Who are in need of lifesaving medical procedures that can be performed on the spot
- Who have been exposed to **nerve agents**—decontamination as soon as possible may be lifesaving

Posttriage Organization

After evaluation and prioritizing victims into treatment groups and providing immediate lifesaving measures, clients will be transported to three locations: Immediate Treatment, Delayed Treatment, and the Morgue.

Treatment area personnel will then:

1. Perform additional *triage* as needed.
2. Complete *physical assessment* (head to toe) to determine extent of injuries.
3. Render *first aid* if needed.

After this posttriage assessment, personnel will provide immediate treatment for burns, open wounds, fractures, sprains, hypothermia, frostbite, and so on. After triage and posttriage assessment, it is essential to document the number of victims in each category (immediate, delayed), as well as the dead victims. See Unit 15.3 for skills in posttriage.

The number of victims may exceed local capacity for treatment. Survivors will assist others, but they may not know lifesaving or postdisaster survival techniques.

Outside resources will be requested. The U.S. government has an action plan in place.

This federal response plan includes a stockpile of specialized medical supplies assembled in secret warehouses nationwide. More than 100 air cargo containers (each one fills a Boeing 747) are ready to be sent to any city in the United States within 12 hours. State and local officials can track the cargo sent by ground transport to a final, local destination.

When the CDC, in consult with local officials, agrees that an attack has occurred and the local system is insufficient to cope, a container of supplies is dispersed, as well as healthcare providers and health personnel, if needed.

Weapons of Mass Destruction

Biological Agents

Biological terrorism is the use of specific agents to cause harm or kill people. It includes the use of organisms such as bacteria, **viruses**, and **toxins** (Table 15-4 ■). The use of biological agents as weapons poses a difficult problem for public health officials, because these agents present with an insidious onset and mimic natural epidemics of influenza. Symptoms may take days to develop before victims seek medical care.

These agents are classified as a threat to national security because they possess unique characteristics:

- They are easily disseminated or transmitted from individual to individual and could be dispersed over a wide geographical area.
- They cause high mortality with the potential for major public health impact.
- They require specific actions in order to secure public health preparedness.

Biological weapons have a history that goes back as far as the sixth century. Recent history reveals that many nations have biowarfare capability with agents such as anthrax, plague, and smallpox. In spite of the fact that the Geneva Convention prohibits use of biological and chemical warfare, and in 1972 many nations agreed to stop research, the United States remains vulnerable to a biowarfare attack.

A biological agent cannot be detected directly. The way it will be identified is when victims arrive at clinics and hospitals and, either through the awareness and perception of professionals who correlate the unusual influx of victims with similar symptoms, or through a review of surveillance and "putting the pieces together," the biological cause will be identified.

To accomplish the goal of identifying a biological attack, several steps need to be taken.

1. Set up bioterrorism education programs and training for healthcare professionals to teach how to recognize signs and symptoms of a biological attack.

2. Prepare and distribute educational materials to inform and remind healthcare professionals of the signs and symptoms of various biological weapons.
3. Establish communication systems to ensure that accurate information is delivered.
4. Recognize the signs and symptoms of major high-priority agents.

Chemical Agents

Chemical terrorism is the deployment of chemical weapons with the intention of causing havoc, harm, and death to the recipients. Their release quickly causes death, especially if released in an enclosed space. The U.S. Army Medical Research Institute of Chemical Defense has classified these agents as potential weapons:

- Choking agents (phosgene, chlorine)
- Blood agents (hydrogen cyanide)
- Mustard agents (mustard, oxime)
- Nerve agents (tabun, sarin, VX)
- Incapacitating agents (agent 15, BZ)

These weapons inflict painful external and internal injuries, psychological devastation, and death. An act of chemical terrorism is overt, because the effects of these agents on people are immediate and obvious as the agents are absorbed through the skin, mucous membranes, or pulmonary system.

Perhaps the most dangerous of these are the nerve agents (sarin, tabun, VX), which are extremely toxic and easy to disseminate in the air. The nerve agents kill people by binding up the compound acetylcholinesterase, which is the body's "off" switch. When acetylcholinesterase is significantly decreased or absent in the body, the glands and voluntary muscles continue to be stimulated, eventually wear out, and the body can no longer sustain healthy function.

Decontamination of some chemical agents is time- and labor-intensive and requires tremendous resources. However, if chemical agents are widely dispersed, every one of thousands of individuals affected cannot be individually decontaminated. In some cases, decontamination may not be required for certain chemical incidents. The triage team may remove victims to an uncontaminated area and/or send victims home to shower.

Radiation

The threat of nuclear or radioactive terrorism in the United States is considered to be real. While we cannot predict the form this terrorist event might take (Box 15-5 ■), we can prepare to cope with the situation should it arise.

Radiation is unique, in that exposure may occur without individuals coming in direct contact with the radiation source through inhalation, ingestion, or absorption through the skin.

Radioactive substances emit radiation in the form of rays (waves) or extremely small particles. *Waveforms* are x-ray and gamma rays; *particle forms* are alpha, beta, and neutron.

Table 15-4 Bioterrorism Agents

Disease	Signs and Symptoms	Incubation Period	Individual-to-Individual Transmission
Anthrax (**inhalational**) Organism—*Bacillus anthracis*	Nonspecific flulike, with fever, malaise, fatigue, cough Delayed symptoms—severe respiratory distress	1–7 days (usually 48 hr) Can be 6 weeks	No
Botulism (inhalational) Organism—*Clostridium botulinum* toxin	Increasing muscle weakness, drooping eyelids, blurred vision, difficulty speaking and swallowing; progresses down body to paralysis	12–36 hr after exposure	No
Pneumonic Plague Organism—*Yersinia pertis*	Sudden onset of high fever, chills, chest pain, headache, and cough with bloody sputum; possible vomiting and diarrhea Advanced: skin lesions, respiratory failure	2–3 days (1–6 days after exposure)	Yes, through droplet, aerosol
Smallpox Organism—*Variola major* virus	Sudden onset of high fever, headache, and backache; then painful rash of small, red spots starts on face and spreads over entire skin surface; progresses from macules to papules.	7–17 days after exposure (average is 12 days)	Yes, airborne, droplet or direct contact with skin lesions (until scabs fall off in 3–4 weeks)
Typhoid Tularemia Organism—*Francisella tularensis*	Sudden onset of high fever, weakness, weight loss, chest pain, and cough	3–5 days after exposure	No
Viral Hemorrhagic Fevers (Filoviruses, such as Ebola and Marburg; arenaviruses, such as Lassa and Junin)	Sudden onset of fever, muscle aches, and profound weakness, followed by circulatory compromise	2–21 days after exposure	Yes, risk higher during late stages of disease

---

Box 15-5 RADIATION EXPOSURE EVENTS

Possible terrorist events involving radiation dispersal could be:

- An attack on a nuclear facility or detonated nuclear weapon
- A radiation dispersal device: "dirty bomb" (embedding radioactive material in a conventional explosive)
- Radioactive material dispersal

Ionizing radiation is radiation that has enough energy to cause atoms to lose electrons and become ions. Charged particles are emitted from ionizing radiation. These particles (alpha and beta) are the most likely to be dispersed after a terrorist attack. They may adhere to airborne dust particles or attach to clothing; they could be inhaled, causing internal contamination. Beta rays are found in "fallout" and alpha particles are emitted from plutonium. Gamma rays, also an example of ionizing radiation, are emitted in a nuclear blast and have high penetration potential. They cause severe damage to the individual but do not require decontamination. In the event of a nuclear attack, both rays and particle forms are likely to be dispersed.

A cell that has been exposed to any type of radiation is damaged and may die. If a terrorist event causes radiation to be released, it could result in either external or internal hazards ranging from major to insignificant.

Internal–External Exposure   Exposure to radiation from a source outside the body is external exposure; internal exposure occurs when radioactive material is assimilated into body tissues and causes damage from the inside. Internal exposure occurs from inhalation, ingestion, or insertion, such as a radioactive implant of iodine-131.

A critical point of discrimination is whether the victim was exposed to or contaminated by radiation. If exposed, the victim is *not* a hazard to others. The radiation is absorbed by or passes through the body, but does not result in radioactive contamination.

Radioactive contamination as radioactive particulate material is a major cause for concern. The source of contamination, resulting from spillage, leakage, deliberate dispersal, or attachment to dust particles in the air, can be passed on to healthcare workers. If this were to occur, external exposure

Treatment	Death Rate if Untreated	Death Rate if Treated	Isolation Precautions/ Standard Precautions
Antibiotics, including ciprofloxacin 500 mg PO q12 hr Doxycycline 100 mg PO q12 hr; also, combined IV and PO	High	Improved chance for survival. Once symptoms appear, treatment is less effective.	Standard Precautions
Antitoxin—requires skin testing; Supportive care and ventilation until victim can breathe independently	High	Low, if breathing can be supported for duration of illness (weeks to months, in some cases)	Standard Precautions
Antibiotics, including ciprofloxacin 400 mg IV q12 hr Doxycycline 200 mg PO, then 100 mg PO q12 hr	Almost always fatal	Low; treatment highly effective if taken within 24 hr of first symptoms	Bubonic form: Standard Precautions Pneumonic form: Standard Precautions plus Droplet Precautions until 48–72 hr after antibiotic treatment
Vaccination is effective if given within 3–4 days of exposure; passive **immunization** with VIG if 3 days postexposure.	3%–30%	If vaccinated, less than 1%	Strict **Isolation** Precautions: Airborne (includes N95 mask) and Contact, in addition to Standard Precautions
Antibiotics, including doxycycline and ciprofloxacin	33%	1%–3% if treated within 24 hr of exposure	Standard Precautions
Little is known. Antiviral agents, such as ribavirin, may be useful. Development of hemorrhagic bioweapons is frightening to consider but impractical to accomplish. These agents are far more hazardous to the perpetrators than other agents. They are fragile to transport. Their effects are slower and more prone to fail than agents with short **incubation periods** and airborne agents.	15%–90%	Unknown	Strict Isolation Precautions including negative-pressure room with anteroom

could also become internal exposure as radiation is incorporated into the body.

The 2011 Great East Japan Earthquake in Fukushima, Japan, brought the world's attention to the potential for widespread radiation exposure resulting from a natural disaster. The earthquake (measuring 9.0) and its aftershocks did considerable damage, but the tsunami it caused did far more. It shut down power to all of the 11 nuclear power plants in the region. Eight had backup generators and achieved "cold shutdown" within 4 days. The backup generators at the three Fukushima plants, however, were destroyed by the tsunami, and radioactive waste was swept directly into the sea. In addition, venting of the nuclear units and hydrogen explosions discharged radioactive materials into the atmosphere. According to Reuters news service of March 17, 2015, more than 1 million tons of debris from Fukushima was still afloat in the Pacific 4 years after the disaster and was expected to continue to wash ashore on the west coast of the United States for another 3 years.

Measuring Radiation   The term **RAD** (radiation absorbed dose) is a unit of measure for radiation exposure; 1 RAD results in absorption of 100 ergs of energy/gram of tissue exposed. The international system now measures the unit of exposure by **Gray** (Gy); (1 Gy equals 100 RADs).

Radiation dose is a specific calculated measurement of the amount of energy deposited in the body. The unit of dose is called **REM**, which takes into account the type of radiation. The technical specifics of exposure and dose are not necessary for the reader to understand, but it is important to know the dangers of exposure and understand how to measure external radiation levels.

A survey instrument measures radiation levels. The readout is in units of R (which can be either RAD or REM), which is exposure or dose. An instrument reading of 50R/hr means that a healthcare worker staying in the exposed area for 1 hr will receive a 50-RAD exposure. Some instruments, called radiation dosimeters, measure dose over time; these should be worn by personnel working in a contaminated area. A radiation detection device (film badge) should be worn by personnel who come in contact with the exposed area or victims. Both survey instruments and dosimeters have limitations. Survey instruments need to be recalculated at regular intervals, and their batteries must be checked and replaced periodically. Dosimeters also must be calibrated and checked at regular intervals.

Health Effects of Radiation A victim contaminated by radiation is at risk—how much risk is dependent on how much radiation is absorbed. Victims who absorb less than 0.75 Gy will not experience symptoms of exposure. Those who absorb 8 Gy could die. Between 0.75 and 8 Gy, the victim could develop acute radiation syndrome (ARS). See Box 15-13, Acute Radiation Syndromes in Skill 15.2.5 for further information.

Low exposures do not cause major damage. High exposure may kill cells, cause bone marrow damage or birth defects, and significantly increase the incidence of cancer. Regardless of the type of exposure, triage must focus on life-threatening injury before radiological injury.

Background Radiation We are all exposed to a certain amount of radiation from our daily environment. This is known as background radiation and is derived from natural sources such as radiation from outer space; industrial, academic, or military uses of radiation; and radiation used in medicine. All these sources combine to give us a background radiation dose of 0.360 REM per individual per year.

Ethical Considerations

When we consider the profession of nursing, a central theme must be the ethical considerations of nursing practice. In the chaotic and challenging conditions of a terrorist event, ethics may seem unimportant. However, while they may not be addressed overtly during a disaster, ethical considerations form the bedrock of nursing interventions.

In the midst of a crisis, decision making, nursing judgments, indeed, even functioning ability will rest on one's code of ethics. To review the Code of Ethics for Nurses, see Chapter 1.

Diversity Considerations

If a mass casualty terrorist event were to occur in the United States, it would likely affect people of every class and culture. It is important for nurses to be aware of the impact of culture, beliefs, and values on responses to a disaster. Cultural competence in disaster nursing should be addressed because nurses may be called upon to perform in areas where they are not familiar with the diverse client population. They may not speak the language of the ethnic groups and may not be familiar with the cultural components. They can, however, convey concern, empathy, and the willingness to communicate with the victims who are sustaining the effects of a disaster. Nurses who travel to a disaster area should learn from and model local helpers so that their actions are culturally sensitive. Simply being aware of diversity within populations will help the emergency team

to accept different responses to a MCI and relate in a sensitive, appropriate manner.

During the initial assessment after a disaster, the nurse should be aware of the following cultural components:

- Language—(non–English-speaking) communication
- Cultural background and beliefs
- Values, patterns relating to health practices
- Religious practices—limitations
- Nutritional parameters
- Assessment variances for people of color

Summary

After the terrorist attacks of 9/11, 800 public health and military professionals participated at a joint conference. They identified the chief challenge in formulating a strategic plan for preparedness response as "lack of training among frontline responders—healthcare providers and nurses—and inadequate planning at the local, state, and federal levels." Combining these deficit areas—lack of planning, identified skills, and training—helps us to design a framework for nurses to acquire the knowledge necessary for strategic planning and preparedness. Nurses are a vital part, along with physicians and other healthcare professionals, of preparedness programs throughout the country. Nurses must identify their own skill level and the skills necessary to participate as members of the medical response team (Box 15-6 ■).

The term *skill* may be applied to performance. A complex series of actions to accomplish a task may be called skilled performance. A skill can be learned, but it takes experience in performing step-by-step actions before a well-defined response pattern is accomplished (Box 15-7 ■). In addition, the change from hesitant responses in the middle of performing a skill to a competent, automatic response takes place only with practice. Thus, the skills necessary to participate in a medical response to a disaster caused by a WMD must be identified, practiced, and mastered.

This chapter identifies certain skills, drawn from performance-based learning objectives, that nurses must acquire to become contributing members of a disaster response team.

Box 15-6 PREPLANNING FOR RESPONSE TO DISASTER

- RN should notify employer in writing of any disaster or emergency preparedness education.
- RN should request written approval for participation on an emergency response team.
- RN should provide employer with ongoing documentation of all continuing education related to disaster preparedness.
- RNs who are preapproved members of emergency preparedness team should give written notice to employer of deployment to emergency team.

Box 15-7 **TERRORISM RESPONSE DRILL: RECOMMENDATIONS FOR FUTURE EVENTS**

1. Appoint an individual as "point" who will maintain communication between command center and ED. Secure two-way radios for hospital staff.

2. Implement a client tracking form and use ID bands to track unidentified clients.

3. Use ID bands and instant photos to identify children and match with parents.

4. Request extra social workers.

5. Create an up-to-date clinical protocol of all potential bioterrorism agents and their treatment, and distribute to all staff in the ED and hospital.

6. Have necessary supplies on hand and develop standardized procedures for obtaining extra supplies during disaster.

7. Plan to call in extra security immediately after a disaster is recognized; assign extra space for dead victims.

CLINICAL ALERT

Although the skills in this chapter have been formulated according to the latest information and protocols available at the time of publication, events change. Nurses must check periodically with the appropriate government sources (i.e., CDC, DHS, NIOSH, AHA, APIC, The Joint Commission, FEMA, and so on) for the latest information and updates on procedures and protocols.

Nursing Diagnoses

The following nursing diagnoses are appropriate to use on client care plans when the components relate to a client who requires treatment related to a disaster.

NURSING DIAGNOSIS	RELATED TO . . .
Ineffective Community Coping	Disaster-overwhelmed community resources Lack of access to healthcare facilities Infrastructure (services) not functioning at 100% Deficits in social support
Deficient Knowledge	Lack of information about bioterrorism agent, triage, decontamination methods, treatment
Ineffective Protection	First responders' and healthcare personnel protection not appropriate for identified bioterrorism agent
Ineffective Role Performance	First responders and healthcare personnel unclear or unable to function in designated roles
Ineffective Health Management	Communication network inadequate for crisis

Natural Disasters

Nursing Process Data

ASSESSMENT Database

- Identify need for information on creating a safety plan for disasters.
- Determine components of a safety plan, including a disaster supply kit.
- Assess need for teaching earthquake safety.
- Identify epidemiologic features of diarrhea-related diseases.
- Assess knowledge of preventive techniques for diarrhea-related diseases.

PLANNING Objectives

- To assist client to create a safety plan for disasters
- To include components of a disaster supply kit
- To identify major challenges (medical or health and infra-structure) after a natural disaster
- To teach disaster safety to appropriate clients
- To prevent diarrhea-related diseases

IMPLEMENTATION Procedures

DOCUMENTATION AND EVALUATION

Expected Outcomes

- Clients are taught how to create a safety plan for disasters.
- Clients learn how to prepare for an emergency.
- Clients know what to include in a disaster kit.
- Disaster safety principles are taught to nurses and clients.
- Diarrhea-related diseases are identified early with subsequent interventions.

Unexpected Outcomes/Alternative Actions

Pearson Nursing Student Resources

Find additional review materials at
nursing.pearsonhighered.com.
Prepare for success with NCLEX®-style practice questions and Skill Checklists.

Skill 15.1.1 | Creating a Safety Plan for Disasters

Procedure

1. Hold a meeting with family members to make a plan in case a disaster occurs.
2. Pick two places to meet, one outside the home and the other outside the neighborhood.
3. Choose someone in another state whom all members of the family can contact during a disaster.
4. Formulate an evacuation plan so that everyone will know how to leave the area.
5. Prepare your home for an emergency.

   a. Teach family how to turn off all utilities (especially gas).
   b. Post emergency numbers in a central location.
   c. Put smoke detectors in every room and have fire extinguishers accessible.
   d. Fix potential hazards in the home (anchor water heater and heavy bookcases in earthquake areas, repair frayed wires, prune trees, and remove dead branches in hurricane areas).
   e. Learn first aid and take a CPR course and have first aid supplies available.
   f. Have emergency supplies and a disaster kit available.

6. Include the basics in a disaster supply kit (Box 15-8 ■).

Box 15-8 DISASTER SUPPLY KIT

- Water—1 gallon/individual/day for a minimum of 1–2 weeks
- Food—selection of ready-to-eat foods, high in protein, for 1–2 weeks
- First aid kit with bandages, gloves, soap, H_2O_2, OTC medications for pain, stomach ills, and so on
- Prescription drugs (with copies of prescriptions) that are essential for health (insulin, heart meds [1 month supply], and the like)
- Supplies—radio (battery-operated) with extra batteries, flashlights or oil-burning lamps, wood for heat in a fireplace, personal maintenance items (contact lens supplies, feminine products, denture needs, extra glasses, and such)
- Clothing and bedding supplies—warm clothing for winter, blankets, sleeping bags, rain protection gear, and the like
- Family documents—personal identification, all records that are essential (passport, wills, trusts, insurance records)
- Credit card and cash

Check and replenish supplies and kits once a year, practice evacuation procedures, and check your disaster plan.

Skill 15.1.2 | Teaching Clients Earthquake Safety

Note: Different regions are more susceptible to specific types of disasters (e.g., earthquakes on the San Andreas fault, wildfires in dry parts of the Rocky Mountains, floods in low-lying coastal areas or river valleys, tornadoes in the Midwest, and hurricanes on the East Coast and Gulf regions). This skill can be used as a template for disasters of different types.

Procedure

1. Make a plan for you and your family if an earthquake should occur. Create a disaster preparedness plan.
2. Create a disaster kit, for both the home and car (see Box 15-8).
3. Identify potential hazards in the home and have them fixed.
   ➤ **Rationale:** A toppled water heater could cause a fire; loose, large furniture could be a hazard.
4. Teach how to protect oneself during severe shaking.

   a. Indoors: Drop to floor, take cover, and hold on; find a space beside a couch or table. ➤ **Rationale:**

Earthquake specialists advise taking cover beside the item, not under it (such as a car) because when items fall they create a "triangle safe space" beside the large object.

   b. Avoid exterior walls, windows, hanging objects, and cabinets filled with items.
   c. Outdoors: Move to a clear area; avoid buildings, power lines, trees.
   d. Driving: Pull over and stop; set the brake. Wait beside the car (not under it) until shaking stops.

5. Taught that, after a quake, to check for injuries and damage (fire, gas leaks, damaged electrical wiring, downed utility lines, chemical spills, damaged structures).
6. Taught to follow the disaster plan after an earthquake: Listen to communication for safety advisories (Box 15-9 ■), pay attention to safety precautions, and check food and water supplies.

(continued)

Skill 15.1.2 | Teaching Clients Earthquake Safety *(continued)*

Box 15-9 MAJOR CHALLENGES FOLLOWING A NATURAL DISASTER

Medical and Health

Contaminated food and water (sewage)

Sanitation—decomposing bodies

Interruption of existing/traditional medical/health care

Ease of disease transmission

Infections such as malaria and cholera and secondary
  infections (pneumonia)

Insect infestation

Skin infections from open wounds and dirty water

Diseases from animal carcasses and spilled chemicals in homes
  and businesses

Contamination from gas or oil in water

Possible epidemics—malaria, cholera, typhoid, and hepatitis A

Mental health concerns—posttraumatic stress disorder (PTSD)

Infrastructure

Destroyed infrastructure contributing to the above issues

Structural damage to homes, hospitals, and other structures

Downed power lines; no electricity

No public transportation

No communication on landlines; cell towers down

Skill 15.1.3 | Preventing Diarrhea-Related Diseases After a Natural Disaster

Procedure

1. Recognize early clinical features.

   a. Early symptoms include abrupt, painless watery stool,
      vomiting; diarrhea may be mild or fulminating.

   b. Delayed symptoms include water and electrolyte
      depletion leading to thirst, oliguria; if untreated, circulatory
      collapse.

2. Identify organism (e.g., cholera)

   a. Know that incubation period is 1–3 days.

   b. Mode of dissemination is most commonly ingestion of
      contaminated water.

3. Teach preventive techniques.

   a. Purify all drinking water; boil, chlorinate, or use water
      purification tablets.

   b. Wash all vegetables, fruit, and fish in clean water and
      cook thoroughly.

   c. Properly dispose of human excrement.

4. Monitor survivors for other manifestations of illness
   (Table 15-5 ■).

Table 15-5 Monitoring Survivors of Natural Disasters for Signs of Illness*

Potential Illness	Causative Conditions	Occurrence of Symptoms	Manifested Symptoms	Mode of Transmission
West Nile Virus	Standing water (3–4 weeks for mosquito production)	3–14 days after mosquito bite	Meningitis, encephalitis, fever, headache, rash, fatigue, muscle aches	Not spread from individual to individual
Leptospirosis	Exposure to infected animals (dogs, rodents, etc.) or water contaminated with urine of infected animals	2 days to 4 weeks	Symptom range: none to high fever, severe headache, jaundice, muscle aches	Not spread from individual to individual
Vibrio vulnificus	Bacteria living in brackish water	Short time after exposure; rapid progression	Pain, redness, swelling, infected wounds, shock	Not spread from individual to individual; those with weakened immune systems are susceptible
Norovirus	Cramped spaces of shelters	Acute onset after exposure	Vomiting, diarrhea, fever, headache, cramps (lasts 3–4 days)	Acutely contagious, spreads from individual to individual
Tuberculosis	Cramped spaces of evacuation centers	4–12 weeks after exposure	Cough lasting more than 3 weeks, chest pain, fatigue, weight loss, fever, night sweats, chills	Spread through droplets of infected individual

Note: These are the most commonly detected conditions or illnesses following a disaster where thousands of survivors are gathered.

Unit 15.1 Documentation and Evaluation

DOCUMENTATION for Natural Disasters

- Safety plan presented to clients
- A basic disaster supply kit discussed and presented to clients

- Principles of disaster safety taught to clients
- Clinical features and preventive techniques for diarrhea-related diseases

EVALUATION/Critical Thinking

Expected Outcomes

- Clients are taught how to create a safety plan for disasters.
- Clients learn how to prepare for an emergency.
- Clients know what to include in a disaster kit.
- Earthquake safety principles are taught to nurses and clients.
- Diarrhea-related diseases are identified early with subsequent interventions.

Unexpected Outcomes	Alternative Actions
Clients and staff do not acknowledge need for a safety plan.	Hold meetings and bring in consultants to present rationale and need for a safety plan for both man-made and natural disasters.
Clients and staff do not have a disaster supply kit.	Discuss need for a supply kit and the components so that clients and staff will follow through and implement the plan.
Staff and clients are not aware of the major challenges after a natural disaster.	Hold meetings to discuss the major challenges so that all are prepared.
People do not understand the need to learn about disaster safety.	Hold discussion groups about the components of disaster safety for both clients and hospital staff.
Diarrhea-related diseases occur after a natural disaster.	• Include the signs and symptoms of these diseases in the preparedness plan so that staff will be able to recognize them. • Institute preventive measures to combat these diseases immediately after a disaster. • Hold meetings to discuss preventive techniques and have the necessary items available (e.g., water purification tablets).

Bioterrorism Agents, Antidotes, and Vaccinations

Nursing Process Data

ASSESSMENT Database

- Identify epidemiologic features:
  - Rapidly increasing incidence of specific signs and symptoms
  - Unusual number of clients seeking care, especially with flulike symptoms, fever, and respiratory complaints
  - An endemic disease that rapidly emerges
  - Clusters of clients from one area
  - Large numbers of fatalities
- Identify mode of dissemination and incubation period.
- Assess the appropriate therapy/antidotes necessary to treat victims of a bioterrorist attack.
- Assess need for collecting a clinical specimen to identify a specific bioterrorism agent.
- Identify ARS.
- Assess **radiation dose** exposure of client.

PLANNING Objectives

- To recognize a possible terrorist attack
- To provide clinical knowledge to recognize features of a biological–chemical–nuclear attack
- To enhance ability to detect a biological attack by distinguishing signs and symptoms of various agents
- To participate in an effective medical response to a terrorist attack
- To provide focused educational content for healthcare professionals as knowledge base
- To possess the skills to initiate an effective response to a terrorist event
- To be able to respond to a nuclear disaster

IMPLEMENTATION Procedures

DOCUMENTATION AND EVALUATION

Expected Outcomes

- Epidemiologic features of disease are identified.
- Preparedness plans for hospitals are in place and staff are aware of the components.
- Radiation dose remains at safe levels.
- Healthcare workers learn how to respond safely to a nuclear event.
- Victims of a manmade disaster (chemical, biological, or nuclear) are treated according to protocols.

Unexpected Outcomes/Alternative Actions

Pearson Nursing Student Resources

Find additional review materials at
nursing.pearsonhighered.com.
Prepare for success with NCLEX®-style practice questions and Skill Checklists.

Skill 15.2.1 | Identifying Agents of Biological Terrorism

Note: Nurses must understand the danger of biologically toxic agents (Box 15-10 ■).

ANTHRAX

Definition: An acute infectious disease caused by *Bacillus anthracis*, a spore-forming gram-positive bacillus. Human anthrax occurs in three forms: inhalation (the form most dangerous), cutaneous, or gastrointestinal.

Procedure

1. Recognize clinical features. The first line of defense for an outbreak of anthrax is rapid identification.

   a. Inhalation or pulmonary form

      1. Early signs and symptoms: developing within days, nonspecific flulike illness with malaise, dry cough, mild fever, and headache
      2. Delayed signs and symptoms: severe respiratory distress, hemodynamic collapse—victim may die, even with antibiotic treatment

   b. Cutaneous form

      1. Early signs and symptoms: local skin involvement with intense itching; painless, papular lesions (commonly seen on head, forearms, or hands)
      2. Delayed signs and symptoms: papular lesion turned vesicular, developing into black eschar with edema

   c. Gastrointestinal form (from contaminated meat)

      1. Early signs and symptoms: abdominal pain, nausea and vomiting, severe diarrhea
      2. Delayed signs and symptoms: gastrointestinal bleeding and fever; usually fatal after progression to toxemia and sepsis

---

Box 15-10 UNDERSTANDING THE DANGER OF BIOLOGICALLY TOXIC AGENTS

1. Biological incidents will be the most difficult of all attacks for the community to recognize and effectively coordinate a response.
2. Most viruses are useful as bioterror agents—they cause unique signs and symptoms that require intervention and isolation of the victims to prevent spread.
3. Specific incapacitating viral or bacterial agents slowly produce signs and symptoms.

   a. Signs and symptoms are nonspecific and difficult to recognize; onset of incident may remain unknown for days before symptoms appear.
   b. It may be necessary to identify "clusters" of illness—many victims in one location become sick within a short period of time.

4. If agents are detected early, most can be treated with antibiotics or antivirals.
5. The most common form of agents that could be used in a bioterror attack are bacteria.

---

2. Know mode of dissemination and incubation period.

   a. Inhalation of spores: aerosol—no individual-to-individual transmission; Incubation: 2–60 days (usually 48 hr)
   b. Cutaneous: direct contact with skin lesions; 1–7 days
   c. Gastrointestinal ingestion of contaminated food: no individual-to-individual transmission; incubation: 1–7 days

3. Manage decontamination.

   a. Remove contaminated clothing.
   b. Instruct clients to shower thoroughly with soap and water.
   c. Instruct personnel to use **Standard Precautions.**
   d. Decontaminate environment with 0.5% diluted bleach (1 part to 9 parts water), or EPA-approved germicidal agent.

4. Institute isolation precautions. ❶

   a. Inhalation—Standard Precautions; Wash victim thoroughly (use 0.5% diluted bleach for visible contamination); store clothing in sealed plastic bag with biohazard label.
   b. Cutaneous—contact precautions (gown and gloves)
   c. Gastrointestinal—Standard Precautions

5. Assign client placement.

   a. Private room placement *not* necessary.
   b. Airborne transmission does *not* occur.
   c. Skin lesions may be transmitted by direct skin contact only.

6. Implement therapy for anthrax infection.

   a. Ciprofloxacin 400 mg IV q8–12 hr, 500 mg PO q12 hr; doxycycline 200 mg IV (1 dose), 100 mg IV q8–12 hr, or 100 mg PO q12 hr; or amoxicillin may also be ordered.
   b. Continue treatment for 60 days.
   c. Mass casualty—oral therapy with standard doses.

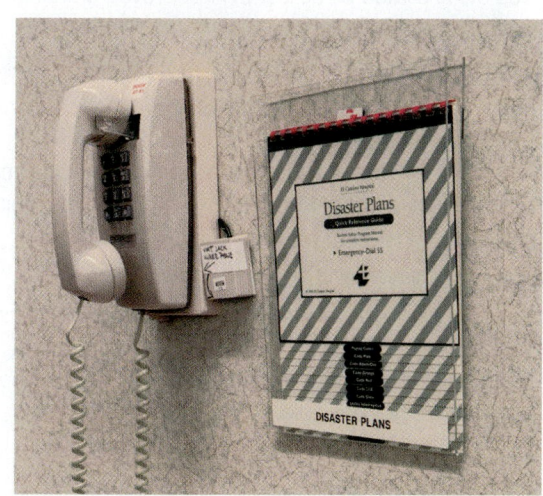

❶ Be familiar with disaster and preparedness plan in the hospital. Perform mock disaster scenarios to maintain skill level and knowledge of procedures if disaster occurs.

(continued)

Skill 15.2.1 | Identifying Agents of Biological Terrorism *(continued)*

PLAGUE

Definition: Acute, severe bacterial infection, caused by gram-negative bacillus. Seen in bubonic or pneumonic form; caused by bacillus *Yersinia pestis*. A bioterrorism outbreak could be airborne, causing pneumonic plague.

Procedure

1. Recognize clinical features.

   a. Bubonic form

      1. Swollen, tender lymph nodes (femoral or inguinal most commonly involved)
      2. High temperature (103.1–105.8°F [39.5–41°C]), chills
      3. Pulse rapid, hypotension
      4. Extreme exhaustion

   b. Pneumonic form

      1. High fever, chills, tachycardia, headache
      2. Cough with foamy hemoptysis
      3. Tachypnea and dyspnea

2. Know mode of dissemination and incubation period.

   a. Transmitted from rodents to humans by infected fleas; incubation 2–8 days
   b. Human-to-human transmission occurs by inhaling droplets through cough; incubation 1–6 days
   c. Bioterrorism outbreak through dispersion of aerosol; incubation: 1–3 days

3. Manage decontamination—procedure should be done in a room designed for this purpose or at a special site outside the hospital.

   a. Instruct clients to remove clothing and store in closed plastic biohazard bags.
   b. Instruct clients to shower thoroughly with soap and water—include all crevices.
   c. Home decontamination: Employ Standard Precautions (gloves, gown, face shield when necessary).
   d. Use 0.5% diluted bleach or EPA-approved germicidal agent.

4. Institute isolation precautions.

   a. Bubonic form—routine aseptic (Standard Precautions).
   b. Pneumonic form—add droplet precautions to Standard Precautions (eye protection and surgical mask when within 3 feet of client) until 72 hr of antimicrobial therapy.

5. Assign client placement.

   a. Bubonic form—private isolation room or cohort clients with similar symptoms.
   b. Maintain at least 3 feet distance between clients when cohorting is not possible.
   c. Do not place client with immunosuppressed client.

6. Implement therapy.

   a. Doxycycline 100 mg 2× daily
   b. Ciprofloxacin 500 mg 2× daily

BOTULISM

Definition: A muscle-paralyzing disease caused by an anaerobic gram-positive bacillus that produces a potent neurotoxin. Food-borne botulism is the most common form; inhalational botulism is most likely to occur through a bioterrorist release of aerosol.

Procedure

1. Recognize clinical features.

   a. Food-borne botulism

      1. Gastrointestinal symptoms: nausea, vomiting, diarrhea
      2. Leads to symptoms of inhalational botulism

   b. Inhalational botulism

      1. No fever—client is responsive.
      2. Symmetric cranial nerve paralysis: drooping eyelids, blurred vision, diplopia, difficulty swallowing, dry mouth.
      3. Symptoms progress to paralysis of arms, respiratory muscles, and legs.
      4. Symptoms may be confused with Guillain–Barrè syndrome or myasthenia gravis.

2. Know mode of dissemination and incubation period.

   a. Food-borne botulism: It is generally transmitted through toxin-contaminated food; incubation is 12–36 hr after ingestion.
   b. Inhalational botulism: It is transmitted through aerosolization of the toxin. Incubation is 24–72 hr postexposure.

3. Manage decontamination.

   a. Client does not require decontamination.
   b. Wash contaminated clothing with commercial soap.

4. Institute isolation precautions.

   a. No evidence of individual-to-individual transmission
   b. Standard Precautions for clients

5. Assign client placement: client room selection and care according to facility policy. Client-to-client transmission does not occur.

6. Implement therapy.

   a. Early recognition of botulism important for administration of antitoxin that may stop or reduce paralysis.
   b. Administer trivalent botulinum antitoxin (per CDC orders); it requires skin testing due to 95% hypersensitivity reactions.
   c. Monitor client for respiratory failure and provide supportive care.

TYPHOIDAL TULAREMIA

Definition: A disease caused by *Francisella tularensis* bacterium. It is extremely infectious and can be transmitted via aerosol or contaminated water or food.

Procedure

1. Recognize clinical features.

   a. Early symptoms: headache, cough, fever, chills, and malaise

   b. Delayed symptoms: pharyngeal ulcers, pleuritic chest pain, pneumonia, and pericarditis—may progress to respiratory failure

2. Know mode of dissemination and incubation period.

   a. Bioterrorism mode is aerosol.

   b. This disease may not be recognized unless a bioterrorist attack is suspected.

   c. Incubation period is 2–12 days (average 3–5 days) after exposure.

3. Manage decontamination: general decontamination measures for clothing of infected individual—shower with soap or use 0.5% diluted bleach. Because there is no individual-to-individual transmission, no other measures are necessary.

4. Institute isolation precautions.

   a. This disease is not transmitted from individual to individual, so isolation measures are not required.

   b. Standard Precautions are recommended.

5. Assign client placement: Cohort clients and do not place with immunosuppressed clients.

6. Implement therapy: ciprofloxacin 250 mg PO q12 hr × 14 days, streptomycin 15 mg/kg BID IM × 10–14 days, or gentamicin 1.5 mg/kg q8 hr IV × 10–14 days.

VIRAL HEMORRHAGIC FEVER

Definition: An infection caused by agents such as Ebola, Marburg, Lassa, Argentine, yellow, and dengue fevers. These viruses could be life-threatening (moderately high lethality) and could be delivered by aerosol in a biological attack. An outbreak of Ebola in West Africa in 2014 caused major concern in this country when an infected individual became symptomatic after traveling to the United States and died. A few subsequent cases occurred in the United States; these clients recovered. The threat of this deadly virus led to new guidelines for healthcare workers and reinforcement of infection control procedures.

Procedure

1. Recognize clinical features.

   a. Each illness has unique clinical manifestations; however, some features are similar.

   b. It is characterized by abrupt onset of fever, myalgia, headache, and prostration.

   c. Other signs and symptoms are nausea and vomiting, diarrhea, pain in abdomen and chest, cough, and pharyngitis.

   d. A maculopapular rash, prominent on the trunk, develops in most clients 5 days after onset of illness.

   e. Bleeding manifestations may occur as the disease progresses. Even though it is rare for this life-threatening condition to occur, bleeding (intracranial hemorrhage) could result, hence the term *hemorrhagic fever*.

2. Know mode of dissemination and incubation period.

   a. Viruses are zoonotic (animal-borne) but can spread from individual to individual.

   b. All viruses (except dengue fever) can spread by aerosol in a biological attack.

   c. Incubation period is usually 5–10 days, with a range of 2–21 days.

3. Manage decontamination: The virus is transmitted from individual to individual; decontamination with overt attack: victim undresses, showers with soap or 0.5% diluted bleach.

4. Institute isolation procedures.

   a. Communicable from individual to individual; risk is highest after infection has progressed. Isolation precautions (including airborne and contact), including respirators, face shields, gowns, gloves, shoe, and head covers.

   b. Negative-pressure ventilated rooms with an anteroom.

5. Assign client placement.

   a. Clients should be under strict isolation precautions, including a negative-pressure room with anteroom.

   b. Only clients with the same form of hemorrhagic infection should be cohorted.

6. Implement therapy.

   a. Primarily supportive.

   b. Ribavirin 30 mg/kg IV × 1 dose; 15 mg/kg IV q6 hr 3 4 days.

RICIN TOXIN

Definition: Produced from the castor in castor bean plant and secreted seeds; *Ricinus communis* is a cytotoxin that blocks protein synthesis, killing the cell.

Procedure

1. Recognize clinical features.

   a. Signs and symptoms depend on route of exposure. Diagnosis is difficult. ELISA test of blood will identify ricin.

      1. Ingestion: Nausea, vomiting, diarrhea, and severe abdominal cramps occur before vascular collapse (GI bleeding), leading to death on third day.

      2. Aerosol—inhalation: cough, fever, hypothermia, and hypotension (usually nonspecific symptoms); cardiovascular collapse leads to death in 36–48 hr.

2. Know mode of dissemination and incubation period.

   a. Ricin will be delivered via the castor bean through a chemical process (ingested) or through inhalation method.

   b. Incubation period is within hours to days (ingestion: 3 days; inhalation 3–4 days).

3. Manage decontamination.

   a. Ingested biotoxin does not require decontamination.

   b. Aerosol exposure—victim should shower with soap or use 0.5% diluted bleach.

4. Institute isolation precautions. This toxin is not transmitted to others, but Standard Precautions should be implemented.

(continued)

Skill 15.2.1 | Identifying Agents of Biological Terrorism *(continued)*

5. Assign client placement. There is no communicability from individual to individual or transport through the skin, so placement is planned to protect client's immune system.

6. Implement therapy. There is no approved antitoxin treatment or prophylaxis (vaccination) at this time.

   a. Therapy is supportive; give oxygen and hydration.
   b. If there is ingestion, GI decontamination would be implemented.

SMALLPOX

Definition: An acute viral disease caused by the *variola virus.* It was eradicated worldwide in 1977, and in the early 1980s, routine vaccinations were discontinued. Because there is a large nonimmune population, authorities fear it could be a bioterrorism weapon, transmitted via the airborne route as aerosol or by infected human vectors.

Procedure

1. Recognize clinical features.

   a. Initially, symptoms resemble an acute viral illness like influenza with high fever, myalgia, headache, and backache.
   b. Rash appears (when smallpox becomes most contagious), progressing from macules to papules (in 1 week) to **vesicles**, and scabs over in 1–2 weeks.
   c. Distinguishing rash from varicella (chickenpox): Smallpox has a synchronous onset on face and extremities, rather than arising in "bunches" starting on the trunk.

2. Know mode of dissemination and incubation period.

   a. Smallpox is transmitted by large and small respiratory droplets; thus both respiratory and oral secretions spread the disease, as well as lesion drainage and contaminated objects such as bed linens.
   b. Clients are considered more infectious if they are coughing or have a hemorrhagic form of the disease.
   c. Vaccination is effective if given within 3–4 days.
   d. Incubation: 7–17 days; average is 12 days.

3. Manage decontamination.

   a. Decontamination of clients is not indicated with smallpox.
   b. Careful management using contact precautions of potentially contaminated equipment and environmental surfaces is needed—clean, disinfect, and sterilize when possible.
   c. Dedicated or disposable equipment for each client should be used.

4. Institute strict isolation precautions *immediately.*

   a. Airborne and contact precautions are needed in addition to Standard Precautions: gloves, gown, eye shields, shoe covers, and correctly fitted masks (very important).
   b. Airborne precautions: **microorganisms** transmitted by airborne droplet nuclei (particles 5 μm or smaller).

      1. Respiratory protection needed when entering client's room (particulate respirators, N95) must meet National Institute for Occupational Safety and Health (NIOSH) standards for particulate respirators.
      2. Isolate in room under negative pressure with high-efficiency particle air filtration.

   c. Contact precautions: Clients known to be infected or colonized with organisms that can be transmitted by direct contact or indirect contact with contaminated surfaces.

      1. Wash hands using antimicrobial agent when entering and leaving room.
      2. Don gloves when entering room.
      3. Wear gown for all client contact or contact with client's environment.
      4. Wear gown when entering room and remove before leaving isolation area.

5. Assign client placement.

   a. Rooms must meet ventilation and engineering requirements for airborne precautions.

      1. Monitored negative air pressure with 6–12 air exchanges/hr
      2. Appropriate discharge of air to outdoors or high-efficiency filtration of air

   b. Door to room must remain closed; private room is preferred. Clients with same diagnosis may be cohorted.
   c. Limit transport of clients; use appropriate mask if unavoidable.

6. Notify CDC for therapy.

   a. Check with CDC for up-to-date recommendations. Only highly trained healthcare providers under strict conditions and training can administer the smallpox **vaccine**. Administration of this vaccine is outside the scope of this text.

Skill 15.2.2 | Identifying Chemical Agent Exposure

Procedure

Note: Chemical agents may be solid, liquid, or gas; there are numerous ways of disseminating the agent.

CLINICAL ALERT

Suspect a chemical agent exposure if a healthcare facility is presented with several nontrauma clients with similar symptoms.

1. **Choking agents** such as chlorine, chloropicrin, or phosgene, when inhaled, produce pulmonary edema with little damage to other pulmonary tissues (with resulting hypoxemia) and hypovolemia.

   a. Immediate symptoms are irritation of eyes, nose, and upper airways—often not distinctive enough to be recognized as chemical agent exposure.

   b. Two to 24 hr later, victim develops chest tightness and shortness of breath with exertion (later, at rest).

   c. Cough produces clear, frothy sputum, fluid that leaked into lungs.

   d. If symptoms begin soon after exposure, death may occur within hours.

   e. Victim may experience delayed effects up to 48 hours after exposure.

   f. Remove clothing if contaminated; do not remove shirt over the head.

2. **Blood agents (cyanide)** may be gases or solids, such as hydrogen cyanide or cyanogens chloride; with high concentrations, death occurs in 6–8 min.

   a. Initial symptoms are burning irritation of eyes, nose, and airways, and may smell of bitter almond. There may be dizziness, headache, and nausea and vomiting.

   b. Victim's skin may be acyanotic, cherry-red (oxygenated venous blood), or normal.

   c. Large amount of gas inhaled can cause hyperventilation, convulsions, cessation of breathing (3–5 min), and no heartbeat (6–10 min).

3. **Mustard agents (vesicants)** cause vesicles or blisters. Common agents are sulfur mustard and lewisite. More lethal than pulmonary agents and cyanide.

   a. Mustard—initial symptoms are not observable. Effects begin hours after exposure: erythema, burning and itching with blisters, burning of eyes, airway pain, sore throat, and nonproductive cough.

   b. Lewisite—oily liquid that results in topical damage. Vapor causes immediate pain, burning, and irritation of eyes, skin, and upper airways.

Note: This is distinguishing feature of lewisite versus mustard when initial symptoms are not observable. Cellular damage occurs that can result in hypovolemic shock.

4. **Nerve agents** are liquids or vapors that are the most toxic of all chemical agents. Common agents are Sarin, tabun, Soman, GF, and VX.

   a. Nerve agents block the enzyme acetylcholinesterase, so activity in organs, glands, muscles, smooth muscles, and central nervous system cannot turn off; body systems wear out.

   b. Effects of nerve agent depend on route (vapor or droplet) of exposure and amount; it is felt within seconds.

   1. Felt first on face: eyes, nose, mouth, and lower airways—watery eyes, runny nose, increased salivation, constriction of airways, and shortness of breath.

   2. Large concentration of vapor causes loss of consciousness, convulsions, no breathing.

CLINICAL ALERT
The most common sign of nerve vapor exposure is constricted pupils (miosis) with reddened, watery eyes.

Skill 15.2.3 | Triaging for Chemical Agent Exposure

Note: Box 15-11 ■ provides notes on triage for chemical agents.

Procedure

1. **Choking agents**

   a. Victim complaining of dyspnea within 6 hr of exposure requires immediate intervention—bed rest (no exertion) and oxygen.

   b. Continued care

   1. Continue airway support with oxygen.
   2. Monitor for hypovolemia and correct acidosis.
   3. If symptoms are not present within 12 hr, and x-ray, physical exam, and ABGs normal, client may be discharged.

2. **Blood agents**

   a. **Antidotes** should be administered within minutes of inhalation if client has seizures or respiratory symptoms.

   b. Mild symptoms: give supportive care and monitor.

3. **Mustard agents**

   a. Almost all victims will have delayed treatment for skin, eyes, and airway injuries.

   b. Clients with severe airway injury (dyspnea) require intensive pulmonary care.

Box 15-11 **TRIAGE IN THE HOT ZONE AFTER A CHEMICAL AGENT TERRORIST ATTACK**

- First responders will probably not be able to identify the exact agent.
- Early intervention is critical for nerve agents and cyanide.
- Choking agent exposure will be treated later.
- Intervention in the hot zone generally has to do with airway, breathing, and circulation (ABCs); add antidotes for nerve agents.

(continued)

Skill 15.2.3 | Triaging for Chemical Agent Exposure *(continued)*

4. **Nerve agents**

   a. Victims exposed to liquid nerve agent who show signs of nerve exposure must be decontaminated immediately.

      ▶ *Rationale:* Rapid decontamination will decrease reaction, but not prevent it.

   b. Administer antidotes immediately according to symptoms—multiorgan involvement, respiratory difficulty, convulsions.

   c. Victims suspected of exposure, but who present with no symptoms, may have delayed treatment.

Skill 15.2.4 | Managing Care After Chemical Agent Exposure

Procedure

1. **Choking agents:** Clients with pulmonary edema must be on immediate bed rest with no exertion and receive oxygen.

2. **Blood agents:** Administer antidotes.

   a. Client inhales amyl nitrite or is given sodium nitrite IV (10 mL; 300 mg); frees bound cyanide from hemoglobin to allow O_2 transport.

   b. Sulfur thiosulfate IV (50 mL; 12.5 g); sulfur converts cyanide to form a nontoxic substance.

   c. Give antidotes sequentially and slowly, titrated to monitor effects; ventilate with oxygen and correct acidosis.

3. **Vesicant agents**

   a. Mustard: Immediate decontamination (within 1 min) will minimize damage; longer will be too late. Irrigate affected skin areas and eyes frequently and apply antibiotics to skin 3–4 times/day.

   b. Lewisite: Similar to mustard. Immediate decontamination is important. An **antidote** for systemic lewisite is British anti-Lewisite (BAL), a drug given IV for heavy metal **poisoning**.

   c. Exposure is usually not fatal.

4. **Nerve agents** (organophosphates) (Box 15-12 ■)

   a. PPE is necessary when decontaminating victims. Decontamination must take place first, before management begins. The extent of poisoning depends on the amount of exposure.

Box 15-12 **CHEMPACKS**

Chempacks are packages that include chemical weapon antidotes. They have been distributed to secure locations around the United States near where they might be needed. There are about 2,000 Chempacks distributed. Because nerve gas antidotes must be administered quickly in order to save lives, they are packaged for rapid unpacking and use.

Source: Centers for Disease Control and Prevention (2015)

---

   b. Antidotes:

      1. *Atropine* 2–6 mg (average dose 2–4 mg) IM; 2 mg more may be administered in 5–10 min if no improvement. A high initial dose is necessary to block excess neurotransmitter, especially if victim is unconscious.

      2. *Valium* might be used for prolonged convulsions.

   c. The military has a device (Mark I Auto-Injection Kit) that holds two spring-powered injectors containing two antidotes, atropine and Protopam, that can be used effectively and quickly to administer antidotes.

Skill 15.2.5 | Identifying Acute Radiation Syndrome

Equipment

Film badge for signaling excess exposure to radiation ❶

Procedure

1. Assess for an acute illness characterized by manifestations of cellular deficiencies. ▶ *Rationale:* Early recognition of the body's reaction to ionizing radiation is important.

   a. Prodromal period: loss of appetite, nausea, vomiting, fatigue, and diarrhea occur.

   b. Latent period: symptoms disappear for a period of time.

   c. Overt illness follows the latent period—infection, electrolyte imbalance, diarrhea, bleeding.

   d. The final phase is a period of recovery or death.

❶ Wear film badge when likely to be exposed to radioactive material.

2. Determine the radiation dose, if possible.
3. Attempt to identify dose exposure of client. ➤ *Rationale:* Treatment is according to dose exposure.

   a. Dose less than 2 Gy (200 RADS) is usually not severe; nausea and vomiting seldom experienced at 0.75–1 Gy (75–100 RADS) of penetrating gamma rays.

      1. Hospitalization unnecessary at less than 2 Gy, thus outpatient care indicated.
      2. Closely monitor and administer frequent CBC with differential blood tests.

   b. Dose greater than 2 Gy (200 RADS).

      1. Signs and symptoms become increasingly severe with increased dose.
      2. See Box 15-13 ■ for description of four ARSs.

   c. Give supportive care—treat gastric distress with H$_2$ receptor antagonists (Tagamet, Pepcid, and the like).

> **CLINICAL ALERT**
>
> The higher the radiation dose, the greater the severity of early effects and possibility of late effects.

   d. Prevent and treat infections—monitor viral prophylaxis.
   e. Consult with hematologist and radiation experts.
   f. Observe for erythema, hair loss, skin injury, mucositis, weight loss, and fever.

4. Identify if radiation dose includes radioactive iodine. ➤ *Rationale:* Uptake of this isotope could destroy thyroid tissue.
5. Administer potassium iodide before exposure, if possible, or as soon as available (within 4 hr). ➤ *Rationale:* It blocks uptake of specific damaging isotope, which protects thyroid tissue.

Box 15-13 **ACUTE RADIATION SYNDROMES**

- *Bone marrow or hematopoietic syndrome:* Characterized by deficiencies of red blood cells, lymphocytes, and platelets, with immunodeficiency; increased infectious complications, including bleeding, anemia, and impaired wound healing.
- *Gastrointestinal syndrome:* Characterized by loss of cells lining intestinal crypts and loss of mucosal barrier with alterations in intestinal motility; fluid and electrolyte loss with vomiting and diarrhea; loss of normal intestinal bacteria, sepsis, and damage to the intestinal microcirculation, along with the hematopoietic syndrome.

- *Cardiovascular (CV)/Central nervous system (CNS) syndrome:* Primarily associated with effects on the vasculature and resultant fluid shifts. Signs and symptoms include vomiting and diarrhea within minutes of exposure, confusion, disorientation, cerebral edema, hypotension, and hyperpyrexia. It is fatal within a short time.
- *Cutaneous radiation syndrome:* Most types of ARS cause some skin damage. It is possible for damage to occur even in the absence of symptoms of ARS. Damage to the basal cell layer can result in desquamation and temporary or permanent hair loss with "radiation burns."

Source: Centers for Disease Control and Prevention (2013)

Skill 15.2.6 | Dealing With a Nuclear Disaster

Procedure

1. Move away from blast area as soon as possible. ➤ *Rationale:* Downwind contamination and dispersed radioactive material will contaminate.
2. Travel in a direction that keeps wind to left or right. ➤ *Rationale:* If wind is blowing from blast toward you, this will give you the most exposure.
3. Cover your face with cloth or mask. ➤ *Rationale:* This will help you avoid inhaling radioactive dust.
4. Remove your outer clothing and shower as soon as you are in a safe area. ➤ *Rationale:* Fallout dust is dangerous because it emits radiation energy that can go through clothing.
5. Find a shelter with enough mass (thickness) to shield you from penetrating radioactive dust. ➤ *Rationale:* The denser the shelter mass or walls, the more effective at blocking (thickness required to stop 99% of radiation is 5 in. of steel, 16 in. of brick or concrete blocks filled with sand or mortar, 2 feet of packed earth, or 3 feet of water).

Unit 15.2 Documentation and Evaluation

DOCUMENTATION for Bioterrorism Agents, Antidotes, and Vaccinations

Agents of Bioterrorism Identified

- Clinical features of agent (anthrax, plague, botulism, typhoid, VHF, smallpox, ricin)
- Incubation period
- Decontamination, if necessary

- Client placement and isolation precautions implemented
- Therapy–treatment implemented

Chemical Agents Identified (Choking, Blood, Mustard, Nerve)

- Triaging, if necessary, for chemical exposure
- Treatment administered to chemically exposed client

EVALUATION/Critical Thinking

Expected Outcomes

- Epidemiologic features of disease are identified.
- Preparedness plans for hospitals are in place and staff are aware of the components.
- Radiation dose remains at safe levels.
- Healthcare workers learn how to respond safely to a nuclear event.
- Victims of a man-made disaster (chemical, biological, or nuclear) are treated according to protocols.

Unexpected Outcomes

- Epidemiologic features of disease cannot be identified.

Alternative Actions

- Examine clusters or unusual numbers of clients with similar signs and symptoms by communicating with other hospitals in the community.
- Gather specimens and send them to the appropriate laboratory.
- Institute Standard Precautions plus airborne and contact precautions until specific agent is identified.

- An effective community response to a terrorist attack is unlikely (hospital does not have a Preparedness Plan in place).

- Form a hospital committee to prepare a Preparedness Plan.
- Collect educational materials to fill in areas of content the response team requires to function effectively in the event of a disaster.
- Set up practice sessions with postevaluation to increase response effectiveness.
- Establish a communication network so it is already in place in the event of a terrorist attack; assign roles and a command center spokesman.

Personal Protective Equipment and Decontamination

Nursing Process Data

ASSESSMENT Database

- Identify clients who present risk to healthcare professionals.
- Assess need for special equipment (biohazard bags, specimen bags, and such).
- Determine type of protection equipment required according to an identified biohazard (biological, chemical, or radiological).
- Assess need for decontaminating victims before triage.
- Assess strategy for decontamination at site of incident.
- Assess need for mass casualty decontamination.

PLANNING Objectives

- To select and utilize appropriate PPE
- To demonstrate Standard Precaution techniques
- To demonstrate behaviors that help to ensure personal safety
- To understand containment principles to avoid spreading contamination
- To prevent further spread of biological–chemical–radiological agents with appropriate decontamination procedures
- To understand principles of decontamination via triage
- To prevent spread of bioterrorism agents by following guidelines of mass casualty decontamination

IMPLEMENTATION Procedures

DOCUMENTATION AND EVALUATION

Expected Outcomes

- Infection control protocols are followed.
- Staff is familiar with protective equipment and the protocols to use it.
- Staff knows decontamination procedures and implements them safely.
- Decontamination procedures for mass casualty disasters are implemented.
- Radiation exposure is controlled.

Unexpected Outcomes/Alternative Actions

Pearson Nursing Student Resources

Find additional review materials at **nursing.pearsonhighered.com.**
Prepare for success with NCLEX®-style practice questions and Skill Checklists.

Skill 15.3.1 | Implementing Hospital Infection Control Protocol

Equipment

Hand washing material/Hand rubbing material
Gloves (Box 15-14 ■)
Masks (HEPA or N95 for respiratory problems, pneumonia, plague, smallpox, and such)
Eye shields or face shields
Gowns
Disinfecting material

Procedure

1. Utilize Standard Precautions (Table15-6 ■) for all clients admitted to or arriving at the hospital. ➤ *Rationale:* Agents of bioterrorism are generally not transmitted from individual to individual.

2. Follow routine client placement for normal number of admissions. ❶

    a. Isolate suspicious cases.

    b. Group similar cases.

3. Utilize alternative placement for large numbers of clients.

    a. Group clients with similar syndromes in a designated area.

    b. Establish designated unit, floor, or area in advance.

    c. Place clients based on patterns of airflow and ventilation with respirator problems, smallpox, or plague. ➤ *Rationale:* Transmission is through droplets (touching).

    d. Place clients after consultation with engineering staff. ➤ *Rationale:* Adequate plumbing and waste disposal must be available.

4. Control entry to client-designated areas. ➤ *Rationale:* This minimizes possibility of transmission to other clients and staff.

5. Transport bioterrorism clients as little as possible—limit to essential movement. ➤ *Rationale:* This practice will reduce opportunity for microorganism transmission within facility.

Box 15-14 GLOVE PROTECTION FROM TOXIC CHEMICALS

- OSHA's new PPE standard requires companies to perform a hazard assessment to determine the need for protective clothing.
- Wide variations in chemical resistance of gloves and protective clothing make equipment selection difficult.
- Many factors affect the performance of gloves during actual use. Toxic chemicals such as pesticides, aromatic amines, and isocyanates can permeate gloves and protective clothing. In addition, flexing, stretching, pressure, and abrasion are physical factors that can cause premature breakthrough.
- A new generation of products produces a color change when permeation occurs, thus providing a method for field validation of the efficacy of protective clothing.
- PERMEA-TEC sensors (Colormetric Laboratories Inc., 2014) are one sensor product that is attached to the hands before gloving to monitor for contamination. Detectors are placed on areas with most contact, abrasion, and risk of perforation (thumb, middle finger, and palm).
- Sensors should be checked hourly to determine when breakthrough occurs, indicating gloves must be changed.

6. Clean, disinfect, and sterilize equipment according to principles of Standard Precautions. ❷

    a. Use procedures the facility has in place for routine cleaning and disinfection.

    b. Have available approved germicidal cleaning solutions.

    c. Contaminated waste should be sorted and disposed of in accordance with biohazard waste regulations. See Box 14-5, Proper Handling of Biohazard Waste.

    d. For clients with bioterrorism-related infections, use Standard Precautions for cleaning unless infecting organism indicates special cleaning.

❶ Clients who are placed in isolation require a room with a directional airflow, negative-pressure ventilation system with minimum of 6–12 air exchanges per hour. An anteroom entry is preferred to maintain isolation protocol.

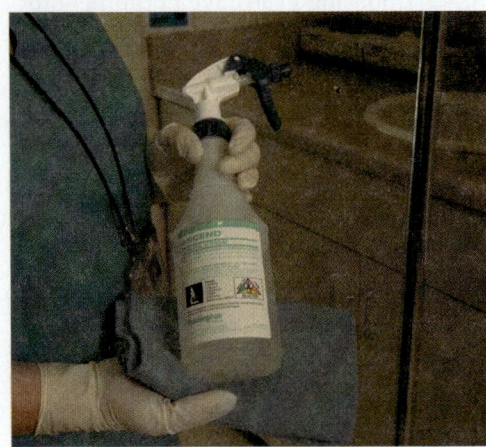

❷ Clean all reusable large equipment thoroughly with antimicrobial or antiseptic agent as required by hospital policy.

Table 15-6 Standard Precautions

Hand hygiene	Use antimicrobial soap or waterless antiseptic agent to clean hands. When hands are not visibly soiled, alcohol gel is the preferred method of hand hygiene when providing health care to clients. Hand washing (40–60 sec) Wet hands and apply soap; rub all surfaces; rinse hands and dry thoroughly with a single towel; use towel to turn off faucet. Hand rubbing (20–30 sec) Apply enough product to cover all areas of the hands, rub until dry.	
Donning gloves	Wear clean, nonsterile gloves to protect healthcare personnel from touching blood, body fluids, secretions, excretions, and contaminated items.	
Donning a gown	A clean, nonsterile gown will protect skin and prevent soiling of clothes.	
Wearing a mask Wearing special masks: HEPA or particulate filter respiratory mask	When bioterrorism agent is suspected and is transmitted via aerosol or airborne, special masks are indicated. Individually fit each mask. Wear a mask to protect mucous membranes of nose and mouth: for workers and victims.	
Wearing eye or face shield	Shield will protect mucous membranes of eyes from splash or spray of victim's body fluids.	

Skill 15.3.2 | Decontaminating via Triage

Equipment

PPE including clothing
Water source
Soap
0.5% **sodium hypochlorite** (HTH chlorine or diluted bleach) cleaning solution
Towels
Waste container for contaminated clothes
Masking tape, 2 in. wide
Body bags
Film badge or chemical agent detector

Procedure

1. Decontaminate at scene of incident (hot zone).
   ➤ *Rationale:* This prevents hospital system from absorbing contaminated victims and protects healthcare providers and uncontaminated casualties.
2. Familiarize emergency personnel with stages of decontamination. ➤ *Rationale:* Effective decontamination is essential for victim and staff protection.

   a. Gross decontamination

   1. Decontaminate those who require assistance. For prioritizing victims of contamination, see Box 15-15 ■.
   2. Remove and dispose of exposed victim's clothing.
      ➤ *Rationale:* This will remove 70%–80% of contaminant.
   3. Perform a thorough head-to-toe tepid water rinse.
      ➤ *Rationale:* Cold water can cause hypothermia and hot water can result in vasodilation, speeding distribution of the contaminants.

   b. Secondary decontamination

   1. Perform a full-body rinse with clean, tepid water.
      ➤ *Rationale:* Water is an effective decontaminant because of rapidity of application.
   2. Wash rapidly from head to toe with cleaning solution (HTH chlorine is effective) and rinse with water.
      ➤ *Rationale:* HTH chlorine can decontaminate both chemical and biological contaminants.

   Note: Undiluted household bleach is 5.0% sodium hypochlorite.

   c. Definitive decontamination

   1. Perform thorough head-to-toe wash and rinse.
   2. Dry victim and don clean clothes.

3. Initial decontamination may be accomplished by the fire department with hoses spraying water at reduced pressure.
   ➤ *Rationale:* This will remove a high percentage of contaminant at an early stage.
4. Decontaminate salvageable clients first (Box 15-16 ■).
   ➤ *Rationale:* The goal is to decontaminate victims who have been exposed, yet are salvageable. Clients who are dead or unsalvageable have lowest priority for decontamination.

5. Reduce extent of contamination in facility by decontaminating clients before receiving in healthcare facility. ➤ *Rationale:* This is necessary to ensure safety of clients and staff.

   a. Establish decontamination site outside facility using a decontamination tent before needing it. ➤ *Rationale:* This is to protect clients and staff inside facility.
   b. Set up procedures for decontamination, depending on infectious agent.

6. Implement procedure for decontaminating client.

   a. Don appropriate personal protective gear before assisting clients to decontaminate.
   b. Remove contaminated clothing and place in appropriate double biohazard bags.
   c. Instruct or assist client to shower with soap and water.
      ➤ *Rationale:* Bathing clients in bleach may be potentially harmful. For specific infections, diluted bleach (0.5%) is indicated.
   d. Use clean water, normal saline, or ophthalmic solution for rinsing eyes.

Box 15-15 PRACTICE GUIDELINES: SETTING UP DECONTAMINATION SITE

- Establish upwind from contamination area.
- Set up site on a downhill slope, if possible, or on flat ground (so that runoff can be captured).
- Have water source available and, if possible, decontamination solution.
- Have decontamination equipment available, if possible.
- Supply PPE for healthcare personnel.
- Notify healthcare facilities nearby to be available, if possible.
- Maintain security and privacy for site.
- Institute postdecontamination monitoring and checks.

Source: Centers for Disease Control (2014c)

Box 15-16 SALVAGEABLE VICTIMS

First Priority: Decontaminate exposed victims with no symptoms.
Second Priority: Decontaminate exposed victims with minor injuries who require minimal resources.
Third Priority: Decontaminate exposed victims needing maximum medical care.
Last to decontaminate are deceased victims.

Skill 15.3.3 | Choosing Protective Equipment for Biological Exposure

Equipment
Listed below in procedure

Procedure
1. Plan for protection from biological hazards.
   a. First responders to a biological hazard may be exposed to bacteria, viruses, or toxins via inhalation (through respiratory tract) or ingestion (contact with mucous membranes of eyes, nasal tissues, or open cuts).
   b. Biological weapons are particles and will not penetrate proper protective equipment.
   c. Respirators—type selected according to hazard identified and its airborne concentration.
      1. High level of protection: Self-contained breathing apparatus (SCBA) with full facepiece. Provides highest level of protection against airborne hazards when used correctly. ➤ *Rationale:* This reduces exposure to hazard by a factor of 10,000.
      2. Minimal level of protection: Half-mask or full facepiece air-purifying respirator with particulate filters like N95 (used for TB) or P100 (used for hantavirus). **❶**
   d. Protective clothing includes gloves and shoe covers—necessary for full protection. ➤ *Rationale:* These prevent skin exposure and/or contamination of other clothing.
      1. Level A Protective Suit used when a suspected biological incident occurs and type, dissemination method, and concentration are unknown.
      2. Level B Protective Suit used when biological aerosol is no longer present.
      3. Full facepiece respirator (P100 or HEPA filters) used if agent was *not* aerosoled or dissemination was by letter or package that could be bagged.
   e. If possible, have biological detection equipment in place—SMART tickets are a handheld point detection system developed by the Navy Medical Institute.

Instrument captures antigen and changes color according to eight different biological agents detected.

2. Identify *anthrax* precautions.
   a. Implement and maintain Standard Precautions (gowns, gloves, and mask). Use Contact Precautions for cutaneous anthrax.
   b. Isolation or decontamination is not implemented. ➤ *Rationale:* Anthrax is not transmitted by individual-to-individual contact.
   c. If client has been exposed and clothing may be contaminated, decontamination is advised.

3. Identify *plague* precautions.
   a. In a bioterrorist attack, bacterium (*Y. pestis*) may be spread by inhalation of droplets, aerosols, or disseminated via infected fleas or other biting insects. ➤ *Rationale:* Droplet precautions are used until client has been treated for 2–3 days (gown, gloves, and mask).
   b. Strict isolation is necessary until client has been treated for 2–3 days. ➤ *Rationale:* This is so that airborne contaminants do not spread throughout the hospital or community.
   c. Decontamination precautions include soap and shower; 0.5% diluted bleach for visible contamination.
   d. Disinfect environment with 0.5% diluted bleach or EPA-approved detergent.

4. Identify *botulism* precautions.
   a. A bioterror attack could disseminate an aerosol of the bacterium or purified neurotoxins. Therefore, use Standard Precautions. ➤ *Rationale:* If toxin is used, there is no danger of individual-to-individual transmission.
   b. Decontamination procedures: Toxin may be removed from skin by soap and water.
   c. Place contaminated clothes in sealed plastic bag for biohazard disposal.

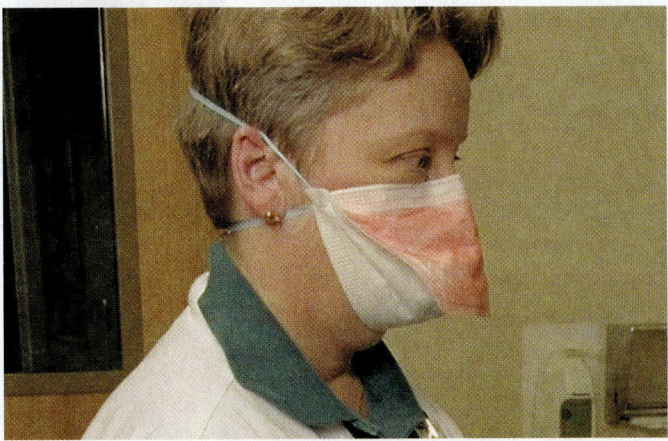

❶ For minimal protection, use particulate filter N95 or HEPA filter respirator when you may be exposed to an unknown biological hazard.

(continued)

Skill 15.3.3 | Choosing Protective Equipment for Biological Exposure *(continued)*

d. Other precautions:

1. Environment: Use diluted bleach 0.5%, 15–20 sec, or EPA-approved germicidal detergent.
2. Boil water for 15 min.
3. Cook food at 176°F (80°C) for 30 min.

5. Identify *smallpox variola* virus.

   a. It is spread through airborne or direct contact with skin lesions or secretions. Use Standard Precautions with airborne (respiratory isolation; N95 or P100 mask) and contact precautions (gown and gloves). ➤ *Rationale:* Virus is spread through droplet or contact; therefore, isolation decontamination precautions are used.

   b. Isolate and quarantine victim immediately and place in negative pressure room with HEPA filtration or direct exhaust to the outside.

   c. All direct contacts are quarantined for at least 17 days. ➤ *Rationale:* Incubation period is 7–17 days.

   d. Cleanse with soap and shower; use 0.5% diluted bleach for gross or visible contamination.

e. Place mask on victim, if not in isolation. ➤ *Rationale:* Virus is spread through airborne method, so mask will protect others.

f. Healthcare workers maintain Standard, airborne, and contact precautions for a minimum of 17 days (until all scabs separate). ➤ *Rationale:* When scabs separate, client is no longer contagious.

g. All bedding and clothing must be autoclaved or laundered in hot water and bleach.

6. Identify *typhoidal tularemia* precautions.

   a. Bioterrorism mode of dissemination would probably be aerosol with nontransmission. Use Standard Precautions.

   b. Isolation and decontamination precautions: Victim should undress, use soap, and shower. For visible contamination, use 0.5% bleach.

   c. Environment: Use 0.5% bleach.

Skill 15.3.4 | Choosing Protective Equipment for Chemical Exposure

Equipment

Listed below in procedure

Procedure

1. Identify victims who were exposed to chemical substance. ➤ *Rationale:* Early identification is essential to save lives, especially from nerve agents or cyanide.

2. Cover all skin surfaces with protective clothing impervious to chemicals. ➤ *Rationale:* This is necessary for protection until exact chemical agent is identified.

   a. Use Mission-Oriented Protective Posture (MOPP) suit, if available (chemical protection suit).

   b. Use fire department chemical suits as alternative.

3. Don masks with filtered respirator. (HEPA filter respirator—P100 with full facepiece—and fit-tested N95 meet CDC performance criteria for chemical exposure.) ❶ ➤ *Rationale:* Chemicals can be inhaled.

4. Wear boots or boot covers. ➤ *Rationale:* Feet should be covered to prevent tracking contaminant.

5. Initiate decontamination procedures with trained personnel.

   a. Decontaminate at site, if possible.

   b. Otherwise, decontaminate outside of facility.

6. Use chemical detection devices, if available. ➤ *Rationale:* Devices would validate presence or absence of agent.

   a. M8 Paper: Sheet of chemically treated paper—if colored spots appear within 20 seconds, chemical agent is present.

   b. M9 Tape: Affix adhesive-backed paper to equipment or protective clothing—color changes when exposed to chemical agent.

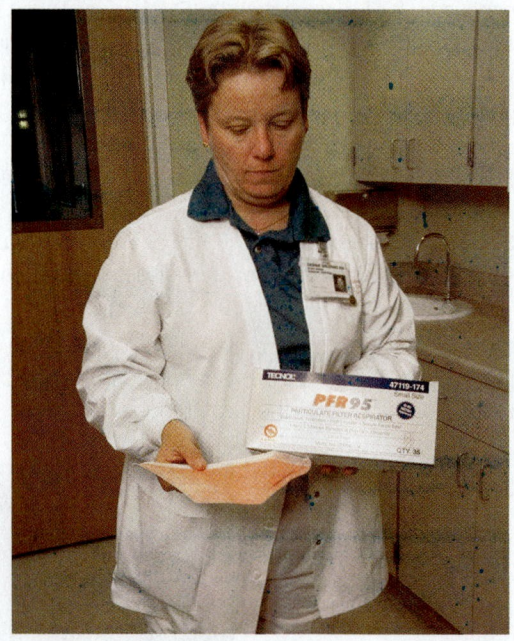

❶ For chemical or certain biological exposure, masks with HEPA filtered respirator or N95 should be used.

   c. M2S6A1 Chemical Agent Detector Kit: Can detect nerve, blister, or blood agent vapors; a glass ampule contains substance that, when placed on test spot, changes color.

   d. Chemical Agent Monitors (CAMs): These contain a microprocessor chip that identifies presence of certain nerve and blister agents.

Skill 15.3.5 | Choosing Protective Equipment for Radiological Attack

Equipment

Listed below in procedure

Procedure

1. Identify victims contaminated by radiation. ➤ *Rationale:* If victim is contaminated, clothes, skin, and more can transmit contamination to others.

    a. If victim was exposed to ionizing radiation (most common are alpha, beta particles, and gamma rays), contamination occurred.

    b. The higher the dose of radiation, the greater the severity of contamination.

2. Don protective clothing: Basic gear will stop alpha and some beta particles, not gamma rays. ➤ *Rationale:* These are necessary to protect responders from exposure and to prevent cross-contamination, exposing other clients.

    a. Scrub suit

    b. Gown and cap

    c. Mask

    d. Eye shield

    e. Double gloves—one pair under cuff of gown and taped to close all entry; second pair can be removed and/or replaced ❶

    f. Masking tape, 2 in. wide

    g. Shoe covers with all seams taped

    h. Radiation detection device able to detect energy emitted from a radiation source: Several detectors are available: Geiger counters, dosimeters, and others. (Box 15-17 ■).

    i. Film badge

3. Transport victim to facility.

    a. If victim is not decontaminated at site, set up portable decontamination unit before entering facility.

    b. Double bag all victim's clothing in sealed biohazard plastic bags marked "Radioactive."

4. Institute decontamination procedures.

    a. Open wounds or nonintact skin: Irrigate with sterile water or normal saline (NS); cover with dry, sterile dressing.

    b. Eyes: Irrigate with sterile water or NS.

    c. Intact skin: Wash skin with soap and warm water. Bleach, 0.5%, may also be used.

    d. Radiation burns: Treat as other burns are treated.

Box 15-17 TINY RADIATION DETECTOR SAVES LIVES

Because the greatest threat to our national security is the use of a nuclear device, this matchbook-size detector that you keep on your keychain could save your life. The device, called a NukAlert, measures levels of radiation (like a Geiger counter) and lets you know which areas are dangerous by emitting a chirp sound. The more chirps, the greater the danger. This device is reasonably priced.

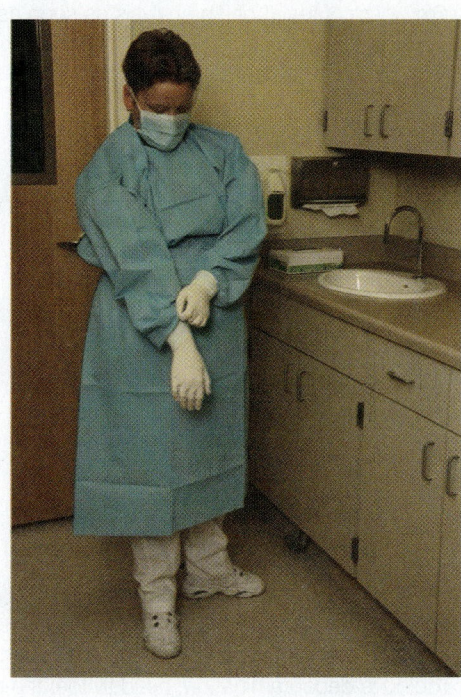

❶ When exposed to radiological material, double gloves that cover all skin exposure should be worn.

5. Recheck radiation levels at each stage of treatment until reduced to background levels.

6. Dispose of used protective gear appropriately. ➤ *Rationale:* This gear is radiologically contaminated waste, and to prevent cross-contamination, it must be treated as such.

Skill 15.3.6 | Decontaminating Victims After a Biological Terrorist Event

Equipment

Protective clothing for healthcare worker
Biohazard bags
Soap and water; diluted sodium hypochlorite (bleach)

Procedure

1. Don protective clothing and adhere strictly to Standard Precautions for emergency personnel. ➤ *Rationale:* This will prevent secondary contamination of personnel.

(continued)

Skill 15.3.6 | Decontaminating Victims After a Biological Terrorist Event (continued)

2. Identify dermal exposure, if possible. ➤ *Rationale:* Biological agents are difficult to detect.

3. Remove victim's clothing as soon as possible and place in biohazard bags. ➤ *Rationale:* If victim was exposed, clothing is contaminated. ❶

4. Cleanse exposed areas using soap and tepid water (large amounts) or diluted sodium hypochlorite (0.5%).

5. Send victims home, if possible, to continue decontamination procedure by washing thoroughly with soap and water.

   a. Instruct victims to monitor for signs and symptoms of agent.

   b. Inform victim of result of lab analysis as soon as possible.

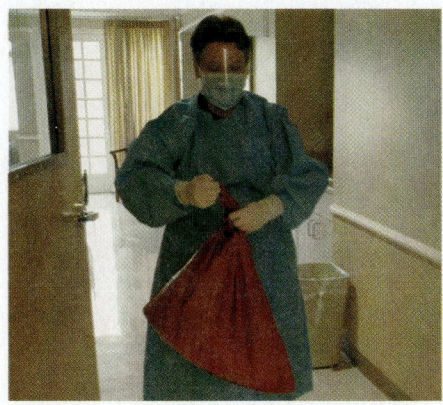

❶ Dispose of all contaminated clothing in appropriate biohazard bags.

Skill 15.3.7 | Decontaminating Victims After a Chemical Terrorist Event

Equipment
Protective equipment for healthcare workers
Biohazard bags
Soap and water; diluted sodium hypochlorite (bleach)
Saline or isotonic bicarbonate
Chemical agent monitor or M8 paper

Procedure

1. Know general principles to guide actions after a chemical agent incident.

   a. Expect a 5:1 ratio of unaffected to affected casualties.

   b. Decontaminate immediately (ASAP).

   c. Disrobing is decontamination, head to toe; the more removal, the better. ❶

   d. Large-volume water flush is best decontamination method.

   e. After exposure, first responders must decontaminate immediately to avoid serious effects.

2. Practice triage guidelines for Mass Casualty Decontamination.
   ➤ *Rationale:* Chemical exposure can be deadly, so early decontamination is critical. Decontaminate according to:

   a. Casualties closest to point of release

   b. Casualties reporting exposure to vapor or aerosol

   c. Casualties with liquid deposits on clothing or skin

   d. Casualties with serious medical conditions

   e. Casualties with conventional injuries

3. Decontaminate victims as early as possible.
   ➤ *Rationale:* Requirements differ according to type of chemical agent used: Sarin dissipates quickly in the air; VX remains lethal for hours.

   a. Nerve agents may be absorbed on all body surfaces—must be removed quickly to be effective.

   b. Vesicant (blister) agents are not always identified due to latent effects.

❶ Place contaminated clothing in bins or biohazard bag labeled "RADIOACTIVE" if that is source of contamination.

4. Treat eyes and mucous membranes with special protocol.

   a. Flush with copious amounts of water. ➤ *Rationale:* Eyes and mucous membranes are too sensitive to use other skin decontaminant solutions.

   b. If available, isotonic bicarbonate (1.26%) or saline (0.9%) may be used as a flushing agent.

5. Monitor victim for remains of agent or contaminant using chemical agent monitor (CAM) or M8 paper for chemical agents. ➤ *Rationale:* This validates removal of contaminant.

Note: Skin decontamination kits (M258A1) designed for chemical decontamination are available. They hold wipes that contain a solution that neutralizes most nerve and blister agents.

Source: U.S. Army Research, Development, and Engineering Command (2013)

Skill 15.3.8 | Decontaminating Victims After Radiation Exposure

Equipment

PPE including self-contained breathing equipment and flash suits, if indicated

Surgical attire or disposable garments, shoe covers, eye shield, gloves, and masks with respirators

Water source and container to catch runoff

Bins for contaminated clothing

Biohazard bags

Vacuum cleaner with HEPA filter

Radiation dose meter

Procedure

1. Determine cause of incident to identify radiation exposure or contamination. ➤ *Rationale:* Exposure does not necessarily indicate need for decontamination.

   a. First responders may be told by those requesting assistance that there has been a radiation-exposure event.

   b. First responders may recognize radiation exposure from observation at incident site.

2. Understand the difference between exposure and contamination.

   a. Exposed victim presents no hazard, requires no special handling, and presents no radiological threat to personnel. ➤ *Rationale:* This is no different from client who has had diagnostic x-rays.

   b. Externally contaminated victim may have come in contact with unconfined radioactive material. ➤ *Rationale:* Any individual or object contaminated by radioactivity must be considered contaminated. Steps should be taken to minimize contamination.

   c. Internal contamination occurs by inhalation or ingestion (airborne radioactive particles) or through an open wound. *Usually* this form of contamination is not a hazard to others.

3. Use appropriate PPE. ➤ *Rationale:* This will protect personnel who may come in contact with contaminated victim.

   a. If radiation incident is suspected, self-contained breathing apparatus (SCBA) and flash suits are indicated. ➤ *Rationale:* This will reduce potential exposure of healthcare providers. Inhalation of radioactive particles is cross-contamination hazard.

   b. If SCBA suits are not available:

      1. Use surgical attire or disposable garments (such as those made of Tyvek).

      2. Use eye protection and double gloves.

      3. Use masks with respirators. ➤ *Rationale:* These will protect healthcare workers from inhaling radioactive particles leading to internal contamination.

   c. It is important to recognize that external radiation (such as penetration by gamma rays) is *not* dangerous to emergency personnel—the only exception to this rule is a rare neutron radiation exposure. ➤ *Rationale:* Gamma ray radiation is absorbed by or passes through the body, but does not leave radioactive contamination.

   d. If monitoring for radiation is not available, consider all clients contaminated.

   e. Personnel should minimize time in radiation zone. ➤ *Rationale:* Radiation exposure depends on time, distance, and shielding.

4. Triage client's medical condition first, regardless of radiation exposure. ➤ *Rationale:* First priority is delivery of emergency medical services (EMS), including transport.

   a. Administer emergency medical treatment to radiation-exposed clients.

   b. Decontaminate clients who have been contaminated on the scene before transport.

5. Complete decontamination of victims. ➤ *Rationale:* Until decontamination is complete, victims are an exposure risk to selves, staff, and others.

   a. Remove client's clothing and have client do a total body wash, scrubbing skin with soap and soft brush. ➤ *Rationale:* Removal of victim's clothing will reduce 80% of the contamination.

   b. Place contaminated clothing in bins or biohazard bag labeled "Radioactive."

   c. Capture runoff of water; contain and label "Radioactive."

   d. Wash area down between washing victims. ➤ *Rationale:* This will prevent transfer of contaminated material.

   e. Capture material with vacuum cleaner with HEPA filter, if appropriate. ➤ *Rationale:* This prevents release of radioactive material into the air.

   f. Monitor client with radiation meter to measure radiation.

6. Implement isolation techniques for contaminated victims. ➤ *Rationale:* This confines contamination and protects personnel.

7. Determine source of radiation, type of radioactive material, and length of time of exposure, if possible. ➤ *Rationale:* This is valuable data for long-term interventions but does not alter immediate handling and transport of victim.

Skill 15.3.9 | Controlling Radiation Contamination

Equipment
Soap and water
Disposable client equipment
Biohazard bags
Wide tape
White tape
Heavy, wide paper
Plastic-lined containers
Radiation meter

Procedure
1. Decontaminate all victims; remove all clothing and complete a full body wash. ➤ *Rationale:* This will reduce most of the contamination.
2. Institute isolation techniques. ➤ *Rationale:* This will confine contamination and protect others.
3. Decontaminate equipment touched by client.
   a. Gurney used to transfer client
   b. Equipment used in client care (BP cuff, stethoscope, and such)
   c. Ambulance
4. Decontaminate care providers who touched or moved client. ➤ *Rationale:* Protective clothing may be contaminated.
5. Examine surrounding area (walls, floor that client may have touched).
6. Control entry and exit of victims. ➤ *Rationale:* Radioactive particles adhere to dust, may become airborne, and can contaminate other clients and personnel.
   a. Mark entry area with white tape to differentiate areas.
   b. Restrict access to controlled area.
   c. Monitor everyone leaving controlled area—have individuals cleared by radiation safety officer.
7. Cover floor areas with rolls of heavy, wide paper and tape securely to floor. ➤ *Rationale:* This prevents tracking of contaminants.
8. Control waste by using large plastic-lined containers for contaminated articles.
9. Monitor radiation by using meter.

Unit 15.3 Documentation and Evaluation

DOCUMENTATION for Personal Protective Equipment and Decontamination

- Specific infection control protocols implemented (i.e., Standard or Airborne Precautions)
- Personal protection gear and equipment used
- Decontamination site established
- Decontamination procedure used for biological or chemical event
- Radiation exposure decontamination procedure

EVALUATION/Critical Thinking

Expected Outcomes
- Infection control protocols are followed. Staff is familiar with protective equipment and the protocols to use it.
- Staff knows decontamination procedures and implements them safely.
- Decontamination procedures for mass casualty disasters are implemented.
- Radiation exposure is controlled.

Unexpected Outcomes	Alternative Actions
• Mass casualty disaster occurs with hundreds of victims affected in one area.	• Don protective gear before approaching WMD site. • Identify weapon or agent used to create disaster, if possible. • Institute field triage (triage first done at site before victims sent to community healthcare facilities). • Decontaminate victims at site before transporting to treatment facility.
• Type of PPE is unknown for agent exposure.	• It is critical that response team be fully protected; thus choose highest level of equipment; that is, assume you need: 1. airborne protection with respirators—self-contained breathing apparatus (SCBA) with full facepiece 2. full Level A protective suit 3. shoe covers and double gloves 4. biological detection device, if available
• Clients are admitted with potential radiation exposure.	• Determine if radiation is exposure or contamination; if the latter, use protective gear and radiation dose meter. • Decontaminate clients by removing all clothing and giving a full body wash—institute isolation techniques. • Decontaminate all equipment, surfaces, and personnel that came in contact with client. • Administer treatment according to dose exposure: supportive care, frequent blood tests (CBC and differential), and prevent infection.

Nursing Process Data

ASSESSMENT Database

- Assess the need to establish triage treatment areas.
- Validate that public health parameters are established.
- Observe that the steps of triage are followed.
- Assess that victim is not in immediate danger or, conversely, requires immediate intervention.
- Assess vital signs of victims.
- Assess the treatment steps necessary to treat life-threatening conditions.
- Observe for signs of respiratory distress.
- Assess need for establishing an airway.
- Observe for amount and source of bleeding and need for intervention.
- Recognize shock state and need for intervention.
- Assess victims posttriage and observe for any signs or symptoms that indicate major injury.
- Identify victims having a severe psychological reaction to bioterrorist event.
- Assess possibility of posttraumatic stress syndrome developing.
- Assess that lines of communication are established and activated.
- Assess that Federal Response Plan is activated.
- Assess that external, internal, and collaborative communication networks are in place.

PLANNING Objectives

- To establish a triage site taking into account public health parameters
- To establish triage treatment areas appropriate to number and injuries of victims
- To follow steps of triage
- To observe for any signs or symptoms that indicate major injury
- To treat life-threatening conditions
- To care for clients with major psychological reactions to bioterrorist event
- To prevent postterrorism trauma
- To develop a communication network including external, internal, and collaborative communication

IMPLEMENTATION Procedures

DOCUMENTATION AND EVALUATION

Expected Outcomes

- Triage treatment areas are established within public health parameters.
- Staff follows appropriate steps of triage protocol.
- Life-threatening conditions are identified and treated.
- Posttriage assessment is completed.
- PTSD is identified and clients are referred appropriately.

Unexpected Outcomes/Alternative Actions

Pearson Nursing Student Resources

Find additional review materials at **nursing.pearsonhighered.com.**
Prepare for success with NCLEX®-style practice questions and Skill Checklists.

Note: In the event of a true disaster, trained disaster management teams are typically deployed to the site. As a trained healthcare worker, you may be called to assist as a first responder.

Skill 15.4.1 | Establishing Triage Treatment Areas

Procedure

1. Assign roles to personnel in treatment areas.
2. Select a site as soon as possible—advance planning is essential.

   a. Select safe area, free of hazards and debris.
   b. Position site upwind of hazard zone.
   c. Determine whether site is accessible to transportation vehicles (ambulances, trucks, helicopters).
   d. Be sure site is able to expand.

> **CLINICAL ALERT**
>
> Survey entire scene, including area above you, for threats to your safety before beginning triage or team work.

3. Protect treatment area and delineate area using tarps and such. If possible, do not contaminate a crime scene.
4. Set up signs to identify subdivisions of area.

   a. I = Immediate care
   b. D = Delayed care
   c. DEAD = Delivery to morgue

5. Establish I and D areas close together. ➤ *Rationale:* This facilitates verbal communication between workers who can also share medical supplies and transfer victims quickly when status changes.
6. Position victims in head-to-toe configuration, with 2–3 feet between victims. ➤ *Rationale:* This system will use space and personnel effectively.
7. Establish morgue site secure and away (and not visible) from medical treatment areas.

Skill 15.4.2 | Establishing Public Health Parameters

Equipment

Soap and water; antibacterial gel
Gloves
Mask and goggles
Biohazard waste disposal containers
Plastic bags
Water purification equipment
Search and rescue equipment

Procedure

1. Assign personnel to monitor public health concerns where disaster victims are sheltered. ➤ *Rationale:* This can help avoid or minimize the disease spreading.
2. Have available search and rescue safety equipment.

   a. Helmet or hardhat
   b. Goggles
   c. Sturdy work gloves and shoes
   d. Clothing appropriate for weather conditions
   e. Dust mask or appropriate filtered mask (see Protection section)
   f. Rescue whistle

3. Maintain proper hygiene by washing hands and using gloves.

   a. Wash hands with soap and water if dirty or antibacterial gel between victims.
   b. Wear gloves at all times.
   c. Change gloves between victims if possible. If not, clean them between victims in a bleach and water solution (1 part bleach to 9 parts water).

4. Wear a mask and goggles.
5. Avoid direct contact with body fluids.
6. Maintain sanitation.

   a. Mark and have available specific biohazard waste disposal containers where bacterial sources (gloves, dressings, and such) are discarded.
   b. Place waste products in plastic bags and bury them in designated area.
   c. Bury human waste.

7. Purify water for drinking, cooking, and medical use, if potable water is not available.

   a. Boil water at rolling boil for 10 min.
   b. Use water purification tablets.
   c. Use unscented liquid bleach (16 drops per gallon of water or 1 teaspoon per 5 gallons; mix and let stand for 30 min).

Skill 15.4.3 | Developing a Communication Network

Procedure

1. Understand lines of communication. ➤ *Rationale:* When lines of communication are compromised, effective triage and intervention cannot take place.

   a. MCI occurs.
   b. Local public health official notifies FBI, the lead agency for crisis plan.
   c. **FBI** notifies DHS, HHS, Centers for Disease Control (CDC), and FEMA.
   d. State health agency requests CDC to deploy response teams if needed.

2. Understand the network of communication that will be activated in response to a suspected or actual bioterrorist event.

   a. Emergency response team:
      Local and state public health officials
      Infection control personnel in notified facilities
      FBI field offices (DHS)
      CDC
      Local EMS
      Local police and fire departments
   b. In turn, the Federal Response Plan will be activated.

3. Activate Federal Response Plan. ➤ *Rationale:* When the local area cannot cope with the disaster, federal assistance is available.

   a. Department of HHS is primary agency.
   b. Office of Emergency Preparedness is action agency.
   c. Emergency Support Function N8 coordinates federal assistance to supplement state and local resources (directed by HHS).
   d. Federal Response Plan is implemented when state requests assistance and FEMA agrees.

EVIDENCE-BASED PRACTICE
Prosocial Behavior After a Disaster
Research has consistently demonstrated that prosocial behavior is increased in the days and weeks following a disaster. This is evidenced in cooperation with recovery efforts, helping others, and putting one's own self-interest aside. Interestingly, people are more expressive of the desire to help than to be helped, even if they have sustained losses as a result of the event.

Source: Cherry (2009)

Skill 15.4.4 | Establishing Viable Communication

Procedure

1. Set up *external communication* system designated spokesperson.

   a. A viable system will minimize disruption.
   b. All communication goes through designated spokesperson—no staff will communicate with the public, press, or outside individuals.

2. Report to appointed community-wide regional spokesperson or small group designated as being in command throughout the incident. Spokesperson will be in charge of coordinating all media relations. ➤ *Rationale:* One individual or small group in charge will minimize confusion.

3. Set up a single community site for family and friends to obtain victim-locator information. ➤ *Rationale:* More than one site will lead to mass confusion.

   a. Provide clear, consistent, and verifiable information to clients and general public.
   b. Plan in advance methods and channels of communication to be used to inform the public.

4. Establish *internal communication*.

   a. Determine position (not individual) that will be in charge (e.g., ED supervisor, called "incident commander").
      ➤ *Rationale:* Position, rather than individual, will negate confusion when there is staff turnover, multiple shifts, or reassignment of staff.
   b. Communicate only through established lines of communication with designated commander or liaisons.

5. Establish a collaborative communication system.

   a. Establish ongoing, open channels of communication with emergency response teams. ➤ *Rationale:* Response teams may have first awareness of the disaster and will need to communicate with the hospital.
   b. Appoint individual (reporting to spokesperson) to collaborate with response team and link to community representative.
   c. Develop a community-wide communications network.
      ➤ *Rationale:* If different organizations cannot communicate with each other, precious time will be lost.
   d. Test the communications network so that overload does not occur in the event of an MCI.

6. Develop clear communication systems that have access to telecommunications as well as an individual-to-individual communication system. ➤ *Rationale:* This position-to-position or individual-to-individual system is necessary if telecommunications are overwhelmed or unavailable.

   a. Use pagers, walkie-talkies, and text messaging as substitutes for communication network during a disaster.
   b. Develop horizontal and vertical relationships between organizations, governmental and private, that will have to work together in a mass casualty event.

CLINICAL ALERT
The goal of disaster medical interventions is to do the greatest good for the greatest number of victims.

Skill 15.4.5 | Carrying Out Steps of Triage

Procedure

1. Evaluate the disaster area: Stop, look, listen, check safety, and identify designated treatment areas.
2. Don protective gear (based on type of disaster) for your safety.
3. Quickly assess conditions for triage before beginning.

4. Conduct voice triage—tell victims to move, if they are able, to designated areas of triage.
   a. Immediate triage for life-threatening conditions
   b. Delayed triage for those who can wait to be treated
5. Treat immediate victims (airway, bleeding, and shock).
6. Tag all victims, even those who are dead.
7. Document results.

Skill 15.4.6 | Treating Life-Threatening Conditions

Equipment

Protective gear
Dressings and bandages
Tourniquets
Stethoscope
Tongue blades
Automated external defibrillator (AED), if available

Procedure

1. Implement Simple Triage and Rapid Treatment (START).
   ➤ *Rationale:* This is the first step for treating multiple casualties in a disaster (Box 15-18 ■).
2. **Check breathing immediately.**
   a. Open airway. ➤ *Rationale:* If airway is obstructed, victim cannot get oxygen.
   b. Move fast—time is critical. ➤ *Rationale:* Heart function will be affected within minutes, and brain damage is possible after 4 min.
   c. Check if tongue is obstructing airway. ➤ *Rationale:* This is the most common airway obstruction (especially when victim is positioned on back).

Box 15-18 STEPS OF TRAUMA ASSESSMENT APPLIED TO TRIAGE

1. Perform a rapid systematic assessment. ➤ *Rationale:* Trauma is a multisystem condition so all systems must be assessed.
2. Complete a primary trauma assessment. ➤ *Rationale:* This is necessary to identify victim's primary and critical problem.
   a. Airway
   b. Breathing capability
   c. Shock—circulation and bleeding
   d. Neurologic status—level of consciousness, mental status
   e. Exposure to contaminant
   f. Disability
   g. Evacuation necessity
3. Complete a secondary assessment (posttriage) that includes a focus assessment.

---

3. Use head-tilt/chin-lift method if victim is not breathing and airway is not obstructed.
   a. Touch victim and shout, "CAN YOU HEAR ME?"
      ➤ *Rationale:* This is to ensure victim has not fainted.
   b. If victim does not respond, place one hand on forehead, two fingers of other hand under chin, and tilt jaw upward and head back slightly. ➤ *Rationale:* This position opens airway.
   c. Look for chest to rise, listen for air exchange, and feel for abdominal movement. ➤ *Rationale:* Reliable indicator of open airway is feeling or hearing air movement.
   d. If no response (victim does not start breathing), repeat procedure. (If AED is available, may apply to victim.)
   e. If victim does not respond after second attempt, move on to next victim. ➤ *Rationale:* Goal of disaster intervention is to do the greatest good for the greatest number of victims.
   f. If the victim begins breathing, maintain airway (hopefully with a volunteer holding airway open) or place soft object under victim's shoulders to elevate him or her, keeping airway open.
4. **Control bleeding.** ➤ *Rationale:* If bleeding is not controlled within a short period of time, victim will go into shock. Loss of 1 L of blood—out of a total of 5 L in the human body—will present risk of death.
5. Identify type of bleeding.
   a. Arterial bleeding (spurting blood)
   b. Venous bleeding (flowing blood)
   c. Capillary bleeding (oozing blood)
6. Choose appropriate method to control bleeding.
   a. Direct local pressure—place direct pressure over wound (using clean or sterile pad) and press firmly. ➤ *Rationale:* 95% of bleeding can be controlled by direct pressure with elevation.
   b. Maintain compression by wrapping wound firmly with pressure bandage.
   c. Elevate wound above level of heart.
   d. Use pressure point to slow blood flow to wound, brachial point for arm, and femoral point for leg. ➤ *Rationale:* Using pressure on a pulse point on a major artery will slow blood flow.

(continued)

Skill 15.4.6 | Treating Life-Threatening Conditions *(continued)*

7. Use tourniquet if bleeding cannot be controlled by other methods (consider this a last resort). ➤ *Rationale:* Tourniquets can pose serious risks to affected limbs.

   a. Incorrect material or application can cause more damage and bleeding; if too tight, nerves, blood vessels, or muscles may be damaged.
   b. If tourniquet is left in place too long, limb may be lost.
   c. If tourniquet is applied, leave in plain sight and affix label to victim's forehead, stating time tourniquet was applied.
   d. Notify healthcare provider to remove tourniquet.

8. **Recognize and treat shock**. ➤ *Rationale:* If the victim remains in shock, it will lead to death of cells, tissue, and organs.

   a. Body will initially compensate for blood loss, so signs of shock may not be observable.
   b. Continually evaluate victim's condition.

> **CLINICAL ALERT**
>
> Most disaster victims could be saved by providing simple medical care for life-threatening conditions: airway obstruction, bleeding, and shock.

9. Observe for signs/symptoms of shock:

   a. Rapid, shallow breathing
   b. Cold, pale skin (capillary refill)
   c. Failure to respond to simple commands

10. Administer treatment for shock:

    a. Position victim supine with feet elevated 6–10 in. (15–25 cm).
    b. Maintain open airway.
    c. Maintain body temperature (cover ground and victim).
    d. Avoid rough or excessive handling, and do not allow victim to eat or drink.

Skill 15.4.7 | Assessing Victims Posttriage

Procedure

1. Perform head-to-toe assessment, always in the same order. ➤ *Rationale:* Performing assessment in the same way every time will enable you to complete it more quickly and accurately.

   a. Head
   b. Neck
   c. Shoulders
   d. Chest
   e. Arms
   f. Abdomen
   g. Pelvis
   h. Legs
   i. Back

2. Complete assessment before beginning any treatment. ➤ *Rationale:* In order to prioritize treatment interventions, a complete assessment must be done.

3. Observe for any sign or symptom that indicates major injury.

   a. How individual received injury (mechanism of injury)
   b. Airway obstruction
   c. Signs of shock
   d. Labored or difficult breathing
   e. Excessive bleeding
   f. Swelling/bruising
   g. Severe pain

4. Provide immediate treatment. During treatment, reclassify victim, if necessary.

5. Assess that victim is not in immediate danger. If available staff, continue to assess for signs of head, neck, and spinal injury.

   a. Change in level of consciousness (unconscious, confused)
   b. Unable to move body part
   c. Severe pain in head, neck, or back
   d. Tingling or numbness in extremities
   e. Difficulty breathing or seeing
   f. Heavy bleeding or blood in eyes or nose
   g. Seizures
   h. Nausea, vomiting
   i. Possible closed compression injury (e.g., victim found under collapsed structure)

6. Immobilize head, neck, or spine by keeping spine in straight line, putting cervical collar on neck, or placing victim on board—if equipment is available.

7. Document who the individual is and relevant medical information.

   a. Available identifying data
   b. Description, clothing
   c. Injuries
   d. Treatment
   e. Transfer location

Skill 15.4.8 | Caring for Those Who Died

Procedure

1. Tag victims pronounced DOA (dead on arrival).
   a. Add special tag "not to remove personal effects."
   b. Incorporate special instructions for people performing autopsies or preparing bodies for burial or transportation. Be particularly sensitive to religious or cultural implications when caring for survivors.
2. Place bodies in cordoned-off area for field triage. ➤ *Rationale:* Decontamination may have to be completed before transport.

3. Notify those performing postmortem care of victim's diagnosis. ➤ *Rationale:* This protects staff who are handling postmortem care.
   a. Autopsies performed carefully using all PPE and Standard Precautions, including use of masks and eye protection.
   b. Incorporate any special instructions about biological–chemical–radiological agent present.
4. Complete a record for all bodies, including identification, name of individual declaring death, diagnosis, if known, name of agency removing body, and so on.

Skill 15.4.9 | Caring for Clients and Staff With Psychological Reactions

Procedure

1. Expect major psychological reactions of fear, panic, anger, horror, paranoia, unrealistic concerns about infection, fear of contagion, social isolation, demoralization, and more, after a bioterrorist event.
2. Plan prior to such an event for professional and educated volunteers to be on site.
3. Minimize fear and panic in staff.
   a. Provide educational materials that include risks to healthcare workers, accurate information of bioterrorism facts, plans for protecting workers, and how to use PPE.
   b. Encourage team participation in disaster drills. ➤ *Rationale:* Experience in handling a disaster will build confidence and allay anxiety.

> **CLINICAL ALERT**
> If a disaster occurs, be alert to signs of caregiver burden and burnout in yourself and your coworkers. Take steps to alleviate stress before it becomes incapacitating.

4. Cope with psychological reactions of fear and anxiety.
   a. Minimize panic by clearly explaining care given with explanations.
   b. Offer rapid evaluation and treatment and avoid isolation, if possible. ➤ *Rationale:* Waiting for evaluation and treatment (as well as isolation) will cause anxiety.
5. Treat major anxiety reactions in unexposed individuals with factual information, reassurance, and medication, if indicated. ➤ *Rationale:* Anxiety is communicable;

prompt intervention will allay group anxiety. ("Worried well" individuals could overwhelm hospitals if they leave the disaster area and go to the closest healthcare facility.)
6. Prevent postterrorism trauma. ➤ *Rationale:* Early intervention may reduce stress disorder.
   a. Identify resources available to address the psychological impact (e.g., Critical Incident Stress Debriefing [CISD] teams, counselors, Psychiatric/Mental Health Nurse Practitioners [P/MHNPs]).
   b. Gather victims into a group with a skilled therapist soon after event (within 24 hr) to prevent a major posttrauma reaction.
      1. Early opportunity for catharsis will help prevent suppression of traumatic event emotions.
      2. Group victims according to age and experience.
   c. Ensure victims continue to meet with a skilled therapist in the aftermath of the event. ➤ *Rationale:* Continued group meetings after a traumatic event help significantly to eliminate PTSD.

EVIDENCE-BASED PRACTICE
Older Adults Demonstrate Greater Resilience
Researchers explored the level of posttraumatic stress (PTS) experienced by older adults after the 2001 attack on the World Trade Center and again after Superstorm Sandy in 2012. They found that older adults confronted by natural disasters are generally more resilient than younger adults. Older age has been associated with lower overall levels of general distress and a decline in PTS symptoms over time.

Source: Shrira, Palgi, Hamama-Raz, Goodwin, & Ben-Ezra (2014)

Skill 15.4.10	Identifying Posttraumatic Stress Disorder

Procedure

1. Recognize possibility of existing condition.
   a. Traumatic event occurs and is re-experienced as flashbacks, dreams, or memory state.
   b. Abreaction occurs: vivid recall of painful experience with original emotions.
   c. Individual cannot adjust to event.
2. Assess signs and symptoms of anxiety and depression. ➤ *Rationale:* Early recognition will assist in therapeutic intervention.
   a. Emotional instability, withdrawal, and isolation
   b. Nightmares, difficulty sleeping
   c. Feelings of detachment or guilt
3. Assess aggressive or acting-out behavior; possible explosive or impulsive behavior.
4. Assist client to go through recovery process. ➤ *Rationale:* Client may need to be assisted through recovery steps to reach adjustment.
   a. Recovery—reassure client that he or she is safe after experience of the traumatic event.
   b. Avoidance—client will avoid thinking about traumatic event; support client.
   c. Reconsideration—client deals with event by confronting it, talking about it, and working through feelings.
   d. Adjustment—client rehabilitates and adjusts to environment after event; client functions well and is able to view future positively.

Unit 15.4 Documentation and Evaluation

DOCUMENTATION for Triage, Treatment, and Communication Matrix

- Triage treatment areas established—note site and subdivisions
- Triage format for assessing victims
- Public health parameters followed
- Protection equipment used for site selection and maintenance:
  Sanitation procedures
  Purified water procedure
  Search and rescue procedures
- Protection gear and equipment used for triaging victims

- Procedures implemented for individual life-threatening conditions
- Posttriage assessment of victim
- Assessment of psychological reactions
- Interventions for identifying PTSD
- Communication network established:
  Internal communication lines
  External communication lines
  Collaborative communication lines

EVALUATION/Critical Thinking

Expected Outcomes

- Triage treatment areas are established within public health parameters.
- Staff follows appropriate steps of triage protocol.
- Life-threatening conditions are identified and treated.
- Posttriage assessment is completed.
- PTSD is identified and clients are referred appropriately.

Unexpected Outcomes	Alternative Actions
• Triage site does not conform to public health requirements.	• Assign additional personnel to monitor for public health concerns (in addition to triage and treatment). • Collect waste in disposable containers for human waste or place in plastic bags and bury. • Boil water or use water-purifying tablets if potable water is not available. • Use diluted bleach (0.5%) to decontaminate surfaces.
• Multiple casualties exhibit life-threatening conditions.	• Implement triage principles—simple triage and rapid treatment (START)—check breathing, control bleeding, and treat shock. • Assess and treat victims posttriage and postinitial interventions, and then refer to community facility.
• Large group of victims are experiencing major psychological reactions of fear, panic, and horror.	• Assign personnel and/or volunteers to separate and group victims according to age and degree of reaction. • Assign skilled therapist to work with group at least 15–30 min, allowing them to talk about their fears and feelings. • Refer victims to post-trauma group to prevent PTSD.

Chapter Wrap-Up

GERONTOLOGIC Considerations

Under the circumstances of a bioterrorist event, all victims will be triaged and treated according to the system established. The older adult will be included in general triage decisions according to their injuries, not age.

For natural disasters, older adult victims will be treated according to the triage system used. The first responders will, however, have to take into account certain principles when dealing with older adult casualties.

• Number of older adult residents in nursing homes expected to double by 2030 to 3.2 million

• Older adults are more vulnerable to disaster conditions—aging immune system, mobility, and physical limitations
• Special concerns for older adults in disaster situations due to:
Mobility impairment
Chronic health issues
Slowed response time
Need for multiple meds
Sensory changes
Memory changes
Communication barriers

MANAGEMENT Guidelines

Delegation

• Pre-emergency and disaster planning and coordination will have (should have) occurred before the terrorist event.

• Personnel roles and lines of authority will have been previously delineated, so healthcare workers will refer to the Preparedness Plan posted in each facility and report to the designated superior or Incident Command Center.

- Each member of the responder team should have an identified role, have practiced actions necessary to perform in this role, studied the educational materials, and demonstrated knowledge necessary to perform in this designated role.
- Role responsibilities must be decided before a disaster occurs. For example, in one disaster scenario, the nursing supervisor is responsible for setting up the command center, the administrator will be in contact with outside resource organizations, and the director of nursing will do the administrator's functions.
- Because emergency response teams must work together as a team, be flexible and adapt to the requirements of a changing situation, team response must have practice sessions.
- Duties of command center designated individual:

  Find adequate nursing personnel and assign roles and responsibilities.

  Assign responsible individual to switchboard.

  Limit all routine nonemergency admissions.

  Refer all public information calls and media to designated place.

Interprofessional Communication

Once a disaster has been declared, the information flow is delineated in the Preparedness Plan.

- Reporting of the incident takes place (see Figure 15-2).
- The community liaison notifies Community Emergency Response Team (CERT) team leader (out-of-hospital staff), who notifies medical–nursing group (in-hospital staff).
- Federal agencies are notified.
- A community-wide network is established—all using the same channels of communication.
- Position-to-position (not individual) cascade of communication (community liaison ▶ command center individual ▶ team leader) is established.
- A single off-site communication center for family and friends of victims must be established to avoid overloading system.

CASE STUDY Applications

Scenario 1

Your hospital has not developed a total Preparedness Plan, including specific recommendations and strategies.

1. What are the implications of this situation under disaster conditions? Include a list of several consequences.
2. What strategies would you suggest to increase hospital administration awareness?
3. Describe the steps you would suggest to alter this situation so that a viable Preparedness Plan is in place.

Scenario 2

An organized crime syndicate has stolen radioactive **isotopes** from an unprotected nuclear research facility and sold the material to a terrorist group. This group smuggled the material into the United States via Canada. At a professional football game, this group detonates the weapon, creating a small explosion that rapidly spreads radiological material. The firefighters and police who rushed to the site had no radiation detectors, so they were exposed to radiological fallout. HAZMAT teams were sent to the area, detected radiation, and set up decontamination equipment.

You are part of the Preparedness Plan team for the local hospital in charge of the command center. Upon being notified of the disaster:

1. What additional information does your team need to make decisions about coping with this disaster?
2. What are the priority actions you would take?
3. What further assessment of contamination is necessary?
4. Describe the special protective equipment your team would require.

Scenario 3

You are tasked with developing a disaster kit for people to carry in their cars in case of a disaster that occurs when they are away from home.

1. What items would you suggest be included in a car disaster kit?
2. Add a rationale for including each item.

NCLEX® Review Questions

Unless otherwise specified, choose only one (1) answer.

1. During an earthquake, what is the best rationale for finding a space *beside* a large piece of furniture or a car (rather than *under* it)?

   A. It will protect your head if the furniture or car collapses.

   B. Research has shown this will be a triangle of safe space.

   C. A large piece of furniture may not completely cover you.

   D. It is easier and quicker to get beside the item rather than under it.

2. What is the best definition of a disaster?

   A. It is an event that is unexpected and occurs with little warning.

   B. It is an event that is of great magnitude that disrupts and overwhelms current resources.

   C. It places the public and environment in danger.

   D. It carries an immediate threat to public health.

3. If a weapon of mass destruction strike occurs in the United States, what is the most difficult type of agent to identify?

   A. A nuclear attack

   B. Smallpox

   C. Sarin gas

   D. A biological agent

4. What are the most Grays (units of exposure to radiation) that an individual can absorb before experiencing symptoms of radiation poisoning?

   A. Over 8 Gy

   B. Between 0.75 and 8 Gy

   C. Less than 0.75 Gy

   D. Over 10 Gy

5. Which of the following biological agents might be used by terrorists to cause a mass casualty incident?
   Select all that apply.

   A. Anthrax

   B. Botulism

   C. Radiation

   D. Smallpox

   E. Typhoid

   F. Sarin gas

6. In triage, what would the rationale be for choosing a five-level system over the more common three-level system?

   A. The five-level system decreases ambiguity of the middle level of emergency cases.

   B. More rapid identification of the client condition can be made.

   C. There is more variety in categorizing client conditions.

   D. This method is more appropriate for categorizing large numbers of victims.

7. You are assigned to establish a site for decontaminating victims. Place the steps for setting up the site in correct order.

   A. Set up the site on a downhill slope.

   B. Establish the site upwind from the contamination area.

   C. Supply personnel protection equipment for all health personnel.

   D. Find a source for water.

8. When managing a client exposed to a chemical agent, the nurse is aware that atropine is an antidote for which of the following agents?

   A. Choking agents

   B. Nerve agents

   C. Blood agents

   D. Vesicant agents

9. Which of the following weapons of mass destruction would fall into the category of chemical agent?

   A. Tularemia

   B. Cyanide

   C. Ricin

   D. Smallpox

10. When distinguishing a smallpox rash from varicella (chickenpox), which of the following is accurate?

    A. Smallpox has a synchronous onset, appearing on face and extremities at the same time.

    B. Smallpox has an asynchronous onset, starting with the face and then appearing on the trunk.

    C. Smallpox arises in bunches starting on the trunk.

    D. Smallpox arises distally and progresses proximally.

QSEN Activity

Domain: Client-Centered Care

KSA: Knowledge

Activity:

You are a home health nurse in the community where there were numerous hurricanes during the last season. One of your goals for the upcoming hurricane season is to assist your clients in developing a disaster kit. Your first client is a socially isolated female with a history of diabetes and coronary artery disease. She has a limited income and one relative who resides outside the state. During your discussion with her, she admits she would not leave her home in the event of a disaster because she could not leave five cats. She takes the following medications: glipizide 10 mg twice a day, captopril 50 mg twice a day, digoxin 125 mcg twice a day, and warfarin sodium 5 mg once a day. As you assist her in developing her disaster kit, what are special considerations for this client in terms of medications, lack of social support, and pets?

Bibliography

American Red Cross. (2015). Plan & prepare. Retrieved from http://www.redcross.org/prepare

Anderson, D. A. (2012). Using disaster exercises to determine staff educational needs and improve disaster outcomes in rural hospitals: The role of the nursing professional development educator. *The Journal of Continuing Education in Nursing, 43*(6), 284–288. doi: http://dx.doi.org/10.3928/00220124-20120201-24

APIC (Association for Professionals in Infection Control and Epidemiology). (2013). *Infection prevention for ambulatory care centers during disasters*. Washington, DC: APIC. Retrieved from http://apic.org/Resource_/TinyMceFileManager/Emergency_Prep/2013_Ambulatory_Care_during_Disasters_FINAL.pdf

APIC (Association for Professionals in Infection Control and Epidemiology). (2012). Mass casualty disaster plan checklist: A template for healthcare facilities. Retrieved from http://apic.org/Resource_/TinyMceFileManager/Education/EPI-201-resources/EPI201_2012_resource_Emergency_Preparedness.pdf

Baack, S., & Alfred, D. (2013). Nurses' preparedness and perceived competence in managing disasters. *The Journal of Nursing Scholarship, 45*(3), 281–287. doi:10.1111/jnu.12029

Barnett, D. J., Thompson, C. B., Semon, N. L., Errett, N. A., Harrison, K. L., Anderson, M. K., Ferrell, J.L., Freiheit, J.M., Hudson, R., McKee, M., Mejia-Echeverry, A., Spitzer, J., Balicer, R.D., Links, J.M, Storey, J. D. (2014). EPPM and willingness to respond: The role of risk and efficacy communication in strengthening public health emergency response systems. *Health Communication, 29*(6), 598. Retrieved from http://www.ncbi.nlm.nih.gov/pubmed/23799806

Cavaliere, V. (2015, Mar. 17). Japanese tsunami debris still washing on U.S. shore. Retrieved from http://www.reuters.com/article/2015/03/17/us-usa-tsunami-debris-idUSKBN0MD2ET20150317

Centers for Disease Control and Prevention. (2014a). Cases of Ebola diagnosed in the United States. Retrieved from http://www.cdc.gov/vhf/ebola/outbreaks/2014-west-africa/united-states-imported-case.html

Centers for Disease Control and Prevention. (2014b). Emergency preparedness and response. Retrieved from http://www.bt.cdc.gov/

Centers for Disease Control. (2014c). Emergency preparedness and response: Public health planning for radiological and nuclear terrorism. Retrieved from http://www.bt.cdc.gov/radiation/masscasualties/publichealthplanning.asp

Centers for Disease Control and Prevention (2015). CDCs Chempack program : The stockpile that may protect you from a chemical attack. Retrieved from http://blogs.cdc.gov/publichealthmatters/2015/02/cdcs-chempack-program-the-stockpile-that-may-protect-you-from-a-chemical-attack/

Cherry, K. E. (Ed.). (2009). Lifespan perspectives on natural disasters. Coping with Katrina, Rita, and other storms. New York: Springer Science + Business Media.

Christensen, D. (2013). The medical basis for radiation-accident preparedness: Medical management: Proceedings of the Fifth International REAC/TS Symposium on the Medical Basis for Radiation-Accident Preparedness and the Biodosimetry Workshop, September 2011, Miami, Florida. Oak Ridge, TN: Oak Ridge Associated Universities.

Clemens, L. (2006, Spring). Culturally competent disaster nursing. *Minority Nurse.com, 40*, 41–43.

College of Registered Nurses of Nova Scotia. (2007). Position statement. Retrieved from http://www.nursing.vanderbilt.edu/incmce/competencies.html

Colleran-Santos, C. (2014). Innovative teaching method in emergency response education of undergraduate nursing students. *Journal of Nursing Education, 53*(8), 483. doi: http://dx.doi.org/10.3928/01484834-20140722-11

Colormetric Laboratories Inc. (2014). PERMEA-TEC TM sensors. An important breakthrough in glove selections. Retrieved from http://www.clilabs.com/index.php/products/permea-tec-sensors.html

Department of Homeland Security. (2014, Jan. 29). Make a plan. Retrieved from www.READY.gov

Federal Emergency Management Agency (FEMA). (2014). National disaster recovery framework. Retrieved from http://www.fema.gov/national-disaster-recovery-framework

Federal Emergency Management Agency. (2014a). Basic disaster supplies kit. Retrieved from http://www.ready.gov/kit

Federal Emergency Management Agency. (2014b). Caring for animals. Retrieved from http://www.ready.gov/caring-animals

Harvard School of Public Health. (2013). Hospital decontamination self-assessment tool. Retrieved from http://www.hsph.harvard.edu/policy-translation-leadership-development/files/2013/01/Hospital-Decontamination-Self-Assessment-Tool-2013.pdf

Khan, A. S., & Nicole L. (2014). Health security in 2014: Building on preparedness knowledge for emerging health threats. *The Lancet, 384*(9937), 93–97.

Late, M. (2014). National public health week tells communities to 'start here. *The Nation's Health, 44*(5), 1–18. Retrieved from http://search.proquest.com/docview/1538578798?accountid=3588

Mukherji, A., Ganapati, N. E., & Rahill, G. (2014). Expecting the unexpected: Field research in post-disaster settings. *Natural Hazards, 73*(2), 805–828. doi: http://dx.doi.org/10.1007/s11069-014-1105-8

Nature Medicine. (2013, Sep.16). Spoonful of Medicine. In wake of Syrian chemical attacks, scientists seek to improve sarin antidotes. Retrieved from http://blogs.nature.com/spoonful/2013/09/in-wake-of-syrian-chemical-attacks-scientists-seek-to-improve-sarin-antidotes.html

Oak Ridge Institute for Science and Education. (n.d.). Guidance for radiation accident management: Managing radiation emergencies. Retrieved from www.orau.gov/reacts/syndrome.htm

Palgi, S., Palgi, Y., Ben-ezra, M., & Shrira, A. (2014). "I will fear no evil, for I am with me": Mentalization-oriented intervention with PTSD patients. A case study. *Journal of Contemporary Psychotherapy, 44*(3), 173–182. doi: http://dx.doi.org/10.1007/s10879-014-9262-3

Raphael, B., & Ma, H. (2011). Mass catastrophe and disaster psychiatry. *Molecular Psychiatry, 16*(3), 247–251. doi: http://dx.doi.org/10.1038/mp.2010.68

Shrira, A., Palgi, Y., Hamama-Raz, Y., Goodwin, R., & Ben-Ezra, M. (2014). Previous exposure to the World Trade Center terrorist attack and post-traumatic symptoms among older adults following hurricane Sandy. *Psychiatry, 77*(4), 374–385.

Sifferlin, A. (2012) Lessons from storm Sandy: When hospital generators fail. *Time*. Retrieved from http://healthland.time.com/2012/10/30/lessons-from-storm-sandy-when-hospital-generators-fail/

Tillman, P. (2011). Disaster preparedness for nurses: A teaching guide. *The Journal of Continuing Education in Nursing, 42*(9), 404–8. doi: http://dx.doi.org/10.3928/00220124-20110502-02

Trocchio, J. (2013). Strategies for disaster readiness. *Health Progress, 94*(6), 4–5.

U.S. Army Research, Development, and Engineering Command. (2013). Guidelines for mass casualty decontamination during an hazmat/weapon of mass destruction incident. Retrieved from http://www.nfpa.org/~/media/Files/Research/Resource%20links/First%20responders/Decontamination/ecbc_Guide_MassCasualtyDecontam_0813.pdfhttp://orise.oran.gov/reacts/resources/guide/management.htm

Veenema, T. (Ed.). (2012). *Disaster nursing and emergency preparedness: For chemical, biological, and radiological terrorism and other hazards* (3rd ed.) New York: Springer.

Walsh, L., Subbarao, I., Gebbie, K., Schor, K.W., Lyznicki, J., Strauss-Riggs, K., Cooper, A., Hsu, E.B., King, R.V. (2012). Core competencies for disaster medicine and public health. American Medical Association *6*(1) 44–52.

Chapter 16
Pain Management

 Learning Objectives

16.1 Discuss what is meant by the experience of pain.

16.2 Explain how natural endorphins work for pain control.

16.3 Describe the body's physiologic response to pain.

16.4 Identify the most important information elicited from the client regarding pain.

16.5 Discuss what it means for the nurse to be the client's advocate in relation to pain control.

16.6 Discuss the main components of The Joint Commission's Standards for Pain Management.

16.7 Compare how you would assess quality of pain versus intensity of pain.

16.8 Outline the main points of one nonpharmacologic method of relieving pain.

16.9 Select a comfort measure for a client in acute pain and for a client in chronic pain.

16.10 Describe two different pain scales.

16.11 Describe the behavioral responses to mild versus severe pain.

16.12 Describe the potential side effects of narcotic medications via IV or epidural route.

16.13 List three criteria for client selection for patient-controlled analgesia (PCA).

16.14 Describe the steps of teaching PCA to a client.

16.15 Discuss two advantages of epidural narcotic analgesia.

Chapter Outline

Terminology

Acupressure Chinese method of treatment that involves compression of certain areas of the body by following a system of meridians or energy flow.

Adaptive reaction a response by which the individual attempts to improve or alter his or her condition in relation to the environment.

Alleviate to make more bearable; reduce pain, grief, or suffering.

ATC around-the-clock medication for persistent pain.

Biofeedback a training technique that uses monitoring instruments to assist people to control stress-related disorders through self-regulation of internal functions.

Bradycardia slowed heart action, below 60 beats/min.

Capnography module a module attached to a PCA pump to detect client hypoventilation or a change in respiratory status.

Coping mechanisms means by which an individual adjusts or adapts to a threat or a challenge; actions that assist in maintaining homeostasis.

Diaphoresis profuse sweating.

Endorphins a naturally occurring body chemical similar to morphine but many times stronger.

Fight or flight immediate response to stress; also called acute stress response.

General adaptation syndrome a general theory of stress response formulated by Dr. Hans Selye; describes the action of stress response in three stages: the alarm reaction, the stage of resistance, and the stage of exhaustion.

ISMP Institute for Safe Medication Practices; a nonprofit organization that focuses on preventing medication errors by providing medication safety information to healthcare practitioners.

Opioid (narcotic) addiction pattern of compulsive drug use characterized by continued craving for the substance—creates both a psychological and physiologic dependence.

Pain a sensation in which an individual experiences discomfort, distress, or suffering. There are three main types of pain: acute, chronic, and malignant.

Parasympathetic nervous system a division of the autonomic nervous system that regulates acetylcholine and conserves energy expenditure; it slows down the system.

PCA—Patient-controlled analgesia a method of delivering pain medication via IV pump. Within healthcare provider-ordered parameters, the client can control the medication amount necessary to manage his or her pain level.

Physiologic concerning body function.

Psychogenic of mental origin; starting in the mind.

Referred pain pain felt in a part removed from its point of origin.

Regression a turning back or return to a former state or stage of development.

Stress a nonspecific response of the body to any internal or external event or change that impinges on an individual's system and creates a demand.

Stressor a specific demand that gives rise to a coping response.

Tachycardia abnormal rapidity of heart action; above 100 beats/min.

TENS—Transcutaneous electrical nerve stimulation a noninvasive method to relieve pain that involves stimulation to the skin via a mild electric current.

Tolerance need for larger and larger doses of an opioid to achieve the same effect.

Coping With Pain

Pain is now considered the fifth vital sign and, according to The Joint Commission's Standards for Pain Management, is essential to regularly assess and manage in order to maintain the client's homeostasis and quality of life.

The experience of pain is direct and personal. In this culture, we tend to view pain as a negative condition and often go to any lengths to avoid the sensation. The positive aspect of pain is that it is an early warning system; its presence triggers an awareness that something is wrong in the body (Box 16-1 ■). Without the sensation of pain we could not survive, because pain provides the cues that allow us to modify our reactions and direct our behavior. One perspective of pain is that it is a message to our conscious self to check out any pain sensation before it gets worse, for that is the nature of pain. Without intervention, the condition may well get worse.

Box 16-1 TYPES OF PAIN

Acute pain	Pain that occurs only in a defined period of time (6 months or less) and is caused by specific stimuli that damage the tissue. Usually of recent onset and varies in intensity.
Chronic/persistent pain	Ongoing or recurrent pain that occurs over a 3–6-month period or longer (lasts beyond the acute illness or injury). Adversely affects the individual's well-being.
Cancer pain	Pain associated with cancer or its treatments. It can be acute or chronic/persistent. Often requires treatment different from that for other types of acute or chronic/persistent pain.

Note: There are many more descriptors to identify locations or characteristics of pain (e.g., **referred pain**, throbbing pain).

In 1999, Margo McCaffery, a nurse–researcher who writes about caring for the client in pain, established a premise in nursing care of the client in pain. It was that pain is what the client says it is and exists when the client says it does. The nurse must rely on the client to describe the sensation of pain, identify its location, and tell about what kind of pain is being experienced. The Joint Commission Standards recognize the rights of clients to an appropriate assessment and management of their pain.

The most important information in pain assessment is the client's report, because the pain experience is totally subjective. The onset of acute pain stimulates the sympathetic nervous system's **fight-or-flight** response, resulting in certain signs or symptoms (Figure 16-1 ■). While observation of these symptoms provides objective data, it cannot be considered conclusive evidence to the identification of pain—that information must come from the client.

The sensation of physical pain arouses some specific responses in the client. The sympathetic nervous system response is usually stimulated by superficial pain; the **parasympathetic nervous system** response is usually stimulated by deeper pain which results in the slowing down of all the systems to conserve energy.

PHYSICAL PAIN SENSATION

Sympathetic Nervous System	Psychological Response	Parasympathetic Nervous System
Elevation of Blood Pressure	Anxiety	Decrease in Blood Pressure
Increased Heart Rate	Apprehension	Decrease in Heart Rate
Increased Respiratory Rate	Focus of Attention on Pain Sensation	Slowed Respirations
Increased Blood Sugar	Irritability	Decreased Blood Sugar
Increased Perspiration	Arousal of Belief Systems	Decreased Perspiration
Increased Muscle Tension	Anger / Depression	Increased Muscle Tension
Skeletal Muscles / Facial Grimacing	Moaning / Crying	Repose, Discrete Response
Restlessness	Verbalize Need for Relief / Silent Endurance	
Guarding of Painful Area	Utilization of Coping Mechanism	

FIGURE 16-1 Comparison of sympathetic, psychological response, and parasympathetic nervous system.

Theories of Pain

The neurophysiologic basis of pain can be explained by several theories, none of which is mutually exclusive or totally comprehensive.

Specificity Theory This theory suggests that certain pain receptors are stimulated by a specific type of sensory stimuli that sends impulses to the brain. The theory deals with the **physiologic** basis for pain but does not take into account the psychological components of pain or the degree of pain **tolerance**.

Pattern Theory This theory attempts to include factors that were not adequately explained by the specificity theory. It suggests that pain originates in the dorsal horn of the spinal cord. A certain pattern of nerve impulses is produced and results in intense receptor stimulation that is coded in the central nervous system (CNS) and signifies pain. Like the specificity theory, the pattern theory does not explain the psychological factors of pain.

Gate Control Theory This theory was developed in an attempt to bridge the gap between the specificity and pattern theories and is based on aspects of each. The first premise of the gate control theory is that the actual existence and intensity of the pain experience depends on the particular transmission of neurologic impulses. Second, gate mechanisms along the nervous system control the transmission of pain. Finally, if the gate is open, the impulses that result in the sensation of pain are able to reach the conscious level. If the gate is closed, the impulses do not reach the level of consciousness and the sensation of pain is not experienced.

Three primary types of neurologic involvement affect whether the gate is open or closed. The first type involves activity in the large and small nerve fibers that affects the sensation of pain. Pain impulses travel along small-diameter fibers. The large-diameter nerve fibers close the gate to the impulses that travel along the small fibers. The technique of using stimulation of the skin, which has many large-diameter fibers, may help to close the gate to the transmission of painful impulses, thereby relieving the sensation of pain. Interventions that apply this theory to practice include massage, hot and cold applications, touch, **acupressure**, and transcutaneous electric nerve stimulation. These interventions are described in detail later in this chapter.

The second form of neurologic involvement is the impulses from the brainstem that affect the sensation of pain. The reticular formation monitors in the brainstem regulate sensory input. If the individual receives adequate or excessive amounts of sensory stimulation, the brainstem transmits impulses that close the gate and inhibit pain impulses from being transmitted. If, on the other hand, the client experiences a lack of sensory input, the brainstem does not inhibit the pain impulses, the gate is open, and pain impulses are transmitted. Interventions that apply to this part of the gate control theory are those related in some way to sensory input, such as techniques of distraction, guided imagery, and visualization.

The third type of neurologic involvement consists of neurologic activities or impulses in the cerebral cortex and thalamus. An individual's thoughts, emotions, and memories may activate certain impulses in the cortex that trigger pain impulses, which are transmitted to the conscious level. Past experiences relating to pain affect how the client responds to current pain. For this reason, it is important to explore the client's previous experiences and teach the client what to expect from the present situation. Interventions that apply to this part of the gate control theory include using and teaching various relaxation techniques, teaching the client about what expectations to have about pain as related to a specific illness, allowing the client to feel he or she has some control over the taking of medication for pain relief, and giving medications properly (i.e., preventively, before the pain is so severe that the client fears he or she will receive no relief).

Endorphins, Natural Opiate Theory A relatively recent theory of pain relief was developed when Avron Goldstein, looking for morphine and heroin receptors, discovered receptors in the brain that fit only morphine or morphine-like molecules. He asked himself why these receptors were located in the brain, when opiates are not naturally found in this area. The answer, learned through diligent research, is that the brain produces natural brain opiates. These substances are hormones, chemicals produced by different parts of the body to regulate certain biological processes. At present, five of these natural opiates have been found. Three are called **endorphins**, one dynorphin, and one enkephalin. Endorphins fit into special cells, called receptors, and thereby activate their regulating powers. In addition to endorphin "keys" and receptor "locks," researchers have found antilocks, called antagonists, that keep endorphins from working. Endorphin receptors and antilocks have been found throughout the body—in the stomach, intestines, pancreas, spinal cord, and bloodstream, as well as the brain.

Pain Pathways

The pathway to pain is a complicated, fascinating expression of how our amazing bodies work. First, there is the source of pain, a direct causative factor. Stimulation of a pain receptor may be mechanical, chemical, thermal, electric, or ischemic. The sensation travels along the sensory pathways and ascends the spinal cord to the thalamus. The autonomic nervous system is activated, and sensations travel to the sensory area of the cerebral cortex. Pain reception occurs in the thalamus, where awareness and integration take place, and pain interpretation occurs in the cerebral cortex. Once awareness of pain takes place and it has been interpreted by the cerebral cortex, the individual becomes aware and the response patterns are activated.

The Pain Experience

The pain experience is a mixture of physical sensations, physiologic changes, and psychosocial (including psychological, sociocultural, and environmental) factors. The client's interpretation of the physical sensation is influenced by the client's culture, previous experiences with and without pain, beliefs about self, interpretation of the future, present environment, and the individuals in that environment. Pain is assessed based on location, duration, intensity, and etiology. The intensity of pain is influenced by what the sensation means to the client, the client's level of anxiety, degree of fatigue, and the number of **stressors** in the client's environment.

There are several methods of assessing the intensity or level of pain a client may be experiencing. Note the examples of pain scales you may use to assess your client's pain (Figure 16-2 ■). After explaining the scale you are using, ask your client what level of pain he or she is experiencing at the moment. You may use a numeric scale of 0–10, an intensity scale with three or more categories to rate client pain, a pain distress scale, or a pain scale showing facial images from relaxed and happy to extremely distressed and uncomfortable. A visual pain scale (Figure 16-3 ■) is very useful with pediatric clients, since children may have difficulty verbalizing the degree of pain they are experiencing. Different facial expressions help them relate to pain by how sad the face appears, thus identifying for the nurse the level of pain they are feeling. The FLACC scale is also used to assess pain in

FIGURE 16-2 Pain scales for acute pain management: Operative or medical procedures and trauma.
Source: U.S. Department of Health and Human Services, Public Health Service.

FIGURE 16-3 A visual pain scale, especially useful for pediatric clients. Child selects the image that most reflects his or her pain level.
Source: From Cerner Electronics Health Record. Copyright © by Cerner Corporation. Pearson has restricted permission to reproduce and distribute this copyrighted work. Further reproduction or distribution is strictly prohibited without written consent of Cerner Corporation.

children who are cognitively impaired or in infants who are preverbal (Figure 16-4 ■). Whichever scale is chosen, maintain its use throughout the course of pain control to provide the best data for observing changes in the client's condition.

The Joint Commission Standards for Pain Management

In 2001, The Joint Commission implemented pain management standards for all accredited healthcare agencies. These standards require:

- Recognizing that clients have the right to appropriate assessment and management of pain (Box 16-2 ■)
- Screening clients for pain during their initial assessment; periodically reassessing their pain when *clinically required* (Figure 16-5 ■)
- Educating clients who are suffering from pain, and their families, about pain management

The Joint Commission website provides resources for clients, encouraging them to speak up about their pain and providing tips on how to help them talk to their doctor or nurse about their pain management needs. These can be found on the Joint Commission website under Pain Management. Some recommendations for pain management are provided in Box 16-3 ■.

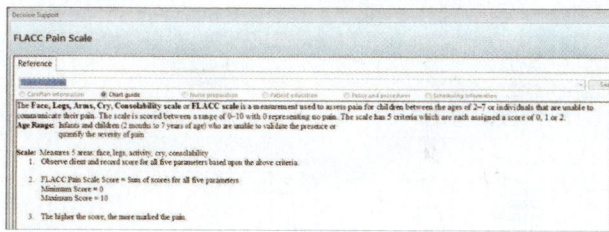

FIGURE 16-4 FLACC pain scale.
Source: From Cerner Electronic Health Record. © Cerner Corporation. Pearson has restricted permission to reproduce and distribute this copyrighted work. Further reproduction or distribution is strictly prohibited without written consent of Cerner Corporation.

Box 16-2 ASSESSING CHARACTERISTICS OF PAIN

Location

- Where exactly is it felt? Is it diffuse or localized? Does it radiate and what area is involved?

Duration

- When did the pain start? How long did/does it last?

Quality

- Stabbing, knifelike
- Throbbing
- Cramping
- Viselike, suffocating
- Searing, burning
- Superficial, deep

Intensity

- How much does it hurt? Use a visual scale or a scale of 0–10 (0 = no pain, 10 = most pain ever experienced)

Pattern

- How does the pain change? What is the timing of the pain (continuous, steady, intermittent, transient)?

Factors Associated With Pain

- Nausea
- Vomiting
- **Bradycardia**, **tachycardia**
- Hypotension, hypertension
- Profuse perspiration
- Apprehension or anxiety

Precipitating Factors

- Motion affecting incision area (e.g., coughing, turning, deep breathing)
- Fear and emotional distress
- Inflammation or infection
- Trauma
- Disease state

Aggravating Factors

- Position changes
- Environmental stressors
- Fatigue
- Inadequate pain-relief measures

Alleviating Factors

- Position change
- Medications
- **Biofeedback**
- Visualization
- Relaxation techniques
- **TENS**
- Massage

Box 16-3 RECOMMENDATIONS FOR PAIN MANAGEMENT

Guidelines for acute pain management include these major recommendations:

- Complete a baseline pain assessment, including pain level.
- Educate client and family about pain management.
- Monitor the acute pain the client is experiencing, including intensity, duration, and effect of pain.
- Follow guidelines of pharmacologic management.
- Implement nonpharmacologic management.
- Assess the effectiveness of pain management.

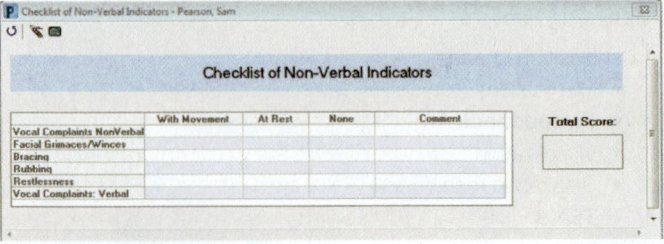

FIGURE 16-5 Pain assessment form.
Source: From Cerner Electronic Health Record. © Cerner Corporation. Pearson has restricted permission to reproduce and distribute this copyrighted work. Further reproduction or distribution is strictly prohibited without written consent of Cerner Corporation.

Noninvasive Pain Relief

When a method to relieve pain is noninvasive, it is safer and results in fewer potential side effects for the client. Such measures are becoming the pain control choice of the future.

Current practice for controlling pain is to use both drugs and nondrug options because both, separately or combined, meet the objectives of relieving pain and making the client more comfortable.

Nondrug options may include:

- Specific cognitive–behavioral techniques: deep breathing, visualization, imagery
- Physical agents: electric stimulators massage–vibration, and biofeedback systems
- Various adjunct therapies: cold therapy, heat therapy, or counterirritants.

EVIDENCE-BASED PRACTICE
Effectiveness of Acupressure on Relieving Pain

Acupressure is a complementary treatment in which pressure is applied to specific points of the human body, generally by fingers or elbows. A recently published systematic review article has established some solid evidence that shows acupressure is effective in relieving pain in clients with dysmenorrhea (menstrual distress), labor pain, low back pain, chronic headache, and other traumatic pain. This has implications for nursing since acupressure is a technique that nurses can learn and apply at the bedside to help provide pain relief to their clients as a primary or adjunctive method of pain control.

Source: Chen & Wan (2014)

The nonpharmacologic approach (Table 16-1 ■) is appropriate for clients who are receptive to alternative methods, who have a high level of anxiety around the issue of pain, who would benefit from reducing dependence on drug therapy, who anticipate or have long-term chronic pain, or who receive inadequate pain relief from pharmacologic interventions. It is always based on individual assessment of the characteristics of the pain (see Box 16-2).

The Nurse's Role

Pain reduction methods include a wide range of techniques and medications. Rarely is pain relief successfully achieved with only one method. Even large doses of narcotics do not always control pain effectively—especially when it has been allowed to escalate.

One of the most important influences on pain relief is the relationship that exists between nurse and client. With most methods (the exception is **PCA**), the nurse has the power to relieve pain or to withhold pain relief. This knowledge creates anticipatory anxiety for the client. The client may request less medication when the nurse is supportive, caring, and assists with pain management.

Table 16-1 Nonpharmacologic Approaches to Pain

Physical Methods	Advantages
TENS—stimulating skin with mild electric current—provides pain relief by blocking pain impulses to the brain	Noninvasive method Allows client mobility Studies show effective for postoperative pain. Gives staff confidence they can assist client with pain. Choice for chronic pain
Acupuncture—ancient Chinese form of treating diseases and pain through insertion and manipulation of needles at specific points on the body	Insertion of thin needles is not painful to the client. Pain-relieving capacity extends beyond actual procedure. Method may provide relief when no other method works.
Biofeedback—electric monitoring device that feeds back effect of behavior so client can control internal processes (e.g., heartbeat)	Noninvasive method Completely controlled by client Promotes **stress** reduction as well as pain relief After mastery, instruments are not needed to achieve result.
Vibration or massage—hands-on manipulation of muscles or electrical form of massage (vibration)	Noninvasive method—electrically **alleviates** pain by numbness or paresthesia, or through touch Increases circulation and endorphins to area Relaxes muscles and reduces tension on nerves and promotes relaxation Useful only for light to moderate pain
Cold therapy—cold wraps, gel packs, cold therapy, ice massage; do not use on irradiated tissue or when clients have peripheral vascular disease	Relieves pain faster than heat therapy Numbs nerves and decreases inflammation and spasms Effective for nerve, abdominal, and lower back pain Alters pain threshold Decreases tissue injury response
Heat therapy—hot wraps, dry heat, moist heat; do not use on irradiated tissue or tumors	Noninvasive method Decreases pain by reducing inflammation Promotes relaxation of muscles Increases vasodilation and blood flow to area Facilitates clearance of tissue toxins and fluids
Counterirritants—mentholated ointments or lotions (Ben-Gay or Icy Hot)	May contain salicylates (reduces inflammation) but dangerous if client has potential bleeding problems May be irritating to the skin—potential skin breakdown
Acupressure application—based on the ancient Chinese method of acupuncture, this method involves using specific points located on meridians at various places on the body	Noninvasive method Redirection of energy flow through pressure on meridian points Reduces pain and increases endorphins
Chiropractic adjustment	Manipulation of muscles and realignment of spinal column Nerve function is restored. Structural integrity and balance are restored.
Relaxation—body relaxation of muscles used with imagery, therapist instruction	Relaxes tense muscles and reduces stress Effective in reducing pain Easy to learn and implement techniques for self-mastery Reduces fear and anxiety connected to pain
Imagery—visualization technique of forming sensory images, or seeing in the "mind's eye" an image that distracts from the sensation of pain	Effective in reducing pain Client can control use and timing of technique. Reduces high-level anxiety connected to pain
Deep breathing—techniques using breath to control pain	Effective in reinforcing body relaxation and visualization Reduces pain through breath control; increases oxygen utilization
Hypnosis—creating a state of altered consciousness so that client is susceptible to instruction	Effective with a client who is suggestive and who experiences tension and anxiety accompanying pain

Note: Other alternative techniques are presented in Chapter 17.

> **CLINICAL ALERT**
>
> The single most critical factor in achieving pain relief is for the nurse to be the client's advocate. The comfort of the client is the nurse's primary concern.

Nursing interventions that provide effective pain relief, in addition to pain medication, are those that encourage behaviors that assist the client not to focus on pain. For example, when the client is talking about something of great interest or pleasure, he or she is not thinking about pain. Slow breathing and deliberate relaxation lessen pain, whereas muscle tension and anxiety increase it. If the nurse teaches pain-relief techniques before surgery, the client can more easily implement them when the pain is intense. The nurse may also encourage the client to use techniques that he or she has found effective in the past, no matter how "unscientific" they may be. Whatever method or technique the nurse uses to assist the client with relieving pain, the single most critical intervention is a caring and supportive attitude.

To provide effective pain management to clients from cultures other than one's own, it is helpful for the nurse to understand a client's culture and how it affects the client's response to pain as well as the client's preferred methods of pain management. Clients with various cultural backgrounds and beliefs have ways of treating pain that may be different from those of the nurse who is caring for the client. To accomplish this, the nurse must ask clients how they would prefer their pain to be managed and make sure they are the ones in control of their care.

Techniques for Pain Control

IV Patient-Controlled Analgesia

One of the most successful methods of pain relief, introduced in the 1970s, was patient-controlled analgesia (PCA). The primary purpose of PCA is to allow the client to self-administer an analgesic dose of medication predetermined by the healthcare provider (Figure 16-6 ■). PCA enables the client to assess and control his or her own pain level. This method of pain control has been found to be very effective because the client feels in more control of his or her life situation, there is no significant difference in the amount of analgesic medication used (if anything, it is usually less), there is better pain control than IV injections, and this method of pain control is less time consuming for the nurse.

Epidural Pain Control

An effective technique for controlling pain is the use of an epidural catheter inserted into the epidural space. The advantage of epidural pain control is that the narcotic moves directly from the epidural space into the spinal fluid and binds with opiate receptors in the spinal cord, blocking reception of pain. Administered by this method, the required drug dose is considerably lower because it is not metabolized in the liver.

FIGURE 16-6 Continuous IV narcotic drip for pain control.

Breakthrough Pain Control

There are two major types of pain—continuous and breakthrough. Many clients with cancer experience long periods of persistent pain and may also experience severe flare-ups that occur even when the client is on around-the-clock (**ATC**) medication. Studies suggest that nearly 70% of cancer clients experience breakthrough pain. These episodes typically last about 30 min, but tend to totally decimate the client.

Generally, breakthrough pain occurs as two types:

- Incident pain—caused by movement or activity (e.g., sitting up, walking, or coughing)
- Spontaneous pain—does not seem to be linked to any specific source but occurs with no warning or relation to activity or movement.

Breakthrough pain can be managed by different protocols, some of which are listed below:

- Increasing the dose of ATC medication so that breakthrough pain is eliminated—this method is not always advisable because sedation and other side effects of the drug may occur.
- Changing the ATC medication so that relatively constant analgesia occurs (use long-acting oral opioids or fentanyl patches).
- Prescribing a supplemental dose of a short-acting morphine-like drug so that it is taken 30 min before incident pain when this type of pain is predictable.
- When spontaneous pain occurs, instruct the client to take the dose as soon as possible after onset.
- An effective delivery method, oral transmucosal, delivers fentanyl citrate via a sucker or lollipop (Figure 16-7 ■). This has the advantage of being quickly absorbed through the mucous membrane of the mouth and working rapidly to control breakthrough pain. This medication should be taken only by clients already taking prescription opioid (narcotic) drugs on a regular schedule.

FIGURE 16-7 The oral transmucosal method for managing breakthrough pain delivers medication via a lozenge on a stick.

Transdermal Patches

Transdermal patches are a useful alternative to oral medication, particularly for people with chronic pain. They deliver medication over several days and come in a variety of units of dosage-strength combinations, frequency of administration, shapes, and sizes. They deliver a uniform plasma drug concentration and encourage client compliance because they are easy to use.

However, some serious adverse events have occurred, so nurses must educate their clients about the potential dangers associated with use of transdermal patches. The Institute for Safe Medication Practices (**ISMP**) has had several safety alerts for Fentanyl transdermal patches because of adverse events. This patch contains high doses of the drug and should only be used for clients who have previously taken large doses of opioids. Problems associated with transdermal patches are failure to remove the existing patch before applying a new one, failure to dispose of patches properly, not storing patches safely, and serious adverse events such as respiratory depression when using the patch.

SAFETY ALERT

A recent ISMP alert (2013) reported another incident in which a child died after apparently ingesting a transdermal fentanyl patch. The child had been sleeping on his mother's chest while they were both taking a nap. The mother had been wearing the patch for chronic pain related to multiple sclerosis. When the mother awoke, the child was unresponsive and, despite efforts to revive him, he died in the emergency room. An autopsy revealed acute fentanyl intoxication.

Cultural Awareness

Healthcare personnel working in a variety of settings maintain that pain is a culturally influenced phenomenon. How pain is experienced and expressed varies by cultural group (Spector, 2012). For example, some cultures (such as the Italian and Jewish people) encourage open expression of feelings like pain, while others (the stoic English, Irish, and Chinese) believe that pain is something to be ignored or endured in silence. This was demonstrated by Zborowski's study done as early as the 1950s. While these general conclusions may lead to stereotyping, it is important to consider the impact of the individual's culture in the assessment of pain level, while ensuring individualized care based on input from the client. A multilingual pain assessment form can be useful (Figure 16-8 ■).

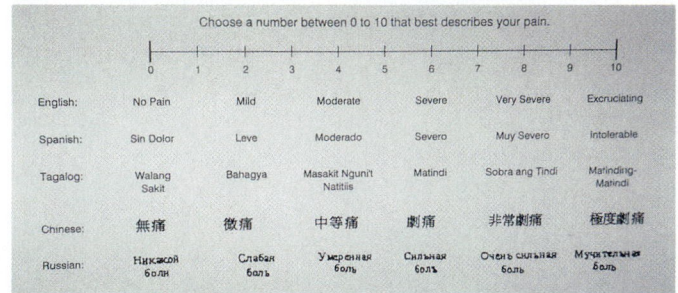

FIGURE 16-8 A multilanguage pain chart helps in obtaining an accurate description of pain.

Nursing Diagnoses

The following nursing diagnoses may be appropriate to include on client care plans when the components are related to alleviating pain in a client.

NURSING DIAGNOSIS	RELATED TO . . .
Anxiety	Anticipation of discomfort, fear, helplessness, inability to relax
Compromised Family Coping	Family members have difficulty dealing with client's pain, functions as proxy for pain relief.
Ineffective Coping	Poor adjustment to pain/illness, fear
Fear	Long-term disability, terminal disease, hospitalization, invasive procedures, lack of knowledge, surgery and its outcome
Acute Pain or Chronic Pain	Trauma, immobility, surgery, chronic illness

Source: Herdman, T. H. & Kamitsuru, S. (Eds.) *Nursing Diagnoses – Definitions and Classification 2015-2017*. Copyright © 2014, 1994–2014 by NANDA International. Used by arrangement with John Wiley & Sons Limited. Companion website: www.wiley.com/go/nursingdiagnoses. In order to make safe and effective judgments using NANDA-I nursing diagnosis it is essential that nurses refer to the definitions and defining characteristics of the diagnoses listed in this work.

Pain Assessment

Nursing Process Data

ASSESSMENT Database

- See Skill 16.1.1, Assessing Pain.

PLANNING Objectives

- To determine the presence of pain in terms of type, location, quality, intensity, and level of discomfort
- To identify associated symptoms
- To identify a database that will assist in formulating a plan for pain management
- To increase client's satisfaction with pain management

IMPLEMENTATION Procedures

DOCUMENTATION AND EVALUATION

Expected Outcomes

- Pain level is assessed adequately.
- Pain level in a cognitively impaired or nonverbal client is adequately assessed.
- Pain in a young child is assessed correctly.

Unexpected Outcomes/Alternative Actions

Pearson Nursing Student Resources

Find additional review materials at
nursing.pearsonhighered.com.
Prepare for success with NCLEX®-style practice questions and Skill Checklists.

Skill 16.1.1 | Assessing Pain

Procedure

1. Assess type of pain, and ask client to describe pain using his or her own words. ❶

   a. Acute pain: short duration of a few seconds/minutes to 6 months
   b. Chronic/persistent pain: prolonged, persistent pain, 6 months to years
   c. Cancer pain

2. Assess location.

   a. Ask client to point to area of the body or verbalize location of pain.
   b. Ask if pain is superficial or deep.
   c. Ask if pain is diffuse or localized.
   d. Ask if pain radiates and where it goes.

3. Assess quality.

   a. Stabbing, knifelike
   b. Throbbing
   c. Cramping
   d. Viselike, suffocating
   e. Searing or burning

4. Assess intensity.

   a. Ask client to indicate intensity of pain using a pain scale; for example, a scale of 0–10. Use the same pain scale to compare intensity before and after interventions.
   b. Ask client what measures have reduced the level of pain on the scale.

5. Assess onset of pain and aggravating factors.

   a. What triggers the pain?
   b. How does movement affect pain?
   c. Does coughing affect pain?
   d. How does emotion affect pain?
   e. How does position or fatigue affect pain level?

6. Assess associated factors.

   a. Nausea and vomiting
   b. Hypotension/hypertension
   c. Profuse perspiration
   d. Apprehension or anxiety
   e. Respiratory and heart rate

7. Assess alleviating factors.

   a. Position
   b. Elevation of extremity
   c. Techniques used at home for pain relief
   d. Pain medications the client uses

8. Assess client's behavioral responses to pain.

   a. No pain—relaxed, calm, and alert (0)
   b. Mild pain—stressed, tense, occasional grimace or frown (1–3)
   c. Moderate pain—stoicism, squirming, grimacing, more reassurance to comfort (4–6)
   d. Severe pain—moaning, restless, muscle twitching, difficult to comfort (7–9)
   e. Worst pain—crying, constant moaning, withdrawal, inability to be comforted (10)

9. What is the client's level of sedation and is it safe to administer the next pain medication (Box 16-4 ■)?

Box 16-4 POSS (PASERO OPIOID-INDUCED SEDATION) SCALE

S = Sleep, easy to arouse
Acceptable; no action necessary; may increase opioid dose if needed

1 = Awake and alert
Acceptable; no action necessary; may increase opioid dose if needed

2 = Slightly drowsy, easily aroused
Acceptable; no action necessary; may increase opioid dose if needed

3 = Frequently drowsy, arousable, drifts off to sleep during conversation
Unacceptable; monitor respiratory status and sedation level closely until sedation level is stable at less than 3 and respiratory status is satisfactory; decrease opioid dose 25%–50% or notify prescriber or anesthesiologist for orders; consider administering a nonsedating, opioid-sparing nonopioid, such as acetaminophen or an NSAID, if not contraindicated.

4 = Somnolent, minimal or no response to verbal or physical stimulation
Unacceptable; stop opioid; consider administering naloxone; notify prescriber or anesthesiologist; monitor respiratory status and sedation level closely until sedation level is stable at less than 3 and respiratory status is satisfactory.

Source: Pasero (2009)

❶ Assist client to describe pain in detail so that your assessment is complete.

(continued)

Skill 16.1.1 | Assessing Pain (continued)

10. When to reassess for follow-up pain medication administration.

    a. Postop client—every 2 hr or until pain is controlled
    b. Client experiencing pain—at least every 4 hr

11. After pain medication is given, the appropriate follow-up time for reassessment is as follows:

    a. Injection—5–30 minutes
    b. Oral medication—60–90 minutes
    c. Sustained-release analgesic or transdermal patch—4 hr

Skill 16.1.2 | Assessing Pain in a Cognitively Impaired or Nonverbal Client

Procedure

1. Assess client's level of understanding.
2. Assess nonverbal cues if you are unable to obtain a verbal response.

   a. Facial expressions
   b. General behavior

   c. Unusual movements, twisting or turning, restlessness, pacing, immobility
   d. Vocal sounds—moaning, crying, gasping, groaning
   e. Muscle contractions, especially around the eyes

3. Evaluate changes after pain-relief intervention to determine whether further assessment is indicated.

Skill 16.1.3 | Assessing Pain in Young Children

Procedure

1. Use a standardized pain assessment tool such as the FACES or FLACC scale to assess level of pain (see Figures 16-3 or 16-4).
2. Assess other indicators of pain including:

   a. Physiologic indicators

      (1) Increase in heart rate
      (2) Elevation in blood pressure
      (3) Sweating
      (4) Changes in skin color

   b. Behavioral indicators

      (1) High-pitched cry
      (2) Inability to be consoled
      (3) Awake continuously—inability to sleep
      (4) Fussy
      (5) Grunting sounds

3. Assess behavioral responses.

   a. Facial movement
   b. Bulging of area between eyebrows
   c. Tightly closed eyes
   d. Rigid mouth and tongue

Unit 16.1 Documentation and Evaluation

DOCUMENTATION for Assessing Pain Level

- Describe client's pain, including all of the assessment parameters, and document client's pain score based on the pain rating scale used.
- Describe pain level, including behavioral and verbal manifestations used to determine level for the cognitively impaired or nonverbal client.

- Describe behavioral cues used to assess pain level in a young child.
- Use a pain scale for children, such as FACES or FLACC.
- Describe response to pain-management intervention using same assessment parameters and pain scale as were used for initial assessment.

EVALUATION/Critical Thinking

Expected Outcomes

- Pain level is assessed adequately.
- Pain level in a cognitively impaired or nonverbal client is adequately assessed.
- Pain in a young child is assessed correctly.

Unexpected Outcomes	Alternative Actions
• Pain level is incorrectly or inadequately assessed.	• Assess client's pain level according to standards. • Pay close attention to client's report of pain level.
• Client reports new level of pain or pain not relieved by previously effective strategies.	• Do not attribute this report to preexisting cause. Instead, let this report trigger a diagnostic evaluation.
• Pain level in a cognitively impaired or nonverbal client is not assessed correctly as behavior and facial expressions indicate.	• Reassess according to the steps of assessment. • Request a consult from a pain expert. Try an alternative method of pain control.
• Pain level in a child is not assessed adequately.	• Reassess pain level, paying close attention to behavioral expressions. • Request a consult with the healthcare provider to change pain medication.

Pharmacologic Pain Management

Nursing Process Data

ASSESSMENT Database

- Assess client's type, description, rating (use a pain-intensity scale), and level of pain.
- Assess vital signs for baseline comparison.
- Assess allergy to ordered pain medication.
- Assess risks of opioid therapy.
- Assess ability of client to self-administer PCA.
- Assess insertion site for drainage, inflammation, and such.
- Assess client throughout PCA/epidural therapy.
- Assess patency of IV lines or epidural catheter.
- Assess sedation level of client on PCA or epidural analgesia.

PLANNING Objectives

- To implement strategies to decrease pain
- To prevent pain from delaying recovery
- To prevent pain from causing nausea and vomiting, a decrease in fluid intake that results in fluid and electrolyte imbalance
- To prevent pain from causing undue fatigue
- To prevent pain from inhibiting moving, ambulating, turning, and coughing; pain increases the possibilities of secondary problems from inactivity (e.g., pneumonia, emboli)
- To provide a consistent level of pain control without unacceptable side effects
- To enable the client to feel in control of his or her pain management
- To decrease the client's anxiety around the pain control issue
- To allow the client, according to needs for pain control, to self-administer pain medication via PCA

IMPLEMENTATION Procedures

DOCUMENTATION AND EVALUATION

Expected Outcomes

- Client feels competent to self-administer pain medication via PCA.
- IV site or epidural site remains free of complications.
- Pain is controlled to client's satisfaction.
- Client's anxiety level remains low or manageable around issue of pain control.
- Family and friends (proxy) are educated not to interfere with pain-relief protocols.

Unexpected Outcomes/Alternative Actions

Pearson Nursing Student Resources

Find additional review materials at **nursing. pearsonhighered.com**.

Prepare for success with NCLEX®-style practice questions and Skill Checklists.

Skill 16.2.1 | Administering Pain Medications

Equipment
Pain-Assessment Scale
Sedation Scale
Ordered pain medication
Electronic Health Record

Procedure
1. Introduce self to client and perform hand hygiene.
2. Identify client using two client identifiers.
3. Assess pain according to the parameters of pain assessment and select a pain tool based on client's preference and cognitive status (e.g., numeric, FACES, FLACC).
4. Check EHR for healthcare provider order and perform medication safety checks (right drug, right client, right dose, right time, right route, right documentation).
5. Check chart for any allergy to pain drug and healthcare provider's orders for changes in pain medication.
6. Administer ordered pain medication or request change in dosing schedule of infusion, PCA, or other method. (Table 16-2 ■).
7. Ensure analgesic is individualized to the client, taking into account type of pain, intensity, and potential for toxicity (age, renal impairment, peptic ulcer, and other factors).
8. Document in EHR.
9. Reassess pain at the appropriate time interval using the appropriate parameters of pain assessment.

Table 16-2 Pain Management

Effective Pain Management	Barriers to Effective Pain Control
Listens to and believes clients when they describe the level of pain they are experiencing. This is the single most important pain assessment tool.	Insensitive response or not believing the client's subjective experience of pain.
Intervenes or administers the pain medication when it is needed.	Nurse wants reassurance the pain really requires medication—does not just respond to the client's request.
Does not allow the pain to escalate but anticipates when pain medication will be needed.	Believes drug tolerance will make the medication less effective, so the less medication given, the better.
Works with the client to control the pain and requests different medications or dosages from the healthcare provider when needed.	Believes the healthcare provider knows best about the amount of pain medication for the client.
Is not concerned about addiction when administering pain medication.	Is concerned about drug dependence or addiction—believes it is more important than effective pain management.
Understands the various actions of drugs and their role in pain control.	Has inadequate knowledge about pain medications, so miscalculates dosage, duration of action, or synergistic drug interactions.

Skill 16.2.2 | Improving Client Satisfaction With Pain Control

Procedure
1. Identify client receiving pain medication using two forms of client ID.
2. Inform client you will be asking questions to determine his or her level of satisfaction with pain medication protocol.
3. Ask, on a scale of 1–5, with 1 being very satisfied, "Can you tell me how satisfied you are with our pain-control program?"
4. Ask, on the same scale, 1–5, "How do you rate nurse intervention for your pain control?"
5. Determine how often in hours during a 24-hr period the client experiences pain.
6. Ask, "During which shift of the three 8-hr shifts do you experience the most pain?"
7. Ask, "How long does it take you to receive pain relief when you have requested it?"

Note: These are only guideline questions. Your hospital may wish to develop its own short questionnaire to increase client satisfaction with pain control and meet The Joint Commission Pain Standards.

EVIDENCE-BASED PRACTICE
Client Attitudes and Beliefs Regarding Pain Management
Nurses need to understand client's beliefs and attitudes about pain medications in order to adequately provide them with appropriate pain medication after surgery. Clients who do not complain about pain may do so for reasons other than a lack of pain. A survey conducted with clients undergoing cardiac surgery found 31% of the 379 clients indicated they thought it was easy to become addicted to the pain medication. Another 36% of the clients believed that the pain medication should be saved just in case the pain got worse, and 20% thought good clients should not speak about their pain. This study underscores the need for nurses to be diligent in educating their clients about the use of pain management therapies after surgery.

Source: Cogan, Ouimette, Vargas-Schaffer, Yegin, Deschamps, & Denault (2014)

Skill 16.2.3 | Managing Pain With Patient-Controlled Analgesia (PCA)

Note: PCA is usually initiated in PACU when ordered by a physician or anesthesiologist.

Equipment

Specific healthcare provider's orders for PCA
Gloves
PCA central unit, infuser pump, and PCA module
PCA administration tubing
IV start kit, tubing, catheter, and ordered fluid
Extension set with Luer-Lok adapter
Analgesic medication cartridge and injector (vial injector)
Electronic Health Record

Procedure

1. Introduce yourself to the client and perform hand hygiene.
2. Identify client using two client identifiers.
3. Determine whether client is a candidate for PCA by evaluating the client's cognitive ability and willingness to use this method of pain control (Box 16-5 ■).
4. Assess pain according to the parameters of pain assessment and select a pain tool based on client's preference and cognitive status (e.g., numeric, FACES, FLACC).
5. Check EHR for healthcare provider order and perform medication safety checks (right drug, right client, right dose, right time, and right route); see Table 16-3 ■.
6. Assess any allergy to prescribed pain medication.
7. Perform basic physical assessment before initiating PCA.
   a. Establish baseline vital sign chart.
   b. Specifically assess client's respiratory system for ongoing evaluation during PCA therapy using a sedation scale (POSS, SAS, RASS) per agency protocol.
8. Assess patency of IV and skin integrity of IV site.
9. Program the pump according to the PCA orders (drug, basal dose, lockout time, demand).
10. Assemble the tubing.

Box 16-5 CRITERIA FOR CLIENT SELECTION FOR PCA

- Clients requiring parenteral analgesic treatment
- Clients requiring postoperative pain relief
- Trauma clients who have clear sensorium
- Clients suffering from chronic pain (terminal cancer)
- Clients who are mentally alert and able to understand and comply with procedure instructions
- Clients without a handicap that impairs ability to use PCA
- Clients with no prior addiction to drugs or alcohol and no allergy to pain medication prescribed—usually morphine, hydromorphone, Dilaudid, or fentanyl
- Usual minimum age of 18 for PCA use, but has been used in children as young as 7 years of age

11. Attach drug syringe to tubing and prime the tubing.
12. Attach a needleless port to the end of the PCA tubing.
13. With alcohol, wipe the injection port of the maintenance IV nearest the client.
14. Attach the PCA tubing using the needleless adapter.
15. Deliver a bolus dose, if ordered, by programming the pump to deliver the bolus.

SAFETY ALERT

Most institutions require an independent double-check by a licensed healthcare practitioner of all PCA administration when the PCA is first administered, when the syringe is changed, when a loading dose is given, and when the rate or drug is changed or there are any other changes in the PCA administration orders.

16. Monitor the client according to agency protocol.
17. Observe closely for signs of allergic reaction and respiratory depression.
18. Document all relevant information in the EHR.

Table 16-3 PCA Risks and Strategies

PCA Risks	Risk Reduction Strategies
Wrong or improper drug or dose	Standardizing the drugs for PCA use Standardizing PCA order sheets Using prefilled syringes and bags with standardized concentrations Integrating bar coding on medications for PCA use Limiting the concentration of drugs Implementing new protocols for infusion of meds
Side effects of medication—toxicity, respiratory distress, oversedation	Continual respiratory monitoring Adding pulse oximetry (S_pO_2) and capnography ($EtCO_2$) to the same module, monitoring adverse responses, monitoring level of consciousness
Improper client selection	Using standard protocol for client selection
Programming errors of meds	Using safety software for dosing and safety limits Having nurses annually demonstrate entering correct PCA settings from standard orders Double-checking all PCA initiation and dosage/syringe changes
PCA by proxy	Intervening in established pain-relief protocols; proxy is usually family and friends' intervention, so better education of family and client is indicated.

Skill 16.2.4 | Ongoing Assessment of the Client With PCA

Procedure

1. Perform hand hygiene.
2. Identify client using two client identifiers.
3. Check pulse oximetry readings—when SpO$_2$ is less than 90% with decreased respiratory rate (less than 10), client status requires intervention.
4. Monitor respiratory status often with a prescribed time interval. ➤ *Rationale:* It is a key indicator of adverse response to opioid infusion.
5. Monitor sedation levels often using a standardized sedation tool such as the POSS or SAS. ➤ *Rationale:* It is a key indicator of early respiratory depression.
6. Check heart rate, respiratory rate, oxygen level, end-tidal CO$_2$ if PCA has **capnography module** (Box 16-6 ■).
   ➤ *Rationale:* These criteria are important to assess and monitor status of the client.

Note: Intermittent monitoring may not pick up ventilatory depression that occurs between monitoring times.

Box 16-6   **PCA CAPNOGRAPHY**

Due to PCA sentinel event warnings, recent studies suggest using side-stream capnography (together with pulse oximetry) to provide continuous recordings of heart rate, oxygen saturation, respiratory rate, and end-tidal CO$_2$ from which they can monitor for respiratory depression. A change in respiratory status is a leading indicator of adverse client response to opioid infusion, and capnography can detect hypoventilation. Most CA pumps have integrated capnography and pulse oximetry.

Skill 16.2.5 | Teaching PCA to a Client

Preparation

1. Determine whether client is a candidate for PCA.
2. Allow client to handle equipment directly and practice using a "dummy" PCA button. ➤ *Rationale:* This reduces fear of technology and teaches basic steps of PCA.

Procedure

1. Perform hand hygiene.
2. Identify client using two client identifiers.
3. Demonstrate how PCA device works. ❶

   a. Set the pump's controls to deliver pain medication.
   b. Instruct client that if amount of medication is not sufficient to control pain, he or she may press a button to deliver an additional bolus.

   c. Dose may be adjusted to maintain pain control.
      ➤ *Rationale:* When clients control their own medication dose, studies indicate usage is not excessive.
   d. Have client explain and demonstrate PCA use before initiating therapy.

4. Clarify with client how he or she administers medication dose when pain is felt.➤ *Rationale:* Self-control of pain medication has been found to be very successful with clients and less time-consuming for the nurse. There is no significant difference in amount of medication used.
5. Program PCA infuser for continuous infusion plus a bolus dose.

   a. Establish amount of narcotic needed to control client's pain (i.e., give 1–5 mg morphine every 10 min until pain is relieved).
   b. Set pump's hourly infusion rate to equal total milligrams per hour needed to control pain.

6. Reassure client that PCA will control, but not totally abolish, pain. ➤ *Rationale:* Continuous infusion supplemented by small boluses provides steady relief (more so than IM injections) but does not eliminate pain.
7. Teach client how to evaluate pain level on a 5-point scale. If client's pain is not sufficiently relieved, medication dose is increased. ➤ *Rationale:* When clients know they can control their pain level, they feel less helpless and more empowered.

   1 = Pain relieved
   2 = Occasional discomfort
   3 = Decreased pain intensity, for example, able to walk, cough
   4 = Minimal pain relief
   5 = No pain relief

❶ Teach PCA procedure to client.

(continued)

Skill 16.2.5 | Teaching PCA to a Client (continued)

8. Evaluate client's response to medication schedule.
   ➤ *Rationale:* It is important to check for adverse effects of sedation to avoid complications or necessity of revising dose parameters.
9. Reassess client's ability to control pain level and effectiveness of medication dosage to control pain.
10. Teach client importance of not letting family member (or anyone other than client) activate PCA pump.
    ➤ *Rationale:* PCA by proxy (family members) has caused critical events of overdosing.

11. Teach client potential adverse effects (sedation, respiratory depression) if anyone other than client activates pump.
12. Instruct client to notify staff if machine malfunctions (alarm sounds or message display indicates a problem), pain is not controlled or changes in severity, or if he or she has any questions.

Skill 16.2.6 | Monitoring a Client Receiving an Epidural Infusion

Preparation
1. Introduce yourself to client and perform hand hygiene.
2. Check that catheter is labeled "epidural catheter," and place the IV line as far as possible from the epidural catheter.
   ➤ *Rationale:* Identifies catheter and avoids confusing epidural catheter with IV tubing.

> **CLINICAL ALERT**
> Confusion of IV line and epidural line could lead to a fatal mistake.

3. Check that Narcan is available on the unit. ➤ *Rationale:* Respiratory depression can be treated with IV Narcan, a narcotic antagonist.
4. Check that there is IV access for administration of Narcan.
   ➤ *Rationale:* It may be necessary to administer a narcotic antagonist quickly if respiratory depression occurs.

Note: *IV should be accessed with a needleless syringe.*

5. Check that Ambu bag is available on the unit. ➤ *Rationale:* This is necessary to mitigate complication of respiratory depression.
6. Check if an apnea monitor or pulse oximeter is ordered. Pulse oximeter alarm should be set at 92%. ➤ *Rationale:* It is important that clients be monitored closely (at least for the first 12 hr) because of dangerous side effects, especially respiratory depression.
7. Check two forms of client identification. Check that there is a sign over the bed stating "Epidural Protocol Client." ❶

Box 16-7 NARCOTICS COMMONLY ADMINISTERED VIA EPIDURAL CONTINUOUS INFUSION
- Preservative-free morphine sulfate (Duramorph: 0.2–1.0 mg/hr)
- Hydromorphone hydrochloride (Dilaudid: 0.05–0.3 mg/hr)
- Fentanyl (50–150 µg/hr)

EVIDENCE-BASED PRACTICE
Use of Range Orders for Opioid Analgesics in Management of Pain

A consensus statement published by the American Society for Pain Management Nurses and the American Pain Society supports safe medication practices and use of range or "prn" orders for opioid analgesics in the management of pain. This statement outlines clear recommendations and conditions for prescribers, institutions, and registered nurses to ensure these medications are given safely. These included the use of pain assessment tools that are valid and reliable, basing decisions on thorough pain assessments, and communicating with the client. This set of guidelines can be found on the American Society for Pain Management Nurses' website.

Source: Drew, Gordon, Renner, Morgan, Swensen, & Manworren (2014)

❶ When a client is receiving epidural analgesia, there should be a sign over the bed stating "Epidural Protocol Client."

Procedure

1. Check healthcare provider's orders for epidural narcotic indicating concentration, basal dose rate, demand dose, and lockout interval. (Box 16-7 ■ names narcotics commonly administered via epidural infusion.)

2. Perform an independent double check of pump settings and narcotic ordered with another healthcare professional.
   ➤ *Rationale:* Narcotic drugs can have serious side effects such as respiratory depression if giving too large a dose.

3. Assess client's vital signs, pain score, and sedation score according to agency protocol using the appropriate pain and sedation tools.

4. Check that a sterile, occlusive dressing is over insertion site. Inspect the dressing every shift, and report any evidence of infection, redness, pain, swelling, or leakage to anesthesiologist. Dressing is changed every 72 hr or per agency policy.

5. Closely monitor respirations every 1 hr for 24 hr or per agency protocol or use apnea monitor or pulse oximeter.
   ➤ *Rationale:* Due to risk of respiratory depression, close monitoring after administration of an epidural narcotic is essential.

6. Monitor vital signs: BP and pulse every 30 min for 1 hr after initial epidural dose, then every 4 hr or per agency policy.

7. Monitor for possible side effects of narcotic administration: respiratory depression, urinary retention, nausea and vomiting, and pruritus.

8. Document dose and client status.

9. Repeat steps for nurse-initiated medication bolus through the infusion device or changes to initial epidural infusion pump settings if allowed in your agency (see Box 16-8 ■).

Box 16-8 WHAT'S A SMART PUMP?

Infusion pumps have revolutionized the way nurses administer IV therapy. Now they have become "smarter." The pump's "brain" includes software that contains a drug library and alerts you if a medication is outside the recommended parameters, such as dose, dosing unit, rate, or concentration. Smart pumps also log data about all these alerts. As required by The Joint Commission, smart pumps include safety features that will prevent unintentional overdoses of a medication or fluid. The smart pumps available include Alaris System with Guardrails Safety Software (Cardinal Health), Colleague CX with Guardian feature (Baxter), Outlook 100-400 Safety Infusion Systems with Dose Guard (B. Braun Medical), PlumA+ and Life Care infusion system with Hospira MedNet Software (Hospira).

Smart Pump Protocol

- Turn on the smart pump and designate the specific client care area where you're going to use it. (The pump will automatically configure itself to give you the infusion parameters for that area, e.g., Pediatrics.)
- Program the pump by choosing the intended drug and concentration from the pump's list.
- Enter the ordered dose and infusion rate. (The pump checks this information against the drug library.)
- If what you've programmed is outside the allowed parameters, the pump will alert you. The pump will sound a "soft" alarm, which you can override to allow the infusion to begin, or a "hard" alarm. This will require you to reprogram the pump to be within the facility's specified limits.
- The pump logs and tracks all alerts to provide the hospital with data to shape current practice guidelines.

Integrating a Smart Pump With Bar Coding

When a hospital integrates a smart pump with a bar-code medication administration system (BCMA), it will address all five "rights" of medication administration.

The FDA mandated that, by 2006, drug manufacturers must label most prescription drugs and certain OTCs with a machine-readable bar code.

General Steps of Using a Bar Code

- Check the client's electronic medication record (which tells you which IV meds were ordered and time of administration).
- Enter client's room with scanning device and scan bar codes on the medication, the client's ID, and your own ID badge.
- The bar-code label on the drug is then programmed into the pump. Software ensures medication in bar-coded drug vial is consistent with hospital guidelines. When all scanned information is received, the pump will allow you to begin the infusion.
- The pump will automatically communicate with a computer in the pharmacy so that an up-to-date status of your client is available.

Alaris Smart Pump with attached modules.

(continued)

Skill 16.2.6 | Monitoring a Client Receiving an Epidural Infusion *(continued)*

Note: Many hospitals require specific certification before the RN can administer narcotics via an indwelling epidural catheter. A student nurse should not administer solutions via epidural catheter. Verify the regulations and role parameters for each healthcare worker. All nurses should be aware of the safety precautions. Epidural catheters are generally placed by specially trained healthcare providers for the treatment of postoperative pain, labor and delivery, or cancer pain. Nurses will manage the client care during the delivery of the epidural pain medication, which is done through an infusion device. In some agencies (if they have received training), they may change the analgesic and make changes to the infusion pump after it is initially programmed. Only certified individuals or those specially trained, such as nurse anesthetists or anesthesiologists, may initiate epidural infusions or administer epidural anesthesia through a bolus injection.

Unit 16.2 Documentation and Evaluation

DOCUMENTATION for Pharmacologic Pain Management

- Pain assessment: onset, pattern, description, location, intensity
- Amount and type of pain medication administered
- Sedation level of client
- Interventions, level of pain relief
- Side effects—pruritus, nausea, and vomiting
- Vital signs

For Epidural Analgesia

- Pain relief from medication
- Side effects—pruritus, nausea, and vomiting
- Condition of insertion site
- Vital signs

For PCA

- Assess and chart on client using PCA infuser every 4 hr (after initial 24 hr), unless otherwise ordered.
- Describe respirations every 2 hr and compare to baseline assessment sheet.

- Record sedation and pain legend every 4 hr. Include degree of pain relief obtained from PCA.
  1 = Wide awake
  2 = Drowsy
  3 = Dozing intermittently
  4 = Mostly sleeping
  5 = Only awakens when disturbed
- Initiate new PCA administration record for each narcotic vial injector used.

For PCA Record

- Chart appropriate entries throughout your shift.
- Document medication per agency policy in the electronic health record.
- Chart wasted narcotic—cosigned per hospital policy.
- Verify and document that calculated volume remaining and actual volume remaining in syringe are the same. Report and follow hospital procedure for any narcotic discrepancies.

EVALUATION/Critical Thinking

Expected Outcomes

- Client feels competent to self-administer pain medication via PCA.
- PCA infuser works efficiently to administer medication.
- IV site used to administer PCA remains free of complications.
- Pain is assessed at the appropriate level and controlled to client's satisfaction.

- Medication administration for pain is monitored at an appropriate level.
- Client's anxiety level remains low or manageable around issue of pain control.
- Family and friends are educated not to interfere with pain-relief protocols.

Unexpected Outcomes	Alternative Actions
For Administering Pain Medication	
• Client says that pain medication is not helping the pain.	• Reassess tolerance level of client (check if client has previously been on high doses of a narcotic, thus developing a high tolerance level). • Check that pain dose is adequate for pain management. • Request consultation with healthcare provider to increase or change pain medication (remember, the nurse is the client's advocate).
• Client appears overly sedated.	• Evaluate the client's respiratory status, sedation score, and notify the healthcare provider. • Check other drugs client is taking—there may be a synergistic effect. • A narcotic or opioid antagonist may need to be administered per agency protocol.
• Client develops constipation from regularly administered narcotic preparations.	• Obtain order for and administer stool softener and peristaltic stimulant. • Encourage intake of high-fiber diet, if not contraindicated. • Encourage adequate fluid intake.
• Client develops nausea and vomits.	• Assess cause of problem—consider pain, ileus, as well as reaction to drug. • Administer antiemetics as ordered, and protect client from aspiration.
• Client complains of numbness in legs and motor weakness but has no pain.	• Notify healthcare provider. • Manage epidural infusion per agency protocol. • Chart nursing actions and client response.
• Catheter insertion site is red and warm to touch, and drainage is noted.	• Check temperature and vital signs and notify healthcare provider.
• Client is insecure and anxious about using PCA mode of pain control.	• Determine which steps client feels insecure about completing, and reteach procedure while demonstrating steps.

Note: Refer to Table 16-3, PCA Risks and Strategies.

Nursing Process Data

ASSESSMENT Database

- Assess type of pain.
  Acute pain: short duration of a few seconds to 6 months
  Chronic/persistent pain: longer duration of 3–6 months or longer
- Choose a pain-intensity scale and identify the level or degree of pain the client is experiencing.
- Assess nonverbal indications of pain.
- Assess client's behavioral responses to pain.
  Depression, withdrawal, or crying
  Stoicism or expressive
- Assess location, quality, intensity, onset, duration, pattern, aggravating factors, associated factors, and relief or alleviating factors. (See Figure 16-1.)

PLANNING Objectives

- To relieve pain or prevent pain from escalating by relaxing muscles; muscle tension increases the pain
- To decrease client's anxiety that present and future pain relief will not be achieved
- To bring pain relief to a level acceptable to the client
- To educate clients to communicate their pain level
- To improve client satisfaction with pain management

IMPLEMENTATION Procedures

- **Skill 16.3.1** Alleviating Pain Through Touch (Massage) 538
- **Skill 16.3.2** Using Relaxation Techniques 539

DOCUMENTATION AND EVALUATION

Expected Outcomes

- Pain is controlled through nonpharmacologic methods such as massage, relaxation techniques, or TENS.
- Client is satisfied with level of pain control.
- Client receives adequate pain medication; pain level does not interfere with client's activity.
- Client's anxiety level is lowered in relation to pain.

Unexpected Outcomes/Alternative Actions

Pearson Nursing Student Resources

Find additional review materials at **nursing.pearsonhighered.com**
Prepare for success with NCLEX®-style practice questions and Skill Checklists.

| **Skill 16.3.1** | Alleviating Pain Through Touch (Massage) |

Equipment
Body lotion
Massage oil
Towel or drape

Procedure
1. Establish a quiet, private environment.
2. Determine whether client achieves more relief from pain with massage over painful area, near painful area, or from foot rub, back rub, or hand rub.
3. Warm your hands by rubbing them together or rinsing in warm water.
4. Warm lotion to be used by holding closed bottle under warm running water.
5. Massage area of client's choice with slow and steady motion. ❶
6. Use deep pressure or light stroking motion, whichever is more comfortable for the client. ➤ *Rationale:* Relaxed muscles result in a decreased pain level.

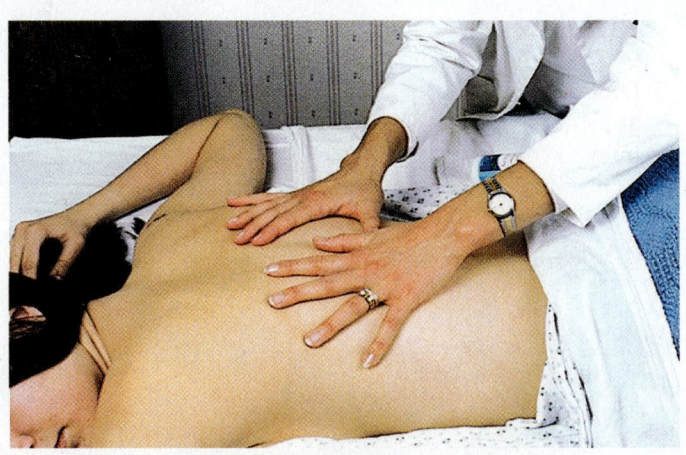

❶ Massage is a valuable nonpharmacologic method of assisting pain relief.

Skill 16.3.2 | Using Relaxation Techniques

Equipment

A printed relaxation technique (the nurse can read slowly until client learns technique)

CD or MP3 player

Procedure

1. Help client assume a comfortable position.

   a. If lying, place support under knees, lower legs, and under head. Be sure body is in good alignment.

   b. If sitting, sit comfortably positioned with both feet on the floor, hands on knees, back straight, and head balanced comfortably straight.

2. Instruct client to inhale deeply, hold breath for a moment, and then exhale deeply. Repeat several times.

3. Give the following instructions to client, using a slow, soothing voice:

   a. Continue to breathe in and out slowly. Concentrate on my voice and follow my words.

   b. Find a point of tension in your body.

   c. As you identify the tension, tense the area up even more.

   d. Then relax the area, letting all the tension drain out.

4. Continue with these instructions until the client has had time to relax all points of tension.

5. To end the process, instruct the client to open eyes slowly and say, "I feel relaxed and awake."

Note: For more relaxation skills, see Skill 17.1.7, Teaching Controlled Breathing; Skill 17.1.8, Teaching Body Relaxation; and Skill 17.1.9, Using Meditation.

EVIDENCE-BASED PRACTICE

Meditation Can Provide Immediate Relief for Migraine Headaches

A study published found that clients who suffered from migraine headaches found pain relief through the use of meditation. They participated in 20-min guided meditation sessions based on the "loving kindness" approach. After the session, the participants experienced a 33% decrease in their pain and a 43% decrease in their emotional tension. Nurses can use this simple yet powerful modality to help clients manage both stress and pain.

Source: Tonelli & Wachholtz (2014)

Unit 16.3 Documentation and Evaluation

DOCUMENTATION for Nonpharmacologic Pain Relief

- Describe the client's pain, including onset, pattern, location, quality, intensity, precipitating factors, associated factors, and aggravating factors.

- Describe alleviating factors, including what the client does to relieve pain as well as nursing assistance.

- Describe behavioral changes due to pain relief or the absence of objective changes in response to nursing interventions.

- If there is a poor response to therapy, state what other measures will be attempted, and chart results.

- Continue to document attempts to relieve pain until relief occurs and the client is satisfied.

EVALUATION/Critical Thinking

Expected Outcomes

- Pain is controlled through nonpharmacologic methods such as massage, relaxation techniques, or TENS.
- Client is satisfied with level of pain control.
- Client's anxiety level is lowered in relation to pain.

Unexpected Outcomes

- Client achieves no relief from massage.

- Client cannot focus on relaxation technique.

Alternative Actions

- Try combining method with use of medications (i.e., while waiting for the medication to take effect).
- Client has to trust the technique before it can be effective. Have client talk to another individual who has found the technique helpful.

- Start with very simple breathing techniques and progress slowly to relaxation and visualization (see Chapter 17 for specifics).

Chapter Wrap-Up

GERONTOLOGIC Considerations

The Incidence of Pain in Older Adults Has Not Been Well Studied and This Population Presents Several Pain Management Problems

- Older adults often suffer acute and chronic painful diseases or have multiple diseases. Thus, they often have more than one source of pain.
- Older adults are at increased risk for drug as well as disease interactions.
- Studies show the incidence of pain is twofold higher in those over 65. Acutely painful conditions affect older adults disproportionately (herpes zoster, arthritis, polymyalgia rheumatica, peripheral vascular disease).
- Older adults may have impaired senses (vision, hearing) and an impaired ability to express themselves.
- Older adults are at increased risks for falls when taking multiple drugs (polypharmacy), so care must be taken when administering opioids to them.

Pain Assessment Is More Complex and Difficult With Older Adults

- The older adult may report pain differently than (not as clearly as) younger clients due to physiologic, psychological, and cultural changes associated with aging.
- Older adults often present with multiple pain etiologies, so a comprehensive assessment is needed to gather complete information.
- Clinicians often hold the mistaken belief that older adults have increased pain thresholds; they may be more stoic about experiencing, and thus reporting, pain.

- Cognitive impairment (which may occur in as many as 50% of institutionalized older adults) may interfere greatly with the assessment of pain. Even though behavior may be assessed (restlessness, groaning, agitation), it is nonspecific and subject to interpretation (Herr, 2011).
- See Gerontologic Considerations for Medications in Chapter 18 for specific guidelines for drug use with older adults.

Traditional Approaches to Pain Control May Not Work With Older Adults

- Universal use of pain protocols may not be possible with visual, hearing, and motor impairments.
- Clients may report pain initially, but recall (due to cognitive impairment) may not be possible.
- Pain assessment may require frequent monitoring. Monitoring may have major implications for quality of care and quality of life, so facilities with limited staff may have poor pain control among the older adults.
- Older adults are at risk for over- and undertreatment. Adverse drug reactions are more prevalent with older adults.
- Attitudes among healthcare professionals may also impede appropriate care (partially due to belief that acute and chronic pain are a normal component of aging).

MANAGEMENT Guidelines

Each state legislates a Nurse Practice Act for RNs and LVN/LPNs. Healthcare facilities are responsible for establishing and implementing policies and procedures that conform to their state's regulations. Verify the regulations and role parameters for each healthcare worker in your facility.

Delegation

- Noninvasive pain management techniques can be delegated to any staff member who feels comfortable performing or has experience in using touch (massage) or relaxation techniques. If TENS is used for pain control, the nurse must understand the basic principles of how this method works.

- The nurse, RN or LVN/LPN, is the primary individual who is responsible for pain management. He or she does this through the nurse–client relationship by becoming the client's advocate. Therefore, a professional nurse must manage the client's pain in order to identify the intensity, codify the degree, and evaluate the response to pain medication and intervene as necessary with the healthcare provider to change the medication protocol.

- Administration of epidural narcotic analgesia *must* be done by an RN and, in many hospitals, the nurse must have special certification. This skill may *not* be delegated to a nonprofessional staff member.

- Initial administration of PCA must be done by an RN or experienced LVN/PN. It may not be delegated to a unlicensed assistive personnel (UAP), nor may the UAP administer a booster dose.

- PCA may be managed and taught to the client by an RN or LVN/LPN *if* two parameters exist: (1) The Nurse Practice Act and agency protocol in the state allow it, and (2) the nurse has the information and experience to qualify the client and teach the procedure (under healthcare provider's orders). Nonprofessional staff may *not* perform this skill.

Interprofessional Communication

- It is critically important that the RN inform all staff where epidural narcotic analgesia is being used.

- Clients receiving opioids through epidurals and PCAs should be monitored carefully for signs of respiratory depression and treated appropriately with naloxone (Narcan) or other antagonist drugs to prevent respiratory arrest.

- It is also imperative that the RN communicate to other nurses through the client's written records, label the IV line and place it as far as possible from the epidural catheter to prevent a potentially fatal mistake, and share in verbal report that the client is receiving epidural anesthesia.

- Because the nurse is the client's advocate in pain control, he or she must receive adequate feedback from all staff who interact with the client so that a viable pain management program can be implemented. It is the nurse's responsibility to inform the auxiliary staff caring for the client to report how the client is managing pain.

CASE STUDY Applications

Scenario 1

The client assigned to you has a diagnosis of advanced Alzheimer disease and cancer with bone metastases. He is a 65-year-old man recently hospitalized. You know he is in pain, but he is unable to relate the degree of pain clearly to the staff or his family.

1. What is the most appropriate method of assessing pain in this client?
2. When considering this client, what is unique about the pain assessment in this situation?
3. What are some possible plans or goals to deal with this client's pain?
4. What are some of the risks in implementing the plan?

Scenario 2

The client has a PCA in place but constantly complains that the pain medication is not working. When asked if he uses the bolus dose, he says that he is constantly "locked out."

1. What further assessment, if any, is necessary with this client?
2. Describe the goals and strategies you would devise to handle this situation.
3. What are the best actions you can carry out to meet these goals?

Scenario 3

A female client has been admitted to the nursing unit with the diagnosis of acute abdominal pain. You are assigned to admit her to room 113. The chart only contains the following demographic data: Lives locally, is 28 years old, recently married. Her husband is at the bedside and is very concerned with his wife's pain. As you walk into the room to complete the admission process, she is writhing in pain and crying loudly.

1. To prepare for the admission interview, what will you do first? Why?
2. State how you will ask the client to describe her pain.

3. What questions might be appropriate to ask regarding the abdominal pain?

4. What assessment data are priority for this client?

5. How will this information be utilized in the development of a client plan of care?

NCLEX® Review Questions

Unless otherwise specified, choose only one (1) answer.

1. Which of the following theories of pain is the most recent and accepted as the most likely explanation of pain?
   A. Pattern theory
   B. Specificity theory
   C. Endorphin theory
   D. Gate control theory

2. Which of the following characteristics are most important when measuring the degree of pain?

   Select all that apply.
   A. Location
   B. Intensity
   C. Quality
   D. Pain pathway
   E. Pattern
   F. Amount of pain relief needed

3. What is the best explanation of why pain is now considered the fifth vital sign?
   A. Pain is as important to assess as blood pressure and other vital signs.
   B. Considered as a vital sign, pain will be measured and documented when other vital signs are taken.
   C. As a vital sign, the presence of pain will result in an intervention.
   D. As a vital sign, assessing pain allows the effectiveness of pain management to be measured.

4. What is the primary purpose of using a nonpharmacologic method of pain relief over a pharmacologic one?
   A. It is noninvasive.
   B. It works better.
   C. It works faster.
   D. It is preferred by clients and healthcare providers.

5. When a client is receiving epidural narcotic analgesia, what is the priority safety issue?
   A. Respiratory depression
   B. Checking that the apnea monitor is working
   C. Assessing for migration of the catheter
   D. Mistaking the epidural catheter for an IV catheter

6. Which of the following is the most important rationale for qualifying a client for patient-controlled analgesia (PCA)?
   A. To determine whether this pain method will relieve the client's pain
   B. To evaluate whether the client is mentally alert and able to comply with the instructions
   C. To assess the level of pain the client is experiencing
   D. To assess whether the client's pain is chronic

7. You are assigned to care for a client receiving PCA. When you assess the client, you find that he is experiencing bradypnea, hypotension, and nausea. What is the priority intervention?
   A. Assess the medication level.
   B. Determine whether the medication is relieving the client's pain.
   C. Monitor the client's sedation level and request that the healthcare provider evaluate dose parameters.
   D. Terminate the PCA.

8. When monitoring a client with PCA, which of the following are common dangers when IV pumps are involved?

   Select all that apply.
   A. Improper dose and quantity
   B. Unauthorized/wrong drug
   C. Poor pain-relief results
   D. Omitting a dose
   E. Drug administration by proxy

9. You have a client who is to receive epidural narcotic analgesia. As a team leader, you may safely assign this client to which of the following staff members?
   A. An LVN/LPN or an RN
   B. A UAP
   C. Any staff member
   D. Only an RN

10. A client with recurrent acute pain is instructed on pain management. Which of the following statements reflects successful compliance with the plan?
    A. "I take the pain medication faithfully every 4 hours."
    B. "The best time to take my medication is after I shower and dress."
    C. "The medication works best when I take it soon after the pain begins."
    D. "I take the pain medication whenever the pain is a 7 on a scale of 10."

QSEN Activity

Domain: Safety Competency

KSA: Skill: Participate appropriately in analyzing errors and designing system improvements

Activity:

Your nursing unit has recently had a sentinel event where a client was receiving hydromorphone (Dilaudid) through a PCA. The mistake occurred when the nurse was interrupted during the initial set up of the PCA. The client ended up receiving too much medication and went into respiratory arrest and died. You are part of a committee that is looking at creating a process to avoid similar errors in the future. What type of process might your committee put into place that would reduce the likelihood of this type of error?

Bibliography

Chen, Y., & Wan, H. (2014) The effectiveness of acupressure on relieving pain: A systematic review. *Pain Management Nursing, 15*(2), 539–550.

Cogan, J., Ouimette, M., Vargas-Schaffer, G., Yegin, Z., Deschamps, A., & Denault, A. (2014) Patient attitudes and beliefs regarding pain medication after cardiac surgery: Barriers to adequate pain management. *Pain Management Nursing 15*(3), 574–579.

Drew, D., Gordon, D., Renner, L., Morgan, B., Swensen H., & Manworren, R. (2014). The use of "as-needed" range orders for opioid analgesics in the management of pain: A consensus statement of the American Society of Pain Management Nurses and the American Pain Society. *Pain Management Nursing 15*(2), 551–554.

Herr, K. (2011). Pain assessment strategies in older patients. *The Journal of Pain, 12*(3), S3–S13.

Hockenberry, M.J. (2011). Wong's nursing care of infants and children. (9th ed.). St. Louis, MO: Mosby.

Institute for Safe Medication Practices. (2007, Jun. 14). Safety issues with patient-controlled analgesia. Available at www.ismp.org

Institute for Safe Medication Practices. (2013, Aug. 8). Acute care ISMP medication safety alert! FentaNYL patch fatalities linked to "bystander apathy." We ALL have a role in prevention! Retrieved from http://www.ismp.org/newsletters/acutecare/showarticle.aspx?id=55

Jarzyna, D., Jungquist, C. R., Paser, C., Willens, J. S., Nisbet, A., Oakes, L., ... & Polomano, R. C. (2011). American Society for Pain Management Nursing guidelines on monitoring for opioid-induced sedation and respiratory depression. *Pain Management Nursing, 12*(3), 118–145.

McCaffery, M., & Pasero, C. (1999). *Pain: Clinical manual* (2nd ed.). St. Louis, MO: Mosby. [classic work]

Pasero, C. (2009). Assessment of sedation during opioid administration for pain management. *Journal of PeriAnesthesia Nursing, 24*(3), 186–190.

Richmond Agitation Sedation Scale. (n.d.). Retrieved from https://app.box.com/files/0/f/2185877057/1/f_18882452925

Spector, R. (2012). *Cultural diversity in health and illness* (8th ed.). Upper Saddle River, NJ: Prentice Hall Health.

The Joint Commission. (2012). The Joint Commission Sentinel Event Alert, *49*(8). Retrieved from http://www.jointcommission.org/assets/1/18/SEA_49_opioids_8_2_12_final.pdf

The Joint Commission. (2013). Improving the quality of pain management through measurement through measurement and action. Retrieved from http://www.npcnow.org/system/files/research/download/Improving-the-Quality-of-Pain-Management-Through-Measurement-and-Action.pdf

The Joint Commission. (2015). Pain management. Retrieved from http://www.jointcommission.org/topics/pain_management.aspx

Tonelli, M. E., & Wachholtz, A. B. (2014). Meditation-based treatment yielding immediate relief for mediation-naïve migraineurs. *Pain Management Nursing, 15*(1), 36–40.

Chapter 17
Alternative Therapies and Stress Management

Learning Objectives

17.1 Define the term *stress* according to Hans Selye.

17.2 Discuss the psychological effect of stress on the body.

17.3 Describe the body's physiologic response to stress, and include at least two body systems.

17.4 List at least three different categories of stressors.

17.5 Identify at least five danger signals of stress.

17.6 Discuss a specific alternative method used to control stress.

17.7 Discuss complementary and alternative medicine (CAM) and how it can be applied to nursing.

17.8 Choose two alternative therapies, discuss the major components, and relate how you use them with clients.

17.9 Practice breathing techniques and discuss how you would teach this to a client.

17.10 Discuss why herbs could be dangerous.

17.11 List two herbs that could be dangerous when taken with a specific medication.

Chapter Outline

Terminology

Adaptive reaction a response by which the individual attempts to improve or alter his or her condition in relation to the environment.

Alleviate to make more bearable; reduce (pain, grief, or suffering).

Anxiety a state of uneasiness and distress; diffuse apprehension.

Apathy indifference; insensibility; without emotion; sluggish.

Apprehension a fearful or uneasy anticipation of the future; dread.

Autonomic nervous system the part of the nervous system that regulates the functioning of internal organs and glands; it controls such functions as digestion, respiration, and cardiovascular activity.

Cerebral cortex the extensive outer layer of gray tissue of the cerebral hemispheres (brain), responsible for higher nervous system functions.

Complementary and alternative medicine (CAM) a set of practices that encompasses many treatments and ideologies outside of mainstream medicine.

Coping mechanisms means by which an individual adjusts or adapts to a threat or a challenge; actions that assist in maintaining homeostasis.

Defense mechanisms conscious or unconscious processes used to protect oneself from threats or to alleviate anxiety.

Dynamics of homeostasis danger or its symbols, whether internal or external, resulting in the activation of the sympathetic nervous system and the adrenal medulla. The organism prepares for fight or flight.

Emotional related to strong feelings, as of joy and sorrow.

Fight or flight a body's immediate response to stress that, although often inappropriate, is part of our central nervous system's biological makeup.

General adaptation syndrome a general theory of stress response formulated by Dr. Hans Selye; describes the action of stress response in three stages: the alarm reaction, the stage of resistance, and the stage of exhaustion.

Hallucination false perception having no relation to reality and not accounted for by external stimuli.

Health the state of physical, psychological, and sociologic well-being.

Herbal preparations medicines made from plants used for healing various conditions.

Holistic a way of looking at individuals and organisms as a whole rather than a sum of the parts.

Homeostasis the maintenance of a constant state in the internal environment through self-regulatory techniques that preserve an organism's ability to adapt to stress.

Hypertension a condition in which the client has a higher blood pressure than judged to be normal.

Illness a state characterized by the malfunction of the biopsychosocial organism.

Insomnia inability to sleep.

Lifestyle the manner in which an individual is accustomed to living.

Meditation the act of reflecting on or pondering; contemplation.

Musculoskeletal pertaining to the muscles and the skeleton.

Pain a sensation in which an individual experiences discomfort, distress, or suffering.

Parasympathetic nervous system a division of the autonomic nervous system that regulates acetylcholine and conserves energy expenditure; it slows down the system.

Perspective subjective evaluation of relative significance; a view.

Psychogenic of mental origin.

Relaxation a lessening of tension or activity in a part.

Stamina constitutional energy; strength; endurance.

Stress a nonspecific response of the body to any internal or external event or change that impinges on an individual's system and creates a demand.

Stressor a specific demand that gives rise to a coping response.

Sympathetic nervous system a division of the autonomic nervous system that controls energy expenditure and mobilizes for action when confronted with a threat.

Tachycardia abnormally rapid heart action; above 100 beats/min.

Tranquilizer a drug that acts to reduce tension and anxiety without interfering with normal mental activity.

Wellness a state of physical, psychological, and sociologic well-being of a whole individual. Synonym for health.

Stress

Stress is a universal phenomenon; all human beings in all cultures experience it as a part of their everyday existence. Although stress is a natural component of life, it can sap energy and contribute to the presence of disease. The concept of stress has been with us since the beginning of time, but it was not until William Osler and Walter Cannon began their investigations in the early 1900s that stress was actually linked to illness. By 1950, Hans Selye, a Canadian endocrinologist and biologist, scientifically demonstrated that stress plays a major role in certain diseases, such as heart disease and cancer (Box 17-1 ■). Since Selye's early research, authorities from medicine as well as all areas of science have studied and written thousands of articles on this subject. Since it is an undeniable fact that stress affects an individual's total life, nurses should have a basic understanding of this phenomenon, its effect on humans, how humans cope and adapt to stress, and how the nurse can deal with his or her own stress and help clients deal with theirs. To examine stress and its influence on human beings in this culture, we have to examine the total scope of life experience.

Stress is a difficult term to define precisely, for it does not have a single specific source or one definite response. Selye stated that stress may be viewed as the common denominator of all the body's adaptive reactions. Stress may be grief as well as joy, pleasure as well as unhappiness, cold as well as heat, and fear as well as elation. In fact, stress covers the total range of mental, **emotional**, and physical demands on the body and causes the body to respond with predictable biochemical and general adaptation changes. If the body is in a state of balance and the whole organism functions in harmony, the body is healthy. Stress can be defined as a state of arousal or agitation that throws the body out of balance.

Although a certain amount of stress is necessary for survival, when it becomes prolonged and intense, our adaptive responses become weary, and the negative aspects begin to take their toll on our bodies and our minds. When this occurs, it can be said that disease has overtaken the body and an unhealthy state exists.

The Effect of Stress

Physiologically, stress may be viewed as the experience an individual has when the demands placed on the body exceed the ability to cope, and the body is thrown out of balance. Chemically, stress initiates certain bodily processes, such as the **fight-or-flight** mechanism, which result in a threat to homeostasis. According to Walter Cannon, the Harvard physiologist who coined the term *homeostasis*, the stress response resulted in these mechanisms being activated, which in turn threw the body out of balance (Goldstein, 2010). As a result of Cannon's work, certain adjustment mechanisms of the body, such as blood sugar level, temperature, and hydration, were identified.

Rather than a specific response, Hans Selye focused on a general adaptation process as a response to stress. This process is the body's attempt to adapt and maintain homeostasis. Selye further defined stress as the rate of wear and tear on the body and stated that the only freedom from stress is death.

Selye's **general adaptation syndrome** occurs in three stages (Table 17-1 ■). The first stage, the *alarm stage*, occurs when the generalized response throughout the body

Table 17-1 Selye's Stress Adaptation Syndrome

Stage	General Function	Interpersonal	Behavioral	Affective	Cognitive	Physiologic
1 Alarm reaction	Mobilization of body defenses	Interpersonal communication effectiveness decreases	Task oriented Increased restlessness **Apathy** Regression Crying	Feelings of anger, suspicion, helplessness Anxiety level increases	Alert thinking becomes narrow and concrete. Symptoms of thought blocking, forgetfulness, and decreased productivity	Muscle tension Increase in epinephrine and cortisone Stimulation of adrenal cortex and lymph glands Increase in blood pressure, pulse, and blood glucose
2 Stage of resistance	Adaptation to stresses Resistance increases	Interpersonal communication self-oriented Uses interpersonal relationships to meet own needs	Automatic behaviors Self-oriented behaviors Fight or flight behavior apparent	Increased use of **defense mechanisms** Emotional responses may be automatic or exaggerated	Thought processes more habitual than problem-solving oriented	Hormonal levels return to prealarm stage if adaptation occurs Physiologic responses return to normal or are channeled into psychosomatic symptoms
3 Stage of exhaustion	Depletion or exhaustion of organs and resources Loss of ability to resist stress	Disintegration of personal interactions Communication skills ineffective and disorganized Self-oriented	Restless, withdrawn, agitated; may become violent or self-destructive Diminished productivity	Depressed, flat or inappropriate affect Exaggerated or inappropriate use of defense mechanisms Decreased ability to cope	Thought disorganization, **hallucinations**, preoccupation Reduced intellectual processes	Exhaustion, with increased demands on organism Adrenal cortex hormone depletion Death, if stress is continuous and excessive

responds to stressors, such as trauma, infection, pain, cold, heat, and fear. The purpose of the alarm reaction is to mobilize the body's defenses to meet the stressor. Biochemically, during the alarm stage, the adrenal cortex produces the anti-inflammatory hormones, the adrenocorticotropin hormones (cortisone and cortisol), and the proinflammatory hormones (aldosterone and desoxycorticosterone). This is also called the shock phase because it is when the **autonomic nervous system** comes into full play.

The second stage, *resistance*, occurs when the body's defenses are mobilized to produce hormones to cope with the alarm stage. The body chemistry either repels or adapts to the stressor. During this phase, the organism may be successful in adapting to the stressor, and, if so, the biochemical changes resulting from the alarm phase return to the pre-alarm stage. Any life change causes alarm and resistance, and the stress accrued through life reduces the body's adaptive abilities.

The *final stage* occurs when the stress is prolonged and the body can no longer cope effectively. The result is exhaustion, and the body may become ill with disease. The organism's adaptive abilities are depleted, and the organism loses its ability to deal with the stress. The organism goes into shock, and if the stress is not **alleviated**, the result may be death of the organism. The general adaptation syndrome varies widely in intensity. Reaction to positive stimuli, such as getting married or a job promotion, also activates a stress response. The response may, however, result in less damage than a negative stressor, even though it does temporarily throw the body out of balance. Furthermore, an individual does not respond with the same intensity to all negative stressors. For example, the response to jumping into a cold pool would not have the same degree of intensity as turning a corner and seeing a man with a gun.

The *local adaptive syndrome* is the manifestation of stress in a limited part of the body. The body responds locally to the stressor, such as a burn or cut to a finger. The local response may also trigger a general response if the ability of the body to respond to the specific area is greatly affected by the condition of the whole organism. An upper respiratory infection causes a much different response within a healthy child than in a child with cystic fibrosis. The better the organism as a whole adapts to stress, the more effective the local adaptive response.

Individual Responses to Stress

Responses to stress, then, can be categorized into several different patterns: the *physiologic response*, in which there is loss or gain in weight over time, hormone levels increase, blood pressure increases, or possibly a somatoform (psychosomatic) symptom appears; the *psychological response*, which may also result in a psychosomatic illness or psychiatric manifestations, such as depression, mania, withdrawal from reality, or **anxiety**; and, the *behavioral response*, in which an individual hits out, becomes aggressive (fights), or withdraws; he or she may also become immobilized, or turn inward (physical or emotional flight). The *interpersonal*

mode can reflect stress when communication effectiveness decreases, relationships deteriorate, trust in others diminishes, and the ability to form and maintain close, intimate, loving ties with another individual decreases. Finally, the affective response may be present when someone's emotions are affected so that anxiety is high and emotions are unstable, labile, unpredictable, and inappropriate to the situation. All of the above-mentioned modes of response relate to the negative elements of response patterns. Of course, these modes can be used in a positive way so that stress becomes nondetrimental. There is no way to eliminate stress completely, but individuals can learn to minimize the harmful effects and use their response modes in a positive way.

Stressors may be chemical, physical, developmental, and emotional. Graduating from nursing school, being promoted, failing to be promoted, having arguments, and playing a tough game of racquetball are all stressful events and require adaptation and change at some level. By understanding stress, we can more easily identify stress factors and their effects on clients who need or seek **health** care. Whether a client is having a baby, undergoing open-heart surgery, or seeking counseling for emotional problems, each of these individuals is experiencing stress in his or her own particular manner. How the individual adapts or fails to adapt depends on several factors: personality and emotional makeup and past experiences in dealing with stress (response repertoire).

People are able to create many different forms of disease as well as emotional and spiritual scars. And the more we use up our reserves of adaptation energy, the more likely we are to age and hasten our death. In fact, Selye warned that there is no evidence that the basic reserves of energy for adaptation can be restored. These may be genetically programmed. The more reserves we use for handling everyday stress, the less we have for major crises or for growing older. The latest research indicates that there is a direct relationship between the amount of stress encountered in everyday life and aging.

Stress and Disease

Stress and an individual's method of handling it have been associated with the risk of developing heart disease, cancer, and other illnesses. Although stress is an inevitable part of life, excessive amounts of it can contribute to poor health (Table 17-2 ■). When an individual goes through a very stressful period, it is important to work through that stress, rather than ignore it.

The mechanisms by which stress leads to disease may differ for heart disease and cancer. Perceived stress leads to a release of adrenaline, cortisol, and other hormones within the body. These substances, in turn, increase the heart rate, blood pressure, cholesterol level, and platelet stickiness. When stress becomes chronic, these physiologic changes can accelerate atherosclerosis, the process that causes coronary heart disease.

Individuals with Type A behavior are known to be at increased risk of heart disease. Type A behavior is defined as having a constant sense of time urgency and

Table 17-2 Signals of Stress

Physiologic	
Fatigue, lethargy	Pain—backache, teeth grinding
Muscle tension—neck, back, legs, and so forth	Excessive sweating
Frequent headaches—tension, migraine	Heart problems—palpitations, racing, variable heartbeat, chest pain
Shaking, trembling, spasms	Breathing complications—hyperventilation
Cold extremities, poor circulation	High blood pressure
Digestion disturbances—acid, nausea, gas, cramps, colitis	Skin eruptions—rash, hives, itching, eczema, acne
Eating disorders—compulsive eating, loss of appetite	Sexual difficulties—impotence, low libido (desire), nonorgasmic, elimination disorders—diarrhea, constipation, vaginitis
Sleep problems—insomnia, nightmares, excessive sleep, early awakenings	Amenorrhea (absence of menstrual period)
Psychological	
Anxiety	Confusion
Panic disorder	Helplessness
Depression	Apathy
Pessimism	Alienation
Melancholy	Isolation
Impatience	Numbness
Anger	Self-consciousness
Irritability	Purposelessness
Boredom	
Behavioral Indicators	
Restlessness	Indecisiveness
Loss of memory, poor concentration	Tardiness
Nervous mannerisms—tics, grimaces, finger tapping, hair twisting	Inflexibility
Speech difficulties—stuttering, stammering	Nonproductivity
Hyperactivity	Poor problem solving
Disorganization	Alcohol and drug abuse
Passivity	Phobic responses
Aggressiveness	Overeating

a feeling of free-floating anger at the world in general. These behavior patterns can be seen as a maladaptive way of dealing with chronic stress. The famous study of the causative factors in heart disease, the Framingham study, examined many aspects of heart disease. Results revealed that males who were classified as Type A developed chest pains three times as often as their more peaceful Type B counterparts. Another fascinating conclusion was that those who remained calm and serene (Type B personalities) rarely developed high cholesterol levels regardless of their diet.

Chronic stress causes changes in the immune system that can interfere with its ability to recognize and destroy cancerous cells. Several researchers have shown that cancer clients have a characteristic personality pattern years before the cancers are diagnosed. Part of this personality pattern involves difficulty dealing with stress and turning conflict inward instead of confronting it directly.

It is important to remember that the stress syndrome can be both positive and negative. Any change or alteration in the balance of life can create stress. The Holmes and Rahe stress scale is an excellent example of the varying conditions in life that result in stress. We are all unique individuals, and we respond differently to various stressors. Thus, it does not matter whether the stress is positive or negative, light or severe. What matters is how we develop adaptive mechanisms to cope with these stressors (Box 17-2 ■). The ability to cope or solve a problem can be translated as the ability to withstand stress and create life experiences that do not work against us. The implications of stress theory—that by being able to withstand stress, by coping with it, diluting it when it occurs, or eliminating it, we can actually affect our life—are tremendously exciting. It means that we are not doomed to inevitable illness later in life, nor are we preprogrammed for premature aging. In fact, every individual controls his or her own health.

Box 17-2 STRESS AND A SATISFYING LIFE

The following critical principles suggest how to use the stresses of life to increase your positive advantage:

- **Stress does not come from the outside; you generate it totally within yourself.** In Hans Selye's definition, stress is the nonspecific reaction to any demand. Consider the stressor of an upcoming exam. A specific response to the exam, such as studying extra hard, is likely to help resolve internal stress. But nonspecific reactions, such as bingeing on junk food, smoking cigarettes, or reducing sleep by several hours a night, will not serve to resolve the stress imbalance. In either case, it is you yourself, not the exam, who generated these reactions. Coping with stress requires self-knowledge so that you can learn to address its symptoms.

- **You cannot see stress directly; you can only experience its symptoms.** No one can see love, but we all know what it feels like to us personally: butterflies in the stomach, inability to concentrate, or a tendency to think about a loved one all the time. Similarly, characteristic symptoms of stress are personal. One individual might overeat; someone else may find it hard to eat. One individual might have trouble sleeping, while another has trouble staying awake and focused. These symptoms are not actual problems but bodily warning lights that signal an imbalance. Seeking relief from the symptoms through drugs, sex, or other distractions covers up, but won't resolve, the imbalance. To correct the imbalance, you need to look inside yourself and identify what is happening.

- **Attitude plays a significant role in illness and wellness.** A positive attitude, even when people are under constant pressure, is a primary factor separating those who become ill and those who stay well. Other key elements in staying healthy are: commitment to a task, tackling problems as challenges (not obstacles), and believing your actions and presence make a difference. Attitude affects people's internal reaction to events and, therefore, their stress level. To maintain good health, it is important to actively shift your attitude to look for the positive side of events and maintain a "can-do" attitude.

- **Stress is essential to everything you enjoy.** We all love the feeling of victory, and the feeling of achievement generally matches the level of challenge. For example, winning a football game in the final 2 min is more exciting and memorable than winning by a large margin over a poor team. Similarly, when you learn a subject well, it can feel more satisfying to succeed on a challenging final exam than on low-level, multiple-choice questions that reflect only the basic information in the course. Stressful events are opportunities to reach a new level; they actually help us make the most of our lives. Celebrating success after overcoming a stressor increases our joy, personal satisfaction, and enthusiasm.

- **A healthy life is a balance of stress and relaxation.** In nature, stress and tension alternate with relaxation. Your heart contracts and relaxes to keep your blood flowing. Your breath enters and leaves. There is no shortage of stressors in daily life. Our job is to find methods of relaxation that work for us and to make those techniques a part of our lives so that we are in balance. Each individual needs to make this happen. Can you imagine a professor asking if you remembered to do your 20-min meditation last night?

- **You must take responsibility for your own life, including its stress.** Only you can really make your life better. No one else can feel or deal with your symptoms of stress. Take responsibility for dealing effectively with stressors. Focus on wellness, not illness. Practice self-awareness, self-education, and self-responsibility. Find stress management methods that work for you and practice them until they are an automatic part of your life.

Guidelines for Implementing Stress Objectives in Nursing

The nurse must have an understanding of the role of stress.

- Understand and accept the theory of stress—what it is and what effect it has on the body (Box 17-3 ■).
- Be aware of how stress manifests: tiredness, apathy, frequent illness, lack of interest or liveliness, unwillingness to seek out new challenges, inability to cope with change, and many other symptoms.

Along with coping with your own stress, it is the responsibility of the nurse to be aware that clients have stress phenomena and that part of the nurse's role is to assist clients to adapt and cope with stress (Box 17-4 ■).

- Recognize the factors that increase stress, both positive and negative (illness, hospitalization, pain, marriage, family pressures, and so on).

- Assist in making a plan and implementing it, designing specific actions to reduce stress, such as relaxation methods, meditation, or exercise.
- Work out a plan with the individual about how to control, alter, or change stressors in his or her life.

The nurse may carry out specific behaviors in the hospital setting to reduce stress.

- Identify the stressors affecting the client now.
- Counsel the client and family on the theory of stress; together, examine how the client's particular stressors affect his or her lifestyle.
- Reinforce the client's adaptive process by meeting his or her needs, listening to concerns, administering care, and providing emotional support.
- Assist the client to alter adaptive behaviors to cope more effectively with stress.
- Remember that laughter decreases stress, so maintain a light rather than a depressed or morbid attitude.

A New Paradigm for Health

The way the Western world views health has undergone a change. Even the terms we use to describe health are changing; terms like *holistic health* and *alternative, unconventional,* or *complementary medicine* are heard more frequently in both medical and nonmedical circles. In the past, good health meant the absence of disease. The commonly accepted definition of health now goes beyond physical health to encompass the health of the whole individual, including mental, emotional, and spiritual health. The World Health Organization (WHO) definition of health developed in 1970 has significantly influenced the medical model of health care. WHO described health as "a state of complete physical, mental, and social well-being, not merely the absence of disease or infirmity." What made this definition innovative is that it took into account the mind as well as the body. In fact, this new interpretation of health almost enters the spiritual dimension. Though critics have pointed out that by this definition no one is truly healthy, it changes the view of health to one of an open system in a holistic framework. A holistic redefinition of health emphasizes high-level wellness or going beyond the absence of disease toward the individual's maximum health potential. This section focuses on the connection among mind, body, spirit, and environment and discusses how we can use this connection to reach the highest possible level of health and wellness.

A Holistic Approach to Health

The term *holistic* implies wholeness; a harmonious individual that integrates mind, body, and spirit into a functioning unit. A holistic stress model implies modifying all parts of an individual's life so that stress is both encountered and alleviated from an integrated perspective.

The current literature, much of it authored by prominent healthcare providers, exemplifies today's trend toward the holistic, or alternative, model.

The holistic paradigm suggests that the body, psyche, and environment are one and interact as an open system. This idea can assist us to view our client's health as well as our personal health from a new dimension. In the holistic view, health care includes three types of actions: disease and injury prevention, treatment, and health promotion.

There are more than 200 alternative modalities—from bee sting therapy for multiple sclerosis to essential healing oils. Some probably do not work, except for a placebo effect, but others definitely are being shown by research to work. An example is stress reduction for heart disease and angina.

Alternative treatments may include treatments that require involvement on the client's part, such as changes in eating patterns and other lifestyle behaviors; or physical treatments, such as acupuncture or vitamin therapy. The client is counseled to take the initiative and assume responsibility for his or her own health, and the role of the nurse and healthcare provider is to guide clients to various healthcare options. Truly holistic treatment involves an integrated assessment of all aspects of health.

Complementary and Alternative Medicine

CAM refers to treatments or medical products that are not part of standard care. Complementary medicine is used along with standard care, and alternative medicine is used in place of standard care. It is important for clients to discuss with their healthcare providers when they are using CAM therapies, because many of these treatments can have side effects or can interfere with standard care. Clients should also research treatments thoroughly and choose their CAM practitioners carefully.

The importance of CAM therapy is growing. The National Institutes of Health (NIH), a conservative, scientifically based organization, gave nearly $130 million in 2010 to the National Center for Complementary and Integrative Medicine. This office was founded because of congressional pressure to investigate new approaches to the degenerative diseases killing Americans. It is one of 27 NIH centers. Several national insurance companies now reimburse their clients for selected alternative treatments.

Complementary Health Approaches

Following is a short sampling of the more than 200 complementary health approaches that may be used alone or in tandem with conventional medical treatments. These methods may be classified as lifestyle (holistic medicine; nutrition), botanical (homeopathy, herbal, aromatherapy), energy/manipulative (chiropractic, acupressure and acupuncture, reflexology, massage), and mind–body (meditation, guided imagery, biofeedback, color healing, and hypnotherapy).

Acupuncture An ancient Chinese method of relieving pain and treating disease, acupuncture is based on the belief that energy, or *qi*, flows along 12 lines or meridians in the body, creating a balance between two principles of nature called yin and yang. Each meridian is connected to a particular organ or system. It is believed that lack of energy flow or blocked energy along the meridians leads to illness or disease. Acupuncture treatment involves inserting sharp needles under the skin along the meridian lines, thereby unblocking energy, stimulating flow, and restoring balance and health of internal organs. Since the 1960s in the United States, Chinese doctors, as well as some in the U.S., have performed major surgery with acupuncture as the only anesthetic.

Applied Kinesiology Applied kinesiology is a form of evaluation based on the theory that the condition of an individual's muscles reflects certain internal disorders or problems. Body imbalances or disorders are identified when certain muscle groups are tested and appear weak. Certain foods, medications, or herbs are held in an individual's hand or placed next to his or her skin. If the substance is not appropriate for the body, the muscles respond to test-

ing by appearing weak. When the substance is removed, the muscles regain their strength. Based on identifying weak muscles, various treatments, such as vitamins, herbs, diet therapy, acupressure, or chiropractic, are suggested.

Aromatherapy Essential oils are the aromatic liquids extracted from herbs, plants, and flowers. These oils have been used to treat various conditions and have been an important part of medical lore for thousands of years. For example, there are 188 references to essential oils in the Bible. Modern aromatherapy became known in the 1930s, but it was not until the 1990s that aromatherapy emerged as a major mode of alternative treatment.

Essential oils can be included in the genre of vibrational therapy because specific oils have their own vibrational level or life force and, as such, work differently in the body. Dr. Robert Becker, in his book *The Body Electric*, discussed the fact that the human body has an average electrical frequency and the health of an individual depends on his or her particular body frequency. Research at the State University in Cheny, Washington, determined that the average body frequency is 62–68 hertz (Hz). When the frequency drops, the immune system is compromised and various illnesses may ensue. Based on this research, scientists found that pollutants lower the body frequency. For example, canned or processed foods have a frequency of 0, fresh produce 15 Hz, and essential oils start at 52 Hz and go as high as 320 Hz (which is organic, pure rose oil). Essential oils have the ability to penetrate the human body through either the skin or olfactory receptors. Supporters of this form of alternative therapy believe that essential oils are a most effective healing agent, and they are noninvasive. Examples of commonly used oils are lemon and thyme oil, used to kill strep, staph, and TB; lavender, used as a relaxing or sleep-enhancing oil; and peppermint, used to aid digestion. This mode of treatment would be used to supplement, not replace, other treatment methods.

Ayurveda A form of medicine that originated in India, Ayurveda, meaning the science of life, has been practiced in India for over 5,000 years and has just recently become known in the West. This system is based on the concept of three metabolic body types: slim, athletic, and heavy. Each body type utilizes food and herbs in a different way; thus, treatment includes dietary changes, herbs, and exercise, as well as specific practices, such as yoga, meditation, massage with herbal remedies, and medicated inhalations. This form of medicine has recently gained popularity in the West after several Indian healthcare providers opened clinics based on this system of treatment. Notable among them is Dr. Deepak Chopra, an endocrinologist, who has written many popular books on the subject.

Biofeedback This technique employs an instrument to monitor physiologic processes of the body and to "feedback" measurements to the individual being monitored. A scale, thermometer, and pulse monitor are common feedback devices, as are more technically sophisticated machines having electronic sensors and digital readouts. Recent research has confirmed that many people can influence or control their autonomic processes (heart rate, blood pressure, temperature, digestive functions, and others). As the client becomes more adept at controlling body responses, the need to use monitoring devices decreases—and the mental skills can be used independently.

Chiropractic   Originating in ancient Greece and literally meaning "done by the hands," chiropractic suggests that one cause of disease and dysfunction in the body is a misalignment of the spinal column that interferes with proper nerve function. These conditions cause or contribute to some diseases and lower the body's resistance to others. Spinal adjustments and manipulation restore structural integrity, thus enabling the body to heal itself. Studies have shown that chiropractic can relieve pain and structural disorders in the joints and muscles. The focus of treatment is general and includes correction of such disorders as headaches; allergies; pain in the back, hip, or spinal column; or gastrointestinal problems.

Energy Medicine   This contemporary aspect of health views the human body as comprised of electronic vibrations. Interventions involving the energy field will interface with environmental, spiritual, and vibrational aspects of healing. Special high and low frequencies of sound and light are already being used for healing. For example, sound therapy is used to speed healing through a cast; full-spectrum light frequencies are being used to affect moods such as seasonal affective disorder (SAD). Other examples of energy/vibrational/frequency healing are Reiki healing, in which the healer has progressed through two or three weekend education levels; Therapeutic Touch, the founders of which are Dolores Krieger and Janet Mentgen, also entails learning the techniques via a seminar or educational program; and energy healing, which may be the transmission of the healer's energy into the client's body, or the empowerment of the client to heal herself or himself. Documented studies have shown that certain individuals have this ability to transmit healing energy to others. In fact, a special photographic process called Kirlian photography has shown the energy moving from healer to client.

Herbal Medicine   There is a growing interest in herbal products, as more and more clients become interested in healing themselves.

All cultures from ancient times onward have used herbs to cure illness. Indeed, many drugs commonly used today are derived from herbs. Nearly one-fourth of all medications have at least one ingredient that is plant-based. The WHO estimates that 80% of the world population includes herbal medicines as part of their health practices.

Other countries are far ahead of the United States in integrating herbal products into mainstream medicine. WHO's *Guidelines for the Assessment of Herbal Medicine* (2014) state that historical use is a valid way to document safety and efficacy in the absence of scientific evidence to the contrary. European herbs are among the world's best-studied medicines. Some are even prescribed by healthcare providers in Europe because they are so effective in treating diseases. In the United States, more and more holistic healthcare providers are incorporating herbs into their medical practice, both because they are effective and because they have far fewer side effects than drugs. For more information on herbs and plants, see Table 17-3 ■.

Homeopathy   Based on the work of the German physician Dr. Samuel Hahnemann in the early 1800s, homeopathy is a system of treatment that rests on the theory that extremely minute doses of certain substances, usually herbal or chemical, cause a response in an individual that mimics a particular disease. These substances, or homeopathic remedies, are administered to an individual with a disease exhibiting a similar symptom pattern, stimulating the body's natural healing response. This is called "treatment by similars, or like cures like." The practice of homeopathy is becoming more popular; there is even a software package designed to assist healthcare providers in the homeopathic diagnosis and treatment of disease.

Massage   Of all the alternative treatments, massage may be the oldest form of medicine known to man. Historical records indicate that the Chinese, in 3000 B.C., wrote about massage, and both the Greeks and Romans considered massage a therapy. Massage was introduced to the United States in 1877 by Dr. S. Mitchell, and schools of massage proliferated in both the United States and Britain.

With the introduction of electrical treatments, the application of massage began to diminish as a part of recommended physiotherapy. However, today, the application of touch to the skin to relieve tension in muscles, ligaments, tendons, and joints is an accepted nonpharmacologic approach to decrease pain.

Naturopathy   Founded almost 100 years ago, this form of medicine includes natural therapeutics such as nutrition, herbs, homeopathy, massage, exercise, and even acupuncture. Drugs are not in this repertoire. Naturopathy school of thought believes that diseases are the body's attempt to heal itself through release of impurities. Treatments are designed to increase the client's "vital force" by eliminating toxins, thus allowing the body to heal.

Nutrition   The holistic approach dictates that an individual pay close attention to nutritional status as a critical component of wellness. Research strongly points to diet as a major contributor to health or disease. This is especially so when an individual has a diet of high saturated fat, refined sugars, additives, preservatives, or junk food. It is also current thinking that a high-carbohydrate diet contributes to obesity. Nutrition can also play a major role in prevention of disease; more and more emphasis is currently being placed on the role of antioxidants (vitamins C, E, beta-carotene,

Table 17-3 Most Common Herbs and Plants and What They Can Do for You

Aloe
A plant that has been used for centuries. It is a proven healer for skin problems and burns and has been used for gastrointestinal distress and as a daily tonic.

Bilberry
A European berry used by British Royal Air Force pilots flying night missions during World War II for improving night vision. This berry also relieves eye strain and helps to prevent eye disorders.

Black Cohosh
A remarkable herb for females because it helps to maintain normal hormone balance, especially during menopause. This herb is powerful and will increase the effect of synthetic hormones.

Cayenne
Anyone who has eaten a chili pepper has experienced the power of cayenne pepper. Capsaicin, the main ingredient, is used topically as a pain reliever and is useful for arthritis. This herb also reduces inflammation and increases circulation.

Chamomile
Produced from the chamomile flowers, this herb renews the skin or, used in a tea, is helpful for digestive upset or insomnia.

Echinacea
A favorite herb because of its immune-boosting properties. It is very effective for colds, flu, and coughs. It is not good to use on a long-term basis.

Elderberry
An ancient remedy for colds and one of the best herbal medicines for the flu. It is available in capsule, tincture, or extract form.

Feverfew
Many holistic healthcare providers recommend this herb as a preventive measure for migraine headaches. Studies have shown that feverfew decreases the severity and intensity of headaches.

Garlic
A common plant Italians love to use in cooking, but it is also a remedy for many disorders. Garlic keeps immunity high, lowers cholesterol, and can be used for ear infections.

Ginger
A medicinal as well as a cooking herb that is useful for nausea, stomach upset, and intestinal gas. Also, taken after meals, it helps digestion and reduces allergies.

Ginkgo
Traced back in time to the age of dinosaurs, this amazing tree is the oldest known species in existence. The many uses include improving circulation, helping memory in individuals with cognitive deficits, relieving tinnitus, and accelerating stroke recovery.

Ginseng
American, Chinese, and Siberian are all forms of this famous root. The Chinese form (Panax) is a warming herb that can increase energy and sex drive. American and Siberian forms are cooling herbs that fight fatigue and decrease stress. This herb also helps to normalize blood pressure and cholesterol.

Goldenseal
Extracted from a root, this bitter herb is excellent for colds, sore throats, ear infections, and as a cream useful for skin infections.

Green Tea
The leaves of this plant have become very popular because they contain some of the most powerful antioxidants known that help the body to eliminate free radicals. Used as a tea, tincture, tablet, or capsule, this herb can be taken as a cancer preventative or detoxification agent.

Hawthorn
A tonic made from berries, hawthorn can be used for a variety of heart disorders—lowering blood pressure, congestive heart failure, angina, and cardiomyopathy. Clients should seek medical consultation when using it with other heart medications.

Milk Thistle
Liver disease is one of the country's major health problems. This seed, known for its restoration of liver function, is one of the best-studied herbs for liver disease. Silymarin is the main ingredient in milk thistle. It is one of the most liver-protecting substances known to protect intact liver cells.

Pau D'Arco
Extracted from the bark of a tree in the Amazon Rain Forest, this potion in tea or capsule form has amazing uses—for infections, cancer, killing parasites, or *Candida* overgrowth.

Saw Palmetto
Made from berries grown on a small palm tree, this extract is a popular substance for men with an enlarged prostate. It relieves symptoms of benign prostatic hyperplasia and has been confirmed as the most researched and helpful substance for the prostate.

St. John's Wort
This herb, from which both the flowers and whole plant are used, enhances the production of key neurotransmitters. It works for mild to moderate depression and to decrease stress. With considerably fewer side effects than antidepressant drugs, it should not be used with pharmaceutical medications.

Turmeric
Known and used for centuries as a basic ingredient in Indian cooking, turmeric (from curcuma) is best used as an anti-inflammatory herb. It is also useful for arthritis, as a digestive aid, and for its antitumor qualities.

Valerian
A root that is used to relax nerves, promote peaceful feelings, and assist in sleeping. It is also used for spasms and pain.

pycnogenol, and the like) in preventing such diseases as cancer and heart disease.

There is much controversy today over whether the average American consumes a diet that provides enough of the essential nutrients to prevent disease and aging. The pro argument group says that if you follow the USDA Revised Food Pyramid, you do not need to supplement your diet. (See Chapter 19.) The opposing argument says that the quality of food today (unless you are eating a majority of organic and natural foods) is so deficient in nutrients that you cannot sustain a healthy diet.

To follow preventive guidelines for better health, most alternative healthcare providers and healthcare workers advocate supplementing diet with a broad-based multiple vitamin and mineral capsule daily, preferably with natural, food-based (not synthetic) nutrients. This prescription would include basic vitamins, all the minerals (including trace minerals), antioxidants, essential fatty acids (Omega 3 and 6), the carotinoids, coenzyme Q10, nutrients for the eyes such as lycopene and lutein, and bioflavonoids.

Prayer and Spirituality in Health   People have used both prayer and spiritual practices for thousands of years. These two areas are currently included in the arena of alternative medicine because it is built on a foundation of mind–body–spirit.

In a major survey of complementary medicine, when prayer was included in the definition, 62% had used this practice for dealing with a health problem. In fact, research shows that it is the therapy most commonly used among all alternative therapies. In one study at Harvard Medical School, analyzed data on the use of prayer showed that among 3,055 participants, 57% used prayer for health concerns or specific medical conditions and 75% prayed for wellness. (See Evidenced-Based Practice, Prayer as Alternative Medicine.)

Reflexology   Also called "zone therapy," reflexology is a method of treatment that proposes that diseases and organ dysfunction can be both diagnosed and treated by pressing on certain areas of the hands or feet. Each area of the body is represented by a corresponding area on the feet or hands; pressing on specific points is said to stimulate blood, nutrient, and energy flow to the diseased area of the body.

Relaxation and Visualization   Stress experts have carefully studied the effects of deep relaxation on the mind and body (Figure 17-1 ■). They found that individuals who regularly practice relaxation exercises experience less stress than people who don't. The relaxation response is actually the physiologic opposite of the stress response. People adept at invoking the relaxation response use their minds to control their autonomic nervous system—oxygen consumption, respiratory rate, heart rate, blood pressure, and muscle tension. Their alpha brain waves, the waves associated with feelings of well-being, increase. Effective body relaxation

techniques have existed for centuries. Several have gained significant popularity in recent years. In the United States, about 12% of adults use deep breathing exercises and 8% use meditation as complementary to their health care. The following short descriptions should familiarize you with the leading techniques.

1. *Deep Breathing:* Emphasized by virtually all relaxation exercises, deep breathing is a key to reducing stress. When you are tense, your breathing becomes rapid, irregular, and shallow. Healthy *deep* breathing increases the amount of oxygen in your blood, cleanses your system of carbon dioxide and other waste chemicals, relaxes your muscles, increases the endorphin release, and encourages your heart rate to return to normal. Learning to take deep, slow, full breaths and exhale completely effects mastery of this key relaxation technique. The following is a breathing technique that can be used for stress reduction. Try it and instruct your clients in this technique.

   - Inhale as you normally do.
   - Exhale as you normally do.
   - Pause as long as comfortable.
   - Repeat the first three steps.

   Simple? Yes. Effective? Yes. This technique allows lungs to empty more completely, continuing the normal exhalation process. Why is this simple exercise effective? Because the completed exhalation enables the mind to quiet—a rest from the jumble of one thought upon another.

2. *Autogenic Training:* In this form of relaxation, warmth and heaviness are visualized: two physical sensations associated with the relaxed state. The warmth represents increased blood flow throughout the body, and heaviness is perceived as relaxation of the skeletal muscles. During progressive relaxation, specific muscles or groups of

FIGURE 17-1 Sound and visualization are alternative treatment methods.

muscles are tensed and released throughout the body. This technique is especially effective for clients who are fearful and stressed.

3. *Meditation:* Originating thousands of years ago, meditation is based on Eastern cultures and religions. The effects of meditation are similar to those associated with deep relaxation. Meditation is the process of bringing the mind to stillness. It sounds easy, but if you have tried meditation, you know that the process can be difficult and requires practice. There are many methods of meditation, from the traditional transcendental meditation (TM) and Zen meditation to the repetition of a word or phrase. In TM, a mantra (a word or sound) is selected and is repeated mentally while the individual is seated quietly in a tranquil place.

   Perhaps the easiest meditation technique is to sit in a comfortable position with the spine straight (the lotus position is perfect if the legs can stand it), eyes closed, and to relax. While meditating, you concentrate on relaxing the muscles and organs throughout the body, and then focus on breathing. Inhale fully, then exhale, watching the breath come out "in your mind's eye." If a thought comes in, make it slip away and continue inhaling and exhaling. No thoughts should be allowed to rush in to break the concentration.

4. *Visualization:* Visualization is a proven technique for healing, stress management, and positive goal attainment. When a mental picture is created, the body responds as if it were a real experience. Visualization can assist a client to feel more confident in circumstances filled with uncertainties. It can also assist with reducing pain. Teach the client first to relax (through one of the techniques mentioned in this chapter), then to breathe deeply, and finally to see the pain in the mind's eye becoming less and less severe.

T'ai Chi Ch'uan This slow, graceful Chinese technique for relaxation is actually a system to both stimulate and balance subtle life energies. Thirty minutes a day devoted to the gentle, flowing movements of t'ai chi is relaxing, centering, and invigorating—a great way to relax and an interesting alternative to energetic Western exercise.

Yoga Yoga is an ancient Indian discipline that begins with postures, or asanas, that stretch and strengthen muscles. It progresses to meditative relaxation or breathing techniques. Yoga is not sport or exercise as such; nor does it have to be a religion. The system is devised completely for health and well-being. The best way to begin yoga is to find an experienced teacher who can correct postures and guide the individual through the breathing and relaxation exercises.

Herb–Drug Interactions

Millions of Americans are using **herbal preparations** instead of prescription and over-the-counter drugs. Other millions are combining herbs and medications.

Since use of herbs among nonprofessionals has greatly increased in the past few years, healthcare professionals must be aware of the potential danger, especially when combined with medications. In addition, there is no regulation, standardization, quality control, or even efficacy with herbal preparations. When nurses are completing admission assessments, questions should include asking about herbal preparations the client is now taking (Box 17-5 ■).

The following table of herb–drug interactions will cover some of the most popular herbs and their interactions with specific drugs (Table 17-4 ■).

Cultural Awareness

Allowing for a religious or spiritual component in the care plan will enhance the client's ability to cope. Each client should be asked about any cultural or religious practices they have that they would like to use as part of their care. Nurses need to be careful not to introduce their own biases into the care of their clients.

Box 17-5 **TOP COMPLEMENTARY AND INTEGRATIVE APPROACHES USED BY AMERICANS**

- In 2012, 33.2% of U.S. adults used complementary health approaches.
- The most commonly used complementary approach was natural products (dietary supplements other than vitamins and minerals).
- Fish oil was the number-one natural product used by adults, with 7.8% using it in 2012, followed by glucosamine and/or chondroitin, probiotics and prebiotics, melatonin, and coenzyme Q10.
- The mind and body approaches most commonly used by adults include yoga, chiropractic or osteopathic manipulation, meditation, and massage therapy.

Source: NCCIH (2012)

Table 17-4 Herb–Drug Interactions Chart

Herb	Action	Side Effects	Drug Interaction	Drugs Affected
Black Cohosh	An herb for females, especially during menopause for hot flashes—maintains healthy levels of luteinizing hormone Decreases menstrual discomfort Sedative, diuretic Lowers blood pressure	Overdose may cause nausea, vomiting, headache, dizziness, tremors, and depressed heart rate.	Increases effects of drugs—especially synthetic hormones **Clients with congestive heart failure and pregnant women should not use this herb.**	Hormone replacement therapy (HRT) Contraceptives Cardiac medications
Echinacea	Immunostimulant Treatment for colds (URIs) and influenza Bladder infections Blood purifier Helps preserve white cells during radiation treatment	Possible, but not common: nausea, vomiting, diarrhea, heartburn, skin rash, allergic reactions	Stimulates immune system—may alter effect of certain drugs; do not use with clients using immunosuppressants, or those who have AIDS, TB, or are pregnant.	Anabolic steroids Amiodarone Methotrexate Ketoconazole
Ephedra (Ma Huang)	Promotes weight loss and acts as a stimulant (asthma) Considered toxic by FDA	Stimulant, insomnia, headaches, nervousness, seizures, death	Heart attack, seizure, or death Additive effect; increased thermogenesis (related to stimulants/coffee) Elevation of BP (related to MAO inhibitors) Reduces drug action—may cause arrhythmias Increased steroid drug clearance may reduce effectiveness	Decongestants (Actifed, Dristan, Sinutab, Sudafed) Stimulants—caffeine MAO inhibitors Beta-blockers Cardiac glycosides Steroids (anti-inflammatories)
Feverfew	Eases pain and nausea of migraine headaches Prevents blood vessel spasms Interferes with action of platelets (which clump together to form clots) Lowers blood pressure	Gastrointestinal symptoms, nervousness, insomnia, and tiredness	Severe bleeding **Pregnant women, children under age 2, and people taking drugs as listed should not take this herb.**	Anticoagulants—Warfarin, aspirin, NSAIDs (ibuprofen)
Garlic	Contains allicin, a natural antibiotic—effective against bacteria and viruses Lowers total cholesterol and increases HDL Reduces blood pressure Reduces blood clot formation (when arteries are narrowed)	Intestinal problems—upset stomach, heartburn, garlic odor	Excessive thinning of blood (bleeding) when used with blood thinners Those who have blood disorders should use this herb conservatively.	Anticoagulants—Warfarin, Coumadin, aspirin Antihypertensives Saquinavir
Ginger	Relieves nausea associated with seasickness, motion sickness, or anesthesia Digestive aid; increased secretion of bile Reduces side effects of chemotherapy Reduces congestion and fevers Supports cardiovascular system	Heartburn	Excessive thinning of blood (bleeding) when used with blood thinners Interferes with platelet action Increases gut absorption (may increase drug bioavailability)	Anticoagulants—Warfarin Take cautiously with all cardiac or diabetic medications. Antihypertensives
Ginkgo Biloba	Improves circulation by thinning blood Enhances flow of oxygen and blood to brain Improves memory and mental function in clients with dementia May delay progression of Alzheimer (unproven) Asthma	Headache Indigestion, nausea, vomiting Nervousness Allergic skin reactions	Anticoagulant effect—may cause spontaneous or excessive bleeding **Those with blood clotting disorders should not take this drug.**	Anticoagulants—Coumadin, Warfarin, aspirin, NSAIDs Cox-2—inhibitors Anticonvulsants Vitamin K antagonists Diuretics, Thiazides

Table 17-4 Herb-Drug Interactions Chart *(continued)*

Herb	Action	Side Effects	Drug Interaction	Drugs Affected
Siberian Ginseng	Tonic, boosts energy and stamina Reduces stress, fatigue Improves sexual performance, regulates hormones Strengthens immune system Raises "good" cholesterol, HDL Protects against heart attacks Preventative for aging Improves blood sugar and diabetic symptoms (could reduce amount of insulin needed)	Insomnia, hypertension Diarrhea Low blood glucose Allergy symptoms Increased alcohol clearance Affects insulin level	Increases anticoagulant effect and bleeding Headache, manic behavior may occur when other drugs are taken. Monitoring effect of drug may be difficult—may increase digoxin levels. Stimulates alcohol metabolism **Those who have blood clotting problems, high blood pressure, asthma, emphysema, and children and pregnant women should not take this herb.**	Anticoagulants— Warfarin, Coumadin, aspirin, NSAIDs Nardil (MAO inhibitor) Digoxin (Lanoxin) Alcohol Insulin Antidepressants (phenelzine sulfate)
Kava Kava	Sedative effect that treats anxiety	GI problems, liver problems (even liver failure reported) Allergic skin reaction	Sedation, and even coma when taken with certain drugs	Alprazolam Sleeping meds Antipsychotics Alcohol, Xanax (antidepressant) Drugs treating Parkinson disease
Licorice Root	Helps steroid drug withdrawal Helps to heal gastric ulcers Diuretic effect	Raises blood pressure Headache Lethargy Cardiac dysfunction	Potentiates drug levels and offsets effects of NSAIDs Antibiotics reduce herb activity. Diuretic effect could result in decreased potassium, leading to electrolyte imbalance. Increased sensitivity to digoxin or other cardiac glycosides **Women who are pregnant or nursing, and people with glaucoma, hypertension, stroke, or heart disease should not take this herb.**	Corticosteroids Thiazides Oral contraceptives Antibiotics
Saw Palmetto	Supports health of prostate gland, benign prostatic hypertrophy (BPH) Improves urine flow Maintains healthy testosterone metabolism Anti-inflammatory	Relatively few: mild nausea, gastrointestinal disturbance, hypertension, headache	The safety profile of this herb is very good—no known drug interactions.	
Silymarin (Milk Thistle)	Increases liver detox capacity in general Supports liver function Protects liver from drug Damage	Nausea, GI disturbance	Reduces drug toxicity to liver and protects liver from drug damage Reduces toxic side effects of chemotherapy Potentially dangerous for transplant clients—reduces levels of immunosuppressives	Aspirin Alcohol Chemotherapy
St. John's Wort	Relieves mild to moderate depression by countering monamine oxidase (avoid same foods as if taking MAO inhibitor drug) Immune-stimulating properties—useful with AIDS because it is antiviral Helps bruises and hemorrhoids	Dry mouth, dizziness, fatigue, digestive problems (fewer side effects than prescription antidepressants) Sensitivity to light	Decreases immunosuppressant therapy Additive serotonin-like effects—serotonin syndrome (serious condition: fever, dizziness, sweating, and such) Could affect action of epilepsy drugs **Clients with hypertension and those on immunosuppressive therapy should not use this herb.**	Tetracyclines Cyclosporin Digoxin Oral contraceptives Zoloft and antidepressants Other SSRIs Anticonvulsants Warfarin
Valerian	Quiets and calms neurologic system Promotes sleep Used for headache, anxiety, and nervousness	Restlessness, headache, giddiness, nausea, and blurred vision	Effect may be altered by alcohol or barbiturates—use cautiously. Not for children under 2 years Effect may be enhanced with sleeping tablets Additive effect—may be used to wean off drugs (diazepam)	Alcohol Barbiturates Sleeping tablets Benzodiazepines

Source: Adapted from Herb/Drug Interaction Chart in Smith (2009)

Nursing Diagnoses

The following nursing diagnoses may be appropriate to include in a client care plan when the components are related to decreasing stress and promoting adaptation.

NURSING DIAGNOSIS	RELATED TO . . .
Anxiety	Increased stress; for instance, illness, trauma, loss
Defensive Coping	Denial of problem; rationalization of failure, such as increased demands on individual
Ineffective Coping	High stress on individual; for example, inability to adapt, length and duration of stressor
Ineffective Health Maintenance	High stress level from illness, abuse, or psychological factors
Deficient Knowledge	Lack of exposure to alternative methods, lack of interest in change (relaxation techniques)
Acute or Chronic Pain	Trauma, immobility, illness, or disease
Trauma, Risk for	Re-experiencing a traumatic event, exhibiting altered lifestyle, psychic numbness
Disturbed Sleep Pattern	Stressful thoughts, anxiety
Social Isolation	Maladaptive coping to stressor, such as long-term or high level of stress

Source: Herdman, T. H. & Kamitsuru, S. (Eds.) *Nursing Diagnoses – Definitions and Classification 2015-2017.* Copyright © 2014, 1994–2014 by NANDA International. Used by arrangement with John Wiley & Sons Limited. Companion website: www.wiley.com/go/nursingdiagnoses. In order to make safe and effective judgments using NANDA-I nursing diagnosis it is essential that nurses refer to the definitions and defining characteristics of the diagnoses listed in this work.

Stress and Adaptation

Nursing Process Data

ASSESSMENT Database

- Identify the client who demonstrates stressed behavior.
- Evaluate, with the client, the past and present stressors that the client has experienced.
- Evaluate the stressors' effect on the client's body and signs of distress in the body.
- Examples of physiologic stress effects:

    Cardiovascular system: increased pulse and blood pressure, evidence of angina, arrhythmias, migraine headaches, disturbance of heat and cold mechanisms

    Gastrointestinal system: ulcers, ulcerative colitis, constipation or diarrhea, imbalance in sugar absorption

    Musculoskeletal system: backache, tension headaches, arthritis, proneness to injuries

    Autoimmune system: infections, flu, allergies, rheumatoid arthritis, cancer

- Assess client's level of energy and the degree to which it is depleted.
- Evaluate client's awareness of thoughts, attitudes, values, and beliefs that influence stress response and adaptation.
- Assess present level of distress in the client's body.
- Assess possible causes of stress that are affecting client:

    Environmental stressors: input overload, such as sights, sounds, smells; actions and demands of others in the environment; or monotony

    Physical stressors: hunger, heat or cold, dangerous environment, injury, or pain

    Emotional stressors: loss of something of value, frustrations of needs and drives, threats to self-concept

    Psychosocial stressors: conflicting cultural values (e.g., the American values of competition and assertiveness versus the need to be dependent)

    Future shock: physiologic and psychological stress resulting from an overload of the organism's adaptive systems and decision-making processes brought about by too rapidly changing values and technology

    Cultural shock: stress developing in response to the transition from a familiar environment to unfamiliar one; involves unfamiliarity with communication, technology, customs, attitudes, and beliefs (e.g., immigrating, being confined in a hospital or prison); crowding, and urban life

    Job choice and the work environment: challenges in the workplace, concerns over healthcare costs and job-related stressors, hostile work environments, and bullying in the workplace

- Assess the factors that influence how the client responds to stress:

    Characteristics of the stressful event: magnitude, intensity, duration

    Client's biological and psychological inclinations

    Appropriateness of support system

- Life changes according to a stress scale (Holmes & Rahe, 1967)
- Assess current coping strategies.

PLANNING Objectives

- To identify presence of stress in client
- To identify how stress affects the body
- To identify the current sources that result in stressed behavior
- To determine the client's response to stress
- To evaluate stress interventions that have a positive effect on stressed client

IMPLEMENTATION Procedures

DOCUMENTATION AND EVALUATION

Expected Outcomes

- Client is able to evaluate the general stressors and identify sources of stress in his or her life.
- Client is aware of response patterns to stress and is able to alter patterns appropriately.
- Client is aware of body–mind stress and its influence on his or her body.
- Client is able to reduce environmental stressors.
- Client is able to identify and alleviate stress caused by mental concerns.

Unexpected Outcomes/Alternative Actions

Pearson Nursing Student Resources

Find additional review materials at
nursing.pearsonhighered.com.
Prepare for success with NCLEX®-style practice questions and Skill Checklists.

Skill 17.1.1	Determining the Effect of Stress

Procedure

1. Identify client's stress tolerance level.
   a. Recognize the body's alarm signals (see major signals in assessment).
   b. Assess signal correctly as signifying high level of stress.
2. Discuss the concept of stress to elicit understanding of its effect on the client (see Box 17-1). ➤ *Rationale:* Stress may be physical, chemical, or emotional and may cause bodily or mental tension that may be a factor in disease causation.

3. Encourage the client to feel free to discuss life patterns that relate to stress.
4. Discuss the effect of stress. ➤ *Rationale:* Directing the conversation to the emotional, mental, and social sources of stress assists the client in examining its total effect and promotes self-awareness.
5. Assist the client in formulating a plan to reduce or eliminate at least some sources of stress. ➤ *Rationale:* This promotes client self-empowerment.

Skill 17.1.2	Determining Response Patterns

Procedure

1. Evaluate adaptation factors that influence stress management.
   a. *Age:* Adaptation is greatest in youth and young middle life and least at the extremes of life.
   b. *Environment:* Does environment support managing stress?
   c. *Time:* The client can more easily adapt to stress over a period of time than suddenly.
   d. *Flexibility:* The degree of flexibility of the individual influences survival.
   e. *Expenditure of energy:* The individual usually uses the adaptation mechanism that is most economic in terms of energy.
   f. *Presence of illness:* Disease decreases the individual's capacity to adapt to stress.
2. Assess the effects of stress on the client.
   a. Feelings resulting from stress:
      1. Anxiety
      2. Anger

   3. Helplessness and hopelessness
   4. Guilt, shame, and disgust
   5. Fear and frustration
   6. Depression
   b. Behaviors resulting from stress:
      1. Apathy, regression, and withdrawal
      2. Crying and demanding
      3. Physical illness
      4. Hostility and manipulation
      5. Senseless violence and lashing out

EVIDENCE-BASED PRACTICE

The Opposite of a Stress Response

The seminal work on the stress response, *The Relaxation Response*, was published in 1984 by Herbert Benson, MD. In his studies, Dr. Benson found that the opposite of a stress response (physiologic response) can be achieved by completing only two steps: repeating a prayer, word, sound, phrase, or movement, and disregarding all other thoughts (as in meditation, yoga, and the like).

Skill 17.1.3 | Managing Stress

Procedure

1. Discuss the client's body response to stress.

   a. The body's response to stress is a self-preservation mechanism that automatically and immediately becomes activated in times of danger.

   b. Assist client to understand response patterns.

2. Teach client to be aware of stress sensations in his or her body—recognize physical symptoms.

3. Suggest that client frequently monitor thought patterns to identify those thoughts that cause automatic tensing responses (tight muscles, increase in heartbeat, butterflies in stomach).

4. Assist client to decide whether these thoughts are essential to survival or if they can be changed, eliminated, or replaced.

5. Assist client in planning to set aside periods each day for self-stress evaluation.

EVIDENCE-BASED PRACTICE
Managing Stress

A recent meta-analysis looked at the effectiveness of cognitive behavior therapy (CBT) at managing a variety of problems including stress management. The findings indicate that CBT is an effective treatment for both general anxiety disorders and general stress. There were several well designed studies to support the use of CBT for the management of stress.

Source: Hofmann, Asnaani, Vonk, Sawyer, & Fang (2012)

---

6. Provide problem-solving assistance, so the client can examine new, more appropriate response patterns.

7. Refer client to resources (therapy classes, books, relaxation tapes) that will assist in developing new responses.

Skill 17.1.4 | Manipulating the Environment to Reduce Stress

Procedure

1. Modify client's external environment so that adaptation responses are within his or her capacity. ❶

2. Support the efforts of the client to adapt or to respond.

3. Provide client with the materials required to maintain constancy of his or her environment.

4. Understand the body's mechanisms for accommodating stress.

5. Prevent additional stress.

6. Reduce external stimuli and input through senses.

7. Reduce or increase physical activity depending on the cause of and response to stress.

❶ Closing curtains and turning off the television are two ways of reducing stimuli in the client's environment.

Skill 17.1.5 | Teaching Coping Strategies

Procedure

1. Analyze client's stress status.

   a. Estimate total amount of stress client is experiencing—too high a level of stress indicates need for intervention.

   b. Recognize where in body or mind the stress is manifesting.

2. Discuss various options for reducing stress—which alternatives fit with client.

3. Suggest client use diversion methods of coping (Box 17-6 ■).

   a. *Physical diversion:* jogging, swimming, cooking, cleaning

   b. *Mental diversion:* reading, painting, going to a movie, or simply thinking about a pleasant memory

4. Plan with client how to use rest as a way to cope with stress.

   a. Vacation, leave of absence from job, frequent naps.

   b. Eliminate or decrease major stressors so that result is rest from stress input.

   c. Plan with client how to manage time so that input can be reduced and goals limited.

Skill 17.1.5 | Teaching Coping Stratgies (continued)

5. Teach client how to use concentration, body relaxation, breathing, or meditation techniques to relieve mind stress.

6. Remind client that laughter is a great tranquilizer and healer as well as a stress reducer, and assist client to plan how to use this method.

Box 17-6 SUGGESTIONS FOR COPING WITH STRESS

- Rank tasks to be completed, and identify activities that need to be accomplished.
- Forget unimportant details; do not try to remember too many things. Concentrate on the essential issues and details.
- Eliminate past unpleasant events from the mind and focus on the present.

- Do not cling to unpleasant experiences and emotions that impair emotional ability to respond to here and now.
- Discard habit of anticipating negative outcomes, which is often worse than the actual event.
- Do not yearn for things relating to the past or the future; focus attention on present desires.

Skill 17.1.6 | Managing Stress Using a Holistic Model

Procedure

1. Manage stress through exercise.

   a. Poor physical condition becomes a stressor—this state contributes to lethargy, a constant fatigue level, and low resistance for illness and lessens adaptive responses.

   b. Good physical condition results in stamina, reserves necessary to withstand stress, and protection against unpredictable stress periods.

   c. Exercise prepares the body physically for stress caused by environmental conditions.

   d. Consistent exercise prepares body to handle stress emotionally.

2. Manage stress through diet.

   a. Certain foods and drug substances (caffeine, alcohol, sugar, junk foods, preservatives, tobacco) are potent stressors to our bodies.

   b. Consuming high-stress foods results in negative body changes, such as hypertension, high cholesterol, labile blood sugar levels, and a rapid, bounding pulse rate.

   c. Consuming a low-stress diet results in more energy and stamina to cope with stress. Teach client that a low-stress diet includes reducing saturated fat and limiting protein intake to 10%–15% of consumed calories. Remainder of intake should be raw or barely cooked vegetables, fruits, whole grains, nuts, low-fat dairy

products, and plenty of liquids. Eliminate sodas, caffeine products, and most alcohol. Exclude refined sugars and carbohydrates and convenience or processed foods.

   d. Encourage the use of vitamin supplements: vitamin C, B-complex, mineral supplements. Assist client to examine diet and experiment with different vitamin–mineral supplements.

3. Manage stress by altering lifestyle patterns.

   a. Counsel clients to eliminate unnecessary stressors in their life—change parts of life that are particularly stressful.

   b. Assist client to develop personal methods for coping with stress: walking in the woods, painting, listening to music, reading, or practicing yoga.

   c. Encourage client to assess lifestyle periodically and alter habits as necessary to reduce stress.

4. Manage stress through use of prayer and/or meditation.

EVIDENCE-BASED PRACTICE

Music Therapy in Terminally Ill Clients

A review of the literature on the effects of music therapy in terminally ill clients found music therapy is effective in managing pain and controlling breathlessness and that it acts as a medium to allow clients to express their emotions.

Source: Leow, Drury, & Poon (2010)

Skill 17.1.7 | Teaching Controlled Breathing

Procedure

1. Instruct client to sit so that his or her back is well supported, with spine straight but not rigid.
2. Have client place feet flat on floor and place hands on legs.
3. If client is lying down, have him or her place hands at side.
4. Suggest client find a comfortable position, close eyes, and take a deep, slow breath through nostrils.
5. Continue giving the client the following instructions.

   a. Extend your abdominal muscles.
   b. Hold your breath for the count of four. Then very slowly release the air through slightly parted lips, making a "whoosh" sound.
   c. When you think that all the air is out, hold your stomach in to push out even more air.
   d. Repeat this breathing pattern several times so that your body relaxes.
   e. Breathe in through your nostrils to the count of four—1-2-3-4. Hold it—1-2-3-4—and expel the breath all the way out slowly, slowly releasing the air through your mouth.
   f. As the air goes out, feel all of the tension drain out with it.
   g. Now double the count and breathe in slowly, filling your lungs all the way to the top to the count of eight.1-2-3-4-5-6-7-8. Hold it—1-2-3-4—and now slowly release the breath—5-6-7-8.
   h. Again breathe in slowly to the count of 10 and count for the client—1-2-3-4-5-6-7-8-9-10. Hold it to the count

of eight—1-2-3-4-5-6-7-8—and slowly release the air through your mouth to the count of 10—1-2-3-4-5-6-7-8-9-10. Pause.

   i. Continue with your regular breathing pattern, letting the air breathe for you.

6. Stop the process by having the client open his or her eyes.

1 Find a quiet room to teach relaxation process.

CLINICAL ALERT

If you are motivated to learn CAM techniques, there are numerous classes available. In fact, to implement certain CAM therapies such as Reiki, therapeutic touch, acupressure, or acupuncture, you will need specialized classes/training.

Skill 17.1.8 | Teaching Body Relaxation

Procedure

1. Place client in a comfortable position.

   a. Have client sit so that back is well supported and spine is straight. Have client put both feet on the floor and hold hands comfortably in lap.
   b. If sitting is uncomfortable, have client lie on a bed and support areas of the body so that he or she is comfortable.

2. Instruct client to concentrate on each key muscle of the body, tensing and relaxing each muscle until it is totally relaxed.

3. Ask client to tense and release the muscles in the left toes, left foot, left calf, left thigh, and left leg.
4. Now have the client continue the process on the right leg, trunk, upper torso, arms, shoulders, neck, and face. Then have the client check to see that every muscle is relaxed.
5. Ask the client to check for tight areas, any tension, any uncomfortable areas or sensations and then to let it all go. Ask the client if he or she is willing to let all of the tension go.
6. Ask client to practice being totally relaxed.

Skill 17.1.9 | Using Meditation as an Alternative Therapy

Procedure

1. Meditation is the process of relaxing the body and focusing and quieting the mind. The essence of this method depends on the ability to concentrate on an object, a word, or nothing at all.
2. The process of meditation begins with slow, quiet breathing and deep muscle relaxation.
3. Instruct the client in meditation techniques—suggest books or tapes that focus on meditation.

4. Encourage the client to begin meditation—suggest positive outcomes.

   a. During meditation, there is a decrease in oxygen consumption, blood pressure, pulse rate, respiration, brain wave activity, and blood lactate level (high in anxious people).

   b. Research indicates that meditation has a measurable effect on stress-related conditions.

Unit 17.1 Documentation and Evaluation

DOCUMENTATION for Stress and Adaptation

- Identification of stressed behavior observed in client
- Separation of physical from emotional and environmental stressors
- How client is responding to stress
- Pertinent verbalizations of client related to stress
- Nursing interventions related to stress reduction

EVALUATION/Critical Thinking

Expected Outcomes

- Client is able to evaluate the general stressors and identify sources of stress in his or her life.
- Client is aware of response patterns to stress and is able to alter patterns appropriately.
- Client is aware of body–mind stress and its influence on his or her body.
- Client is able to reduce environmental stressors.
- Client is able to identify and alleviate stress caused by mental concerns.

Unexpected Outcomes	Alternative Actions
• Client moves into the stage of exhaustion, and stress becomes dangerous to health.	• Immediately take measures to remove stressors through medication, complete rest, and so forth. • Implement specific stress-reducing measures, such as the relaxation processes, visualization, and biofeedback.
• Client refuses to acknowledge that stress is affecting his or her life.	• Attempt to elicit feelings of client before giving information about the role of stress and effect on the body. • Refer client to resources, articles, and knowledgeable individuals who can discuss the effect of stress and the importance of eliminating stressors.

Chapter Wrap-Up

GERONTOLOGIC Considerations

The Influence of Stress on Aging is Significant and Affects Response and Coping Ability

- Nearly 23% of older people living in the community have some degree of disability.
- Older adults have less resistance to stressors: mental, emotional, environmental, and physical.
- Homeostatic imbalance is more common in the older adult and causes additional stress on the body.
- Adaptation to stress lessens with age (depends in part on genetic makeup and personal learning to deal with life crises).
- Many older adults have depression.
- Nursing care should focus on adaptive responses to stress—assist client to develop mechanisms to deal with the stress of illness and hospitalization.

Risk Factors That Influence Stress Levels and Psychosocial Adaptation

- Lowered economic resources
- Unanticipated events such as death of a spouse
- Poor **coping mechanisms**
- Unrealistic appraisal of conditions
- Physical illness

Symptoms to Evaluate That Indicate High Stress Levels

- Insomnia
- High anxiety level
- Abuse of drugs, alcohol, or tobacco
- Hypertension, tachycardia, irregular heartbeat
- Depression, chronic fatigue
- Chronic pain
- Physical complaints
- Lack of any pleasure in life

MANAGEMENT Guidelines

Each state legislates a Nurse Practice Act for RNs and LVN/LPNs. Healthcare facilities are responsible for establishing and implementing policies and procedures that conform to their state's regulations. Verify the regulations and role parameters for each healthcare worker in your facility.

Delegation

- Stress assessment should be completed by an RN or LVN/LPN with experience evaluating stress in clients and one who understands Selye's model of stress.
- An LVN/LPN assigned to a client who needs coping strategies for stress should check the care plan with an RN or team leader.

- Teaching a client body relaxation, controlled breathing, or meditation should be done by an experienced nurse—RN or LVN/LPN.

Interprofessional Communication

- Integrating stress reduction and coping strategies into a client's care plan should be shared by the total staff interacting with the client to maintain a consistent approach.
- The staff approach should have outcome behaviors designated so that the strategies can be evaluated as to effectiveness and efficacy for the client.

CASE STUDY Applications

Scenario 1

Robert Warren is 40 years old and works as an administrative assistant for a senator in Washington, D.C. Before his admission to the hospital, he had no history of heart trouble and had no other major health problems. He is overweight by 30 lb, has complained of difficulty sleeping for several years, and has admitted to several brief depressive episodes that he has handled by either working longer hours or becoming intoxicated with alcohol. He does admit to overuse of alcohol on a daily basis.

Robert complains of burnout related to his work. Although he admires and supports his boss, he also competes with him and secretly believes he would make a better senator. Another area of concern is his marriage, which he says is dull except for an explosive argument every few weeks. Robert has been having affairs with other women regularly for the past few years. He and his wife have no children. Robert's admission diagnosis is acute myocardial infarction.

1. What are the consequences of Robert's adhering to this lifestyle behavior?

2. Which assessment parameters for stress are important for this client? Be specific about the areas of stress in the assessment.

3. In what ways can you assist this client to improve his coping with stress? (Robert's nutrition and exercise plans are deferred because he is currently in a cardiac rehabilitation program that monitors his diet and exercise daily.)

4. How might you test the result of stress reduction behaviors?

Scenario 2

The nurse is admitting a 60-year-old client to the unit. He is scheduled to undergo a series of tests to determine why he is fatigued, dizzy, and has constant digestive complaints. He had one seizure and was started on Dilantin until a diagnosis is made. As the admitting RN, you are completing an assessment.

1. Excluding the physical assessment parameters and signs and symptoms, what additional assessments will you make?

2. Based on the information you receive from the client, what teaching does this client require?

NCLEX® Review Questions

Unless otherwise specified, choose only one (1) answer.

1. Which of the following indicate signals of stress the nurse should recognize?

    Select all that apply.

    A. Fatigue, lethargy
    B. Eating disorder
    C. Anxiety
    D. Anger
    E. Restlessness

2. Which of the following is the best definition of *holistic* when referring to a holistic approach to health?

    A. The term implies wholeness.
    B. Holistic refers to the whole body, including mind and psyche.
    C. The term parallels wellness and means that if the individual is holistic, he or she is healthy.
    D. The term suggests that the body, mind, and spirit are one and interacts as an open system with the environment.

3. The World Health Organization (WHO) estimates that 80% of the world's population uses which of the following alternative practices as a part of their health care?

    A. Herbal medicine
    B. Chiropractics
    C. Energy medicine
    D. Homeopathy

4. Which of the following adaptation factors influence stress management?

    Select all that apply.

    A. Age
    B. Environment
    C. Degree of flexibility of the individual
    D. Religion
    E. Presence of illness
    F. Expenditure of energy needed

5. Which of the following is a therapeutic suggestion for coping with stress?

    A. Pay attention to unimportant details.
    B. Rank tasks to be completed in order of importance.
    C. Consider unpleasant past events and figure out what went wrong.
    D. Anticipate negative outcomes before they occur.

6. What is the best rationale for including nutrition or diet as an alternative treatment method?

    A. Diet is a major contributor to health or disease.
    B. Nutrition influences how long we live.
    C. Diet can cure disease.
    D. The quality of food influences well-being.

7. A client requests information about alternative treatments. Choose the most appropriate response.

   A. "I think that you should ask your doctor about this."

   B. "Perhaps it would be better to stick to mainstream medicine."

   C. "Let's get your doctor and my supervisor together to discuss your question."

   D. "I'll bring you information about alternative treatments."

8. Which of the following statements does not fit into Hans Selye's definition of stress?

   A. Stress is a specific syndrome.

   B. Stress is manifested by specific changes in the body.

   C. Stress can only be controlled by changes in thought patterns.

   D. Stress causes a multiplicity of changes in the body.

9. Which one of the following statements about stress is inaccurate?

   A. Chronic stress causes changes in the immune system.

   B. Stressors may be chemical, physical, developmental, or emotional.

   C. The stress syndrome can be both positive and negative.

   D. The danger signals of stress are easy to observe.

10. A client tells the nurse that he is constantly under stress. Which stress reduction technique could the nurse teach the client?

    A. Counting to 10 before getting angry

    B. Sitting relaxed and quiet, clearing the mind, and breathing deeply

    C. Jumping up and down on a trampoline

    D. Saying a mantra or one word over and over again

QSEN Activity

Domain: Client Centered Care

Describe how diverse cultural, ethnic, and social backgrounds function as sources of client, family, and community values.

- Diversity in all its dimensions
- Impact of culture on the client experience

Activity:

You are caring for a client who has requested CAM therapies to be delivered along with traditional medication therapies. Determine how you will integrate that into the plan of care. Select a client you are currently familiar with and some appropriate CAM therapies that would integrate well.

Bibliography

Becker, R., & Selden, G. (1998.) *The body electric: Electromagnetism and the foundation of life*. New York: Harper Collins.

Benson, H. (1984). *The relaxation response*. New York: Times Books.

Complementary and Alternative Medicine. (2005, Winter). *Prayer and spirituality in health: Ancient practices, modern science*. Washington, DC: NIH.

Goldstein, D. S. (2010). Adrenal responses to stress. *Cellular and Molecular Neurobiology, 30*(8): 1433–1440.

Hofmann, S. G., Asnaani, A., Vonk, I. J., Sawyer, A. T., & Fang, A. (2012). The efficacy of cognitive behavioral therapy: A review of meta-analyses. *Cognitive Therapy and Research, 36*(5), 427–440.

Holmes, T. H. & Rahe, R. H. (1967). The social readjustment rating scale. *Journal of Psychosomatic Research, 11*(2), 213–221.

Leow, Q., Drury, V., & Poon, W. (2010). Experience of terminally ill patients with music therapy: A literature review. *Singapore Nursing Journal, 37*(3), 48–52.

National Center for Complementary and Integrative Health. (2012). What complementary approaches do Americans use? Retrieved from https://nccih.nih.gov/research/statistics/NHIS/2012/key-findings

National Library of Medicine. (2015). Complementary and integrative medicine. Retrieved from http://www.nlm.nih.gov/medlineplus/complementaryandalternativemedicine.html

Selye, H. (1965). *The stress of life*. New York: McGraw-Hill.

Selye, H. (1974). *Stress without distress*. New York: Signet.

Shealy, N. (2002). *90 days to stress-free living: A day-by-day health plan, including exercises, diet, and relaxation techniques*. London, U.K.: Vega.

Simonton, O. C., Henson, R. M., & Hampton, B. (2002). *The Healing Journey*. Lincoln, NE: Authors Choice Press.

Singh, P., & Chaturvedi, A. (2015, Jan.–Apr.). Complementary and alternative medicine in cancer pain management: A systematic review. *Indian Journal of Palliative Care, 21*(1), 105–115.

Whitaker, J. (2009). *Target your health concerns with potent herbal remedies*. Baltimore, MD: Healthier News.

World Health Organization (WHO). (2014). Guidelines for the assessment of herbal medicine. Retrieved from http://apps.who.int/medicinedocs/en/d/Jh1813e/3.html#Jh1813e.3.1

Chapter 18
Medication Administration

 Learning Objectives

18.1 Explain the concepts of drug absorption, distribution, biotransformation, and excretion.

18.2 List the seven parts of a medication order.

18.3 State the "six rights" for administering medications.

18.4 Describe the use of an automated dispensing unit.

18.5 Identify three nursing actions to prevent medication errors.

18.6 Outline steps for applying a transdermal medication.

18.7 List factors to assess before applying medications to the skin or mucous membranes.

18.8 Describe steps for instilling eyedrops.

18.9 Outline the process of eye and ear irrigations.

18.10 Contrast the procedure for instilling ear medication in adults and children.

18.11 Outline steps used when preparing parenteral medications.

18.12 Demonstrate correct calculation and preparation of a complex medication order.

18.13 Compare insulin types, their onset, peak, and duration of action.

18.14 List four important factors to assess when administering parenteral medications.

18.15 State four techniques to alleviate pain with parenteral injections.

18.16 Describe the Z-track method of intramuscular injection.

18.17 List steps for inserting a rectal or vaginal suppository.

Chapter Outline

Note: Intravenous (IV) medication administration is discussed in depth in Chapter 28.

Terminology

Absorption the passage of a substance from administration site into the bloodstream.

Actuation propellant-driven medication dose.

Adverse reaction undesirable, usually unpredictable medication effect; may be immediate or take months to develop.

Aspirate to remove by suction.

Biotransformation metabolic conversion of a drug into inactive metabolites that are readily excreted from the body.

Buccal administration placement of a medication between the gum and the cheek.

Compatible able to mix with another substance without destructive changes.

Contraindication any circumstance indicating the inappropriateness of a form of treatment otherwise advisable.

Dosage the amount of medicine to be administered to a client at one time.

Enteral administration through the gastrointestinal tract via a tube, catheter, or stoma to deliver nutrients/medications distal to the oral cavity.

Generic common or general name for a drug, as opposed to a brand name.

Instillation slowly pouring or dropping a liquid into a cavity or onto a surface.

Intradermal within the dermal layer of the skin; injection here used for testing allergies or immune responses.

Intramuscular within a muscle; injected medication is rapidly absorbed due to rich vascular supply.

Intravenous administration into a vein for immediate drug action.

Medicine a drug or remedy.

Metabolism the biological process of changing a substance so that it (a) is less active, and (b) can be excreted.

Narcotic a controlled substance that depresses the central nervous system, thus relieving pain and producing sedation.

Nebulizer a device for breaking a drug into small particles to produce a mist or fog for inhalation.

Ophthalmic relating to the eye; topical route for administering eye medications.

Otic relating to the ear; topical route for administering ear medications.

Parenteral absorption route for administering medications other than the GI tract; requiring injection.

Subcutaneous third layer of skin, which contains fat, with few blood and lymph vessels; route for injected medication that results in slower absorption.

Sublingual under the tongue.

Systemic pertinent to the whole body rather than one specific area.

Therapeutic having medicinal or healing properties.

Pharmacologic Agents

The term *medication* refers to approved **therapeutic** (pharmacologic) agents applied to or introduced into the body to produce specific local or **systemic** physiologic effects. Medications are chemical compounds that are produced in a pharmaceutical laboratory and prescribed by a healthcare provider to be administered to a client to prevent, treat, or cure illness. These agents should be differentiated from over-the-counter (OTC) products such as vitamins, minerals, nutritional supplements, and botanical agents (herbs, phytomedicines), which also affect the body. While such OTC products are available to the public and commonly used for self-treatment, they are not officially regulated or monitored in the United States. It is important to assess the client's use of pharmaceutical agents as well as over-the-counter products or supplements, since there is potential for dangerous interactive effects.

Pharmacologic agents have a **generic** (patented official) name (e.g., acetaminophen), and a trade or brand name (created by the particular manufacturer), which is capitalized (e.g., Tylenol). Generic formulations are usually less expensive than brand-name products.

Biological Effects of Drugs

The ultimate effect of a drug is influenced by four biological processes: **absorption**, **distribution**, **metabolism** (**biotransformation**), and excretion. These processes determine the onset, duration, and intensity of a drug's action.

Absorption   This process refers to the movement of the drug from the administration site into the bloodstream.

The route of administration determines whether or not a drug is confined to one area of the body to exert a *local effect*, or is absorbed by the vascular system and distributed to body tissues for a *systemic effect*. The oral route (PO, *per os* [Latin], or by mouth) is most frequently used for drug administration. Drugs may be given PO to exert a local effect (e.g., cough **medicine**, antacid), but more commonly the drug dissolves and is absorbed by the GI tract to exert a systemic effect. Liquid forms are absorbed more quickly. Most drugs are absorbed in the small intestine via the large vascular mucosal surface. The alkaline environment of the intestines enhances this absorption process. GI absorption is influenced by the pH, the presence or absence of food, concomitant ingestion of other drugs, solubility of the drug, and blood flow to the absorption site. In general, bioavailability of oral drugs is decreased because after absorption, the drug is circulated to the liver (first pass) and metabolized before reaching the circulation.

Medications applied "topically" to the skin (dermal) or eye (**ophthalmic**) or into the ear canal (**otic**) are often administered for local action. The skin is also used for transdermal (percutaneous) absorption of drugs by diffusion via patches, which release a medication continuously into capillaries of the epidermis for a systemic effect.

Mucous membranes provide a variety of convenient sites for drug administration to achieve a local or systemic effect by absorption. Sites include **sublingual** and **buccal** areas, the nose or respiratory tract (by inhalation), the eye, vagina, and rectum.

The **parenteral** route (by injection) provides the most direct, reliable, and rapid drug absorption. Methods of parenteral administration include **intradermal** (ID), **subcutaneous** (Sub Q), **intramuscular** (IM), intraosseous, and intravenous (IV). Site selection depends on the drug, its action, and client factors. For example, a client with a severe allergic reaction receives epinephrine IV (directly into the bloodstream) because this route bypasses the process of absorption and provides immediate distribution and drug action in an emergency situation.

Distribution   Distribution refers to the process by which a drug is transported by the blood to the site of action. Some of the drug binds to plasma protein and may compete with other drugs for this storage site. The rest is transported in "free" form through the circulation. It is the "free" form that is pharmacologically active. The "free" drug crosses cell membranes and as it is metabolized and excreted, the protein-bound drug is freed for action. Lipid-soluble drugs are distributed to and stored in fat and then released slowly into the bloodstream when drug administration is discontinued. The distribution process requires adequate cardiac output and tissue perfusion, while the rate of diffusion is influenced by the drug's protein-binding capacity, its solubility, the amount of drug in the plasma, and the presence of physiologic barriers such as the blood–brain and placental barriers.

Metabolism   Metabolism or biotransformation refers to the enzymatic process by which a "free" drug is converted to an inactive and harmless form that can be excreted. Most drugs are metabolized in the liver, where some drugs are converted into metabolites that are more pharmacologically effective than their "parent" form. Some drugs given orally are significantly inactivated by "first passing" through the liver before entering the general circulation to be transported to the site of action. Oral doses of these drugs must be higher than parenteral doses, and some drugs totally inactivated by "first pass" must be given parenterally. Other sites of drug metabolism include the lungs, kidney, plasma, and intestinal mucosa.

Excretion   This is the final process by which the drug is eliminated from the body. The kidneys are the most important route of excretion because they eliminate both the pure drug as well as metabolites of the parent drug. During excretion, substances are filtered through the glomeruli, secreted by the tubules, and then either reabsorbed by the tubules or directly excreted and eliminated through urine. Other routes of excretion include the lungs (by exhalation), GI tract, saliva, sweat, and breast milk.

Medication biodynamic processes and the individual client's response to drug therapy are influenced by many factors, including a client's body weight, body mass index, age, gender, acid–base and fluid and electrolyte balance, biorhythms, and general health and nutritional status. In addition, ethnic origin and genetic and immunologic factors affect biodynamics, as do psychological, emotional, and environmental influences. The term *drug polymorphism* is applied to these variations in clients' response to medications.

Administering Medications Safely

A medication must have healthcare provider's order or prescription before it can be legally administered to a client. If a written order is illegible or is questionable for any reason, the healthcare provider must be notified for clarification. In many agencies, it is the pharmacist's responsibility to contact the prescriber to clarify unclear or questionable orders. As institutions move towards electronic health records and computerized provider order entry (CPOE), illegible orders have become less of a problem.

Since medication orders may be written or spoken, it is important to specify the mode of communication. If a medication order is spoken aloud as a voice order (VO) or as a telephone order (TO), there is greater risk of error than if it is written. Verbal orders should not be taken if the prescriber is present, and they are never appropriate for complex therapeutic protocols (e.g., chemotherapy). Verbal orders are taken only in emergency situations such as a code in which the client's life depends on having the orders carried out immediately.

If an order is communicated by telephone, always repeat the order to avoid misinterpretation. Remember the acronym TORB, *Telephone Order Repeat Back*. Have the prescriber spell out the name of the medication and **dosage**, and then repeat the order back to the healthcare provider. This has been part of the Joint Commission's National Patient Safety Goals to improve safety in healthcare communication around TOs. After verification, the order is then entered into the EHR and cosigned by the healthcare provider.

Often the healthcare provider is able to enter the order directly into the system if he or she has access to a computer. Medication orders may be *routine* (administered as ordered until discontinued by the prescriber), *one-time-only*, *stat* (immediate), or *prn* (administered when the client needs the medication within the specified time interval, e.g., q4h). The continued validity of any medication order should be evaluated, since prescribers sometimes forget to discontinue medications that are no longer appropriate for the client's condition (Box 18-1 ■).

While the healthcare provider prescribes the medication and the pharmacist dispenses it, the nurse is responsible for validating, preparing, and administering medications safely and in accordance with agency policies and procedures. The nurse should understand why the medication is prescribed for the particular client and clarify concerns about its use. The nurse who prepares the medication must also give it to the client, and then document the medication, time, dosage, and route on the client's record. In addition, the nurse assesses and documents the client's response to the drug administered. If the client is allergic to a medication, an anaphylactic reaction may occur. This is a life-threatening medical emergency requiring immediate administration of epinephrine.

PARTS OF MEDICATION ORDERS AND COMMUNICATION ISSUES

- Client's name
- Date medication was ordered
- Name of medication
- Medication dosage
- Route of administration and any special instruction for administration
- Time and frequency medication is to be given
- Signature of individual ordering the drug

Common communication breakdowns leading to medication errors include:

- Unapproved or unclear abbreviations (see Legal Considerations)
- Illegible writing
- Misplaced or unnoticed decimals (e.g., .2 rather than 0.2)
- Verbal orders
- Incomplete orders

Source: Institute for Safe Medication Practices (2013); website provides updated list of abbreviations to avoid.

Safety Precautions

When administering medications, follow established safety rules, known as the "six rights." These rules are to be carried out each time you give a medication to a client.

The Six Rights

- **Right medication.** Compare medication container label to the medication sheet (MAR) **three** times (when obtaining the medication, when preparing the medication, and after preparation). Note medication expiration date. Know action, dosage, and method of administration. Know side effects of the medication and any *allergies* the client might have.
- **Right client.** Check the room and bed number and client's identification band: Validate correct client with two identifiers other than room number (e.g., stated name and date of birth).
- **Right time.** Give medication within a range of 30–45 min before or after time ordered (according to agency policy).
- **Right method or route of administration.** If a change in route is indicated, request new orders from healthcare provider.
- **Right dose.** Validate appropriate dosages for your client. Perform independent calculation of doses with another nurse for critical drugs such as insulin. Know the usual dose, and question any dose outside safe range.

- **Right Documentation.** Document the name of the drug, the dose and route, time administered, and the client's response to the medication administered. Documentation after administration is considered to be the sixth "right" action.

Medication Errors and Near Misses Medication errors and adverse events are serious safety concerns that can lead to poor client outcomes if not identified and proper actions taken. Besides these, it is also important to identify events called "near misses." These are events that did not go as planned but that did not result in harm or injury. The National Coordinating Council for Medication Error Reporting and Prevention (2015) recommends using a standard definition for medication error, which includes classifying a medication error as any preventable event that may cause client harm. In the event of a medication error, the healthcare provider must be notified immediately so that potential adverse client outcomes can be prevented or minimized. This includes an investigation of the cause of error and what steps need to be taken to prevent the error or adverse event. When an error does occur, the nurse then follows the agency's unusual occurrence or variance reporting procedure to facilitate audits that help identify and rectify sources of medication errors.

Cultural Awareness

Cultural factors including values and beliefs, educational level, previous experiences, family influence, and healthcare provider–client relationship may affect how the client views medication therapies. Physiologic rhythms, use of alcohol, and stress may either inhibit or accelerate drug biodynamics. The concomitant use of "natural" remedies can also alter the client's response to drug therapy.

It is thought that the pathophysiology of various disease states may differ among populations based on genetic determination (as in thalassemia among people of Mediterranean descent). One genetic factor noted to differ among ethnic groups is variation in metabolic pathways that may accelerate or slow drug metabolism. For example, Black clients respond differently to certain antihypertensive drugs than White clients do. Hispanics generally need lower doses of antidepressants than other groups and may experience more serious adverse effects from these drugs. Chinese Americans appear to have more lithium receptors than the general population, and so require a lower dose to achieve therapeutic effect. Controlled studies on various ethnic groups have identified some useful similarities, but they have also shown subgroups with divergent reactions. In addition, interethnic mixing is becoming more common. So, even as more individualized dosing becomes possible, it is clear that global judgments cannot safely be made based on race or ethnicity (Aschenbrenner, 2012).

Nursing Diagnoses

The following nursing diagnoses are appropriate to use on client care plans when the components relate to a client who requires treatment with medications.

NURSING DIAGNOSIS	RELATED TO . . .
Ineffective Health Maintenance	Lack of education or readiness to learn, cognitive impairment, lack of equipment, inadequate support systems, inadequate financial resources, religious beliefs, cultural beliefs or values
Enhanced Health Management, Readiness for	Client who seeks supervision and practices self-administration of metered dose inhaler/dry powder inhaler (MDI/DPI)
	Client who expresses interest in use of insulin pump or delivery system and seeks counseling for diabetes management with Certified Diabetes Educator
	Client who seeks supervision and practices self-injection of anticoagulant before discharge
Risk for Injury	Altered clotting factors due to anticoagulant therapy
	Altered regulatory function due to side effects of medications (e.g., drowsiness)
	Altered biochemical function due to interactive effects of prescribed or nonprescribed medications, herbal supplements, or vitamins
	Allergic or anaphylactic reaction to administered medication
	Medication error on part of nursing staff
Deficient Knowledge	Inadequate understanding of condition, medication regimen, or self-care skills
	Inadequate understanding of rationale for follow-up laboratory monitoring related to prescribed medications
Ineffective Health Management	Impaired ability to perform tasks, side effects of therapy, nontherapeutic environment, denial of condition, lack of information or finances, poor self-esteem, and nonsupportive family

Nursing Process Data

ASSESSMENT Database

- Validate medication to be given with healthcare provider's order and client's MAR.
- Know desired therapeutic action of the drug, side effects, and adverse reactions.
- Assess for potential drug interaction with client's other medications or **contraindication** to administration (allergy, lab data, vital signs, unsafe dose).
- Identify route for drug administration.
- Recognize need to calculate drug dosage and seek verification of calculation by another nurse when indicated.
- Validate drug and dosage of certain critical drugs with another nurse or pharmacist.

PLANNING Objectives

- To understand the drug's action and rationale for administration to the client (desired therapeutic effect)
- To prepare the appropriate medication to be given by the correct route
- To have another nurse double-check dosage calculations and preparation of high-alert medications
- To anticipate potential side effects or adverse client reactions and be prepared to take corrective actions

IMPLEMENTATION Procedures

DOCUMENTATION AND EVALUATION

Expected Outcomes

- Rationale for medication administration is clear.
- Client's MAR matches healthcare provider's orders.
- Dosage calculations are accurate.
- Medication is administered according to the "six rights."

Unexpected Outcomes/Alternative Actions

Pearson Nursing Student Resources

Find additional review materials at
nursing.pearsonhighered.com.
Prepare for success with NCLEX®-style practice questions and Skill Checklists.

Skill 18.1.1 | Preparing for Medication Administration

Equipment

Reference resource (e.g., *Physicians' Desk Reference*,
   pharmacology textbook, drug handbook)
Calculator (if indicated)
Medication administration record sheet (MAR) ❶

Procedure

1. Check's healthcare provider's orders and client's MAR ❷
   for medications client is to receive (drug, dosage, route of
   administration, time intervals).
2. Identify any unfamiliar drugs.
3. Research unfamiliar drugs using appropriate reference.

   a. Generic and trade name
   b. Drug classification and major uses
   c. Pharmacologic actions
   d. Safe dosage, route, and time of administration
   e. Side effects; adverse reactions
   f. Nursing implications
   g. Client teaching as needed

> **CLINICAL ALERT**
>
> Individual drugs are designed to be administered by specific
> route—be sure to check drug labels for appropriate route of
> administration.

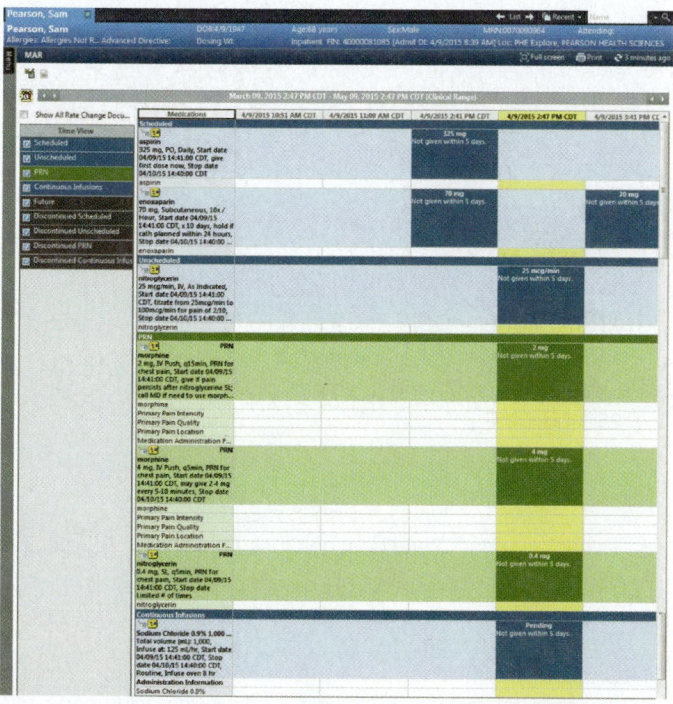

❶ Example of a medication administration record. *Source:* From
Cerner Electronic Health Record. © Cerner Corporation. Pearson
has restricted permission to reproduce and distribute this copyrighted work. Further reproduction or distribution is strictly prohibited without written consent of Cerner Corporation.

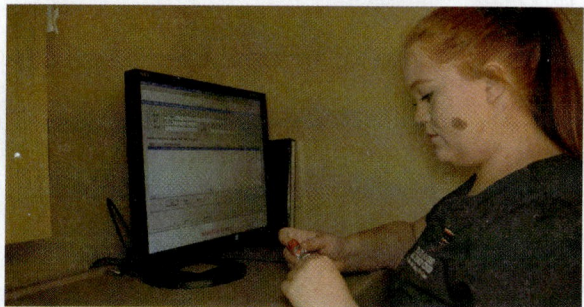

❷ Check healthcare provider's order against medication
administration record (MAR).

4. Review client's record for allergies, lab data, any factor
   (e.g., NPO status, planned procedures) that contraindicates
   administration of ordered medications.
5. Check client's MAR with previous 24 hr for each drug's
   dosage, route, and time to be given. ➤ *Rationale:* Any new
   medications, discontinued medication, or altered dosage must
   be identified and verified with the healthcare provider's orders.
6. Validate carefully that MAR is consistent with healthcare
   provider's most recent order for each medication.
   ➤ *Rationale:* Some medication dosages are adjusted on
   a daily basis. Errors in transmission of intentions may occur
   between healthcare provider, pharmacy, and client's MAR.
7. Perform hand hygiene.
8. Obtain client's medication from automated dispensing unit
   or medication cart. ❸
9. Determine if any calculation is necessary to prepare the
   correct dosage.
10. Calculate client's dosage based on strength of medication,
    if indicated. Have another nurse double-check your
    calculation if necessary. (See Skill 18.1.3 for formulas to
    calculate dosage.)
11. Prepare medication as indicated for nonparenteral or
    parenteral route, checking drug label before, during, and
    after preparation.
12. Check each medication in order against the MAR. ❹
13. Reverify the first five rights of medication (right medication,
    right client, right dose, right route, and right time).
14. If you have prepared medications in a medication room and not
    at the client's bedside, label medications with client identifiers
    and medication information before leaving the medication room.
15. Do not document until *after* administering medication (sixth
    "right"). ➤ *Rationale:* If client is unable to take the
    medication, your documentation would need to be corrected.

> **CLINICAL ALERT**
>
> Check medication label three times before administering the
> medication:
>
> • When retrieving the medication from storage area
> • When preparing the medication
> • At the client bedside before administering the medication

(continued)

Skill 18.1.1 | Preparing for Medication Administration *(continued)*

❸ Locate medications in client's drawer. Retrieve medication to be given and inspect label.

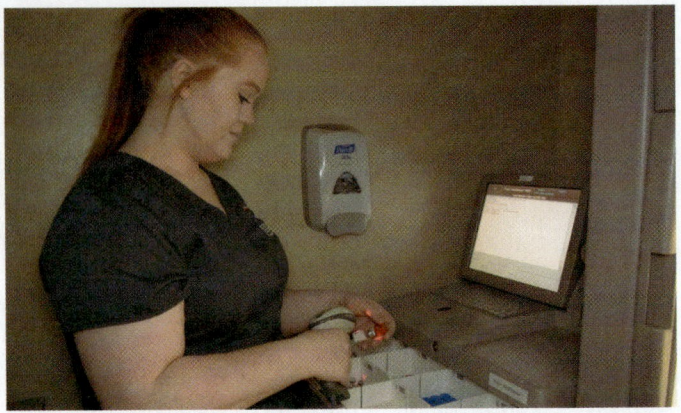

❹ Check individually wrapped medication against client's MAR.

Skill 18.1.2 | Converting Dosage Systems

Procedure

1. To make conversions from the metric to apothecaries' or household systems, it is necessary to memorize or refer to equivalency tables.
2. To convert milligrams to grains, use the following formula:

$$\frac{1 \text{ grain}}{\text{Milligrams per grain}} = \frac{\text{Dose desired}}{\text{Dose on hand}}$$

$$\frac{1}{60} = \frac{X}{180}$$

$$60X = 180$$

$$X = 3 \text{ grains}$$

3. You may also use ratio and proportion to calculate dosage:

1 gr: 60 mg : : X gr: 180 mg

60X = 180

X = 3 gr

4. To convert milligrams to milliliters, you can set up a direct proportion and, following the algebraic principle, cross multiply.
5. Check Conversion Tables in the Drug Supplement at the end of the chapter.

Skill 18.1.3 | Calculating Dosages

Equipment

Orders for dosage of medication needed
Dosage of medication on hand

Procedure

1. To calculate oral dosages, use the following formula. (D and H must be in same unit of measure.)

$$\frac{D}{H} = X$$

where D = dose desired; H = dose on hand; and X = dose to be administered.

Example: Give 500 mg of ampicillin sodium when the dose on hand is in capsules containing 250 mg.

$$\frac{500 \text{ mg}}{250 \text{ mg}} = 2 \text{ capsules}$$

2. To calculate dose when in liquid form, use the following formula:

$$\frac{D}{H} \times Q = X$$

where D = dose desired; H = dose on hand; Q = quantity; and X = amount to be administered.

Example: Give 375 mg of ampicillin when it is supplied as 250 mg/5 mL.

$$\frac{375 \text{ mg}}{250 \text{ mg}} \times 5$$

$$1.5 \times 5 = 7.5 \text{ mL}$$

3. To calculate parenteral dosages, use the following formula:

$$\frac{D}{H} \times Q = X$$

Example: Give client 40 mg gentamicin C complex sulfate. On hand is a multidose vial with a strength of 80 mg/2 mL.

4. To calculate dosages for infants and children using body surface area (BSA*):

$$\frac{BSA^*}{1.7} \times \text{Adult dose} = \text{Pediatric dose}$$

*A number of internet resources provide details and formulas and a complete description of methods of determining body surface area.

5. To calculate dosages for infants and children using Clark's weight rule:

$$\text{Child's dose} = \frac{\text{Child's wt. in lbs.}}{150} \times \text{Adult dose}$$

6. Check your calculations before drawing up the medications.

Note: Calculation of Solutions is in the Drug Supplement section at the end of this chapter.

Skill 18.1.4 | Using the Controlled Substance System

Equipment
Medication Administration Record
Medication

Procedure

1. Check client's MAR for medication order. Validate that client's MAR matches selected medication and dose on screen.
2. Check dose and time last medication was administered.
3. Retrieve controlled substance. ❶
4. Count the number of pills, ampules, or prefilled cartridges in container.
5. Check the controlled substance record, and check that the number of **narcotics** in drawer matches the number on specific controlled substance record. ➤ *Rationale:* Laws on controlled substances require careful monitoring of narcotics.
6. Correct any discrepancy before proceeding with medication administration (Box 18-2 ■).
7. Record the amount of medication removed.
8. Lock unit after removing medication. ❷
9. Administer medication.
10. Document medication on client's MAR according to agency procedure. Include client's sedation level and pain rating (e.g., 8/10, 3/10) before and after medication administration according to agency policy. ❸

> **CLINICAL ALERT**
>
> If the narcotic depresses breathing, note client's level of sedation and respiratory rate before administering, and document assessment.

> **CLINICAL ALERT**
>
> All Joint Commission–accredited agencies must have protocols developed for documenting and reconciling medications across the continuum (admission, transfer, discharge). A list of the client's home medications is compared with the admitting medication orders. Upon transfer, medications being taken are compared with orders in the new unit. Upon discharge, medications taken in the hospital are compared with the discharge medication orders. Verification, clarification, and reconciliation of discrepancies help prevent adverse drug events throughout the client's hospitalization.

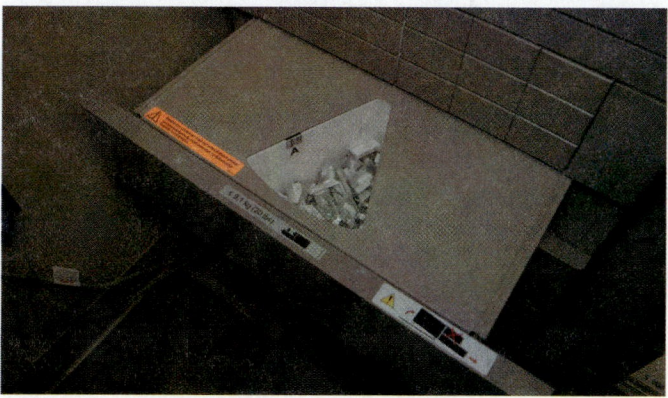

❷ Lock narcotic drawer after removing medication. Keep key with you at all times.

❶ User ID and password for scanned fingerprint control access to medication.

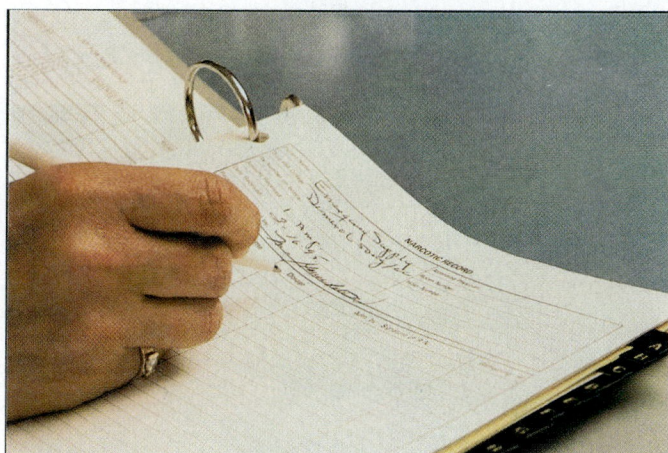

❸ If using paper documentation, sign on specific narcotic sign-out sheet after taking narcotic out of drawer

(continued)

Skill 18.1.4 | Using the Controlled Substance System *(continued)*

Box 18-2 MEDICATION SAFETY MEASURES

- Accurately and completely reconcile the client's medications across the continuum of care.
- Keep all medications in locked carts or cabinets.
- Limit access to and use special safeguards with "high-alert" drugs (those causing significant client harm if used in error; e.g., hypoglycemic, anticoagulant, anesthetic agents, narcotics, paralytic agents, chemotherapy drugs, and certain cardiac drugs). This list is periodically updated by the Institute for Safe Medication Practices (ISMP).
- Keep narcotics in locked cabinet and follow agency protocols for securing and managing narcotics.
- Separate topical medications from parenteral or oral medications.
- Clearly label all prepared medication containers (syringes, medicine cups, solutions).
- Check with another nurse (1) mathematical calculations for dosages and (2) dispensed/prepared "high-alert" drugs and those for high-risk clients (e.g., insulin, anticoagulants, concentrated electrolytes, digoxin, and hemodynamic agents if not premixed).

- Do not leave any medication at client's bedside unless there is a specific healthcare provider's order to do so.
- Report any errors in drug administration to charge nurse and client's healthcare provider immediately. Monitor the client closely for adverse effects. Document the drug given, and complete an incident report per agency protocol. Reporting of medication errors to Institute for Safe Medication Practices online or at 1-800-FAIL-SAF(E) is strongly encouraged to improve client safety by increasing knowledge about medication errors. The site forwards data to the FDA, ISMP, and the product manufacturer.
- Provide complete instruction to clients regarding medications to be used at home.

Remember:

- No technology system eliminates the risk for error.
- Never become complacent about what technology can do to support safe practice.
- No computer has your ability to think critically to understand whether an ordered drug is appropriate for your client.

Skill 18.1.5 | Administering Medication Protocol

Equipment
Prepared medication
Gloves (if indicated)
Stethoscope and sphygmomanometer, if indicated

Preparation
See Skill 18.1.1 for all procedures.

Procedure
1. Introduce yourself to the client and perform hand hygiene.
2. Check client's identification band and ask client to state name and birth date. ❶❷ See (Box 18-3 ■) for bar code system.

3. Provide privacy.
4. Explain procedure and purpose of medication to client.
5. Assist client to appropriate position for medication administration.

> **CLINICAL ALERT**
> Use at least two client identifiers when administering medications or providing treatments (e.g., stated name and birth date or medical record number).

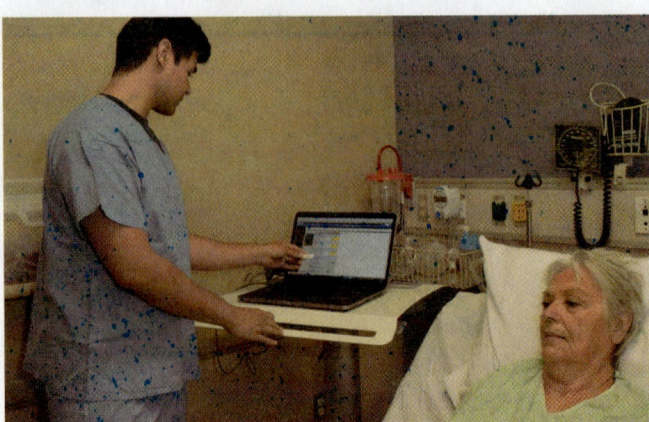

❶ Check client's name and birth date against medication record.

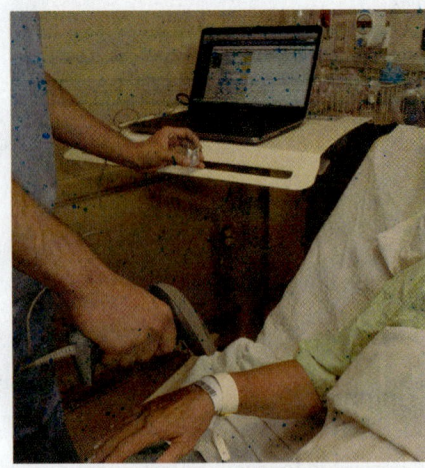

❷ Check client's identification band and ask client to state name and birth date.

6. Check client's vital signs if indicated before administering medication. ➤ *Rationale:* Medication's effects may cause hemodynamic instability if client's vital signs are at the high or low extreme of normal.

7. Perform hand hygiene and don gloves if indicated. ➤ *Rationale:* Parenteral and **enteral** medication administration may require the use of gloves, as well as preparation and administration of oral antineoplastic agents.

8. Administer medication according to route procedure and adhering to the "six rights" of medication administration. Verify medications against MAR if there is a computer at the bedside or scan medication bar code if that system is used.

9. Dispose of equipment appropriately; then remove gloves, if used, and wash your hands.

10. Record administered medications in client's MAR; the time, medication given, dosage, and route (including site of injection); and any relevant assessment findings.

Box 18-3 BAR CODE MEDICATION ADMINISTRATION

Medication administration errors are a serious safety concern and contribute to client error and adverse events. Bar code medication administration (BCMA) technology can improve client safety by reducing these errors. The central feature of this point-of-care system is bar code labeling of medications and client wristbands. In order to facilitate implementation, vendors and hospitals usually customize these systems to interface with existing electronic medical records.

Failure to adhere to the steps of the BCMA process may expose the nurse to fraud charges. Hazardous shortcuts ("workarounds") may lead to client harm and legal pitfalls.

Steps to take before medication administration:

- Compare the medication order in the client's medical record against each medication on the eMAR.
- Obtain medication from the automated dispensing unit.

- Perform a "five rights" check against the eMAR while removing the medication.

Note: The sixth "right" is *documentation* and does not apply here.

Steps to perform at the client's bedside:

- Check client's identification band and ask client to state name and birth date.
- Perform a second "five rights" check of selected medications against the eMAR.
- Scan bar code on client's identification band, and then scan bar code on *unopened* medication packaging.
- Obtain confirmation of bar code matching by the software system and attend to any alarms or cues.
- Prepare scanned medication.
- Administer the medication promptly.
- Document medications administered (sixth "right").

Scan the bar code on the client's ID band.

Scan the bar code on the unopened medication packaging to confirm matching.

CLINICAL ALERT

Report any actual or potential error (e.g., look-alike or sound-alike drug names, confusion over abbreviations) to the Institute for Safe Medication Practices at 1-800-FAIL-SAF(E) or complete the form at the Institute for Safe Medication Practices website. All communications are kept confidential. This agency publicizes warnings and notices in response to submitted information to help alert other professionals to potentially dangerous medication pitfalls.

(continued)

Skill 18.1.5 | Administering Medication Protocol *(continued)*

EVIDENCE-BASED PRACTICE

Wristband Placement

It is best to place all wristbands on the same arm, but best practice requires the nurse to check both arms and also the ankles, since placement here may be required.

Source: Cizek, Estrade, Allen, & Elsholz (2010)

Medication Errors—A Growing Problem

Medication errors originate across the spectrum of care: prescribing, 39%; transcribing, 17%; dispensing, 11%; and administering, 38%. Nurses must identify errors before administering medications: both the mistakes of others and their own.

Source: Cohen (2008)

Medication Administration Errors

Medication errors continue to be a significant threat to client safety. A recent study investigated the relationship between the characteristics of the nursing practice environment, nurse staffing levels, nurses' error interception practices, and rates of nonintercepted medication errors in acute care hospitals. The study found that a supportive practice environment was positively associated with error interception practices among nurses and that those practices were inversely associated with medication error rates. When nurses work in a unit that is supportive, they can intercept medication errors before they reach their clients.

Source: Flynn, Liang, Dickson, Xie, & Suh (2012)

Interruptions Linked to Medication Errors

This study of 98 nurses administering 4,271 medications to 720 adult clients showed that nurses who are interrupted while preparing and administering medications may have increased risk of making medical errors. Interruptions require switching from one task to another, completing the interrupting task, and then returning to the interrupted task. For each interruption, there is an increase in procedural error (e.g., technique) and clinical error (e.g., dosage). Frequency of interruption was associated with increased severity of error. While some interruptions are necessary when directed toward provision of safe client care, there is a need to better understand the reasons for high interruption rates to determine if there are solutions to better manage these interruptions.

Source: Barclay (2010)

LEGAL CONSIDERATIONS

Transcription Error and Reconciliation Failure (*Robert Ferguson v. Baptist Health System, Inc.,* 2005)

Robert Ferguson brought medical malpractice action against Baptist after experiencing drug toxicity due to a medication (Dilantin) transcription error on the part of the pharmacist and failure on the part of the nurse to conduct reconciliation between the MAR entry and the healthcare provider's order. The order was for Dilantin, 300 mg "po QHS." The MAR was generated by pharmacy for Dilantin, 300 mg, "t.i.d." The agency policy dictated that any time a new medication order was entered, the nurse initially undertaking to administer the medication was responsible for comparing the MAR to the actual order to "reconcile" the two. In this case, the pharmacy error was not detected by the reconciliation process. Subsequent erroneous doses were administered, but none of the nurses administering the Dilantin detected the error "due to the fact that there were no additional checks, balances, or other safeguards in place to prevent the repetition of the error." No one ever checked the original order "despite the unusually large amount of Dilantin being administered." None of the nurses suspected that Ferguson's symptoms represented Dilantin toxicity. Ferguson was awarded compensatory damages and punitive damages.

McMunn v. Mount Carmel Health et al., 1998

Plaintiff was awarded $433,415.00 for wrongful death of William Muncey, age 39, resulting from improper administration of morphine and failure to monitor and guard the client from adverse effects of the drugs he received, those known to cause respiratory depression. The client presented to Mount Carmel ED at 1635 with severe pain due to kidney stones. He received 5 mg of morphine IV at 1653, at 1700, and again at 1740. His respiratory rate was 24 and SpO_2 was 92%.

He then received additional 5 mg of intravenous morphine at 1805 and 1820, whereupon his SpO_2 dropped to 86%. The client was placed on oxygen therapy and by 1835 his SpO_2 had increased to 94%.

At 2015, he was admitted as an inpatient. His vital signs were taken at that time, but not again for the evening shift. The nurse had not been advised that the client's O_2 saturation had dropped while he was in the ED. At 2215, the nurse administered 15 mg of morphine sulfate and 50 mg Phenergan by injection. At 2300, it was documented that the client was sleeping, but no vital signs were taken.

At 0105, the nurse was notified that Mr. Muncey was unresponsive and had no pulse or respirations. A "Code Blue" was called, Narcan was given, but the client died. At autopsy, spinal fluid and blood levels of morphine were supportive of death from a respiratory depressant effect of morphine, with unusually high levels explained by the *combination* of depressant drugs he had received.

Three areas of nursing care were found to fall below the accepted standard: coordination and communication of assessment and care, monitoring of a client receiving narcotics, and documentation of assessments for a client receiving narcotics.

Unit 18.1 Documentation and Evaluation

EVALUATION/Critical Thinking

Expected Outcomes

- Rationale for medication administration is clear.
- Client's MAR matches healthcare provider's orders.
- Dosage calculations are accurate.
- Medication sign-out sheet matches remaining stock.
- Medication is administered according to the "six rights."

Note: Six rights is correct here because it includes documentation.

Unexpected Outcomes	Alternative Actions
Medication or dosage on MAR does not fit client's clinical picture.	• Consult with healthcare provider. • Discuss concerns with agency pharmacist. • Contact healthcare provider for clarification.
Nurse is unsure of dosage calculation.	• Utilize helpful calculation formulas. • Use a calculator. • Request that another nurse check calculation or conversion.
Medication sign-out sheet does not correspond to remaining stock.	• Seek agency pharmacist's assistance. • Check with other nurses who may have dispensed stock medication. • Check MARs for unclaimed stock that may have been administered. • Complete discrepancy report if sign-out sheets and stock cannot be reconciled.
Client receives the wrong medication.	• Document the medication administered on client's MAR. • Monitor client closely for potential undesired effects and document findings. • Notify client's healthcare provider and document. • Complete incident report according to agency policy. • Always check two client identifiers before administering medication.

Oral Medication Administration

Nursing Process Data

ASSESSMENT Database

- Check that medication is to be given by oral route.
- Determine that client is not NPO.
- Determine that client is able to take medication orally.
  - Client is alert.
  - Swallow–gag reflex is present.
  - No risk of aspiration exists.
  - Client is not nauseated or vomiting.
- Determine that medication can be safely altered if necessary for administration.

PLANNING Objectives

- To provide an easy, inexpensive, and convenient route for administering medications
- To ensure that client is able to take oral medication
- To safely administer an altered oral medication
- To facilitate administration of oral medication to the client with swallowing difficulty (dysphagia)
- To administer oral medication to an adult or child

IMPLEMENTATION Procedures

DOCUMENTATION AND EVALUATION

Expected Outcomes

- Client takes medication orally without difficulty.
- Client experiences intended therapeutic drug effect.

Unexpected Outcomes/Alternative Actions

Pearson Nursing Student Resources

Find additional review materials at
nursing.pearsonhighered.com.
Prepare for success with NCLEX®-style practice
questions and Skill Checklists.

Skill 18.2.1 | Preparing Oral Medications

Equipment

Oral medication: tablet, capsule, or liquid from bottle or unit dose
(Medications should remain in their unopened packages unless
the nurse needs to prepare them in the medication room.)

Client's preference of water, juice, milk, or other vehicle
(e.g., jelly, yogurt, pudding) to assist swallowing (if not
contraindicated for drug absorption)

Mortar and pestle to crush or pill cutter to divide medication if
necessary

Measuring spoon, *calibrated* dropper, syringe, or medicine cup

Gloves, for oral antineoplastic agents

Preparation

1. Follow all steps for Medication Preparation, Skill 18.1.1.
2. Perform hand hygiene.

Procedure

Liquid Medications Not Available in Unit Dose Packaging

1. Remove bottle lid and place topside down to avoid
   contamination.
2. Hold bottle with label facing palm to avoid dripping
   medication onto label. ❶
3. Set medication cup on firm surface and pour liquid
   medication; read fluid dispensed at eye level, *read at lowest
   point of meniscus.* ❷ ➤ *Rationale:* This reading ensures
   accurate dose of medication.
4. Wipe bottle lip before replacing cap. Check medication label
   again. ➤ *Rationale:* This safety check ensures correct drug
   and dosage.
5. Return multidose bottle to storage area. Sign out for any
   narcotic dispensed on narcotic sheet with date, client's
   name, room number, healthcare provider's name, dosage,
   your signature, and any wasted narcotic (cosigned by
   another nurse or witness).
6. Remember to check the label three times:
   a. When taking the medication container from storage place
   b. When placing medication into medicine cup
   c. When returning medication container to storage place

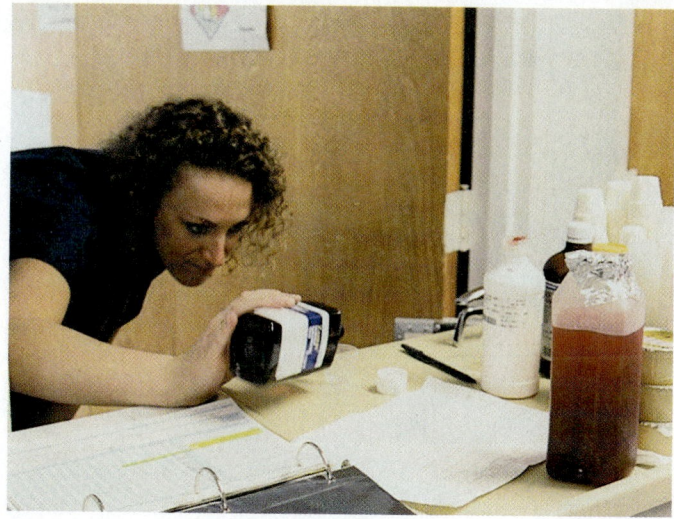

❷ Pour liquid at eye level to read dose correctly.

Crushing or Altering Medications

1. Leave pill in unit dose packaging and place on firm surface.
   ➤ *Rationale:* Labeled packaging maintains identity
   and prevents loss of medication. If client does not take
   medication, it can be returned to drawer.
   Or:
2. Place pill between two soufflé cups ❸ and pound with pestle
   or other tool to crush ❹, pulverizing thoroughly ➤ *Rationale:*
   The cups confine the medication. ***Note:*** *This is the preferred
   method for crushing medication to be given enterally.*
3. Remove any uncrushed pill coating if medication is to be
   given per feeding tube. ➤ *Rationale:* This safeguards
   against clogging the tube.
4. If giving orally, mix pulverized medication (or powder from
   opened capsule) carefully in small amount of soft food (pudding,
   jelly, applesauce). ❺ ➤ *Rationale:* For many clients with
   swallowing difficulty, soft food is easier to swallow than liquid.
5. Check orders for partial dose medication. ❻ Place tablet in
   pill cutter or break tablet if scored.

❶ Palm the label while pouring liquid medication.

❸ Place tablet between med cups to pulverize with crusher.

(continued)

Skill 18.2.1 | Preparing Oral Medications (continued)

❹ Place pill in crusher to crush tablet, or pulverize pill in unit dose container.

❺ Mix pulverized medication (or powder from opened capsule) carefully in *small* amount of soft food (pudding, jelly, applesauce).

❻ If partial dose is ordered, place tablet in pill cutter to be cut in half.

6. Open capsule and sprinkle "beads" over soft food to administer. Warn client not to chew the "beads" (Box 18-4 ■).
   ➤ *Rationale:* Beads are formulated for a sustained timed release therapeutic effect.
7. Ensure client has received all of the medication.
8. Offer liquid or food to cleanse palate.

Box 18-4 GENERAL PRECAUTIONS FOR ALTERING ORAL MEDICATIONS

Unsafe Actions

- *Do not* crush enteric coated or gel-coated tablets.
  ➤ *Rationale:* Coatings allow intestinal absorption of the drug, protect the medication from stomach acid, or protect the stomach from the medication.
- *Do not crush* long-acting tablets. ➤ *Rationale:* Sustained action over hours is the advantage of extended-release versions of drugs. Crushing could yield a toxic dose and eliminate the sustained action needed through the day.
- *Do not* try to open sealed capsules.
- *Do not* crush contents of capsules (e.g., spansule) with beads or pellets. ➤ *Rationale:* These are intended for sustained-release action.
- *Do not* give sublingual formulations orally. ➤ *Rationale:* Ingredients may be inactivated by stomach acid.
- *Do not* crush sublingual formulations.
- *Do not* give oral medications sublingually. ➤ *Rationale:* This could yield a toxic dose since the medication would be absorbed directly into the bloodstream and skip intended first pass through the liver for early metabolism before entering the bloodstream.
- *Do not* alter (crush, split) tablets or open capsules of anti-neoplastic agents. ➤ *Rationale:* This avoids sending drug particles into the air where they could be inhaled.

Safe Actions

- Scored tablets may be split. Unscored tablets may be cut unless they are:
  - extended release
  - a combination product
  - a critical dose product
  - film-coated
  - crumbled with cutting

Note: Dispose of unused medication in the Medication Waste receptacle.

- Chewable medications *can be* crushed safely.
- If a capsule opens easily, powder from the capsules *can be* mixed with food or liquid.
- Liquid-filled capsule contents *can be* (a) squeezed out through a hole punched with a large gauge needle, or (b) aspirated, then mixed with food or liquid. *Liquid-filled capsule contents should not be administered sublingually.*
- Beads from readily opened capsules *can be* sprinkled over soft food to administer, *but should not be chewed.*
- A sublingual formulation still *can be* given sublingually if the client is NPO.

Skill 18.2.2 | Administering Oral Medications to Adults

Equipment
See Equipment for Skill 18.2.1, Preparing Oral Medications.

Preparation
1. Follow steps for Skill 18.1.5, Administering Medication Protocol.
2. Follow procedure for Skill 18.2.1, Preparing Oral Medications.
3. Perform hand hygiene.

Procedure
1. Take labeled medications or medications in their unopened packages to client's room.
2. Perform hand hygiene.
3. Check client's identification band and ask client to state name and birth date so you are sure you have the correct client, or if client is nonverbal, identify client using two client identifiers.
4. Perform medication safety rights, check medication against the MAR if there is a computer in the room, or use the bar code scanner if that system is used.

5. Assist client to sitting position.
6. Explain type of medication you are giving and purpose.
7. Determine if specific assessment is indicated before administering medication (e.g., vital signs) and assess client.
8. Remove medication from packet and place into medication cup.
9. Hand medication cup to client if assessment findings do not contraindicate administration.
10. Offer water or other liquid. ➤ *Rationale:* The liquid aids swallowing, dilution, and absorption of medication.
11. Make sure client swallows medication.
12. Discard used medicine cup.
13. Record medication on client's record, including assessment findings, if indicated.
14. Continue to assess client for desired drug action and possible side effects or adverse reactions.

Skill 18.2.3 | Administering Medications per Enteral (NG or NI) Feeding Tube

Equipment
See Equipment for Skill 18.2.1, Preparing Oral Medications.
Sterile water for diluting and flushing
50-mL irrigating piston (oral) syringe
Clean gloves

Preparation
1. Follow steps for Skill 18.1.5, Administering Medication Protocol.
2. Stop any continuous tube feeding and flush tube with 15 mL of water. ❶, ❷
3. Follow procedure for Skill 18.2.1, Preparing Oral Medications. Determine if medications are **compatible** with enteral tube feeding solution.

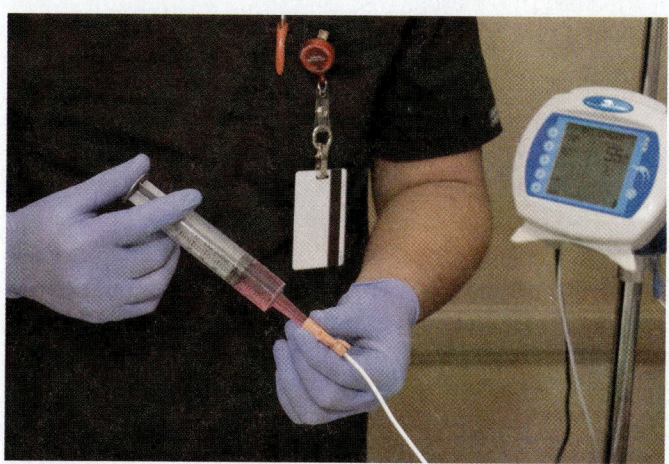

❷ Flush tube with 15 mL sterile water after each medication and record total amount on I&O sheet.

4. Obtain liquid dosage form of medication if available.
5. Dilute each medication (crushed tablet, powder from capsule, or liquid medication) separately in 30 mL of warm water (*considering client's fluid balance status*).

Note: Do not mix medications together. Do not add medication directly to an external feeding formula. ➤ *Rationale:* This reduces the risk of physical and chemical incompatibilities, tube obstruction, and altered drug responses.

6. Perform hand hygiene.

❶ Administer each medication separately, flushing before with 15 mL water. Allow to flow through tube by gravity, and then flush tube again with 15 mL water.

(continued)

Skill 18.2.3 | Administering Medications per Enteral (NG or NI) Feeding Tube *(continued)*

CLINICAL ALERT

Consult with pharmacist before deciding to alter the form of *any* medication. Have pharmacist substitute liquid form of medication if available, or substitute a short-acting formulation that can be safely crushed for administration. Contact the healthcare provider for a substitute medication if formulation alternatives are unavailable.

CLINICAL ALERT

Never use a parenteral (Luer-Lok) syringe for enteral tube administration. It may then be mistakenly administered IV. Oral syringes are incompatible with IV ports to prevent this hazard.

Procedure

1. Don gloves.
2. Disconnect feeding tube from feeding delivery system or select port for decompression.
3. Verify tube placement. Review skills for large-bore or small-bore feeding tube in Chapter 19.
4. Insert 50-mL oral syringe into NI tube or NG tube decompression port, and **aspirate** to check residual volume. Return residual and flush tube with 15 mL of water. ❸ ➤ *Rationale:* This validates enteral capacity for receiving medication.

Note: Do NOT administer medication through blue pigtail of Salem sump tube (see Chapter 19).

5. Administer each medication separately, allowing to flow through tube by gravity.
6. Flush tube with 15 mL of water after each medication, monitoring amount of flush to record on I&O sheet. ➤ *Rationale:* Flushing reduces risk of drug incompatibilities and tube clogging.

❸ For closed system, use medication/irrigation port. Administer each medication separately, flushing before and after with 15 mL water.

7. Restart tube feeding at appropriate time. ➤ *Rationale:* It is important to avoid altering bioavailability of medication and to avoid compromising client's nutritional therapy.
8. Rinse and replace syringe to storage area at client's bedside.
9. Remove gloves and perform hand hygiene.

LEGAL CONSIDERATIONS

Nimodipine capsules were dispensed to the clinical area, where they were used for clients who could not swallow. In one case, a nurse softened the gelatin capsule in hot water, withdrew the medication into a parenteral syringe, and the dose was inadvertently administered as IV instead of via a feeding tube. Subsequently, the client died. A boxed warning has now been added to the nimodipine labeling to caution about this type of administration error.

Source: ISMP (2010)

Unit 18.2 Documentation and Evaluation

DOCUMENTATION for Oral Medications

Client's Medication Record

- Name of medication
- Vital signs if indicated
- Dosage
- Route
- Time administered

- Initials of nurse administering medication
- *Intake and Output record: Amount of water used for medication dilution and administration.*
- Signature of nurse identifying initials

Nurses' Notes

- Client's assessment parameters
- Documentation of prn, STAT, and one-time-only medications

- Name of medication, dosage, route, time administered
- Client's response
- Signature of nurse

EVALUATION/Critical Thinking

Expected Outcomes

- Client takes medication orally without difficulty.
- Client experiences intended therapeutic drug effect.

Unexpected Outcomes	Alternative Actions

• Client has an allergic or anaphylactic response to medication.	• Immediately stop or hold medication.
	• Notify healthcare provider at once; prepare to administer epinephrine to dilate bronchi and support blood pressure.
	• If reaction is severe:
	  • Keep client flat in bed with head elevated.
	  • Take vital signs every 10–15 min; stay with client.
	  • Assess for hypotension or respiratory distress.
	  • Establish airway if necessary.
	  • Have emergency equipment available.
	  • Provide psychological support to client to alleviate fears.
	  • Record type and progression of reactions.

• Client has difficulty swallowing medication.	• Offer water before administering oral medication. • Crush medications if appropriate and administer mixed with food such as applesauce, pudding, or jelly. • Consult pharmacist to dispense same medication in liquid form. • If difficulty continues, consult healthcare provider for altered route of medication delivery (rectal, parenteral). • Request swallow study.
• Client is nauseated and oral medications have not been taken.	• Hold medication. Notify healthcare provider for antiemetic medication order and alternate route for administering necessary medications. • Administer antiemetic if ordered, then administer medication when client's nausea is relieved.

Topical Medication Administration

Nursing Process Data

ASSESSMENT Database

- Assess for proper route of medication administration.
- Observe skin for open lesions, rash, or redness.
- Determine drug manufacturer's recommended site for transdermal application.
- Assess that area for transdermal application is dry, hairless, and intact.
- Assess for allergies as reported by client or noted in client's chart.
- Assess condition of ear or eye and surrounding area.
- Determine purpose for eye or ear irrigation.
- Assess client's ability to cooperate with eye or ear medication administration or irrigation.

PLANNING Objectives

- To provide local anesthetic, anti-inflammatory, or anti-infective effect to a specified part of the body
- To provide slow, continuous transdermal absorption of medication
- To decrease intraocular pressure
- To prevent unwanted systemic effect of topically applied eye medication
- To provide pupil dilation to facilitate eye examination or therapeutic procedure
- To remove debris or neutralize chemical action and minimize eye injury
- To soften and remove cerumen (ear wax)

IMPLEMENTATION Procedures

DOCUMENTATION AND EVALUATION

Expected Outcomes

- Topical medication has intended effect.
- Client self-administers eye medication according to instructions.
- Ear canal irrigation removes cerumen.

Unexpected Outcomes/Alternative Actions

Pearson Nursing Student Resources

Find additional review materials at **nursing.pearsonhighered.com.**
Prepare for success with NCLEX®-style practice questions and Skill Checklists.

Skill 18.3.1 | Applying Topical Medications

Equipment

Medication container (tube or jar)
Soap and water to cleanse skin
Clean gloves
Tongue blade
Gauze or transparent dressing (as indicated)
Tape
Pen (to label dressing, if indicated)

Preparation

See Skill 18.1.1, Medication Preparation.

Procedure

1. Take medication container and dressing supplies to client's room.
2. Perform medication safety checks, including verification against MAR.
3. Identify client using two client identifiers.
4. Provide privacy.
5. Explain procedure and purpose to client.
6. Perform hand hygiene and don clean gloves.
7. Cleanse skin site with soap and water and dry thoroughly.
8. Squeeze medication from tube or use a tongue blade to take cream/ointment from medication container.
9. Spread small quantity of medication smoothly and evenly with gloved hand over client's skin following direction of hair follicles. ➤ *Rationale:* Gloves facilitate smooth application.
10. Apply dressing if indicated. ❶ ➤ *Rationale:* Dressing may ensure that medication is not rubbed off.
11. Label dressing with date, time, and your initials.
12. Remove gloves and perform hand hygiene.
13. Check that client is comfortable.
14. Return medication container to storage area.

CLINICAL ALERT

Systemic absorption of topical medication from open lesions can result in toxic reactions.

---

❶ Apply dressing; then label with date, time, and initials.

Skill 18.3.2 | Applying Creams to Lesions

Equipment

Medication container (tube or jar)
Sterile normal saline for cleansing
Sterile gauze for cleansing site
Sterile tongue blade
Mask (see agency policy)
Sterile gloves
Sterile gauze or transparent dressing (or commercially prepared burn dressing)
Gauze roll or stretch net to secure dressing
Pen for labeling dressing

Preparation

See Skill 18.1.1, Medication Preparation.

Procedure

1. Take medication to client's room.
2. Perform medication safety checks, including verification against MAR.
3. Identify client using two client identifiers.
4. Provide privacy.
5. Perform hand hygiene, don mask (as appropriate) and clean gloves.
6. Remove previous dressing if present.
7. Note characteristics of site and cleanse area as ordered with sterile gauze pads and saline. Remove gloves.
8. Open medication container.
9. Don sterile gloves.
10. If no dressing is ordered, use gloved hand to apply medication directly to lesion; apply medication sparingly to ¹⁄₁₆-in. (0.2-cm) thickness. ➤ *Rationale:* This provides an occlusive effect.
11. If dressing is ordered, apply thin layer of medication to sterile gauze and then apply dressing to lesion area.
12. Secure dressing with gauze roll or net if large area is involved.
13. Label dressing with date, time, and your initials.
14. Check to ensure that client is comfortable after procedure.
15. Remove gloves and perform hand hygiene.
16. Return medication container to appropriate storage area.

Skill 18.3.3 | Applying Transdermal Medications

Equipment
Medication patch or tube
Gloves
Premeasured medication administration paper
Soap and water
Clear plastic wrap (optional)
Tape and pen for labeling dressing

Preparation
See Skill 18.1.1, Medication Preparation.
1. Obtain transdermal patch or premeasured paper that accompanies medication tube. ❶
2. Carefully read the manufacturer's directions for application.
   ➤ *Rationale:* Directions as well as application areas of the body differ.

Procedure
1. Take medication to client's room, and perform medication safety checks, including verification against MAR.
2. Identify client using two client identifiers.
3. Provide privacy.
4. Perform hand hygiene.

> **CLINICAL ALERT**
> **Fentanyl Transdermal Route**
> - Use exactly as directed by the healthcare provider.
> - Use only on skin that is not irritated or injured.
> - Do not cut or tear the patch, as it will allow the medication to release into the skin too quickly and potentially cause an overdose.
> - If the patch becomes loose, tape can be used around the edges to resecure it in place.
> - If you need to apply more than one patch, place the patches far enough apart to make sure they do not touch or overlap.
> - Remove the patch after 3 days or as recommended by the healthcare provider. When you apply the new patch, choose a different area—preferably on the other side of the body. Wait at least 3 days before using the first area again.
>
> *Source:* Mayo Clinic (2015)

5. Don gloves. ➤ *Rationale:* Gloves prevent you from absorbing transdermal medication. ❷
6. Alternate areas with each dose of medication to prevent skin irritation. Remove previous medicated paper or patch, fold patch in half with sticky side in, and discard in biohazard container (Box 18-5 ▪).
7. Cleanse area before applying new dose at another site.
8. Place prescribed medication directly on paper (usually ½–1 in. strip).
9. Apply medicated paper to clean, dry, hairless, intact skin.
10. Use paper to spread medication paste over a 2-in. area. Secure paper with tape or cover medicated area with plastic wrap and tape.

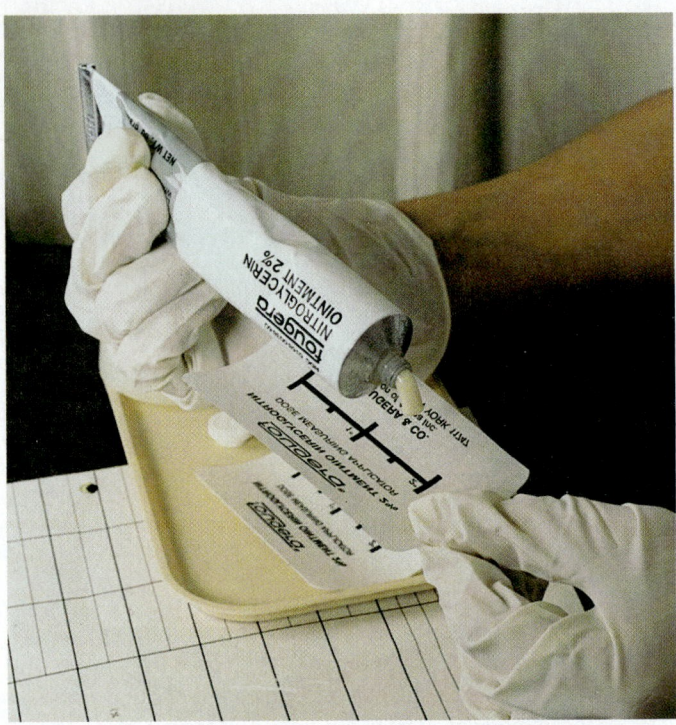
❶ Use premeasured paper to measure medication dosage.

❷ Wear gloves to prevent drug absorption through fingertips.

The use of heating pads or hot tubs can increase the absorption rate of transdermal medications.

The nonadhesive backing of some drug patches contains metal that may not be visible. These may become heated during MRI and can cause second-degree burns. Warnings may be missing from patch labels. Patches may need to be removed before MRI.

Self-improvement patches purporting to deliver herbs or other substances (marketed on TV or the internet) are not FDA regulated. Counterfeit patches also endanger clients. Refer clients to the FDA website for information on counterfeit medication.

11. For patch, remove protective covering and immediately apply patch to clean, dry, hairless, intact skin.
12. Press patch with palm for 30 sec to attain a good seal.
13. Remove gloves and perform hand hygiene.

Dispose of used transdermal patch by folding sticky sides together and discarding in a medical waste receptacle to protect others from exposure to medication. Do not flush used patches down the toilet because trace amounts of the drug may appear in treated water.

14. Label patch or paper with date, time, and your initials.
15. Return medication tube to appropriate storage area.

Box 18-5 HAZARDOUS WASTE DISPOSAL

Health care produces biohazardous waste, chemical waste, pharmaceutical waste, and other toxins, with each source having environmental consequences. Scientists have found concentrations of antibiotics, hormones, antineoplastic agents, and other chemical products in our water supplies due to improper disposal of pharmaceuticals into the sink, toilet, or trash. Best practice waste management is consistent with regulations mandated by the Environmental Protection Agency:

- Discard pharmaceutical waste into a Medical Waste receptacle (black box):

  1. Any unused oral medication not in package
  2. Unused IV medication that has been partially infused (unused IV fluid with electrolytes and TPN are excluded)
  3. Unused medication in syringes or vials (empty vials, empty IV bags, and tubing are discarded in the trash)

- Chemotherapy Waste Container (yellow) is used to discard any trace chemotherapy (containers, tubing, contaminated PPE).

Discard pharmaceutical waste into Medical Waste receptacle (black box).

Skill 18.3.4 | Instilling Ophthalmic Drops

Equipment

Eye medication ocumeter
Gloves
Tissues

Preparation

1. See Skill 18.1.1, Medication Preparation.
2. Gather necessary equipment.
3. Compare the label on the medication container to the medication record. ▶ *Rationale:* This is a safety check to ensure that medication is for ophthalmic **instillation**.

Procedure

1. Take medication to client's room; perform medication safety checks, including verification against MAR.
2. Identify client using two client identifiers.
3. Perform hand hygiene and don gloves.
4. Explain procedure and purpose of medication to client.
5. Tilt client's head slightly backward and ask client to look up. ▶ *Rationale:* The cornea is protected as client looks up.
6. Uncap eye medication container, placing cap on its side.
7. Give tissue to client for wiping off excess medication.

Apply pressure to inner canthus for 2 min to prevent rapid drug absorption if eyedrops have potential systemic effects (e.g., bradycardia due to timolol maleate [Timoptic] drops for glaucoma).

(continued)

Skill 18.3.4 | Instilling Ophthalmic Drops (continued)

CLINICAL ALERT

Occult blood developer bottles are the same size and shape as eyedrop bottles. Never leave occult blood developer in the client's room where it could be confused with the client's ophthalmic drops.

8. Place eyedrop medication container ½–¾ in. (1.3–1.9 cm) above eyeball with dominant hand. ➤ *Rationale:* This position reduces risk of dropper touching eyeball and causing injury.
9. Place nondominant hand on cheekbone and hand holding dropper on top. ❶
10. Expose lower conjunctival trough by pulling lower lid down on cheek.
11. Drop prescribed number of drops into center of conjunctival trough. ➤ *Rationale:* Placing medication directly on the cornea could cause injury to it.
12. Apply pressure to inner canthus, if indicated.
13. Ask client to close eyelids and move eyes. ➤ *Rationale:* This distributes solution over the conjunctival surface.
14. Very gently massage closed lid for client who cannot cooperate (e.g., comatose client).
15. Remove excess medication with tissue.
16. Remove gloves and perform hand hygiene.
17. Replace medication in appropriate place.

❶ Use nondominant hand to pull lower lid down. Drop eye medication in the center of lower conjunctival trough.

CLINICAL ALERT
Promoting Safe Practice

Abbreviations for eye medication administration should not be used, as they may be mistaken for ear administration (OS as AS, OD as AD, and OU as AU). Always check that the medication label states **ophthalmic** for use in the eye (ISMP, 2013).

Skill 18.3.5 | Administering Ophthalmic Ointment

Equipment
Eye ointment in tube
Tissues
Gloves

Preparation
See Skill 18.3.4, Instilling Ophthalmic Drops.

Procedure
1. Take medication to client's room, and perform medication safety checks, including verification against medical record.
2. Identify the client using two client identifiers.
3. Explain procedure and purpose to client.
4. Perform hand hygiene and don gloves.
5. Take protective guard off medication tube and lay on its side.
6. Expose conjunctival trough by pulling lower lid down on cheek or grasping lower lid below client's eyelashes to form a trough.
7. Instruct client to look upward. ➤ *Rationale:* This keeps cornea out of way of medication administration area.
8. Place medication tube tip ½–¾ in. (1.3–1.9 cm) above exposed conjunctival trough.
9. Squeeze ribbon of ointment along middle third of lower lid trough. ❶
10. Ask client to close eyelids and move eyes or gently massage closed lid to distribute medication.

11. Remove excess medication from client's eye area with tissue.
12. Caution client that ointment will cause vision to be temporarily blurred.
13. Recap and replace medication.
14. Remove gloves and perform hand hygiene.

❶ Squeeze ointment along middle third of lower conjunctival trough and ask client to close eyes.

Skill 18.3.6 | Irrigating The Eye

Equipment
500-mL bag of sterile normal (isotonic) saline *or* bottle of
   sterile pH-balanced commercial eye irrigating solution (e.g.,
   Dacriose)
IV administration tubing
IV fluid pole for elevation
Nasal cannula (as for oxygen delivery)
Tape
Sterile gauze pads
Absorbent pad or towel
Clean gloves

Preparation
1. Check healthcare provider's order for irrigation.
2. Perform hand hygiene.
3. Gather equipment.
4. Warm irrigating solution to body temperature by placing
   container in dry heating pad.

Procedure
1. Take equipment to client's room; perform medication safety
   checks, including verification against medical record.
2. Identify the client using two client identifiers.
3. Provide privacy.
4. Explain procedure and purpose to client.
5. Place client in semi-Fowler's position, turned to side of
   client's affected eye.
6. Have client hold curved basin on cheek under affected eye.
7. Don gloves.

8. Using your thumb and forefinger, open client's eye to
   expose lower conjunctival trough by pulling the lower lid
   down toward cheek.
9. Place eye irrigation bottle spout tip ¾ in. (1.9 cm) above
   client's inner canthus, pointing downward toward the outer
   canthus.
10. Squeeze bottle, allowing irrigating solution to flow into
    client's conjunctival trough to remove debris.
11. Continue irrigating for 10 min or until eye is cleansed
    completely.
12. Note results of debris returned with irrigation.
13. Wipe client's eyelid with gauze, wiping from inner to outer
    canthus.
14. Dispose of equipment in appropriate area.
15. Remove gloves and perform hand hygiene.
16. Assist client to comfortable position.
17. Document irrigation and results.

Bilateral Irrigation
1. Spike saline bag with IV tubing and hang bag on pole.
2. Affix end of IV tubing to nasal cannula, and then fit cannula
   around client's head (or around ears as for oxygen
   administration), securing prongs at bridge of client's nose
   with tape.
3. Start flow of saline solution from IV bag and allow to flush
   client's eyes to neutralize a chemical exposure.
4. Increase flow rate, and then continue wide open irrigation
   until 500 mL has been used over a 10-min period.
5. Follow steps 12–17 above.

Skill 18.3.7 | Administering Otic Medications

Equipment
Ear wick, if ordered
Prescribed ear medication
Dropper for instilling medication
Gloves (optional)

Preparation
1. See Skill 18.1.1, Medication Preparation.
2. Gather necessary equipment.
3. Remove the medication from the medication cart.
4. Compare the label on the medication bottle to the
   medication record. ➤ *Rationale:* This is a safety check.
5. Before preparing medication for administration, warm
   medication bottle to body temperature. ➤ *Rationale:*
   Instillation of cold medication can cause vertigo.

Procedure
1. Take medication to client's room; perform medication safety
   checks, including verification against medical record.

2. Identify the client using two client identifiers.
3. Explain procedure and purpose to client.
4. Perform hand hygiene.
5. Don gloves.
6. Position client on side, with ear to be treated in the
   uppermost position. ➤ *Rationale:* This position allows
   medication to enter external ear canal by gravity.
7. Fill medication dropper with prescribed amount of
   medication.
8. Prepare client for instillation of ear medication as follows:
   a. *Infant to 3 years.* Draw the pinna gently down and back.
      ➤ *Rationale:* This separates the drum membrane from
      the floor of the cartilaginous canal.
   b. *Adult.* Lift pinna upward and backward. ❶ ➤ *Rationale:*
      This position straightens the ear canal.
9. Insert ear wick if ordered. ➤ *Rationale:* Medication is
   absorbed into the ear wick. Ear wick enhances medication
   delivery directly to the entire ear canal.

(continued)

Skill 18.3.7 | Administering Otic Medications *(continued)*

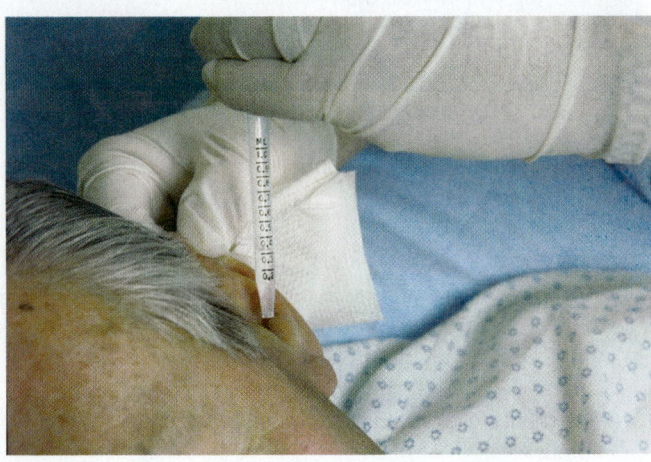

10. Instill medication drops, holding dropper slightly above ear. ➤ *Rationale:* This position protects dropper from contamination.
11. Instruct client to remain on side for 5–10 min after instillation. ➤ *Rationale:* This prevents medication from escaping and facilitates distribution.
12. Dispose of gloves and perform hand hygiene.

Note: The ear wick normally extrudes spontaneously in 12–36 hr (after edema subsides).

❶ Lift pinna upward and backward to instill eardrops in an adult. For a child under 3 years, pull the pinna gently down and back before instilling drops.

Skill 18.3.8 | Irrigating the Ear Canal

Equipment
Asepto or irrigating syringe
Prescribed irrigating solution or tap water
2 basins: round basin, curved basin
Absorbent pad or towel
Cotton ball

Preparation
(Client may have instilled wax-softening eardrops several hours before irrigation.)
1. See Skill 18.1.1, Medication Preparation.
2. Perform hand hygiene.
3. Gather equipment.
4. Warm irrigating solution to body temperature. ➤ *Rationale:* Cold solution can precipitate nausea and vertigo.

Procedure
1. Take equipment to client's room; perform medication safety checks, including verification against medical record.
2. Identify the client using two client identifiers.
3. Provide privacy.
4. Explain procedure and purpose to client.
5. Don clean gloves.

6. Place client in Fowler's position and place absorbent towel over client's chest and shoulders.
7. Pour irrigating solution into round basin.
8. Place curved basin under ear to catch irrigating solution.
9. Fill syringe with irrigating solution.
10. Open and straighten client's ear canal by pulling the pinna up and backward for adult or down and back for an infant or child under 3 years. ➤ *Rationale:* This action allows the solution to flow into ear canal.
11. Hold irrigating syringe at entrance to ear canal without occluding meatus. ➤ *Rationale:* Entering ear canal can cause impaction.
12. Push plunger, directing flow of solution toward the top of the canal. ➤ *Rationale:* This action allows the flow to reach the entire length of the canal.
13. Note return flow throughout procedure.
14. After solution has ceased to flow, dry outside of ear.
15. Return client to comfortable position and place cotton ball in ear canal to absorb excess fluid. ➤ *Rationale:* This reduces risk of external otitis.
16. Return used equipment to appropriate area.
17. Remove gloves and perform hand hygiene.
18. Document irrigation and results.

> **CLINICAL ALERT**
> Ear canal irrigation should be performed only when the tympanic membrane can be visualized because of the risk that debris may cover an unseen perforation.

> **CLINICAL ALERT**
> Ensure that client's tympanic membrane is intact before irrigating the ear. Water should not be used to irrigate the ear to remove an organic foreign body (e.g., insect or bean) since water may cause the object to swell.

Unit 18.3 Documentation and Evaluation

DOCUMENTATION for Topical Medications

Client's Medication Administration Record

- Time administered
- Name of medication
- Dosage
- Route and site of application
- Initials of nurse administering medication
- Signature by nurse which identifies initials

Nurses' Notes

- Documentation of prn, STAT, and one-time-only medications
- Time administered, name of medication, dosage, route, site
- Client's response to application
- Condition of area treated
- Signature of nurse

EVALUATION/Critical Thinking

Expected Outcomes

- Topical medication has intended effect.
- Client self-administers eye medication according to instructions.
- Ear canal irrigation removes cerumen.

Unexpected Outcomes	Alternative Actions
Client develops **adverse reaction** to topical medication (e.g., itching, inflammation).	Rotate sites of medication system application. Consult healthcare provider or pharmacist for alternative route of medication administration (e.g., oral).
Obese client fails to obtain pain relief from topical analgesic patch.	Consult pain management team. Consider weight-based dosage.
Client is reluctant to use eye medication ointment because it causes "blurred vision."	Suggest client apply eye ointment at bedtime. Assist client to create safe means for urination at night (e.g., night lighting, safety rails, bedside commode, urinal).
Client complains of nausea and vertigo after ear irrigation.	Warm irrigating solution to body temperature. Consult healthcare provider to order wax-softening eardrops to instill before irrigation to facilitate removal of cerumen and shorten process.

Mucous Membrane Medication Administration

Nursing Process Data

ASSESSMENT Database

- Assess that drug can be administered sublingually.
- Assess client's ability to understand and follow directions.
- Assess vital signs, SpO_2, relevant to medication action.
- Assess for dyspnea, labored breathing, and wheezing.
- Determine possible undesired systemic effects of inhaled agents (tremor, nausea, tachycardia).
- Review healthcare provider's orders for medication and diluent to be administered, and frequency of treatments.
- Observe amount and character of expectorated sputum.
- Determine need for other respiratory techniques.
- Assess client's breath sounds before and after each treatment.
- Assess client's bowel elimination pattern.

PLANNING Objectives

- To provide appropriate surface for rapid absorption of medication for systemic effect
- To confine drug action to a local area
- To facilitate ease and consistency of self-administration of medication
- To decrease client's work of breathing
- To provide alternate route of medication administration when client is NPO/nauseated
- To promote bowel elimination
- To combat infection
- To deliver aerosolized medications
- To temporarily decrease the work of breathing
- To promote better ventilation
- To loosen secretions

IMPLEMENTATION Procedures

DOCUMENTATION AND EVALUATION

Expected Outcomes

- Chest pain is relieved due to rapid systemic response to sublingual medication administration.
- Desired local effect of medication is achieved without undesired side effects.
- Suppository has desired effects/results.

Unexpected Outcomes/Alternative Actions

Pearson Nursing Student Resources

Find additional review materials at
nursing.pearsonhighered.com.
Prepare for success with NCLEX®-style practice
questions and Skill Checklists.

Skill 18.4.1 | Administering Sublingual Medications

Equipment

Sublingual medication (e.g., nitroglycerin tablets in a dark bottle). *Tablets lose potency when exposed to light; opened bottle should be replaced in 3 months.*

or

Nitrolingual aerosol spray in canister

Preparation

1. See Skill 18.1.1, Medication Preparation.
2. Perform medication safety checks, including verification against medical record.
3. Identify the client using two client identifiers.
4. Perform hand hygiene
5. Assess vital signs if administering sublingual nitroglycerin. (*Systolic BP should not be lower than 90 mm Hg.*)
6. Place client in a sitting position.

Procedure

1. Follow steps for preparing and administering oral medications, *except*:

    a. Explain that client must not swallow drug or eat, smoke, or drink until medication is completely absorbed.

    b. Ask client to place tablet under the tongue or to hold tongue up so tablet can be placed under tongue. ❶
    ➤ *Rationale:* Absorption is rapid and complete due to the vast network of capillaries in this area.

    c. Alternate: Hold nitrolingual canister vertically with spray opening as close to mouth as possible. Deliver 1 or 2 metered sprays onto or under tongue, and then have client close mouth immediately. Tell client not to inhale medication.

2. Evaluate client for drug action and possible side effects (e.g., headache).

❶ Sublingual medication is placed under client's tongue for rapid absorption.

CLINICAL ALERT

Assess client's chest discomfort: quality, location, radiation, intensity, duration, and precipitating factors. When administering rapid-acting (sublingual) nitroglycerin, monitor client's response and vital signs. If chest discomfort is not relieved in 5 min, notify healthcare provider. Obtain order for opiate analgesic (morphine sulfate), EKG, ST-segment monitoring, and cardiac biomarkers. No more than three doses of nitroglycerin should be administered in a 15-min period because of potential hypotensive effect (BP ≤90 mm Hg) or bradycardia (HR 50), as this would preclude adequate dosage of morphine sulfate for pain control.

EVIDENCE-BASED PRACTICE

ACC/AHA Guidelines—Nitroglycerin

It is recommended by the American College of Cardiology and the American Heart Association that clients who have been previously prescribed nitroglycerin be advised to take ONE dose sublingually promptly for chest discomfort or pain. If symptoms *do not* improve, or worsen in 5 min after ONE nitroglycerin dose, the client should call 9-1-1 immediately to access EMS. For clients with chronic stable angina, if symptoms are significantly improved after ONE nitroglycerin dose, repeat nitroglycerin every 5 min for a total of three doses and call 9-1-1 if symptoms have not totally resolved.

Source: O'Gara et al. (2013)

Skill 18.4.2 | Instilling Nose Drops

Equipment

Medication bottle
Dropper
Tissues

Preparation

1. See Skill 18.1.1, Medication Preparation.
2. Perform hand hygiene.

Procedure

1. Take equipment to client's room; perform medication safety checks, including verification against medical record.
2. Identify client using two client identifiers.
3. Place client in sitting position with head tilted back ❶, ❷ or in supine position with head tilted back over pillow.

4. Fill dropper with prescribed amount of medication.
5. Place dropper just inside the naris and instill correct medication dosage. Repeat procedure in other naris.
6. Wipe away any excess medication with tissue.
7. Instruct client not to sneeze or blow nose and to keep head tilted back for 5 min to prevent medication from escaping.
8. Check to see that client is comfortable before leaving room.
9. Perform hand hygiene.
10. Return medication to appropriate storage area.

Ethnoid and Sphenoid Sinuses

❶ Instruct client to tilt head backwards and place dropper inside nares when instilling nose drops.

❷ Tilt client's head back for nose drops to reach maxillary and frontal sinuses.

Skill 18.4.3 | Administering Metered-Dose Inhaled (MDI) Medications

Equipment

Prescribed medication canister
Metered-dose inhaler (MDI) dispenser (actuator or holder)
Spacer or holding chamber (if ordered)
Tissues

> **CLINICAL ALERT**
>
> Check inhaler medication label for number of **actuations** (propellant-driven medication doses, e.g., 200). Have client maintain a record of actuations and discard after the number indicated. Final puffs may be nothing but propellant, which would not dilate airways in an emergency situation.

EVIDENCE-BASED PRACTICE

MDI Dose Counters and Client Satisfaction

Clients have often struggled with knowing how many doses they have left in their metered-dose inhalers (MDIs). New MDIs are now available with integrated dose counters. Clients are finding them easy to use and are overall satisfied with the product.

Source: LaForce, Weinstein, Nathan, Weinstein, Staudinger, & Meltzer (2011)

Preparation

1. See Skill 18.1.1, Medication Preparation.
2. Perform hand hygiene.

3. Gather equipment.
4. Compare label of drug canister to client's medication record.

Procedure

1. Take medication canister and MDI dispenser to client's room. Perform medication safety checks, including verification against medical record.
2. Identify client using two client identifiers.
3. Provide privacy.
4. Explain procedure and purpose to client.
5. Assist client to standing or sitting position.
6. Insert canister (stem down) into longer part of metered-dose dispenser. (For new canister, test spray [prime] MDI into air one or more times. ➤ *Rationale:* This is done with new canister to ensure patency of the unit, following directions on the package.)
7. Shake MDI with canister to mix medication and propellant. *(Shake canister before each MDI puff)*. See Box 18-6 ■.
   ➤ *Rationale:* Without shaking propellant, little or no medication will be delivered.

Note: Canisters typically contain propellants and other inert ingredients in addition to the actual drug; a client may believe a canister contains medication when none is actually present.

8. Instruct client to remove mouthpiece and hold inhaler 2 in. away from mouth (following manufacturer's instructions). Mist is to be *inhaled* into airways. ❶ Alternatively, place mouthpiece into the mouth, holding the canister upright.
9. Instruct the client to exhale through pursed lips.
   ➤ *Rationale:* Exhaling through pursed lips increases exhaled volume, allowing room for a greater *inspiratory* volume.
10. Instruct the client to depress the inhalation device, releasing a puff of medication while inhaling slowly and deeply (3–5 sec). ➤ *Rationale:* With slow deep inhalation, medication goes to lower respiratory tract.
11. Tell client to hold breath for 10 sec, then remove the unit and slowly exhale through pursed lips. ➤ *Rationale:* Holding the breath allows time for the medication to be absorbed.
12. Assess client's breathing and reaction to medication.
    ➤ *Rationale:* With certain drugs, heart rate may increase.

❶ Depress inhalation device while inhaling slowly (3–5 sec) and deeply through mouth.

13. Provide tissues. ➤ *Rationale:* Inhaled medication may stimulate coughing.
14. Instruct client to wait 1 or 2 min between inhalations and to *shake canister* before each puff. ➤ *Rationale:* Waiting between doses helps prevent paroxysmal bronchospasm.
15. Have client replace mouthpiece cap.
16. Caution client not to increase the dose without a healthcare provider's order. ➤ *Rationale:* Potential side effects of an increased dose could be serious.
17. Instruct client to rinse the mouth after using MDI that contains steroids and not to swallow the water. ➤ *Rationale:* Rinsing prevents oral candidiasis.
18. Teach client to remove canister and to clean mouthpiece *daily*, washing with soap and water and allowing to air dry. ➤ *Rationale:* These devices are sites for microbial growth.
19. Review information about the inhaled medication and possible side effects with client (Box 18-7 ■). ➤ *Rationale:* Client continues home therapy and should be aware of self-monitoring needs.
20. Perform hand hygiene.
21. Document procedure and results.

Box 18-6 CLIENT TEACHING ABOUT METERED-DOSE INHALERS

- Canister must be shaken before each puff so that propellant and medication are adequately combined. Priming sprays are performed with a new canister or when a canister has not been used for a long period of time.
- Prime new MDI by spraying into the air one or more times. Check the directions on the package to see how to prime your MDI.
- Tell client to keep track of number of puffs (actuations) used in order to plan for refill of prescription if the MDI does not have a built-in dose counter.

Box 18-7 INHALED MEDICATIONS

- Inhaled medications provide relief for bronchospasm, wheezing, asthma, or allergic reactions.
- Medications include bronchodilators, steroids, and antimediators.
- Common systemic side effects include tremors, nausea, tachycardia, palpitations, nervousness, and dysrhythmias.

Skill 18.4.4 | Using MDI with Spacer

Equipment
See Skill 18.4.3, Administering Metered-Dose Inhaled (MDI) Medications.

Preparation
1. See Skills 18.1.1, Medication Preparation, and 18.4.3, Administering Metered-Dose Inhaled (MDI) Medications.
2. Perform hand hygiene.

Procedure
1. Assemble medication canister in MDI.
2. Insert MDI mouthpiece into spacer. ➤ *Rationale:* Research indicates an MDI inhaler fitted into a spacer improves airway delivery of medication because large drops do not fall into the mouth.
3. Remove mouthpiece cover from spacer.
4. Hold upright and shake MDI with spacer to mix medication and propellant.
5. Instruct client to exhale slowly through pursed lips.
6. Instruct client to close lips around spacer mouthpiece. ❶
   ➤ *Rationale:* Spacer eliminates need for simultaneous hand action and mouth inspiration coordination.
7. Activate MDI canister, pressing down with fingers, pushing it farther into plastic adapter. ➤ *Rationale:* This releases metered dose of medication into spacer.
8. After activation, instruct client to inhale slowly and deeply through mouth and hold breath for 10 sec.
9. Instruct client to exhale and relax.
10. Provide water mouth rinse after inhaled corticosteroids.
    ➤ *Rationale:* Rinsing prevents oral candidiasis.

❶ Hold canister upright when using MDI with spacer.

11. Remove drug canister and clean mouthpiece and spacer daily, washing with soap and water.

> **CLINICAL ALERT**
> If several types of medications are used, follow this sequence: quick-acting bronchodilator (e.g., albuterol sulfate); slower-acting bronchodilator (e.g., ipratropium bromide [Atro-vent]); antimediators (e.g., steroids).

Skill 18.4.5 | Administering Dry Powder Inhaled (DPI) Medications

Equipment
Dry powder capsule intended for oral inhalation
Medication package insert (instructions)
Handheld inhalation device intended for medication to be given

Preparation
1. See Skills 18.1.1, Medication Preparation, and 18.4.3, Administering Metered-Dose Inhaled (MDI) Medications.
2. Review medication package insert instructions.
3. Perform hand hygiene.

Procedure
1. Take dry powder capsule package and inhalation device to client's room. Perform medication safety checks, including verification against medical record.
2. Identify client using two client identifiers.
3. Provide privacy.
4. Explain procedure and purpose to client.

5. Assist client to a sitting position.
6. Remove capsule from package, peeling back foil cover to expose only one capsule. ➤ *Rationale:* Capsules should be used immediately; unused capsules exposed to air may lose effectiveness.
7. Open the outer cap of inhaler device (pull cap upward).
8. Open the mouthpiece.
9. Insert the capsule into center of chamber of the inhalation device. ❶
10. Hold the device upright, and, leaving the outer cap open, close mouthpiece/lid firmly until a click is heard and leave the outer cap open.
11. Press the side-mounted piercing button in completely, then release. ➤ *Rationale:* The piercing button punctures the capsule, allowing medication to be released upon inhalation.
12. Have the client breathe out completely.
13. Have the client keep his or her head in upright position and place lips tightly round the mouthpiece.

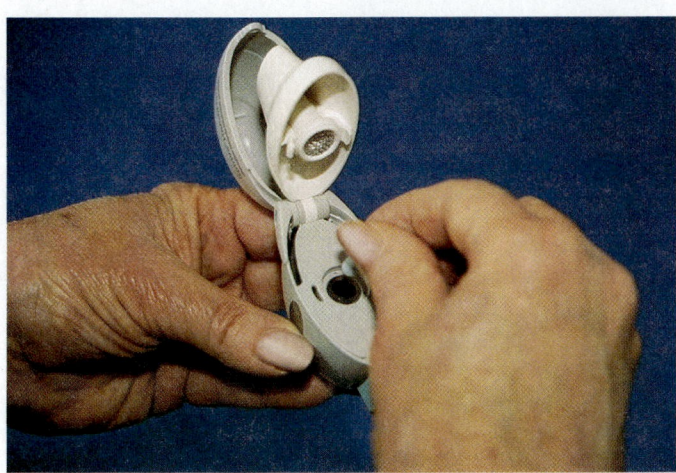

❶ Insert capsule into center of chamber of the inhalation device.

14. Have client breathe slowly and deeply with sufficient energy to hear the medication capsule vibrate. ➤ *Rationale:* As long as the capsule rattles, the client's inhalation is fast enough.

Note: Some DPIs require a fast initial inhalation to activate the medication distribution.

15. Have the client hold the deep breath as long as comfortable, and then return to normal breathing.
16. Have client repeat Steps 12–15 if indicated in medication package insert. ➤ *Rationale:* Repeating the steps may be necessary to get the full dose of medication.
17. Open mouthpiece and discard remaining capsule.
18. Close mouthpiece and outer cap and store at client's bedside.
19. Clean unit only as necessary, using warm water and allowing device to air dry thoroughly before next use. ➤ *Rationale:* No cleaning agents should be used and the device should not be wet when used.

Skill 18.4.6 | Administering Medication by Nonpressurized (Nebulized) Aerosol (NPA)

Equipment
Nebulizer medication chamber
T-piece, mouthpiece or mask
Corrugated tubing
Air flow tubing
Prescribed medication (e.g., bronchodilator)
Prescribed diluent (normal saline)
Wall source (or other source) for compressed air, or oxygen with flowmeter

Preparation
1. See Skill 18.1.1, Medication Preparation.
2. Perform medication safety checks, including verification against medication administration record.
3. Identify client using two client identifiers.
4. Perform hand hygiene.
5. Dilute medication as ordered and place in nebulizer chamber.
6. Attach one end of tubing to compressed air source.
7. Attach other end of tubing to nozzle at side or bottom of nebulizer.
8. Keep nebulizer chamber vertical, and connect top of chamber to mask or T-piece sidearm.
9. Hold mouthpiece in its protective cover, and attach to one end of T-piece.
10. Attach corrugated tubing to other end of T-piece.

Procedure
1. Turn on air or oxygen (8 L/min) source, and observe for mist flow.

   a. If the client is receiving 3 L/min or less of oxygen therapy, deliver aerosolized medications with compressed air (yellow wall outlet).

   b. If the client is receiving 4 L/min or more of oxygen therapy, deliver the aerosol medication with the oxygen flowmeter (green wall outlet) set at 8 L/min.

> **CLINICAL ALERT**
> The plastic containers with respiratory medications for nebulizers are similar to the plastic containers for single-dose eyedrops. Both products have the drug name molded into the plastic, but it is difficult to see.

2. Have client place mouthpiece in mouth and close lips. ❶
3. Instruct client to breathe normally in and out of mouthpiece or mask.
4. Have client take a deep breath and hold for several seconds, and then exhale slowly every 3–5 breaths. (Treatment is complete when all medication is used and no mist is seen.)
5. Turn power (air or O_2 flow) off, and unplug compressor (if used), or reset prescribed O_2 flow rate.
6. Clean mouthpiece, and place equipment in plastic bag at bedside. (Dispose of and replace components according to agency policy.)

❶ Client preparing for nonpressured aerosol (NPA) treatment.

Skill 18.4.7 | Administering Rectal Suppositories

Equipment
Suppository as ordered from refrigerator
Clean gloves
Water-soluble lubricant
Paper towel

Preparation
1. See Skill 18.1.1, Medication Preparation.
2. Compare the medication record with the most recent health-care provider's order.
3. Perform hand hygiene.
4. Gather necessary equipment.
5. Retrieve medication from refrigerator if indicated.
6. Compare the medication label with client's MAR.
7. Place suppository, lubricant, and paper towel on a tray if not using medication cart.

Procedure
1. Take medication and equipment to client's room.
2. Perform medication safety checks, including verification against medication administration record.
3. Identify client using two client identifiers.
4. Explain procedure and purpose to client.
5. Provide privacy.
6. Place client in dorsal-recumbent or side-lying position.
7. Squeeze dollop of lubricant onto paper towel.
8. Remove foil wrapper from the suppository.
9. Moisten suppository tip with warm water or lubricant to facilitate insertion.

10. Don clean gloves and inspect anal area for hemorrhoids.
11. Instruct client to bear down to identify anal opening and insert the suppository about 1½ in. (4 cm) into the rectal canal beyond the anal sphincter. ❶ ➤ *Rationale:* This prevents suppository from slipping out.
12. Instruct client to lie quietly for 15 min while medicine is absorbed and that suppository may take up to 1 hr to be effective.
13. Dispose of equipment and gloves and perform hand hygiene.
14. Return after 15 min to ensure client is comfortable.
15. Document medication and results obtained.

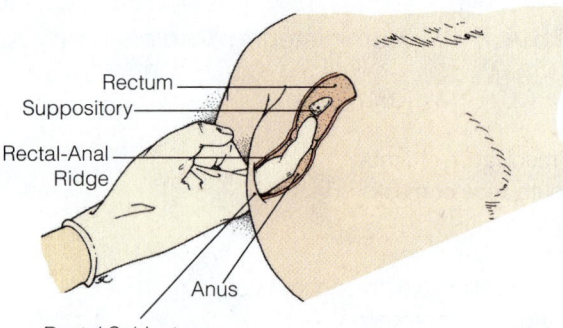

Rectum
Suppository
Rectal-Anal Ridge
Anus
Rectal Sphincter

❶ Insert rectal suppository beyond the anorectal ridge to ensure it is retained.

Skill 18.4.8 | Administering Vaginal Suppositories

Equipment
Prescribed vaginal suppository
Client's applicator (should be kept in client's room)
Clean gloves

Preparation
1. See Skill 18.1.1, Medication Preparation.
2. Compare the medication record with the most recent health-care provider's order.
3. Perform hand hygiene.
4. Gather necessary equipment.
5. Remove the medication from medication cart.
6. Compare the medication label to the client's MAR.

Procedure
1. Take medication and equipment to client's room.
2. Perform medication safety checks, including verification against medication administration record.
3. Identify client using two client identifiers.
4. Provide privacy.
5. Explain procedure and purpose to client.

6. Don gloves.
7. Place client in dorsal-recumbent or side-lying position.
8. Remove foil wrapper from suppository. Insert into applicator.
9. Don clean gloves.
10. Insert applicator with suppository into the vaginal canal at least 2 in. (5 cm). ❶ ➤ *Rationale:* This prevents suppository from slipping out.

❶ Insert vaginal suppository at least 2 in. (5 cm) into vaginal canal using applicator as shown.

11. Instruct client to lie quietly for 15 min until the suppository is absorbed.
12. Discard equipment, wash applicator, and return to appropriate place in client's room.
13. Remove gloves and perform hand hygiene.
14. Chart medication and assessment findings (e.g., discharge, odor).

Unit 18.4 Documentation and Evaluation

DOCUMENTATION for Mucous Membrane Medications

Client's Medication Record
- Time
- Medication administered
- Route of administration
- Initials of nurse administering medication
- Signature of nurse identifying initials

Nurses' Notes
- Time
- Name of medication, dosage, route pre- and postadministration assessment findings (chest discomfort, vital signs, SpO_2, breath sounds)
- Healthcare provider notification, if done
- Results of suppository action

EVALUATION/Critical Thinking

Expected Outcomes
- Angina is relieved with ONE dose of sublingual nitroglycerin.
- Chest pain is relieved due to rapid systemic response to sublingual medication administration.
- Desired local effect of medication is achieved without undesired side effects.
- Suppository has desired effects or results.

Unexpected Outcomes
- Client's chest discomfort is not relieved with ONE dose of sublingual nitroglycerin.

Alternative Actions
- Provide anticipatory instructions.
- Check bottle for expiration date—potency is lost 3 months after opening bottle.
- Recognize associated symptoms of acute MI such as dyspnea, nausea, cold sweat, and lightheadedness.
- Do not take a "wait and see" approach or deny symptoms indicative of acute MI.

(continued)

Unexpected Outcomes	Alternative Actions
• Client's discomfort is not relieved with sublingual nitroglycerin.	• Check bottle for expiration date—potency is lost 3 months after opening bottle. • Administer second tablet in 5 min—if discomfort continues, administer opiate analgesic, call Rapid Response Team, notify healthcare provider, and obtain stat ECG. • Administer no more than three tablets/sprays in a 15-min period. • Monitor for blood pressure effect—hold medication if systolic BP is less than 90 mm Hg. • Consult with healthcare provider for blood test for possible myocardial injury and need for continuous cardiac monitoring.
• Client states that breathing has not improved after using inhaler.	• Place client in Fowler's position. Validate that MDI/spacer/NPA device is functioning properly (e.g., canister shaken before use). • Check number of actuations left in MDI canister. • Validate that client's lips have tight fit around MDI mouthpiece, so mist is inhaled. • Instruct client to hold breath for 10 sec after MDI use and to wait 2 min between puffs.
• Client using MDI reports painful white patches in mouth.	• Instruct client to use spacer with MDI steroid medication. • Instruct client to rinse mouth with water and expectorate after administering MDI steroid. • Notify healthcare provider of findings.
• Client fails to have BM postlaxative suppository administration.	• Reassess abdomen and check client for rectal fecal impaction. • Consult with healthcare provider to order oil-retention enema or cleansing enema. • Teach client ways to prevent constipation.
• Client is unable to retain vaginal suppository.	• Administer vaginal suppository at bedtime to prevent medication leakage.

Nursing Process Data

ASSESSMENT Database

- Check that appropriate method for administration of drug was ordered.
- Assess condition of administration site for presence of lesions, rash, inflammation, lipid dystrophy, and ecchymosis.
- Assess client's understanding of medication action.
- Check client's written history and ask for oral history for past allergic reactions. (Do not rely solely on client's chart.)
- Review client's chart noting previous injection sites.

PLANNING Objectives

- To ensure proper route of drug administration
- To protect self from harm when administering parenteral injections
- To administer medication parenterally according to the "six rights"
- To reduce discomfort with medication injection
- To alternate injection sites for consistent absorption of medication
- To observe and report side effects/adverse reactions of drug administration

IMPLEMENTATION Procedures

DOCUMENTATION AND EVALUATION

Expected Outcomes

- Injection is administered without complications.
- Injection is as painless as possible.
- Medication therapeutic effect is achieved.

Unexpected Outcomes/Alternative Actions

Pearson Nursing Student Resources

Find additional review materials at
nursing.pearsonhighered.com.
Prepare for success with NCLEX®-style practice questions and Skill Checklists.

Skill 18.5.1 | Preparing Injections

Equipment

Medication in vial or ampule
Vial of compatible diluent (if necessary)
Syringe of closest capacity to hold medication ❶
Filter needle for withdrawing medication from ampule or rubber-topped vial
Appropriate-size safety needle for injection ❷ ❸
Antimicrobial wipe
Dry gauze sponge
Label for prepared injection

Preparation

See Skill 18.1.1, Medication Preparation.

Procedure

1. Perform hand hygiene.
2. Obtain equipment.
3. Assemble the syringe and filter needle, maintaining sterility.
4. Fill syringe with medication.
5. Attach appropriate-size needle (Box 18-8 ▪) for injection, considering route, desired site (Box 18-9 ▪), client's size, and viscosity of medication. ➤ *Rationale:* The larger the gauge number, the *smaller* the needle lumen. Larger gauges produce less tissue trauma and are used for aqueous solutions. Smaller gauges are required for viscous solutions such as hormones.
6. Unless administering immediately, apply identifying label to prepared syringe. ➤ *Rationale:* Lack of labeling has been cited as a major risk for medication administration errors.

EVIDENCE-BASED PRACTICE

Education and Safety Syringes

To date, there are two factors that have had a positive impact on reducing needlestick injuries in any setting: ongoing education and the use of safety syringes. Additionally, fixed-needle safety devices should be used routinely to decrease the incidence of accidental needlesticks.

Source: Higginson & Parry (2013)

CLINICAL ALERT

Do Not Use These Sites

- The dorsogluteal site is no longer recommended for IM injection. There is a high risk for injury to the sciatic nerve and major blood vessels due to difficulty palpating appropriate bony landmarks in this area. Variation of thickness of subcutaneous tissue at this site makes inadvertent injection into subcutaneous tissue, altered drug absorption, and tissue injury possible.
- Do not use the rectus femoris (anterior thigh) muscle for injection.

❶ Three types of syringes: tuberculin, insulin, and 3-mL. The type of syringe should be close in capacity to the amount of medication ordered.

❷ Healthcare facilities must use safety needles to conform to needlestick safety legislation.

❸ Safety syringes with retractable needles.

Box 18-8 **SELECTING THE APPROPRIATE-SIZE NEEDLE FOR INJECTION**

- *Subcutaneous injections*: 0.5–3 mL syringe with 25–29 gauge, ⅜–⅝ in. needle.
- *Intramuscular injections*: 1–5 mL syringe with needle gauge and length appropriate for muscle site and fat thickness; deltoid muscle requires 23–25 gauge, ⅝–1 in.

- needle; needle sizes for the vastus lateralis and ventro-gluteal muscle vary from 18 to 23 gauge, needle lengths, 1–1½ in.
- *Intradermal injections*: 1 mL tuberculin syringe with short bevel, 25–27 gauge, ⅜–½ in. needle.

(Left) Subcutaneous injection: Insert needle at 45- or 90-degree angle into tissue for subcutaneous injection. *(Right)* Insert needle at 15-degree angle just under the epidermis for intradermal injection.

Note that needle color matches the gauge.

Box 18-9 **SITES FOR INJECTIONS**

Site is the single most consistent factor associated with complications and injury. The client's age, size, medication type, and medication volume must be considered.

Intradermal Injections

- Injection sites: inner aspect of forearm or scapular area of back; upper chest; medial thigh
- Purpose: to test for antigens (tubercle bacillus, allergens)
- Amount injected: ranges from 0.01 to 0.1 mL
- Absorption rate: slow

Subcutaneous Injections

- Injection sites: fatty tissue of abdomen, lateral and posterior aspects of upper arm or thigh, scapular area of back, upper ventrodorsal gluteal areas
- Purpose: for medications that are absorbed slowly
- Amount injected: variable—no more than 2 mL. If repeated doses are necessary, alter site accordingly.

Intramuscular Injections

- Purpose: to promote rapid absorption of the drug; to provide an alternate route when drug is irritating to subcutaneous tissues
- Amount injected: variable—may be large amount of fluid. If more than 5 mL for adult, or 3 mL for child, and 1 mL for infant, divide dose into two syringes.
- Absorption rate: depends on circulatory state of client

- Injection sites:

Ventrogluteal Injection Site (preferred site for IM injection for all clients over age 7 months)

1. Place client in side-lying or supine position.
2. Use right hand for left anterior hip, or left hand for right anterior hip.
3. Identify greater trochanter and place palm at site.
4. Keep palm on greater trochanter and point index finger toward client's anterior superior iliac spine and fan out other three fingers.
5. Form "V" area with index finger separated from other three fingers.
6. Inject medication at 90-degree angle within "V" area.

Vastus Lateralis Injection Site

1. Place client in supine position with thigh exposed.
2. Identify greater trochanter and lateral femoral condyle.
3. Using middle third and anterior *lateral* aspect of thigh, select site.
4. Inject medication directly into muscle at 90-degree angle.

Deltoid Injection Site (solution must be nonirritating)

1. Expose client's upper arm.
2. Deltoid site is two fingerbreadths below acromion process.
3. Place left hand on acromion process and right index finger two fingerbreadths below.
4. Inject limited medication volume (0.5–1 mL) in deltoid IM site at 90-degree angle.

Withdrawing Medication From a Vial

1. Remove the vial cap.
2. Open antimicrobial wipe, and cleanse the rubber top of the vial. ► *Rationale:* Manufacturer does not guarantee sterility of rubber top.

3. Tighten needle to syringe. Remove needle guard.
4. Pull back on plunger to fill syringe with an amount of air equal to amount of solution to be withdrawn. ► *Rationale:* The displacement of solution with air is necessary to prevent the formation of a vacuum in the sealed vial.

(continued)

Skill 18.5.1 | Preparing Injections *(continued)*

5. Insert needle into upright vial. Inject air into vacant area of vial, keeping needle bevel above surface of medication. **4**
   ➤ *Rationale:* Air creates positive pressure within vial, allowing accurate withdrawal of medication.
6. Invert vial, and pull plunger to extract desired amount of medication. **5** Touch only syringe barrel and plunger tip.
   ➤ *Rationale:* This prevents contamination of the plunger, inside of barrel, and medication.
7. Expel any air bubbles from syringe at this time by tapping the side of syringe sharply with your finger or pen below the air bubble. ➤ *Rationale:* Air bubbles form in syringe due to dead air space in needle hub. Removing air bubbles while needle remains within the inverted vial avoids accidental contamination of needle and facilitates easy removal of air and accurate withdrawal of solution.
8. Recheck amount of medication in syringe.

9. Turn vial to upright position and remove needle.
   ➤ *Rationale:* Removing needle from inverted vial may cause leaking of medication from needle insertion site.
10. Replace needle with appropriate size needle for injection.
11. Recheck medication label and dosage against medication record and any dosage calculation. ➤ *Rationale:* This is a second safety check.
12. Replace or dispose of medication vial, checking label once again. ➤ *Rationale:* This is a third safety check. See Box 18-10 ∎.

Combining Medications in One Syringe Using Two Vials

1. Prepare both vials by removing caps and cleansing tops with separate antimicrobial wipes.
2. Draw air into syringe equal to amount of solution to be removed from *second* vial. Inject air into *second* vial. Do not withdraw medication at this time. ➤ *Rationale:* Air creates positive pressure within the vial, allowing withdrawal of solution.

CLINICAL ALERT

If multiple-use vials are opened, they must be marked with the date and time the container is entered and nurse's initials. Consult the product label or package insert to determine whether refrigeration is necessary. Unless contamination is suspected, the Centers for Disease Control and Prevention (CDC) recommends that the vial be discarded either when empty or on the expiration date set by the manufacturer.

5 Invert vial to extract desired amount of medication.

4 Inject prescribed amount of air into vial.

Box 18-10 **RECONSTITUTING POWDERED MEDICATION**

- Insert needle into upright powdered medication vial.
- Remove the amount of air equal to desired quantity of diluent; this provides space for the diluent.
- Inject diluent into upright powdered medication vial.
- Remove needle and cover with guard.
- Rotate powdered medication vial with diluent between palms. Do not shake vial because shaking creates air bubbles and may cause difficulty withdrawing medication dose.
- Withdraw medication from vial.
- Replace needle with appropriate size needle for injection.

3. Draw air into syringe equal to amount of solution to be removed from *first* vial and inject it into *first* vial.
4. Invert first vial and withdraw ordered amount of medication without removing syringe.
5. Expel all air bubbles from syringe.
6. Recheck amount of solution and remove syringe from vial.
7. Insert needle into *second* vial, invert, and carefully withdraw exact amount of solution ordered. ➤ *Rationale:* Withdrawing excess solution from second vial results in an inaccurate dosage of medication. If this occurs, syringe must be discarded and procedure begun again.
8. Replace needle with needle for injection.

Withdrawing Medication From an Ampule

1. Move solution from neck to body of ampule by tapping stem sharply or holding neck of ampule between thumb and forefinger and flicking wrist.
2. Using a pad, grasp neck (stem) of ampule between thumb and forefinger of one hand and grasp body of ampule with other hand. Break stem away from you. ❻ (If ampule is not scored, partially file neck of ampule.) ➤ *Rationale:* Gauze pad protects hands, and breaking away from you prevents injury from glass fragments. Alternatively, slip a nipple from a baby bottle over the stem to prevent injury.
3. Set the ampule upright. It is not necessary to add air before withdrawing the medication.
4. Use a special filter needle to withdraw solution. ❼ ➤ *Rationale:* Filter needle prevents aspiration of glass when withdrawing solution from ampule, especially if the ampule is inverted.
5. Remove needle guard and insert filter needle into ampule without touching sides of ampule and withdraw medication. ❽ Alternatively, invert ampule and withdraw appropriate amount of medication. ➤ *Rationale:* Surface tension prevents solution from leaking out of inverted ampule.
6. Withdraw filter needle with ampule in upright position.
7. Tap syringe barrel below bubbles to dislodge air bubbles to hub of syringe.
8. Eject air with syringe in an upright position. If amount of solution is overdrawn, invert syringe and remove excess solution into the Medical Waste (black box) receptacle. ➤ *Rationale:* Appropriate waste disposal is mandated by the EPA.
9. Cover needle with guard, using scoop method.
10. Remove filter needle and replace with appropriate-sized needle for injection. ➤ *Rationale:* Filter needles cannot be used to give injections into the client.

Combining Medications Using Alternative Method

1. Draw up ordered dose from each vial or ampule into two separate syringes. First, syringe must be able to hold entire volume of combined medications.

❻ Using alcohol swab or dry gauze square, grasp and snap off stem of ampule, breaking away from you.

❼ A special filter needle should be used to prevent aspirating particulate matter when withdrawing solution from an ampule or vial.

❽ Tilt or invert ampule to withdraw appropriate amount of medication, using filter needle.

(continued)

Skill 18.5.1 | Preparing Injections (continued)

2. Remove needle from first syringe.
3. Pull back plunger of first syringe to allow space for volume of second medication to be added.
4. Insert needle of second syringe into hub of first syringe.
5. Slowly inject medication of second syringe through first syringe hub, and then withdraw needle.
6. Attach new needle to first syringe.
7. Discard needles and second syringe.

Preparing Prefilled Medication Cartridge

1. Hold barrel of cartridge syringe (e.g., Tubex) in one hand and pull back on plunger with other hand.
2. Insert prefilled medication cartridge, needle first, into cartridge barrel. ❾
3. Twist cartridge syringe flange clockwise until it is secure.
4. Screw plunger rod onto screw at bottom of medication cartridge until it fits firmly and tightly into rubber stopper.
5. Remove needle guard and any air bubbles.
6. Determine if dosage in cartridge is greater than required amount. If so, invert Tubex and gently expel excess medication into Medical Waste receptacle, being careful to maintain sterility of needle. ➤ *Rationale:* If permanent needle is contaminated, the cartridge becomes contaminated and must be discarded.
7. Replace needle guard, using scoop method.

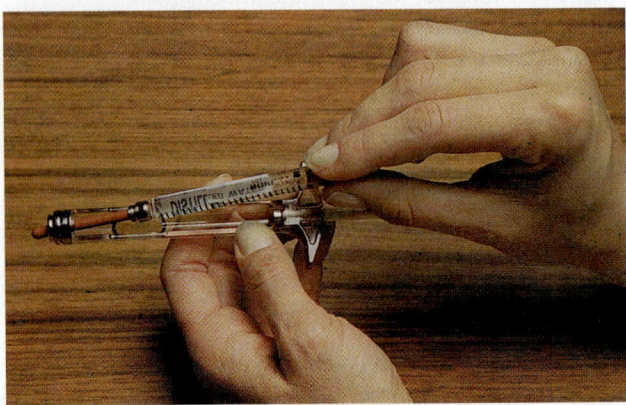

❾ Slide prefilled, sterile cartridge into syringe barrel; then turn and lock.

Skill 18.5.2 | Administering Intradermal Injections

Equipment
Medication (e.g., 0.1 mL Purified Protein Derivative Antigen for tuberculin testing)
Unit dose (1 mL) tuberculin syringe with ¼- to ⅜-in. 27-gauge needle
Antimicrobial wipes
Gauze sponge
Clean gloves (if indicated)
Pen to mark injection site

Preparation
Follow steps for Skill 18.5.1, Preparing Injections.

Procedure

1. Take prepared injection to client's room, perform medication safety checks using medication administration record.
2. Identify client using two client identifiers.
3. Explain procedure and purpose to client.
4. Perform hand hygiene and don gloves if exposure is anticipated.
5. Select lesion-free injection site on undersurface, upper third of forearm for skin testing.
6. Cleanse area with antimicrobial wipe and allow to dry.
7. Remove needle guard.
8. Grasp the client's dorsal forearm to gently pull the skin taut on ventral forearm.
9. Holding syringe almost parallel to skin, insert needle at a 10- to 15-degree angle with bevel facing up, about ⅛ in. ❶ Needle point should be visible under skin. DO NOT ASPIRATE.

❶ Insert needle with bevel up for intradermal injection.

10. Inject medication slowly, observing for a wheal (blister) formation ❷ and blanching at the site. ➤ *Rationale:* This indicates that the medication was injected within the dermis. If no wheal develops, injection was given too deeply.
11. Withdraw needle at same angle as inserted. Pat area gently with dry gauze sponge, but DO NOT MASSAGE. ➤ *Rationale:* Massaging could disperse medication.
12. Activate needle safety feature and discard syringe unit in puncture-proof container.

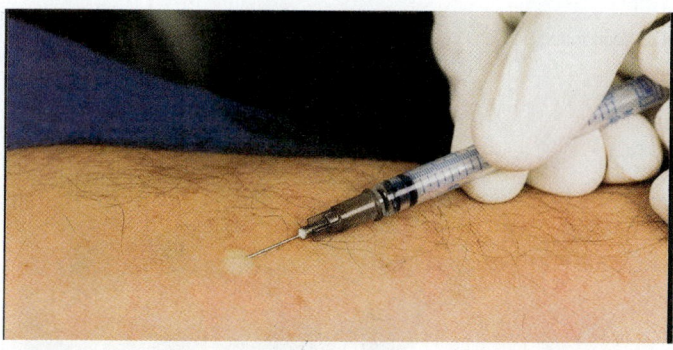

❷ Inject solution to form wheal on skin.

13. Mark injection site with pen for future assessment.
14. Return client to comfortable position.
15. Dispose of gloves and perform hand hygiene.
16. Record site and antigen in client's record.

> **CLINICAL ALERT**
>
> For tuberculin testing, instruct client to return and have the site checked by the healthcare provider in 48–72 hr.

Skill 18.5.3 | Administering Subcutaneous Injections

Equipment

Nonirritating medication
3-mL syringe with ⅝-in. needle (usually 25–27 gauge)
Antimicrobial wipe
Dry gauze sponge
Nonsterile gloves if indicated (Box 18-11 ▪)

Preparation

See steps for Skill 18.5.1, Preparing Injections.

Procedure

1. Take prepared injection to client's room. Perform medication safety checks using medication administration record.
2. Identify client using two client identifiers.
3. Explain procedure and purpose to client.
4. Perform hand hygiene and don gloves.
5. Select fatty site for injection (e.g., abdomen, avoiding 2-in. radius around umbilicus), alternating sites for each injection.
   ➤ **Rationale:** This prevents repeated trauma to tissue.

6. Cleanse area with antimicrobial wipe and allow to dry.
7. Remove needle guard.
8. Use thumb and forefinger and gently grasp loose area ("pinch an inch") of fatty tissue on appropriate site (e.g., posterior-lateral aspect, middle third of arm).
   ➤ **Rationale:** This ensures insertion of medication within subcutaneous tissue, not muscle.

Note: This action is not necessary when there is substantial fatty tissue.

9. Hold syringe like a dart between the thumb and forefinger.
10. Insert needle at a 45- or 90-degree angle. A 90-degree angle is used more commonly due to short needles on prepackaged syringes. ➤ **Rationale:** Angle varies with the amount of subcutaneous tissue, selected site, and needle length.
11. Inject medication slowly, 10 sec/mL.
12. When injection is complete withdraw needle and activate needle safety feature.

Box 18-11 **GLOVING PROTOCOL FOR INJECTIONS**

The CDC has no regulations concerning the wearing of gloves during injections. OSHA recommends that gloves are not necessary when administering IM or subcutaneous injections, as long as bleeding that could result in hand contact with blood (or other potentially infectious material) is not anticipated.

The practice of whether or not to wear gloves for subcutaneous or IM injections is based on judgment. Hospital policy may dictate gloving protocol for injections.

If wearing gloves for mass inoculations, nurses must change gloves between clients and perform hand hygiene. Therefore, nurses may choose not to wear gloves in these situations (CDC, 2011).

(continued)

Skill 18.5.3 | Administering Subcutaneous Injections (continued)

CLINICAL ALERT

Irritating medications such as Vistaril must not be administered subcutaneously, or tissue necrosis may result. Such medications should be administered intramuscularly in the ventrogluteal site using the Z-track method.

13. Discard needle/syringe unit in a puncture-proof container. ❶
14. Return client to position of comfort.
15. Discard gloves and perform hand hygiene.
16. Record medication and site used.

❶ Discard syringe in biohazard container following injection.

Skill 18.5.4 | Preparing Insulin Injections

Note: Insulin pumps are discussed later in this chapter; see Box 18-13.

Equipment
Insulin(s) vials

    Unopened vials of insulin should be stored in refrigerator. Opened vial of insulin may be refrigerated or kept at room temperature; recommend discard after 28 days.

    Insulin should not be exposed to light or to temperatures over 80°F.

Do not use insulin that has clumping, frosting, or precipitation.

Insulin syringe: available in 3/10 mL, 1/2 mL, and 1 mL sizes (**Note:** Syringes are no longer called U40, U100, etc.)

Needles: 29- to 31-gauge short needles

Antimicrobial swab

Dry gauze sponge

Clean gloves if indicated

Preparation
1. Follow steps for Skill 18.5.1, Preparing Injections.
2. Obtain client's blood glucose level *before preparation* to determine appropriate administration of insulin. See Chapter 20 (Specimen Collection) for finger stick blood.

Newly Diagnosed Client with Diabetes
a. Explain to client that the dose of short-acting insulin must be adjusted according to blood glucose test results.
b. Explain that there is a variation in levels—the lowest blood glucose level is before meals and highest 1–2 hr after meals.
c. Goal of treatment is to eliminate wide swings in glucose levels.

Procedure
One Insulin Solution
1. Perform hand hygiene.
2. Turn intermediate or long-acting (cloudy) insulin vial top-to-bottom 10 times. ➤ *Rationale:* This brings cloudy insulin

solution into suspension. Clear insulins do not require this. See Table 18-1 ■ for types of insulin.
3. Wipe top of insulin bottle with antimicrobial swab.
4. Remove needle guard and place on tray.

CLINICAL ALERT

Hypoglycemia is the most common adverse effect of insulins. Client should wear Med-Alert bracelet/ID to alert others. The client should be instructed to carry at least 15 g of fast-acting sugar (e.g., glucose tablet, 1 tbsp sugar, jelly, honey) to be taken in the event of a hypoglycemic reaction.

CLINICAL ALERT

Do not shake insulin vial, as this destroys insulin potency. Rolling the vial fails to bring insulin into suspension. Turn the vial top to bottom 8–10 times instead.

5. Pull plunger of syringe down to desired amount of medication (e.g., 12 units). With vial upright, inject amount of air into air space, not into insulin solution.
    ➤ *Rationale:* Injecting air directly into insulin solution causes bubbles.
6. Withdraw ordered amount of insulin into syringe.
7. Validate medication record, insulin bottle, and prepared syringe with an RN for accuracy. ➤ *Rationale:* Double-checking insulin helps safeguard against errors.
8. Remove needle from vial and expel air from syringe.
9. Replace needle guard.
10. Take medication to client's room.
11. Follow steps for administration of medications by subcutaneous injection. ❶–❹

Two Insulin Solutions
1. Check medication orders.
2. Perform hand hygiene.

3. Follow steps for combining medications in one syringe using two vials.
4. Turn cloudy insulin **Bottle (A)** top to bottom 8–10 times.
   ➤ *Rationale:* This brings cloudy solution into *suspension*.
5. Wipe top of both insulin bottles with alcohol swab.
6. Take needle guard off and place on tray.

> **CLINICAL ALERT**
> The IV route is superior for administering RAPID OR SHORT-ACTING insulin to an obese client. Adipose tissue slows onset of insulin action.

> **CLINICAL ALERT**
> Long-acting insulin, LANTUS (glargine) and Levemir (detemir), are clear solutions. These are *not* to be mixed with any other type of insulin or solution. They are administered subcutaneously and are not intended for IV use.

❶ Select site on lateral aspect of mid-upper arm for subcutaneous injection.

❸ Sites for subcutaneous injections given routinely. (Avoid umbilicus area.) Abdomen site preferred for insulin injection as absorption is more predictable.

❷ Insert needle at 45- or 90-degree angle, using short needle for subcutaneous injection.

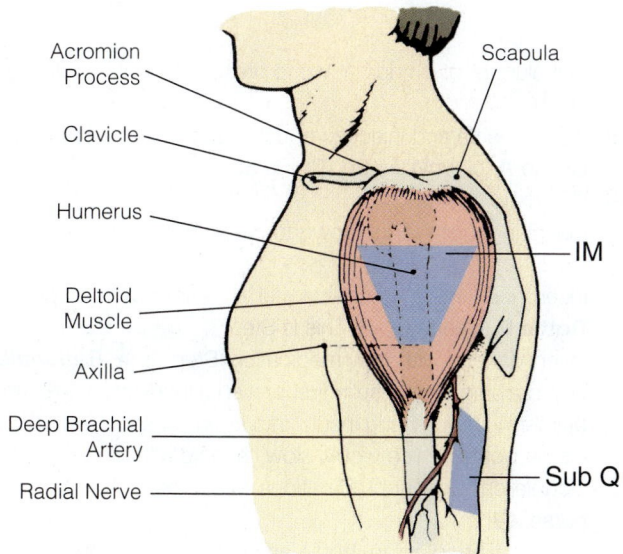

❹ Use upper shaded triangle for IM injection in upper arm; use lower shaded area for subcutaneous injection.

(continued)

Skill 18.5.4 | Preparing Insulin Injections (continued)

Table 18-1 Insulin Types and Therapeutic Action (in Minutes/Hours)

Types	Inject	Onset	Peak	Duration
Very Rapid Acting (clear solution)				
Humalog (lispro)	Within 15 min AC* or immediately PC* NovoLog (aspart) Within 5–10 min AC	5–15 min	30–90 min	3–5 hr
Apidra (glulisine)	15 min AC or within 20 min after *starting* a meal			
Short Acting (clear solution)				
Novolin R	Per order	0.5–1 hr	2–4 hr	5–7 hr
Humulin R	Within 30–60 min AC			
Intermediate Acting (cloudy solution)				
Humulin N (NPH [neutral protamine Hagedorn])	Per order	1–2 hr	6–10 hr	16–24 hr
Novolin N (NPH)	Per order			
Mixtures (cloudy solution)				
Novolin 70/30 (70% NPH, 30% Regular)	Per order	30 min	R-2–4 hr	24 hr
Humulin 70/30 (70% NPH, 30% Regular)	Within 30–60 min AC		N-6–10 hr	
Humulin 50/50 (50% NPH, 50% Regular)		15 min	1 hr	
Humalog 75/25 *(75% lispro protamine suspension, 25% lispro)*	Within 15 min AC			
Humalog 50/50 *(50% lispro protamine suspension, 50% lispro)*	Within 15 min AC			
NovoLog 70/30 *(70% aspart protamine suspension, 30% aspart)*	Within 15 min AC			
Long Acting				
Lantus (glargine) *(clear solution)*	Daily	4–6 hr	No peak	24 hr
Levemir (detemir) *(clear solution)*				

Note: Insulin is biologically engineered through the process of recombinant DNA technology. Insulin is produced by various companies who use different names for short-, intermediate-, or long-acting forms of insulin or their mixtures.
*AC = before meals; PC = after meals

7. Pull plunger of syringe down to prescribed units of cloudy insulin.
8. Insert needle and inject air equal to cloudy dose into upright **Bottle A** (*cloudy*) insulin. This is Step 1. ❺
9. Withdraw needle.
10. Pull plunger of syringe down to prescribed units of clear insulin.
11. Insert needle and inject air equal to clear dose into upright **Bottle B** (*clear*) insulin. This is Step 2.
12. Invert vial and withdraw medication (Step 3). ➤ *Rationale:* Withdrawing *clear* insulin first prevents inadvertent injection of intermediate-acting insulin into rapid- or short-acting insulin bottle, which would slow its rapid action.
13. Double-check your preparations with another nurse. ❻
14. Withdraw needle from bottle and expel all air bubbles.
15. Invert **Bottle A** and insert needle (Step 4). Take care not to inject any rapid or short-acting (*clear*) insulin into

intermediate-acting (*cloudy*) insulin bottle. This can be avoided by holding steady pressure on plunger when inserting needle into bottle.
16. Pull back on plunger to obtain exact prescribed amount of intermediate or long-acting insulin. The total insulin dose now includes both the clear insulin, previously drawn up into syringe, and the intermediate cloudy insulin you have just drawn up.

CLINICAL ALERT
Do not massage site after injection of certain drugs such as insulin or heparin because this hastens absorption and drug action and may cause tissue irritation.

17. Withdraw needle from bottle and replace needle guard.
18. Follow protocol for administration of medications by subcutaneous injections.

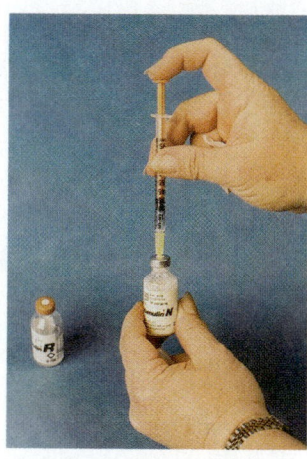

⑤ Step 1: Inject prescribed amount of air into intermediate-acting (cloudy) insulin vial—withdraw needle without needle touching solution. See Box 18-12 ■ for information on premixing insulins.

Step 2: Inject prescribed amount of air into rapid- or short-acting (clear) insulin vial. Do not withdraw needle.

Step 3: Invert vial of rapid or short-acting insulin; withdraw prescribed amount of medication and withdraw needle from vial.

Step 4: Invert intermediate-acting insulin vial and withdraw exact amount without injecting insulin into bottle.

Box 18-12   **PREMIXING TYPES OF INSULIN**

- Mixtures of rapid-acting (Humalog) and intermediate- or long-acting insulin should be administered within 10 min before a meal.
- Mixtures of NPH and regular (short-acting) insulin should be administered 20–30 min before a meal.
- Mixtures may be stored in refrigerator for up to 30 days and should be gently inverted before injection.

CLINICAL ALERT

Insulin type and brand should remain consistent for an individual client.

⑥ Double-check insulin dose with a second nurse to help prevent errors in preparation.

Skill 18.5.5 | Using an Insulin Pen

Equipment

Insulin delivery device labeled with client's name: prefilled pen or cartridge with correct insulin type with instructions for use
Device-compatible needle
Antimicrobial swab

Preparation

1. Perform hand hygiene.
2. Identify client.
3. Complete the first "five rights" validation again before administering insulin. **Note:** The sixth right is documentation and is not indicated here. ➤ **Rationale:** The client may be receiving more than one type of insulin.

Procedure

1. Remove pen cap and insert insulin cartridge (if indicated).
2. Turn pen up and down at least 10 times if indicated. ➤ **Rationale:** This creates suspension of cloudy insulin.
3. Wipe pen's rubber stopper with antimicrobial swab before placing pen needle.
4. Remove needle cap and screw needle onto the pen immediately before injecting.

(continued)

Skill 18.5.5 | Using an Insulin Pen *(continued)*

CLINICAL ALERT

Insulin injection "dial a dose" pens contain a prefilled multidose cartridge available with various types of insulin.

- The pen is intended for single-client use.
- Do not aspirate contents out of the pen cartridge with a needle, because then pen calibration will no longer be accurate.
- A sterile disposable needle is attached for each injection.
- An "air shot" primes the needle before the appropriate dose (units) of insulin is dialed for injection.

After initial use, device may be kept for 28 days. Most devices are not to be stored in the refrigerator nor to be exposed to excessive heat.

5. Pull cover off needle.
6. Hold pen with needle up and tap cartridge to move air bubbles to top of cartridge.
7. Dial pen dose selector to 2 units.
8. Keeping needle pointing upward, press push button until dose selector returns to "0." ▶ **Rationale:** This will allow an "air shot" to clear cartridge of air and prime needle before injection. ❶ A drop of insulin should show at the needle tip. *Do not recap after priming needle.*
9. Check that dose selector is set at "0," and then dial required number of insulin units to be injected; listen for a click for each unit dialed.
10. Swab client's injection site.
11. Insert needle perpendicular (90-degree angle) to the skin, maintaining constant pressure. The needle is in the subcutaneous tissue when the shield completely retracts (½ in.) and touches the insulin reservoir. ❷

12. Using your thumb, press pen "push button" completely and keep depressed, counting to 10 after plunger has returned to "0" position before removing needle from skin.

Note: There may be a drop of residual fluid left on skin after injection due to fall back into shield with priming.

13. Do not massage the area.
14. Remove retracted pen needle from device and dispose in sharps container. ▶ **Rationale:** A new needle must be used for each injection.
15. Replace pen/device cap and store according to directions.

CLINICAL ALERT

An FDA alert reminds healthcare providers that single-client insulin pens and insulin cartridges must not be used for multiple clients, even if needles are changed, due to risk of transmitting bloodborne pathogens.

Note: Insulin pumps are another method of delivery of insulin (Box 18-13 ■).

CLINICAL ALERT

Insulin pump management and education should be done by a certified diabetes educator who is also a certified insulin pump trainer.

CLINICAL ALERT

If insulin must be discontinued (e.g., for MRI, CT scan), the pump should be disconnected. Blood glucose level should be checked before disconnecting and upon reconnecting. Ketoacidosis can occur within 2 hr if insulin delivery is interrupted.

❶ Air shot clears cartridge and needle of air and primes needle for injection.

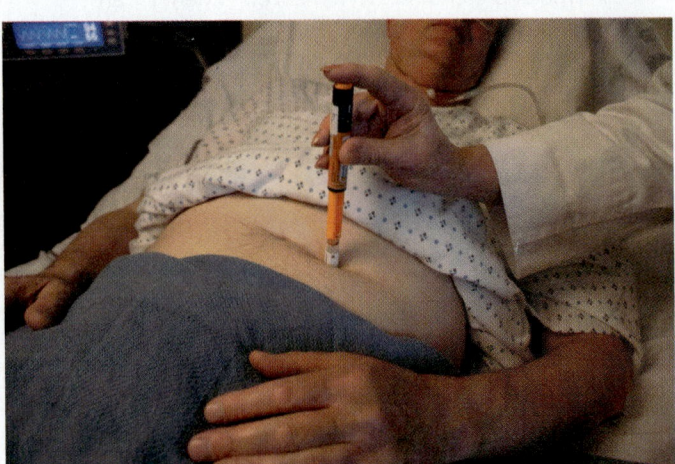

❷ Press pen firmly on client's abdomen to engage needle; inject dialed units and hold 10 sec before releasing. Remove needle, dispose in sharps receptacle. Recap and return pen to storage area for future use.

Box 18-13 THE CLIENT WITH AN INSULIN PUMP

- Continuous Subcutaneous Insulin Infusion (CSII) is a form of intensive insulin therapy utilized as an alternative to multiple daily injections in an attempt to achieve optimal glycemic control and decrease risk of long-term complications of diabetes. Insulin pumps are manufactured by a number of companies that provide 24-hr emergency and clinical specialists to assist clients with start-up of their pump. All models consist of a battery-powered pump with insulin reservoir, an infusion catheter, and microcomputer that allows programming to deliver basal and bolus doses according to the healthcare provider's orders. Only rapid- or short-acting insulin is used.
- CSII more closely mimics release of insulin by the pancreas with continuous-delivery basal and bolus insulin infusions.
- Basal rate or rates refers to the amount of insulin delivered (units per hour) to keep blood glucose levels in target range between meals and overnight.
- A bolus is an additional amount of insulin delivered immediately before meals or for episodes of hyperglycemia, the greatest risk associated with insulin pump therapy.
- The client should be referred to a certified diabetes educator before the start of pump use. Insulin boluses will be based on blood glucose readings and carbohydrate grams intake.

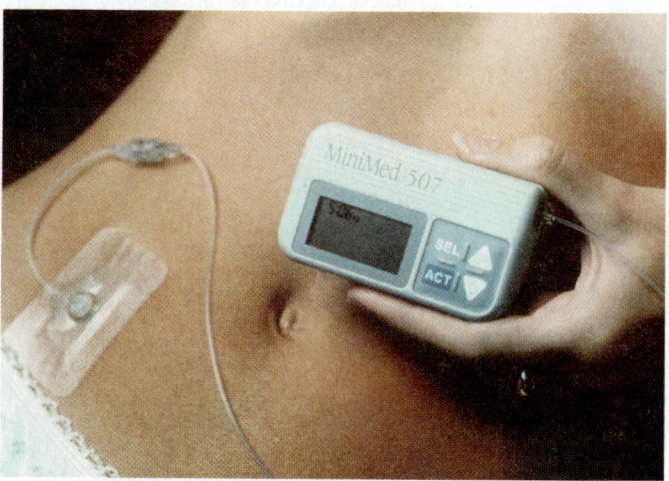

MiniMed 507 Insulin Pump attached to infusion set. Abdominal site is preferred because insulin absorption is faster and most predictable.

- The client performs frequent fingerstick blood glucose checks: before adjusting any insulin dose, fasting, before meals, 2 hr after eating, at bedtime, and at 3 a.m. once weekly.
- A lifestyle advantage is flexibility: Insulin needs can be tailored to changes in schedule (meal time, exercise, or sleep).

Skill 18.5.6 | Administering Subcutaneous Anticoagulants (Heparin, Low-Molecular-Weight Heparin [LMWH])

Equipment

Heparin in vial (*carefully note units per mL*)
1-mL tuberculin syringe or unit-dose syringe with small (25–29)-gauge needle ❶
or
Low-molecular-weight heparin (LMWH) in prefilled syringe
Antimicrobial swab
Dry gauze sponge
Gloves (if indicated)

Preparation

1. See Skill 18.5.1, Preparing Injections.
2. Double-check heparin calculated dose with another nurse.
3. Perform hand hygiene.

Note: To avoid loss of drug, do not clear prefilled syringe needle of air before injecting LMWH.

❶ Low-molecular-weight heparin and needle.

(continued)

Skill 18.5.6 | Administering Subcutaneous Anticoagulants (Heparin, Low-Molecular-Weight Heparin [LMWH]) *(continued)*

CLINICAL ALERT

Heparin is available in a variety of strengths (e.g., 1,000, 2,500, 5,000, 10,000, 25,000 units per mL vials). *Carefully* check vial units per mL before drawing into syringe and have another nurse double-check your calculations and prepared injection.

CLINICAL ALERT

Subcutaneous injection of low-molecular-weight heparin (LMWH) involves low doses that help prevent clot formation but do not alter blood coagulation studies and do not require coagulation monitoring as does unfractionated heparin.

Procedure

1. Check client's record for site of previous injection.
   ➤ *Rationale:* Injections should be rotated to prevent local postinjection complications.
2. Take prepared injection to client's room, and perform medication safety checks against medication administration record.
3. Identify client using two client identifiers.
4. Provide privacy.
5. Explain procedure and purpose to client.
6. Don gloves (if indicated).
7. Assist client to supine position.
8. Select site on client's lower abdomen (at least two fingerbreadths from umbilicus) or select area of fatty tissue above iliac crest.➤ *Rationale:* Anticoagulants should not be administered IM or in the extremities.
9. Avoid ecchymotic area or lesions.
10. Cleanse site gently with antimicrobial swab, and allow to dry.
11. Gently pinch an inch of subcutaneous tissue (fat roll) between thumb and forefinger of nondominant hand and hold fat pad throughout injection.
12. Hold syringe between thumb and forefinger of dominant hand and insert full length of needle into skinfold at a 90-degree angle.
13. Inject medication slowly. *Do not aspirate first.* ➤ *Rationale:* Aspiration can rupture small vessels and increase risk of bleeding into tissue.

Note: Press prefilled syringe plunger rod firmly as far as it will go.

14. Wait 10 sec before gently withdrawing needle at same angle in which it entered skin. ➤ *Rationale:* This allows medication to absorb into tissue and minimizes bruising.

Note: Release of plunger will cause needle to retract into the security sleeve as it automatically withdraws from the skin.

15. Press and hold dry gauze sponge over injection site.
    ➤ *Rationale:* This prevents backtracking of medication.
16. Do not massage area. ➤ *Rationale:* Massaging the site may cause bruising. ❷

17. Activate needle safety feature and discard syringe in puncture-proof container. ❸
18. Return client to position of comfort.
19. Remove gloves and perform hand hygiene.
20. Document injection.

❷ To prevent tissue damage and bruising, *do not aspirate or massage* anticoagulant injections.

❸ Activate needle safety feature; then, dispose of syringe in sharps container.

Skill 18.5.7 | Administering Intramuscular (IM) Injections

Equipment
Medication vial or ampule
3-mL syringe with 1–1½ in. needle (21–23 gauge)
Antimicrobial swab
Dry gauze sponge
Gloves (if indicated)

Preparation
See Skill 18.5.1, Preparing Injections.

— Epidermis
— Dermis

— Subcutaneous Tissue

— Muscle

Intramuscular

1 Insert needle at 90-degree angle for IM injections into muscle.

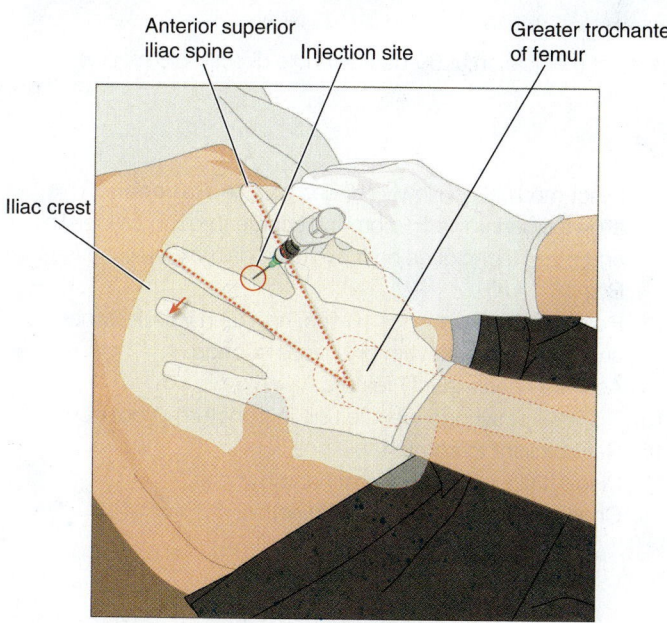

Anterior superior iliac spine   Injection site   Greater trochanter of femur

Iliac crest

2 Overlay of hand shows area of injection into ventrogluteal site for IM injections (client's right side).

Procedure
1. Check client's record for site of previous IM injections.
   ➤ *Rationale:* IM injections should be rotated to prevent local postinjection complications.
2. Take prepared injection to client's room; perform medication safety checks against medication administration record.
3. Identify client using two client identifiers.
4. Explain procedure to client.
5. Provide privacy for client.
6. Perform hand hygiene and don gloves, if indicated.
7. Select injection site, identifying bony landmarks. Consider client's size and amount and viscosity of medication being injected. Alternate sites each time injections are given. **1**–**8**
8. Cleanse area with antimicrobial swab and allow to dry.
9. Spread skin taut between thumb and forefinger (grasping muscle is acceptable in pediatric and geriatric clients with less fatty tissue) to ensure needle placement in muscle belly.
10. Insert needle perpendicular (90-degree angle) to the muscle, using a quick, darting motion. ➤ *Rationale:* This angle facilitates medication reaching muscle.

3 Locate greater trochanter and anterior superior iliac spine.

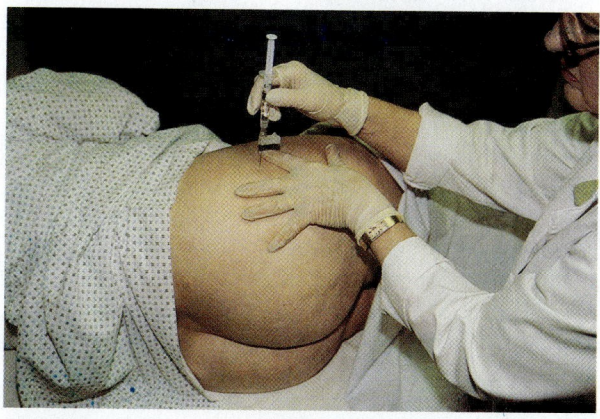

4 Place palm at trochanter and index finger at anterior superior iliac spine; fan remaining fingers posteriorly.

(continued)

Skill 18.5.7 | Administering Intramuscular (IM) Injections (continued)

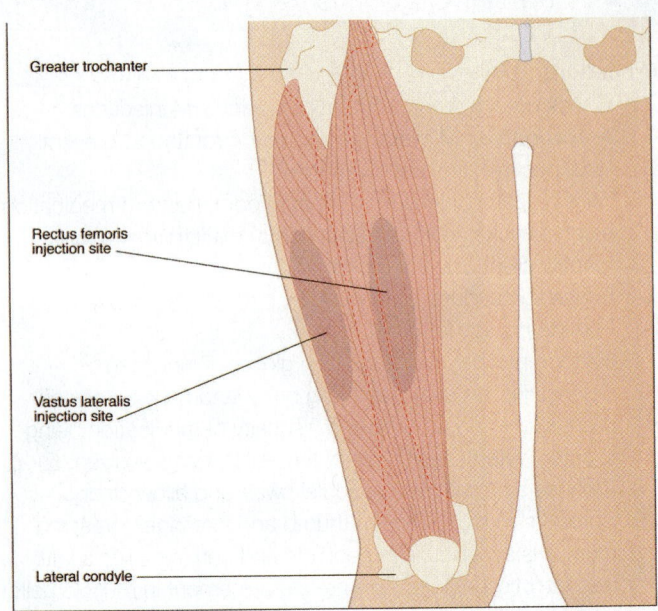

Greater trochanter

Rectus femoris injection site

Vastus lateralis injection site

Lateral condyle

5 Shaded area indicates site location for vastus lateralis injection.

6 Select site one hand's breadth below greater trochanter and one hand's breadth above knee for vastus lateralis injection.

7 Site is middle third of anterior-lateral aspect of thigh. Avoid the rectus femoris muscle (anterior thigh).

8 Inject medication at 90-degree angle directly into muscle.

11. Decision Point: Although aspiration is not indicated for IM injections of vaccines and immunizations, it is indicated for certain medications to check for blood (see Evidence-Based Practice box). It is strongly recommended to check with facility policy before aspirating any IM injection. To aspirate, pull back on plunger for 5–10 sec; if blood returns, discard the needle and prepare a new injection. ➤ *Rationale:* Aspiration causes discomfort and should be avoided unless necessary. The appearance of blood indicates needle has entered a blood vessel. IM medication must not be injected directly into bloodstream.

12. Inject medication slowly (10 sec/mL). ➤ *Rationale:* This allows time for medication to disperse through tissue. This and other techniques help minimize pain on injection (see Box 18-14 ■).

13. Hold needle in place for 10 sec, and then withdraw needle and massage area with dry gauze sponge.

14. Activate needle safety feature.

15. Dispose of syringe–needle unit in puncture-proof container.

16. Return client to comfortable position.

17. Discard gloves and perform hand hygiene.

18. Chart medication and site of injection.

Box 18-14 **TECHNIQUES FOR MINIMIZING PAIN DURING IM INJECTIONS**

- Encourage client to relax.
- Use a new needle for injection.
- Place client on side with upper knee flexed for ventrogluteal injection.
- Have client place hand on hip to relax deltoid muscle.
- Avoid injecting into sensitive or hardened tissue.
- Apply pressure to site for 10 sec before injecting.
- Ensure that needle length reaches muscle for IM injection.

- Prevent antiseptic from clinging to needle during insertion by waiting until skin prep is dry.
- Reduce puncture pain by "darting" needle quickly into muscle.
- Use as small a gauge needle as possible.
- Inject medication slowly (10 sec/mL).
- Hold needle in place for 10 sec after injecting medication.
- Maintain grasp on syringe; do not move needle once inserted.
- Withdraw needle quickly after injection.
- Use Z-track technique.
- EMLA cream may be applied 30–40 min before injection.

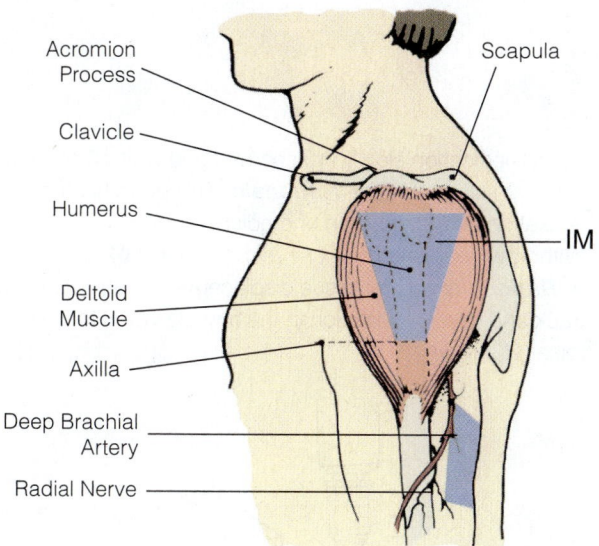

Locate deltoid site in the area between two fingerbreadths below the acromion process and anterior axillary fold.

Inject medication into deltoid area site.

EVIDENCE-BASED PRACTICE

Blood Aspiration

Crawford and Johnson (2012) performed an integrative review to seek clarity about the need for blood aspiration in vaccinations and immunizations. They immediately identified a history in which aspiration was taught or not over the past 40 years depending on several variables. They found there were two camps among nurses. In an informal poll of 40 nurses, about 50% aspirated and 50% did not. Those who had learned to aspirate continued to aspirate, and those who had not learned to aspirate, continued to omit this step. They found no association between age or demographics and whether a nurse did or did not aspirate before injecting. (*Aspiration for blood* is 5–10 sec of slow withdrawal of tissue fluid followed by 5–10 sec of slow administration of medication and slow withdrawal of the needle.)

Leading authorities, including the American Academy of Pediatrics (2012), the Advisory Committee on Immunization Practices (2011), and the World Health Organization (2004), have stated that the practice of aspirating for blood is not necessary for IM or subcutaneous immunizations and vaccines, because large blood vessels are not present at the recommended injection sites (CDC, 2011). The AAP, ACIP, and WHO do not recommend aspiration for subcutaneous immunizations or administration of heparin or insulin.

Crawford and Johnson (2012) and Rishovd (2014) found no evidence to indicate that—for subcutaneous or IM immunizations—aspiration with or without blood return confirmed correct needle placement and therefore eliminated the possibility of injecting an IM medication into the bloodstream. They did find suggestions that eliminating the discomfort of aspiration had no harmful effects and that omitting aspiration in this setting especially benefited young children who receive numerous immunizations. Reviewers determined that complications of injections generally resulted from incorrect site, needle size, needle gauge, or needle angle. They suggest that correct angle and correct placement for immunization injections virtually eliminate the possibility of injection into a vein.

These reviewers state that aspiration with certain medications such as penicillin may still be needed. They also state that aspiration is used as a precaution for administration of allergy medications, because inadvertent entry of those drugs into the bloodstream could lead to systemic reaction.

Based on their review of the evidence in outpatient settings, the authors make the following recommendations:

- Aspiration is not indicated for IM injections of vaccines and immunizations.

(continued)

Skill 18.5.7 | Administering Intramuscular (IM) Injections *(continued)*

- Aspiration is not indicated for subcutaneous injections of immunizations, heparin, and insulin.
- Aspiration may be indicated for IM injections of medications such as penicillin.
- Until a standard can be established, injection techniques must be individualized to the client, the equipment, and the medication being administered.

The researchers acknowledge that as-yet-unreported data could surface indicating that aspiration is effective. They suggest that conflicting best practice guidelines reflect the need to study this process further.

Sources: Crawford & Johnson (2012) and Rishovd (2014)

Skill 18.5.8 | Using Z-Track Method

Equipment
Syringe
Filter needle for preparation
2-in. needle for injection
Medication
Antimicrobial swab
Dry gauze sponge
Gloves (if indicated)

Preparation
See Skill 18.5.1, Preparing Injections.

Procedure
1. Use filter needle to draw up prescribed medication into syringe.
2. Attach new 2-in. sterile needle to syringe. ➤ *Rationale:* A new needle prevents introducing medication that could be irritating to tissue. A long needle allows medication to go deep into the muscle.

> **CLINICAL ALERT**
> The Z-track method prevents "tracking" (leakage of medication upward along the track of the injection) and is recommended for administering medications into the ventrogluteal or vastus lateralis sites.

3. Take prepared injection to client's room. Perform medication safety checks using medication administration record.
4. Identify client using two client identifiers.
5. Provide privacy.
6. Explain procedure and purpose to client.
7. Perform hand hygiene and don gloves (if indicated).
8. Position client for ventrogluteal or vastus lateralis injection.
9. Cleanse site with antimicrobial swab.
10. Pull skin 1–1.5 in. (2.5–3.8 cm) laterally away from injection site. ➤ *Rationale:* This tissue displacement creates a track that keeps medication from seeping into subcutaneous tissue.
11. Maintain displacement and insert needle at a 90-degree angle. Aspirate by pulling back on plunger (5–10 sec) to see if needle is in blood vessel. If so, discard and prepare new injection.

12. Inject medication slowly (10 sec/mL) and wait 10 seconds, keeping skin taut. ❶ ➤ *Rationale:* This permits muscle relaxation and absorption of medication.
13. Withdraw needle and release retracted skin. ❷
    ➤ *Rationale:* Lateral tissue displacement interrupts needle track and seals medication in the muscle when the tissue is released.

Z-Track Injection

❶ Z-track injection. Maintaining displacement, insert needle at 90-degree angle. Aspirate by pulling back on plunger, checking to see if needle is in blood vessel. If blood is aspirated, discard and prepare new injection.

Medication

❷ Z-track injection, after displacement released. Method is used to prevent backflow of medications into subcutaneous tissue.

14. Apply light pressure with dry gauze sponge. Do not massage. ➤ *Rationale:* Massage may disperse medication into subcutaneous tissue and cause tissue irritation.
15. Activate needle safety feature.
16. Return client to a position of comfort and safety.
17. Discard gloves and equipment in appropriate area.
18. Perform hand hygiene.

19. Document administration of medication in the medication record.

> **CLINICAL ALERT**
>
> If client is obese, use a 2- to 3-in. needle so that medication is absorbed into muscle (not fat) tissue and blood level of drug is achieved.

Unit 18.5 Documentation and Evaluation

DOCUMENTATION for Parenteral Medications

Client's Medication Record

- Time administered
- Name of medication
- Dosage
- Route
- Injection site
- Initials of nurse administering medication
- Signature by nurse (to identify initials)

Nurses' Notes

- Documentation of prn, STAT, intradermal, and one-time-only medications
- Name of medication, dosage, route, site, time administered
- Client's pre- and postinjection assessment findings (sedation and pain rating, any relevant laboratory data)
- Signature of nurse
- For vaccines and immunizations, the lot number and expiration date must be documented

EVALUATION/Critical Thinking

Expected Outcomes

- Injection is administered without complications.
- Injection is as painless as possible.
- Medication therapeutic effect is achieved.

Unexpected Outcomes	Alternative Actions
Ecchymosis occurs after heparin injection.	• Rotate injection site. Do not inject medication into ecchymotic area. • Do not aspirate before injection or massage site after needle withdrawal. • Do not pinch tightly when forming fat pad in preparation for injection site. • Apply ice to area before injecting heparin.
Client experiences pain with IM injection.	• Use Z-track method for ventrogluteal or vastus lateralis sites to prevent medication from leaking into subcutaneous tissue. • Use new needle for injection. • Inject medication slowly (10 sec/mL) to allow medication to diffuse. • Hold needle in place for 10 sec after injection. • Use a dry gauze sponge to apply pressure to site after withdrawing needle.

(continued)

Unexpected Outcomes	**Alternative Actions**
• Medication is administered using wrong parenteral route.	• Notify healthcare provider; medications may need to be administered to reverse the action of the medication. • Monitor client's response closely and report adverse findings immediately. • Medication administered IM or IV rather than subcutaneous route leads to faster absorption rates; therefore, ongoing assessment must be done to determine effects. (IV administration has immediate action.) • Complete unusual occurrence report according to agency policy.
• Client has allergic or anaphylactic response to medication.	• Call rapid response team immediately. • Maintain a patent airway and follow ABCs of emergency care. • Notify client's healthcare provider. • Document incident; place allergy alert bracelet on client. • Complete unusual occurrence report according to agency policy.
• Obese client fails to obtain pain relief from subcutaneous injection.	• Consult pain management team. • Consider weight-based dosage. • Obtain order to change to IV route for analgesic administration since adipose tissue has decreased perfusion and subcutaneous medication uptake is unpredictable.

Chapter Wrap-Up

GERONTOLOGIC Considerations

Older clients take more medications than any other age group, largely because of chronic illness. Risk of adverse drug events rises with comorbidity. *Major problems with prescriptive drugs in older adults include the following:*

• Drug–drug interactions—older adults may use multiple healthcare providers and pharmacies, each unaware of what others have prescribed, creating risk of taking two or more medications to treat the same condition.

• Medication errors—the more medications an individual takes, the greater risk of medication error (people over age 75 take an average of 17 prescriptions annually).

• Poor adherence—not taking right dose at right time or discontinuing drug without consultation; common due to lack of understanding about reason to take drug and general knowledge base of drug action. Older adults may have difficulty reading labels and directions and opening medicine containers.

• Unpredictable drug action—age-related physiologic changes and comorbid conditions affect drug utilization (absorption, distribution, metabolism, and elimination).

• Drug side effects not recognized—older adults are not aware or do not understand potential dangerous side effects of drugs.

- Inadequate monitoring—older adults are often alone or not monitored consistently, so drug problems are not identified.
  - Cost of drugs—multiple medications are costly for many older adults, so they may reduce the frequency of dosing or stop taking a drug.

Older Adults Are at Risk for Drug Toxicity.

- Drug absorption is altered; oral route is slower, but complete; topical route absorption may increase due to thin skin.
- Drug distribution is altered; increased percentage of body fat in older adults results in longer storage of fat-soluble medications. Older adults have proportionately less body water, so blood levels of a water-soluble drug may be higher than usual.

- Decreased blood flow through the liver slows medication metabolism.
- Altered renal excretion slows drug excretion.
- Reduced protein level (increased ratio of fat to muscle) decreases medication binding and increases free circulating drug levels.
- Increased CNS sensitivity to drugs that interfere with neurotransmitters that regulate brain function.

Drugs Older Adults Should Avoid:

- Sedative/hypnotics
- Tranquilizers (antianxiety medications)
- Anticholinergics (belladonna alkaloids, antispasmodics)

MANAGEMENT Guidelines

Each state legislates a Nurse Practice Act for RNs and LVN/LPNs. Healthcare facilities are responsible for establishing and implementing policies and procedures that conform to their state's regulations. Verify the regulations and role parameters for each healthcare worker in your facility.

Delegation

- Registered and licensed vocational nurses are responsible for administering oral and parenteral medications to clients. In some nonacute facilities, such as residential homes, geriatric technicians may administer medications following standard procedures.
- Individuals administering medications must be knowledgeable about the RATIONALE for their use. This insight cues the need for specific pre- and postadministration individual client assessment (responses such as vital signs, lab values, adverse reactions) as an integral part of this deceptively simple skill.
- Unlicensed assistive personnel are not trained (or expected) to obtain and interpret essential client data

necessary for decision making when administering medications. However, if they are assigned to administer daily care, they should be informed what to observe for and report to the RN or LVN/LPN.

Interprofessional Communication

- *Immediately report to healthcare provider:*
  All errors in medication administration (and complete agency variance report)
  Ineffective client responses to medication including adverse responses (vital signs, rash, paradoxical reaction, and the like)
  Reports of abnormal relevant lab data (e.g., toxic drug levels)
- *Report to relief staff:*
  All of the above PLUS:
  Any new or discontinued medication orders prn or STAT, and one-time-only medications given
  Effectiveness of medication therapy

DRUG Supplement

Calculations of Solutions
Types of Solutions

- Volume to volume (vol/vol): A given volume of solute is added to a given volume of solvent.
- Weight to weight (wt/wt): A stated weight of solute is dissolved in a stated weight of solvent.
- Weight to volume (wt/vol): A given weight of solute is dissolved in a given volume of solvent, which results in the proper amount of solution.

Preparing Solutions
Solutions of Varying Strengths

Determine the strength of the solution, the strength of the drug on hand, and the quantity of solution required.

Use this formula for preparing solutions:

$$\frac{D}{H} \times Q = X$$

Where, D = desired strength; H = strength on hand; Q = quantity of solution desired; and X = amount of solute.

Example: You have a 100% solution of hydrogen peroxide on hand. You need a liter of 50% solution.

$$\frac{50}{100} \times 1{,}000 \text{ mL} = 500 \text{ mL (solute)}$$

If the strength desired and strength on hand are not in like terms, you need to change one of the terms.

Example: You have 1 L of 50% solution on hand. You need a liter of 1:10 solution. 1:10 solution is the same as 10%.

$$\frac{10\%}{50\%} \times 1{,}000 \text{ mL} = 200 \text{ mL (solute)}$$

Add 200 mL of the drug to 800 mL of the solvent to make a liter of 10% solution.

Volume-to-Volume Solutions

Use the formula:

$$\frac{D}{H} \times Q = X$$

Example: Prepare a liter of 5% solution from a stock solution of 50%.

$$\frac{5\%}{50\%} \times 1{,}000 \text{ mL} = 100 \text{ mL (solute)}$$

Add 100 mL to 900 mL of diluent to make 1 L of 5% solution.

Solutions From Tablets

Use the formula:

$$\frac{D}{H} \times Q = X$$

where X = amount per number of tablets used.

Example: Prepare 1 L of a 1:1000 solution, using 10-gr tablets.

$$\frac{1/1000}{10 \text{ gr}} \times 1{,}000 \text{ mL} = X$$

First convert 10 gr to grams, so the numerator and denominator are in the same unit of measure. 1 g = 15 gr; therefore 10 gr = 2 mg. Now substitute the new numbers in the formula and solve for X.

$$\frac{1/1000}{2/3} \times \frac{1000}{1} \text{ mL} = X$$

$$\frac{3}{2000} \times \frac{1000}{1} = X$$

$$X = \text{⅔ or 1½ tablets.}$$

Place tablets into the liter of solution and dissolve.

Abbreviations and Symbols

Aa	of each
a.c.	before meals
ad lib.	freely, as desired
BID	twice each day
C	with
C	carbon
Ca	calcium
Cl	chlorine
Et	and
GI	gastrointestinal
gt *or* gtt	drop(s)
H_2O	water
H_2O_2	hydrogen peroxide
IM	intramuscular
K	potassium
lb *or* #	pound
M	meter
mcg	microgram
mEq	milliequivalent
mg	milligram
mL	milliliter
mmol	millimole
Na	sodium
NA	not applicable
NG	nasogastric
NPO	nothing by mouth (Latin *nil per os*)
oob	out of bed

oz	ounce
p.c.	after meals
per	by, through
PO	by mouth (Latin *per os*)
prn *or* PRN	whenever necessary
q.h.	every hour
q.i.d.	four times each day
q.s.	as much as required, quantity sufficient
q2h	every 2 hr
q3h	every 3 hr
q4h	every 4 hr
R_X	treatment, "take thou"
STAT	immediately
S	without
TID	three times each day
tsp	teaspoon
WBC	white blood count
°	degree
−	minus, negative, alkaline reaction
+	plus, positive, acid reaction
%	percent
v	Roman numeral 5
vii	Roman numeral 7
ix	Roman numeral 9
xiii	Roman numeral 13

ABBREVIATION ALERT

Abbreviations to Avoid: Entries marked * are prohibited by The Joint Commission

@ (at) misinterpreted as a 2. Write out "at."

AU (each ear) misinterpreted as OU (each eye). Do not use AU. Also avoid AD (right ear) and AS (left ear).

cc (cubic centimeter) misinterpreted as units. Write "mL" for milliliters.

D/C misinterpreted as discharge or discontinue. Write out "discharge" or "discontinue."

Per os (orally) misinterpreted as OS (left eye). Use "PO."

IN (intranasal) misinterpreted as IM (intramuscular) or IV (intravenous), or as inhaled. Write out "intranasal" and "inhaled."

*IU (international unit) misinterpreted as IV. Write "international unit."

Large doses without properly placed commas (e.g., 100000). Place commas appropriately.

*MS, MSO4, or MgSO4 confused with one another. Write "morphine sulfate," "magnesium sulfate."

*Q.D. (each day) misinterpreted as qid (four times a day). Write "daily."

*Q.O.D., (every other day) misinterpreted as four times a day. Write "every other day."

qhs (at bedtime) misinterpreted as qh (every hour). Write "at bedtime."

SC or SQ, sub q (subcutaneous) misinterpreted as SL for sublingual. "sub q 2 hours before surgery" has been misinterpreted as "every 2 hours before surgery." Write "subcutaneously."

ss (one-half) misinterpreted as 55. Write "one-half" or "½."

SSRI (sliding scale regular insulin) misinterpreted as selective-serotonin reuptake inhibitor. Write out.

*Trailing zero after a decimal point (e.g., 5.0). Use a zero before a decimal point, never after.

*U (unit) misinterpreted as cc, or 0. Write "unit."

µg (microgram) mistaken for milligram. Write "mcg."

X4d (for 4 days) misinterpreted as times three doses. Write out "for four days" or "for 4 days."

Conversion Tables

Household Equivalents (Volume)		
Metric	**Apothecary**	**Household**
0.06 mL		1 drop
5 mL		1 teaspoonful
15 mL		1 tablespoonful
30 mL	1 fluid ounce	2 tablespoonfuls
240 mL	8 fluid ounces	1 glassful

Apothecary Equivalents (Volume)	
Metric	**Apothecary**
30 mL	1 fluid ounce
500 mL	1 pint
1,000 mL (1 L)	1 quart

Metric Equivalents (Weight)	
Metric	**Apothecary**
1.0 g	1,000 mg
0.6 g	600 mg
0.5 g	500 mg
0.3 g	300 mg
0.2 g	200 mg
0.1 g	100 mg
0.06 g	60 mg
0.05 g	50 mg
0.03 g	30 mg
0.015 g	15 mg
0.010 g	10 mg
0.008 g	8 mg

CASE STUDY Applications

Scenario 1

Your client has recently sustained a "brain attack" (stroke), which has caused him to have difficulty swallowing (dysphagia) and places him at risk for aspiration. When the previous shift nurse attempted to have him take his oral medications with water, he coughed and choked violently, so the nurse discontinued efforts to complete his medication administration. One of this client's most important medications is Inderal LA 80 mg, a timed-release capsule that is given once a day. This long-acting capsule cannot be opened and its contents emptied for convenient administration without interfering with the timed-release property of its formulation.

1. What types of consult would provide assistance in decision making about this client's swallowing problem and medication administration?

2. What actions would facilitate this client's swallowing and decrease the risk of aspiration?

3. What alternative method is there for administering the Inderal LA?

4. How will the nurse communicate adjustments in administration to the other staff members?

Scenario 2

This is Nancy Dalaney's third hospitalization for diabetic ketoacidosis this year. She has been an insulin-dependent diabetic for 5 years (since age 9). For several years, Nancy has controlled the condition using two daily insulin injections, a combination of regular and NPH (intermediate-acting) before breakfast and dinner.

This year Nancy made the cheerleading A squad—quite an achievement and an honor—requiring practice before and after school, enrollment in gymnastics class, and participation at evening and weekend games, some of which were out of town. In addition, Nancy must attend cheerleading camp this summer and is preparing for all-state competition trials.

Nancy's condition is stabilized during hospitalization, and shortly before discharge she confides in you that she hates needles, that "the shots really hurt," and, in fact, she prepares the syringes and sometimes just throws them away. In addition, she has experienced low blood sugar on occasion while cheerleading and knows that something happens with her insulin "overreacting" at these times; it makes her uncoordinated and "confused," but she just can't take time out to ingest sugar. She is afraid of losing her position on the A squad—she worked so hard to get there.

1. Based on this data, identify Nancy's psychosocial needs and developmental tasks at age 14.
2. What are the implications of insulin absorption and action as influenced by exercise and site of administration?

3. Describe actions that can decrease pain associated with medication injections.
4. Suggest an alternative way for Nancy to maintain her insulin coverage without discomfort and erratic absorption rates.

Scenario 3

Your older adult client takes many medications at the same time, all for a variety of chronic disorders. She sees several healthcare providers for these various conditions and uses several pharmacies to have prescriptions filled.

When you visit her, she asks you how she can remember to take all her medications, states that she does not take all the pills she should each day, and says that she feels fine anyway, without taking her medications.

1. Why do older adults take so may medications (polypharmacy)?
2. Identify drugs that frequently cause adverse effects in the older adult.
3. Why are older adults more susceptible to adverse drug events?
4. Identify some ways to protect older adult clients from adverse drug events due to polypharmacy.
5. How can the client's medication regimen be simplified to help prevent adverse drug events?

NCLEX® Review Questions

Unless otherwise specified, choose only one (1) answer.

1. What type of medication error is the most common cause of injury?
   A. The wrong client
   B. The wrong medication
   C. The wrong dosage
   D. The wrong route

2. Before administering a medication that appears to be inappropriate for the client, what should the nurse do?
   A. Consult the pharmacist.
   B. Consult the ordering healthcare provider.
   C. Consult the drug manufacturer.
   D. Recheck the medication against the MAR.

3. In general, at what systolic blood pressure should agents that lower blood pressure be held?
   A. Less than 110 mm Hg
   A. Less than 100 mm Hg
   B. Less than 95 mm Hg
   C. Less than 90 mm Hg

4. Which of the following alterations of oral medications are acceptable?

Select all that apply.
   A. Capsules should never be opened.
   B. Beads from capsules may be chewed.
   C. Liquid from capsules can be mixed with food.
   D. Sublingual tablets may be given to the client who is NPO.
   E. Gel-coated tablets can be dissolved to ease swallowing.

5. For what type of eyedrop is the inner canthus pressed to slow absorption?
   A. Those that can cause systemic effects
   B. Those that cause a burning sensation
   C. Those that dilate the pupil
   D. Those that treat eye infections

6. When administering ear drops to an adult, how does the nurse position the pinna?
   A. Upward and backward
   B. Downward and backward
   C. Upward and forward
   D. Downward and forward

7. What are bony landmarks for administering a ventrogluteal injection?

   Select all that apply.

   A. Acromion process

   B. Anterior superior spine of iliac crest

   C. Posterior superior spine of iliac crest

   D. Greater trochanter

   E. Gluteal fold

   F. Upper outer quadrant of buttocks

8. Why should clients keep track of the number of MDI actuations performed?

   A. The canister's remaining contents may have expired.

   B. The canister's remaining contents may be active ingredient only.

   C. The canister's remaining contents may be propellant only.

   D. Clients become drug tolerant before the canister is empty.

9. When preparing an insulin injection using two solutions, what is the proper order of steps to be used?

   A. Add equivalent amount of air to the clear insulin.

   B. Add equivalent amount of air to the cloudy insulin.

   C. Withdraw the cloudy solution.

   D. Withdraw the clear solution.

10. What is the greatest risk associated with use of an insulin pump?

    A. Site infection

    B. Lipodystrophy

    C. Insulin shock

    D. Ketoacidosis

QSEN Activity

Domain: Safety

KSA: Describe the benefits and limitations of selected safety-enhancing technologies:

- Bar codes
- CPOE
- Medication pumps
- Automatic alerts/alarms

Activity:

You are a nurse on a unit and you have been selected to participate on a committee to implement the new medication bar code and computerized order entry system. You have been asked help with the rollout of the new system. Develop an education plan to assist the nurse on the unit as he or she begins to use this new type of technology. Consider some of the barriers to using the new technology and workarounds some nurses might employ if they are in a hurry and the system is not working well.

Bibliography

Adams, M. A., & Urban, C. Q. (2016). *Pharmacology: Connections to nursing practice* (2nd ed.). Hoboken, NJ: Prentice Hall.

Aschenbrenner, D. (2009). Unsafe injection practices put patients at risk. *American Journal of Nursing, 109*(7), 45–47.

Aschenbrenner, D., & Venable, S. (2012). *Drug therapy in nursing* (4th ed). Philadelphia, PA: Wolters Kluwer/Lippincott Williams & Wilkins.

Barclay, L. (2010, Apr. 26). Interruptions linked to medication errors by nurses. *Archives of Internal Medicine, 170*(4), 683–692.

Boullata, J. (2009). Drug administration through an enteral feeding tube. *American Journal of Nursing, 109*(10), 34–41.

Carter-Templeton, J. & McCoy, T. (2008). Are we on the same page? A comparison of intramuscular injection explanations in nursing fundamental texts. *MEDSURG Nursing, 17*(4), 237–240.

Centers for Disease Control (CDC). (2011). General recommendations on immunization: Recommendation of the Advisory Committee on Immunization Practices (ACIP) *MMWR 60*(2) 1–64.

Cescon, D. & Etchells, E. (2008). Barcoded medication administration. *Journal of the American Medical Association, 299*(18), 2, 200.

Cizek, K. E., Estrade, N., Allen, J., & Elsholz, T. (2010). A crystal clear call to standardize color-coded wristbands. *Nursing, 40*(5), 57–59.

Crawford, C. L., & Johnson, J. A. (2012). To aspirate or not: An integrative review of the evidence. *Nursing, 42*(3), 20–25.

Clinical Rounds. (2009, Oct.). Bar codes reduce errors … sometimes. *Nursing, 39*(10), 29–31.

Clinical Rounds. (2009). Hidden hazard in transdermal patches. *Lippincott Nursing Center.* Retrieved from http://nursingcenter.com/JournalArticle?Article_ID=858639&Journal_ID=54016&Issue_ID=858618

Cohen, H. (2008, Apr.). Let's work together to improve medication safety. *Nursing, 38*(4), 6.

Dittrich, K. (2007, Dec.) ACLS update: A new role for medications. *Nursing, 37*(12), 56cc1–56cc3.

Eliopoulos, C. (2009). *Gerontological nursing* (7th ed.). Philadelphia, PA: Lippincott Williams & Wilkins.

Flynn, L., Liang, Y., Dickson, G. L., Xie, M., & Suh, D. C. (2012). Nurses' practice environment, error interception practices, and inpatient medication errors. *Journal of Nursing Scholarship, 44*(2), 180–186.

Food and Drug Administration. (2015) Counterfeit medication. Retrieved from http://www.fda.gov/Drugs/ResourcesForYou/Consumers/BuyingUsingMedicineSafely/CounterfeitMedicine/default.htm

Getting started with an insulin pump. (2009). *PediatricConsultantLive*. Retrieved from http://www.pediatricsconsultantlive.com/articles/getting-started-insulin-pump.

Grissinger, M., & Globus, N. (2004). How technology affects your risk of medication errors. *Nursing, 34*(1), 36.

Higginson, R., & Parry A. (2013). Needlestick injuries and safety syringes: A review of the literature. *British Journal of Nursing, 22*(8), S4–S12.

Hunt, C. (2008). Which site is best for an I.M. injection? *Nursing, 38*(11): 62.

Institute for Safe Medication Practices. (2013). ISMP's list of error-prone abbreviations, symbols, and dose designations. Retrieved from http://www.ismp.org/tools/errorproneabbreviations.pdf

ISMP Medication Safety Alert. (2010, Apr.). *Nurse Adviser 8*(4), 1–2.

Institute for Safe Medication Practices. (2013). Reporting an error. Retrieved from https://www.ismp.org/orderforms/healthcaremerp.asp

Kuehn, B. (2009). FDA warns against shared insulin pens. *Journal of the American Medical Association, 301*(15), 1527.

LaDuke, S. (2009). Playing it safe with bar code medication administration. *Nursing, 39*(5), 32–34.

LaForce, C., Weinstein, C., Nathan, R., Weinstein, S. F., Staudinger, H., & Meltzer, E. O. (2011). Patient satisfaction with a pressurized metered-dose inhaler with an integrated dose counter containing a fixed-dose mometasone furoate/formoterol combination. *Journal of Asthma, 48*(6), 625–631.

Lynn, P. (2008). *Lippincott's photo atlas of medication administration* (3rd ed.). Philadelphia, PA: Wolters Kluwer/Lippincott Williams & Wilkins.

Mattox, E. (2010). Identifying vulnerable patients at heightened risk for medical error. *Critical Care Nurse, 30*(2), 61–68.

Mayo Clinic. (2015). Fentanyl (transdermal route). Retrieved from http://www.mayoclinic.org/drugs-supplements/fentanyl-transdermal-route/proper-use/drg-20068152

Miller, D. K. (2009). Are you ready to care for a patient with an insulin pump? *Nursing, 39*(10) 57–60.

National Coordinating Council for Medication Error Reporting and Prevention. (2015). Medication errors. Retrieved from http://www.nccmerp.org/about-medication-errors

O'Gara, P. T., Kushner, F. G., Ascheim, D. D., Casey, D. E., Chung, M. K., de Lemos, J. A., … & Zhao, D. X. (2013, Jan. 29). 2013 ACCF/AHA guideline for the management of ST-elevation myocardial infarction. *Journal of American College of Cardiology, 61*(4), e78–e140.

Olsen, J. E., Giangrasso, A. P., & Shrimpton, D. (2016). *Medical dosage calculations* (11th ed.). Hoboken, NJ: Prentice Hall.

Poon, E. G., Keohane, C. A., Yoon, C. S., Ditmore, M., Bane, A., Levtzion-Korach, O., … & Gandhi, T. K. (2010). Effect of bar-code technology on the safety of medication administration. *New England Journal of Medicine, 362*(18), 1698–1707.

Rishovd, A. (2012). Pediatric intramuscular injections: Guidelines for best practice. *Maternal Child Nursing, 39*(2), 107–112.

Rutecki, G. W. (2008). Statins and stroke: A compelling reason for medication reconciliation. *Consultant-Greenwich, 48*(2), 82.

Turkiski, B. (2009). Improving patient safety by improving medication communication. *Orthopaedic Nursing, 28*(3), 150–154.

Woolever, D. (2008). Achieve better glucose control for your hospitalized patients. *Journal of Family Practice, 57*(12), 782–787.

Chapter 19
Nutritional Management and Enteral Intubation

 ## Learning Objectives

19.1 List the essential nutrients necessary to sustain life.

19.2 Describe the functions of the gastrointestinal system and accessory organs.

19.3 Identify the categories important for a total nutritional assessment.

19.4 Discuss feeding techniques and precautions used for dysphagic clients.

19.5 Identify clients who are candidates for modified diets.

19.6 List foods that are restricted or supplemented for clients who are receiving modified diets.

19.7 Outline steps for inserting a nasogastric tube.

19.8 Describe ways to determine placement of a nasogastric/intestinal tube.

19.9 Outline the steps of administering a tube feeding.

19.10 List possible complications of GI tract decompression.

19.11 Describe emergency management to decontaminate the GI tract of toxins/poisons.

19.12 Compare and contrast aspects of gastric versus intestinal tube feedings.

19.13 Discuss problems that may occur with tube feedings.

Chapter Outline

Terminology

Alimentary of or pertaining to nutrition.

Anorexia loss of appetite for food.

Aspirate to remove fluids or gases by suction.

Aspiration accidental inspiration of fluid or a foreign body into the airway.

Calorie the amount of heat necessary to raise the temperature of 1 kg of water by 1°C. This is the "small" calorie. The dietary, or large, calorie represents 1,000 of these calories, or 1 kilocalorie.

Carbohydrates a group of chemical substances, including sugars, glycogen, starches, dextrins, and celluloses, that contain only carbon, oxygen, and hydrogen.

Carina point at which the trachea divides into the right and left bronchi.

Cardiovascular term that pertains to the heart and blood vessels as cardiovascular system.

Diabetic related to an individual who has inadequate production and/or use of insulin.

Diet liquid and solid food substances regularly consumed.

Digestion the process by which food is broken down mechanically and chemically in the gastrointestinal tract.

Diverticulosis diverticula of the colon without inflammation or symptoms.

Dumping syndrome symptoms (weakness, cramping, diarrhea) that develop due to rapid entry of undigested food into the jejunum.

Dysphagia difficulty swallowing.

Emesis the act of vomiting.

Enteral nutrition provision of nutrients via the gastrointestinal tract (includes oral feedings).

Enterostomy opening into the stomach or jejunum through which a feeding tube can be inserted.

Fat substance made up of carbon, hydrogen, and oxygen, occurring naturally in most foods but especially in meat and dairy products.

Gastrointestinal term that pertains to the stomach and intestines.

Hematemesis vomitus containing blood.

Hyperglycemia condition characterized by an increase in blood sugar.

Hypoglycemia condition characterized by a deficiency of sugar or glucose in the blood.

Ileus obstruction of the intestine caused by paralysis of the intestinal muscles.

Ingest to take material into the gastrointestinal tract.

Jejunostomy surgical creation of a permanent opening into the jejunum.

Kwashiorkor a type of protein–energy malnutrition primarily associated with hypermetabolic acute illness such as burns, trauma, and sepsis.

Lavage to wash.

Lumen the inner open space of a tube.

Malnutrition a condition characterized by a lack of necessary food substances or improper absorption and distribution of food substances in the body.

Marasmus a type of protein–energy malnutrition due to long-term calorie and protein deprivation, resulting in cachexia or severe muscle/fat depletion (COPD, heart failure, cancer, AIDS).

Minerals inorganic elements or compounds.

Nasogastric tube a tube that is passed through the nose and into the stomach.

Nasointestinal tube small-bore flexible tube passed through the nose and advanced to the proximal intestine to be used for short-term feeding.

Nausea a feeling of sickness accompanied with the urge to vomit.

Nutrient nourishment; food item that supplies the body with necessary elements.

Obstruction blocking of a structure that prevents it from functioning normally; obstacle.

Parenteral nutrition process of providing nutrition via a route other than the alimentary canal, such as intravenously.

PEG percutaneous endoscopic gastrostomy.

Polyunsaturated term usually referring to a fat, indicating that the carbon chain has more than one double bond.

These fats tend to have higher densities (HDL) than saturated fats.

Proteins substances that contain amino acids essential for growth and repair of tissues.

Renal pertaining to the kidney.

Saturated fatty acid fatty acid carrying the maximum possible number of hydrogen atoms.

Sepsis systemic inflammatory response to an infection or cellular injury process.

Trans fat a partially hydrogenated mono- or polyunsaturated fat.

Unsaturated fatty acid fatty acid that lacks hydrogen atoms and has at least one double bond between carbons (includes polyunsaturated and monounsaturated fatty acids).

Vitamin organic substance essential for life.

Nutritional Management

Food is undeniably necessary for maintenance of life, and is, as a symbol, equally important to man's psychological health. Food has powerful social meaning as it promotes hospitality, companionship, and kinship, and perpetuates ethnic heritage and traditional customs. While these emotional and social aspects are influential in food choices, they are not necessarily based on an awareness of the importance of nutrition in health.

Nutrition is the science of foods, the **nutrients** and other substances they contain, and how they act in our body. These include carbohydrates, **fats**, **proteins**, fat-soluble and water-soluble vitamins, minerals, and water, all of which are necessary for life. The body requires a proper balance of nutrients, vitamins, and minerals for energy, growth and development, tissue repair and regulation, and maintenance of body processes. Box 19-1 ■ lists essential body nutrients. **Malnutrition** occurs when this balance is disrupted.

The body can make some but not all nutrients, and some are made in insufficient amounts. Therefore, it is essential that an individual obtain and consume the essential nutrients from exogenous sources. A deficiency of one nutrient causes abnormalities that will usually disappear if the deficiency is corrected. Deficiencies may be the result of decreased dietary intake, a disease condition, or even drug interactions.

Dietary Reference Intakes and Recommended Dietary Allowances

Standards have been established that recommend the amounts of energy, nutrients, other dietary components, and physical activity that best support health. These recommendations are called Dietary Reference Intakes (DRIs), which consist of several component values such as Recommended Dietary Allowances (RDAs). Established Energy Recommendations for dietary energy intake

Box 19-1 ESSENTIAL BODY NUTRIENTS

- Carbohydrates
  - Monosaccharides
    - Glucose, fructose, galactose
  - Disaccharides
    - Sucrose, lactose, maltose
  - Polysaccharides
    - Starch, dextrin, glycogen, cellulose, hemicellulose
- Fats
  - Linoleic acid, linolenic acid, arachidonic acid
- Proteins
  - Amino acids
    - Phenylalanine, lysine, isoleucine, leucine, methionine, valine, tryptophan, threonine, and (required only by infants) histidine
- Vitamins
  - Fat soluble
    - Vitamins A, D, E, and K
  - Water soluble
    - Vitamins B and C
- Minerals
  - Calcium, chloride, iron, magnesium, phosphorus, potassium, sodium, sulfur
- Water
  - Trace elements

(kilocalories per day) have also been established. These recommendations are based on the requirements of an average healthy individual of a particular age, gender, weight, height, and physical activity level so that energy intake does not exceed energy needs in order to help prevent obesity (excess amount of body fat). Obesity is associated with increased morbidity and mortality. It is recommended that body mass index (weight in kilograms, divided by height in meters squared, or weight in pounds multiplied by 704,

Table 19-1 Body Mass Index (BMI) Table

	Normal						Overweight						Obese				
BMI	**19**	**20**	**21**	**22**	**23**	**24**	**25**	**26**	**27**	**28**	**29**	**30**	**31**	**32**	**33**	**34**	**35**
Height								Weight (in pounds)									
4'10" (58")	91	96	100	105	110	115	119	124	129	134	138	143	148	153	158	162	167
4'11" (59")	94	99	104	109	114	119	124	128	133	138	143	148	153	158	163	168	173
5' (60")	97	102	107	112	118	123	128	133	138	143	148	153	158	163	168	174	179
5'1" (61")	100	106	111	116	122	127	132	137	143	148	153	158	164	169	174	180	185
5'2" (62")	104	109	115	120	126	131	136	142	147	153	158	164	169	175	180	186	191
5'3" (63")	107	113	118	124	130	135	141	146	152	158	163	169	175	180	186	191	197
5'4" (64")	110	116	122	128	134	140	145	151	157	163	169	174	180	186	192	197	204
5'5" (65")	114	120	126	132	138	144	150	156	162	168	174	180	186	192	198	204	210
5'6" (66")	118	124	130	136	142	148	155	161	167	173	179	186	192	198	204	210	216
5'7" (67")	121	127	134	140	146	153	159	166	172	178	185	191	198	204	211	217	223
5'8" (68")	125	131	138	144	151	158	164	171	177	184	190	197	203	210	216	223	230
5'9" (69")	128	135	142	149	155	162	169	176	182	189	196	203	209	216	223	230	236
5'10" (70")	132	139	146	153	160	167	174	181	188	195	202	209	216	222	229	236	243
5'11" (71")	136	143	150	157	165	172	179	186	193	200	208	215	222	229	236	243	250
6' (72")	140	147	154	162	169	177	184	191	199	206	213	221	228	235	242	250	258
6'1" (73")	144	151	159	166	174	182	189	197	204	212	219	227	235	242	250	257	265
6'2" (74")	148	155	163	171	179	186	194	202	210	218	225	233	241	249	256	264	272
6'3" (75")	152	160	168	176	184	192	200	208	216	224	232	240	248	256	264	272	279

Source: National Heart, Lung, and Blood Institute (1998)

divided by height in inches squared) should be kept within the range of 18.5–24.9 (Table 19-1 ■).

Energy-producing nutrients, called macronutrients, include carbohydrates, fats, and proteins. The percentage of each macronutrient range recommended to provide adequate energy and nutrients, and to reduce risk of chronic diseases, follows:

45%–65% from carbohydrate	(4 kcal/g)
20%–35% from fat	(9 kcal/g)
10%–35% from protein	(4 kcal/g)

The recommended intakes for nutrients are generous and probably should not be exceeded. Food labels now incorporate a column providing macronutrient and micronutrient (vitamins A and C, calcium, and iron) "% Daily Value." This assists in calculating the particular food's stated serving size energy-yielding nutrient contribution to the total **diet** (based on a 2,000-kcal daily recommendation).

Macronutrients

Carbohydrates

Carbohydrates are the chief source of energy and contain carbon, hydrogen, and oxygen. Carbohydrates include simple sugars, starches, and cellulose. Simple sugars (refined carbohydrates) such as white sugar, white rice, and white flour are easily digested. They cause fluctuations in blood sugar and create a feeling of hunger that can lead to overeating. Starches, which are more complex, require more sophisticated enzyme processes and are more slowly reduced to glucose, the end product of carbohydrate metabolism. Examples include whole grains and some fruits and legumes.

Glucose (converted sugars and starches) appears in the body as blood sugar and is "burned" as fuel by the tissues. Glucose is the only energy source for red blood cells and is the preferred energy source for the central nervous system, placenta, and fetus. A minimum of 100 g of carbohydrate is essential for daily brain function and to prevent ketosis. Some glucose is processed by the liver, converted to glycogen, and stored by the liver for later use.

The acceptable macronutrient range for carbohydrate is 45%–65% of total **calories**. Ingesting too many carbohydrates (sugars) supplies calories, but few if any nutrients. The greater the number of high-carbohydrate foods consumed, the more difficult it is to take in essential nutrients without weight gain. It is recommended that individuals select fiber-rich fruits and vegetables and whole grains often, and prepare food with little added sugar. Too few carbohydrates may lead to loss of energy, depression, ketosis, and a breakdown of body protein.

Fats

Fats or lipids are the second important group of nutrients. When oxidized, fats are the most concentrated sources of energy and, as such, furnish the calories necessary for survival. Fats also act as carriers for the fat-soluble vitamins, A, D,

E, and K. The optimal percentage of fat in the diet is 20%–35% of our daily caloric intake. Consuming too much fat can lead to weight problems. High-fat diets may increase the risk of developing atherosclerotic cardiovascular disease and cancer.

Fatty acids are the basic components of fat and comprise two main groups: **saturated fatty acids** and **unsaturated fatty acids**. Saturated fatty acids usually come from animal sources. It is recommended to limit total fat and **trans fat** intake and *substitute* saturated (hydrogenated) fats with **polyunsaturated** and monounsaturated fats. Saturated fats typically are solid at room temperature and should not exceed 10% of calories; cholesterol and trans fat consumption should be limited to less than 300 mg daily. Unsaturated fatty acids primarily come from vegetables, nuts, or seed sources. The unsaturated group provides two essential fatty acids: linoleic and linolenic acid. These acids are called "essential" because they are necessary for health and growth and the body cannot manufacture them. They must therefore be obtained from the diet.

Proteins

Proteins, the third essential group of nutrients, are complex organic compounds that contain amino acids. Proteins are critical to all aspects of growth and development, necessary for building muscles, blood, skin, internal organs, hormones, and enzymes, and are also a source of energy when there is insufficient carbohydrate or fat in the diet. Protein is either used for tissue repair and maintenance or converted by the liver and stored as fat.

When digested and broken down, proteins form 20 amino acids. Amino acids are then absorbed from the intestine into the bloodstream and carried to the liver for synthesis into tissues and organs of the body. If just one amino acid is missing, protein synthesis is impaired. All but nine of the amino acids are produced by the body. These nine must be obtained from the diet. Eight essential amino acids are required by all, while infants require one more, histidine. If all are present in a particular food, the food is a "complete protein." Foods that lack one or more of these essential amino acids are called "incomplete proteins." Most meat and dairy products are complete proteins, and most vegetables and fruits are incomplete. When several incomplete proteins form the major portion of an individual's diet, they should be combined carefully so that the result is a balance yielding complete protein. For example, the combination of beans and rice is balanced to give a complete protein food.

It is difficult to determine the exact amount of protein needed to supply all of the essential amino acids because there are many variables. Height and weight, level of activity, and nutritional and health status all influence the amount of protein necessary for any individual. The National Research Council recommends that 0.42 gram (g) of protein be consumed per day per pound of body weight or 56 g/day for men and 45 g/day for women. The optimal healthy diet should be 10%–35% protein.

Protein deficiency can affect the entire body—organs, tissues, skin, and muscles—as well as certain body processes. If a child is deficient in protein, he or she may have **kwashiorkor,** a disease resulting in physical and mental impairment and, if severe enough, death. If an adult is deficient in protein, ability to recover from illness or surgery may be affected.

Protein is very plentiful in the body. It is an integral part of all cells and essential for growth and development. Just like fats and carbohydrates, adequate protein must be consumed in balance with other nutrients for human survival.

Water

Although not specifically a nutrient, water is essential for survival. Water is involved in every body process, from **digestion** and absorption to excretion. It is a major portion of circulation and is the transporter of nutrients throughout the body.

Body water performs three major functions: It gives form to the body, constituting 50%–75% of the body mass; it provides the necessary environment for cell metabolism; and it maintains a stable body temperature.

Almost all foods contain water that is absorbed by the body. The average 75-kg (165-lb) adult has 42 L of water and loses 2.8 L/day. If an individual sustains severe water depletion, dehydration can result and can eventually lead to death. An individual can survive several weeks without food, but only days without water. In order to prevent dehydration (water loss exceeding water intake), a general requirement is to drink 2–3 L of water daily, or 1 mL/kcal expenditure. Measures of intake and output assist the healthcare team in identifying and correcting body water imbalances.

Micronutrients

Vitamins

Vitamins are organic food substances and are essential in small amounts for growth, maintenance, and the functioning of body processes. Vitamins are found only in living things—plants and animals—and usually cannot be synthesized by the human body.

Vitamins can be grouped according to the substance in which they are soluble. The fat-soluble group includes vitamins A, D, E, and K. Excessive amounts of vitamins A and E can be quite toxic. The water-soluble vitamins include eight B complex vitamins, vitamin C, and the bioflavonoids. These are usually measured in milligrams.

Vitamins have no calorie value, but they are as necessary to the body as any other basic nutrient. Currently, there are about 20 substances identified as vitamins, but recent research suggests that more substances could be essential to survival.

Minerals

Minerals are inorganic substances, widely prevalent in nature, and essential for metabolic processes. Minerals are grouped according to the amount found in the body. *Major minerals* include calcium, magnesium, sodium, potassium, phosphorus, sulfur, and chlorine, all of which are measured in milligrams. A second group—*trace minerals*—include iron, copper, iodine, manganese, cobalt, zinc, fluorine, selenium, and molybdenum. These minerals are measured in micrograms. Minerals form 60%–90% of all inorganic material in the body and are found in bones, teeth, soft tissue, muscle, blood, and nerve cells.

Minerals act as catalysts for many metabolic processes, and all minerals work synergistically with other minerals; their actions are interrelated. A deficiency of one mineral, therefore, affects the action of others in the body. It is essential that adequate minerals be ingested because a mineral deficiency can result in serious illness. A balanced **diet** that includes a variety of foods provides most fat-soluble and water-soluble vitamins and minerals.

Refined foods such as rice, pasta, cereals, and products that include these may sustain loss of nutrients during processing. To compensate for these losses, many foods are *enriched* with iron, thiamin, riboflavin, and niacin. Since the 1940s, all grain products are enriched, with folate being added in 1996 to help prevent birth defects. Food labels indicate such enrichment. Additionally, some foods are *fortified* by the addition of nutrients that are not present or are present in insignificant amounts in a food, such as orange juice fortified with calcium and vitamin D.

While some nutritionists and biochemists recommend taking a daily basic vitamin–mineral supplement to ensure adequate levels, the intake of supplements in excess of the Tolerable Upper Level Intake can have toxic systemic effects. Tolerable Upper Intake levels represent the maximum amount of a nutrient that is safe for most people on a daily basis.

As new knowledge surfaces about the importance of nutrients for basic health, the recommended intake reflects this increased awareness.

Nutritional Assessment

Healthy individuals can satisfy essential nutrient recommendations by following a personalized approach to healthy eating and exercise. The *Dietary Guidelines for Americans 2015*, published by the U.S. Department of Agriculture, provide sound advice for making food and physical activity choices that promote good health and a healthy weight. These choices also help prevent disease for Americans ages 2 years and over. This includes Americans at risk for chronic disease. In 2011, First Lady Michelle Obama, in conjunction with the USDA, released the federal government's new food icon, MyPlate, to remind consumers to make healthier food choices (Figure 19-1 ■). MyPlate emphasizes the fruit, vegetable, grain, protein, and dairy groups. This unique public service is also available in Spanish, *MiPlato*. The USDA Center for Nutrition Policy and Promotion has two primary goals: (1) to advance and promote dietary guidelines for all Americans; and (2) to conduct applied research and analysis in nutrition and consumer economics.

FIGURE 19-1 The illustration provided by MyPlate emphasizes food proportions that lead to a nutritious diet.

In today's technology-oriented environment, many people are relying on applications (apps) for their smartphone or mobile device to assist them with weight loss and diet management. Many of these apps are free to download and provide ongoing support features such as a daily log entry, weight tracking, and social support. One such app is *MyFitnessPal*.

No single parameter is sufficient to determine a client's nutritional status. Initial screening of the hospitalized client is performed by the professional nurse on admission. In general, the nurse asks the client about a recent change in body weight of 10 lb or more in the last 6 months, **nausea**, vomiting, diarrhea lasting more than 5 days, any declining food intake, difficulty chewing or swallowing, and the time and duration of recent hospitalizations. If results of this initial screening (within 24 hr of hospital admission) classify the client at "nutrition risk," a dietician consult is indicated. Unfortunately, many clients are unable to provide the essential subjective information.

Objective measures of nutritional status include weight in relation to height (body mass index), monitoring dietary intakes with calorie counts, examination for signs of micronutrient deficiencies, and laboratory tests such as serum albumin, transferrin, and prealbumin; tests of cellular immunity; and total lymphocyte count. Other measures include evaluation of body composition by visual inspection or anthropometric measurements (triceps skin fold, mid-arm muscle circumference). See Nutritional Assessment Parameters, Table 19-2 ■.

EVIDENCE-BASED PRACTICE
Mini Nutritional Assessment
The Mini Nutritional Assessment (MNA) is an assessment tool (Table 19-2) that helps identify older adults who are at risk of malnutrition.

Source: DiMaria-Ghalili & Guenter (2008)

Table 19-2 Nutritional Assessment Parameters

Clinical Assessment	Normal	Abnormal
Dietary Data		
Appetite	Remains unchanged	Increased or decreased recently Particular cravings
Nutritional intake	Adequate foods and fluids to supply body nutrients Nonallergic response to major food groups	Elimination of certain food categories that result in limited nutrients Emphasis on some food groups (sugar) to the exclusion of others (vegetables) Allergic response to certain foods
Caloric intake	Average 28 kcal/kg/day	Constant use of fad diets to lose weight Use of drugs or chemicals that interfere with appetite or nutrient assimilation
Meal patterns	3–6 home-prepared meals per day Adequate time and calm atmosphere for meals	Fast-food or packaged foods Missed meals, constant snacking, or overeating Eating "on the run" or hurriedly
General Appearance		
Affect	Alert, responsive, healthy-appearing eyes and skin	Listless, dull, nonresponsive Skin and eyes appear unhealthy.
Physical factors	Adequate chewing and swallowing capability Mouth and gums healthy so food can be ingested Physical exercise adequate for calorie intake	Teeth or gums in poor condition or ill-fitting dentures Swallowing impairs ingestion. Inadequate physical exercise to burn calories
Presence of disease	No disease process that interferes with nutrient assimilation No congenital condition or postsurgery condition that interferes with nutrient assimilation	Disease present that interferes with ingestion, digestion, assimilation, or excretion Congenital condition, rehabilitation phase, or postsurgery that interferes with food assimilation
Elimination schedule	Regular, adequate elimination of foods Absence of constant flatus, discharge, or mucus	Irregular or painful elimination Presence of constant flatus Presence of discharge, blood, or mucus
Anthropometric Measurements		
Height	For bedridden clients, measure arm span—fully extend arms 90-degree angle to body and measure from tip of one middle finger to the tip of other middle finger for estimated height.	Loss of 2–3 inches in height may indicate osteoporosis.
Weight—compared to ideal and usual body weight.	Ideal body weight 100 lb (female); 106 lb (male) for 5 feet height + 5 lb for each 1 in. over 5 feet (female) and 6 lb for each 1 in. over 5 feet (male). Small frame minus 10% Large frame plus 10%	Changed—markedly increased or decreased recently: important indicator of changed nutritional status Loss of more than 10% weight for prior 6 months should be clinically evaluated.
Body Mass Index Ratio of weight in kilograms and height in meters	18.5–24.9	Less than 18.5—underweight 25–29—overweight 30–39—obese
Triceps skinfold measurement (mm)	Standard values—male to female 12.5–16.5	If values change over months, may indicate a chronic condition.
Length of upper arm (cm)	35.8–39.1	Less than 33; more than 37
Mid-arm muscle circumference (cm)	31.9–34.2	Hydration status may influence results.
Biochemical Assessments*		
Serum albumin	3.5–5.0 g/dL	Examples of possible disease conditions: Decrease signifies lowered nutritional status—protein deficient.
Serum transferrin binds iron to plasma and transports to bone marrow.	200–430 mg/dL	Reduced levels may indicate chronic diseases and protein deficiency. Elevated levels—anemias, liver damage, lead toxicity
Hemoglobin	Male—13.5–17 g/dL Female—12–15 g/dL	Decreased related to iron deficiency (anemias and leukemia)

(continued)

Table 19-2 Nutritional Assessment Parameters *(continued)*

Clinical Assessment	Normal	Abnormal
Prealbumin (PA) serum	20–50 mg/dL	Decreased—protein wasting diseases, malnutrition (<10.7 indicates severe nutritional deficiency.) Elevated—Hodgkin disease
Blood urea nitrogen/creatinine	10:1–20:1	Nitrogen imbalance, inadequate **renal** functioning; ratio increased in heart failure, decreased renal perfusion
24-hr urinary nitrogen	Positive balance	Inadequate protein intake
Sociocultural Data		
Cultural–religious factors	Ability to afford adequate foods in all food categories Cultural beliefs that do not eliminate whole food groups Religious beliefs that do not eliminate whole food groups	Economic position that precludes purchase of adequate food Religious or cultural beliefs that interfere with receiving balanced diet (macrobiotic diets) Inadequate knowledge, experience, or intelligence to prepare healthy meals
Ethnicity	Traditional foods that do not eliminate whole food groups	Beliefs and ethnic preference that eliminate major nutrients from the diet
Lifestyle	Well-balanced meals that include all nutrients Food does not lose all nutrient value in preparation.	Fast-paced, stressful lifestyle that incorporates fast food or convenience foods deficient in nutrients or imbalanced (high-fat)

*Laboratory test parameters differ among laboratories. Check the reference range for the specific lab where the client's blood or urine was tested.

Assimilation of Nutrients

Nutrients must be broken down by the body. This process is called **digestion**. It starts in the mouth and continues in the stomach and small intestine.

The total daily energy requirement of an individual is the number of calories needed to replace the energy loss from the metabolic rate, plus loss from an individual's physical, emotional, and mental output. The number of calories ingested should be directly related to maintaining an adequate energy level and supporting the body's metabolic processes.

Gastrointestinal System

The **gastrointestinal** system is comprised of the mouth, esophagus, and intestines, plus accessory organs. The main functions of the gastrointestinal system are the secretion of hormones, enzymes, and hydrochloric acid to digest ingested materials; the movement of the ingested contents through the system; their absorption into the blood; and the storage or elimination of the end products of digestion.

Mechanical digestion begins with chewing of food. When food reaches the stomach, both mechanical and chemical digestive processes occur.

The average meal remains in the stomach for 3 hr, where digestion continues. The stomach's secretion of hydrochloric acid and pepsin break down proteins, while the *acid pH* environment helps protect against ingested pathogens. Vomiting or suction removal of *acid* gastric contents (primarily HCl, Na, and K) can lead to fluid and electrolyte imbalance with metabolic *alkalosis* (high bicarbonate and elevated pH on arterial blood gases [ABGs]). H_2 receptor antagonists (e.g., cimetidine) make gastric secretions less acidic, so their administration reduces the risk of metabolic alkalosis and

electrolyte disturbance in clients who require gastric secretion suction (decompression).

The stomach's mechanical processes occur with intervals of peristalsis and relaxation of the pyloric sphincter as gastric content (chyme) moves into the small intestine (duodenum). Digestive processes continue within the small intestine (duodenum, jejunum, ileum) as enzymes break down protein to amino acids, fats to glycerol and fatty acids, and carbohydrates to monosaccharides. Here, most nutrients and water are absorbed into the circulation. While 7–10 L of electrolyte-rich secretions mix with the chyme, only 600–800 mL enters the large intestine. Small intestine secretions have an *alkaline pH*, making this environment more vulnerable to bacterial invasion. *Alkaline* intestinal fluid loss (e.g., due to diarrhea, intestinal decompression) can lead to fluid and electrolyte imbalance with metabolic *acidosis* (low bicarbonate and low pH on ABGs).

The ileocecal valve separates the small intestine from the large intestine. In the large intestine, fluids and electrolytes continue to be absorbed to solidify the stool, and mucus is secreted to lubricate waste as it moves toward the rectum for storage and final elimination of stool, which contains approximately 200 mL water.

The Accessory Organs

The accessory organs of the gastrointestinal tract also play an important role in the utilization of nutrients.

The liver has a major role in the metabolism of carbohydrates, fats, and proteins. In carbohydrate metabolism, the liver converts glucose to glycogen and stores it. The liver then can reconvert glycogen to glucose when the body requires higher blood sugar. The process of releasing carbohydrates (end products) into the bloodstream is called glycogenolysis.

The liver metabolizes fats through the process of oxidation of fatty acids and the formation of acetoacetic acid. Also, the liver forms lipoproteins, cholesterol, and phospholipids and converts carbohydrates and protein to fats.

The liver metabolizes proteins by deamination of amino acids. In this process, the urea and plasma proteins are formed.

The gallbladder functions as a reservoir for bile, which is produced by the liver. When food enters the duodenum, it releases cholecystokinin, which causes the gallbladder to contract and release bile, while the sphincter of Oddi relaxes so that bile enters the duodenum. Here, the bile acids emulsify and digest lipids, which are then absorbed by the intestine.

The pancreas secretes enzymes into the small intestine for the digestion of carbohydrates, fats, and proteins. The enzyme trypsin acts on proteins to produce peptones, peptides, and amino acids. Pancreatic amylase acts on carbohydrates to produce disaccharides, and pancreatic lipase acts on fats to produce glycerol and fatty acids.

In summary, the gastrointestinal tract's primary function is to provide the body with a continuous supply of nutrients by the processes of ingestion, digestion, and absorption.

Gastrointestinal Dysfunctions

Dysphagia

The voluntary and involuntary actions of swallowing require coordination of several muscles and brain areas. **Dysphagia** (difficulty swallowing) commonly affects the older adult population, especially those in nursing home facilities. Difficulty may be due to dysfunction of neurologic pathways or from dysfunction of muscles of the swallowing tract such as occurs with stroke, dementia, and Parkinson disease. Dysphagia resulting from stroke is usually temporary, whereas it progresses as part of a general decline in those with dementia or Parkinson disease. Others who experience dysphagia are those with esophageal obstructive disorders or reflux, and chronic neurologic disorders such as cerebral palsy, multiple sclerosis, polio, amyotrophic lateral sclerosis, and myasthenia gravis.

The most serious complication of dysphagia is **aspiration** of oropharyngeal secretions, liquid, or food into the lungs, creating an environment conducive to bacterial growth (aspiration pneumonia). This occurs in more than 50% of those with dysphagia. A protective cough normally prevents aspiration, but 50% of clients who **aspirate** do so silently, *without* coughing, so aspiration goes undetected until pneumonia develops. A complex disorder, dysphagia, requires an individualized diagnosis and management by collaborative experts: speech–language pathologist, dietitian, radiologist, and occupational therapist.

GI Hemorrhage

The gastric blood from GI hemorrhage is an irritant that usually triggers vomiting, which may aggravate the bleeding. Clients with impaired liver function are an example of those

most likely to experience a gastric bleed, but these clients are also unable to process the protein load created by digestion and absorption of blood. The digestion of blood can cause a precipitous rise in serum ammonia, which can lead to altered neurologic function (somnolence, loss of coordination, coma). **Lavage** (to wash) per gastric intubation removes blood to prevent this "metabolic encephalopathy," and also allows estimation of the client's acute blood loss.

Intestinal Obstruction

When gastrointestinal processes are disrupted, intestinal **obstruction** develops. Cessation of peristalsis (**ileus**) due to neurogenic impairment (traumatic stress), abdominal pathology, electrolyte imbalance (hypokalemia), or bowel manipulation (as in surgery) may alter GI movement and absorption, allowing secretions and gas to accumulate. The small intestine is the first site to regain motility after surgery (24 hr), then the stomach (2–4 days), and finally the colon (3–7 days). The presence or absence of bowel sounds, however, does not relate to feeding tolerance. Early postoperative nasointestinal or direct small bowel feeding is thought not only to be safe, but also important for maintaining bowel integrity and preventing **sepsis**. Temporary decompression to remove fluids and gas *may* be necessary in some instances because progressive accumulation of gases and fluid distends the bowel, compresses bowel wall capillaries, and can lead to septic shock, as well as hypovolemic shock. Decompression *may* also alleviate pain, nausea, and vomiting, and reduce the possibility of aspiration.

Decompression Decompression requires the insertion of a **nasogastric tube** (NGT), which is connected to continuous or intermittent negative pressure suction while the client is kept NPO and given IV fluids. Since gastrointestinal secretions are isotonic with extracellular fluid, a guideline for fluid replacement is to administer a volume of normal saline (or one-half normal saline with KCl) equivalent to the previous day's drained secretions. A unique feature of the GI tract is that its nutrition is derived directly (rather than from the bloodstream), so early ambulation, termination of decompression, and resumption of PO intake are recommended. The passage of flatus, bowel movement, and tolerance of oral intake are indicators that GI function has returned and is able to accommodate PO intake.

Normal and Therapeutic Nutrition

Normal nutrition is based on recommended daily dietary allowances designed for the maintenance of health. While these standards have been established for nutrition requirements of an average healthy individual, therapeutic modification of nutritional needs may be based on a client's disease condition associated with an excess or deficiency of a particular nutrient. Therapeutic diets may include alterations of minerals, vitamins, proteins, carbohydrates, fats, and fluids, as well as alterations of their consistency to facilitate the client's intake. Whether a normal or therapeutic diet has been ordered based on the client's physiologic status, the client's cultural, socioeconomic, and psychological influences must also be taken into account. The nutritional requirements must be considered within the context of the total needs of the individual client.

Eating and mealtime are considered by many to be a "social" event. Hospitalized clients, however, may be isolated from others so that eating is not a pleasure. Painful or uncomfortable procedures should be planned so that they are not immediately before or after meals. The client should be in a position as near to normal as possible: sitting in a chair or with the head of the bed elevated 90 degrees. The environment should be bright and free of offensive odors. Client allergies should be noted; personal preferences and cultural or religious restrictions should be honored. Food trays should be checked for compliance with the healthcare provider's order. If the client is NPO, a sign may be posted on the unit door so that the client does not receive a tray.

When you are preparing to assist the client to eat, lower the side rail and place the tray table over the client's lap low enough so that he or she can see what is on it. If the tray is not neatly arranged, rearrange it. Food appearance and presentation influence appetite. Assist the client with whatever is needed, such as cutting meat. If the client is unable to drink from a glass, provide a straw or adaptive cup.

Be sensitive to the client's response to food, and continually attempt to orient feeding to meet the client's needs. If the client has impaired vision but is able to self-feed, tell the client what is on the tray and the position of each item. Often, it is clearer to describe position of foods by a clock; for example, chicken at 12 o'clock, green beans at 3 o'clock.

When therapeutic diets are ordered, it is critical to be sensitive to the client's acceptance of any restrictions or supplements and to help the client understand their purpose. The nurse is most closely involved with the client and can best determine the client's actual intake. The nurse should ensure that the client is not receiving inappropriate foods from other sources and that the client is actually eating the foods prescribed.

Nutrition Problems in the Hospital

Nutrition may be overlooked as a vital component of a hospitalized client's care. For clients who seem to be stable on admission and give no history of nutrition-related problems, the usual hospital diet is adequate; however, all clients must be reassessed periodically to detect and prevent nutritional problems. Fear, anxiety or depression, poorly fitting dentures, and even medications and therapies may limit a client's ability to eat or may interfere with his or her appetite. Some clients may have the desire to eat and have a good appetite, but shortly after eating certain food, experience cramps, pain, or diarrhea or feel nauseated or vomit. This may lead to decreased food intake. Clients may become more malnourished the longer they remain in a hospital for a variety of reasons that limit food intake.

Well-nourished clients can tolerate a short period of caloric balance deficit such as that occurring with a brief illness or surgery, because the body's fat stores provide calories during such periods. Nutrient guidelines for healthy individuals, however, are not meant to meet the needs of clients whose nutritional status is altered by illness that affects oral intake and nutrient digestion, absorption, or utilization. Protein–energy malnutrition is widely seen in hospitalized clients due to acute illness and protein-deficient diets (kwashiorkor) or long-term calorie and protein deprivation with cachexia or severe muscle/fat depletion (**marasmus**). Protein–energy malnutrition is commonly seen in the obese or **diabetic** client as well, and while the client may not appear to be malnourished visually, nutrition parameters reveal a malnourished state.

Studies indicate that malnutrition (protein–energy deficiency) is present in as many as 50% of hospitalized clients and that clients become more malnourished the longer the hospital stay. Clients with negative nitrogen balance (reduced serum albumin, reduced prealbumin) have already lost structural and functional proteins and have poor surgical outcome, increased infection rates, and prolonged hospital stays. As **malnutrition** progresses, all major organ systems, fluids and electrolytes, and immune system dysfunction develops.

EVIDENCE-BASED PRACTICE
Oral Intake During Hospitalization

Several studies have documented that inadequate oral intake is prevalent among hospitalized clients. Inadequate oral intake during hospitalizations increases the prevalence and worsens the degree of malnutrition, which is known to increase morbidity and mortality. In one study of ventilated ICU clients ($N = 2,772$), overall mean caloric intake was 59% of estimated needs. Researchers found that an oral intake of 1,000 cal/day had a protective effect and improved outcomes (Peterson, Sheean, & Braunschweig, 2011).

Enteral Feeding for Nutritional Support

Enteral nutrition may be prescribed for clients who are unable or unwilling to eat or those who need a supplement to ingested food, as well as for clients in catabolic states with intensive caloric requirement (e.g., burn, trauma clients).

Enteral feeding is preferred over parenteral (intravenous) nutrition because it is safer, less expensive, and associated with fewer complications. It helps to maintain GI function and speeds regeneration of the small intestine, which receives its nutrition from food directly rather than from the bloodstream. Enteral nutrition preserves production of humoral antibodies, reduces gut bacterial overgrowth, and, by helping to maintain the gut's protective mucosal barrier, promotes gut motility and reduces risk of sepsis. Since the small intestine is less prone to ileus than the stomach and large intestine, postoperative feeding into the small intestine is feasible even though the client is NPO.

Enteral formulas come in powder form to reconstitute or as ready-to-use liquids. They contain all or just one of the following: protein, carbohydrates, fat, electrolytes, and vitamins and minerals, depending on the client's needs. Isotonic formulas provide 1 cal/mL and are most commonly used.

Modified formulas are available for clients with specific nutritional requirements: lactose-free or lactose-containing, fiber-containing, elemental (predigested), or modular formulations that provide additional macronutrient components (lipid, carbohydrate, or protein). Specialized formulas are also available for trauma clients or those with pulmonary disease, renal failure, diabetes, liver failure, or immune deficiency.

Many types of nasogastric and **nasointestinal tubes** are available for enteral feeding. Large-bore nasogastric tubes are inserted for short-term (1 week) intermittent feedings that are delivered by gravity through a syringe or by an infusion pump 4–6 times daily. If nutritional support is indicated for an extended period (4 weeks), a long, soft, flexible, small-bore tube made of silastic or polyurethane is placed naso- or orointestinally (advanced beyond the pylorus). Small-bore tubes are more comfortable for the client. Since feeding is by continuous infusion using a pump, the client's position must be kept with head of bed elevated 30 degrees or greater to decrease risk of aspiration. Feeding into the small intestine is associated with greater risk of infection due to the intestine's alkaline (less protected) environment.

For clients with a history of gastric reflux or tube feeding–related aspiration pneumonia, a small-bore **jejunostomy** tube may be placed surgically or by laparoscopy. Special "dual-purpose tubes" (e.g., Moss tube) can be placed at the time of surgery to provide gastric decompression and simultaneous (early postoperative) feeding into a functional small intestine while the client is NPO.

For *extended nutritional support* (feeding over 4 weeks), tube enterostomies are created surgically through the abdominal wall, directly into the stomach (gastrostomy, percutaneous endoscopic gastrostomy [PEG], or small intestine jejunostomy). Directly placed tubes are secured by stabilizing bars (bumpers), a large mushroom tip, or a balloon inflated with water (similar to a urinary retention catheter).

Parenteral Nutrition (PN)

Parenteral nutrition (PN) is a modality that provides nutrients, multivitamin supplementation, and calories intravenously to clients who cannot be fed orally or who are unable to meet their caloric requirements via the enteral route. PN is invasive and costly, and it can contribute to infectious complications (line sepsis), volume overload, and **hyperglycemia**. Despite these complications, PN has been shown to decrease morbidity and mortality in critically ill and severely malnourished clients. For additional information on PN, see Chapter 29.

Cultural Awareness

- American acculturation tends to replace traditional habits, tastes, and preferences with a detrimental switch to highly processed foods.
- This may account for increased rates of illness and death from heart disease and cancer in some populations.
- While not all cultural food habits are healthy, they are usually higher in fiber and vitamins than the typical American diet and should be encouraged.

General Recommendations

- Food preferences should be maintained. When a special diet is prescribed, it should be consistent with the client's cultural preferences and religious practices. For example, Jewish people do not combine certain foods; so, to comply with kosher laws, do not combine meat and dairy products at the same meal.
- Focus education on food practices and preparation, possible health hazards, and importance of role modeling for children.

Nursing Diagnoses

The following nursing diagnoses are appropriate to use on client care plans when the components are related to nutritional problems or nutritional health maintenance.

NURSING DIAGNOSIS	RELATED TO . . .
Aspiration, Risk for	CVA, neuromuscular disease, NG intubation, artificial airway, decreased level of consciousness, oral/cervical surgery
Impaired Dentition	Poor oral hygiene, oral surgery, injury, ill-fitting dentures
Deficient Knowledge	Lack of appropriate dietary information, misinterpretation of information, cognitive limitation, inadequate motivation
Imbalanced Nutrition: Less Than Body Requirements	Impaired swallowing, faulty metabolism, altered level of consciousness, inadequate absorption, eating disorders
Overweight Obesity	Lack of basic nutritional knowledge, excessive intake in relation to metabolic requirements, decreased activity patterns, decreased metabolic needs, eating disorders
Impaired Swallowing	Esophageal obstructive disorder, chronic neurologic disorder (multiple sclerosis, ALS, myasthenia gravis), muscle dysfunction (stroke, dementia, Parkinson disease)

Source: Herdman, T. H. & Kamitsuru, S. (Eds.) *Nursing Diagnoses – Definitions and Classification 2015-2017*. Copyright © 2014, 1994–2014 by NANDA International. Used by arrangement with John Wiley & Sons Limited. Companion website: www.wiley.com/go/nursingdiagnoses. In order to make safe and effective judgments using NANDA-I nursing diagnosis it is essential that nurses refer to the definitions and defining characteristics of the diagnoses listed in this work.

Modified Therapeutic Diets

Nursing Process Data

ASSESSMENT Database

- Refer to general assessment parameters (physical and laboratory findings) in chapter introduction.
- Assess client's dietary preferences.
- Assess client's health status that necessitates diet modification.
- Identify disease state, which may necessitate dietary modification (e.g., cardiac, pulmonary, renal disease).
- Determine whether registered dietician has consulted to assist with diet design.

PLANNING Objectives

- To meet nutritional needs of clients with altered health status
- To provide a therapeutic diet that is acceptable to client's taste and cultural orientation
- To provide specialized dietary information to promote client's adherence

IMPLEMENTATION Procedures

DOCUMENTATION AND EVALUATION

Expected Outcomes

- Therapeutic diet assists in management of client's altered health status.
- Client accepts therapeutic diet prescribed to help manage altered health status.
- Client demonstrates understanding (verbalized knowledge) of dietary information provided.

Unexpected Outcomes/Alternative Actions

Pearson Nursing Student Resources

Find additional review materials at
nursing.pearsonhighered.com.
Prepare for success with NCLEX®-style practice questions and Skill Checklists.

Skill 19.1.1 | Restricting Dietary Protein

1. A **restricted protein diet** is used for clients with renal insufficiency, hepatic coma, and cirrhosis (according to individual requirements).

   a. Control end products of protein metabolism (nitrogenous waste) by limiting protein intake.

   b. Protein allowance is decreased to 0.5–0.6 g/kg/day (predialysis).

   c. Limit high-protein foods, such as eggs, meat, milk, and milk products.

2. A **PKU diet** is an amino acid metabolism abnormality diet used for phenylketonuria (PKU), galactosemia, and lactose intolerance.

   a. Reduce foods that contain compounds that cannot be metabolized correctly.

   b. Avoid milk and milk products.

   c. Provide substitutes to meet daily allowances.

Skill 19.1.2 | Restricting Dietary Fat

1. A **restricted fat diet** is used to reduce risk for and to manage cardiovascular diseases, diabetes mellitus, and high serum cholesterol levels. It focuses on restriction of saturated (hydrogenated) fats, trans fats (found in fast and fried foods), and cholesterol to treat dyslipidemia and reduce risk for atherosclerosis. These fats are solid or semisolid at room temperature.

   a. Lipid levels goals = total cholesterol <200 mg/dL, LDL-C <100 mg/dL, HDL-C >45 mg/dL for males and 55 mg/dL for females, and triglycerides <150 mg/dL.

   b. Restrict total fat to less than 30% of calories, achieve normal body weight by reducing calorie intake; restrict saturated fat to 7% of calories and reduce cholesterol to 200 mg/day.

   c. Higher percentage may be allowed if saturated and trans fats are substituted with monosaturated fats found primarily in plant products (olive oil, canola oil, avocados, pecans, almonds); use low-fat or nonfat products; increase intake of fruits and vegetables, whole grains, legumes, and seeds.

   d. Limit high-cholesterol foods found in animal products, such as egg yolk, red meat, shellfish, organ meats, bacon, and pork.

2. A **modified-fat diet** is used according to individual tolerance in malabsorption syndromes (cystic fibrosis, gallbladder disease, obstructive jaundice, pancreatitis, and liver disease).

   a. Attempt to lower fat content in diet when there is inadequate absorption of fat or when excessive fat aggravates a condition.

   b. Avoid such foods as gravies, fatty meat and fish, cream, fried foods, rich pastries, whole milk products, cream soups, salad and cooking oils, nuts, and chocolate. Allow eggs (3–5 per week), lean meat, and small amount of butter or butter substitute.

Skill 19.1.3 | Restricting Mineral Nutrients (Sodium, Potassium)

1. A **restricted sodium diet** is used to manage hypertension, liver disease, heart failure (edema), and renal insufficiency (Box 19-2 ■).

   a. Correct or control the retention of sodium and water in the body by limiting sodium intake. May include restriction of salt in the diet or in combination with medications.

   b. Sodium restriction may allow lower dosage of diuretic.

   c. Restrict salt in cooking or at the table. May prohibit any product containing sodium, such as soda bicarbonate (typical diet provides 4–6 g of sodium/day).

   d. Explain sodium restrictions in diet.

   Mild: 2–3 g of sodium (no added salt—provides 2–3 g of sodium/day)

   Moderate: 1,000–1,500 mg of sodium

   Strict: 500 mg of sodium

   Be aware of sodium content of some medications (e.g., antacids).

2. Potassium may be restricted for the renal client (see Box 19-2).

(continued)

Skill 19.1.3 | Restricting Mineral Nutrients (Sodium, Potassium) *(continued)*

Box 19-2 FOODS HIGH IN SODIUM AND POTASSIUM

Foods High in Sodium

- Table salt and all prepared salts, such as celery salt
- Smoked meats and salted meats
- Most frozen vegetables or canned vegetables with added salt
- Butter, margarines, and cheese
- Quick-cooking cereals
- Shellfish and frozen or salted fish
- Seasonings and sauces
- Canned soups
- Chocolates and cocoa
- Beets, celery, and selected greens (spinach)
- Anything with salt added, such as snack chips and popcorn

Foods High in Potassium

- Fruit juices, such as orange, grapefruit, banana, raw apple
- Instant, dry coffee powder
- Eggs, legumes, whole grains
- Fish: fresh halibut, codfish
- Pork, beef, lamb, veal, chicken
- Milk, skim and whole
- Dried dates, prunes
- Bouillon and meat broths
- Salt substitute

Skill 19.1.4 | Providing Consistent Carbohydrate Diets

1. Nutrition is one of the cornerstones of treatment for diabetes.
   a. Foods included on the diet are balanced and provide protein, fat, and carbohydrates in relation to an individual's needs.
   b. Foods limited are refined or simple sugars.
   c. Counting grams of carbohydrates and using the glycemic index (describes how much blood glucose level rises with a specific food when compared with an equivalent amount of glucose) are nutritional tools for managing diabetes.
   d. Equal (consistent) amount of carbohydrate is provided at each meal to ease management of blood sugars.

2. Reactive **hypoglycemia** occurs when the pancreas oversecretes insulin postprandially and most of the glucose moves from the blood into cells, resulting in abnormally low blood glucose levels.
   a. Foods prescribed are a combination of foods high in protein and a variety of complex carbohydrates, consumed in five or six small meals per day.
   b. Foods restricted are simple carbohydrates; for example: juices, white sugar, white rice, and white flour.

Skill 19.1.5 | Providing Nutrient-Enhanced Diets

1. An **increased potassium diet** is used to compensate for potassium loss due to certain diuretics or steroids, burns, vomiting, fever, and COPD and may have an antihypertensive effect.
   a. Replace potassium loss from the body with specific foods high in potassium or a potassium supplement. Severe loss is managed with intravenous replacement therapy.
   b. Avoid no specific foods unless there is a sodium restriction (some foods high in potassium are also high in sodium).
   c. Reduced sodium intake reduces potassium loss.

2. A **high-iron diet** is used to manage anemias (blood loss, nutritional) and malabsorption syndrome.
   a. Replace a deficit of iron caused by inadequate intake or chronic blood loss.
   b. Include foods high in iron content, such as meats (especially organ meats), egg yolks, seafood (especially

shellfish), and plant-based sources such as whole wheat products, leafy vegetables, nuts, dried fruits, and legumes.
   c. Vitamin C enhances absorption of plant-based iron.

3. A **high-calcium diet** is used to prevent osteoporosis and prevent and treat hypertension.
   a. Increases normal adult intake of 1 g/day to 1.5 g/day for postmenopausal female.
   b. Recommends use of *fortified* low-fat and nonfat dairy products, fruit juices, and oatmeals.
   c. Clients who are lactose intolerant should use leafy green vegetables and nonliquid dairy products (cheese, yogurt) or lactose-free dairy products, fish products, and almonds.

4. Clients receiving nutritional therapy must be watched for complications (Box 19-3 ■).

Box 19-3 REFEEDING SYNDROME

Refeeding syndrome typically occurs within 2–5 days after the reintroduction of parenteral, enteral, or even oral feedings. It affects semistarved or fasting clients, and those with morbid obesity, anorexia nervosa, or chronic alcoholism. These clients' bodies have adapted to using free fatty acids and ketone bodies for energy. As a result, they can develop hypophosphatemia, hypokalemia and hypomagnesemia, altered glucose metabolism, and fluid shifts associated with hematologic, neuromuscular, cardiac, and respiratory dysfunction when large amounts of carbohydrate feedings are reintroduced. Sudden expansion of extracellular (intravascular) fluid can result in cardiac decompensation, and administration of dextrose can result in hyperglycemia with osmotic diuresis and dehydration.

When nutritional support therapies are initiated in malnourished clients, caloric goals should be achieved gradually over 3–4 days while the client's cardiopulmonary response, serum electrolytes, and glucose are monitored closely.

Source: Parli, Ruf, & Magnuson (2014)

Skill 19.1.6 | Providing Progressive Diets

Dietary Fiber

1. There are two types of fiber: Insoluble fiber, found in cell walls of plants, does not dissolve in water, so it speeds elimination of waste products, and soluble fiber (oat bran), which dissolves in water and decreases intestinal speed, decreases blood cholesterol levels, and slows absorption of glucose, so blood sugar levels are reduced in diabetes.

2. A *low-fiber diet* is used during phases of intestinal diseases and may be used preoperatively and postoperatively during transition to a regular diet.

   a. Long-term fiber restriction is discouraged.

   b. Inform client that low-fiber foods are ground meat, fish, broiled chicken without skin, limited fat, refined strained cereals, white bread, and possibly limited milk products.

3. A *high-fiber diet* is prescribed to treat constipation and **diverticulosis.**

   a. Includes foods high in fiber such as beans, fruits, vegetables, nuts, whole grain breads and cereals, and especially unrefined bran.

   b. Fluid intake should be increased as fiber is increased in the diet.

Postoperative Diet Progression

1. A special postoperative surgical diet may be necessary to promote wound healing (Box 19-4 ■) to avoid hypovolemia due to decreased plasma proteins and circulating red blood cells and to prevent edema.

   a. For tissue repair and extensive stress states, energy needs should be determined by a specialist.

   b. Fluid intake is 2–3 L/day for uncomplicated surgery and 3–4 L for sepsis. Clients with extensive wound drainage may require more fluid intake.

2. Diet progression may consist of nothing by mouth (NPO) the day of surgery and advance to a regular diet as soon as tolerated. A progressive diet may include the following diets:

   a. **Clear liquid diet** 1,000–1,500 mL/day of liquid foods such as water, tea, broth, gelatin, and pulp-free juices or clear carbonated beverages.

   b. **Full liquid diet** lacks many nutrients, so is used temporarily. Includes any food that is liquid at room temperature—clear liquids, milk and milk products, custard, puddings, creamed soups, sherbet, ice cream, and any fruit juice.

Box 19-4 NUTRIENT REQUIREMENTS FOR HEALING*

- Total calories per day:
  1. 2,800 for tissue repair
  2. 6,000 for extensive repair
- Protein:
  1. 40–50 g/day average individual
  2. 50–75 g/day early in postoperative period
  3. 100–200 g/day if needed for new tissue synthesis
- Carbohydrates:
  1. 55%–60% of calories—sufficient in quantity to meet caloric needs and allow protein to be used for tissue repair
- Fat:
  1. 25%–30%—not excessive as it leads to poor tissue healing and susceptibility to infection

- Vitamins:
  1. Vitamin C—up to 1 g/day for tissue repair
  2. Vitamin B—increased above normal for stress management
  3. Vitamin A—adjuncts autoimmune system
  4. Vitamin E—increases O_2 to tissues
- Minerals:
  1. Zinc—tissue repair
  2. Selenium—cell repair
  3. Calcium/magnesium—relaxes nerves and maintains electric function

*This is an example of nutrients necessary for healing. Each diet should be individualized and a dietary consult is required.

(continued)

Skill 19.1.6 | Providing Progressive Diets *(continued)*

c. A **surgical soft diet** is full liquid plus pureed vegetables, eggs (not fried), milk, cheese, fish, fowl, tender beef, veal, potatoes, and cooked fruit. Include foods that are easy to chew and digest and limited in fiber; do not include gas formers.

d. **General diet:** Take into consideration client's tolerance and preferences.

Skill 19.1.7 | Providing Altered Food Consistency Diets

Bland Diet

1. A bland diet is used to promote the healing of the gastric mucosa by eliminating food sources that are chemically and mechanically irritating. Bland diets may be used to manage duodenal ulcers, gastric ulcers, and postoperative gastric surgery.

   a. Instruct client that bland diets are presented in stages with the gradual addition of certain foods.
   b. Provide frequent, small feedings during active stress periods.

2. Establish regular meals and food patterns when condition permits.
3. Foods allowed include:

   a. Milk, butter, eggs (not fried), custard, vanilla ice cream, cottage cheese
   b. Cooked refined or strained cereal, enriched white bread
   c. Gelatin; homemade creamed, pureed soups
   d. Baked or broiled potatoes

4. Examples of foods that are eliminated include:

   a. Spicy and highly seasoned foods
   b. Raw foods
   c. Very hot and very cold foods
   d. Gas-forming foods (varies with individuals)
   e. Coffee, alcoholic beverages, carbonated drinks
   f. High-fat-content foods (some butter and margarine allowed)

Mechanical Soft Diet

1. A mechanical soft diet is used when clients

   a. Are edentulous
   b. Have poorly fitted dentures
   c. Have difficulty chewing
   d. Do not chew food thoroughly

2. Any food that can be easily digested can be included in this diet. It allows clients variations in tastes that are not allowed on a soft diet (chili beans).

Pureed Diet

1. A pureed diet provides food that has been mashed, minced, or ground.

   a. Used for clients with dysphagia
   b. Used for clients with limited chewing ability

2. When assisting clients with this type of diet, talk with them about the meal, describing the different foods. When the texture is all the same, distinguishing between foods is difficult.
3. Do not mix all pureed food together or feed out of one bowl or dish. Try to keep foods separate and feed alternately, with dessert last.

Blenderized Liquid Diet

1. Contains food and liquid that are blenderized to liquid form
2. Used for individuals who cannot chew, swallow, or tolerate solid food; or may be used for gastrostomy feeding.

Unit 19.1 Documentation and Evaluation

DOCUMENTATION for Modified Therapeutic Diets

- Type of diet provided
- Client's daily weight
- Intake and output
- Client's understanding of dietary restriction

- Any client or family teaching provided
- Nutritional consult requested
- Client's tolerance of diet progression
- Community agency referral offered

EVALUATION/Critical Thinking

Expected Outcomes

- Therapeutic diet assists in management of client's altered health status.
- Client accepts therapeutic diet prescribed to help manage altered health status.
- Client demonstrates understanding (verbalized knowledge) of dietary information provided.

Unexpected Outcomes	Alternative Actions
• Client does not adhere to diet.	• Elicit client's feelings to determine reason for nonadherence. • Check method of diet preparation and administration to see if it is attractive and appealing. • Ensure that environment is conducive to eating. • Notify dietician to discuss diet with client.
• Client with sodium-restricted diet states that food has no taste.	• Recommend use of lemon, herbs, and spices to add flavor to foods. • Encourage client to avoid processed foods, frozen entrees, and salty snacks. • Inform client that salt craving decreases over time with change in diet. • Consult healthcare provider for recommendation of potassium-containing salt substitute.
• Client states that fat is fat and all fats are to be avoided in preference to carbohydrates.	• Suggest client remove all visible fat from and limit intake of red meats. • Encourage to substitute poultry (skin removed) and fish for red meat. • Limit intake of butter, salad dressings, and trans fat (partially hydrogenated) products. • Use low-fat or nonfat products. • Increase intake of fruits, vegetables, and legumes.
• Postmenopausal client has lactose intolerance but is concerned about need for increased calcium to prevent osteoporosis.	• Consult with registered dietitian. • Encourage intake of nonliquid dairy products (yogurt, cheese) or lactose-free dairy products. • Suggest intake of leafy vegetables and canned fishes. • Calcium carbonate supplements are best absorbed. • Recommend calcium carbonate supplement in low dose (500 mg or less), several times/day for better absorption and efficacy.

Nutrition Maintenance

Nursing Process Data

ASSESSMENT Database

- Check healthcare provider's or consultant's diet order.
- Determine client's sociocultural orientation.
- Obtain client's diet history and determine eating habits and food preferences.
- Determine if client is candidate for dietitian or speech pathologist consultation.
- Assess client's risk for aspiration.
- Check for specific instructions for positioning and feeding technique for the dysphagic client.

PLANNING Objectives

- To provide a diet that meets nutritional requirements and is acceptable to client
- To assist the visually impaired client to self-feed
- To assist the dysphagic client to eat

IMPLEMENTATION Procedures

DOCUMENTATION AND EVALUATION

Expected Outcomes

- Diet meets nutritional requirements and is acceptable to client's taste and cultural orientation.
- Visually impaired client is able to self-feed.
- Dysphagic client is able to eat using adaptations to prevent aspiration.

Unexpected Outcomes/Alternative Actions

Pearson Nursing Student Resources

Find additional review materials at
nursing.pearsonhighered.com.
Prepare for success with NCLEX®-style practice questions and Skill Checklists.

Skill 19.2.1 | Serving a Food Tray

Equipment
Diet tray
Overbed table
Utensils
Protective covering (e.g., towel)

Preparation
1. Check client's record for healthcare provider's diet order.
2. Obtain dietary consult, if necessary, to meet client's needs.
3. Elicit food preferences of the client.
4. Check all diet trays before serving to ensure the diet provided is the one ordered.

> **CLINICAL ALERT**
>
> Clients sensitive to latex have potential for serious allergic reactions to some plant proteins. Cross-reactivity to latex has been shown with foods such as avocado, banana, papaya, chestnuts, kiwi, potatoes, and tomatoes. Clients with allergy to these foods may have latex allergy and vice versa.

5. Ensure that hot food is hot and cold food is cold. ❶
6. Keep food trays attractive. Avoid spilling liquids on tray.
7. Assist client to empty bladder (if needed) and perform hand hygiene.
8. Remove unpleasant objects from area such as bedpan or urinal.

Procedure
1. Identify client by checking two forms of ID such as having client state name and birth date.
2. Perform hand hygiene and assist client to do so.

❶ Serving a food tray. *Source:* Monkey Business Images/Shutterstock

3. Assist client to sit in a chair, or elevate the head of the bed to 90 degrees.
4. Place protective covering over client's chest.
5. Place food tray on overbed table and adjust the table, so client can see the food.
6. Assist client as needed (cut meat, open containers).
7. Leave call light in client's reach and check on client periodically.
8. Reposition tray table at bedside when meal is completed.
9. Assist client with hand and oral hygiene if desired.
10. Position client for comfort.
11. Note percentage and type of food eaten.
12. Remove food tray from room.
13. Document percentage and type of food eaten and, if indicated, amount of liquid intake on I&O record.
14. Perform hand hygiene.

Skill 19.2.2 | Assisting the Visually Impaired Client to Eat

Procedure
1. Check client record for ordered diet.
2. Identify client by checking two forms of ID such as having client state name and birth date.
3. Perform hand hygiene.
4. Raise head of bed to HIGH position, or assist client to sit in chair if possible.
5. Assist client to perform hand hygiene.
6. Place protective covering over client's chest.
7. Place food tray on client's overbed table and adjust to client and caregiver's comfort.
8. Stand or sit facing client.

9. Assist client by using the following technique:
   a. Use the clock face to describe food arrangement on the plate.
   b. Tell the client the time on the clock at which each food item is placed; for example, "The corn is at 4 o'clock; chicken is at 8 o'clock."
   c. Encourage the client to feed self, but remain with client if possible.
10. Encourage the client to hold glass, bread, and finger foods.
11. Allow client time to chew and swallow.
12. Provide fluids throughout meal.
13. Alternate foods; rather than one complete item at a time.

(continued)

Skill 19.2.2 | Assisting the Visually Impaired Client to Eat *(continued)*

14. Allow client to rest at intervals during the meal.
15. Talk with client during meal. ➤ *Rationale:* Talking makes mealtime more pleasant and promotes relaxation.
16. Reposition tray table at bedside when meal is completed.
17. Assist client with hand and oral hygiene if desired.
18. Raise side rail if it has been lowered.
19. Position bed for comfort. Lower bed if it is raised.
20. Note percentage of food eaten.
21. Remove food tray from room.
22. Perform hand hygiene.
23. Document amount eaten. If necessary, record fluid intake on the I&O record.
24. Place call bell within client's reach.

Skill 19.2.3 | Assisting the Dysphagic Client to Eat

Equipment
Provision for oral care and hand hygiene
Towel
Penlight to inspect oral cavity
Oral suction catheter connected to suction source

Preparation
1. Note specific instructions for feeding technique (diet and positioning) prescribed by speech or swallowing specialist; for example, cornstarch, Thickit, or rice cereal to thicken food, as prescribed. ➤ *Rationale:* Clients with swallowing problems find it easier to swallow thickened liquids.
2. Check if client is receiving both oral and enteral feeding; stop the enteral solution about 1 hr before oral feeding.
3. Check that client has not recently received sedating medication.
4. Eliminate environmental distractors such as television and radio.
5. Provide a 30-min rest period before mealtime.
6. Ensure that temperature of food is appropriate.

Procedure
1. Complete hand hygiene.
2. Identify client by checking two forms of ID such as having client state name and birth date.
3. Provide client privacy.
4. Maintain bed in LOW position.
5. Assist client to sit upright (90 degrees) in a chair, or in bed with hips flexed, shoulders and face slightly forward, and chin parallel to the floor or slightly tucked. ➤ *Rationale:* Gravity assists proper bolus movement to the stomach.

Note: Prescribed position is different for specific forms of dysphagia. Some types of dysphagia necessitate client positioning to one side, or with head rotated toward the stronger or weaker side, or even side-lying. Instructions should be placed in client's record, care plan, and posted at client's head of bed.

6. Assist client to perform hand hygiene before eating.
7. Place towel over client's chest.
8. Place tray on overbed table and towel under plate.
   ➤ *Rationale:* This stabilizes the plate while feeding.
9. Suction oral secretions before feeding, if necessary.
10. Sit at client's side, or sit facing client.

11. Encourage self-feeding.
12. Instruct client to take (or offer) small portions of food at first (0.5–1 tsp at a time), bites manageable in size but large enough to require chewing.
13. Instruct client to eat food first, without accompanying liquid, reserving *all* liquid intake until after finishing food. ➤ *Rationale:* Using liquids to wash down boluses of food pushes the food down too rapidly, although some authorities recommend alternating solids with liquids.

> **CLINICAL ALERT**
> The use of a straw increases risk of aspiration because the dysphagic client has less control over the amount of fluid intake. Similarly, the dysphagic client should not be fed with a syringe.

14. Instruct client to perform an exaggerated sucking motion at the beginning of each swallow with chin tucked slightly. ➤ *Rationale:* This decreases risk of aspiration.

Note: Clients with advanced dementia may not remember how to chew or swallow. Demonstrating chewing and gently stroking the area under the client's chin with a downward motion during swallowing may be helpful cues.

15. Allow client to concentrate on swallowing *without* distractions such as conversation or television. ➤ *Rationale:* For the dysphagic client, swallowing takes concentration; talking increases risk for aspiration.
16. Avoid rushed or forced feeding and make sure client is swallowing every mouthful.
17. Visually inspect oral cavity and under dentures for retained food. ➤ *Rationale:* Buildup may occur on weak side of mouth or pharynx.
18. Observe client closely for evidence of aspiration (e.g., cough, drooling, voice change such as hoarseness or a gurgling noise after swallowing), and suction oropharynx if indicated.
19. Help with feeding only if client shows signs of weakness and fatigue.
20. Provide positive reinforcement for accomplishment.

21. Assist with oral care and hand hygiene after meal.
    ➤ *Rationale:* This reduces oral colonization with pathogens and risk of aspiration pneumonia.
22. Remove food tray and raise side rails as indicated.
23. Place call bell in reach.

24. Record percentage of food eaten and amount of liquid intake (if indicated).
25. Maintain client's sitting position for 30 min after eating.
26. Carefully observe client with impaired communication for 30 min after the first few servings.

Unit 19.2 Documentation and Evaluation

DOCUMENTATION for Nutrition Maintenance

- Appetite
- Food intake (percentage eaten)
- Tolerance to diet

- Weight
- Liquid intake
- Feeding techniques for the dysphagic client

EVALUATION/Critical Thinking

Expected Outcomes

- Diet meets nutritional requirements and is acceptable to client's taste and cultural orientation.
- Visually impaired client is able to self-feed.
- Dysphagic client is able to eat using adaptations to prevent aspiration.

Unexpected Outcomes	Alternative Actions
• Client is nauseated and vomits.	• Withhold food if client is nauseated or vomiting. • Provide antiemetic or client's preferred comfort measures (cold cloth to throat, soda drink if not contraindicated). • Identify potential sources for nausea: specific foods or odors, experience of pain, side effects of medication (e.g., morphine sulfate), or positional changes.
• Visually impaired client only eats food on one half of food tray.	• Client may have *homonymous hemianopia* due to stroke and may be unable to see the half of the tray on paralyzed side. • Move food tray so that ignored side is within client's restricted range of vision (move tray leftward if client has had a left CVA and right side of tray has been ignored). • Encourage client to turn head so that client's visual field includes the half of tray with food that has not been seen or eaten.
• Client has signs of aspirating food (coughing, drooling, hoarseness, noisy breathing).	• Request speech pathologist consult for swallow evaluation. • Ensure that assistive personnel are following individualized feeding instructions and precautions (e.g., client positioning, use of thickening agents, and avoiding use of straws). • Remind client not to talk while eating and to concentrate on swallowing.

Nasogastric Tube Therapies

Nursing Process Data

ASSESSMENT Database

- Validate order for NG tube type and purpose.
- Assess overall status necessitating NG decompression (gastric surgery, intestinal obstruction).
- Assess status of GI function (presence of nausea, vomiting, abdominal distention, presence/absence of passage of flatus or bowel movement).
- Assess patency of nares.
- Assess risk for aspiration.
- Assess client's I&O balance and relevant lab data (electrolytes, hemoglobin and hematocrit, coagulation studies).
- Assess type of IV fluid replacement therapy client is receiving.

PLANNING Objectives

- To remove fluid and gas from the gastrointestinal tract
- To maintain decompression tube patency
- To perform gastric lavage to remove blood, fluid, or particles, or to prevent digestion and absorption of poison

IMPLEMENTATION Procedures

DOCUMENTATION AND EVALUATION

Expected Outcomes

- NG tube is placed without complication.
- NG tube functions effectively (gastric contents are decompressed).
- Toxic substances are removed by lavage or not absorbed.

Unexpected Outcomes/Alternative Actions

Pearson Nursing Student Resources

Find additional review materials at **nursing.pearsonhighered.com.**
Prepare for success with NCLEX®-style practice questions and Skill Checklists.

Skill 19.3.1 | Inserting a Large-Bore Nasogastric (NG) Tube

Equipment

Tapered plug for tube (if indicated for single-**lumen** tube)

Single-lumen Levin tube or double-lumen Salem sump tube with antireflux valve (30–36 in. [76–91 cm]) (Box 19-5 ■)

Water-soluble lubricant

Tape (1 in. or 2.5 cm) or commercial tube holder

pH chemstrip or Gastroccult test card and developer

Towel

Emesis basin

Tissues

Safety pin and rubber band

Tongue blade

Glass of water with straw

50-mL catheter-tip syringe

Clean gloves

Indelible pen or piece of tape for marking tube

Spindle adapter

Suction tubing and suction source

Preparation

1. Check healthcare provider's order and client care plan for inserting an NG tube.

2. Check client's identification using two forms of ID such as having client state name and birth date.
3. Discuss procedure with client. ➤ *Rationale:* Demonstration of items to be used helps to allay client's fear and to gain cooperation.
4. Provide privacy.
5. Gather equipment.

Procedure

1. Perform hand hygiene.
2. Don clean gloves.
3. Position client at a 45-degree angle or higher with head of bed elevated.

Box 19-5 GASTRIC (SALEM) SUMP TUBE AND SALEM SUMP TUBE WITH GiENTRI PORT

This gastric tube is a double-lumen radiopaque plastic tube. One lumen is used for decompression. The blue lumen with a blue pigtail provides an air vent to allow atmospheric pressure to enter the stomach to prevent tube adherence to gastric mucosa when the tube is attached to suction. It is NOT used for irrigation, obtaining a specimen, and so on. However, if the vent lumen is blocked and requires flushing, after the flush, the pigtail should be cleared with an injection of 20 mL air. The pigtail should be kept above the level of the client's stomach to prevent stomach contents from siphoning into the air vent lumen, making it dysfunctional.

One specific type of nasogastric system is the Salem sump tube with GiENTRI port. This nasogastric tube has selector knobs to allow a change in modes for suctioning (decompression), feeding, irrigating, and medication administration, all through one closed port. The antireflux valve/air vent lumen allows atmospheric air to enter the stomach similar to the way the double lumen tube with blue pigtail functions.

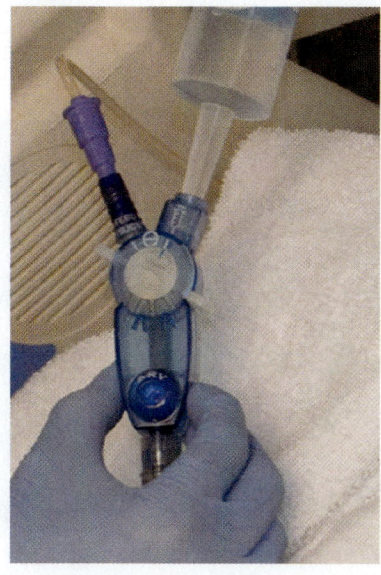

Salem sump with GiENTRI port.

(continued)

Skill 19.3.1 | Inserting a Large-Bore Nasogastric (NG) Tube *(continued)*

4. Examine nostrils, and select the most patent nostril by having client breathe through each one. ➤ *Rationale:* The nostril with greater airflow should be chosen for insertion.

5. Place a towel over client's chest, an emesis basin and tissues within reach; establish a cueing signal for client to use to stop you momentarily. ➤ *Rationale:* Client may experience discomfort or gag during tube insertion.

6. Measure from tip of client's nose to earlobe to xiphoid (NEX) process of sternum to determine appropriate length for tube insertion. ❶

7. Mark determined distance on tube with tape or pen if tube does not have markings.

8. Coil end of tube over fingers. ➤ *Rationale:* This softens tube and facilitates insertion.

9. Lubricate first 4 in. (10 cm) of tube with water-soluble lubricant. ➤ *Rationale:* Oil-based lubricant could cause respiratory complications. ❷

10. With client's head slightly extended, carefully insert tube through nostril to back of throat. ❸ Aim the tube toward the ear on that side and downward toward the nasopharynx. ➤ *Rationale:* Advancing tube this way conforms to anatomic passageways.

11. Instruct client to flex head forward. ❹ ➤ *Rationale:* This position helps prevent the tube from entering client's airway.

> **CLINICAL ALERT**
> Coughing and choking are normal responses for some clients. However, choking and coughing *plus cyanosis* or inability to speak indicate that the tube may be in the airway.

12. Suggest client sip water while advancing tube until predetermined mark is reached. ❺ ➤ *Rationale:* Swallowing opens the upper esophageal sphincter and allows the tube to enter the esophagus.

13. Listen at tube end for air exchange at 10-in. (25-cm) (**carina**) level; if no sound is heard, advance tube. ➤ *Rationale:* If sound is heard, the tube may be advancing into the airway and should be removed.

14. Continue advancing tube, having client dry swallow or giving client sips of water, until mark is reached.

15. Obtain radiographic confirmation of correct tube placement of any blindly inserted tube before its initial use for feeding or medication administration.

16. Verify tube placement by aspirating gastric contents with 50-mL syringe to check color and pH. ❻ See Skill 19.4.2, Determining Gastric pH; if it is 5 or less, color is green or clear with tan *mucus shreds*, tube is in stomach. (Small bowel aspirate indicates a pH range of 6–7 and color is golden

A

B

❶ NG tube measuring **(A)** Nose to earlobe, **(B)** Earlobe to xyphoid.

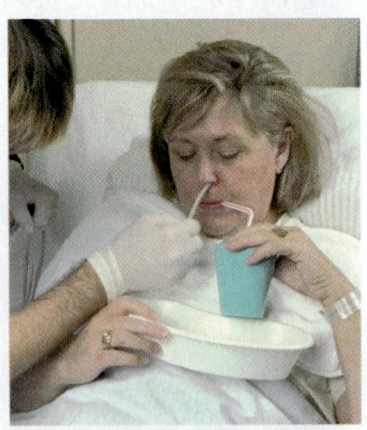

❷ Lubricate first 4 inches of NG tube with water-soluble lubricant.

❸ Insert NG tube through client's more patent nostril.

❹ Instruct client to flex head forward and take sips of water as tube is advanced.

yellow to brownish green, consistency is thick. Pulmonary tree aspirate has pH of 6 or greater and color is white or pale yellow and watery consistency.) ➤ *Rationale:* The outcome of pH testing is useful only if the fluid aspirated tests acidic (<5.5).

Note: The pH and capnography methods are inconclusive for *initial* verification of feeding tube placement.

❺ NG tube inserted through naris to stomach.

❻ Aspirate gastric contents to check color and pH.

❼ Tape tube securely to client's nose to prevent tube migration.

EVIDENCE-BASED PRACTICE
Determining Proper NG Tube Placement

In adults, nasogastric tube placement errors vary considerably from 1.3% up to 50%. A number of methods have been proposed to determine whether a tube has been inadvertently placed into the pulmonary tree, including air insufflation, observation of respiratory symptoms, pH testing of aspirated fluid, visual inspection of aspirated fluid, detection of carbon dioxide in the tube, and x-ray tube location verification. Radiographic confirmation is the gold standard. The use of capnometry or capnography (measurement of the concentration of carbon dioxide in exhaled air) is a reliable method in differentiating between respiratory and GI tube placement after the initial verification. Spring gauge pressure manometer is also highly sensitive and specific identifying tube location. Visual inspection of aspirate and auscultation are *unreliable* and should.

Testing Blood in Gastric Specimen

a. Note *color* of secretions. ➤ *Rationale:* Coffee-grounds appearance may represent digested blood, while bright red color may indicate active bleeding or ingestion of red food.

b. Place one drop of aspirate onto Gastroccult test area. (See photo in Skill 19.4.2, Determining Gastric pH.)

c. Apply two drops of Gastroccult developer directly over the sample in the Gastroccult test area.

d. Read occult blood results within 60 sec; any blue color indicates presence of blood.

Note: To determine if reagents in developer are functioning properly, add one drop of developer between positive and negative areas. The positive Performance Monitor area should turn blue within 10 sec and the negative area should not turn blue.

17. Tape tube securely to nose or use an attachment device. ❼ (StatLock-NG Securement Device is flexible, yet resistant to tearing and adheres strongly to skin.) ❽ ➤ *Rationale:* When tube is taped securely, tissue trauma caused by pull on sides of nostril will be minimized.

a. Cut tape about 3 in. (7.6 cm) long.

b. Split half of tape lengthwise.

c. Place unsplit end of tape over bridge of nose, with bifurcated ends hanging free.

d. Wrap each end of tape around the tube where it exits from the nose.

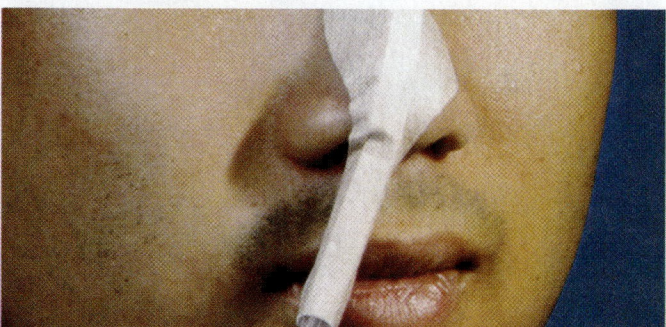

❽ StatLock-NG Securement Device prevents tissue trauma.

(continued)

Skill 19.3.1 | Inserting a Large-Bore Nasogastric (NG) Tube (continued)

18. Plug end of tube or connect it to suction tubing using tapered adapter. ❾
19. Mark tube at client's nostril. ➤ *Rationale:* This is to note possible tube migration.

Decompressing the GI Tract

a. Connect suction tubing to suction source. ❿ ⓫
b. Set suction on *intermittent low* (40 mm Hg) for decompression. ➤ *Rationale:* Intermittent suction allows gastric tube suction force to be intermittently released, thereby reducing risk of mucosal erosion.
   Or
c. Connect clear lumen of Salem sump tube to *continuous low* suction (30–40 mm Hg) or to *intermittent high* suction (120 mm Hg). ➤ *Rationale:* Continuous suction can be used because air vent lumen prevents excessive negative pressure from developing in stomach.

20. Secure tube with tape or rubber band pinned to client's gown, leaving slack for head movement. ⓬

❾ Tapered adapter is inserted to connect NG tube to suction tubing.

⓫ Closed all-in-one enteric system port allows feeding, suctioning, irrigating, and medication administration. The built-in antireflux valve prevents gastric wall invagination during suction, replacing blue "pigtail" function.

❿ Connect suction tubing to suction source.

⓬ Secure tube by pinning to client's gown so that blue pigtail is stabilized.

Box 19-6 **ORAL/NASAL HYGIENE FOR NG/NI TUBE CLIENTS**

- Clients who are unable to **ingest** food or take fluids by mouth should receive regular oral and nasal hygiene to keep mucous membranes moist and to help prevent infection of the parotid glands.
- Oral hygiene also reduces the risk of aspiration pneumonia, as it decreases the number of pathogens in oropharyngeal secretions.
- Chewing gum or sucking on sugar-free candy also helps stimulate salivation, but excessive use can stimulate gastric secretions and cause electrolyte imbalance.

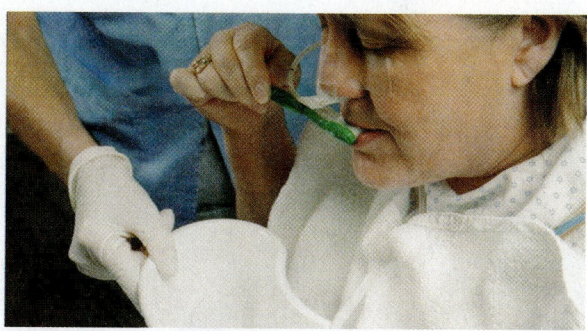

Provide regular nasal and oral hygiene to keep mucous membranes moist and help prevent parotiditis and bacterial colonization of the upper respiratory tract.

21. Implement procedure below when double-lumen (Salem sump) tube is used.

   a. Stabilize blue pigtail above level of stomach.
      ➤ **Rationale:** This helps to prevent siphoning into sump (pigtail) tubing.

   b. Insert antireflux valve (blue tip) into blue pigtail of Salem tube. ⑬ ➤ **Rationale:** Antireflux valve allows air to enter tube, yet prevents leakage of gastric secretions.

22. Provide oral and nasal hygiene. (Box 19-6 ▪)
23. Remove gloves and perform hand hygiene.
24. Position client for comfort.

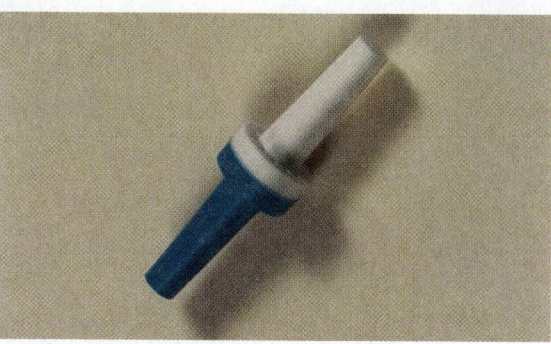

⑬ Insert blue side of antireflux valve into Salem sump tube blue pigtail.

Skill 19.3.2 | Flushing and Maintaining Nasogastric (NG) Tube

Equipment
Disposable irrigation set with 50-mL syringe with catheter tip
Emesis basin
Towel
Normal saline irrigation solution
I&O record sheet
Clean gloves

Preparation
1. Check orders and client care plan.
2. Perform hand hygiene.
3. Check client identity with two forms of ID such as having client state name and birth date.
4. Provide privacy.
5. Explain procedure to client.
6. Place client in semi-Fowler's position.

Procedure
1. Don clean gloves.
2. Disconnect NG tube from suction source if used.
3. Place towel under NG tube to protect sheets and place emesis basin nearby.

4. Check for NG tube placement by obtaining a radiograph if tube placement is in doubt. ❶ ➤ **Rationale:** Solution could be instilled in lungs if NG tube is not in the stomach.
5. Draw up 20–30 mL normal saline into irrigating syringe. ❷

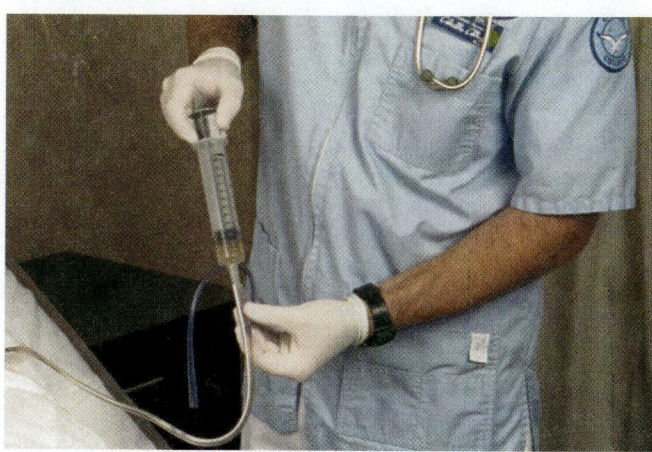

❶ Aspirate secretions to check tube placement before instilling saline solution.

(continued)

Skill 19.3.2 | Flushing and Maintaining Nasogastric (NG) Tube *(continued)*

❷ For irrigating NG tube, draw up 20–30 mL normal saline into irrigating syringe.

❸ Gently instill normal saline into NG tube by syringe, or allow to flow by gravity.

CLINICAL ALERT

- If water rather than normal saline is used to flush enteral decompression tubes, the production of gastric secretions will increase and increasing amounts of electrolytes will be washed out. Similarly, if the client is NPO but ingests ice chips ad lib, electrolyte imbalance due to washout can occur, causing metabolic alkalosis.
- Limit the use of ice chips by substituting chips made from an electrolyte solution, and provide oral hygiene to keep the client's mucous membranes moist for comfort.
- If the client is receiving adequate parenteral hydration (IV fluids), excessive thirst should not be experienced.

6. Gently instill normal saline into NG tube or remove syringe plunger, pour NS into syringe barrel, and allow solution to flow in by gravity. ❸ ❹
7. Repeat procedure if necessary.
8. Reconnect NG tube to suction or plug tube.
9. Record instilled amount on I&O record.
10. Remove gloves and perform hand hygiene.
11. Reposition client for comfort.

CLINICAL ALERT

If secretions siphon into blue vent lumen, clear it by instilling 20 mL of normal saline followed by 20 mL of air. Air vent must be cleared of secretions to restore proper functioning.

❹ Follow Salem tube irrigation with injection of air into blue pigtail to clear; then reinsert blue end of antireflux valve.

Skill 19.3.3 | Performing Gastric Lavage

Equipment
Large-bore (37–40 Fr) soft Ewald or orogastric tube (Client must
  have cuffed endotracheal tube in place if comatose.)
Large irrigating syringe with adapter
Container for aspirate
Lavage fluid, normal saline, or lukewarm water
Container for specimen
Water-soluble lubricant
Standby suction available
Towel
Pen and tape
Gloves

Preparation
1. Check healthcare provider's orders for gastric lavage and
   solution to be used.
2. Identify client using two forms of ID.
3. Determine if client is alert or comatose.
4. Gather equipment.
5. Perform hand hygiene and don gloves.

Procedure
1. Per agency protocol (healthcare provider may insert)
   measure for tube insertion using the following guidelines:
   a. Measure distance from bridge of nose to earlobe to
      xiphoid process (NEX).
   b. Mark with pen or tape.
2. Place client in head-down, left side-lying position.
   ➤ *Rationale:* This reduces risk of aspiration if client
   vomits.
3. Lubricate tube with water-soluble lubricant.
4. Insert tube nasogastrically or orogastrically (about 20 in.
   [50 cm]).

5. Aspirate gastric contents with syringe and confirm pH, before
   instilling solution. **Save specimen for analysis.**
6. Obtain radiographic confirmation of correct placement of
   any blindly inserted tube before its initial use for medication
   administration.

> **CLINICAL ALERT**
> Gastric lavage used to remove unabsorbed poison or
> drug ingestion is generally ineffective if more than 60 min
> have passed, and the procedure may delay administration
> of activated charcoal or antidotes; therefore, it is not
> recommended to manage an overdose. It is not used
> for corrosive agents or petroleum distillates due to
> risk of aspiration, and induced vomiting is no longer
> considered safe.

7. Repeatedly instill 50–100 mL normal saline or water
   and aspirate contents. ➤ *Rationale:* Some authorities
   recommend water to lavage the stomach of blood since
   it breaks up clots more easily than saline solution, is less
   expensive, and is readily available.
8. Carefully monitor volume instilled and character and volume
   of aspirated contents. ➤ *Rationale:* This will assist in
   determining net volume if there is blood loss.
9. Continue repeating process until gastric return is clear, or as
   ordered.
10. Stomach will be left empty for decontamination. See Skill
    19.3.4, Administering Poison Control Agents.
11. Pinch tube for removal, wrap in towel, and dispose of
    equipment.
12. Remove and dispose of gloves and perform hand hygiene.
13. Record vital signs frequently and monitor client's response
    closely.

Skill 19.3.4 | Administering Poison Control Agents

Equipment
Large (37–40 Fr) Soft Ewald tube (healthcare provider may insert);
  comatose client must have endotracheal tube in place.
Lukewarm tap water or saline for lavage
Container for aspirated contents
Large irrigating syringe with catheter tip
60–100 g of activated charcoal in aqueous slurry consistency to
  administer orally or through gastric tube (Box 19-7 ■)
  Or
Balanced polyethylene glycol–electrolyte solution (e.g.,
  GoLYTELY) for mechanical bowel cleansing

Preparation
See Skill 19.3.1, Inserting a Large-Bore Nasogastric Tube.

Box 19-7 **ACTIVATED CHARCOAL FOR INGESTED POISONS**
Activated charcoal absorbs significant amounts of certain poisons
in the stomach and intestines. The earlier charcoal is given, the
more effective it is. The amount given is 60–100 g orally or per gastric tube. Repeated doses (20–30 g) may be given every 3–4 hr.

Procedure
1. Identify client using two forms of ID such as having client
   state name and date of birth.
2. Place comatose *intubated* client in a head-down, left side-
   lying position. Place cooperative alert client on commode
   and monitor client for safety.

(continued)

Skill 19.3.4 | Administering Poison Control Agents *(continued)*

3. Insert large-bore (37–40 Fr) flexible tube nasogastrically or orogastrically.
4. Aspirate gastric contents with syringe and confirm pH, before instilling activated charcoal. Consider capnometry to confirm placement. **Note**: This is a critical step if client is not intubated. Save specimen for analysis.

5. Lavage repeatedly with 50–100 mL of fluid until return is clear.
6. Administer activated charcoal slurry and repeat if ordered or, for cooperative client, administer balanced electrolyte solution per NG tube at a rate of 1–2 L/hr until rectal run-out is clear.

Skill 19.3.5 | Removing an NG or Nasointestinal (NI) Tube

Equipment
Towel, paper towel
Stethoscope
Container of sterile normal saline solution
50-mL syringe with catheter tip
Tissues
Gloves
Tube plug

Preparation
1. Check healthcare provider's orders for NG tube removal.
2. Verify client's identity using two forms of identification.
3. Assess client to determine the presence of bowel sounds (auscultate to right of umbilicus as alternative to all four sites). Signs more indicative of GI function include passage of flatus, bowel movement, absence of nausea or vomiting, and presence of hunger. ❶
4. Prepare client for tube removal by explaining that it may cause some nasal discomfort, coughing, sneezing, or gagging.
5. Perform hand hygiene and don gloves.

Procedure
1. Provide tissues and place towel over client's chest.
2. Disconnect NG tube from suction tubing if indicated.

3. Flush NG tube with 20 mL normal saline (sterile water or saline for NI tube). ➤ *Rationale:* This clears the tube so that GI contents do not inadvertently drain into esophagus on tube removal.
4. Follow saline flush with a bolus of air. ➤ *Rationale:* This frees tube from stomach and intestinal lining.
5. Unpin tube from client's gown and loosen tape that secures tube to client's nose. ❷
6. Plug tube or clamp it by folding it over in your gloved hand.
7. Pinch tube close to client's naris, have client take a deep breath and hold it while you withdraw the tube in one continuous motion. ❸ ➤ *Rationale:* Holding breath closes the glottis and helps prevent aspiration.
8. Wrap tube in paper towel to remove from client's view.
9. Offer oral and nasal hygiene. ❹
10. Empty and record amount and character of drainage.
11. Discard disposable equipment and return reusable equipment to appropriate area.
12. Remove and dispose of gloves and perform hand hygiene.

❶ To determine return of GI function, assess client for presence of bowel sounds, passage of flatus or bowel movement, absence of nausea, presence of hunger.

❷ Clamp tube, unpin tube from gown, and loosen tape on nose securing NG tube.

❸ Have client hold breath. Remove NG tube with continuous steady pull.

❹ Offer oral and nasal hygiene after removing tube.

EVIDENCE-BASED PRACTICE
Postoperative Ileus

Postoperative Ileus (POI) occurs almost universally among clients worldwide after abdominal surgery. Historically, nurses and physicians have been trained to auscultate for 5 min in each quadrant. Bowel sounds were an indicator of POI resolution. This practice has been questioned, since bowel sounds reflect the normal activity of the small intestine alone but do not represent return of functional GI motility. Primary indicators of the return of GI motility include return of flatus, bowel movement, client's tolerance of oral intake without nausea or vomiting, return of appetite, and absence of abdominal distension, bloated feeling, and cramps. Auscultation of bowel sounds after surgery may be an antiquated practice and should be replaced with more reliable indicators.

Source: Massey (2012)

Unit 19.3 Documentation and Evaluation

DOCUMENTATION for Nasogastric Tube Therapies

- Type of tube inserted
- Technique used to assess NG tube placement
- Character and amount of drainage
- Type of suction and pressure setting used
- Frequency and solution used for flush or irrigation
- Gastrointestinal assessment findings (e.g., passage of flatus, bowel movement)
- Net return for lavaged client (amount of irrigant instilled subtracted from amount of aspirated return)
- Frequent vital signs (if indicated)
- Nasal and oral hygiene measures
- Client's tolerance of decompression
- Results of gastric specimen testing (blood, pH)
- Decontaminating agents instilled

EVALUATION/Critical Thinking

Expected Outcomes

- NG tube is placed without complication.
- NG tube functions effectively (gastric contents are decompressed).
- Toxic substances are removed by lavage or not absorbed.

Unexpected Outcomes	Alternative Actions
• NG tube is difficult to advance.	• Select more patent nostril: Have client compress each nostril and breathe in to determine which is more patent. Ask about previous fractures. • Rotate tube or withdraw slightly, then try to advance, but do not force. • Relubricate tube and try again. • Curl tube around fist and hold under warm running water to soften for easier insertion. • Have client hold ice chips in mouth for a few minutes to numb nasal passage and suppress gag reflex.
• Client coughs, is unable to speak, and becomes cyanotic during tube insertion.	• Remove tube immediately, as these indicate that tube is being advanced into client's airway.
• Salem sump pigtail leaks gastric contents.	• Flush pigtail with normal saline, then with air to clear. • Keep blue pigtail at level above client's stomach. • Maintain antireflux valve plug insertion (blue side into blue pigtail lumen).
• Client has ingested a large number of tablets that cannot be removed by lavage.	• Whole bowel irrigation is more effective for ingestion of enteric-coated or sustained-release tablets. • Repeated dose of activated charcoal may be indicated to speed drug elimination. • Prepare for possible arrangement for hemodialysis.

Nursing Process Data

ASSESSMENT Database

- Assess client's nutritional status.
- Check healthcare provider's order for enteral feeding.
- Determine rationale for prescribed enteral feeding.
- Ensure appropriate placement of NG/NI tube using a variety of means.
- Assess client's gastrointestinal status (passage of flatus, bowel movement).

PLANNING Objectives

- To provide nutrients to the client who is temporarily unable to ingest food
- To correct nutritional deficiency in selected clients
- To provide nutrients to the client who requires continuous enteral feeding
- To maintain gastrostomy tube site

IMPLEMENTATION Procedures

DOCUMENTATION AND EVALUATION

Expected Outcomes

- Client's nutritional needs are met with nasogastric feeding.
- Client's nutritional needs are met with continuous enteral feeding.
- Gastrostomy tube site is free of signs of irritation or inflammation.

Unexpected Outcomes/Alternative Actions

Pearson Nursing Student Resources

Find additional review materials at
nursing.pearsonhighered.com.
Prepare for success with NCLEX®-style practice questions and Skill Checklists.

Several guidelines exist for the provision and assessment of nutrition support therapy in the adult critically ill client:

1. Traditional nutrition assessment tools (albumin, prealbumin, and anthropometry) are not validated in critical care. Before initiation of feedings, assessment should include evaluation of weight loss and previous nutrient intake prior to admission, level of disease severity, comorbid conditions, and function of the GI tract.

2. Nutrition support therapy in the form of enteral nutrition should be initiated in the critically ill client who is unable to maintain volitional intake.

3. Enteral nutrition is the preferred route of feeding over PN for the critically ill client who requires nutrition support therapy.

4. Enteral feeding should be started early, within the first 24–48 hr following admission. The feedings should be advanced toward goal over the next 48–72 hr.

5. In the setting of hemodynamic compromise (clients requiring significant hemodynamic support including vasoactive agents, alone or in combination with large volume fluid or blood product resuscitation to maintain cellular perfusion), enteral nutrition should be withheld until the client is fully resuscitated and/or stable.

6. In the ICU client population, neither the presence nor absence of bowel sounds nor evidence of passage of flatus and stool is required for the initiation of enteral feeding.

7. Either gastric or small bowel feeding is acceptable in the ICU setting. Small bowel access should be used in clients at high risk for aspiration, or those with repeated high gastric residual volumes.

8. Inappropriate cessation of enteral nutrition should be avoided. Holding enteral nutrition for gastric residual volumes <500 mL in the absence of other signs of intolerance should be avoided. NPO periods for diagnostic tests or procedures should be minimized to prevent inadequate delivery of nutrients and prolonged periods of ileus.

9. If there is evidence of protein–calorie malnutrition on admission and enteral nutrition is not feasible, it is appropriate to initiate PN as soon as possible (McClave, Martindale, Vanek, McCarthy, Roberts, Taylor, Ochoa, … & Cresci, 2009).

Skill 19.4.1 | Administering an Intermittent Feeding via Large-Bore Nasogastric Tube

Equipment
Pen to mark date and time on equipment
Prescribed nutritional formula/product (check expiration date)
Calibrated container for measuring formula
Irrigating syringe (50 mL) with catheter tip (date and discard in 24 hr)
pH indicator strip
Warm water for flushing, towel
Antimicrobial swab
Gloves
Clean dressing for gastrostomy site, if needed

Preparation
1. Check healthcare provider's order for type, amount, and frequency of feeding (Table 19-3 ■).
2. Wipe unopened formula container top with swab.
3. Pour prescribed amount of formula into container (if refrigerated, warm formula by placing container in hot water; do not use microwave to warm formula).
4. Cover, date, and refrigerate opened formula (discard in 24 hr).
5. Perform hand hygiene.
6. Maintain artificial airway cuff inflation during feeding (if indicated).

Procedure
1. Check client identity using two forms of ID such as having client state name and birth date.
2. Provide privacy and explain procedure and purpose to client.
3. Assess that client does not have abdominal distention, nausea or pain, and has bowel elimination or flatus.
4. Check mark on tube at exit site. Obtain an x-ray to confirm tube position if the tube's location is in doubt. ➤ *Rationale:* Tube may migrate.
5. Don gloves.
6. Elevate client's head of bed 30–45 degrees or high Fowler's.
7. Place towel under work area.
8. Remove white tip of antireflux valve from NG tube if indicated.
9. Insert syringe into NG tube to validate gastric placement. ➤ *Rationale:* Tube could have migrated between feedings.
   a. Check color, character, and test pH of aspirate (once every 4 hr after first 24 hr of tube placement).
   b. Aspirate gastric contents to determine residual volume. ❶ ➤ *Rationale:* Further client assessment is indicated if residual volume is greater than 500 mL and client shows other signs of intolerance (Box 19-8 ■).
   c. Return aspirated contents to stomach. ➤ *Rationale:* This helps prevent electrolyte imbalance.
10. Pinch tubing. ➤ *Rationale:* This procedure prevents air from entering stomach.

Table 19-3 Comparison of Enteral Tube Feeding Methods

	Advantages	Disadvantages
Nasogastric	• It is easily placed. • Intermittent feeding is possible (not recommended), so client is less confined. • Large-volume feeding may be delivered less often. • Acidic environment may reduce infection. • There is less risk of **dumping syndrome**. • It uses normal gastric emptying, preventing intestinal overload. • It is less expensive; no feeding pump required.	• Limited to 1 week use. • Gastric retention, reflux, and aspiration are possible. • It requires x-ray confirmation of placement before feeding unless aspirate is definitely acidic (<5.5 pH). • Large tube is uncomfortable and visible to others. • Naris ulceration may occur. • It allows regurgitation by interfering with normal upper and lower esophageal sphincter function. • Gastric ulceration or fistulae may occur.
Gastrostomy or PEG	• Long-term use is possible. • It allows intermittent feeding. • Normal gastric emptying occurs. • Tube is not visible to others. • Medication administration is easier. • There is less risk of infection. • Client can ambulate. • Esophageal irritation is avoided.	• It requires surgical placement with sedation or local anesthetic. • It requires local skin care. • It may ulcerate gastric mucosa.
Nasointestinal tube	• Smaller tube is more comfortable. • There is less risk of reflux and aspiration.	• It requires x-ray confirmation before feeding or flushing. • Tube is more difficult to place. • Client is still at risk for aspirating nasopharyngeal and gastric contents. • Elevated position must be maintained. • Constant infusion is used; intermittent feeding is not recommended because of osmotic response of small intestine. • Cramping, vomiting, distention, and diarrhea are more common. • It requires a pump and is more expensive. • Tube can displace back into stomach (with constant infusion, this increases risk of aspiration). • Medication administration is difficult (liquid form preferred). • There is greater risk of infection due to alkaline environment. • It is limited to 4-week use.
Jejunostomy	• Tube position is guaranteed. • Tube is not visible. • There is possibly less risk of reflux and aspiration.	• It requires general anesthesia for placement. • Continuous infusion is required. • Local skin care is required. • Cramping, vomiting, distention, and diarrhea are more common. • It has other disadvantages associated with nasointestinal feeding.

❶ Aspirate gastric contents to determine residual volume; then return contents to stomach to prevent electrolyte imbalance.

Box 19-8 RESIDUAL VOLUME CONSIDERATIONS

Gastric residual volumes do not correlate well to incidence of pneumonia, to measures of gastric emptying, or to incidence of regurgitation and aspiration. There is potential for inadequate nutrition support when feedings are delayed or withheld based on residual volumes under 500 mL. Assessment of tolerance should include absence of abdominal distention, nausea, and pain, and presence of bowel elimination and flatus.

Source: Metheny, Mills, & Stewart (2012)

CLINICAL ALERT
Always flush the NG tube with warm water after checking residual volume to prevent tube clogging.

(continued)

Skill 19.4.1 | Administering an Intermittent Feeding via Large-Bore Nasogastric Tube (continued)

11. Remove plunger from barrel of syringe, and attach barrel to NG tube.
12. Flush tube before feeding with 30 mL of warm water.
13. Fill syringe barrel with formula.
14. Hold container no more than 18 in. (46 cm) above client's stomach. ➤ *Rationale:* Holding container too high increases flow rate; rapid infusion can cause diarrhea or aspiration.
15. Allow formula to infuse slowly by gravity (between 20 and 35 min) through the tubing. Clamp tubing or continue to fill syringe before syringe empties; do not allow syringe to "run dry." ❷ ➤ *Rationale:* If syringe runs dry before the addition of more formula, air enters stomach.
16. Follow tube feeding with 30 mL warm water flush.
    ➤ *Rationale:* Water cleans tube and prevents obstruction with formula.
17. Reinsert antireflux valve.
18. Maintain head of bed elevation at least 1–2 hr.
19. Wash, rinse, and dry equipment after each feeding. Mark date and *change syringe daily.*
20. Return equipment to client's bedside.
21. Give prescribed amount of water between feedings, if tube feeding is the sole source of nutrition.
22. Provide regular oral hygiene.
23. Remove gloves and perform hand hygiene.

Note: An NG tube is meant to be used only on a short-term basis. Using a temporary NG tube for too long can lead to sinusitis, infections, and ulcerations on the tissue of your sinuses, throat, esophagus, or stomach.

Intermittent Feedings via Gastrostomy Tube

1. Check length of exposed tubing.
2. Aspirate to check residual volume. ➤ *Rationale:* Increased residuals may indicate delayed gastric emptying or migration of gastrostomy tube's internal stabilizer and pyloric outlet obstruction.
3. Hold syringe no higher than 18 in. (46 cm) above client's stomach and administer 30 mL of warm water to flush and test patency of tubing. Clamp tubing by folding before syringe empties. ➤ *Rationale:* This prevents administering air into client's stomach.
4. Remove plunger, insert empty syringe barrel into gastrostomy tube, and administer feeding no higher than 18 in. above client's stomach, allowing formula to flow slowly by gravity.
5. Proceed as with flushing, and then reinsert tube plug.
6. Remove dressing (if present) around gastrostomy site.
7. Wash, rinse, and dry skin. Assess skin condition.
8. Apply clean dressing. (See Skill 19.4.3, Dressing the Gastrostomy Tube Site.)
9. Maintain head of bed elevation for 1–2 hr.

❷ Allow feeding to flow by gravity through gastrostomy tube.

EVIDENCE-BASED PRACTICE
Safety Issues for Gastric Feeding
Studies show that clients receiving gastric feedings require intact gag and cough reflexes and adequate gastric emptying. Small bowel access for continuous enteral nutrition should be obtained for clients with tracheal aspiration, reflux esophagitis, gastroparesis, gastric outlet obstruction, or previous gastric surgery. Prokinetic drugs (metoclopramide and erythromycin) or narcotic antagonists (naloxone, alvimopan) should be initiated to promote motility when clinically feasible.

Source: McClave, Martindale, Vanek, McCarthy, Roberts, Taylor, ... & Cresci (2009)

Skill 19.4.2 | Determining Gastric pH

Note: Gastric pH is used to help determine NG tube placement, to assess gastric contents, and to evaluate and treat certain disease conditions. It is useful to determine placement only if aspirated secretions are acidic.

Equipment
50-mL syringe with catheter tip
Emesis basin
Applicator
pH test paper (e.g., Gastroccult card)

Procedure

1. Complete initial steps as for any procedure: gather equipment, explain procedure to client, perform hand hygiene, and don gloves.

Note: When testing for pH, wait at least 1 hr after administering medication or an NG feeding.

2. Attach a 50-mL syringe with catheter tip to the NG tube and flush with 20 mL of air.
3. Aspirate 5–10 mL of gastric secretions. **❶**
4. Note color of secretions—gastric secretions are greenish to tan or off-white; respiratory secretions are clear to light yellow with mucus; duodenal samples are usually deep yellow. *Color of secretions does not guarantee correct placement.*
5. Place 5 mL of gastric aspirate into a small cup or emesis basin and dip test pH paper into the cup, place a sample on the pH test paper, or using applicator, apply one drop of gastric sample to pH test area on Gastroccult card. **❷ ❸**
6. Read chemstrip pH within 30 sec by comparing the color of the paper with the pH color guide.
7. Gastric contents are usually pH ≤5.5. If the NG tube is in the pulmonary tree, it will be 6 or more. If the NG tube has passed into the small intestine, the pH is more than 6 and could be 7.0–8.0.

8. If clients are receiving medications that raise gastric pH, or have gastric bleeding or esophageal reflux, pH measurement may be unreliable.
9. Document result of gastric specimen (pH).

Note: Gastrostomy site may be left open to air.

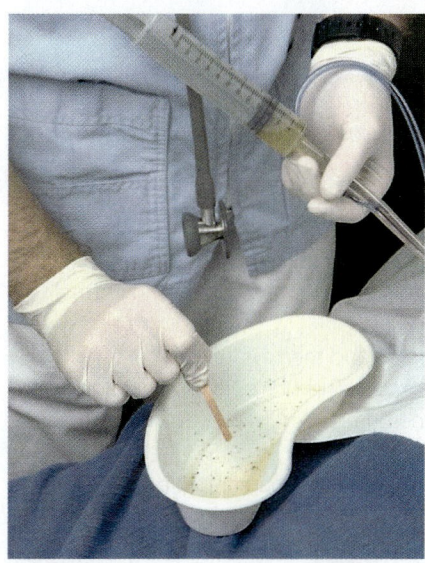

❷ Dip test paper into gastric secretion to test pH.
Note: Normal gastric pH is 1.5–3.5.

❶ Aspirate 5–10 mL of gastric secretions to test pH.

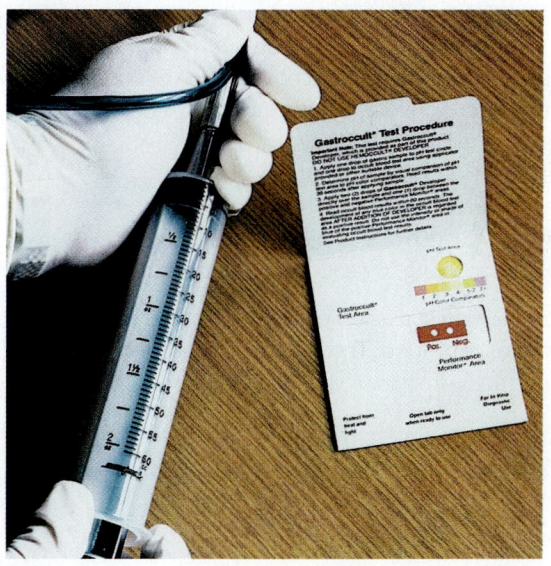

❸ Place small drop of secretion on card to check pH.

Skill 19.4.3 | Dressing the Gastrostomy Tube Site

Equipment

Normal saline; dated and initialed container left at client's bedside.

4×4 gauze squares or swabs

Protective skin barrier (if indicated)

Prepared split gauze dressing (occlusive dressing encourages fungal growth)

Gloves

Tape

Pen to label dressing

(continued)

Skill 19.4.3 | Dressing the Gastrostomy Tube Site *(continued)*

Preparation

1. Gather equipment.
2. Perform hand hygiene.

Procedure

1. Check client identity using two forms of ID such as having client state name and birth date.
2. Provide privacy and explain procedure and purpose to client.
3. Don gloves.
4. Remove old dressing and discard.
5. Inspect exit site for signs of irritation or leakage.
6. Open packet of gauze squares and saturate with normal saline.
7. Cleanse around exit site, and then rotate external bumper 90 degrees. ➤ *Rationale:* This prevents skin irritation and ulceration beneath the bumper.
8. Dry site.
9. Apply thin layer of protective skin barrier paste to site (if irritated). ➤ *Rationale:* This protects the skin from leakage.
10. Place split dressing over (*not under*) external bar. ❶
    ➤ *Rationale:* Dressing placed under the external bar can cause erosion of gastric tissue or abscess of the abdominal wall due to pressure on the internal bar within the stomach.
11. Secure dressing with tape (if necessary) and if external tube is long, secure it to dressing with tape. ➤ *Rationale:* This prevents tube drag and erosion or ulceration of the internal mucosa from tension on the inner retaining piece.
12. Mark dressing with initials, date, and time.
13. Remove gloves and perform hand hygiene.
14. Change tube dressing when wet, or daily.
15. After 1 week, cleanse site with soap and water and leave open to air, according to healthcare provider's orders.

Note: Clients requiring *sustained* enteral feeding may prefer a low-profile gastrostomy tube. These tubes are inserted several (3+) months after the gastrostomy tract (stoma) has healed. They fit close to the skin, so are less apt to be pulled out or get in the way of daily activities. In addition, some incorporate a one-way antireflux valve that opens for feedings and also prevents backflow of gastric contents. Since products differ, refer to the manufacturer's instructions for the specific tube your client has had inserted.

EVIDENCE-BASED PRACTICE
Blind Placement of Small-Bore Feeding Tubes

Small-bore feeding tubes (SBFT) placed blindly can cause bronchopulmonary injury related to misplacement. Estimates suggest more than 1.2 million SBFT are placed each year. If these were placed blindly, it could result in 3,600–8,400 pulmonary injuries and up to 3,600 deaths in the United States. There is discussion to abolish bedside SBFT insertion (Krenitsky, 2011).

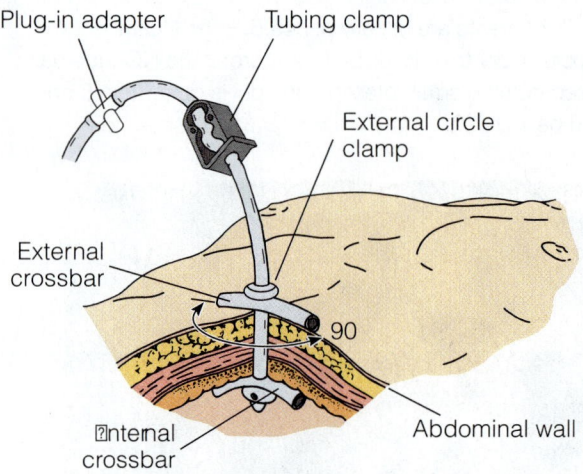

❶ Change tube dressing when wet, or daily, placing dressing over external crossbar.

Skill 19.4.4 | Inserting a Small-Bore Feeding Tube

Equipment

Small-bore (8–12 Fr) radiopaque enteral feeding tube (43–60 in. [110–150 cm]) with stylet
Administration set with pump or controller
60-mL catheter tip syringe
Sterile water or saline
Clean gloves
Water-soluble lubricant (if needed)
Tape or other device to secure tube
Cup with water and straw, if appropriate
Towel and tissues
Safety pin or clip
Emesis basin
pH chemstrip

Pen for marking tube
Prepared prokinetic agent (metaclopramide by IV injection or erythromycin by IV infusion) if ordered
Antimicrobial swab

Preparation

1. Validate healthcare provider's orders.
2. Gather equipment.
3. Identify client using two forms of ID, such as having client state name and birth date.
4. Provide privacy.
5. Administer prokinetic agent injection or infusion (if ordered for duodenal advancement) 10 min before tube insertion.

Procedure

1. Perform hand hygiene.
2. Explain procedure to client.
3. Elevate head of bed at least 45 degrees. Place towel over chest; provide tissues and emesis basin.
4. Determine length of tube for insertion into stomach. Use distal end of feeding tube, and measure from tip of nose to earlobe to xiphoid process (NEX) for gastric placement.

Note: For small bowel placement, all but 4 in. (10 cm) of tube is inserted.

5. Note NEX marking on tube and place tape or mark with pen.
6. Seat stylet connector firmly into tube connector.
7. Check that guidewire does not protrude through holes in feeding tube. Reposition guidewire if necessary. ❶ ➤ *Rationale:* This prevents trauma to mucosa during placement.

Note: Use of stylet is optional and may not be necessary in a conscious, cooperative client.

8. Don clean gloves.
9. Lubricate tip of feeding tube with water-soluble lubricant, or for tube with surface lubricant, moisten tip in water to activate lubricant.
10. Assess nares to determine patency. ➤ *Rationale:* The more patent nare is selected for tube insertion.
11. Instruct client to momentarily hyperextend neck.

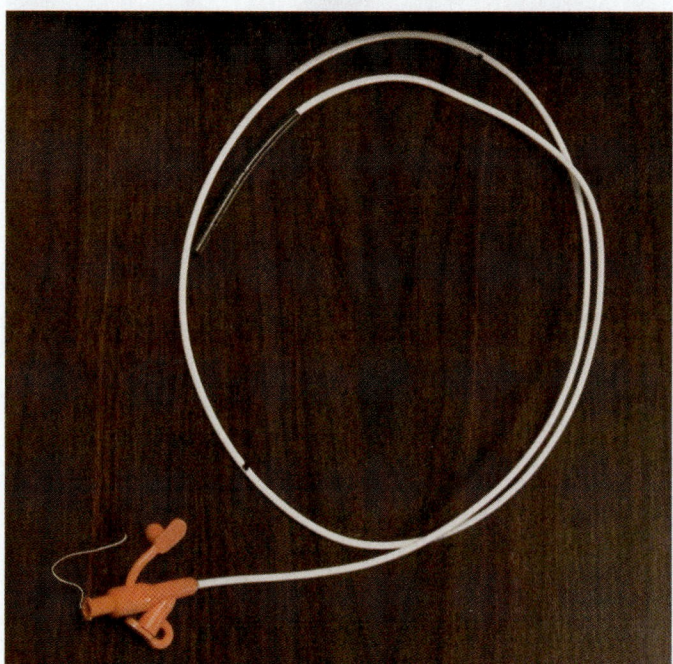

❶ Check that guidewire (stylet) does not protrude through holes in feeding tube. Reposition guidewire if necessary.

12. Insert feeding tube through patent nostril, gently advancing tube—advance parallel to nasal septum.
13. Ask client to flex head forward and swallow when tube reaches pharynx. ➤ *Rationale:* Hyperextension at this stage may open airway, and tube could advance into the trachea.
14. Pull back on tube if client begins to cough or shows signs of respiratory distress or cyanosis. ➤ *Rationale:* Tube may have entered trachea. Wait several seconds, and then advance tube asking client to swallow sips of water with tube advancement.
15. Listen at tube end for air exchange at carina level. ➤ *Rationale:* If air exchange is heard, tube may be in respiratory tract. If no sound is heard, advance tube.
16. Advance tube to premeasured (NEX) position.
17. Tape tube securely in place.
18. Flush tube side port with 30–50 mL of AIR and then attempt to slowly aspirate gastric contents; reposition client to *left side* and repeat aspiration if necessary to obtain a specimen.
19. Test aspirated specimen for color, character, and pH. ➤ *Rationale:* Gastric specimen should have pH ≤5.5. As tube advances into small intestine, pH becomes higher (>5.5).
20. Obtain x-ray to determine feeding tube placement.
21. Once gastric placement is confirmed, use a rotating motion to gently advance tube to all but 4 in. (10 cm) and retape securely.

Note: This may be facilitated by injections of 30 mL of air to free the tube away from the intestine.

22. For stylet removal, activate internal lubricant before removing stylet. Cap access port and flush tube through the stylet connector with 10 mL sterile water. ➤ *Rationale:* Reinsertion of stylet into the enteral tube should never be attempted because this can perforate tube and client's esophagus.
23. Once desired position is validated, swab feeding tube port, and attach administration set.
24. Swab port, and then *gently* flush feeding tube (side port) with 20 mL of sterile water (using 60-mL catheter tip syringe) every 4 hr, and before and after each medication administered. ➤ *Rationale:* This maintains patency of the tube. Smaller syringe and vigorous flushing could cause pressure exceeding bursting pressure of the tube.
25. Check tape that secures tube to nose daily. Keep nares clean. Provide slack, securing tube by pinning or clipping to client's gown.
26. Replace small-bore tube every 4 weeks or as ordered, alternating nostrils. ➤ *Rationale:* Small-bore tubes can become contaminated or obstructed.
27. Provide frequent and regular oral hygiene. ➤ *Rationale:* This prevents parotiditis and respiratory complications.
28. Remove gloves, perform hand hygiene, and make client comfortable.

Equipment

Prescribed formula in closed container ready to infuse system (preferred). Note expiration date. ❶

Antimicrobial swabs

Formula reservoir or bag if necessary for open system (date and replace daily)

Container of ready-to-use sterile formula (cover, label for client, refrigerate unused portion, and discard in 48 hr) or closed system formula

Administration tubing compatible with pump (replace daily)

Infusion pump (not to exceed 40 psi)

Label or pen

60-mL sterile syringe

Sterile water or saline

Gloves

Mask (if caregiver has URI)

Preparation

1. Check healthcare provider's order for feeding formula type and rate of administration.

2. Check x-ray report. ➤ **Rationale:** This validates desired tube placement.

3. Check length of exposed tubing. ➤ **Rationale:** An increase in length may indicate tube tip has dislocated upward, from duodenum to stomach, or from stomach into the esophagus.

4. Perform hand hygiene.

5. Gather equipment.

6. Don clean gloves, and mask if indicated.

Procedure

1. If using reservoir or bag for continuous intestinal feeding, rinse bag with sterile water, and fill with enough formula to limit hang time to 8 hr. **Note:** *Bring unused formula to room temperature before use.* ➤ **Rationale:** This reduces risk of infection. Advancement of tube to intestine places it in less protected (alkaline) environment.

2. Disinfect ports with antiseptic swab before and after handling.

3. Connect administration tubing to formula reservoir (container or bag) and prime tubing per manufacturer's instructions.

4. Thread tubing through pump per manufacturer's instructions. ❷

5. Note mark on client's feeding tube to determine if migration has occurred. Request x-ray if migration is suspected.

6. Connect primed formula tubing to client's small-bore feeding tube. Initiate feeding with isotonic (300 mOsml) or slightly

❶ Closed system formula can hang for 48 hr if sterile technique is used.

❷ Thread tubing through pump per manufacturer's instructions. Pump must not exceed 40 psi.

hypotonic formula. ➤ *Rationale:* This prevents dumping syndrome (cramping and diarrhea).

Note: Alternate method is to connect formula tubing to client's surgically established jejunostomy feeding tube. ❸ ❹

7. Start feeding at slow constant infusion rate (25–50 mL/hr). ➤ *Rationale:* Slow increase in feeding volume is better tolerated. (Maximum rate is 100–150 mL/hr.)
8. If client tolerates feeding, increase rate in 8–24 hr (increase by 25–50 mL/hr to prescribed rate).
9. Keep client's head of bed elevated at 30–45 degrees, or maintain obese client in reverse Trendelenburg position. ❺ ➤ *Rationale:* This lowers intraabdominal pressure and reduces risk of aspiration.

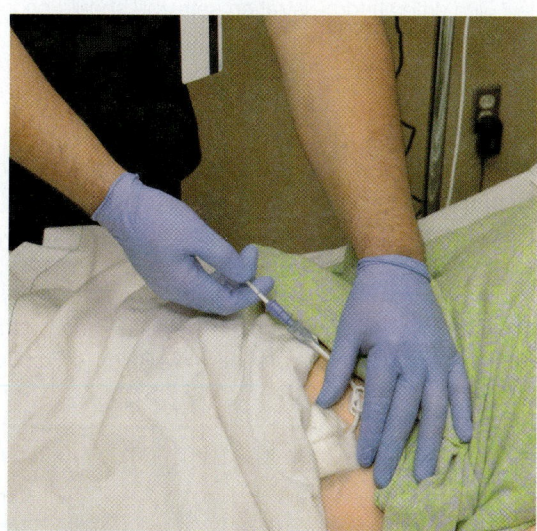

❸ Connect continuous feeding system to client's surgically placed jejunostomy tube.

❹ The Kangaroo enteral feeding pump provides a preset water flush volume at programmed time intervals, reducing need of manual flush and risk of misconnecting various devices.

> **CLINICAL ALERT**
> * If client is receiving continuous feeding, maintain HOB elevation at 30–45 degrees at all times. Turn off feeding 1 hr before client must be repositioned at less than 30-degree elevation for any procedure or transport.
> * Transition from nutrition support to oral feeding requires careful monitoring. Enteral tubes or parenteral access should not be removed until the client has tolerated oral nutrition for 2–3 days.

10. Prep side port with antimicrobial swab and, using 60-mL syringe ❻, flush small-bore continuous feeding tube with 20–30 mL sterile water or saline every 4 hr; flush before and after each medication administered with 15 mL sterile water or saline. ➤ *Rationale:* This is to prevent tube clogging.

❺ Maintain head of bed elevation at 30–45 degrees to reduce risk of aspiration in clients receiving continuous enteral feeding.

❻ Use 60-mL syringe to flush tube with 15 mL sterile water or saline every 4 hr and before and after each medication administered. Do not use tap water.

(continued)

Skill 19.4.5 | Providing Continuous Feeding via Small-Bore Nasointestinal or Jejunostomy Tube *(continued)*

11. Check residual volume regularly. ➤ *Rationale:* Small-bore feeding tube residuals are usually less than 10 mL. Residuals as much as 50 mL may indicate upward displacement from the bowel into the stomach.
12. Monitor for safety and prevention of complications (Box 19-9 ■).

EVIDENCE-BASED PRACTICE
Minimizing Risk of Misconnections

- Only those knowledgeable about the device should make a connection or reconnection.
- Enteral equipment should not mate with female Luer connectors—avoid GI tubes with female Luer connectors.
- Ensure that all connections are made under proper lighting conditions.
- IV and feeding devices should not be modified or adapted (this may compromise the safety features incorporated into their design).
- Trace lines back to their origins when making connections.
- Recheck connections and trace all tubes when the client arrives at a new setting or as part of a handoff process.
- Route IV lines toward the client's head; route enteric lines toward the client's feet.
- "Package" all parts needed for enteral feeding; reduce availability of additional adapters and connectors to reduce risk of improperly connecting dissimilar tubes or catheters.
- Label feeding tubes and connectors.

Source: Guenter, Hicks, & Simmons (2009)

Box 19-9 SAFETY CONCERNS: CONTINUOUS ENTERAL FEEDINGS

- Limit formula hang to 8 hr for an open system and 48 hr for a closed system if sterile technique is used.
- Change administration sets and syringes used for flushing daily.
- Do not add new formula to any formula remaining from previous administration. Flush bag with tap water before refilling.
- Disinfect ports with antiseptic swab before and after handling.
- Prefilled enteral feeding containers should be accompanied with enteral administration sets and should be labeled "Non-IV Compatible."
- Only enteral feeding sets or pumps are used; IV pumps are *not* used for enteral delivery.
- Enteral pumps should feature an automatic flush mode so that there is no need to manually flush lines and to reduce risk of misconnecting adapters or Luer devices.
- Use oral syringes rather than Luer syringes to draw up and deliver medications into the enteral feeding system.
- Identify and confirm a solution's label (e.g., 3-in-1 PN solution may look similar to an enteral nutrition formulation bag).
- Label bags with bold statements **"WARNING! For Enteral Use Only—Not for IV Use."**

Unit 19.4 Documentation and Evaluation

DOCUMENTATION for Enteral Tube Feedings

- Date and time of procedure
- Placement of small-bore enteral tube and x-ray validation of proper placement
- External length of exposed tubing
- Methods of validating tube placement
- Quantity and character of aspirated residuals (color, pH, other tests)
- Amount and type of formula administered
- Head of bed elevation during and after feeding
- Frequency of tube irrigation and irrigant used
- Abdominal assessment findings (distention, nausea, vomiting, flatus, bowel movement)
- Bowel elimination pattern and characteristics
- Daily weight
- Intake and output
- Tube exit site assessment
- Application of dressing to exit site
- Oral hygiene provided

EVALUATION/Critical Thinking

Expected Outcomes

- Client's nutritional needs are met with intermittent naso-gastric feeding.
- Client's nutritional needs are met with continuous enteral feeding.
- Gastrostomy tube site is free of signs of irritation or inflammation.

Unexpected Outcomes	Alternative Actions
• NG tube feedings are delayed or skipped due to large residual volumes.	• Assess for adequate GI function (no abdominal pain or distention; no nausea or vomiting, presence of flatus, bowel movement). If residual is <500 mL, continue feeding but closely monitor client's response. • Change to continuous rather than intermittent feeding. • Continue measures to prevent aspiration. • Consider postpyloric feeding.
• Client develops diarrhea with enteral feeding.	• Use closed system if possible to prevent contamination. • Don clean gloves when setting up or opening system; use sterile technique if client is immunocompromised or critically ill. • Flush bag before refilling with formula. • Use prepackaged, ready-to-use sterile feeding formulas. If using open system, cover, label, and refrigerate unused formula and discard in 24 hr. • Disinfect ports before and after any handling. • Consult dietitian about osmolarity of formula (hyperosmolar or high-fiber formula may cause diarrhea).
• Small-bore feeding tube fails to advance into duodenum.	• Determine if gastric feeding is acceptable (client does not have gastroparesis, reflux esophagitis, high risk for aspiration, and absence of gag or cough reflex). • Administer prokinetic agent before rather than after tube insertion. • Suggest tube be advanced under fluoroscopy.
• Small-bore feeding tube becomes clogged; occlusion alarm sounds.	• Do not let formula bag run dry. • Use warm sterile water in 50-mL syringe with a gentle push–pull technique for flushing tube. Do not use vigorous pressure. • Do not flush with cola or acidic pH juices such as cranberry juice, as this can precipitate protein and cause tube clogging. • Papain, combinations of activated pancreatic enzymes and sodium bicarbonate mixed with water may declog the tube. • Flush tube with sterile water every 4–6 hr and before and after any medication administered. • Crush medications fully—ensure proper dilution and administer each medication separately. • Consider use of papain and sodium bicarbonate with water for flush. • Use declogging system suggested by tube manufacturer— do not reinsert guidewire to unclog tube. • Replace long-term tube every 4 weeks using alternate nostril.

Unexpected Outcomes

- Gastrostomy tube site becomes irritated.

Alternative Actions

- Apply plain antacid (e.g., Mylanta) to area if condition is mild.
- Use skin prep barrier followed by antifungal powder followed by skin prep barrier.
- Request tube with external bar or disc be replaced with plain tube that is sutured into place (bars and discs may embed into skin).

Chapter Wrap-Up

GERONTOLOGIC Considerations

Dietary Needs of Older Adults

- **Energy** (caloric) requirement: 2,000–2,400 kcal/day (may adjust to energy expenditure and physical activity)
- **Protein:** 10% of energy requirement, increases to 20% of energy requirement during periods of stress (surgery, infection, burn)
- **Fiber:** 20–35 g/day of fiber (five servings of fruit per day)
- **Fluids:** 1,500–2,000 mL of water/day or 30 mL/kg body weight (2.7–3.7 L/day if constipation is an issue)
- **Vitamins:** same as for younger adult except for vitamins D, B_6, and B_{12}. *Significant deficiencies in serum levels of vitamins and minerals are rare in healthy older adults.*
  - Vitamin D requirement is 10 mg/day for adults 51–70 and 15 mg/day for those over age 70.
  - Vitamin B_6 intake should be 1.7 mg/day for men and 1.5 mg/day for women over age 51 (25% of older adults are deficient in vitamin B_6).
  - Vitamin B_{12} intake should be 2.4 mg for all adults over age 51 (about 15% of older adults are deficient in vitamin B_{12}).
- **Minerals:** increased need—10 mg/day of iron
- Older adults are at high risk for malnutrition due to age-related physiologic changes, health care status, and lifestyle factors.

Physiologic Changes Associated With Aging

- Between ages 25 and 70, percentage of body fat doubles and lean body mass decreases by about one-third.
- Metabolic rate decreases 20% in men and 13% in older women; energy requirements decrease; there is reduced hunger and increased satiety due to increased levels of cholecystokinin, so food intake decreases.
- Esophageal and intestinal motility decrease.
- Saliva production decreases.
- Gastric secretions decline by 30% in adults over age 65, increasing risk for malabsorption of vitamin B_{12}, calcium, iron, folate, and possibly zinc.
- Lactose intolerance (more prevalent in older adults than younger adults) increases risk for calcium and vitamin D deficiency.
- Gastric emptying is slowed.
- Protein reserves may be inadequate for periods of stress, sepsis, or injury, leading to protein–calorie malnutrition.
- Loss of sense of smell (in more than 50% of those age 65–80 and 75% of those older than age 80).
- Decline in thirst drive (risk for dehydration).

Health Status Factors

- Poor dentition (up to 37% of older adults are edentulous). Loss of dentition is not due to the normal aging process but to improper oral hygiene or inadequate nutrition beginning at an earlier age.
- Ill-fitting dentures causing pain limiting variety and quantity of intake
- Swallowing or self-care deficit disorders (e.g., neuromuscular disorders, Parkinson, Alzheimer)
- Psychological changes (depression, cognitive impairment)
- Effect of medications (altered metabolism, **anorexia**, nausea, diarrhea, cognitive disturbance)
- Inappropriate diet prescription (low-salt, low-cholesterol, or low-calorie diet)
- Medical conditions (e.g., COPD, heart failure, cancer)

Lifestyle Factors

- Alcoholism
- Inadequate income
- Decreased physical activity, lack of transport, isolation
- Cultural values
- Lack of monitoring or caregiving

Assessment parameters for nutritional status of the older adult client in addition to the above risk factors include:

- Body mass index risk for malnutrition:
  - Mild = BMI is 17.0–18.4

- Moderate = 16.0–16.9
- Severe = less than 16.0
- Biochemical indicators of *malnutrition*:
  - Serum albumin below 3.5 mg/L (increased risk for infection, pressure ulcers, prolonged hospitalization)
  - Low serum cholesterol
- Serum creatinine (reflects muscle mass)
  - Moderate deficit if 60%–79% of predicted
  - Severe deficit if less than 60% of predicted

MANAGEMENT Guidelines

Each state legislates a Nurse Practice Act for RNs and LPNs/LVNs. Healthcare facilities are responsible for establishing and implementing policies and procedures that conform to their state's regulations. Verify the regulations and role parameters for each healthcare worker in your facility.

Delegation

- The professional nurse is responsible for the client's basic nutritional assessment (an evaluation tool) if a dietician is not available. The unlicensed assistive personnel (UAP) is not trained to assess this information. A periodic nutritional assessment should be completed for any client who is hospitalized for a long period of time.
- The UAP (unless specifically trained by a swallowing specialist) should not be allowed to feed or assist in feeding the dysphagic client. The licensed professional should monitor and evaluate the UAP's adherence to client-specific feeding instructions.
- Generally, serving a food tray or feeding a client is assigned to the UAP. These staff should be reminded to report any unusual complaints or poor intake of food based on the client's care plan.
- Insertion of NG tubes is performed by a healthcare provider, RN, or an LPN/LVN in accordance with agency policy. The UAP may measure and record drainage from an NG tube and provide oral hygiene.
- Enteral feedings should be given by professional nurses, but some facilities do allow trained nonprofessionals to administer the feedings.
- If medication is administered through a (double lumen) tube, refer to agency protocol to determine who may administer the medication. According to some facilities, it is only an RN or LPN/LVN who may administer medication.

Interprofessional Communication

- Changes in GI therapy or nutritional support orders as well as significant changes in client data regarding tolerance of nutritional therapies (including laboratory data client's elimination pattern) should be communicated to all staff.
- NPO or positioning requirements should be posted at the client's head of bed (HOB) and communicated to all attending staff (orally and by written plan of care).
- Specific instructions and special techniques for feeding the dysphagic client should be posted at the client's HOB.
- The UAP should report to the nurse when a feeding pump alarm sounds, or when additional formula is needed.
- The UAP should report to the nurse if a client's NG tube is leaking or if the client becomes nauseated or vomits.
- The nurse assigned to the client is the essential link between the client and the team; thus both verbal and written reports are important for continuity of care and assessment of the nutritional status of the client.
- It is also important for the nurse to teach the client and his or her family about the need for and aspects of nutritional support through enteral feedings.
- After initial nutrition screening by the admitting nurse or speech pathologist, the Nutrition Support Team for individualized assessment of clients should be contacted. Referral concerns include:
  - Nutrition risk on initial screening
  - Extended ICU stay
  - Any nutrition support (tube feeding, TPN)
  - Latex allergy
  - 75 years and older and having surgery
  - Liquid diet or NPO for more than 72 hr
  - Pregnant or lactating but not admitted for delivery

CASE STUDY Applications

Scenario 1

Mrs. Ramsey, age 62, has been admitted to the hospital with complaints of painful abdominal distention and signs of dehydration after 2 days of vomiting. She is diagnosed with small bowel obstruction due to adhesions (scar tissue) from a remote abdominal hysterectomy.

1. What are the pathophysiologic effects of intestinal obstruction?
2. What potential fluid and electrolyte problems occur with small bowel obstruction?
3. How does the loss of gastric secretions differ from the loss of intestinal secretions?
4. What are the body's normal compensatory mechanisms for acid–base imbalances due to loss of gastrointestinal fluids?
5. What interventions help to correct these imbalances?

Scenario 2

An older adult client (age 64) is admitted to the hospital for a hip replacement. When you are taking a history, you note that she appears to be malnourished.

1. What additional dietary information would be important to include in the database for this client?
2. Evaluate the assessment parameters in terms of the nutritional needs of the older adult and examine how this client fits into the model.

3. Identify the primary parameters to be included in the discharge plan for this client.

Scenario 3

Mr. Bradley has been diagnosed with cancer of the liver and is admitted to the hospital with brain metastases. He complains of no appetite, refuses most meals, and is becoming significantly malnourished with drastic weight loss. Impairment of his hepatic and neurologic status has caused intermittent periods of nonresponsiveness and inability to eat.

Mr. Bradley's family is asking about alternative nutrition options and the healthcare provider is requesting that they make decisions about the treatment options.

1. If nutritional support is indicated, what are the processes normally followed?
2. Who has the primary decision-making power about medical treatments such as nutritional support?
3. Do healthcare providers have an obligation to provide extraordinary care?
4. Once initiated, can healthcare providers discontinue artificial feeding?
5. In what ways can healthcare providers provide symbolically significant care?

NCLEX® Review Questions

Unless otherwise specified, choose only one (1) answer.

1. Trans fats are polyunsaturates and monounsaturates that have what in common?
   A. They have been hydrogenated.
   B. They are unsaturated.
   C. They primarily come from vegetables, nuts, and seeds.
   D. They are liquid at room temperature.

2. Which of the following clients would mostly likely be placed on a potassium-restricted diet?
   A. Heart failure client
   B. Renal failure client
   C. COPD client
   D. Burn client

3. Which of the following are helpful for the dysphagic client?
   Select all that apply.
   A. Swallowing liquid foods
   B. Eating food accompanied by liquids
   C. Swallowing thickened liquids
   D. Eating food without accompanying liquid

   E. Using a straw for liquids
   F. Being fed with a syringe

4. What is the purpose of the Salem NG decompression tube's blue lumen?
   A. Prevent esophageal reflux of gastric contents
   B. Allow siphoning of gastric contents if they stagnate
   C. Provide a port for continuous feeding
   D. Prevent tube adherence to the gastric mucosa

5. Which of the following is the least reliable indicator of the return of bowel function?
   A. Appetite
   B. Bowel sounds
   C. Presence of flatus
   D. Bowel movement

6. What is the best way to determine NG tube placement with continuous feeding?
   A. Auscultate for injected air sound over the epigastrium.
   B. Aspirate secretions and check for an acid pH.
   C. Note the character of aspirated secretions.
   D. Use capnography to detect presence of carbon dioxide.

7. At what amount of residual volume should an intermittent NG tube feeding be withheld?

   A. 50 mL

   B. 100 mL

   C. 150 mL

   D. >500 mL

8. What is the best way to prevent clogging of a small-bore feeding tube?

   A. Flush frequently with cola.

   B. Flush frequently with cranberry juice.

   C. Flush frequently with warm water.

   D. Replace the tube weekly.

9. What is the most effective way to promote small-bore feeding tube advancement into the small intestine?

   A. Place the client in right side-lying position.

   B. Place the client in left side-lying position.

   C. Administer prokinetic medication before tube insertion.

   D. Reinsert the guidewire to advance the tube.

10. What is the most appropriate method for extended nutritional support?

    A. Nasogastric tube feeding

    B. Nasointestinal tube feeding

    C. Gastrostomy tube feeding

    D. Parenteral nutrition

QSEN Activity

Domain: Evidence-Based Practice (EBP)

KSA: Attitude

Activity:

You have been assigned to care for a client who is dysphagic following a hemorrhagic stroke. He is experiencing hemianopsia. He is Hispanic and, during the 24-hr diet recall, his family mentioned a very traditional Hispanic diet consisting of rice, beans, yucca, and malanga. He has been cleared to start oral feedings with caution. You have not cared for him in the past and are unfamiliar with his dietary needs. Develop an individualized care plan based on diagnostic concerns, client values, clinical expertise, and evidence.

Bibliography

American Society for Parenteral and Enteral Nutrition (ASPEN). (2009). Clinical guidelines for the use of parenteral and enteral nutrition in adult and pediatric patients. *Journal of Parenteral and Enteral Nutrition 33*(3), 255–316.

ASPEN (2009). Special report: Enteral nutrition practice recommendations. *Journal of Parenteral and Enteral Nutrition, 33* (2), 122–125.

Baker, H. (2007). Nutrition in the elderly: An overview. *Geriatrics, 62*(7), 28–31.

Bourgault, A. M., Heath, J., Hooper, V., Sole, M., & Nesmith, E. G. (2015). Methods used by critical care nurses to verify feeding tube placement in clinical practice. *Critical Care Nurse, 35*(1), e1–e7.

DiMaria-Ghalili, R., & Guenter, P. (2008). How to try this: The mini nutritional assessment. *American Journal of Nursing, 108*(2), 50–59.

Guenter, P., Hicks, R., & Simmons, D. (2009). Enteral feeding misconnections: An update. *Nutrition in Clinical Practice, 24*(3), 325–334.

Joanna Briggs Institute. (2010, Jan). Methods for determining the correct nasogastric tube placement after insertion in adults. *Best Practice 14*(1): 1–4.

Johnson, A. (2009). Assessing gastric residual volumes. *Critical Care Nurse, 29*(5), 72–73.

Krenitsky, J. (2011, May). Blind bedside placement of feeding tubes. Nutrition issues in gastroenterology, series #93. *Practical Gastroenterology*, 32–42.

Massey, R. (2012). Return of bowel sounds indicating an end of postoperative ileus: Is it time to cease this long standing nursing tradition? *MedSurg Nursing, 21*(3), 146–150.

McClave, S. A., Martindale, R. G, Vanek, V. W., McCarthy, M., Roberts, P., Taylor, B., ... & Cresci, G. (2009). Guidelines for the provision and assessment of nutrition support therapy in the adult critically ill patient: Society of Critical Care Medicine (SCCM) and American Society for Parenteral and Enteral Nutrition (ASPEN). *Journal of Parenteral and Enteral Nutrition, 33*(3), 277–316.

Metheny, N. (2008). Preventing aspiration in older adults with dysphagia. *American Journal of Nursing, 108*(2), 45–49.

Metheny, N., Davis-Jackson, J., & Stewart, B. (2010). Effectiveness of an aspiration risk-reduction protocol. *Nursing Research, 59*(1), 18–25.

Metheny, N., Mills, A. C., & Stewart, B. J. (2012). Monitoring for intolerance to gastric tube feedings: A national survey. *American Journal of Critical Care, 21*(2), e33–e40.

Miller, S. (2011). Capnometry vs. pH testing in nasogastric tube placement. *Gastrointestinal Nursing, 9*(2), 30–33.

National Heart, Lung, and Blood Institute (NHLBI). (1998). *Clinical guidelines on the identification, evaluation, and treatment of overweight and obesity in adults: The evidence report.* Bethesda, MD: Author.

Parli, S. E., Ruf, K. M., & Magnuson, B. (2014). Pathophysiology, treatment and prevention of fluid and electrolyte abnormalities during refeeding syndrome. *Journal of Infusion Nursing, 37*(3), 197–202.

Peterson S. J., Sheean, P. M., & Braunschweig, C. (2011). Orally fed patients are at high risk of calorie and protein deficit in the ICU. *Current Opinion in Clinical Nutrition and Metabolic Care, 14*(2), 182–185 DOI: 10.1097/MCO.0b013e3283428e65.

The Joint Commission Sentinel Event Alert. (2006, Apr. 3). Tubing misconnections—a persistent and potentially deadly occurrence. 36.

U.S. Department of Agriculture. (n.d.). MyPlate. Retrieved from http://www.choosemyplate.gov/about.html

White, G., O'Rourke, F., Ong, B., Cordato, D., & Chan, D. (2008). Dysphagia: Causes, assessment, treatment, and management. *Geriatrics, 63*(5), 15–20.

Chapter 20
Specimen Collection

 Learning Objectives

20.1 Discuss the nursing responsibilities for reporting abnormal laboratory values.

20.2 Describe the major instructions that ensure uncontaminated urine specimens, including midstream urine specimens.

20.3 State the purpose for testing urine for ketone bodies.

20.4 State two objectives for obtaining a stool specimen.

20.5 List four precautions that must be carried out when obtaining a stool specimen for parasite identification.

20.6 Demonstrate the procedure for testing for occult blood.

20.7 State necessary documentation when collecting a stool specimen.

20.8 Explain the objectives for collecting a sputum specimen.

20.9 Outline the steps of collecting a sputum specimen from a suction trap.

20.10 Compare and contrast obtaining an aerobic and anaerobic culture.

20.11 State purpose for obtaining a blood specimen for glucose testing.

20.12 Write two nursing diagnoses that are relevant for specimen collection.

20.13 Demonstrate the removal of blood using a Vacutainer.

20.14 List specimen collections requiring specific consent forms.

20.15 State two critical-thinking solutions for the problem of blood not flowing into the syringe when withdrawing blood.

20.16 State the nursing action when a hematoma occurs at the puncture site.

20.17 Describe procedure for testing for the presence of HIV antibodies.

Chapter Outline

Terminology

Aerobe a microorganism that lives and grows in the presence of free oxygen.

Albuminuria the presence of albumin in the urine.

Anaerobe an organism that lives and grows in the absence of molecular oxygen.

Antimicrobial an agent that prevents the multiplication of microorganisms.

Autolet a small instrument with lancet used to obtain a capillary blood specimen; usually used to measure blood glucose level.

Bacteria unicellular plant-like microorganisms lacking chlorophyll.

Cannula a tube for insertion into a duct or cavity.

Culture to grow microorganisms or living tissue cells in a special medium.

Expectorant an agent that facilitates the removal of the secretions of the bronchopulmonary mucous membrane.

Exudate material obtained from a wound as the result of the inflammatory process.

Glucose a monosaccharide, the end product of carbohydrate metabolism; also known as dextrose; found in the normal blood.

Glycosuria the presence of sugar in the urine.

Granulocyte a white blood cell with secretory granules in cytoplasm, for example, eosinophil.

Hematuria blood in the urine.

HIV antibodies produced by the immune system and present in the blood when individual is exposed to HIV.

Inflammatory process localized response when injury or destruction of tissue has occurred; destroys, wards off, or dilutes the causative agent or the injured tissue.

Micturition the process of emptying the urinary bladder; voiding.

Occult blood blood in minute quantities, can be recognized only by microscopic examination or by chemical means.

Parasite an organism that lives within, on, or at the expense of another organism, known as the host.

Patency the state of being freely open.

Pathogen a disease-producing organism.

Pinworm oxyurid parasite of the intestine, usually *Enterobius vermicularis*. Commonly found in children. Piperazine is drug of choice.

Purulent containing pus, or caused by pus.

Pus an inflammation product containing leukocytes and exudate.

Sepsis a systemic inflammatory response to infection.

Septicemia presence of pathologic bacteria in the blood.

Specific gravity weight of a substance compared with an equal volume of water. Water is 1.000.

Specimen a sample taken to show or to determine the character of the whole, for example, a specimen of urine.

Sputum substance expelled by coughing or clearing the throat.

Stool waste matter discharged from the bowels.

Urinary tract infection (UTI) an infection of the urinary tract, including all or part of the organs and ducts participating in the secretion and elimination of urine.

Vacutainer a plastic adapter that fits onto a double-ended needle for obtaining a venous blood sample.

Venipuncture puncture of a vein with a needle or catheter.

Venous pertaining to the veins; unoxygenated blood.

Viscosity resistance offered by a fluid; property of a substance that is dependent on the friction of its component molecules as they slide by each other.

Laboratory Tests

Laboratory tests are an adjunct for diagnosing healthcare problems and assessing the health status of clients. Test findings can reveal occult problems, determine the stage of disease, estimate the activity of the disease process, and measure the effect of therapy. Multiple laboratory tests are usually ordered not only to assist in diagnosing problems, but also to rule out certain disease states.

Laboratory tests can be analyzed individually or as a part of a screening panel. For example, a routine urinalysis screens for the chemical makeup of the urine, as well as color, clarity, and presence of abnormal cells. Blood chemistry components can be tested individually, as well as in combination through a multiparameter test. These tests provide data on 8, 12, or 16 different elements of blood, depending on the laboratory equipment. It is more cost-effective when all the tests are run simultaneously with one blood **specimen**. For example, a "panel 12" analyzes the following tests: total protein, albumin, calcium, inorganic phosphorous, cholesterol, **glucose**, blood urea nitrogen (BUN), uric acid, creatinine, total bilirubin, alkaline phosphatase, and serum glutamic oxaloacetic transaminase (SGOT). *Note:* Institutions refer to chemistry and blood testing by different names and acronyms; refer to your facility's policy and procedure.

Every laboratory establishes its own normal values for each test. The normal values are generally printed on each laboratory slip to facilitate comparisons with the client's findings. Healthy clients do not always fall within the calculated laboratory norms. The healthcare provider, considering other variables, must judge the value and diagnostic implications of these tests.

Point-of-Care Testing

An important component of client care has always been bedside nursing. Now, and in the future, this will include procedures to obtain laboratory results at the bedside. This testing is often referred to as *point-of-care testing* (POCT). POCT is a type of analysis that is "waived." This means it has been approved for use outside the laboratory, such as at the bedside or in a provider's office or clinic. A laboratory, according to regulatory protocols,

coordinates most POCT in facilities. For example, the Clinical Laboratory Improvement Amendment (CLIA) regulates, at the federal level, who may perform the test and which tests may be included in POCT. The Joint Commission and the College of American Pathologists set additional standards. In the future, more tests will be incorporated into these protocols, because results at the bedside can greatly improve client outcomes. Immediate lab results save crucial time and allow for quick decision making. For example, if the nurse knows through POCT that a critically ill client's glucose level is elevated, an immediate intervention of IV insulin and monitoring may be done to improve the client's status. The most common POCTs performed at the bedside are glucose levels, coagulation, blood gas, electrolytes, pregnancy tests, and urine dipstick tests.

POCT testing has become more commonplace, especially in high-acuity areas such as the emergency department. For instance, the *I-STAT System* provides nurses and clinicians with the ability to run tests at the bedside, providing instantaneous information that could save lives. Common tests include creatine phosphokinase (CPK), troponin, and beta-natriuretic peptide (BNP) used to evaluate chest pain.

Nursing Responsibility

Nursing responsibilities associated with the collection of specimens range from client education to reporting abnormal laboratory findings to the appropriate health team member. When specimens are ordered, it is essential that the client understand the full importance of how and why the specimen is to be obtained. If sterile or clean technique is required, client teaching can provide an understanding of the process. If the client is involved with obtaining the specimen, precise instructions should be given.

To prevent unnecessary lost time and cost to the client, the nurse must be well informed of the correct procedure for obtaining, handling, and processing each specimen. If the nurse is unfamiliar with the procedure, he or she should refer to the nursing procedure or laboratory manual for the healthcare facility. Specific directions are written for most tests performed by the laboratory.

If there is any question about the procedure, the laboratory should be called for directions before obtaining the specimen.

The healthcare provider should be notified immediately of any abnormal laboratory findings that could be potentially life-threatening. With today's technological advances and growing adoption of the EHR, many institutions have the ability to provide data to the providers via smartphone, hand-held device, or electronic tablets. Most laboratory results appear instantaneously in the EHR. There is a significant push to limit documenting in alternative forms (e.g., by text message), because this can increase communication errors and lead to poor client outcomes.

The nurse should also document when abnormal results are reported to the healthcare provider. Documentation should include date, time, tests, and the orders taken. If results were left with another individual, such as office personnel, the name of the individual receiving results should be documented.

It is the nurse's responsibility to be aware of any and all legal implications of specimen collection. Reporting certain tests, such as HIV testing, requires a specific consent; likewise, certain test results are required to be reported to ensure public safety. It is important to remember that all client information is confidential, including laboratory results.

Urine Tests

Nursing responsibilities include collecting, temporarily storing, and performing tests on the urine specimen. Timed urine specimens are usually left in the nursing unit until completion of the test. When urine specimens are retained in the nursing unit, the nurse must take special care in the storing and handling of the specimen to ensure reliable results. Generally, urine specimens collected over a period of hours must be refrigerated, put on ice, or have preservatives added to the specimen to ensure accurate results. Preservatives, such as hydrochloric acid or thymol, prevent deterioration of the specimen.

Most urine specimens are collected as clean-catch (midstream) specimens and sent directly to the laboratory. Single urine specimens are obtained through random sampling. It is best to obtain the first voided specimen in the morning for routine urine tests. This specimen is more concentrated, and the pH is more acidic. The midstream method of urine collection necessitates that proper instructions be given to the client in cleansing the genitalia and obtaining the specimen.

When timed specimens are ordered, the nursing role encompasses not only the handling of the urine specimen, but also precise instructions to the client for collecting the specimen. The collection of urine needs to start and finish at the designated time. Timed tests vary from 2 hr to 24 hr. Assessment for amylase and bilirubin can be done on a 2-hr collection. Creatinine clearance and estriol determination require a 24-hr specimen. A 24-hr urine specimen that is started at 9 a.m. must be finished at 9 a.m. the next day in order to obtain accurate results. Instructions to the client include voiding at 9 a.m., discarding that urine specimen, and collecting the rest of the urine until 9 a.m. the next morning.

Urine reagent strips and the test for **specific gravity** are usually performed by the nurse and are not done by the laboratory. Nurses should follow the specific procedures for each test to obtain accurate results.

Blood Tests

Even though blood studies can be carried out on **venous**, capillary, or arterial blood, the usual sample is obtained from venous blood. Capillary blood specimens are usually used to obtain specimens from infants and neonates. In adult clients, blood glucose and hemoglobin levels can be determined from capillary blood. Arterial samples are obtained for blood gas determination.

In most institutions, nurses are credentialed in performing **venipuncture** and are required to adhere to specific safety principles to prevent potential needlesticks and splashes. Safety needles and apparatuses should be used in all instances. Always refer to the policy and procedure manual of the institution.

Venipunctures must be carried out keeping in mind that hemoconcentration and hemolysis can occur if the procedure is done improperly. Hemoconcentration and hemolysis result from prolonged use of a tourniquet. Hemolysis may occur from using a small-bore needle for the venipuncture of rapidly infusing blood into specimen tubes. Hemolysis can result in false potassium levels.

Note: Use of a needle and syringe for drawing blood increases risk for the provider.

Blood specimens are placed in specific blood tubes according to the type of test ordered (Table 20-1 ■) and sent to the laboratory for analysis. Each healthcare facility has a list of blood tests that are analyzed from blood in a specific color-top test tube (Figures 20-1 and 20-2 ■). The colored top on the test tube indicates whether or not the tube contains a preservative. When whole blood is required for the test, an anticoagulant, such as heparin or trisodium citrate, is placed in the test tube to keep the blood from clotting. When serum is needed for the laboratory test, no preservative is added to the blood, as the clot is used for the test. If the test tube contains a preservative, the tube should be gently rotated back and forth with palms of hands to prevent the blood from clotting.

> **CLINICAL ALERT**
> Order of tube draw is important because there may be a small amount of residual or tube coating, called "carryover," which could invalidate the results. The correct tube order is: Yellow (Sterile), Blue, Red, Green, Purple, Gray.

Table 20-1 Collection Blood Sample Types

Purpose	Common Tests	Tube Color	Draw Volume	Additives
Whole blood studies	Blood culture	Yellow*	12 mL	Acid citrate Dextrose/nutrient broth or preservative
Prothrombin times (PT)	Coagulation studies on plasma	Blue (or black)	3–5 mL	Sodium citrate
Chemistry, therapeutic drug monitoring, blood type	Serum studies	Red	2–20 mL	None
Chemistry (including lipids)	Plasma	Green	2–15 mL	Lithium heparin
Hematology CBC—CSR	Whole blood studies	Purple/ Lavender	2–10 mL	K_2 or K_3 EDTA anticoagulant
Glucose on serum or plasma	Plasma	Gray	3–10 mL	Anticoagulant Sodium fluoride Sodium oxalate

*Requires sterile technique.

FIGURE 20-1 Examples of color-identified blood specimen tubes. Each color indicates the specific test ordered and contains the appropriate additive/preservative.

Some blood tests require that the client fast for several hours before obtaining the specimens. Other blood tests have no special requirements for collection. Blood studies requiring a fasting specimen for accuracy include fasting blood sugar, lipid panels, glucose tolerance tests, and insulin levels.

Cultures

Specimens from the throat, eyes, nose, vagina, wounds, **sputum**, **stool**, urine, and blood are often ordered to be **cultured** for **pathogens**. Special tubes or containers with culture media (such as blood agar plates) are used for organism growth. The culture is prepared in the laboratory according to the type of test ordered. It is essential that the proper technique be used to place the specimen in the appropriate container to ensure accurate results. Specimens obtained for culture and sensitivity require immediate processing and must be sent directly to the laboratory after they are obtained. If a time lapse occurs, the specimen may need to be discarded and a new one obtained. If the specimen is

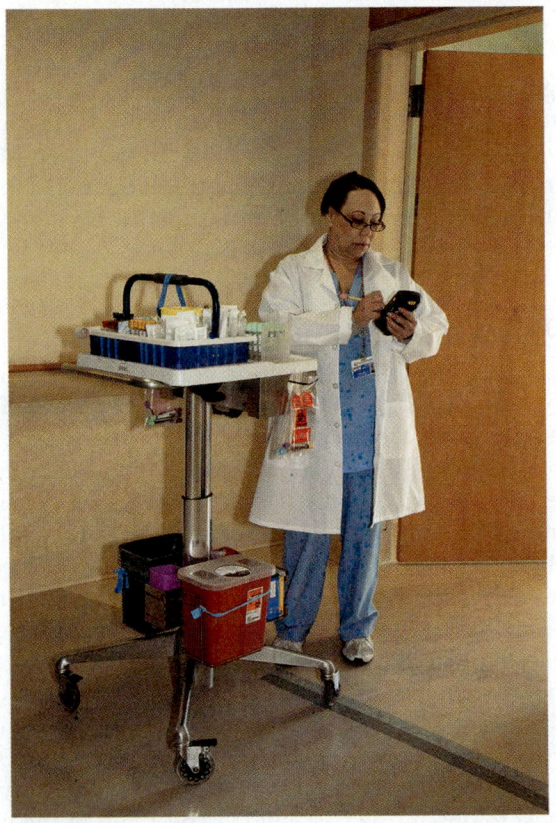

FIGURE 20-2 Blood specimens are usually drawn by a lab technician or phlebotomist according to the healthcare provider's orders.

allowed to dry before the examination, the organism cannot be transferred to the slide and thus to the culture medium.

When collecting and preparing specimens, always consult institutional policy and procedure guidelines. In addition, refer to the manufacturer's guidelines. Failure to collect specimens correctly may result in false positives or negatives, which have the potential to affect client outcomes.

Nursing Diagnoses

The following nursing diagnoses may be appropriate to include in a client care plan when the components are related to collecting specimens.

NURSING DIAGNOSIS	RELATED TO . . .
Anxiety	Dread of unknown outcome, results of specimen tests
Ineffective Coping	Fear, external stress, situational crisis
Infection, Risk for	Invasive procedure, contamination from poor technique of specimen collection
Deficient Knowledge	Inaccurate collection of specimen (e.g., instruction not clear, unable to hear or see well enough to complete collection)
Noncompliance	Inadequate understanding of the purpose or value of diagnostic test (e.g., language and cultural barriers)
Acute Pain	Invasive procedure, altered body function, recent surgery

Source: Herdman, T. H. & Kamitsuru, S. (Eds.) *Nursing Diagnoses – Definitions and Classification 2015-2017*. Copyright © 2014, 1994–2014 by NANDA International. Used by arrangement with John Wiley & Sons Limited. Companion website: www.wiley.com/go/nursingdiagnoses. In order to make safe and effective judgments using NANDA-I nursing diagnosis it is essential that nurses refer to the definitions and defining characteristics of the diagnoses listed in this work.

Nursing Process Data

ASSESSMENT Database

- Assess client's ability to understand instructions and to obtain specimens properly.
- Identify if signs and symptoms of urinary tract infections are present: frequency, urgency, dysuria, **hematuria**, flank pain, fever, and cloudy urine with sediment.
- Determine the purpose for which the specimen is being obtained.
- Determine how the collection is to be obtained.
- Assess parents' understanding of the purpose for collecting infant's urine.
- Assess client's ability to test own urine for ketone bodies.

PLANNING Objectives

- To instruct the client in the method for obtaining a specimen
- To obtain an uncontaminated urine specimen for culture and sensitivity
- To obtain urine specimen for routine hospital admission or as a preoperative urine sample
- To maintain the collection of urine for 24 hr
- To successfully teach client to test urine for ketone bodies

IMPLEMENTATION Procedures

DOCUMENTATION AND EVALUATION

Expected Outcomes

- Client understands rationale and procedure for collecting urine specimen.
- Uncontaminated urine specimen is collected.
- Collection of 24-hr urine specimen is successful.
- Client learns how to test for ketone bodies.
- A clean, uncontaminated urine specimen is collected from a child.

Unexpected Outcomes/Alternative Actions

Pearson Nursing Student Resources

Find additional review materials at
nursing.pearsonhighered.com.
Prepare for success with NCLEX®-style practice questions and Skill Checklists.

Skill 20.1.1 | Collecting Midstream Urine

Equipment

Soap and water or hand cleanser
Cleaning swab or bactericidal soap
Sterile specimen container
Label for container
Clean gloves

Procedure

1. Verify provider's order.
2. Gather equipment.
3. Perform hand hygiene.
4. Identify client by checking two forms of client ID.
5. Explain procedure to client.
6. If client is able, have him or her perform perineal care. Or, don clean gloves and provide perineal care as needed.
7. Instruct client to collect specimen in bathroom or place on bedpan.
8. Instruct client to clean the urinary meatus and obtain urine specimen. (See procedure below: *For a Female*, a–e.)

For a Male

  a. Don clean gloves, and open container.
  b. Cleanse end of penis with cleansing swab using circular motion and moving from middle toward outside.
    ➤ *Rationale:* Always swab from clean to dirty area to decrease **bacteria** levels.

❶ Sterile urine specimen container.

  c. Ask client to initiate urine stream.
  d. After single stream achieved, pass specimen bottle into stream and obtain urine sample. At least 30 mL must be obtained for adequate specimen. ➤ *Rationale:* The microorganisms that accumulate at the urinary meatus have been flushed out with the original stream of urine and are not collected in the specimen.

For a Female

  a. Don clean gloves, and open container.
  b. Spread labia minora with nondominant hand.
  c. Cleanse area with disinfectant swab, beginning above the urethral orifice and moving posteriorly.
  d. Ask client to initiate urine stream. Hold labia open throughout the voiding process.
  e. After single stream achieved, pass specimen bottle into the stream and obtain sample.

9. To prevent contamination of specimen with skin flora, instruct the client to remove the bottle before the flow of urine stops and before releasing the labia or penis.

> **CLINICAL ALERT**
>
> A contaminated specimen is the single most common reason for inaccurate reporting on urinary cultures and sensitivities. To prevent contamination, place cap of container with sterile side up while collecting specimen and do not touch inside of container.

10. Instruct client to empty bladder completely.
11. Wipe off outside of container after replacing cap.
12. Remove gloves and perform hand hygiene.
13. Label the specimen (as appropriate) with client's name, room number, medical record number, date, time, and healthcare provider's name.
14. Take specimen to laboratory within 15 min. If this is not possible, refrigerate specimen in a designated refrigerator or place on ice. ➤ *Rationale:* Delays in testing may decrease glucose ketone, bilirubin, and urobilinogen values. Falsely elevated bacteria counts can also occur if specimen is not refrigerated.

Skill 20.1.2 | Collecting 24-Hour Urine Specimen

Equipment

Urine specimen container
Preservative, if required
Requisition slip
Label for specimen

Sign that urine collection is in progress
Container with ice, if needed

Note: 24-hr urine specimens must be collected for the entire time ordered. To obtain accurate finding, the laboratory needs the

(continued)

Skill 20.1.2 | Collecting 24-Hour Urine Specimen *(continued)*

entire urine specimen. The start and stop dates and times should be reported at change of shift.

> **CLINICAL ALERT**
> Note any dietary restriction or medication precautions in preparation for 24-hr urine collection.

Procedure

1. Verify physician's orders.
2. Explain procedure to client and check two forms of client ID. Stress the importance of saving all urine for 24 hr.
3. Place sign in client's bathroom stating that 24-hr urine specimen is in progress, with start and stop date and time.
4. Collect urine specimen and discard it. ➤ *Rationale:* The first specimen is considered "old urine" or urine in the bladder before test began. Test begins with an empty bladder.
5. Record date and time of first specimen on label, and place bottle in appropriate area. Depending on hospital protocol, specimens may be refrigerated, placed on ice, or left in the client's bathroom.
6. Add preservative, if required.
7. Post sign in appropriate place, if other than client's bathroom.
8. Place all urine voided in specimen container. Instruct client *not* to urinate directly into the large collection container.
9. Request client to void exactly 24 hr after first specimen was obtained. Place voided urine in container.
10. After the last voided specimen is placed in the container, cover and send entire specimen to the lab with the proper requisition.
11. Remove sign, and remind client that the test is completed.
12. If a specimen is accidentally discarded, obtain a new container, note the new date and time, and restart the procedure. Notify lab of lost urine.

Note: For creatinine clearance test: Instruct client to avoid caffeine-containing drinks including coffee, tea, and most soft drinks and to drink plenty of water before and during the 24-hr collection.

Skill 20.1.3 | Collecting a Specimen From an Infant

Equipment

Cleansing solution
Towel
Pediatric urine collector
Diapers
Appropriate specimen containers
Clean gloves (2 pairs)
Clean specimen container
Label for specimen

Procedure

1. Verify provider's orders.
2. Gather equipment.
3. Perform hand hygiene. Don clean gloves.
4. Identify correct child by checking two forms of infant ID.
5. Cleanse and dry child's perineum.
6. Remove paper backing from the adhesive on the urine collector.
7. Apply urine collector to child's perineum, avoiding extension over anus to prevent contamination.
   a. *Male:* Place child's penis through the opening of the collector. ❶
   b. *Female:* Place the opening of the collection bag over the child's urinary meatus.
8. Remove gloves.
9. Place a diaper on the child to help hold the collector in place.
10. Perform hand hygiene.
11. Check the collector every 15 min until a specimen is obtained.
12. Don clean gloves.
13. Remove the collector and place in a urine specimen container.
14. Place clean diaper on child.
15. Send the urine specimen to the lab by either placing the urine collection bag in a urine container or pouring urine from collection bag into the urine container.
16. Remove gloves and perform hand hygiene.
17. Label the container with the child's name, date and time of collection, and the initials of the nurse doing the collection.

❶ Remove adhesive backing from urine collection bag and place securely over penis.

Skill 20.1.4 | Teaching Clients to Test for Urine Ketone Bodies

Note: In certain instances, individuals with Type I diabetes need to have their urine tested for ketone bodies.

Equipment

Urinal or container
Test tube
Urine testing kit (test tube, dropper)
Color charts
Paper towel
Watch for timing

Procedure

1. Instruct client to void in urinal or container to collect urine specimen. ➤ ***Rationale:*** Specimen should be fresh because urine collected overnight will not accurately reveal concentration of ketone bodies.

2. Empty small amount of urine into test tube. Place a drop of urine onto test tablet or dip ketone strip into urine. ❶ Wait 15 sec.

3. Compare strip against color chart and note findings. ❷
   ➤ ***Rationale:*** Instruct the client to notify client's healthcare provider if ketone bodies are present.

> **CLINICAL ALERT**
> Ketones in urine may be negative or present in small, moderate, or large amounts. If there are more than moderate ketones and the client does not feel well or has nausea and vomiting, client should immediately contact a healthcare provider.

❶ Place one drop of urine on Acetest tablet to check for ketone bodies.

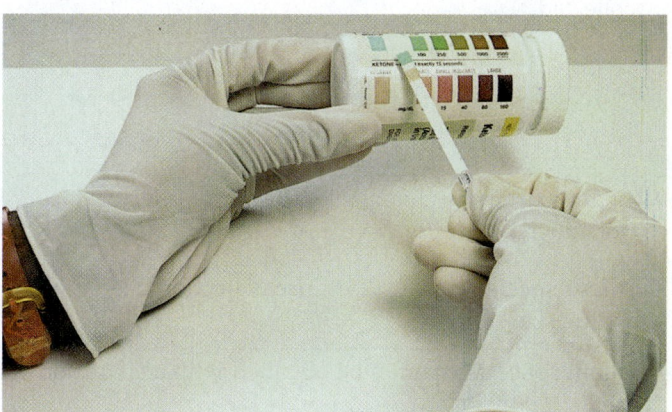

❷ Ketone strips are checked against the chart for ketone bodies.

Unit 20.1 Documentation and Evaluation

DOCUMENTATION for Urine Specimens

- Method used to obtain specimen
- Color, consistency, and odor of urine
- Amount of urine obtained (record this amount on the intake and output record also)

- Time specimen sent to laboratory
- Refrigeration, if required
- Exact time for 24-hr specimen
- Results of client teaching to test for ketone bodies

EVALUATION/Critical Thinking

Expected Outcomes

- Client understands rationale and procedure for collecting urine specimen.
- Uncontaminated urine specimen is collected.

- Collection of 24-hr urine specimen is successful.
- Client learns how to test for ketone bodies.

(continued)

Unexpected Outcomes	Alternative Actions
• Client is unable to assist with obtaining a sterile specimen.	• Place female client in bed and, after cleaning perineum thoroughly, place on clean bedpan. Cleanse perineal area with swab and obtain specimen according to procedure. • Assist client into bathroom. Assist client to cleanse perineum, instruct to start urine stream, and place the sterile specimen container under the stream to collect specimen. • For male clients, cleanse the penis, and place a sterile or clean urinal under the client. Instruct to start stream of urine and then place sterile container under stream. • Notify healthcare provider. Consider catheterization.
• Urine specimen contaminated with feces or toilet paper.	• Instruct client on need for accuracy and compliance to urine collection.
• Client cannot void on command at completion of test.	• Instruct client to void as close to time as possible. • Chart exact time when last specimen collected on both urine bottle and lab slip. Notify lab of findings.
• Urine specimen discarded before 24-hr sample collected.	• If time period is close to 24 hr, call laboratory to determine whether test can be completed on sample collected. • If 24-hr sample must be started again, instruct client of necessity to save all urine. • Place signs indicating 24-hr test collection in progress on bathroom door and client's bedside stand.
• Infant's urine specimen is lost because collector does not adhere.	• Obtain a new collection bag and repeat the procedure. • Tape bag in place with nonallergenic paper tape if necessary.
• Infant specimen is lost because collection bag is the wrong size.	• Obtain appropriate size bag and repeat the procedure.
• Infant specimen cannot be obtained with a collection bag.	• Notify the healthcare provider that you are unable to obtain urine specimen. • If possible, keep diapers off and observe when infant urinates; attempt to obtain specimen.
• Strips or tablets are discolored or moist.	• Sensitivity is lost. They need to be disposed of and new strips or tablets used. • Keep tablets and strips away from moisture by keeping them in tightly covered container (original bottle for tablets and baby food jar for tape). • Always check tablet before using to ensure accurate results.
• Ketones are present in urine specimen.	• Check expiration date on strip; an expired product will not yield accurate results. • Check that client understands what actions to take if moderate or above ketones are present in the urine. • Be sure client is aware that a low-carbohydrate or a high-fat diet may cause false-positive results; certain drugs may also cause a false positive.

Stool Specimens

Nursing Process Data

ASSESSMENT Database

- Determine the purpose for the test.
- Check whether the specimen must be sent to the laboratory immediately.
- Determine the eliminatory status of the client (i.e., liquid versus formed stools).
- Assess gastrointestinal tract dysfunction.

PLANNING Objectives

- To obtain stool specimens for diagnosing dysfunction in bowel elimination
- To assess for perforation or bleeding from a gastric ulcer
- To detect presence of ova and parasites
- To determine presence of pinworms

IMPLEMENTATION Procedures

DOCUMENTATION AND EVALUATION

Expected Outcomes

- Client understands purpose of test.
- Client is able to follow procedure of collection when appropriate.
- Dietary restrictions (if appropriate to test) were adhered to by client before test.
- Specimen collected is adequate for test.

Unexpected Outcomes/Alternative Actions

Pearson Nursing Student Resources

Find additional review materials at
nursing.pearsonhighered.com.
Prepare for success with NCLEX®-style practice
questions and Skill Checklists.

Skill 20.2.1 | Collecting Adult Stool Specimen

Equipment
Waxed cardboard or plastic container with cover
Tongue blade
Label for container
Clean bedpan or bedside commode
Clean gloves
Two signs for over client's bed and in bathroom stating, "Save All Stool."

Procedure
1. Check provider's order.
2. Check two forms of client ID, and explain the procedure to the client.
3. Determine if dietary restrictions are required before specimen collection.
4. Before collecting stool specimen, ask the client to void. Tell client not to void on the specimen. ➤ *Rationale:* This prevents contamination of specimen with urine, which could result in inaccurate test results.
5. Don gloves.
6. Clean out all urine from the bedpan or bedside commode.
7. Perform hand hygiene.

CLINICAL ALERT
Do not allow urine or water to come in contact with the stool specimen.

8. Raise the head of the bed so that client can assume a squatting position on the bedpan, or help client sit on the bedside commode.
9. Provide privacy until client has passed a stool.
10. Remove the bedpan or bedside commode. If necessary, help the client clean perineum.
11. Use tongue blade to obtain and place a small portion (2 teaspoons) of the formed stool in a waxed cardboard or plastic container. (For some tests you may need to collect the entire specimen.) Do not contaminate inside of container.
12. Wrap tongue blade in paper towel, discard remaining stool, and clean bedpan or bedside commode.
13. Remove gloves, and perform hand hygiene.
14. Label container with client's name.
15. Fill out laboratory request for appropriate test.
16. Take specimen to laboratory immediately. ➤ *Rationale:* Specimen may need to be refrigerated or examined immediately after collection.

Skill 20.2.2 | Collecting Stool for Ova and Parasites

Equipment
Waxed cardboard or plastic container with cover
Tongue blade
Label for container
Clean bedpan or bedside commode
Clean gloves

Procedure
1. Follow the steps for Skill 20.2.1, Collecting Adult Stool Specimen. Don clean gloves to collect stool specimen.

① Equipment necessary for collection of ova and/or parasite specimen.

2. Collect **exudate**, mucus, and blood with all specimens.
   a. Place stool into container (with a preservative fluid).
   b. Mash the specimen in the container until mixed well with preservative. ➤ *Rationale:* **Parasites** thrive in this type of medium.
3. Replace and tighten cup. Shake the contents until mixed well.
4. Keep specimens at body temperature to be examined within 30 min. ➤ *Rationale:* Organisms must be seen in their active stages. Loose fluid stools are likely to contain trophozoites or intestinal amoebas and flagellates.
5. There is usually no need to maintain well-formed or semiformed stool specimens at body temperature or to examine them quickly even though they may contain ova or parasites.
6. Collect complete stools after purgative medications are administered.
7. When the presence of tapeworms is suspected, all stools must be examined in their entirety in order to find the head of the parasite.
8. Do not give barium, oil, and laxatives containing heavy metals that interfere with the extraction process for 7 days before stool examination. ➤ *Rationale:* Ova or parasites are not revealed.

9. Use only normal saline solution or tap water if an enema must be administered to collect specimens. Do not use soapsuds or other substances.

10. Do not contaminate the specimen with urine, as it kills amoeba.

11. Collect three random, normally passed stool specimens to ensure accurate test results.

12. Use odor-eliminating spray if needed.

Skill 20.2.3 | Collecting Child or Infant Stool Specimen

Equipment
Diaper
Plastic diaper liner
Waxed cardboard or plastic container with cover
Cotton swabs
Label for container
Clean gloves

Procedure
1. Perform hand hygiene and identify infant using two forms of ID.
2. Place a clean, disposable diaper on the child or infant.
3. Check diaper frequently so that you obtain a specimen that is not contaminated with urine.
4. If child is passing liquid stools, place a plastic liner inside the diaper.
5. Don clean gloves before taking diaper off child and collecting specimen.
6. Use cotton swabs to procure the specimen.
7. Place specimen in stool container.
8. Remove gloves, perform hand hygiene, label with client's name and medical record number, and send the specimen to the lab immediately.
9. Use odor-eliminating spray if needed.

Skill 20.2.4 | Testing for Occult Blood

Equipment
Clean bedpan or bedside commode
Tongue blade
Guaiac test (Hemoccult) or gamma Fe-Cult packet ❶
   Note: Check expiration dates of cards and developer.
Guaiac solution (developer)
Clean gloves

Procedure
1. Verify provider's orders.
2. Explain need for stool specimen to client and check two forms of client ID.
3. Provide privacy.
4. Position client on bedpan or commode.
5. Don clean gloves.
6. Take stool specimen to bathroom or utility room.
7. Prepare slide for testing according to packet instructions.

Gamma Fe-Cult Plus
   a. Smear thin layer of stool on panel number 1.
   b. Obtain second specimen from a different part of stool specimen and smear thin layer on panel number 2.
   c. Turn packet over, and remove perforated flap (marked Not to Be Opened by Client).
   d. Add 2 drops of Fe-Cult developing solution to test area over smear of stool.
   e. Read and record test results within 30 sec. ➤ *Rationale:* Color reaction fades within 2–3 min. Any trace of blue indicates a positive result. No trace of blue indicates a negative result.

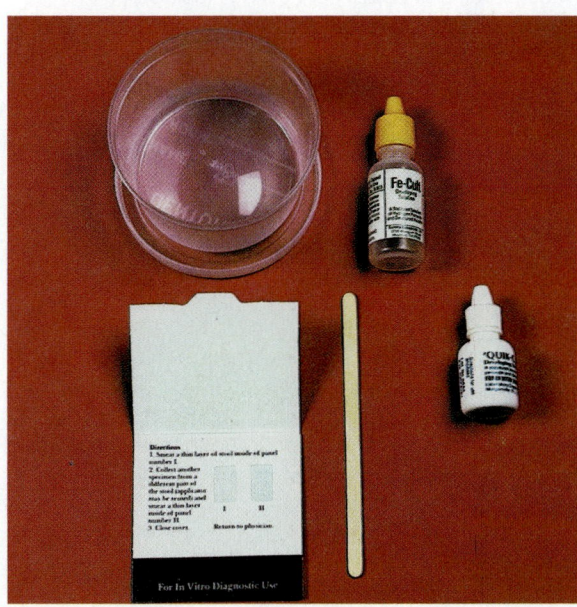

❶ Supplies needed for testing stool for **occult blood**.

(continued)

Skill 20.2.4 | Testing for Occult Blood *(continued)*

Hemoccult

    a. Follow steps a and b for Fe-Cult Plus test.
    b. Wait 3–5 min before processing test.
    c. Turn packet over, and lift flap.
    d. Apply two drops of developer over each smear.
    e. Read and record test results within 60 sec.
    f. Apply 1 drop of developer between the + and – performance monitor test strip (orange section at bottom of packet).
    g. Interpret results within 10 sec. If the positive side turns blue, the test slide is accurate.

  8. Discard filter paper or packet.
  9. Remove gloves and perform hand hygiene.
10. Check facility policy for testing. Some laboratories conduct studies.
11. Document stool smear results and confirm quality monitor test.

> **CLINICAL ALERT**
>
> Overt bleeding from hemorrhoids or menstrual bleeding renders the Hemoccult test inaccurate.

Gastroccult

Note: See Skill 19.3.1, Inserting a Large-Bore Nasogastric (NG) Tube: *Testing Blood in Gastric Specimen.*

> **CLINICAL ALERT**
>
> A Hemoccult processing test cannot be used for gastric contents. A Gastroccult test must be used.

Skill 20.2.5 | Collecting Stool for Bacterial Culture

Equipment
Waxed cardboard container with cover
Tongue blade
Label for container
Clean bedpan or bedside commode
Clean gloves

Procedure
1. Follow steps for Skill 20.2.1, Collecting Adult Stool Specimen.
2. Perform hand hygiene and don clean gloves before collecting stool specimen.
3. Collect exudate, mucus, and blood with all specimens.
4. Place a small amount of feces in a waxed cardboard container (if entire specimen is not needed).
5. Remove gloves, perform hand hygiene, and send entire specimen to the laboratory immediately after collection. If there is any delay, the specimen must be iced.
6. Report and calculate on the basis of daily output any stool specimens that are to undergo chemical analysis.

Skill 20.2.6 | Teaching Parents to Test for Pinworms

Equipment
Specimen container with paddle
Clean gloves

Procedure
1. Explain procedure to child and parent.

Note: This test is rarely done or seen in hospital settings, so if **pinworms** are suspected, the parents can be taught how to obtain specimen at home.

2. Parents may choose to wear clean gloves.
3. Instruct parents to make collection upon arising in the morning before bathing, cleansing, or passing a bowel movement.

Note: For very active children, specimens may be collected a few hours after going to bed, while the child is sleepy and more cooperative. ➤ *Rationale:* Pinworms, when present, migrate out of the anus to lay eggs when clients sleep.

4. Remove cap. Inside it is a plastic paddle with one side coated with a nontoxic, adhesive material and marked "sticky side." Do not touch the sticky side.
5. Separate buttocks and press the sticky side against several areas around anus using moderate pressure.
6. Replace the paddle in tube. Be sure there is no stool on paddle.
7. Label container with child's full name, medical record number, and date.
8. Keep specimen at room temperature until all specimens are collected (on consecutive days). Return all tubes to the healthcare provider.

> **CLINICAL ALERT**
>
> After treatment for pinworms and to prevent reinfection, use meticulous cleaning practices and teach parents of child to do the same.

Unit 20.2 Documentation and Evaluation

DOCUMENTATION for Stool Specimens

- Date and time specimens collected
- Date and time specimens sent to laboratory
- Number of specimens sent to laboratory
- Description of stool: color, amount, odor, and any purulent patches or blood noted

- Dietary restrictions imposed
- Condition of perianal skin, if client is having diarrhea

EVALUATION/Critical Thinking

Expected Outcomes

- Client understands purpose of test.
- Client is able to follow procedure of collection when appropriate.
- Dietary restrictions (if appropriate to test) were adhered to by client before test.
- Specimen collected is adequate for test.

Unexpected Outcomes	Alternative Actions
• Client is embarrassed by having to give stool specimen.	• Place a bedpan or other collection device under the toilet seat in bathroom to obtain specimen. • If client is confined to bed, pull sheets over client's legs and draw curtains around the bed until procedure is completed. • If odor occurs from passage of stool, spray room with odor eliminator sprays.
• Client is unable to pass adequate stool for specimen collection.	• Notify healthcare provider to obtain order to give a normal saline or tap water enema.
• Client passes liquid stools.	• Determine if part or entire specimen is required for test. • Obtain a plastic container with a cover and several large cotton swabs. Dip cotton swabs into the liquid stool. Place swabs in plastic container. After procedure, pay close attention to skin care. A protective ointment may be necessary to protect skin from liquid stools.

Nursing Process Data

ASSESSMENT Database

- Check order for blood withdrawal in client's chart.
- Note specific requirements for the test (e.g., fasting or administration of medications before the test).
- Check to see if the test is routine or urgent.
- Assess veins for venipuncture site.

PLANNING Objectives

- To obtain an uncontaminated blood specimen
- To obtain a blood sample without complications, such as hematoma formation or excessive oozing at the site
- To obtain specimens of blood that can be used to diagnose the client's illness
- To obtain and transfer specimens without destroying red blood cells
- To ensure accurate test results by making sure the client follows all requirements for the test (e.g., fasting)
- To ensure accurate test results by selecting the right tube for the right test
- To ensure that uncontaminated blood specimen for culture is obtained
- To obtain an accurate blood glucose level

IMPLEMENTATION Procedures

DOCUMENTATION AND EVALUATION

Expected Outcomes

- Blood sample is collected without complications. Uncontaminated blood specimen is collected.
- Blood is collected according to designated test tube colored top.
- Client follows all requirements for test (e.g., fasting before collection).
- Client understands and learns steps of procedure when necessary (glucose levels).
- Accurate blood glucose level is obtained.

Unexpected Outcomes/Alternative Actions

Pearson Nursing Student Resources

Find additional review materials at **nursing.pearsonhighered.com.**
Prepare for success with NCLEX®-style practice questions and Skill Checklists.

Skill 20.3.1 | Withdrawing Venous Blood (Phlebotomy)—Needle & Syringe Method

Equipment

5-mL or 10-mL safety engineered device (whenever available)
22-gauge 1-in. needle(s) or less
Antimicrobial wipe (with blood alcohol specimen, use nonalcohol solution such as chlorhexidine or soap and water)
Appropriate plastic laboratory tubes
Dry, sterile sponges
Single-use tourniquet (check for latex allergies)
Absorbent pad or towel
Well-fitting, nonsterile gloves
Gown, if splashing is likely
Laboratory slip

Preparation

1. Check healthcare provider's orders for tests to be obtained.
2. Perform hand hygiene.
3. Gather equipment.
4. Open sterile packages.

Procedure

1. Identify client by two identification methods; introduce yourself and explain the procedure.
2. Don clean gloves.
3. Place extremity straight and in dependent position, if possible.
4. Place absorbent pad or towel under arm. ➤ *Rationale:* This prevents soiling the linen with blood.
5. Place equipment close to work area.
6. Place a tourniquet 8–10 cm (3–4 in.) above insertion site. Tighten the tourniquet and tell the client to open and close fist. ➤ *Rationale:* Muscle contraction increases blood flow to arm.

7. Cleanse antecubital fossa (inner aspect of elbow) with recommended **antimicrobial** wipe (e.g., 70% alcohol) starting at vein site and working downward and outward to cover an area of 2 cm or more. ➤ *Rationale:* A larger vessel is more appropriate than a smaller vessel for blood draw. (In certain instances, vigorous rubbing back and forth of site with 70% alcohol is recommended. Check policy and procedure at institution.)

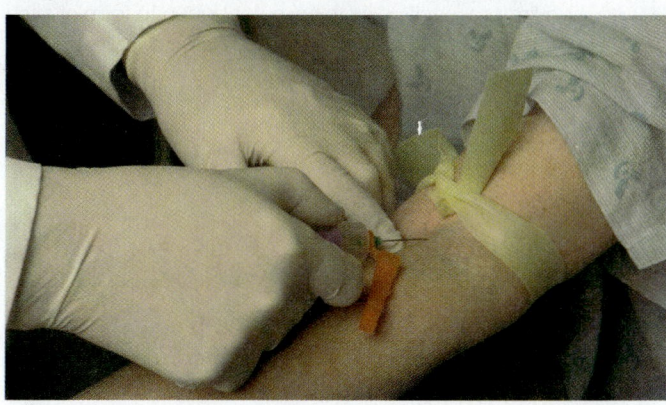

❶ Clamp vein down by placing forefinger below puncture site and insert needle at a 15- to 30-degree angle.

8. Let site dry for 30 sec. ➤ *Rationale:* This reduces bacteria on skin surface when dry.
9. Hold skin taut with nondominant hand. Perform a venipuncture with bevel of needle pointed up at a 15- to 30-degree angle. ❶
10. Lower needle toward skin after needle has entered vein. ➤ *Rationale:* This decreases risk of accidentally penetrating the other side of vein.
11. Thread needle along path of vein. Watch for backflow of blood in syringe.
12. Pull syringe plunger back gently, and check for placement of the needle in the vein. If placement is correct, release tourniquet, wait a few seconds to allow fresh blood to flow into the vein, and then pull back gently on the plunger.
13. Fill syringe to desired amount.
14. Remove needle from vein, cover venipuncture site with a sterile sponge, and press (or have client press) the sponge firmly on the site for 2–3 min.
15. To transfer specimen:
    a. Do not remove top from laboratory tube; vacuum will be lost. Place needle straight through top of laboratory tube. ➤ *Rationale:* Needle can be inserted through rubber stopper of test tube if 20-gauge needle is used.

    b. Gently eject blood down the side of the tube. Do not allow blood to foam or splash. ➤ *Rationale:* Red blood cells can be destroyed if the blood sample is not handled carefully.
    c. Rotate blood gently to mix blood with tube contents.
16. Label tube promptly. Write client's name, date, and time. You may also need to write initials of the individual who drew the specimen if this information is required by facility policy.

(continued)

Skill 20.3.1 | Withdrawing Venous Blood (Phlebotomy)—Needle & Syringe Method (continued)

17. Check client's venipuncture site for oozing. Continue to press sponge firmly over site if clots have not begun to form at site.
18. Dispose of shielded needle and syringe in biohazard receptacle.

19. Remove gloves, and perform hand hygiene.
20. Take blood specimens to a designated station or laboratory according to hospital procedure.

Skill 20.3.2 | Using Vacutainer System

Equipment

Vacutainer assembly with shielded or blunting needle
Antimicrobial wipe (with blood alcohol specimen, use nonalcohol solution such as chlorhexidine or soap and water)
Plastic vacuum blood collection tubes, placed in order of collection
Dry, sterile sponges
Double-ended needle that screws into the adapter
Well-fitting, nonsterile gloves
Single-use tourniquet (check for latex allergies)
Tape
Laboratory slip

Preparation

1. Check healthcare provider's orders for tests to be obtained.
2. Perform hand hygiene.
3. Obtain plastic adapter, double-ended needle that screws into the adapter, and appropriate vacuum specimen tubes.
4. Screw the double-ended needle into the plastic adapter, with the shorter needle facing the plastic adapter.
5. Explain procedure to client.
6. Don clean gloves.

Procedure

1. Follow Steps 1–12 in Skill 20.3.1, Withdrawing Venous Blood.
2. Once the needle is positioned inside vein and blood return is visualized, insert blood collection tube into plastic holder while holding the plastic adapter steady. Press the vacuum

tube firmly into the short needle so that it pierces the top of the tube. Blood should begin to spurt quickly into the tube until the tube is filled or vacuum is used.
3. Instruct client to relax fist and release tourniquet. ❶
   ➤ *Rationale:* Hemolysis occurs with prolonged tourniquet use.
4. Release the tube, and set it aside. Attach another tube to Vacutainer, or prepare to remove needle.

> **CLINICAL ALERT**
> Never remove needles with tube attached. This can increase vacuum and collapse the vein.

5. Place sponge over needle site, and remove needle while applying gentle pressure to site.
6. Hold sponge on site for 2–3 min. Do not have client bend elbow. ➤ *Rationale:* Bending the elbow can facilitate formation of a hematoma.
7. Place Vacutainer with needle in biohazard container. ❷

Note: Never reuse a Vacutainer.

❶ When blood begins to fill tube, tell client to relax fist and release tourniquet.

❷ Place Vacutainer with safety needle attached into biohazard container.

8. Check if tube contains additive, gently invert to mix, and label specimen tubes.
9. Remove gloves, and perform hand hygiene.
10. Complete laboratory slip, and take specimen to designated station or laboratory (Tables 20-2 and 20-3 ■).

Table 20-2 Reference Ranges for Common Blood Chemistry Test

Note: Reference values may vary from institution to institution.

Potassium	3.5–5.1 mEq/L
Sodium	136–145 mEq/L
Chloride	98–107 mEq/L
CO_2	23–30 mEq/L
Glucose	70–110 mg/dL
BUN	7–20 mg/dL
Creatinine	0.6–1.3 mg/dL

Table 20-3 Routine Blood Chemistry Tests

Test	Purpose	Normal Values
Erythrocytes		
Red blood cell count (RBC or erythrocytes)	Determines actual number of formed blood elements in relation to volume; identifies abnormalities; monitors RBC count	Males: 4.6–6.0 million/mm³ Females: 4.0–5.0 million/mm³ Children: 3.8–5.5 million/mm³
Hematocrit (HCT)	Measures percentage of red blood cells per fluid volume of whole blood	Males: 40–54/100 mL Females: 36–46/100 mL Children: 29–54/100 mL
Hemoglobin (Hgb)	Measures amount of hemoglobin/100 mL blood to determine oxygen-carrying capacity; assists in diagnosing anemia	Males: above 13.5–18 g/100 mL Females: above 12–15 g/100 mL
Platelet count	Determines number of platelets	Adults: 150,000–400,000/mm³
Prothrombin time (PT)	Evaluates thrombin generation, or how long it takes for a fibrin clot to form; detects deficiencies in extrinsic clotting mechanism; monitors anticoagulant therapy	10–13 sec Prolonged values seen in liver disease, vitamin K deficiency, specific drugs, and so on
Activated partial thromboplastin time (APTT)	Evaluates adequacy of plasma-clotting factors—intrinsic clotting mechanism	20–35 sec Prolonged values indicate coagulation factor deficiency, cirrhosis, vitamin K deficiency.
Thrombin time	Screening test to detect abnormalities in thrombin fibrinogen reaction (conversion to fibrin in Stage 3 of clotting sequence)	10–15 sec
Leukocytes		
White blood cell count (WBC or leukocytes)	Establishes quantity and maturity of white blood cell elements	Adults: 4,500–10,000/mm³ Children (2 years): 6,000–17,000/mm³ Neutrophils: 2,500–7,000/mm³ Band neutrophils: 0–500/mm³ Basophils: 40–100/mm³ Eosinophils: 100–300/mm³ Lymphocytes: 1,700–3,500/mm³ Monocytes: 200–600/mm³
Erythrocyte sedimentation rate (ESR)	Measures rate of red blood cells settling from plasma—reflects **inflammatory process** or conditions	*Wintrobe Method* Males: 0–9 mm/hr Females: 0–15 mm/hr Children: 0–20 mm/hr *Westergren Method* Males: 0–15 mm/hr Females: (under 50 years) 0–20 mm/hr; (over 50 years) 0–30 mm/hr Children: 0–20 mm/hr

Source: Kee (2013)

Skill 20.3.3 | Withdrawing Arterial Blood

Note: Arterial blood draws are performed by healthcare providers who have been trained or credentialed in the procedure.

Equipment

A commercial arterial blood gas (ABG) kit containing all of the equipment OR 3-mL syringe with 22-gauge 1-in. needle with safety guard

Syringe cap/stopper/Bung

1:1,000 solution heparin, 1-mL ampule (Most institutions have preassembled heparinized syringes. This greatly reduces the chance of heparin-related problems.)

Antimicrobial swabs (2)

2×2 gauze pad

Nonallergenic tape

Plastic bag filled with crushed ice

Clean gloves

Goggles and mask

Laboratory requisition

Label for syringe

Adhesive bandage

Preparation

1. Check healthcare provider's orders for test to be performed (usual test is arterial blood gases).
2. Call laboratory to apprise them of specimen being sent for ABGs according to facility policy.
3. Assemble equipment found in ABG kit.
4. Perform hand hygiene.

Steps 5–9 if NOT using preassembled ABG kit:

5. Wipe top of heparin bottle with antimicrobial swab.
6. Uncap needle and insert into heparin bottle.
7. Withdraw 0.5–1 mL of heparin solution into syringe.
8. Prepare syringe by pulling plunger back the entire length of syringe; rotate syringe to allow heparin to coat syringe sides.
9. Express excess heparin into sink.

Procedure

1. Take equipment into room and place on overbed table and check two forms of client ID.
2. Explain procedure and purpose of test.
3. Ask if client is taking aspirin or anticoagulant therapy. ➤ *Rationale:* These drugs will affect test results and should be documented.
4. Don clean gloves, goggles, and mask.
5. Palpate selected radial site (the site most frequently used) with fingertips. ➤ *Rationale:* You can determine the best site for puncture this way. ❶

Note: Allen's test should precede an arterial puncture if there is a question of poor collateral circulation (Box 20-1 ■).

6. Hyperextend wrist slightly. ➤ *Rationale:* This position will stabilize radial artery.

❶ An arterial blood sample requires puncture of the brachial, radial, or femoral artery or a sample from an arterial line.

Box 20-1 ALLEN'S TEST

Allen's test is performed to determine adequacy of collateral perfusion before arterial blood stick.

- Ask client to rest hands facing upward.
- Observe color changes in palm.
- Ask client to make a tight fist (to force blood from hand).
- Compress the radial and ulnar arteries by applying direct pressure using index and middle fingers (obstructs blood flow to hand).
- Ask client to clench and unclench fist several times.
- Ask client to relax hand in a slightly flexed position. Hand should appear blanched due to absence of blood flow.
- Release pressure on ulnar artery and note if fingers and palm flush within 5 sec. This is a positive test for **patency**.
- If fingers and palm remain pale, do not use this site for arterial puncture; test other extremity.

7. Cleanse puncture site with antimicrobial swab using a circular motion beginning over the artery site. Place swab on inside of packet and in close proximity to site.
8. Keep fingertip of nondominant hand over puncture site. ➤ *Rationale:* This maintains puncture site location.
9. Pick up syringe and hold needle bevel in uppermost position and insert needle into artery at a 30- to 45-degree angle.

10. Do not advance needle once blood is observed flowing into syringe.
11. Hold needle steady and allow blood to fill syringe automatically. Collect 1–5 mL of blood. Pulsations from artery will assist in filling syringe. Do not draw back on syringe.
    ➤ *Rationale:* Drawing back on syringe can cause air bubbles to fill syringe and inaccurate ABGs results will occur.
12. Place 2 × 2 in. gauze next to needle site and withdraw needle when syringe is filled.
13. Immediately apply pressure over site with gauze. Maintain pressure for 5–10 min. ➤ *Rationale:* Prolonged pressure over arterial puncture site will prevent bleeding.

> ### CLINICAL ALERT
> If client is receiving anticoagulant therapy, apply pressure for 10 to 15 min. after arterial puncture.

14. Monitor puncture site for signs of oozing. When bleeding has stopped, place 2 × 2 gauze over site and apply adhesive bandage as you would for a pressure dressing.
15. Expel any air bubbles from syringe. Activate needle guard. Syringe contents should be airtight.
16. Label syringe.
17. Place syringe in plastic bag filled with ice. Close plastic bag.
18. Remove gloves and perform hand hygiene.
19. Complete laboratory requisition slip. Indicate client's temperature and oxygen percentage as necessary.
20. Take specimen to laboratory immediately.
21. ABG values are most often ordered for clients who have the following diagnoses: chronic obstructive pulmonary disease, pulmonary edema, myocardial infarction, pneumonia, or acute respiratory distress syndrome.
22. Check client's values against normal arterial values.

    a. Oxygen saturation   93%–98%
    b. PaO_2 75–100 mm Hg
    c. Arterial pH   7.35–7.45 (7.4)
    d. $PaCO_2$ 35–45 mm Hg (40)
    e. HCO_3^- 24–28 mEq/L
    f. Base excess   –2 to +2 mEq/L (0)

23. Check acid–base imbalances (acid–base balance is the ratio of acids and bases in the body necessary to maintain a chemical balance conducive to life).

    a. Acid–base ratio is 20 base to 1 acid.
    b. Values are measured by an arterial blood sample and recorded as blood pH. Normal range is 7.35–7.45.

Skill 20.3.4 | Collecting a Blood Specimen for Culture

Equipment

Two sets of paired culture media bottles (anaerobic and aerobic)
Blood withdrawal equipment (e.g., tourniquet, two needles, and syringe with attached needle)
Povidone–iodine (Betadine) swab or chlorhexidine swab (check institution policy)
Two antimicrobial swabs (70% alcohol)
Additional needles
Well-fitting nonsterile gloves
Laboratory request form and biohazard transport bag
Small adhesive bandages

Preparation

1. Check healthcare provider's orders.

> ### CLINICAL ALERT
> Check with healthcare provider—blood culture may be ordered prior to client beginning antibiotic therapy.

2. Perform hand hygiene.
3. Gather equipment. Check expiration dates on culture bottles.
4. Don nonsterile gloves.
5. Explain procedure to client and check two forms of client ID.

Procedure

1. Prepare bottles; remove cap and disinfect the top with an alcohol swab; allow to dry. Leave alcohol swab in place.
2. Prepare skin with povidone–iodine (Betadine) or chlorhexidine. Cleanse starting at vein site and moving in circular motion outward 5 cm (2 in.; check facility policy).
3. Allow skin to dry.
4. Perform venipuncture.

❶ Inject blood into both anaerobic and aerobic culture bottles.

(continued)

Skill 20.3.4 | Collecting a Blood Specimen for Culture *(continued)*

5. Withdraw 10–20 mL of blood from vein without IV. Do not draw specimen through catheter. ➤ *Rationale:* Fluid from IV alters results.
6. Remove needle used for venipuncture and replace with new sterile needle. ➤ *Rationale:* Contamination may result if needle used to puncture skin is reused.
7. Gently rotate bottle to mix well. Change needle each time, so new sterile needle is used for each bottle.
8. Draw a second sample of blood after 15 min or according to facility policy. Use percutaneous stick if required by facility policy (follow above procedure).

9. Place in second set of paired blood culture bottles, using single sterile needle technique.
10. Remove gloves and perform hand hygiene.
11. Place bandage over puncture site.
12. Label bottles with your name, date, and time of collection and transport to lab immediately. Include site where blood specimens were obtained.
13. Discard syringes, needles, and gloves in appropriate container.

Skill 20.3.5 | Calibrating a Blood Glucose Meter (One Touch Ultra)

Note: There are many commercially available bedside glucose-monitoring devices. Check your institution's policy.

> **CLINICAL ALERT**
> In many institutions, student nurses and new employees are not allowed to perform bedside glucose monitoring until their competency has been validated.

Equipment
Blood glucose meter
Glucose test strips including calibration strip
Dry cotton ball
Clean gloves

Procedure
1. Obtain container of glucose test strips and remove calibration strip. Check expiration date on strips.

2. Compare lot numbers on calibration strip to lot number on side of glucose test strips bottle. These must match.
3. Place calibration strip in meter by opening door and inserting top of strip into slot on right side of meter.
4. Insert strip until you hear a "click."
5. Close door.
6. Push ON/OFF button. Numbers 888 should appear on screen.
7. Open door of monitor.
8. Push black button on the left side of door, and slide glucose test strip under strip guide with test pads facing up.
9. Close door quickly. Numbers 000 should be displayed on screen indicator. If not, open and close door again.
10. Open door and remove strip. Leave door open.
11. Don clean gloves and prepare to obtain blood specimen.

Skill 20.3.6 | Obtaining Blood Specimen for Glucose Testing (Capillary Puncture)

Equipment
Single-use blood-letting device (**Autolet**)
Soap and water
Cotton ball, sterile sponges
Clean gloves

Preparation
1. Check provider order (Box 20-2 ■).
2. Gather equipment and take to bedside.
3. Perform hand hygiene.
4. Don gloves.
5. Identify client using two forms of client ID.

Procedure
1. Wash client's fingertip (especially side of finger where lancet will puncture, or heel for infant) with soap and water and dry. ❶ ➤ *Rationale:* Use soap and water if repeated sticks are to be done, as alcohol toughens skin.

2. Insert test strip into monitor (you have 30 sec to obtain reading). ❷

Box 20-2 GUIDELINES FOR MEASURING BLOOD GLUCOSE

- Bedside glucose testing is used only to monitor progress of treatment and not to establish a diagnosis of diabetes.
- Specimens used for glucose testing must be whole blood (capillary, arterial, or venous).
- Appropriate nursing actions need to be taken whenever client results exceed critical lab values (check facility policies).
- For a critical value, the FIRST action is to repeat the test.
- Test strip bottle should be dated when opened and recapped firmly between uses to protect strips.
- All unlicensed assistive personnel (UAP) must report all POCT testing blood glucose to RN or LPN/LVN.

(continued)

3. Gently manipulate finger or heel to determine whether good blood supply is available.
4. Adjust Autolet device to depth. ❸
5. Place Autolet on side of finger and release. The lancet punctures the skin immediately.
6. Gently massage the base of the finger, stroking toward the puncture site. Do not squeeze or apply pressure to site.
   ▶ *Rationale:* Massaging increases blood flow to the fingertip.
7. Wait a few seconds to allow blood to collect at puncture site.
8. Place a large drop of blood onto test strip (you have 30 sec to obtain a reading). ❹
9. Wait 30 sec and note reading on monitor. ❺
10. Rotate fingertips when doing capillary punctures.
11. Wipe puncture site with cotton ball to seal.
12. Remove gloves and perform hand hygiene.
13. Document results.

Note: Many hospitals have changed to blood glucose meters that can "download" results, such as the Sure Step Flexx BG meter. The data are immediately entered into the EHR.

❶ Use soap and water or swab to cleanse finger before puncture.

❷ Insert test strip into monitor (you have 30 sec to obtain a reading).

❸ Adjust Autolet depth, place on side of finger, and release.

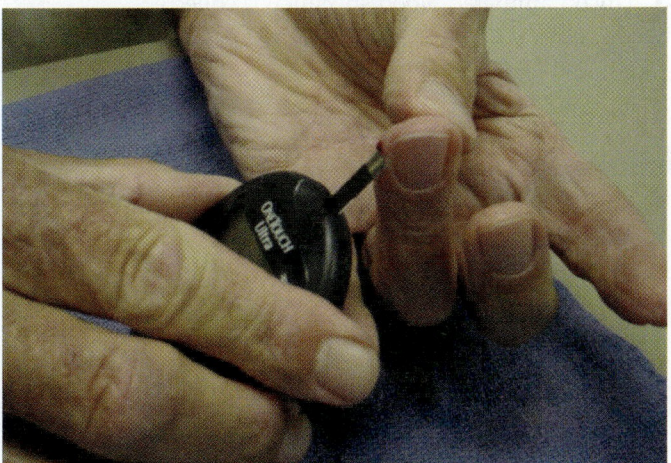

❹ After gently massaging finger, place large drop of blood on test strip.

❺ Wait 30 sec and note reading on monitor.

Unit 20.3 Documentation and Evaluation

DOCUMENTATION for Blood Specimens

- Date and time of blood withdrawal
- Date and name(s) of test(s) for which blood was drawn
- Any unusual conditions in either the client or specimen
- Site where blood cultures were obtained for capillary specimen

- Results of blood glucose reading
- Insulin administered: type, amount, location of injection
- Notification of healthcare provider of critical lab values, orders, or interventions

EVALUATION/Critical Thinking

Expected Outcomes

- Blood sample is collected without complications.
- Uncontaminated blood specimen is collected.
- Blood is collected according to designated test tube colored top.

- Client follows all requirements for test (e.g., fasting before collection).
- Client understands and learns steps of procedure when necessary (glucose levels).
- Accurate blood glucose level is obtained.

Unexpected Outcomes	Alternative Actions
• Veins roll away from needle when performing a venipuncture.	• Stabilize vein by applying traction to skin below needle insertion site. • Common occurrence in older adults. Use a 5- to 15-degree angle when inserting needle into vein as older adult clients' veins are superficial.
• Blood does not flow into the syringe.	• Check the position of the needle in the vein. • Pull needle back slightly away from the wall of the vein. Rotate needle gently. Do not pull excessively on the plunger, especially if the vein is small, since this movement may cause the vein to collapse.
• Blood does not flow into the vacuum tube.	• Check the position of the needle in the vein. If vacuum in the tube is lost or if the vein is not large enough, discard the tube and get another. • If there is pressure on the vein for vacuum pull, select a larger vein or use a syringe and needle instead of the Vacutainer method.
• Unable to get blood sample with Autolet.	• Check that fingertip or heel is not toughened with overuse of alcohol sponges. You should use soap and water to clean area. • Choose an alternative site and repeat the stick. • Stroke gently from base of finger toward the tip. Do not apply firm massage as it can interfere with blood flow.
• Meter shows not enough blood.	• Remove test strip, and insert new strip. • Obtain new blood drop. • Ensure blood drop is sufficient to form a round, shiny drop that covers entire strip. • Complete procedure.

Sputum Collection

Nursing Process Data

ASSESSMENT Database

- Check diagnosis for indication of need for specimen.
- Observe client's ability to cough up specimen. You may need to assist the client while obtaining a specimen, or suction equipment may be necessary.
- Determine the degree of pain the client can tolerate.
- Check client's understanding of procedure, so sputum and not saliva is obtained.

PLANNING Objectives

- To obtain adequate sputum specimen for laboratory examination
- To identify predominant organisms, if respiratory disease is present
- To maintain client's respiratory status during and after procedure

IMPLEMENTATION Procedures

DOCUMENTATION AND EVALUATION

Expected Outcomes

- Client understands and participates in specimen collection.
- Adequate amount of specimen is collected for the test ordered.
- Specimen collected is uncontaminated.

Unexpected Outcomes/Alternative Actions

Pearson Nursing Student Resources

Find additional review materials at
nursing.pearsonhighered.com.
Prepare for success with NCLEX®-style practice questions and Skill Checklists.

Skill 20.4.1 | Obtaining Sputum Specimen

Equipment

Sputum specimen container and label
Biohazard bag for delivery of specimen to laboratory
Tissues
Laboratory requisition slip
Clean gloves
Gown, mask (HEPA or N95 if client has TB),
  goggles, if needed

Preparation

1. Verify provider's orders.
2. Identify client with two forms of ID.
3. Gather equipment.
4. Perform hand hygiene.
5. Provide privacy.
6. Place client in sitting position.

Procedure

1. Explain procedure and rationale to client.
2. Have client rinse mouth before coughing to remove any oral contaminants.
3. Don clean gloves. Don mask, gown, and goggles if client requires assistance with procedure.
4. Instruct client to breathe in and out deeply 2–4 times, and then give a series of low, deep coughs to raise sputum from the lungs. Expectorate directly into container. ❶ ➤ **Rationale:** Deep coughs produce sputum rather than saliva.

5. Obtain 1–2 teaspoons of sputum in container; close and seal lid. ❷
6. Follow directions on specimen container to complete closing system.
7. Label specimen tube directly and place in biohazard transport bag.
8. If client is unable to produce sputum specimen, assist client by splinting the incision area if client is inhibited by pain. ➤ **Rationale:** Wrapping a sheet around chest or abdomen also provides support for body walls during coughing.
9. Remove gloves, gown, mask, and goggles, and perform hand hygiene.
10. Evaluate client's status after procedure.
11. Deliver sputum to the laboratory within 30 min after collection. Obtain specimen during treatment if client is receiving intermittent positive pressure breathing (IPPB).

CLINICAL ALERT

A first specimen obtained in the early morning before eating or drinking provides the best sputum sample. Chest physiotherapy may be helpful in mobilizing secretions just before sputum collection.

❶ Instruct client to lift hinged lid of sputum collection system, and expectorate directly into sterile container.

❷ Instruct client to obtain 1–2 teaspoons of sputum; close and seal lid of container.

Skill 20.4.2 | Using Suction Trap

Equipment

Suction machine
Sterile catheter and glove
Sterile saline
Sterile sputum trap ❶
Culture tube
Biohazard disposal bag
Clean gloves
Gown, mask, goggles

Preparation

1. Check healthcare provider's orders and client care plan for type of equipment needed.
2. Perform hand hygiene.

❶ Two common types of suction traps used in client care.

3. Gather equipment.
4. Explain procedure to client and check client's identity with two forms of ID.
5. Provide privacy.
6. Don clean gloves, goggles, gown, and mask as appropriate.

Procedure

1. Set up suction equipment.
2. Attach sputum trap between suction catheter and tubing. Maintain trap in upright position throughout the procedure.
3. Complete suctioning as for naso-oropharyngeal suctioning using sterile technique.
4. Place your thumb on top of sputum trap to provide suction until 3–5 mL specimen is collected.
5. *Suction no more than 5–10 seconds at a time.* ➤ **Rationale:** This prevents hypoxia.
6. Turn off wall suction.
7. Label specimen container: client's name, date, time, and healthcare provider.
8. Cap suction trap and place it in a biohazard bag. Follow agency protocol for double-bagging specimens before transporting to laboratory.
9. Remove gloves and other equipment (mask, gown, and goggles if used) and dispose of in appropriate receptacle.
10. Send specimen that was collected in trap to laboratory (in many hospitals, suction tube is also sent to the lab with specimen).
11. Place client in a comfortable position.
12. Perform hand hygiene.

Unit 20.4 Documentation and Evaluation

DOCUMENTATION for Sputum Collection

- Date and time of collection
- Amount, color, and consistency of sputum
- Mechanical sputum trap used for collection
- Client's tolerance of procedure

EVALUATION/Critical Thinking

Expected Outcomes
- Client understands and participates in specimen collection.
- Adequate amount of specimen is collected for the test ordered.
- Specimen collected is uncontaminated.

Unexpected Outcomes	Alternative Actions
• Pain inhibits client from coughing.	• If diagnosis permits, support painful area with rolled pillows or tight sheets so that external pressure equals internal pressure, thus minimizing pain and discomfort. • Before beginning procedure, ask client to take several deep breaths. These breaths may trigger the cough reflex and aerate the lungs. • Give client pain medication as ordered 15–30 min before obtaining the specimen.
• Client develops coughing spasms during procedure.	• Press your third finger lightly over the client's trachea in the cricoid hollow. This pressure releases the nerve that innervates the coughing reflex. • Report to healthcare provider to obtain an order for nebulization.
• Unable to obtain sputum specimen.	• Notify healthcare provider for orders: bronchodilator drugs, nebulization treatment. • Perform chest physiotherapy to mobilize secretions for expectoration before obtaining sputum specimen. • Attempt procedure early in the morning when mucus has collected during the night and is more easily expectorated. • Obtain order for aerosol therapy.

Swab Specimens

Nursing Process Data

ASSESSMENT Database

- Identify appropriate container for specimen swabs or material.
- Determine time frame for expediting specimen to lab.
- Assess exact area for specimen.
- Assess client's ability to cooperate with procedure.
- Assess wound and drainage.

PLANNING Objectives

- To obtain an uncontaminated specimen for study
- To place specimen swab or material in container using appropriate techniques
- To send specimen to laboratory within specified time frame

IMPLEMENTATION Procedures

DOCUMENTATION AND EVALUATION

Expected Outcomes

- Uncontaminated specimen is collected.
- The proper container (aerobic or anaerobic) is used for specimen collection.
- Specimen is sent to the lab within specified time.

Unexpected Outcomes/Alternative Actions

Pearson Nursing Student Resources

Find additional review materials at **nursing.pearsonhighered.com.**
Prepare for success with NCLEX®-style practice questions and Skill Checklists.

Skill 20.5.1 | Obtaining a Throat Specimen

Equipment
Tongue depressor
Culture tube with applicator stick
Light source
Clean gloves
Laboratory request form and biohazard transport bag, if indicated

Preparation
1. Verify healthcare provider's orders.
2. Gather equipment.
3. Explain procedure to client and check two forms of client ID.
4. Position client in Fowler's position.
5. Place treatment light or face client toward natural light source to provide good lighting.
6. Perform hand hygiene and don clean gloves.

Procedure
1. Remove the sterile applicator from the culture tube by rotating cap to break seal.
2. Ask the client to tilt head back and open mouth.
3. Use tongue depressor if desired to depress tongue. ➤ *Rationale:* This prevents the tongue from contaminating the swab.
4. Swab the back of the throat along the tonsillar area from left to right. ➤ *Rationale:* Swab only one side of the throat. A second specimen of the other side may be taken; check facility protocol.
5. Remove the applicator stick, and place in the specimen tube. ❶
6. Push the stick into the tube until the swab is saturated with culture medium and cap reaches black dot. ❷ ➤ *Rationale:* This places the applicator tip into the culture medium to preserve bacteria until laboratory can complete test.
7. Position client for comfort.
8. Remove gloves and perform hand hygiene.
9. Label specimen tube, and send to laboratory immediately. ➤ *Rationale:* This is to ensure accurate identification of microorganisms.

❶ After swabbing throat, remove applicator stick, being careful not to touch any part of the mouth.

❷ Push applicator stick into specimen tube, being careful not to contaminate stick.

Skill 20.5.2 | Obtaining a Gum Swab for HIV Antibodies

Equipment
Rapid point of care HIV test (several commercially available), for example, OraQuick Advance Rapid HIV-Antibody Test
Clean gloves

Procedure
1. Verify provider's order.
2. Perform hand hygiene and don gloves.
3. Check two forms of client ID.
4. Swab outer gum with device included in kit. ➤ *Rationale:* Device contains absorbent pad to absorb oral fluid and transudate.
5. Insert swab into vial containing special solution.
6. Check window display on device, and if antibodies are present, two red-purple lines will appear. ➤ *Rationale:* When an individual is exposed to HIV, the immune system will produce antibodies.
7. Following preliminary positive results, instruct client to confirm results with a *Western blot test.*
8. Refer client to appropriate consultation if results are positive.

Skill 20.5.3 | Obtaining Wound Specimen for Aerobic Culture

Equipment
Culture transport swab with transport medium (sterile)
Laboratory slip
Clean gloves, 2 pairs
Sterile gloves
Dressing material
Disposal bag
Biohazard bag

Preparation
1. Check healthcare provider's orders and client care plan.
2. Perform hand hygiene.
3. Gather equipment.
4. Explain procedure to client and check two forms of client ID.
5. Open all sterile dressing material, and arrange for easy access during dressing change.

Procedure
1. Don clean gloves.
2. Remove and discard soiled dressing from wound into disposal bag.
3. Remove gloves, discard into disposal bag, and don clean gloves.
4. Rinse wound thoroughly with sterile normal saline.
   ➤ **Rationale:** This decreases risk of culturing normal flora, exudate, or eschar.
5. Collect specimen by gently rotating swab in a zigzag fashion, avoiding wound edges. ➤ **Rationale:** Touching skin edges or other surfaces will contaminate swab.

> **CLINICAL ALERT**
> Large wounds should have separate cultures taken from different areas of the wound.

6. Return swab to container.
7. Crush transport medium vial, and push swab tip into contact with transport medium. ❶ ➤ **Rationale:** Specimen should be covered by medium.
8. Close container.
9. Place specimen in sealed biohazard bag. Label with specific anatomic site from which culture was taken.
10. Write any recent antibiotic or antifungal therapy on laboratory requisitions. ➤ **Rationale:** These drugs may lead to false-negative results from the culture.
11. Remove clean gloves and perform hand hygiene.
12. Don sterile gloves and replace dressing.
13. Remove gloves, discard, and perform hand hygiene.
14. Transport specimen to laboratory within 30 min. Do not refrigerate. ➤ **Rationale:** This ensures organisms are still viable.

❶ Push tip of swab into liquid culture medium.

Skill 20.5.4 | Obtaining Wound Specimen for Anaerobic Culture

Equipment
Anaerobic transport medium kit with swab
Laboratory slip
Clean gloves
Sterile gloves
Dressing material
Disposal bag
Plastic bag

Preparation
1. Check healthcare provider's orders and client care plan.
2. Perform hand hygiene.
3. Gather equipment.
4. Explain procedure to client and check two forms of client ID.
5. Open all sterile dressing material, and arrange for easy access during dressing change.

Procedure
1. Don clean gloves.
2. Remove dressing from wound, and discard in disposal bag.
3. Remove gloves and don clean gloves.
4. Rinse wound thoroughly with sterile normal saline.
   ➤ **Rationale:** This increases the chance of culturing microorganisms rather than normal flora or other exudate.

(continued)

Skill 20.5.4 | Obtaining Wound Specimen for Anaerobic Culture *(continued)*

5. Remove specimen swab, insert deeply into wound, rotate it gently, and remove. Be sure you do not tip the anaerobic transport medium tube because it contains carbon dioxide (Box 20-3 ■). ➤ *Rationale:* Tipping "spills" the gas out, making it useless to transport anaerobic organisms.

6. Return swab to container. *Do not* touch sides of container with applicator.

7. Fill out or affix label to specimen and place specimen in sealed biohazard bag.

8. Write any recent antibiotic or antifungal therapy on laboratory requisition. ➤ *Rationale:* These drugs can lead to false-negative results.

9. Transport specimen to laboratory *immediately*. Do not refrigerate specimen.

10. *Alternative method:*

    a. Draw up 1–5 mL of exudate in sterile 10-mL syringe with all air expelled or have a healthcare provider aspirate the wound.

    b. Inject drainage into anaerobic culture tube.

    c. Transport specimens to laboratory *immediately*.
       ➤ *Rationale:* Anaerobic organisms may appear on gram stain even though they are not grown in the culture.

11. Remove clean gloves, perform hand hygiene, and don sterile gloves.

12. Replace sterile dressing following protocol.

CLINICAL ALERT

Obtain wound specimen for both aerobic and anaerobic organisms during scheduled dressing change before any medication or antimicrobial agents have been applied.

---

13. Remove sterile gloves.

14. Perform hand hygiene.

Box 20-3 USING AN ANAEROBIC SPECIMEN COLLECTOR

Anaerobic specimens must be transported in tubes filled with carbon dioxide, because most **anaerobes** die when exposed to oxygen. A special carbon dioxide–filled, rubber-stopped container with a small inner tube and a swab attached to a plastic plunger is used.

Before specimen collection, hold the inner tube in place with the plunger rubber stopper. After collecting the specimen, quickly replace the swab into the inner tube and push on the plunger. This will force the inner tube down, away from the plunger and into the carbon dioxide environment of the outer tube. The rubber stopper will maintain the overall tube seal.

Before   After

Anaerobic specimen collector tube.

Skill 20.5.5 | Collecting an Ear Specimen

Equipment

Normal saline solution
2×2 gauze pads
Gloves
Sterile swabs
Labeled sterile culture tube with medium
Laboratory request form
Biohazard transport bag

Procedure

1. Perform hand hygiene and don gloves.
2. Check two forms of client ID.
3. Cleanse ear with normal saline and gauze pad.
4. Insert sterile swab into ear canal and rotate gently along ear walls without pressing on eardrum.
5. Withdraw swab and place into sterile culture tube.
6. Remove gloves and complete hand hygiene.
7. Complete laboratory request form and send biohazard bag to the laboratory.

Note: If a middle ear specimen is ordered, the healthcare provider will puncture the eardrum with a needle and aspirate fluid into a syringe, which will be sent in a container to the laboratory.

Unit 20.5 Documentation and Evaluation

DOCUMENTATION for Obtaining Specimen for Culture

- Assessment of wound and drainage
- Date and time specimen collected
- Type of culture obtained (aerobic or anaerobic)
- Site where culture obtained
- For wound specimens, document an assessment of wound and drainage
- Time specimen sent to lab

EVALUATION/Critical Thinking

Expected Outcomes

- Uncontaminated specimen is collected.
- The proper container (aerobic or anaerobic) is used for specimen collection.
- Specimen is sent to the lab within specified time.

Unexpected Outcomes	Alternative Actions
Inner surface of collection container contaminated while inserting swab into the culture medium container.	Obtain new specimen and send to laboratory.
Swab becomes contaminated.	Touch only sterile items with replaced swab. Obtain new specimen.
Anaerobic specimen not sent to laboratory immediately.	Obtain new specimen and send to laboratory.
Anaerobic specimen sent in incorrect container (**aerobe**)	Obtain appropriate container and send new specimen to laboratory.
Wound culture produces false-negative results.	Check if antibiotics or antifungal medications had been administered. If so, notify laboratory and provide specific drugs administered.
Testing kit for HIV antibodies shows positive.	Counsel client to repeat test. Refer client to appropriate entity for treatment and support.

Chapter Wrap-Up

GERONTOLOGIC Considerations

- Older adult clients may not clearly hear and understand the directions given regarding specimen collection. Ask specific questions to ensure compliance.
- Determine client's ability to follow directions for obtaining specimens such as urine and stool. Hearing and vision may be impaired, thereby interfering with their ability to follow through on specimen collection.

(continued)

- Assess client's ability to accurately use blood glucose–monitoring equipment. Finger dexterity may be altered due to stroke, arthritis, or other chronic conditions, thus preventing him or her from being able to use the equipment or obtain the blood specimen.
- Residual urine may increase as a result of changes in the bladder tone, leading to urinary stasis and potential bacterial proliferation. This leads to bladder infections, necessitating accurate identification of bacteria. This is accomplished through analysis of urine obtained from specimens free of contamination. Ensure client understands the procedure for obtaining an uncontaminated urine specimen. The nurse may need to obtain the specimen if the client is unable to do so without contaminating it.
- Avoid obtaining blood specimens from client's arm if neurologic or vascular alterations are present.
- Clients receiving anticoagulant or antiplatelet therapy require a longer pressure time over the venipuncture site to prevent bleeding.
- Older adult clients have rolling veins that may make it difficult to perform a venipuncture. In fact, the veins tend to collapse and rupture quite easily. Older adult clients may not require a tourniquet for venipuncture.
- Minimize the amount of tape used over IV site to prevent skin breakdown.

MANAGEMENT Guidelines

Each state legislates a Nurse Practice Act for RNs and LPN/LVNs. Healthcare facilities are responsible for establishing and implementing policies and procedures that conform to their state's regulations. Verify the regulations and role parameters for each healthcare worker in your facility.

Delegation
- UAP can be assigned to obtain specimens that are nonsterile and noninvasive. Examples of these specimens include urine and stool collections.
- UAP have been instructed in some areas to take blood measurements using bedside glucose testing. You will need to check with the facility policy and procedure manual for directions. Most states consider this an invasive technique and do not allow this level of healthcare worker to perform the task.
- LVN/LPNs can obtain most specimen collections except withdrawing blood. This task requires that they have additional education and be IV certified in order to obtain the blood specimens.

Interprofessional Communication
- It is very important that all staff members be aware of clients needing specimen collection. Many of the specimens, particularly blood specimens, require fasting. Shift and team reports should identify those clients with special needs relative to obtaining all specimens.
- When 24-hr specimens are being collected, ensure that signs are posted in the client's room to remind all healthcare workers to save the specimens. This is usually for a 24-hr urine specimen collection.
- Remind LVN/LPN to notify the RN of blood glucose findings, even if they are administering the insulin. It is the RN's responsibility to know and document these facts because there are legal aspects to these interventions.
- Remind all healthcare workers to notify the nurse manager when any specimen has been collected. Follow the procedure for the facility for sending the specimen to the laboratory. Some facilities have personnel who pick up specimens from the nursing unit; others require the unit staff to take the specimen to the laboratory.
- Inform the healthcare workers about specimens that must be taken to the laboratory immediately after collection.

CASE STUDY Applications

Scenario 1
You have been assigned to collect specific specimens from several clients. Ms. Saunders is scheduled to have a 24-hr urine specimen collected.

1. When will you start collecting the specimen? List parameters necessary for accurate collection.
2. If the 24-hr urine specimen becomes contaminated with stool, what nursing action is indicated?

Scenario 2
Mrs. Block has orders for a stool specimen to be collected for presence of amoeba. When you collect the specimen from her, urine is mixed with the stool.

1. What is the nursing action?

Scenario 3
Mr. Jarvis has recently been diagnosed with diabetes, and you are assigned to collect a blood specimen for glucose testing.

1. Describe the activities you would perform to complete this assignment.
2. If the results exceed critical lab values, what is the implication of this result?
3. What actions will you take?

NCLEX® Review Questions

Unless otherwise specified, choose only one (1) answer.

1. The nurse is teaching a client how to obtain a sputum sample. Which one of these statements is a critical factor in the instruction?

   A. Rinse the mouth before obtaining the sample.

   B. Obtain the sample in the morning after breakfast.

   C. Have client hold breath before coughing up sputum.

   D. Take an expectorant to help facilitate the cough.

2. When collecting a blood specimen for culture, what should the nurse do?

   Select all that apply.

   A. Draw the blood from the existing IV line.

   B. First wipe the sample site with an antimicrobial wipe.

   C. Wear gloves during the procedure.

   D. Use the venipuncture needle to inject blood into the culture bottle.

   E. Remove needle and replace with sterile needle when transferring specimen to tube.

3. A 4-year-old child with vomiting and diarrhea is admitted to the hospital. Which one of these statements regarding collecting stool specimens for ova and parasites is correct?

   A. Specimen or culture must be from first stool of the day.

   B. Clean-catch technique is used to collect stool sample.

   C. Specimen can be refrigerated up to 24 hr.

   D. Samples can be affected by laxatives containing heavy metals.

4. A client asks the nurse about the purpose of a guaiac test. What would the best response by the nurse be?

   A. A guaiac test detects the presence of bacteria.

   B. A guaiac test tests for fat in the stool.

   C. A guaiac test tests for hidden or occult blood.

   D. A guaiac test determines whether pinworms are present.

5. During a 24-hr urine collection, the client discards a recent void. What action should the nurse take?

   A. Stop the collection.

   B. Extend the collection by 2 hr.

   C. Call the laboratory to report the loss.

   D. Reinforce to the client to save urine.

6. A female client has collected a clean-catch urine sample. The sample is 50 mL, cloudy, odorless, and light yellow. Which one of the specimen's characteristics would be considered abnormal?

   A. Color

   B. Clarity

   C. Amount

   D. Odor

7. The nurse is withdrawing a venous blood sample from the antecubital fossa using a Vacutainer system. Which one of these statements would indicate the nurse is using correct technique in obtaining the sample?

   A. Place tourniquet 2.5–5 cm (1–2 in.) above client's elbow.

   B. Instruct client to keep fist clenched until needle is withdrawn.

   C. After needle removal, have client bend elbow and hold gauze on site.

   D. Preclean the site with antimicrobial wipe and allow to dry.

8. When drawing an arterial blood sample, which of the following should the nurse do?

   A. Flex the wrist to stabilize the vessel.

   B. Draw back on the syringe when blood is observed.

   C. Apply pressure for 1–2 min after needle is withdrawn.

   D. Perform Allen's test before arterial puncture.

9. The nurse is teaching a male client how to monitor his blood glucose using a One Touch meter. When observing his technique, which one of these actions would be cause for further instruction?

   A. The client places the lancet on the lateral side of his finger.

   B. The client washes his hands with soap and water.

   C. The client adds additional blood to the strip after the test begins.

   D. After the stick, the client strokes gently from base of the finger to the tip.

10. A client has a large, draining wound and the nurse is to obtain a specimen for an aerobic culture. When performing this procedure, what should the nurse do?

    A. Collect the specimen by gently rotating the swab along the wound edges.

    B. Cleanse the wound with normal saline solution first.

    C. Place specimen in a paper cup to transport.

    D. Refrigerate specimen if unable to take immediately to lab.

QSEN Activity

Evaluating Complex Wound Dressing Methods

Domain: Evidence-Based Practice

KSA: Knowledge

Activity:

You are a new graduate on the medical surgical unit. Many of your clients require complex dressings and wound management. You recently attended a national conference about best practices to dress complex wounds. You notice on your unit that they are still using some outdated practices to dress wounds. You are concerned and would like to bring this subject up with your preceptor and manager but you are not sure how to go about it.

Identify approaches you can use to convince your institution to explore changes in wound care and dressing changes; document your ideas.

Bibliography

American Diabetes Association. (2009). *Diabetes experts issue new recommendations for inpatient glycemic control—call for systemic changes in hospitals nationwide*. Retrieved from http://www.diabetes.org/newsroom/press-releases/2009/diabetes-experts-issue-new-2009.html

Eliopoulos, C. (2009). *Gerontological nursing* (7th ed.). Philadelphia, PA: Lippincott Williams & Wilkins.

Kee, J. L. (2013). *Pearson handbook of laboratory and diagnostic tests with nursing implications* (7th ed.). Hoboken, NJ: Pearson.

Kuznar, W. (2010). Sepsis: Still tricky to treat: Researchers weigh measuring tissue oxygen, controlling blood glucose. *American Journal of Nursing, 110* (5), 16.

Smith, S. F. (2016). *Sandra Smith's review for NCLEX-RN* (13th ed.). Burlington, MA: Jones & Bartlett Learning, LLC.

Tabloski, P. (2007). *Clinical handbook for gerontological nursing*. Upper Saddle River, NJ: Pearson.

Woolever, D. (2008). Achieve better glucose control for your hospitalized patients. *The Journal of Family Practice, 57*(12), 782–787.

World Health Organization. (2010). *WHO guidelines on drawing blood: Best practices in phlebotomy*. Retrieved from http://apps.who.int/iris/bitstream/10665/44294/1/9789241599221_eng.pdf

Chapter 21
Diagnostic Procedures

Learning Objectives

21.1 Describe the major components of client teaching for diagnostic studies.

21.2 Define interventional radiology (IR) and the nurse's role in IR.

21.3 List at least three preparatory functions for clients undergoing diagnostic studies.

21.4 Explain the importance of determining allergic responses to shellfish before clients undergo contrast media studies.

21.5 List the signs and symptoms that occur when a client experiences an allergic reaction.

21.6 Explain the reason for giving blocking agents before administering radioisotopes to clients.

21.7 Outline the nursing care responsibilities when a client returns from myelography.

21.8 Discuss the nursing care responsibilities when a client returns from arteriography.

21.9 Describe the care necessary after cardiac catheterization to prevent postprocedure complications.

21.10 Explain the steps you would take if a client is given medication before a GI series.

21.11 Describe client positions for at least four diagnostic procedures commonly performed at the bedside.

21.12 Compare and contrast postprocedure nursing observations for clients undergoing liver biopsy, paracentesis, and thoracentesis.

21.13 Explain the nurse's role during procedures that use fiberoptic scopes.

21.14 Describe how ultrasonography is used for diagnostic studies.

21.15 Describe the data that should be included in the charting for clients undergoing diagnostic procedures.

21.16 Describe the preparation clients must complete before an MRI.

Chapter Outline

Terminology

Abscess a localized collection of pus in any part of the body.

Amniocentesis puncturing the amniotic sac, usually by using a needle and syringe, to remove amniotic fluid for assessment of the fetus.

Arteriography study using radiopaque dye injected into an artery to assess arteries.

Barium a radiopaque compound used in roentgenography of the gastrointestinal tract.

Black box warning Federal Drug Administration warning on a drug package with a client instruction sheet for serious or life-threatening risks associated with the drug. Black box name comes from the black border around the information.

Bone densitometry test used to determine bone mineral content and density; used to diagnose osteoporosis.

Bronchoscopy a visualization of the larynx, trachea, and bronchi through a flexible scope.

Catheterization use or passage of a catheter, a tube for evacuating or injecting fluids.

Cholangiography x-ray examination of the bile ducts.

Cholecystogram x-ray picture of the gallbladder.

Computed tomography (CT scan) a scanning technique that provides a series of detailed visualizations of the body or its parts.

Contrast medium a radiopaque substance used during x-ray examination to provide a contrast in density between the tissue being filmed and the medium.

Crepitus a crackling breath sound caused by air pockets in the subcutaneous tissue.

Diagnosis method or art of identifying the disease or condition an individual has or is believed to have.

Doppler diagnostic instrument that emits ultrasonic beam to detect and measure blood flow.

Dyspnea shortness of breath.

Endoscopy visualization of body organs and cavities using an endoscope (tubular instrument with light source and viewing lens).

Enema introduction of a solution through a tube into the rectum or colon.

Fiberoptic scope flexible scope that uses fiberoptic materials for visualization. These materials transmit light along its course by reflecting it from the side or wall of the fiber. Devices using fiberoptic materials are used in endoscopic examinations.

Fluoroscopy type of examination using a screen and x-rays to view internal, moving structures of the body in real time.

Genetic or genomic testing method of examining DNA for disorders with genetic components or vulnerabilities.

Interventional radiology use of minimally invasive image-guided procedures to diagnose and treat diseases.

Lithotomy incision into the bladder for removing a stone.

Lumbar pertaining to the joints and vertebrae of the lower back.

Magnetic resonance imaging (MRI) a noninvasive test that uses a magnetic field with radio frequency waves to produce cross-sectional images of the body.

Mammography x-ray examination of breast used to detect breast cancer.

Myelography x-ray inspection of the spinal cord by the use of radiopaque medium.

Neoplasm a new and abnormal formation of tissue, such as a cancerous tumor or growth.

NPO nothing by mouth.

Oliguria diminished amount of urine formation.

Paracentesis puncture of the abdominal cavity in order to remove fluid.

Peripheral outer part or surface of a body.

PET (positive emission tomography) scan imaging technique using radioactive agent and computed tomography to scan entire body or its various regions.

Pyelography x-ray study of the renal pelvis and ureter.

Radiation the emission of energy, rays, or waves used in the diagnosis and treatment of disease.

Scintillation emissions from radiographic substances; a subjective sensation of seeing sparks.

Septicemia bacteria in the blood that often occur with severe infections.

SPECT (single photon emission computerized tomography) scan type of nuclear imaging test using a radioactive substance or tracer and scanner to create three-dimensional pictures showing body function.

Tachycardia fast pulse above 100 beats/min.

Thoracentesis surgical puncture of the chest wall in order to remove fluid.

Tumor uncontrolled new growth or tissue forming an abnormal mass that performs no physiologic function.

Urticaria a vascular reaction of the skin characterized by the eruption of pale, elevated wheals that are associated with severe itching.

Vertigo sensation of moving or having objects move when they are actually still.

Client Preparation

Diagnostic tests play a major role in the **diagnosis** and care of clients. Diagnostic testing is as important as a thorough history and physical examination. The results from diagnostic tests can confirm or eliminate client diagnoses. Besides assisting with identification of disease states, diagnostic tests also help with monitoring diseases and evaluating responses to interventions and treatment. Both for cost containment and for quality of care, tests need to be scheduled appropriately, the client must be well prepared for the tests, and any necessary specimens must be collected and disseminated efficiently. If tests are completed during inpatient hospitalizations, the nurse must critically evaluate procedure preparation and follow up within the context of overall care and treatment.

Many types of diagnostic tests are used in the healthcare industry today. This chapter covers only a few of the most common tests. It begins with a brief overview of pretest preparation and assessment, followed by common posttest interventions. Nursing interventions during tests are discussed where applicable. Client education, a major role of the nurse, is noted throughout the chapter.

Nurses play a major role in client preparation for diagnostic tests. The responsibility of the nurse starts with the initial scheduling of the test and continues after the results of the test are explained to the client by the physician. At this point, the nurse will answer questions, interpret terminology, listen to client's feelings or apprehensions, and possibly function as a client and family advocate.

Client education is one of the most effective ways of promoting accurate test results. Teaching begins with a discussion of the test itself, then preparation that will be necessary to obtain an accurate result, and finally, any posttest interventions that may be required.

Client preparation for diagnostic tests must be individualized. Some clients arrive well informed about the test they are scheduled to take. Others need to be taught about diet and fluid restrictions, what to expect during the procedure, whether or not there is any discomfort with the test, and how long the procedure takes. Some clients need or want a great deal of explanation; others prefer to be told as little as possible. Nurses need to respect client preferences, unless doing so would in some way endanger the client.

Good client teaching involves attention. On the one hand, the nurse should avoid giving the impression that she or he is in a hurry and has no time to answer questions. On the other hand, the nurse should be aware of the client's ability to pay attention to what is being said. Clients who seem distracted may be worried about finances, about who is watching the children, about whether or not their job will be waiting after discharge from the hospital, or about the impact of test results on lifestyle, level of function, and family. Preoccupied clients may not be able to assimilate information and may then be unprepared for events that follow.

Diagnostic tests can be frightening for clients; they may be unaware of what the procedure involves or be worried about the outcome. Clients probably do not know medical jargon, so procedures should be explained in terms they can understand. If the client looks puzzled and does not ask any questions, evaluate how the information was presented. Therapeutic communication involves an active verbal interchange of information. This includes client and family views and concerns, ideas, and astute observation of the client's nonverbal cues.

One effective way to allow clients time to think about questions is to provide a printed form explaining the diagnostic test. The form may cover information such as how long a test takes, equipment used for the test, and any sensations experienced during the test. Follow-up teaching offers the opportunity to clarify and provide additional information, answer questions, and confirm understanding of preparation and post-procedure activities. (In the ambulatory setting, follow-up may take place by telephone calls or email.) Remember that feedback is the only way in which you can evaluate the learner's knowledge. Feedback can be in the form of direct questioning about certain aspects of the test. Feedback can also be determined through direct observation of facial expressions, posture, and behaviors.

Most diagnostic procedures are done on an outpatient basis. Clients may need to begin preparation 1 or 2 days in advance of the actual test. They must thoroughly understand and be able to comply with instructions in order for the test result to be accurate. This makes it imperative for nurses to give clients explicit information about the procedure or to collaborate with primary care providers or interventional clinicians to ensure appropriate preparation.

Written instructions with preprocedural directions are always sent home with the client.

Identifying medication regimens is an especially important component of preprocedure preparation. For example, it is often necessary to discontinue anticoagulation and hypoglycemic medications prior to procedures.

When the client arrives for the diagnostic test, time should be allotted to answer questions, reassure the client, and determine if the preprocedure preparation was followed. Nurses are often responsible for participating in medication reconciliation processes, identifying a complete list of medications prescribed, PRN medications utilized, and over-the-counter products used. Nurses must understand the impact of medications taken prior to procedures and be able to evaluate them critically. Family involvement is often required, especially when anesthesia or medication is administered for the procedure.

After the procedure has been performed and results obtained, nurses still have responsibility for client care. Initially, they answer questions, restate information that clients request, provide explanations, and identify any necessary follow-up. They also provide verbal and written instructions for discharge and ensure that clients know when to contact the healthcare provider should complications occur.

X-Ray Studies

Many x-rays use the normal contrasts of the body, such as air, water in soft tissues, fat, and bone. These four densities absorb varying degrees of **radiation**. Air has less density, causing dark images on the film, whereas bone has high density, producing light images. Plain radiology (e.g., x-rays of chest, skull, abdomen, and bones) is performed without contrast material.

Some tests do require a **contrast medium**. Types of contrast media that are used routinely include barium sulfate, helium, carbon dioxide, iodized oils, and organic iodides.

Contrast media may cause adverse reactions or sensitivity. This is more common with iodine preparations than with other contrast solutions. The degree of reaction varies from mild (such as nausea) to severe (such as cardiac arrest). Common symptoms include **urticaria**, hives, dyspnea, nausea, vomiting, and decreased blood pressure.

Clients with allergies to food (especially shellfish) or to drugs are often allergic to dyes used in diagnostic studies, particularly those that are iodine-based. Furthermore, injections of iodine dye may cause other tests to get abnormal results for varying lengths of time. Urine sodium, specific gravity, protein, and osmolality are abnormal for 16 hr. Urine catecholamines are also abnormal for 16 hr.

Barium sulfate is a radiopaque substance that blocks the passage of x-rays and provides excellent contrast to body structures. It can cause some uncomfortable feelings and problems with the gastrointestinal tract, but with proper postprocedure care, this condition can be greatly reduced. Barium is not used frequently now due to newer diagnostic equipment and methods.

Fluoroscopy, x-rays that pass through the body creating a continuous x-ray image (similar to a movie), has been very important in diagnosing and confirming client conditions. Two very common uses of fluoroscopy are upper GI barium swallow studies and angiography procedures to guide catheters to predetermined positions, such as in cardiac **catheterization**.

Computed tomography (CT) scans of various organs, particularly abdominal and renal organs, are noninvasive x-ray procedures used to diagnose pathologic conditions such as **tumors**, cysts, **abscesses**, inflammation, perforation, obstruction, and calculi. CT scans are used as a guide to aspirate fluid from organs for cultures and biopsies. The CT scan creates a slice or cross-section that can build a three-dimensional image of anatomic structures and regions, including blood flow and degree of vascularity through organs with injection of contrast agents. The helical CT scan obtains images as the client passes through the scanner. A large advantage of this type of scanning is the speed with which the client passes through the scanner. For example, a CT scan of the abdomen or chest, completed in less than 30 sec, can be done with the client holding only one breath.

Ultrasound Studies

Ultrasonography can be done alone or with other procedures. Sound waves produced by ultrasound differentiate normal from diseased tissue. The sound waves are transmitted through fluid, but not bone, air, or contrast material. It is usually performed in physicians' offices or outpatient settings. Ultrasound is painless, requiring only that the client lie quietly during the 15- to 30-min procedure. There is no risk to the procedure, so it can be repeated frequently without side effects. This procedure needs to precede barium studies because barium impedes transmission of sound waves. It requires that a gel be placed over the site of the organ to be tested. This provides an air-free barrier between the probe (which holds the transducer) and the skin. The probe is passed over the specific body area, and ultrasonic waves are transmitted through the tissue. The transducer converts the echoes to electric impulses and transforms them into visual images. Generally, there is no preprocedural or postprocedural care for the client because it is a noninvasive procedure. The exception is an ultrasound of pelvic organs. In this procedure, the client needs to drink four glasses of water to promote a full bladder. The full bladder enhances transmission of sound waves and thus improves visualization of organs.

Echocardiography is a procedure similar to ultrasound. It is a painless, noninvasive technique that uses transducers and oscilloscopes similar to those used in ultrasound procedures. The echocardiogram records heart motion, not heart outline. There is no preparation or postprocedure alteration in activity for this procedure.

Doppler ultrasonography is used to evaluate blood flow through carotid arteries or **peripheral** blood vessels. Transcranial Doppler procedures can be used to evaluate cranial arteries for spasm or stenosis. Deep vein thrombosis and peripheral vascular disease are diagnosed using this test. A handheld transducer transmits high-frequency sound waves to an artery or vein. The sound waves strike the moving RBCs and are reflected back to the transducer, which amplifies the sound and produces a graphic recording.

Nuclear Imaging

Radioisotopes (radiopharmaceuticals or radiotracers) are injected, administered orally, or inhaled by gas. They accumulate in organs or areas of the body to be examined. The radionuclide atom emits radioactive particles (photons in the gamma radiation range), which have short half-lives. A scanner then detects the energy emitted and, with a computer, creates images offering details of structure and function of organs and tissues.

CT and MRI scans show structure. **PET (positron emission tomography)** scans and **SPECT (single photon emission computerized tomography)** scans show how organs and tissues function. PET and SPECT scans use gamma cameras to detect internal radiation. *Scintigraphy* captures energy emitted externally from the body to form a two-dimensional image. Interestingly, a scanning procedure involves less radiation exposure than a chest **x-ray.**

The most commonly used radiotracers are gallium, thallium, and iodine. Radioisotopes tend to concentrate in specific organ tissues and thus are more effective when administered for scanning a particular organ. For example, technetium-99m is often used for both thyroid and cardiac scanning. Thallium-201 (^{201}Tl) is used to evaluate blood flow through vessels that are too small to visualize with a cardiac catheterization procedure. This is often termed a *myocardial perfusion scan*.

Scanning allows visualization of organs that are unobservable by x-ray alone. Tumors present as areas of reduced radioisotopic activity. Radioisotope studies are contraindicated with pregnancy, breastfeeding mothers, or individuals who are allergic to the radioisotopes.

As noted, the radioactive isotopes are usually administered intravenously or orally to the client. A specified time elapses before the scanning is done. This allows time for the radioactive material to reach the specific tissue under study. Then, a scanning device is used to record the concentration of radiation that emerges from the radioisotope. Equal or gray distribution is normal, but lighter or brighter areas, termed "hot spots," indicate hyperfunction, and darker areas, "cold spots," indicate hypofunction.

Some clients are given blocking agents before the administration of the radioisotope. This prevents the radioactive material from entering organs other than those being studied. A common blocking agent is Lugol's solution, which is given to a client who is having a study done on an organ other than the thyroid gland.

Microscopic Studies

Microscopic studies are necessary for diagnosis and treatment of many diseases and infectious processes. Specimens are collected from tissues, blood, organ biopsies, and secretions, in addition to other sources such as blood and urine.

Biopsies involve the physician taking a piece of tissue from the designated area to be used for microscopic evaluation. Biopsies can be done on endometrial tissue, the lung and liver, and bone marrow aspiration, to name a few areas. Information obtained from the biopsy can indicate pathologic conditions, diseases, and treatment for infections.

Endoscopic Studies

An **endoscopy** refers to inspection of an internal body organ and cavities by introducing an instrument called an endoscope. Biopsies of suspicious tissue, removal of abnormal growths, injection of blood vessels, dilation and stent procedures, and surgical procedures can all be accomplished through the endoscope.

Endoscopes are either rigid or flexible and have a light source and viewing lens that allows the physician to observe the specified area. Scopes can be inserted through body orifices or through small incisions. Rigid scopes are used mostly for operative laparoscopic procedures. Flexible **fiberoptic scopes** are used in pulmonary and GI endoscopy. Because the scope is flexible, light can be transmitted around corners and thus provide a view of body structures not visible by older, rigid scopes.

Fluid Analysis Studies

Normal body fluids can provide information concerning the client's health status. Body fluids frequently studied include cerebrospinal fluid (CSF) analysis and condition of the fetus and its environment (amniotic fluid analysis). Abnormal accumulation of fluids within the body can be analyzed by aspirating the fluid and sending it to the laboratory for studies. The most common areas where fluid needs to be removed include the abdomen and pleural space. Most often, the fluid is removed for therapeutic purposes, although it may be removed for diagnostic purposes. Once fluid is removed, it is measured and samples are sent to the laboratory for analysis.

Magnetic Resonance Imaging

The **MRI** procedure has revolutionized diagnostic medicine. It is a method of looking inside the body that identifies the distribution of hydrogen molecules using a three-dimensional process. The images are translated by computer and differentiate normal from abnormal tissue structure and blood flow. It uses a strong magnetic field in conjunction with radio frequency waves to transmit signals from body cells to the computer. The computer produces cross-sectional images of the body. The procedure is noninvasive and does not involve harmful exposure to radiation. The MRI detects and describes soft tissue abnormalities and yields information about the chemical nature of the cells. Gray and white brain matter can be differentiated and brain tumors and vascular abnormalities, identified. The MRI is the most sensitive technique for defining the structures of internal organs and for detecting edema, infarction, hemorrhage, tumors, and infection. MRI or CT may be used in the diagnosis of stroke.

The MRI scan may require the use of a contrast agent administered IV to assist in visualization of certain structures in the body.

SAFETY ALERT

Always assess for presence of metallic objects to prevent "never events" of death or serious injury associated with the introduction of metallic objects into the MRI area.

Interventional Radiology

With the technological advances and changes in health care, many procedures performed exclusively in the perioperative settings are now being performed in the radiology department. The usual procedures completed in the radiology department are those that have minimal incisions, are low risk, entail low pain, and have a short recovery time.

Interventional radiology encompasses the following: biopsies, cryotherapy, embolization, stenting, thrombolysis, vascular access procedures, and vertebroplasty.

The radiology team consists of the physician, technologist, and nurse. Selected radiology departments employ physician's assistants and nurse practitioners. Some procedures may require more than one nurse.

Role of the RN in Radiology The nurse working in the radiology department is a critical care RN who manages clients during interventional radiology procedures. This nurse must have experience in ICU or ER and be certified in both advanced cardiac life support (ACLS) and administration of moderate sedation. Responsibilities include completing preprocedure assessments and preparation, intraprocedure monitoring, positioning, medication administration, procedural sedation, postprocedure recovery from sedation, and monitored anesthesia care. Other postprocedure activities may include pain management, complication prevention, and client and family education. The RN works in all modalities of radiology, including CT scan, ultrasound, PET, vascular radiology, MRI, and interventional radiology procedures including abdominal, bone, neurovascular, and thoracic.

CLINICAL ALERT

The Nuclear Regulatory Commission (2014) uses the acronym ALARA for "as low as (is) reasonably achievable," which means making every reasonable effort to maintain exposures to ionizing radiation as far below the dose limits as practical.

Assisting the Physician During Tests

Nurses are frequently called on to assist the physician with procedures at the bedside. The procedures presented in this chapter are the most common ones performed in the

hospital unit. It is important that the nurse be aware of the correct client positioning in order to facilitate the procedure, decrease complications, and decrease the time it takes to complete the procedure.

Some diagnostic tests frequently used in the past are used less frequently today. One such procedure is the **lumbar** puncture. Removal of fluid from the spinal tract may cause the brain, because of edema, to herniate down through the tentorium. Because of this complication, a lumbar puncture is not done on a client with head trauma or potential increased intracranial pressure. The CT scan is now frequently used to determine intracranial bleeding. If a lumbar puncture is ordered, the client may have the procedure done in the x-ray department.

Genetic Testing

Tests done on blood or tissue are becoming increasingly common. **Genetic tests** are utilized to identify risks for diseases and disorders, make diagnoses, and to determine medications or dosage most effective for an individual. Testing can help individuals make life decisions but also requires counselor support to understand the pros and cons of testing (NIH, 2014).

Cultural Awareness

A cross-culture assessment questionnaire should be offered to clients who may have difficulty in understanding or following directions in preparation for diagnostic procedures. In some cultures, it is difficult for clients to admit they do not understand what is being said to them. Westerners are bold and direct when asking questions, so they expect the same from clients of different cultures. If there is a question about the client's ability to understand, interpretation services should be utilized. Family and noncertified staff translation should not be used.

With the "push" to get clients in and out of procedure rooms, communication and understanding can be compromised. However, while preparing for the procedure, talking with the client can provide the comforting measures necessary to allow her or him to participate appropriately during the procedure. Ask clients which family member should be included in the discussion and client teaching regarding the diagnostic procedure. Follow facility policies about disclosures of information to families. Pay close attention to what family members say. They can provide valuable information regarding the client's understanding or fear of the procedure. In some cultures, words such as *cancer*, *surgery*, or *death* are not used. In many Middle Eastern cultures, it is not acceptable to speak of death; it is viewed as a breach in the nurse–client relationship. Modesty is an issue with some cultures. This varies greatly among cultures and individuals within those cultures. Be sensitive to this issue, and allow the client to undress in private if at all possible.

Nursing Diagnoses

The following nursing diagnoses may be appropriate to include in a client care plan when the components are related to clients undergoing diagnostic procedures.

NURSING DIAGNOSIS	RELATED TO . . .
Anxiety	Apprehension regarding test or procedure outcome
Fear	Results of diagnostic test, change in health status, threat to self-concept
Deficient Fluid Volume, Risk for	Reaction to contrast media, NPO status, side effects of medication
Deficient Knowledge	Misunderstanding of instructions or information, inadequate data or explanation of procedure (maintaining position after spinal tap, liver biopsy)
Noncompliance	Inability to follow directions as a result of poor health status, cultural influences, or client's value system

Source: Herdman, T. H. & Kamitsuru, S. (Eds.) *Nursing Diagnoses – Definitions and Classification 2015-2017*. Copyright © 2014, 1994–2014 by NANDA International. Used by arrangement with John Wiley & Sons Limited. Companion website: www.wiley.com/go/nursingdiagnoses. In order to make safe and effective judgments using NANDA-I nursing diagnosis it is essential that nurses refer to the definitions and defining characteristics of the diagnoses listed in this work.

Contrast Media and X-Ray Studies

Nursing Process Data

ASSESSMENT Database

- Assess client's knowledge of procedure to be done.
- Identify any history of drug or food allergies.
- Evaluate client's ability to follow directions before and during the test.
- Assess vital signs and document for baseline data.
- Assess medication regimen.

PLANNING Objectives

- To determine if the client is physically prepared for the test
- To determine if the client is psychologically prepared for the test
- To determine if the client is at risk for an allergic reaction
- To determine if the client is able to cooperate with the preparation and completion of the test

IMPLEMENTATION Procedures

DOCUMENTATION AND EVALUATION

Expected Outcomes

- Client acknowledges understanding of the scheduled procedure.
- Client is calm and emotionally prepared for procedure.
- Client is well prepared for x-ray study after client teaching.
- Client completes x-ray study without complications.
- Client did not experience allergic reaction to contrast media.
- Client describes posttest care upon discharge.

Unexpected Outcomes/Alternative Actions

Pearson Nursing Student Resources

Find additional review materials at
nursing.pearsonhighered.com.
Prepare for success with NCLEX®-style practice
questions and Skill Checklists.

Skill 21.1.1 | Preparing for Diagnostic Imaging Studies

Equipment

Signed consent form, if required
Pajama bottoms and hospital gown
Client identification band per facility protocol
Allergy Ident-A-Band, if needed
Wheelchair, if needed for safe client transport

Procedure

All X-Ray Studies

1. Before the procedure is started, identify the specific diagnostic test to be performed (Table 21-1 ■).
2. Determine if any tests must precede others in order to schedule test appropriately.
3. Obtain client's history to determine allergies to food or drugs, and note these on the chart. Identify and describe signs and symptom of allergic reaction. Notify physician of findings.

> **CLINICAL ALERT**
>
> Ensure that female client is not pregnant nor is there a chance of being pregnant before performing any diagnostic tests using x-rays.

4. Complete medication reconciliation form. Based on test ordered, contact and request identification of medications to be held or taken. For example, if test is invasive, anticoagulation therapy could be contraindicated.

> **CLINICAL ALERT**
>
> **Black Box Warning for Interaction Between Metformin and Iodinated Contrast Media**
>
> Metformin has a **black box warning**. Clients taking metformin hydrochloride (Glucophage, Glucophage XR, or Riomet) are at risk for acute renal failure and lactic acidosis with iodinated contrast media. Instruct the client to STOP the metformin for 48 hr before and after the studies or according to facility protocol. Renal function tests may be indicated.

5. Identify specific preparations that need to be carried out before the studies.
6. Monitor food and fluid restrictions that need to be altered for the studies.
7. Obtain special consent forms for all invasive diagnostic studies after the physician has explained the study to the client. The consent form must be signed before any medication is administered (Box 21-1 ■).
8. Provide client teaching regarding the purpose of the study, including any special preparation required and restrictions imposed by the study. (If client will be going home after the test and is unable to drive, transportation should be arranged prior to the test.)
9. Provide psychologic support and reassurance to the client.
10. Obtain orders regarding medications or nutrition for clients with special problems, such as diabetes, anxiety, pain, or seizure disorders.
11. Carry out safety precautions immediately before the study:

    a. Check two forms of client identification; introduce yourself and explain the procedure to client; and perform hand hygiene.

    b. Have client void if necessary.

Box 21-1 INFORMED CONSENT

- Informed consent indicates that clients have received a full explanation of the procedure, including risks, complications, benefits, and alternatives.
- Obtaining informed consent is the responsibility of the healthcare provider. It is the nurse's responsibility to check that the consent is signed before the procedure.
- The nurse can be asked to witness the signature. In order to witness the signature, the nurse should have been present during the client–healthcare provider discussion.

Table 21-1 Contrast Media and X-Ray Studies

Diagnostic Test	Rationale	Contrast Media
Intravenous **pyelography**	To visualize structures of the urinary tract	Yes
Myelography	To visualize the subarachnoid space to identify abnormalities	Yes
Arteriography	To visualize abnormalities or obstructions in specific blood vessels	Yes
CT scan	To visualize a cross-section of the brain, chest, or abdomen to localize lesions precisely	Sometimes, depending on procedure
Cardiac catheterization	To measure oxygen concentration, provide blood samples, determine cardiac output, and visualize coronary arteries	Yes
Bone densitometry	To determine bone mineral density and strength of bone	No
MRI	To visualize inner structures of body	Sometimes, depending on procedure.
Mammography	To determine presence of breast pathology	No

(continued)

Skill 21.1.1 | Preparing for Diagnostic Imaging Studies *(continued)*

c. Remove client's hairpins, jewelry, and dentures if necessary.

d. Chart premedication given.

e. Monitor safe transfer from the bed to gurney or wheelchair if client is not ambulatory.

f. Accompany client to x-ray department if needed. (Usually, nurses accompany critically ill clients.)

g. Utilize handoff communication.

CLINICAL ALERT

Clients scheduled for a diagnostic test using contrast media must have BUN and creatinine tests completed before the scheduled study. Nephrotoxicity is a side effect of the contrast media, particularly iodinated dyes.

Intravenous Pyelography (IVP)

1. Follow steps in the All X-Ray Studies section of this procedure, as appropriate.

   a. Give client clear liquid diet the evening before the IVP and maintain **NPO** status after 12 midnight or per facility protocol and according to scheduled time of procedure. Some facilities allow clear liquid diet in the morning.

   b. Review medications routinely taken, including when last administered or taken. Provide information to physician.

   c. Give laxative or cathartic as ordered, usually the night before test. A cleansing **enema** may be ordered the morning of the test (check facility policy). ➤ *Rationale:* Eliminating feces and gas provides better contrast.

   d. Identify allergies to shellfish or iodine. ➤ *Rationale:* Other contrast material will need to be used in place of iodine contrast media.

   e. Obtain consent.

   f. Take baseline vital signs.

   g. Take client to x-ray department when notified.

2. Explain details of procedure to client.

   a. Client is positioned in supine position.

   b. Flat plate of abdomen taken. ➤ *Rationale:* Ensure no residual stool, which could interfere with visualization of renal system.

   c. Test dose of contrast medium may be injected intradermally for clients with a history of allergies. The contrast material is administered if there is no reaction within 15 min of test dose. Identify location of emergency equipment for availability if needed.

   d. IV is inserted and contrast medium injected as a large single dose.

   e. X-rays are taken over a period of 30 min to 1 hr to determine extent to which dye is filtered through the kidneys.

3. Warn client that contrast medium can cause feelings of nausea, shortness of breath, and a hot, flushed effect.

CLINICAL ALERT

Symptoms of contrast media reactions:

- Urticaria, hives
- Nausea, vomiting
- Respiratory distress
- Decreased blood pressure
- Cardiac or respiratory arrest

Clients allergic to food or drugs may also be allergic to contrast media used for diagnostic studies.

---

4. Instruct client to void at end of test. An x-ray is taken to visualize residual dye in kidneys.

5. Return client to room and resume ordered activity level.

6. Encourage fluids, and resume usual diet. Fluids should include at least 24 oz of water. ➤ *Rationale:* Increasing fluid intake prevents osmotic diuresis from contrast medium.

7. Monitor client for at least 24 hr for signs and symptoms of reactions to contrast medium such as **oliguria**, nausea, and vomiting.

Myelography

1. Follow steps as appropriate in All X-Ray Studies, including medication reconciliation and two client identifiers, and introduce yourself.

   a. Explain procedure to client—test identifies abnormalities of spine and subarachnoid space.

   b. Client may have cleansing enema ordered.

   c. Identify allergies to shellfish, iodine, or other contrast media.

   d. Keep client NPO for 4–8 hr before test.

   e. Obtain baseline levels of motor and sensory function and vital signs.

   f. Assess for signs of increased intracranial pressure (ICP). ➤ *Rationale:* This test is contraindicated for clients with ICP. Brain herniation can occur.

   g. Obtain consent form.

   h. Medicate with sedative if ordered. ➤ *Rationale:* This provides client comfort.

   i. Take client on gurney to x-ray department.

CLINICAL ALERT

Myelograms are performed less frequently today because of the wide use of MRI and CT scanning. The MRI is more accurate for viewing the spinal cord and surrounding structures.

---

2. Explain details of procedure to client.

   a. Client is placed either in prone position with pillow under abdomen, side-lying with knees drawn up to abdomen and chin on chest on fluoroscopic table, or sitting on bed or table and leaning forward against pillows. ➤ *Rationale:* These positions allow the physician to visualize ruptured disc or **neoplasms**.

   b. A lumbar puncture needle is inserted between the vertebrae into the subarachnoid space.

c. A small amount of cerebrospinal fluid is sent to lab for study.

d. Contrast medium is injected, and client is tilted on table to allow flow of dye to designated areas of spine to visualize it by x-rays.

e. Procedure lasts about 1 hr.

f. Client is returned on gurney to room.

3. After the test:

   a. Keep client in prone position or supine position for 4–8 hrs per orders or protocol. May turn side to side. ➤ *Rationale:* This position prevents a headache and CSF leaks.

   b. Keep head of bed elevated 30–50 degrees for 8 hr. Client may be on bed rest for up to 24 hr, although bathroom privileges may be allowed. ➤ *Rationale:* This position reduces rate of upward displacement of dye.

4. Observe for seizure activity if metrizamide is used for procedure. It can precipitate seizures. Do not give medications that can decrease seizure threshold.

5. Monitor vital signs, and motor and sensory function. Monitor for signs and symptoms of infection, nausea, and vomiting.

   a. Cervical myelogram: Check upper and lower extremities and bladder function.

   b. Lumbar myelogram: Check lower extremities and bladder function.

6. Medicate for pain as ordered, usually with a mild sedative.

7. Increase fluids to at least 2,500 mL each day for 2 days. ➤ *Rationale:* Fluids rehydrate and replace cerebrospinal fluid, promote elimination of dye, and may prevent headache after procedure. Offer appropriate diet for client.

8. Monitor output, and observe for distention.

9. Observe puncture site for 24 hr for bleeding, hematoma, or edema.

10. Observe for complication of chemical or bacterial meningitis: fever, stiff neck, photophobia, or delayed reaction to dye.

11. Use comfort measures and relaxation techniques when needed.

Arteriography

1. Follow steps as appropriate in the All X-Ray Studies section of this procedure.

2. Identify client using two identifiers, introduce yourself, and explain purpose of procedure to client—examination of arteries to determine abnormalities in blood flow.

3. Identify allergies to shellfish, iodine, or any contrast media. Ask client if taking anticoagulants.

4. Obtain baseline blood tests, including CBC, PT/PTT, and APTT, BUN, and creatinine. Anticoagulants must be discontinued before procedure.

5. Obtain consent form.

6. Keep client NPO for 2–8 hr or as ordered.

7. Perform hand hygiene and prepare puncture site when ordered.

8. Have client void before procedure. Follow screening protocols for removal of implants, metal objects, and other objects that could produce artifacts.

9. Obtain vital signs and check peripheral pulses, sensation, and movement. Mark pulse palpation site. ➤ *Rationale:* This is to provide comparison data after procedure.

10. Administer preprocedure medications 1 hr before test, if ordered, and transport client to x-ray department.

11. Apply electrocardiogram electrodes and begin monitoring the heart rhythm.

12. Identify location and availability of emergency equipment if needed.

13. Explain details of procedure to client.

    a. Client is positioned supine on x-ray table.

    b. IV for fluid administration will be started. ➤ *Rationale:* This is for use in emergency situations.

    c. Puncture site will be scrubbed and a local anesthetic administered. Catheter is inserted into brachial or femoral artery.

    d. Contrast medium will be injected to visualize abnormalities or obstruction to specific vessels. Inform client that a warm flush may be felt when dye injected.

    e. Client may be instructed to hold breath for x-rays. Procedure takes about 1–2 hr if an automatic film changer is used.

    f. Catheter is removed and pressure dressing applied over site.

14. Monitor vital signs, level of consciousness, pulses and tissue (temperature, sensation, capillary refill) distal to the puncture site, and puncture site (hematoma can occur), as with surgical clients. ➤ *Rationale:* This is done to identify potential complications.

> **CLINICAL ALERT**
> An external mechanical compression device may be utilized at the puncture site. Special training is required prior to managing this device. Its use requires appropriate monitoring and control of blood pressure.

15. Observe for signs of shock and presence of pain; these manifestations indicate hemorrhage or thrombosis.

16. Observe for symptoms of delayed allergic reaction to dye, such as nausea, vomiting, **tachycardia**, sweating, rash, or hives. ➤ *Rationale:* Delayed reactions can occur up to several hours after the procedure.

17. Notify physician immediately if unusual symptoms are present. ➤ *Rationale:* Immediate medical intervention is necessary to prevent anaphylaxis.

18. Do not flex the involved extremity.

19. Maintain bed rest with head elevated slightly for at least 6–8 hr depending on site of puncture. Check hospital policy for time.

20. Offer fluids and diet as ordered and tolerated. Fluids should be 1–2 L. ➤ *Rationale:* This facilitates elimination of contrast media.

21. Provide comfort measures as needed.

Computed Tomography (CT Scan)

1. Explain purpose of procedure to client—CT scans give outlines of bone tissue and fluid structures due to tumors and hematomas. Tomography can be performed on abdomen, brain, chest, or bones and joints.

(continued)

Skill 21.1.1 | Preparing for Diagnostic Imaging Studies *(continued)*

2. Identify allergies to shellfish or iodine if contrast medium is used.
3. Obtain consent if contrast medium is used or facility requires.
4. Client may be NPO if contrast medium is used. Follow protocol for the specific test. ➤ *Rationale:* Dye can cause nausea; NPO prevents emesis and potential aspiration. However, ingestion of fluids supports ease of vascular access and may help support overall well-being, including kidney function.
5. Administer preprocedure medication if ordered. A mild sedative may be ordered for client to alleviate anxiety.
6. Remove all metal objects, such as hair clips, necklace, and jewelry. ➤ *Rationale:* Metal objects block bony structures on the film.
7. Take client on gurney to x-ray department.
8. Explain equipment and procedure to client.
9. Explain client will have IV injection of contrast material if enhanced study is to be done. Explain that a warm, flushed feeling or nausea can occur.
10. Explain that client will be placed in an encircling body scanner.
11. Instruct client to lie very still during the procedure and not to touch area to be scanned. Scan takes 15 min. ➤ *Rationale:* Movement causes artifact on the image.
12. Return client to room.
13. Provide diet and encourage fluids to 3,000 mL or as ordered. ➤ *Rationale:* Increasing fluids assists in eliminating the contrast medium more quickly.
14. Observe for signs of delayed allergic reaction if contrast study was done.

Cardiac Catheterization

1. Explain purpose and risk factors of procedure to client—to visualize heart structures and coronary blood flow and measure oxygen saturation, cardiac output, and heart pressures. Angioplasty or stent placement is done through cardiac catheterization (Box 21-2 ■; see also Box 21-7). It is used most often to determine the cause of chest pain in adult clients. Procedure takes about 1 hr.

Box 21-2 PROCEDURES DONE DURING CARDIAC CATHETERIZATION

Transluminal Coronary Angioplasty: Specially designed catheter is introduced into the coronary arteries and placed across the stenotic area of the artery. The artery is then dilated by controlled inflation of the balloon for a few seconds. Coronary stents can be placed at the site of the stenosis after angioplasty. The stent is used to keep the coronary artery patent.

Laser Arterectomy: Permanent procedure using laser therapy to open coronary arteries that have plaque deposits

Angioplasty: Catheter is placed in a stenotic area and a balloon is inflated, which forcefully dilates the stenotic area. The client is monitored during the procedure using ECG tracings. If myocardial ischemia is present during the procedure, the balloon is removed.

2. Obtain consent form.
3. Identify allergies to drugs, iodine, shellfish, or any other contrast media.
4. Check if client is on anticoagulants. Contact physician for instructions related to drug administration.
5. Complete prep and shave of groin or brachial area (or both). Mark peripheral pulses for postcatheterization assessment.
6. Establish baseline data for vital signs, peripheral pulses, coagulation studies (PTT, PT), ACT, BUN, creatinine, renal function tests, and ECG pattern.
7. Place client on NPO 6–8 hr before test if possible.
8. Keep client NPO for medications 6–8 hr before test, unless physician orders otherwise. Oral anticoagulants are discontinued. ➤ *Rationale:* This prevents bleeding.
9. Before procedure, obtain vital signs, take weight, and have the client void. ➤ *Rationale:* Weight is used to calculate the amount of dye required for the test.
10. Administer preprocedure medication 30 min to 1 hr before procedure.
11. Take client on gurney to cardiac catheterization lab.
12. Explain equipment and details of procedure to client.
    a. Client is strapped onto a table. ECG leads and blood pressure equipment are applied.
    b. IV is started using normal saline unless otherwise ordered at TKO (to keep open) rate. ➤ *Rationale:* This is for use in an emergency.
    c. ECG monitoring is initiated to monitor heart rate and rhythm.
    d. Groin or brachial area is scrubbed and injected with lidocaine (Xylocaine).
    e. Catheter is placed in femoral or brachial artery and advanced to cardiac chambers.
    f. When contrast medium is injected for coronary artery visualization, explain to client that a warm, flushed feeling, shortness of breath, or nausea can occur.
    g. Instruct client to report any chest pain immediately.
    h. Client is asked to hold breath about 10 sec during contrast medium injection.
    i. Reinforce that client will not fall off table as he or she may be turned on side for cineangiography. Total procedure takes 30 min to 3 hr.
    j. After catheterization, pressure is applied to puncture site for 10–15 min or per protocol.
13. Transport client on gurney to room.
14. Provide post–cardiac catheterization care.
    a. Monitor vital signs, puncture site, heart and lung sounds, and peripheral pulses as with a surgical client.
    b. Elevate extremity used for catheterization site. Keep extremity extended. ➤ *Rationale:* This position promotes blood supply back to heart and prevents thrombus formation.
    c. Apply pressure dressing to puncture site if bleeding continues. Monitor client closely.
    d. Encourage fluids and diet when vital signs are stable and no evidence of nausea or drowsiness is present.
    e. Monitor for signs and symptoms of allergic response.

f. Monitor for signs of clot-induced stroke or myocardial infarction.

g. Administer analgesics for pain.

15. Position client for comfort. Place on back for several hours after the procedure, and then turn from side to side.

Bone Densitometry

1. Discuss procedure with client before scheduled test and ask pertinent questions for the record.

 a. Determine whether barium studies have been done within last 10 days. ➤ *Rationale:* Barium may falsely increase bone density of lumbar spine.

 b. Determine if calcium-containing medication has been ingested and provide instructions regarding use per protocols established. ➤ *Rationale:* Calcium may alter bone density measurement results.

 c. Instruct client that no specific pretest fasting, blood work, or sedation needs to be done. A consent form may be required.

 d. Instruct client to go to outpatient x-ray or hospital facility according to instructions (there are no preparations for study, so it is usually not important to come early for test).

 e. Instruct client not to wear jewelry, belt buckles, or zippers to x-ray department and to remove coins and keys from pocket; clothing need not be removed for test.

 f. Determine whether client has had previous bone density tests or fractures. Document findings for physician.

2. Explain that there is no pain or discomfort associated with test. It is used to detect early osteoporosis. The bones usually examined include lumbar spine, neck of femur, and heel. Test takes approximately 30–60 min.

3. Explain that false-positive results can include previous fractures and previous bone scans.

4. Explain procedure to client.

 a. Client will be placed on an imaging table with legs supported on padded box. ➤ *Rationale:* Position flattens pelvis and lumbar spine. Radiation source is below, with detector above the table that measures the bone's radiation absorption.

 b. Images of lumbar and hip bones are projected on a computer monitor.

 c. Each machine scans the bones of the finger, heel, and forearm differently, so specific instructions will be given according to machine descriptions.

 d. After computer screen calculates bone mineral density, it is compared with existing data from healthy 25- to 35-year-old women and a T score is determined. The T score indicates the strength of the bone. The positive T score indicates a bone that is stronger than normal. A negative T score indicates the bone is weaker than normal. Z scores are also obtained. These scores compare clients matched for age, gender, race, height, and weight.

5. Instruct client that no specific postprocedural care is required. There are no side effects or complications associated with the test.

Mammography

1. Instruct client to not wear deodorant, ointments, or talcum powder. ➤ *Rationale:* They can interfere with the reading of the mammogram, and false-positive results can occur.

2. Instruct client not to wear jewelry around the neck.

3. Review client's history regarding breast implants or previous breast surgery, lumps, or unusual findings on monthly examinations. ➤ *Rationale:* These need to be included on health record, so radiologist has an accurate assessment of mammogram findings (Boxes 21-3 and 21-4 ■). The mammogram is contraindicated for pregnant clients.

CLINICAL ALERT

Mammography only suggests a possible diagnosis of breast cancer. The diagnosis must be confirmed with histological examination of breast tissue obtained through a biopsy.

---

4. Explain the procedure to the client: It may cause some momentary discomfort when x-ray cone compresses breast tissue. Discomfort does not last after release of the cone. ➤ *Rationale:* Compression of breast provides better visualization of breast tissue.

5. Explain that there is minimal radiation exposure from this procedure.

6. Instruct client to take off clothing above waist, including bra, and put x-ray gown on so it ties in front.

 a. One breast is placed on x-ray plate and the cone is brought down on the breast to compress it.

 b. The breast will be placed in different positions to view the entire breast tissue.

Box 21-3 DIGITAL MAMMOGRAPHY

Digital mammography, a method of breast imaging in which images are captured electronically and viewed on a computer monitor, is replacing x-ray imaging as the standard. The radiologist is able to manipulate the contrast and brightness of the images, which increases the chance of identifying cancers. Portions of the breast image can be magnified with computer manipulation rather than with repeated films.

Box 21-4 STANDARDIZATION OF MAMMOGRAPHY REPORTS

Class I: Negative

Class II: Benign

Class III: Benign; short-term follow-up suggested

Class IV: Suspicious abnormality; biopsy should be suggested

Class V: Highly suggestive of malignancy; appropriate action should be taken

Class VI: Known biopsy-proven malignancy; appropriate action should be taken (this category is used for findings already confirmed as malignant by biopsy)

Source: American College of Radiology (2013)

(continued)

Skill 21.1.1 | Preparing for Diagnostic Imaging Studies *(continued)*

c. The second breast is done in same manner.

d. The test takes 15–30 min.

7. Instruct client to wait when mammography is finished until films are processed. ➤ *Rationale:* Sometimes additional films will need to be taken (Box 21-5 ■); this prevents client from having to return to the department. Contrast imaging may need to be done if the breasts are dense.

8. Instruct the client in self breast examination, if necessary, and answer questions before the client leaves.

a. Test results are mailed to the client, are available on client health record system, or may be provided by phone call.

b. If the mammography is being done for diagnostic purposes, the mammogram may be read, and results are immediately available for client.

EVIDENCE-BASED PRACTICE

Comparison of Tomosynthesis Plus Digital Mammography *Versus* Digital Mammography Alone for Breast Cancer Screening

Digital tomosynthesis is a method for performing high-resolution, limited-angle tomography at mammographic dosage levels. This method is used in three-dimensional mammography in order to create a three-dimensional image of breast tissue for better examination.

A total of 13,158 clients were screened for mammography, and 6,100 received tomosynthesis. The overall recall rate was 8.4% for clients in the tomosynthesis group and 12.0% for those who had the conventional mammography. The addition of tomosynthesis reduced recall rates for all breast density and client age groups. The cancer detection rate was 5.7 per 1,000 clients receiving tomosynthesis versus 5.2% of clients receiving conventional mammography. Clients undergoing both tomosynthesis and digital mammography had significantly lower screening recall rates. The greatest reductions were for those younger than 50 and those with dense breasts.

Source: Haas, Kalra, Geisel, Raghu, Durand, & Philpotts (2013)

Box 21-5 NUCLEAR MEDICINE BREAST IMAGING (SCINTIMAMMOGRAPHY)

Scintimammography is a nuclear medicine breast imaging test that is considered supplemental to a breast exam and mammography. The test is often referred to as the Miraluma test or Sestamibi breast imaging. It assists the physician to determine the presence of cancer in the breast. It is used in some clients to investigate breast abnormalities, especially if the client has dense breast tissue, which is difficult to interpret. It is also used if the client has a palpable mass or when multiple tumors are suspected. A radioactive tracer is injected intravenously; the dye accumulates differently in noncancerous and cancerous tissue.

Magnetic Resonance Imaging (MRI)

1. Evaluate client for the following conditions. ➤ *Rationale:* These conditions exempt clients from having MRI because the magnet can move and displace metal, such as clips and staples, or cause a malfunction (see Box 21-6 ■).

a. Clients with pacemakers, insulin pumps, nerve stimulating devices, or implanted devices (*e.g.*, Port-a-Cath, PAS Port).

> **SAFETY ALERT**
>
> The MRI is always on, so clients, visitors, the environment, and staff need to be assessed for metal objects. Codes and resuscitation efforts are not allowed in the scanner. If the client has an emergency, he or she must be removed from the scanner.

b. Clients with joint prostheses, cardiac surgery, or metal implants.

c. Clients with vascular clips and staples from recent surgery.

d. Pregnant clients should not be scanned even though there is no definitive evidence of harm to fetus.

e. Clients with cardiac or respiratory complications may be excluded.

2. Check for allergies if contrast medium is to be used. Two common contrast mediums are gadodiamide and gadolinium Magnevist.

3. Instruct client to remove all metal or magnetically sensitive objects: jewelry, glasses, wallets, watches, hair clips, tongue and body piercings, credit cards, and so on. ➤ *Rationale:* The magnetic field can damage watches and credit cards.

4. Describe MRI machine and procedure to client—it provides a clear picture of the inner structures of the extremities, brain, and spinal cord, and it clearly reproduces soft tissue, ligaments, and nerves; it is often used for determining response to radiotherapy and chemotherapy.

Box 21-6 CONTRAINDICATIONS OR POTENTIAL CONTRAINDICATIONS FOR MRI

Cochlear implants: Some cochlear implants employ magnets, and client injury or impairment of implant function may occur.

Gastric reflux devices for controlling GERD: These devices are not compatible with MRI.

Metallic foreign body in the eye: If intraocular metal foreign bodies are of concern, MRI is contraindicated due to the potential for eye damage. For example, sheet metal workers should be examined to rule out foreign bodies.

Bone growth stimulators: These are not designated by FDA as MRI compatible.

Intracranial vascular clips: Some are contraindicated.

Penile implants, shrapnel, stents, halos, pacemakers, implantable cardioverter/defibrillator, implanted drug infusion pumps: These devices may not be compatible with MRI.

Source: University of California, San Francisco Medical Center (2015)

Note: Newer implanted devices may be compatible with the use of MRI. Each client needs to be assessed for type of device (Box 21-7 ■).

CLINICAL ALERT

Clients who are extremely claustrophobic may require conscious (moderate) sedation or may be moved to an open MRI. If sedated, client must be monitored for at least 1 hr before discharge. The open MRI is also used for obese clients, confused clients, or children. Clients must remain still. This MRI uses a lower-field magnet, so it produces lower-quality images than a closed MRI.

---

a. Client is placed in a padded plastic cradle or on a pillow (Box 21-8 ■). The table then slides into the scanner so that the whole body is encased in the machine.
b. Client needs to lie flat, still, and relax inside the tube magnet. ➤ ***Rationale:*** Movement can produce artifacts on the image.
c. The client is instructed to hold his or her breath for up to 30 sec.

d. Explain that during the procedure the client will hear rapidly repeating, loud thumping noises coming from the walls of the scanner. ➤ ***Rationale:*** Noises are caused by changing magnetic fields.
e. During the time the client is in the machine he or she can talk to and hear staff. Prism glasses may be worn so client can see outside the scanner.
f. Inform client he or she will have ear plugs in place but will be able to communicate with MRI staff through a microphone. ➤ ***Rationale:*** This reduces feelings of claustrophobia.
g. Instruct client in relaxation techniques.
h. Procedure lasts 20–90 min.

5. Instruct client to void before procedure. ➤ ***Rationale:*** This prevents the need for client to void while undergoing procedure.
6. Administer premedication as ordered, usually antianxiety agents. Follow infection control protocols (Box 21-9 ■).
7. Place client in a comfortable position on table.
8. Instruct client on feelings of warmth or shortness of breath if contrast medium is used during procedure.
9. Transport client to room after procedure.
10. Observe for symptoms of delayed reaction to contrast material if used during procedure.

Box 21-7 **VESSEL CLOSURE DEVICES**

There are several arterial closure devices on the market. The Perclose ProGlide Suture-Mediated Closure System is one that is commonly used. These devices provide a monofilament suture knot that is easily advanced to the opening in the artery and delivers a pretied knot to close the access site in the femoral artery after a catheterization procedure. If needed, the physician can easily reopen the access site in the vessel for repeat or additional procedures.

This secure stitch provides rapid hemostasis (the cessation of bleeding) and allows a shorter recovery time, which is more cost effective for the facility.

However, not all clients should be considered for early discharge, because suture-mediated closure is not risk-free. There are complications associated with the procedure.

Box 21-8 **DISCOMFORT IN THE MRI**

Claustrophobia is not the only concern preventing clients from lying still while in the MRI. Discomfort with having to lie still on hard or worn cushions may also be a factor. Some facilities now use improved cushions, wedges, and positioners that conform to the body's shape, help prevent movement, and provide greater client comfort.

Box 21-9 **INFECTION CONTROL IN THE MRI SUITE**

Challenges in Preventing MRSA and Other Infections in the MRI Suite

Infection occurs as a result of hospitals prohibiting cleaning crews from entering to clean the pads and the suite due to its high magnetic field. Most facilities just change the sheet on the table and the pillowcase. This will not prevent contamination of the pads. An average MRI scans 3,000–5,000 clients each year. Many of these clients are infected with MRSA, and 30%–50% of all clients carry less virulent staphylococcus on their skin. Direct contact with personnel also leads to the spread of infection. Most clients undergoing an MRI have IVs inserted, which can lead to blood getting onto the sheets.

To prevent the spread of infection, hand hygiene must be completed frequently and the pads cleaned with antiseptic solutions after each client. To check efficacy of the cleansing process, the pads can be visualized under ultraviolet wavelengths, which detect biologic material such as blood, bacteria, and bodily fluids. (The Joint Commission, 2009).

In addition to cleaning the pads in the MRI, the bore (inside of the machine) must be cleaned as it is an area of high risk for MRSA transmission due to clients' touching or close contact with the bore surface. It is very difficult to clean the bore surface as it requires someone climbing into the bore or using a long cleaning tool with a sponge soaked in disinfectant solution to reach the inside of the bore (Rothschild, 2008).

Unit 21.1 Documentation and Evaluation

DOCUMENTATION for Diagnostic Imaging Studies

- Client's history
- Preparation completed (e.g., NPO, clear liquid dinner, medications)
- Client teaching completed
- Medication administered
- Allergies noted
- Unusual anxiety or fears of client
- How client transported to test
- Time sent and returned from test
- Postprocedure care
- Appearance of dressing or puncture sites

EVALUATION/Critical Thinking

Expected Outcomes

- Client acknowledges understanding of the scheduled procedure.
- Client is calm and emotionally prepared for procedure.
- Client is well prepared for x-ray study after client teaching.
- Client completes x-ray study without complications.
- Client did not experience allergic reaction to contrast media.
- Client describes post-test care upon discharge.

Unexpected Outcomes

- Client has allergic reaction.

Alternative Actions

- Follow protocol or standing orders for allergic reactions.
- Start O_2 at 6 L/min unless otherwise contraindicated. Use nasal cannula. If respiratory distress is severe, use mask and increase oxygen delivery
- Place in semi- or high-Fowler's position if not contraindicated.
- Administer medications as outlined in protocol or according to physician's orders.
- Provide reassurance and encouragement.
- Have client take slow, deep breaths.
- If nausea or vomiting occur, obtain an order for an antiemetic from the physician.
- Notify colleagues to be available if condition worsens.
- Identify location of emergency equipment if needed.

- Client is given meal when on NPO status.

- Call x-ray and change time of test. If possible, arrange for test to be done later in the day to avoid additional hospitalization or return visit.
- Instruct client on what NPO means. Place signage to alert other providers of NPO status.

Unexpected Outcomes	Alternative Actions
• Client very apprehensive and refuses test at last minute.	• Identify reasons for anxiety and attempt to allay fears. • Notify physician and ask if he or she wants to cancel or postpone test to later time. Do not attempt to "talk client into it." • Discuss use of sedation during test.
• Bleeding or hemorrhage occurs from arteriogram puncture site.	• Notify physician. • Apply direct pressure until pressure dressing can be applied. • Monitor amount of blood loss and possible signs and symptoms of shock. • Elevate and keep extremity in extension position. Monitor circulation to distal sites. • Monitor vital signs. Apply oxygen if oxygen saturation declines per protocol.
• Client develops irregular pulse after cardiac catheterization.	• Notify physician immediately. • Start IV if not in place. • Prepare for possible code and IV administration of medication. • Monitor vital signs and level of consciousness frequently. • Initiate cardiac monitoring and oxygen. • Notify rapid response team and/or supervisor. • Provide support.
• Bleeding occurs at catheter insertion site after cardiac catheterization.	• Apply pressure dressing and monitor site. • Elevate extremity. • Monitor peripheral pulse and vital signs. • If bleeding does not subside, notify physician. • Monitor ECG findings.

Nursing Process Data

ASSESSMENT Database

- Assess client's understanding of nuclear imaging and the specific diagnostic test he or she is to receive.
- Assess client's ability to tolerate procedure (e.g., swallowing iodine solution, fasting).
- Determine client's psychologic needs in relation to the nuclear scan.
- Identify any allergies the client may have to radioactive materials.
- Assess need to remain with client during procedure.
- Assess vital signs and document for baseline data.

PLANNING Objectives

- To diagnose tumors, metastatic disease, abnormal conditions, and cardiac and other organ abnormalities via noninvasive method
- To prepare the client physically for the nuclear diagnostic test
- To prepare the client psychologically to prevent undue stress
- To complete client teaching to ensure the client understands the procedure

IMPLEMENTATION Procedures

DOCUMENTATION AND EVALUATION

Expected Outcomes

- Client is physically and psychologically prepared for the scan.
- Client demonstrates understanding of the purpose of the test and potential side effects from the radionuclide material.
- Client completes procedure without complications.

Unexpected Outcomes/Alternative Actions

Pearson Nursing Student Resources

Find additional review materials at
nursing.pearsonhighered.com.
Prepare for success with NCLEX®-style practice questions and Skill Checklists.

Skill 21.2.1 | Preparing for Nuclear Scans

Equipment

Signed consent form
IV equipment (for most scans)
Hospital gown and pajama bottoms

Preparation

1. Identify the client using two identifiers and introduce yourself.
2. Perform hand hygiene.
3. Identify the specific diagnostic test that is to be performed (Table 21-2 ■).
4. Determine if any tests must precede others in order to schedule test appropriately.
5. Have client remove all jewelry. Determine other restrictions based on test.
6. Provide client teaching regarding the study, including any special preparation required for the study.
7. Obtain special consent forms if required by facility after the physician has explained the study to the client.
8. Provide psychological support and reassurance to the client.
9. Identify specific preparations that need to be carried out before the studies. Check for recent exposure to radionuclides. ➤ **Rationale:** Such exposure may interfere with current study.
10. Monitor fluid alterations that need to precede the studies.
11. Explain that radiation exposure is minimal and limited.

Note: Technetium-99m, gallium, thallium, and iodine are used commonly for scanning. Technetium-99m is used extensively because it has a 6-hr half-life and emits low levels of gamma rays.

12. Record client's height and weight.
13. Carry out safety precautions immediately before the study:
    a. Check two forms of client identification.
    b. Check for allergies.
    c. Chart premedication if given.
    d. Monitor safe transfer from the bed to gurney or wheelchair.
    e. Accompany client to nuclear medicine department if needed. ❶ (Usually, nurses accompany critically ill clients.)

Table 21-2 Nuclear Studies

Diagnostic Test	Rationale
Bone scan	To diagnose metastatic bone disease, osteomyelitis, or fractures
Lung scan	To diagnose pulmonary embolism or pneumothorax or to assess pulmonary status before lung surgery
PET scan	To scan whole body or its various areas; used in diagnosis; especially useful in diagnosing epilepsy
Cardiology scan	To diagnose coronary artery disease, cardiomyopathy, valvular heart disease, or to assess cardiac status and analyze ventricular function
Thyroid scan	To diagnose thyroid nodules, abnormal function, or thyroid cancer

❶ Magnetom Large Bore MRI, 1.5 magnet strength.

Procedure

Bone Scan

1. Follow steps as appropriate in Preparation section.
   a. Explain purpose of procedure to client—usually done to detect metastatic cancer, early bone disease, osteomyelitis, fractures, or abnormal healing of fractures. If client is of child-bearing age, determine whether she is pregnant. If so, test cannot be done.
   b. No fasting or sedation is required. Drinking extra fluids is often encouraged.
   c. Have client ready for injection of radionuclide material, probably technetium-99m, 2–4 hrs before scan.
   d. Force fluids between injection of isotope and scan.
   e. Have client void before going to x-ray department.
   f. Take client to nuclear medicine department.
2. Explain procedure.
   a. Client is positioned supine under **scintillation** camera (camera records radiation emitted by skeleton).
   b. Instruct client to remain very still for 20 min to ensure observation of bone abnormalities.
   c. Client will be repositioned to prone and lateral positions during scan.
   d. Return client to room.
3. Instruct client to resume activities and diet. ➤ **Rationale:** There is no problem with radiation exposure because only trace doses of radioisotopes are used.
4. Force fluids for 2–3 hr after scan. ➤ **Rationale:** This promotes renal filtering of excess tracer. Trace elements are excreted in 6–24 hr.

Lung Scan

1. Follow steps as appropriate in the Preparation section.
   a. Explain purpose of procedure—used to detect pulmonary embolism or tumors and to assess lung function. Two types of scans are usually done together: ventilation and perfusion scans. Ventilation scans show areas of lungs not receiving adequate air after inhalation of

(continued)

Skill 21.2.1 | Preparing for Nuclear Scans *(continued)*

radioactive mist or gas. Perfusions scans show areas of lungs not receiving adequate blood flow after injection of radioactive tracer.

b. Obtain consent if required.

c. Chest x-ray is usually done the same day, before, or after lung scan.

d. Transport client to nuclear medicine department.

e. Ensure all jewelry is removed.

2. Explain details of procedure.

a. Explain equipment to client:

Closed-breathing system is used when ventilation scan is done.
Scintillation camera

b. Client is injected intravenously with a tracer amount of radioactive material—usually, radionuclide-tagged MAA (macroaggregated albumin with technetium) is used.

c. Client is positioned in several ways to obtain clear images.

d. Client is instructed to breathe through a closed system until all radioactive gas is cleared from the system.

e. Instruct in use of mouthpiece or nose clips if used.

f. Client is instructed to lie quietly for 30 min as radiography is completed—gamma ray detector is passed over client, records radionuclide uptake on film.

3. Transport client on gurney to room.

4. Instruct client to resume prestudy activities.

PET Scan

1. Follow steps as appropriate in Preparation section.

2. Explain the purpose of test. It scans the whole body or its various regions for early detection of recurrent tumor or cancer that has spread. A PET scan can determine what heart tissue is still alive after a suspected heart attack. It aids in determining focal area for seizure activity and is used to help diagnose epilepsy. It is also useful in determining brain region for surgical removal of affected area when medication resistance is present (Box 21-10 ■). It can reveal size, shape, position, and some functions of organs.

3. Assess client and take complete history to determine if client is pregnant. Determine if client is claustrophobic or anxious. ► *Rationale:* Test cannot be performed if client is pregnant. Client must be able to lie still during the entire process, including a minimum of 45 min with his or her head inside scanner.

4. Premedicate with nonaspirin analgesia if client has arthritis or lower back pain that could prevent client from lying still for

Box 21-10 PET SCANS

Unlike CT scans or MRIs, which show only body structure, PET provides information about the body's metabolism. Metabolic change occurs before structural changes. Some studies have shown that up to 60% of invasive tests or surgeries can be eliminated by using the PET scan.

prescribed time. ► *Rationale:* Sedatives are avoided if at all possible because they alter metabolism.

5. Instruct client to stay NPO for 4–8 hr or per protocol.

6. Instruct client to void 1–2 hr before the test.

7. Instruct client to avoid caffeine, alcohol, and nicotine for 24 hr before test.

8. Explain procedure:

a. Reassure client that there is no discomfort except lying on a hard surface for up to 3 hr and insertion of IV.

b. Ensure client has not taken aspirin or other anticoagulants for several days before scan.

c. Explain that an arterial line will be inserted to obtain blood samples.

d. Explain that a peripheral intravenous catheter will be inserted to inject radioisotope. One hour after injection, client will be placed in scanner.

e. Instruct client to lie quietly for 45 min. Lights will be dim. ► *Rationale:* This is time for radioisotope uptake to occur, as isotopes are circulating to the brain.

f. Monitor vital signs as indicated.

g. Explain that actual scan time is about 30–75 min. He or she must remain quiet with head in scanner during this entire time. ► *Rationale:* Any motion, moving, or talking can detract from the quality of image.

h. Explain that arterial blood samples may be drawn from arterial line during scan.

i. Place blindfold on client to keep client from being distracted during certain brain studies. The head is also placed in a holder to restrain movement. Sometimes, immobilizer wedges or pillows are used.

j. Place Velcro straps on clients with heart or abdominal studies. ► *Rationale:* This prevents movement.

9. Provide post-procedural instructions.

a. After scan, IV and arterial lines will be discontinued.

b. Client can resume normal activities and meals.

c. Monitor for signs of seizure activity or adverse effects if seizure did occur during scan.

d. If sedative was given, do not allow client to drive or engage in any hazardous activities until sedative has worn off. Instruct client to have someone drive him or her home.

Nuclear Cardiography

1. Follow steps as appropriate in the Preparation section.

2. Instruct client that radioactive tracer substances are used to detect and evaluate cardiovascular abnormalities (Box 21-11 ■). Alterations of left ventricular muscle function and coronary blood flow are evaluated.

3. Instruct client in specific activities related to the test being given (i.e., exercise on a treadmill, holding certain medications, fasting). See Step 2 for specific cardiology test.

4. Explain that short fasting time may be necessary.

Box 21-11 COMMON TESTS IN NUCLEAR CARDIOLOGY

Technetium pyrophosphate scan. This binds with calcium and creates an area of increased radionuclide uptake. The client receives an injection into the antecubital vein. He or she then waits 2 hr while the renal system clears the drug. A special camera scans the heart to identify areas of increased uptake of the radioisotope. The radioisotope accumulates in damaged areas of the heart and shows any evidence of a recent MI. Scan is also called a myocardial infusion scan.

Thallium scan. A medication (^{201}Tl) is injected into the antecubital vein and scanning is done within 4–10 min. Necrotic or ischemic tissue does not reflect the radioisotope as tissue with normal blood supply as healthy cells do. To detect myocardial scarring and perfusion, an acute or chronic MI, or the evaluation of prior cardiac surgery are the primary purposes for this test.

Thallium scan with exercise. When this test involves exercise, it takes 1 hr and 15 min; 3 hr later, a 30-min resting scan is performed. Imaging with exercise may demonstrate perfusion problems not apparent when the client is at rest.

Gated cardiac blood pool scan. The client receives an intravenous injection of a red blood cell tagging agent, and ECG leads are positioned on him or her. The computer is then synchronized with the ECG reading. This test evaluates left ventricular function.

❷ Nuclear scanner used for cardiac thallium scans.

5. After isotope injection, scan will be performed 15 min to 4 hr later.
6. Instruct client in nuclear medicine department.
    a. Gamma ray detector is placed over heart.
    b. Detector is placed in several positions during scan.
    c. Scan records images of heart ❷.
7. Evaluate client's status after the scan.
    a. Encourage fluids to excrete isotopes.
    b. Apply pressure over venipuncture site if necessary.

Thyroid Scan

1. Follow steps as appropriate in the Preparation section.
2. Purpose of scan is to diagnose thyroid nodules, abnormal thyroid function, or thyroid cancer.
3. Explain procedure to client.
    a. Instruct client not to consume any iodine compounds (vitamin or mineral supplements that may contain iodine or iodized table salt) or eat any foods that contain iodine—especially seafood, which has a high iodine content, for at least 3 days. ➤ *Rationale:* Consuming iodine products interferes with the test.
    b. Instruct client not to take thyroid or antithyroid drugs or x-ray contrast medium before the test, usually 3 days before test. ➤ *Rationale:* These materials interfere with the thyroid scan.
    c. Instruct client to remain NPO for 2 hr after oral iodine administration.
    d. Tell client that after the initial oral radioactive technetium, he or she must return to the lab 24 hr later. Some labs do scanning after 2 hr of ingestion of technetium.
    e. Instruct client that no isolation is needed after scan.

Skill 21.2.2 | Teaching for Nuclear Scans

Procedure

1. Inform client that test is to be performed in the nuclear medicine department.
    a. The department name alone may be frightening to the client.
    b. Taking the client to the department ahead of time may help to decrease anxiety.
    c. Instruct client to remove jewelry or metal objects in the area of the study.
2. Explain to the client that he or she will be receiving an injection of a radioisotope through a vein. The exceptions to

this procedure are a lung scan in which the isotope is administered through an oxygen mask and a gastric-emptying scan in which the isotope is given orally with food.

    a. Inform client that this isotope emits a harmless amount of radiation.
    b. Inform client that the camera used for scanning does not emit radiation. The camera detects a small and harmless amount of radiation from the isotope as it is lodged in the part of the body being imaged.
    c. The radioactive substance usually leaves the body in 6–24 hr.

(continued)

Skill 21.2.2 | Teaching for Nuclear Scans *(continued)*

3. Explain to the client that he or she will be lying on a table (he or she will not be confined in an enclosed space) while the camera is positioned above or below the table. He or she may be asked to change positions during the test.
4. Assure the client that someone will be with him or her throughout the test, contrasting this procedure with x-rays for which the technician must leave the room or with the MRI for which the client enters a tube-like structure.
5. Tell the client that if he or she is in pain, he or she may receive an analgesic during the procedure, as he or she must remain still while the camera is scanning the body.
6. The scanning usually takes 30–60 min.

Unit 21.2 Documentation and Evaluation

DOCUMENTATION for Nuclear Scanning

- Client teaching completed
- Client's emotional state
- Any radioisotopes given on the unit
- Preprocedural preparation completed (i.e., enema or laxative)
- History regarding earlier tests or studies
- NPO status
- Means by which client transported to nuclear medicine department
- Time client sent to and returned from scan

EVALUATION/Critical Thinking

Expected Outcomes

- Client is psychologically and physically prepared for the scan.
- Client demonstrates understanding of the purpose of the test and potential side effects from the radionuclide material.
- Client completes procedure without complications.

Unexpected Outcomes	Alternative Actions
• Client appears not to understand purpose of diagnostic test.	• Observe for nonverbal cues or misunderstandings in order to clarify purpose of the test. • Provide alternative teaching aids. • Show client the equipment if necessary. • Ask client to repeat explanation to you.
• Client is unable to cooperate during the procedure.	• If not contraindicated by condition, ask physician for sedation order. • Nursing staff members may be asked to help client remain quiet. If so, wear lead apron shield.
• Client is uncomfortable during procedure.	• Reposition client for comfort if possible. (It may not be possible depending on area of body to be scanned.) • Provide support by propping client in position needed for scanning. • Assist client to focus on other things (e.g., the ball game, weather, or something pleasant).

Barium Studies

Nursing Process Data

ASSESSMENT Database

- Assess results of laxative and enema administration to ensure a clean colon for the study. Notify physician if client is unable to "hold" enema solution.
- Evaluate client's ability to cooperate with test.
- Evaluate client's knowledge of test.

PLANNING Objectives

- To determine the client's ability to understand the preparatory process
- To clean out colon in order to ensure visualization of colon
- To prepare the client psychologically for the test

IMPLEMENTATION Procedures

DOCUMENTATION AND EVALUATION

Expected Outcomes

- Client is able to cooperate with test.
- Client's bowel is clean and free of stool, promoting an accurate barium study.
- Client is prepared and knowledgeable about what to expect during procedure.
- Client's study is completed without complications.
- Client successfully expels barium following test.

Unexpected Outcomes/Alternative Actions

Pearson Nursing Student Resources

Find additional review materials at **nursing.pearsonhighered.com.**
Prepare for success with NCLEX®-style practice questions and Skill Checklists.

Skill 21.3.1 | Preparing for Barium Studies

Equipment
Signed consent if agency requires
Enema tube and bag
Ordered solution for enema
Laxative
Wheelchair

Preparation
1. Identify client using two identifiers.
2. Introduce yourself.
3. Perform hand hygiene.

Procedure
1. Identify the specific diagnostic test that will be performed (Table 21-3 ■).
2. Explain purpose of procedure to client.
3. Obtain consent for specific test to be performed.

> **CLINICAL ALERT**
> Obtain specific orders for enemas when client has severe abdominal pain, ulcerative colitis, or history of megacolon. Do not follow general preprocedural orders.

4. Instruct client to refrain from smoking for 8–12 hr.
5. Instruct client to withhold medications for 8 hr before test unless otherwise indicated. Narcotics and anticholinergics are withheld for 24 hr. ➤ *Rationale:* This is to avoid intestinal immobility.
6. Instruct client to prepare for test.
   a. Stay on low-residue diet 2–3 days before test and a clear liquid diet from lunch the day before test. No dairy products.
   b. Take one glass of water or clear fluid every hour for 8–10 hr.
   c. Administer one full bottle (10 oz) of magnesium citrate or X-prep at 2 p.m. day before test.
   d. Administer three 5-mg Dulcolax tablets at 7 p.m., evening before test.
   e. Keep NPO after Dulcolax tablets.
   f. Administer a suppository or a cleansing enema (or both if necessary) in early morning on day of test. Ensure bowel is clear; liquid return should be clear. If not, notify x-ray department.

> **CLINICAL ALERT**
> If client has suspected bowel obstruction, no cathartics are given.

7. Carry out safety precautions immediately before the procedure:
   a. Check two forms of client identification.
   b. Monitor safe transfer from bed to gurney or wheelchair.

Barium Enema
1. Transport client to radiology department, usually via wheelchair.
2. Explain details of procedure to client.

> **CLINICAL ALERT**
> Barium studies should follow IVPs, ultrasound examinations, and arteriograms because barium interferes with visualization of other structures. Barium enema should precede barium swallow.

   a. A balloon rectal tube is inserted and balloon is tightly inflated against anal sphincter. ➤ *Rationale:* This keeps barium in rectum during study.
   b. Client is turned side to side while dripping barium into rectum using gravity flow for infusion.
   c. Barium flow is monitored by fluoroscopy continuously and colon is examined as barium goes through colon.
   d. Barium is drained out and an x-ray is taken to determine whether barium has been expelled.
   e. Entire procedure takes 15 min to 1 hr.
3. Transport client to room.
4. Force fluids with electrolytes unless contraindicated.
5. Administer laxative or enema as ordered (Box 21-12 ■).
   ➤ *Rationale:* This is to facilitate bowel evacuation.
6. Ensure client has bowel movement within 2–3 days.

Box 21-12 SMALL-BOWEL ENEMA
Barium is injected into a tube positioned in the small bowel. This procedure provides better visualization of the entire small bowel because the barium solution is not diluted by juices from the GI tract. This test is used when bowel obstruction is suspected.

Table 21-3 Barium Studies

Diagnostic Test	Rationale
Lower GI Studies	
Barium Enema	To visualize the lower GI tract for contour, patency, position, and mucosal pattern of colon
Upper GI Studies	To visualize the upper GI tract; pharynx, esophagus, and stomach
Barium Swallow	To visualize the esophagus
Small Bowel Follow-Through	To visualize the duodenum, jejunum, and ileum

Barium Swallow Study

1. Explain purpose of procedure to client.
2. Instruct client to stay on low-residue diet 1–3 days before procedure, if ordered, and to stay NPO for 8 hr before test.
3. Administer laxative or enema the evening before procedure, particularly if this test follows barium enema study.
4. Instruct client not to smoke. ➤ *Rationale:* Smoking causes an increase in flow of digestive juices.
5. Transport to radiology department.
6. Explain details of procedure to client.

   a. Client is instructed to drink a cup of flavored barium, usually in milkshake-like form, under fluoroscopic exam.
   b. Client is instructed to turn to several positions while x-rays are obtained.

   c. X-rays are taken every 30 min as barium advances. Procedure can take up to 4–6 hr.

Note: Lower GI series, or barium enema, provides better visualization of the bowel. Large tumors and perforations of the bowel can be identified with the CT scan.

Small Bowel Follow-Through

   a. Barium swallow may be extended to examine duodenum and small bowel.
   b. Films can be taken as long as 24 hr later.

7. Transport client to room.
8. Force fluids unless contraindicated.
9. Administer cathartic.
10. Ensure bowel movement within 2–3 days. Enema may need to be administered.

Unit 21.3 Documentation and Evaluation

DOCUMENTATION for Barium Studies

- Laxative administered
- Type, amount of fluid, number of enemas administered
- Enema result, consistency of stool, color of returning enema solution
- Unusual symptoms such as pain, bleeding, or nausea associated with enemas
- Color of stool after test

EVALUATION/Critical Thinking

Expected Outcomes

- Client is able to cooperate with test.
- Client's bowel is clean and free of stool, promoting an accurate barium study.
- Client is prepared and knowledgeable about what to expect during procedure.
- Client's study is completed without complications.
- Client successfully expels barium after test.

Unexpected Outcomes	Alternative Actions
• Barium is unable to be expelled even after administration of laxatives and enemas	• Obtain order for and administer oil-retention enema. • Administer tap water enema following oil-retention enema. • Continue to administer laxatives until barium is expelled.
• Laxatives or enemas (or both) are ordered for clients with ulcerative colitis or severe abdominal pain.	• Do not administer either the laxative or enema without checking with the physician. • If physician confirms order, carefully administer small amount of enema fluid, and observe and document effects on client. • Chart the type of pain, if any, characteristics of stool, and any symptoms noted while enema is administered. • If client complains of excruciating pain, stop procedure and notify the physician.
• Client's medications are administered in error.	• Notify x-ray department, and ask for specific orders regarding what action needs to be taken regarding the test. • Inform physician, complete a medication error form, and send to nursing office. An unusual occurrence report may need to be completed as well. • If this is a frequent problem on the unit or in the hospital, an in-service education program should be given that includes a discussion of when medications should be given and when held.

Unit 21.4
Endoscopic Studies

Nursing Process Data

ASSESSMENT Database

- Assess vital signs before and during studies, if indicated. Some studies require general anesthesia or conscious (moderate) sedation, and scope is used that could result in perforation and bleeding.
- Assess client's knowledge of procedure to be done.
- Evaluate baseline laboratory tests, particularly those for potential bleeding problems, if biopsy is to be done.
- Evaluate if client is at risk for complications, especially infection (antibiotics may need to be ordered).
- Assess biopsy site for indications of bleeding.
- Evaluate for signs of infection after procedure.

PLANNING Objectives

- To provide information regarding procedure to decrease client's anxiety
- To determine if previous studies were completed using barium
- To evaluate potential for complications following procedure
- To position client on table correctly to facilitate optimal visual outcome and aid in diagnosing condition

IMPLEMENTATION Procedures

DOCUMENTATION AND EVALUATION

Expected Outcomes

- Client is prepared psychologically and physically for endoscopic procedure.
- Client experiences no sequelae after moderate sedation.
- Client does not experience pain or discomfort with procedure.
- Client diagnosis is confirmed with endoscopic study.

Unexpected Outcomes/Alternative Actions

Pearson Nursing Student Resources

Find additional review materials at **nursing.pearsonhighered.com.**
Prepare for success with NCLEX®-style practice questions and Skill Checklists.

Skill 21.4.1 | Preparing For Endoscopic Studies

Preparation

1. Identify client using two forms of identification and introduce yourself.
2. Perform hand hygiene.
3. Explain test to client.
4. Obtain signed consent form.
5. Complete preparation according to endoscopic test being performed (Table 21-4 ■).
6. Place on NPO status for 8–12 hr for gastroscopy and as directed for other procedures.
7. Clarify if dentures should be removed for bronchoscopy or gastroscopy procedures.
8. Provide bowel prep for laparoscopy, sigmoidoscopy, or colonoscopy to cleanse all fecal material from colon. ➤ *Rationale:* This allows adequate visualization of mucosa.
9. Obtain lab results for CBC, bleeding and clotting factors, Hgb, Hct, and electrolytes if potential bleeding could occur or possible biopsy will be done with endoscopy.
10. Withhold medications that interfere with coagulation, such as ASA, NSAIDs, iron medications, and alcohol 1 week before test.
11. Complete physical assessment to determine risk factors for possible complications and allergies.
12. Complete medication reconciliation documents for review prior to procedure.
13. Notify special procedure room staff and physician of potential problems with client's condition that could interfere with procedure.

CLINICAL ALERT

Conscious sedation is a preferred method for anxiety and pain relief during therapeutic and diagnostic procedures, particularly in the radiology department.

Versed is the most common drug used for sedation, and fentanyl is commonly administered for pain control. Both are short-acting drugs with duration of 30–60 min.

See also Moderate Sedation, Chapter 26, Unit 4.

Procedure

Arthroscopy

1. Follow steps in the Preparation section as they apply to this procedure.
2. Explain that arthroscopy allows direct visualization of specific anatomic site (e.g., knee joint). Small trocars are placed into joint and surgical procedure is completed with direct vision of a camera attached to arthroscope.
3. Explain that client usually receives local anesthesia and procedure takes 30 min to 2 hr.
4. Instruct client to remain NPO from midnight if general anesthesia is to be given.
5. Instruct client in use of crutches, if necessary.
6. Shave hair 15 cm (6 in.) above and below involved joint, if ordered.
7. Explain procedure to client.

   a. Anesthesia is given, either local or general.
   b. Leg is scrubbed, elevated, and wrapped in elastic bandage from toes to lower thigh. ➤ *Rationale:* This is to reduce blood flow from lower extremity.
   c. Physician places tourniquet or instills saline solution in client's knee before insertion of scope. ➤ *Rationale:* This is to reduce bleeding.
   d. Knee is placed at 45-degree angle.
   e. Small incision is made in skin around knee and scope is inserted into joint space.
   f. Procedure is completed, joint is irrigated, and medication to decrease inflammation is injected into knee.
   g. Sutures or butterfly tapes are placed on skin with pressure dressing applied over site.

8. Assess client's neurovascular status immediately after procedure.
9. Assess vital signs and observe site for potential complications (i.e., bleeding, edema, or excessive drainage).
10. Provide discharge teaching.

    a. Elevate knee at all times when sitting; minimize use of joint for several days.
    b. Apply ice packs according to physician's orders.

Table 21-4 Endoscopic Procedures

Diagnostic Test	Rationale
Arthroscopy	To evaluate meniscus cartilage or ligament injury; to differentiate arthritic inflammation from injury
Bronchoscopy	To visualize larynx, trachea, bronchi, and alveoli; to diagnose bleeding sites and obtain sputum specimens
Colonoscopy	To visualize rectum and colon; to obtain tissue biopsy and remove polyps
Cystoscopy	To visualize urethra, bladder, ureters, prostate; to place stents
Gastrointestinal tract endoscopy (esophagogastroduodenoscopy, or EGD)	To visualize esophagus, stomach, and duodenum; to obtain specimen for cell studies
Laparoscopy	To visualize abdominal cavity; to perform surgical interventions
Sigmoidoscopy	To visualize anus, rectum, sigmoid colon; to remove polyps, obliterate hemorrhoids

c. Instruct client to observe for potential complications: fever, redness around site, excess drainage, or alteration in color of drainage, pain, increased edema.

d. Ambulation with crutches is usually allowed on same day as surgery.

e. Remind client to make postop physician appointment according to orders.

Bronchoscopy

1. Follow steps in the Preparation section as they apply to this procedure.

2. Explain purpose of procedure to client.

3. Explain that test provides endoscopic visualization of larynx, trachea, and bronchi through insertion of flexible fiberoptic bronchoscope. Biopsies may be taken and cultures obtained during procedure. Procedure is done under local anesthetic.

4. Place client on NPO for 6–8 hr before procedure. ➤ *Rationale:* This decreases risk of aspiration while gag reflex is blocked during the procedure.

5. Instruct client to practice good oral hygiene.

6. Remove dentures if ordered. ➤ *Rationale:* This prevents damage or lodging of dentures in the throat during procedure.

7. Remove contact lenses and jewelry.

8. Obtain baseline data: vital signs and respiratory assessment. Identify if there is difficulty swallowing. ➤ *Rationale:* This provides comparison data after procedure.

9. Premedicate client. ➤ *Rationale:* These medications inhibit vagal stimulation, suppress gag reflex, and decrease the client's anxiety.

10. Assist client to relax and decrease anxiety. Instruct client to breathe through nose.

11. Client is placed in sitting or supine position in operating room or special procedure room.

12. Explain procedure to client.

a. Physician sprays nasopharynx and oropharynx with topical anesthetic. ➤ *Rationale:* This prevents laryngospasm, depresses gag reflex, and prevents discomfort when scope is inserted.

b. Client is instructed to avoid swallowing anesthetic agent. Instruct client to expectorate into emesis basin.

c. Bronchoscope is inserted into mouth and advanced to trachea and bronchi.

d. Tissue specimens or secretions are collected and sent to laboratory for study. Lavage may be incorporated into the procedure to facilitate specimen collections and visualization.

e. Bronchoscope is removed. Procedure takes about 1 hr.

13. Cleanse client's nose of lubricant after removal of scope.

14. Provide postprocedure care.

a. Monitor vital signs, respiratory and cardiac status as with a surgical client. ➤ *Rationale:* This is to identify possible complications, such as bleeding or hypoxia.

b. Assess for respiratory difficulties (**dyspnea**, wheezing, apprehension, and decreased breath sounds). Call physician if this occurs.

c. Elevate head of bed, place in side-lying position if not alert.

d. Monitor for bloody sputum. ➤ *Rationale:* Bleeding can occur as a result of the bronchoscopy. Notify physician immediately if this occurs.

e. Instruct client not to eat or drink until gag reflex returns, usually 1–2 hr. ➤ *Rationale:* Aspiration can occur when gag reflex is absent.

f. Explain hoarseness and/or sore throat can occur after procedure.

Colonoscopy

1. Follow steps in the Preparation section as they apply to this procedure.

2. Explain that procedure visualizes rectum, colon, and small bowel to detect pathologic conditions. It is used for cancer screening. Ensure barium studies were completed 10–14 days before fast, although this would not commonly occur. ➤ *Rationale:* Barium can decrease visualization of colon.

3. Place client on liquid diet and Dulcolax tabs 2 days before procedure, if ordered. May use just 1-day prep with Colyte. Maintain NPO status for 8 hr. Complete all preparations.

4. Instruct client to drink electrolyte laxative solution (Go-lytely or Nu-lytely) the day before procedure. Take according to directions, usually 8 oz every 15 min until 1 gallon is taken. Entire gallon should be taken in 4 hr. Solution should be chilled (more palatable) and swallowed quickly. ➤ *Rationale:* This osmotic solution works quickly and produces a clear colon in about 4 hr if directions are followed accurately. Watery diarrhea usually begins 30–60 min after first glass is taken.

Note: If client has diabetes, an implantable cardioverter defibrillator, pacemaker, or prosthetic heart valve, instruct him or her to call physician before buying bowel prep.

5. Explain side effects of nausea and fluid and electrolyte imbalance to client, especially older adult clients.

6. Instruct client to not take any routine or PRN medications when drinking electrolyte solution. ➤ *Rationale:* The medications will not be digested.

7. Obtain baseline vital signs.

8. Start peripheral IV and medicate client with a narcotic analgesic (usually Versed) as ordered.

9. Take client to special procedure room. Procedure takes 15–60 min.

10. Explain procedure to client.

a. Position client on left side with legs drawn up.

b. Flexible fiberoptic or video colonoscope is inserted through rectum and advanced through the sigmoid, descending, transverse, and ascending colon.

c. Client may experience discomfort when air is instilled into colon to open colon and advance scope.

d. Monitor vital signs and oxygen saturation during procedure, if needed.

e. Antianxiety agents may be administered if client is anxious.

(continued)

Skill 21.4.1 | Preparing For Endoscopic Studies *(continued)*

f. Biopsy forceps or brush is inserted through scope to obtain specimens for study.

g. Tissue or secretions obtained are placed in specimen container.

h. Scope is removed and rectal area cleaned and dried.

11. Instruct client in discharge teaching: to report any rectal bleeding, abdominal pain, distention, or purulent rectal drainage. ➤ *Rationale:* These symptoms indicate possible bowel perforation or hemorrhage.

a. Instruct client to resume normal diet and force fluids after test.

b. Instruct client that he or she may experience flatulence from air instillation.

12. Monitor vital signs as with any client. ➤ *Rationale:* Vital sign changes indicate complications, especially increased temperature and pulse and decreased blood pressure.

Cystoscopy

1. Follow steps in the Preparation section as they apply to the procedure. Review assessment to determine if cystitis or prostatitis is present. ➤ *Rationale:* Sepsis could occur, so antibiotics may be ordered.

2. Explain that cystoscopy is used to evaluate conditions associated with the urinary tract: urethra, bladder, lower ureters. It is used for both diagnostic and therapeutic procedures. The test takes 30–60 min.

3. Instruct in bowel prep, if ordered.

4. Keep client NPO for 6–8 hr if general anesthesia is given. Otherwise, a full liquid breakfast can be given. Several glasses of water may also be ordered.

5. Administer preprocedural medications 1 hr before test. Ensure consent form was signed before giving medication.

6. Place client in **lithotomy** position. Provide covering to preserve modesty and prevent chilling.

7. Prepare external genitalia with antimicrobial swabs.

8. Explain procedure to client.

a. If local anesthesia is being used, it may be instilled into the urethra before the scope is inserted.

b. Cystoscope is inserted through the urethra to inspect bladder and urethral wall and facilitate a biopsy.

c. Bladder is filled with sterile irrigating solution to assist in distending the bladder and removing clots. ➤ *Rationale:* Irrigation allows for better visualization of bladder.

d. Biopsy forceps may be passed through cystoscope to obtain tissue.

e. Bladder is emptied, and scope removed.

9. Provide posttest instructions. Instruct client to:

a. Observe closely for signs of **septicemia** (i.e., chills, fever, flushed feeling).

b. Force fluids unless contraindicated.

c. Monitor urine for persistent bright red color. ➤ *Rationale:* Bleeding can occur; if present, notify physician.

d. Assess for severe pain (colicky pain is normal with urethral catheterization), continual burning, and frequency.

10. Monitor vital signs.

11. Palpate client for bladder distention and ensure client voids before discharge. Use bladder scanner to identify bladder contents if client does not void. ➤ *Rationale:* Urinary retention can be caused by edema from instrumentation.

12. Encourage fluids and monitor urine output for 48 hr. If client's output is less than 200 mL in 8 hr, increase fluid intake. ➤ *Rationale:* Anuria can indicate urinary retention due to blood clot obstructions or urethral stricture.

Gastrointestinal Tract Endoscopy

1. Follow steps in the Preparation section as they apply to this procedure.

2. Explain that this procedure is used to visualize upper GI tract by inserting flexible fiberoptic-lighted scope.

3. Keep NPO for 6–12 hr.

4. Remove dentures.

5. Explain procedure to client.

a. Client taken to special procedure room.

b. Client is awake during procedure; usually takes 20–30 min.

c. Cardiac monitoring and pulse oximetry are done.

d. Throat is anesthetized by swabbing with local anesthetic, usually Xylocaine. ➤ *Rationale:* This is used to decrease gag reflex.

e. Client is sedated with intravenous medication (Versed). Metoclopramide (Reglan) or ondansetron (Zofran) may be administered.

f. Client is placed in left lateral recumbent position.

g. Endoscope is passed through esophagus to the duodenum. All structures can be evaluated as scope goes through the GI tract (termed *EGD*). See Box 21-13 ■.

h. Air is introduced through scope to distend upper GI tract. ➤ *Rationale:* This maximizes visualization.

i. Specimens may be taken and sent to lab.

6. Provide postprocedure care.

a. Monitor vital signs as for surgical client.

b. Check for signs and symptoms of bleeding or perforation. ➤ *Rationale:* Sharp, intense pain in stomach or chest and cool, pale skin indicate perforation.

c. Check gag reflex. ➤ *Rationale:* It may take 2–3 hr for gag reflex to return.

d. Keep side rails up until effects of medications have subsided.

e. Provide ice chips or throat lozenges for sore throat.

Box 21-13 EGD AND ERCP

The esophagogastroduodenoscopy (EGD) can be used therapeutically for cautery and injection of sclerosing agents on bleeding varices.

Endoscopic retrograde cholangiopancreatography (ERCP) provides visualization of the bile and pancreatic ducts. Stones can be removed and stents placed in the bile ducts to drain bile.

Laparoscopy

1. Follow steps in the Preparation section as they apply to this procedure. Ensure consent form is signed.
2. Explain that scope is inserted through abdominal wall and into peritoneum to visualize abdominal and pelvic organs—used to assist in diagnosing pathologic conditions of pelvic and abdominal area.
3. Instruct client to discontinue anticoagulant therapy 5–7 days before test.
4. Complete bowel prep as ordered.
5. Instruct in NPO status after midnight. Client receives general anesthesia.
6. Prep abdomen as ordered.
7. Start a peripheral IV as ordered. Medications will be given during procedure.
8. Have client void just before surgery. ➤ *Rationale:* To prevent accidental penetration of distended bladder during procedure.
9. Insert Foley catheter and NG tube before or after anesthesia administration, according to facility policy. ➤ *Rationale:* This is to prevent complications associated with penetration of distended stomach or bladder with needle placement.
10. Explain procedure to client.
    a. Client is placed in supine position on operating room table.
    b. Skin preparation is completed using antimicrobial swabs.
    c. Blunt-tipped needle is inserted through small incision in periumbilical area and into peritoneal cavity.
    d. Peritoneal cavity is filled with CO_2. ➤ *Rationale:* This separates the abdominal wall from intra-abdominal viscera to allow better visualization of pelvic and abdominal structures.
    e. Laparoscope with lighted camera is inserted through trocar and procedure completed.
    f. Scope is removed and CO_2 is allowed to escape. It takes 24 hr to be totally eliminated.
    g. Incision is closed with butterfly tape, spray tape, or sutures, and covered with transparent dressing.
11. Provide general postop care.
12. Instruct client in discharge teaching.
    a. Observe site for signs of infection, bleeding, increased pulse rate or fever. Notify physician immediately if these signs occur.
    b. Instruct client that he or she will have shoulder or subcostal discomfort for 24 hr. Medicate for pain as needed.
    c. Instruct client not to do physical exercise for 4–7 days. Ambulation is encouraged on a limited basis. Immobility is discouraged to prevent complications.

Sigmoidoscopy

1. Follow steps in the Preparation section. Ensure consent form is signed.
2. Explain that test allows for visualization of rectum and sigmoid colon. Used for screening for colon polyps.
3. Ensure barium studies have not been given up to 3 days before test.
4. Administer tap water or disposable enema (e.g., Fleet's) as ordered the morning of the procedure. Clients with ulcerative colitis will not have an enema ordered. Oral cathartic may also be given.
5. Provide light dinner the night before test and then place client on NPO. Avoid heavy meat, vegetables, and fruit for 24 hr before test.
6. Have client void before procedure.
7. Explain procedure to client.
    a. Client is placed on special table in special procedure room or in physician's examining room.
    b. Position in a knee–chest position if using examination table and rigid scope. Place on left side with right leg bent and placed over left leg if using flexible scope.
    c. Drape client to provide for modesty and warmth.
    d. Physician examines the rectum digitally first.
    e. Lubricated flexible sigmoidoscope is advanced through anus into the rectum to visualize any abnormality of rectum, sigmoid colon, and large bowel.
    f. Client may feel pressure and need to have a bowel movement. Assure client this is usual feeling.
    g. Air may be introduced to increase visualization of bowel wall.
    h. Suction equipment passed through the scope may be used to remove secretions for better visualization of colon.
    i. Biopsy may be obtained by passing a snare through scope.
    j. Scope is removed, and client's rectal area is cleaned and dried.
    k. Gloves are applied if nurse is assisting with cleaning. Remove gloves and wash hands.
    l. Have client remain flat for 10–15 min before leaving room. Procedure takes 15–30 min.
8. Instruct client in discharge teaching.
    a. Resume pre-examination activities.
    b. Monitor stools for bleeding. Bloody stools are normal first 1–2 days after test.
    c. Instruct client to avoid enema or barium studies for at least 1 week.
    d. Observe for signs of increased abdominal distention, increased tenderness, or rectal bleeding. ➤ *Rationale:* These are symptoms of bowel perforation.

Unit 21.4 Documentation and Evaluation

DOCUMENTATION for Endoscopic Studies

- Test preparation completed
- Client teaching completed and client's ability to understand procedure evaluated
- Client's tolerance of procedure
- Preprocedure and postprocedure vital signs, if required
- Record type of specimen taken and sent to lab
- Specific postprocedure care given and client's response to treatment
- Specific signs and symptoms indicating potential complications

EVALUATION/Critical Thinking

Expected Outcomes

- Client is prepared psychologically and physically for endoscopic procedure.
- Client experiences no sequelae after moderate sedation.
- Client does not experience pain or discomfort with procedure.
- Client diagnosis is confirmed with endoscopic study.

Unexpected Outcomes	Alternative Actions
• Lower gastrointestinal tract not clear and sigmoidoscopy not completed.	• Repeat laxative and enemas per physician orders. • Observe results of enema; if solution not clear, notify physician.
• Vertigo occurs while maintaining knee–chest position during sigmoidoscopy.	• Have client lie in supine position for few minutes. • Have client assume standing position slowly. • Have client assume Sims position.
• Upper gastrointestinal bleeding begins when scope inserted.	• Insert nasogastric tube, and apply suction or use other suction equipment for upper airway. • Monitor vital signs for evidence of shock. • Place in semi-Fowler's position.
• Potential colon perforation after endoscopic procedure.	• Assess for abdominal distention, tenderness, and pain. • Notify physician immediately. • Ensure client has a patent IV line, if not, insert peripheral line.
• Potential infection after cystoscopy.	• Instruct client to force fluids to maintain constant flow of urine and prevent accumulation of bacteria in bladder. • Instruct client on signs and symptoms of sepsis: fever, flushing, chills, nausea/vomiting, increased pulse rate, and feeling faint. Instruct client to notify physician immediately if any of these occur. Monitor labs. • If client has been given prophylactic antibiotics, instruct in taking them as ordered: Do not stop taking the medication; take entire prescription.

Fluid Analysis and Microscopic Studies

Nursing Process Data

ASSESSMENT Database

- Assess vital signs before, during, and after the procedure.
- Assess client's ability to maintain position necessary for procedure.
- Assess client's knowledge of the procedure to be performed.
- Review pertinent laboratory tests before procedure.
- Review medication reconciliation forms.
- Evaluate signs and symptoms that indicate a potential problem could exist if test performed.

PLANNING Objectives

- To provide reassurance for clients undergoing diagnostic tests
- To position the client in a manner that facilitates the introduction of a needle through the skin surface to obtain a fluid or tissue sample
- To obtain tissue or fluid to determine presence of infection or diseases
- To obtain body fluids for specific disease analysis
- To aspirate fluid to relieve pressure on body organs to prevent complications

IMPLEMENTATION Procedures

DOCUMENTATION AND EVALUATION

Expected Outcomes

- Client is prepared psychologically and physically for procedure.
- Diagnostic tests performed with minimal discomfort and no untoward effects.
- Specimens from studies sent to laboratory according to hospital policy, in appropriate container and in a timely manner.

Unexpected Outcomes/Alternative Actions

Pearson Nursing Student Resources

Find additional review materials at **nursing.pearsonhighered.com.** Prepare for success with NCLEX®-style practice questions and Skill Checklists.

Skill 21.5.1 | Assisting With Lumbar Puncture

Equipment

Diagnostic tray or equipment specific for procedure (Table 21-5 ■)
Bath blanket
Sterile collection bottles or test tubes if indicated and not on tray
Sterile gloves
Xylocaine injection or EMLA cream if not on tray
Examination light
Clean gloves
Dressing or Band-Aid
Waste receptacle at bedside

① Place client in Sims position to facilitate needle insertion for lumbar puncture.

Procedure

1. Identify client using two forms of identification and explain that a lumbar puncture (LP) is used for diagnosis of tumors, hemorrhage, infection, and autoimmune diseases involving CNS.
2. Introduce yourself and explain procedure—a hollow core needle is placed in the subarachnoid space at L3–4 or L4–5 to facilitate measuring CSF pressure and obtaining fluid for testing.
3. Obtain history of client's complaints, including known allergies and current medications.

> **CLINICAL ALERT**
> This procedure is contraindicated in clients with increased intracranial pressure. A reduction in pressure may cause a herniation of the brainstem. It is also contraindicated if infection is present at puncture site or client is uncooperative.

4. Obtain consent.
5. Instruct client to empty bowel and bladder.
6. Perform hand hygiene.
7. Obtain tray and any additional equipment needed, such as sterile gloves and bath blanket.
8. Position client in lateral recumbent position with back at the edge of the examining table. Cover with bath blanket, exposing only client's back. ①
9. Open sterile tray if requested by physician. Pour antiseptic solution into sterile medicine cup if needed.
10. Instruct client to pull knees up to abdomen and flex chin on chest. Assist client to maintain position, by nurse standing in front of the client, reaching across to support client behind

neck and knees. ➤ **Rationale:** This position widens the space between the spinous processes of the lower lumbar vertebrae for ease of needle insertion.

11. Place pillows between knees. ➤ **Rationale:** This prevents upper legs from sliding off lower legs.
12. Assist client in relaxation exercises or instruct in deep, slow breathing through the mouth.
13. Use Xylocaine or EMLA cream around site before needle insertion by physician.
14. Explain that he or she must remain still without movement during test.
15. Assist physician with the Queckenstedt's test when requested. After opening pressure is obtained, apply compression to neck veins with your fingers.

> **CLINICAL ALERT**
> Queckenstedt's test is used to identify blockage of CSF flow in the spinal subarachnoid space. Generally when neck pressure is applied, there is a rapid rise in pressure level on the manometer with a return to normal within seconds when pressure is released.

16. Don clean gloves and assist physician as directed.
17. Label cerebrospinal fluid samples with number and client information on each specimen container. (Label in presence of the client.)

Table 21-5 Diagnostic Procedures

Diagnostic Test	Rationale
Lumbar puncture	To obtain a cerebrospinal fluid specimen to determine presence of microorganisms, RBCs, or WBCs
Liver biopsy	To obtain a specimen to determine presence of tumor or disease
Thoracentesis	To remove fluid from the thoracic cavity; to obtain a specimen for cell study
Paracentesis	To remove fluid from the abdominal cavity; to obtain a specimen for cell study
Bone marrow aspiration	To study cells obtained from the specimen
Vaginal examination and Papanicolaou smear	To determine cell changes through a smear; to obtain a specimen for venereal disease identification
Amniocentesis	To remove amniotic fluid for studies of fetal maturity and genetic abnormalities

18. After removal of needle, apply Band-Aid to the puncture site.
19. Provide for client safety and comfort (side rails, repositioning).
20. Remove gloves and perform hand hygiene.
21. Submit data entry for appropriate test if needed (i.e., cell count, serology).
22. Instruct client to lie flat for 4–24 hr, depending on hospital policy. Head is to remain flat and even with position of body. ➤ *Rationale:* This is to reduce CSF leakage.

23. Encourage fluids if not contraindicated by client's condition. ➤ *Rationale:* This reduces chance of headache.
24. Observe for spinal fluid leak from puncture site.
25. Check for headaches or alterations in neurologic status or symptoms of infection.
26. Document CSF characteristics, including color and clarity. Record opening pressure.

Skill 21.5.2 | Assisting With Liver Biopsy

Equipment
Same as for Skills 21.5.1, Assisting With Lumbar Puncture
Procedure is often done through ultrasound to guide the needle to pathologic site.
Tray with equipment, sterile gloves, 2×2 dressing, and tape

Preparation
1. Obtain lab values before scheduled test: prothrombin time, bleeding time, and platelet count if ordered. ➤ *Rationale:* Liver is vascular and if these lab results are abnormal or client has bleeding disorder, bleeding may occur after the procedure.

> **CLINICAL ALERT**
> A liver biopsy is contraindicated in clients with platelet counts below 50,000/mm³ or prolonged prothrombin time. Bleeding can occur after the procedure.

2. Obtain and review medication reconciliation. Identify anticoagulants and other medications contraindicated per facility protocol.
3. Determine if a blood typing and crossmatching is needed.
4. Determine if client is to be NPO.
5. Identify client using two forms of identification and explain that tissue will be removed after special needle is inserted into liver. Tissue will be studied to determine presence of disease.
6. Obtain and confirm consent.
7. Assess whether client has any allergies to topical anesthetic agents.

Procedure
1. Perform hand hygiene.
2. Take vital signs. ➤ *Rationale:* This provides baseline data to compare with postprocedure data.
3. Administer sedative and pain medications as ordered.
4. Obtain tray and any additional equipment needed, such as sterile gloves, sandbag, and bath blanket.
5. Place client in supine position at the right edge of the bed. Raise right arm and extend it over the left shoulder behind the head. ❶ If possible, turn head to left side. ➤ *Rationale:* This position provides maximal exposure of right intercostal space.

Note: Left lateral position can be used for biopsy.

❶ Instruct client to raise right arm and extend it over the left shoulder behind the head to facilitate needle insertion for liver biopsy.

6. Open sterile tray if requested by physician. (Have waste receptacle at bedside.)
7. Local anesthesia is used around puncture site.
8. Instruct client to inhale and exhale deeply several times and then exhale and hold breath while physician inserts the biopsy needle. ➤ *Rationale:* Holding the breath prevents the needle from tearing the diaphragm or lacerating the liver as it descends during exhalation.
9. Instruct the client to breathe normally after the physician removes the needle.
10. Don clean gloves and place Band-Aid or small dressing over puncture site.
11. Position client on right side for 2–4 hr. A folded blanket may be placed under client's right side to provide hemostasis. ➤ *Rationale:* This position compresses the liver against the chest wall, thereby decreasing risk of hemorrhage.
12. Remove gloves and perform hand hygiene.
13. Instruct client to remain on bed rest for 24 hr.
14. Assess for signs of complications including hemorrhage and infection.
15. Monitor vital signs as you would for a surgical client (e.g., every 15 min for 1 hr).
16. Assess rate, rhythm, and depth of respirations.
17. Assess breath sounds and check for signs of dyspnea and restlessness. ➤ *Rationale:* Lung may be punctured during biopsy.
18. Send specimen to lab.

Skill 21.5.3 | Assisting With Thoracentesis

Equipment

Same as for Skills 21.5.1, Assisting With Lumbar Puncture
Vacutainer
Interventional radiologist may perform biopsies using CT or
ultrasound (paracentesis and thoracentesis) for better
visualization of organs.
Sterile gloves
Sterile pressure dressing and tape
Emergency equipment available

Preparation

1. Identify client using two forms of identification and explain purpose of procedure to client.
2. Explain that needle is inserted into pleural space for removal of fluid for either diagnostic tests or to relieve pleural pressure.
3. Obtain consent.
4. Check if chest x-ray film is to be taken before the procedure. ➤ *Rationale:* This film is used to compare with the film taken after the procedure and to collect baseline data (not as commonly done as in past).
5. Assess if client has any allergies to topical anesthetic agents.
6. Explain that movement or coughing must not be done during procedure to prevent lung or pleural damage.
7. Ensure client has IV access for emergency medication administration.

Procedure

1. Perform hand hygiene.
2. Take vital signs, and complete a respiratory assessment. ➤ *Rationale:* This information provides postprocedure comparisons and early identification of potential complications.
3. Administer sedative or other medication as ordered.
4. Position client on edge of bed with arms crossed and resting on the overbed table. ❶ ➤ *Rationale:* This position provides good access to the intercostal spaces and facilitates fluid removal.

Note: Client can be placed in side-lying position on unaffected side if unable to sit up.

5. Provide adequate warmth and covering for client using bath blanket.
6. Place unwrapped sterile tray on bedside stand.
7. Open sterile gloves as indicated. Maintain sterile technique throughout procedure.
8. Assist physician as needed with skin prep.
9. Don clean gloves. Instruct client not to cough, take a deep breath, or move during placement of needle by the physician. Ultrasound may be used for accuracy of insertion.
10. After insertion of needle into pleural space, observe client for pallor, dyspnea, tachycardia, chest pain, or **vertigo**. Report these findings immediately to the physician. ➤ *Rationale:* These symptoms occur with a pneumothorax.

❶ Place client in a leaning forward position to expose intercostal space for thoracentesis.

11. Connect tubing to Vacutainer, allowing fluid to be drawn from cavity.

Note: Blunt-tip, soft catheter-over-needle is used more often than a needle to prevent pneumothorax.

12. Apply pressure dressing (as determined by policy) after fluid and needle are removed. Remove gloves and perform hand hygiene.
13. Observe client every 5 min for half hour for pulmonary edema (blood-tinged sputum), **crepitus**, cardiac distress (changes in respirations, pulse, or color), or a shift in the mediastinum.
14. Place client on unaffected side with head elevated 30 degrees for at least 1 hr.
15. Monitor vital signs and breath sounds as with postoperative clients for 2 hr and as indicated.
16. Observe dressing; change as needed. ➤ *Rationale:* Drainage is a common occurrence after a "tap."
17. Obtain chest x-ray after procedure, if ordered, to check for pneumothorax.
18. Record color, amount, consistency, and samples of fluid obtained.
19. Complete lab slips or computer data entry, label in presence of client, and send specimen to lab.
20. Post-procedure teaching should include reasons to contact (if ambulatory procedure), when to resume medications, how to manage dressing, activity level, and when activities may be resumed.

Skill 21.5.4 | Assisting With Paracentesis

Equipment

Same as for Skills 25.5.1, Assisting With Lumbar Puncture
Sterile tray
Vacutainer
Chair
Drape
Sterile gloves
Bucket
Dressing-elastic adhesive patch
Blood pressure and emergency equipment
Clean gloves
Waste receptacle

Preparation

1. Identify client using two forms of identification and explain purpose of procedure to client.
2. Explain that needle is inserted into peritoneal cavity and fluid removed for fluid analysis or to remove fluid from cavity to promote comfort and increase respiratory status.
3. Obtain consent.
4. Assess whether client has any allergies to topical anesthetic agents.
5. Assess whether client has coagulation abnormalities or bleeding tendencies. (Procedure is contraindicated in these clients.)
6. Perform hand hygiene.
7. Assess client's abdominal girth, bowel sounds, vital signs, and respiratory status. ➤ *Rationale:* This information provides postprocedure comparisons and early identification of potential complications. Distended abdomen often impedes breathing.
8. Have client empty bladder. ➤ *Rationale:* This prevents accidental puncture of the bladder during the procedure.
9. Weigh client. ➤ *Rationale:* This information can be used to assess fluid loss after the procedure.

Procedure

1. Place client in Fowler's position on chair or on edge of bed with legs spread apart. ❶
2. Drape client, and provide adequate warmth and covering with a bath blanket.
3. Obtain vital signs, and observe client for pallor and vertigo during procedure. ➤ *Rationale:* These symptoms are indicative of shock.
4. Position and open tray on overbed table.
5. Open sterile gloves if needed.
6. Assist physician in preparing skin with antiseptic solution and topical anesthesia or as needed.
7. Don clean gloves.
8. Physician inserts trocar needle or cannula through small incision. Plastic tubing is attached to cannula and other end of tubing is placed in the collection receptacle. Vacutainer may be used to provide gentle suction of fluid from the cavity.

❶ Position client in chair to facilitate trocar insertion and drainage for paracentesis.

9. Observe total amount of fluid aspirated. Usually no more than 2,000 mL (2 L) is removed at one time. ➤ *Rationale:* Removing larger amounts of fluid can lead to hypotension and hyponatremia.
10. Apply pressure dressing after removal of needle. ➤ *Rationale:* This prevents bleeding from puncture site.
11. Remove gloves, and place in appropriate receptacle.
12. Perform hand hygiene.
13. Return client to bed and place in semi- to high-Fowler's position. ➤ *Rationale:* These positions usually are most comfortable for the client and promote lung expansion.
14. Observe for leakage at puncture site or scrotal edema in male client.
15. Monitor vital signs and observe closely for signs of hypotension. Monitor urine output and color and dressing every 15 min for at least 2 hr; every hour for 4 hr; and every 4 hr for 24 hr.
16. Assess bowel sounds, and measure abdominal girth. ➤ *Rationale:* Data are used to monitor for signs of perforated bowel or peritonitis.
17. Weigh client when vital signs are stable. ➤ *Rationale:* This prevents hypotension.
18. Reinforce or change dressings as needed.
19. Monitor serum protein and electrolytes, particularly sodium. ➤ *Rationale:* Fluid contains high levels of protein that is removed with this procedure.
20. Record color, amount, consistency, and samples obtained from paracentesis, and send to laboratory. (Use gloves when handling specimens.)

Skill 21.5.5 | Assisting With Bone Marrow Aspiration

Equipment

Same as for Skills 21.5.1, Assisting With Lumbar Puncture
Specimen containers specific to test performed
Sterile gloves

Procedure

1. Identify client using two forms of identification and explain purpose of procedure.
2. Explain procedure.
3. Inform client that he or she will experience discomfort or pressure when the needle is inserted.
4. Obtain consent.
5. Obtain tray and provide any additional equipment needed, such as specimen container.
6. Assess coagulation studies and report unusual findings to physician.
7. Premedicate client with prescribed drugs.
8. Position client in supine position if sternum or anterior iliac crest is the biopsy site or prone if posterior iliac crest is the biopsy site. Client may also be placed in lateral position with upper leg flexed if iliac crest accessed. Place a sandbag under iliac crest area if physician requires.
9. Open tray on overbed table.
10. Perform hand hygiene and don sterile gloves.
11. Assist physician as needed.
12. Physician injects local anesthetic at site.

Note: A large-bore needle containing a stylus is inserted into bone, about 3 mm deep. Stylus is removed and 10–20 mL syringe is attached to needle. About 0.5–2 mL of bone marrow is removed. Aspirant is placed in specimen container. The type of container used is determined by the test ordered.

13. Apply direct pressure for 5–15 min after removal of needle.
    ➤ *Rationale:* This is to prevent bleeding.
14. Cover puncture site with sterile pressure dressing. Dressing usually remains in place for 48 hr before removal. Ice pack may be applied to help control bleeding.
15. Clean residual antiseptic to prevent skin irritation.
16. Remove gloves and perform hand hygiene.
17. Monitor vital signs, and observe puncture site for drainage, edema, or pain, as with surgical client. ➤ *Rationale:* This is to monitor for signs of infection. Call physician for temperature above 101°F (38°C).
18. Position the client for comfort.
19. Properly label specimens and send to laboratory.
20. Evaluate client for signs of hemorrhage, shock, or infection.

Skill 21.5.6 | Assisting With Vaginal Examination and Papanicolaou (PAP) Smear

Equipment

Two slides
Cytology container
Fixative agent/kit
Vaginal speculum, several sizes
Gloves
Water-soluble lubricant (use approved lubricant; others may interfere with results)
Examining light

Preparation

1. Identify client using two forms of identification and explain purpose of procedure.
2. Explain that test is performed to detect neoplastic cells in cervical and vaginal secretions. Procedure takes 10 min.
3. Instruct client not to douche, insert vaginal medications, or take tub bath for 24 hr before exam.
4. Instruct client that test should be done 2 weeks after start of last menses.
5. Instruct client to refrain from sexual intercourse for 24–48 hr before exam, according to physician's orders.
6. Foods or fluids are not restricted.

Procedure

1. Instruct client to empty bladder.
2. Assist client to examination room.
3. Instruct client to remove clothing including underwear and don gown.
4. Position client on examining table in lithotomy position using stirrups.
5. Provide adequate coverings to preserve modesty and prevent chilling.
6. Open speculum package, gloves, and lubricant. Place on tray. Place cytology slides and container on tray.
7. Position light for good exposure.
8. Stay with client if she is a child or physician is male.
9. Assist physician as needed. A lubricated speculum is inserted into vagina.
10. Instruct client that material is collected from cervical canal by rotating either a cotton swab moistened with saline or a wooden spatula.
11. Wipe swab across a clean glass slide to disperse cells.
12. Affix to slide utilizing facility-approved fixation technique to ensure specimen quality.
13. Label two slides with client's name and area from where specimen is obtained. Place slides in cytology container and send to the lab. Complete all required forms or electronic documentation. Client's medical history and reason for examination are written on request form.
14. Assist client in perineal care.
15. Provide perineal pad if bleeding occurs.
16. Assist client to dress if necessary.

Skill 21.5.7 | Assisting With Amniocentesis

Preparation

1. Identify client using two forms of identification and explain purpose of procedure to client.

Note: Test is to withdraw fluid for analysis to check fetal maturity status, gender of fetus, genetic or chromosomal abnormalities, hereditary metabolic disorders, anatomic abnormalities, or fetal distress.

2. Obtain consent, both client and her partner.
3. Explain that foods and fluids are not restricted. Have client void before test. ➤ **Rationale:** This prevents injury to the bladder. Before 20 weeks of gestation, bladder may be kept full to support the uterus.
4. Transport client to treatment room.
5. Instruct client to lie quietly in supine position for 30 min.
6. Obtain fetal heart tones and mother's blood pressure and vital signs.
7. Open amniocentesis tray and gloves. Place Xylocaine nearby if not included on tray. ➤ **Rationale:** This procedure is performed under sterile conditions to prevent infection.
8. Explain details of the procedure to the client.

Procedure

1. Perform hand hygiene and don gloves. Have extra sterile gloves available if needed. Assist the physician in the procedure:

   a. Physician prepares abdomen with antiseptic solution or alcohol.

   b. Xylocaine injection provides local anesthesia for needle insertion area.

   c. Placenta, umbilical cord, fetus, and pocket of amniotic fluid are located by ultrasound.

   d. A 22-gauge spinal needle with a stylet is inserted through the midabdominal wall and 5–15 mL of amniotic fluid is withdrawn. Amount is determined by test.

   e. Amniotic fluid is placed in light-resistant specimen container and labeled with client's name. Appropriate lab slips are completed. ➤ **Rationale:** This is to prevent breakdown of bilirubin.

   f. Procedure takes about 10 min if access to fluid is obtained without difficulty.

2. Remove gloves, perform hand hygiene, and don new sterile gloves. Place small dressing or Band-Aid over needle site.
3. Remove gloves and perform hand hygiene.
4. Monitor fetal heart tones and observe for signs of labor.
5. Observe puncture site for bleeding or other drainage.
6. Instruct client to notify healthcare provider of any unusual occurrences such as cramping, pain, bleeding or drainage at needle insertion site or vaginally, signs of labor, or signs of infection.
7. Give RhoGAM if woman is Rh-negative. ➤ **Rationale:** There is a risk of immunization against fetal blood (hemolytic disease).
8. Explain that test results will be available in 2 weeks.

Unit 21.5 Documentation and Evaluation

DOCUMENTATION for Fluid Analysis and Microscopic Studies

- Preparation completed for test
- Client teaching completed and client's ability to understand procedure evaluated
- Consent form signed
- Client's tolerance of procedure
- Fluid or specimens sent to laboratory for analysis
- Preprocedure and postprocedure vital signs if required
- Color and amount of fluid withdrawn from paracentesis, thoracentesis, or lumbar puncture

- Fetal heart tones before and after amniocentesis
- Type of dressing applied and postprocedure care.
- Specific position assumed after procedure as indicated
- Abnormal findings after procedure indicating potential complications

EVALUATION/Critical Thinking

Expected Outcomes

- Client is prepared psychologically and physically for procedure.
- Diagnostic tests performed with minimal discomfort and no complications.
- Specimens from studies sent to laboratory according to facility policy, in appropriate container and in a timely manner.

Unexpected Outcomes	Alternative Actions
• Client has spinal fluid leak after lumbar puncture.	• Keep client in supine position or as ordered. • Notify physician. • Keep sterile dressing over puncture site. Do not allow dressing to become wet. • Monitor vital signs and physical complaints.
• Client complains of shortness of breath or expectorates blood-tinged sputum after a thoracentesis.	• Place client in Fowler's position. • Assess vital signs. • Administer oxygen. • Monitor breath sounds. • Notify physician and check on order for chest x-ray. • Have chest tube insertion tray available. • Insert IV if consistent with hospital policy. • Allay client's fears and provide emotional support.
• Urine output is blood-tinged after paracentesis or amniocentesis.	• Notify physician at once; bladder may have been punctured during procedure. • Monitor vital signs for shock. • Establish IV access if consistent with hospital policy. • Maintain client on bed rest. • Observe for urine output.

Chapter Wrap-Up

GERONTOLOGIC Considerations

Older Adult Clients Requiring Diagnostic Tests Are at Risk for the Following Problems:

- Dehydration can result from fluid restriction, use of contrast agents for the tests, and bowel preparation using enemas. Osmolar imbalances and hypovolemia can result from the dehydration.
- Extracellular fluid volume excess can occur if large volumes of fluid are required for the test. Renal studies, which usually require the use of large volumes of fluid, should not be considered if the client is at risk for circulatory overload. Older adult clients may have a compromised cardiorespiratory status. A secondary choice of tests may need to be considered, such as a CT scan.
- Renal dysfunction resulting from multiple tests using contrast agents should be avoided. Acute renal failure can result from multiple tests with contrast agents in older adult clients who already have a compromised renal system. Spacing tests over time helps prevent this problem.

Nursing Responsibilities for Older Adult Clients Requiring Diagnostic Tests Should Include the Following:

- Carefully monitor fluid and electrolyte balance.
- Adequately hydrate client before and after tests unless contraindicated.
- Monitor laboratory tests, such as electrolytes and osmolarity.
- Monitor intake and output frequently.
- Monitor vital signs.
- Assess for fall risk initially and if condition changes. Implement safety measures.
- Weigh clients who are at risk for fluid volume disturbances.
- Complete physical assessment, including mental status, each shift, and report unusual findings to physician.

Each state legislates a Nurse Practice Act for RNs and LVN/LPNs. Healthcare facilities are responsible for establishing and implementing policies and procedures that conform to their state's regulations. Verify the regulations and role parameters for each healthcare worker in your facility.

MANAGEMENT Guidelines

Only RNs can transport clients who have received conscious sedation for a procedure.

Delegation

- LVNs/LPNs and RNs may both be assigned to care for clients undergoing diagnostic tests. Nurses are frequently working in x-ray and diagnostic procedure laboratories today and assisting physicians with invasive procedures. Technicians are also educated to work in areas such as cardiac catheterization labs. These technicians are not nursing personnel. In most cases, radiological technologists assist with the various procedures within the x-ray and diagnostic procedure labs.
- When invasive procedures such as liver biopsy and paracentesis are performed on the nursing unit, either an LVN/LPN or RN is assigned to assist the physician.
- Preprocedure and postprocedure interventions are assigned to the LVN/LPN or RN for direct responsibility. A CNA may assist the nurse by taking vital signs.

Interprofessional Communication

- All staff members must be aware of clients undergoing diagnostic tests. This information is disseminated through shift and team reports. It is also written on the Kardex card or is on the client's information sheet on the computer. If premedication is required, this information is found on the Medication Administration Record as well. If the client is NPO for the test, a sign must be placed in the client's room indicating this status.
- Specific directions must be given to the staff member assigned to the client to inform them of their client care responsibilities both pre- and postprocedure.
- The RN must assess the knowledge base of the staff member assigned to assist the physician with any procedure being performed on the unit. This is to ensure safety for the client.
- The RN collaborates with the physician to identify any specific equipment or needs he or she may have for the procedure being performed on the unit.

CASE STUDY Applications

Scenario 1

Mr. Michael Spicer, a 72-year-old retired fireman, is scheduled for the following diagnostic procedures as an outpatient. He has started his testing with a barium enema. You have been asked to call him and instruct him about the procedures.

Diagnostic Tests to Be Completed

- IV pyelography
- Bone scan
- Sigmoidoscopy
  1. What is the priority question you should ask? Provide rationale for your answer.
  2. When beginning the discussion about the IVP, what is your priority question? Provide rationale for your answer.

3. Identify the most important post-procedure client education regarding the IVP. Provide rationale for your answer.
4. The client asks you if he will be radioactive and a risk to his family after the bone scan. What is your best response?
5. Briefly explain the preprocedure prep for the sigmoidoscopy.

Scenario 2

A young, 30-year-old client has been referred to the surgeon for further evaluation of a lump in the upper, outer quadrant of her left breast. You work with the physician and are obtaining the history from the client. She tells you she noticed the lump about 1 month ago. When you examine the breast you feel a quarter-size lump without dimpling of the nipple.

1. The client asks you how will they know if it is benign or malignant. What is your best response?

2. She is very anxious and asks you questions about the various procedures that they do now to determine whether surgery is necessary. Explain the various diagnostic tests that are completed and prioritize the tests according to usual protocol for completion of the tests.

3. Describe the preprocedural instructions for the procedures listed in question 2.

NCLEX® Review Questions

Unless otherwise specified, choose only one (1) answer.

1. What is the nurse's major responsibility with interventional radiology?
   A. Assisting the radiologists in preparing the client for the procedure
   B. Managing procedural sedation, monitoring, and postprocedure recovery
   C. Monitoring vital signs during the procedure
   D. Providing client education about the procedure

2. How would you best define dynamic CT scanning?
   A. The test visualizes blood flow and degree of vascularity of organs via dye injection to specific organs.
   B. It uses sound waves produced by ultrasound to differentiate normal from diseased tissue.
   C. It is observation of internal body organs and cavities by introducing the endoscope and then obtaining scans of the organs or cavities.
   D. It is a scan that uses a strong magnetic field in conjunction with radiofrequency waves to transmit signals from body cells to the computer.

3. Which one of the following preparations would not be included in the procedure for x-ray studies?
   A. Determine, if several studies are ordered, which one needs to be completed first.
   B. Ensure informed consent form is signed.
   C. Inform the client there is no restriction on food or fluid before the tests.
   D. Determine need for withholding medications before the x-ray.

4. What are the client instructions when undergoing an intravenous pyelography (IVP)?
   Select all that apply.
   A. "You should not eat anything after 6 p.m. but you can take fluids until early morning."
   B. "Do you have any allergies to shellfish or iodine?"
   C. "Dye injection material can cause nausea, shortness of breath, and a hot, flushed feeling."
   D. "Drink at least 24 oz of water immediately after the IVP."
   E. "Monitor for signs and symptoms of reactions to contrast media for 4 hr; if none, discontinue monitoring.

5. Which of the following baseline lab values need to be obtained before an arteriography?
   A. Hemoglobin and hematocrit
   B. WBC, RBC, SGOT, SGPT
   C. BUN, creatinine, PT/PTT, APTT
   D. MVP, platelets, blood smear

6. You are obtaining a history before scheduling the client for a bone scan. What is the most important question to ask?
   A. "Have you had a barium study done in the last 10 days?"
   B. "You have had a bone scan before; do you have any questions?"
   C. "Do you have claustrophobia?"
   D. "Do you have someone who can take you home after the test?"

7. What do printed instructions for a client scheduled for a mammogram include?
   A. Remain NPO for at least 6 hr before the test.
   B. Refrain from wearing deodorant.
   C. Remove jewelry from neck and wrists.
   D. Wear easy-to-remove clothing, as it must all be removed.

8. As you observe the catheter insertion site after a cardiac catheterization, which of the following interventions would be considered a priority to implement?
   A. Apply a pressure dressing over the site.
   B. Call lab to order a CBC, HGB, and HCT.
   C. Elevate the extremity.
   D. Monitor peripheral pulses.

9. What is a major reason why PET scans are used in place of the CT scan or MRI?
   A. It is not necessary to have an IV or dye injection for the PET scan.
   B. Metabolic changes, which are visualized on the PET scan, occur before structural changes.
   C. It takes only a few minutes for a PET scan, whereas it can take up to 75 min for an MRI.
   D. Foods or fluids do not need to be restricted with the PET scan.

10. A client is very fearful and asks you about the arthroscopy he is scheduled to have in the afternoon. Which of the following responses would be most appropriate?

A. "You will receive general anesthesia, not local anesthesia, so you will not experience any pain."

B. "The procedure will take about 2–3 hr."

C. "The incision will probably be under the knee cap and you will have sutures to hold the tissue in place."

D. "You will most likely be able to ambulate with crutches the same day."

QSEN Activity

Medication Administration

Domain: Safety

KSA: Knowledge

Activity:

A student nurse is assigned to work with a registered nurse. One of the clients being cared for is undergoing a bronchoscopy. A physician enters the room as the procedure is beginning, and the registered nurse must leave the room briefly to collect additional supplies requested by the physician. While the nurse is gone, the physician asks the student to draw up and administer an IV medication, something that the student is not authorized to do without a nurse or instructor present. Role-play the interaction with the physician. Describe elements of the student's response.

Bibliography

American College of Radiology (ACR). (2013). BI-RADS assessment categories. Retrieved from http://www.acr.org/Quality-Safety/Resources/BIRADS

Haas, B., Kalra, V., Geisel, J., Raghu, M., Durand, M., & Philpotts, L. E. (2013). Comparison of tomosynthesis plus digital mammography and digital mammography alone for breast cancer screening. *RSNA Journal, 269*(3), 694–700.

Kee, J. (2013). Laboratory and diagnostic tests with nursing implications (7th ed.). Upper Saddle River, NJ: Pearson.

NIH: National Human Genome Research Institute. (2014). Genetic testing. Retrieved from http://www.nlm.nih.gov/medlineplus/genetictesting.html

Nuclear Regulatory Commission. (2014). ALARA. Retrieved from http://www.nrc.gov/reading-rm/basic-ref/glossary/alara.html

Pisano, E. D., Gatsonis, C., Hendrick, E., Yaffe, M., Baum, J. K., Acharyya, S., Conant, E. F., Fajardo, L. L., Bassett, L., D'Orsi, C., Jong, R., Rebner, M. (2005). Diagnostic performance of digital versus film mammography for breast-cancer screening. *The New England Journal of Medicine, 17*(353), 1773–1783.

Pullen, R. L. & Matthias, T. (2010). Fostering therapeutic nurse-patient relationships. Retrieved from http://journals.lww.com/nursingmadeincrediblyeasy/Fulltext/2010/05000/Fostering_therapeutic_nurse_patient_relationships.1.aspx

Rothschild, P. (2008, Jun.). Preventing infection in MRI: Best practices for infection control on or around MRI suites. Retrieved from www.patientcomfortsystems.com/MRI_infection_control_white paper pdf

Spader, C. (2006, Mar. 13). Diagnostic imaging; contrast counts. *Nurseweek*, 18–20.

The Joint Commission. (2009, May 5). The Joint Commission warns of poor infection control in MRIs. Retrieved from http://www.itnonline.com/article/joint-commission-warns-poor-infection-control-mris.

University of California, San Francisco Medical Center. Department of Radiology & Biomedical Imaging. (2015). Magnetic resonance safety policy of UCSF. Retrieved from http://radiology.ucsf.edu/patient-care/patient-safety/mri-safety

Chapter 22
Urinary Elimination

Learning Objectives

22.1 Describe the process of urine production.

22.2 List four alterations that result in urinary elimination problems.

22.3 State two nursing diagnoses that relate to urine elimination.

22.4 Complete an intake and output bedside record.

22.5 Compare and contrast the steps for inserting a straight catheter in a male and female client.

22.6 Describe the major parameters needed to preserve a sterile environment when inserting a catheter.

22.7 Demonstrate the clamping protocol used for clients with suprapubic catheters.

22.8 Explain how a catheter is attached to a leg bag.

22.9 Identify the most important advantages of a suprapubic catheter.

22.10 Outline the steps necessary to obtain a urine specimen from a closed urinary drainage system.

22.11 Outline the steps for applying a urinary diversion pouch.

22.12 Describe rationale for renal replacement therapy.

22.13 List safety precautions for caring for a client with a fistula or graft for vascular access for hemodialysis.

Chapter Outline

Terminology

Albuminuria the presence of albumin in the urine.

Antidiuretic pituitary hormone that causes water reabsorption by the distal tubule of the nephron.

Anuria suppression of urine production (less than 100 mL/day).

Arteriovenous extracorporeal circuit created with arterial to venous blood flow. The client's blood pressure forces blood through a hemofilter and back to a venous return access.

AV fistula anastomosis of an artery with a vein as an access site for hemodialysis.

Azotemia increased levels of BUN and creatinine in the blood.

Calyx cuplike portion of the kidney pelvis.

Catheterization insertion of a tube for the injection or removal of fluids from a vessel or body cavity.

Coudé catheter an elbowed catheter used for draining urine from bladder.

Dehydration use or loss of more fluid in the body than was taken in, which can lead to harm or potential harm to body functioning.

Dialyzer artificial kidney.

Distention stretching or inflating a structure such as the bladder.

Diuresis the excessive production of urine.

Dysuria painful urination.

Edema a condition of excess fluid in the interstitial space.

Electrolytes substances that develop an electrical charge when dissolved in water.

Encrustation the deposit of mineral salts, such as on the surface of and inside an indwelling catheter.

End-stage renal disease the loss of 90% of kidney nephrons resulting in accumulation of nitrogenous wastes in the blood and uremia, necessitating dialysis.

Foley catheter a self-retaining indwelling tube that is used to provide continuous drainage, usually from the bladder.

Genitourinary pertaining to the genital and urinary systems.

Hemodialysis process of removing excess fluid and accumulated wastes and electrolytes from the blood.

Hydrostatic pressure pumping force created by the mean arterial blood pressure, or a pump.

Incontinence inability to retain urine.

Indwelling urethral catheter a retention, or Foley, catheter.

Irrigation the flushing of a tube or area with solution.

Micturition the process of emptying the urinary bladder; voiding.

Nocturia waking up frequently during the night with a need to urinate.

Oliguria diminished production of urine (400 mL/day).

Patency the state of being freely open.

Peri prefix meaning around or about.

Peristalsis a progressive wavelike movement that occurs involuntarily in hollow tubes in the body.

Polyuria the excessive production of urine (output >2 L/day).

Pyuria the presence of pus in the urine.

Renal pertaining to the kidney.

Sediment a substance settling at the bottom of a liquid.

Sepsis presence of pathogens or their toxins in the blood.

Septicemia presence of pathogens in the blood.

Shock a state of inadequate tissue perfusion.

Specific gravity weight of a substance compared with an equal volume of water. Water is 1.000.

Stoma surgically created opening.

Urethra a canal for the discharge of urine from the bladder to the outside.

Urinary diversion an alternate route for urine elimination.

Urinary tract infection (UTI) an infection of the urinary tract, including all or part of the organs and ducts.

Urinary System

The structures of the urinary system are the kidneys, ureters, bladder, and **urethra**. Each kidney produces urine, which is carried to the bladder by a ureter that is about 25 cm (10 in.) long and 0.6 cm (about ¼ in.) in diameter. Peristaltic waves, pressure, and gravity propel urine through the ureters so that it can be discharged into the bladder.

The bladder serves as a reservoir for urine until voiding takes place. When voiding, or urination, occurs, urine passes through two sphincters and is transported from the bladder to the external environment through the urethra. The kidneys are essential to life, but the urine collection system is not.

The anatomic position of the bladder and the structure of the urethra differ in males and females. The bladder is posterior to the symphysis pubis. In a female, the bladder is anterior to the vagina and the neck of the uterus (Figure 22-1 ■). In a male, the bladder is anterior to the rectum (Figure 22-2 ■). The urethra of the female is about 4 cm (1.5 in.) long, and the male urethra is 20 cm (8 in.) long.

The urethra, bladder, ureters, and kidney pelves are lined with a continuous layer of mucous membrane. Because there is continuity of the lining, bacteria introduced into the normally sterile system can spread throughout the urinary tract. When the bladder is empty, its lining falls into folds that provide pockets where bacteria can multiply. Since the membrane is highly vascular, bacteria can easily enter the bloodstream and **septicemia** can result.

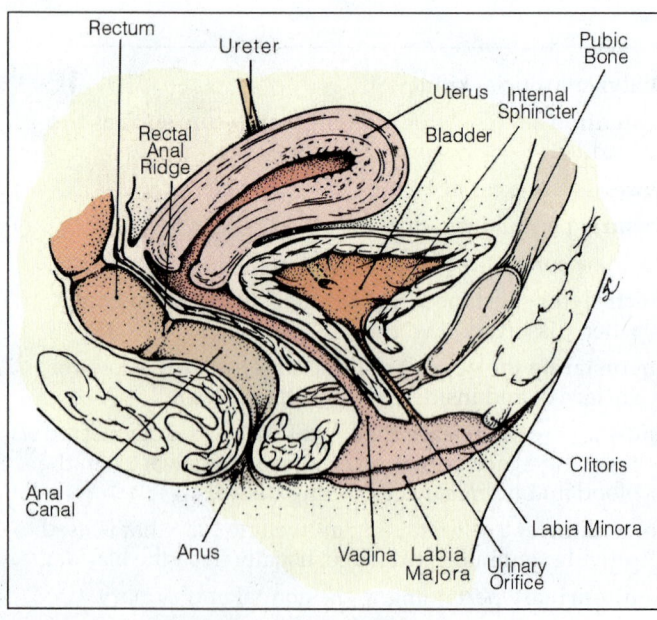

FIGURE 22-1 Female **genitourinary** system.

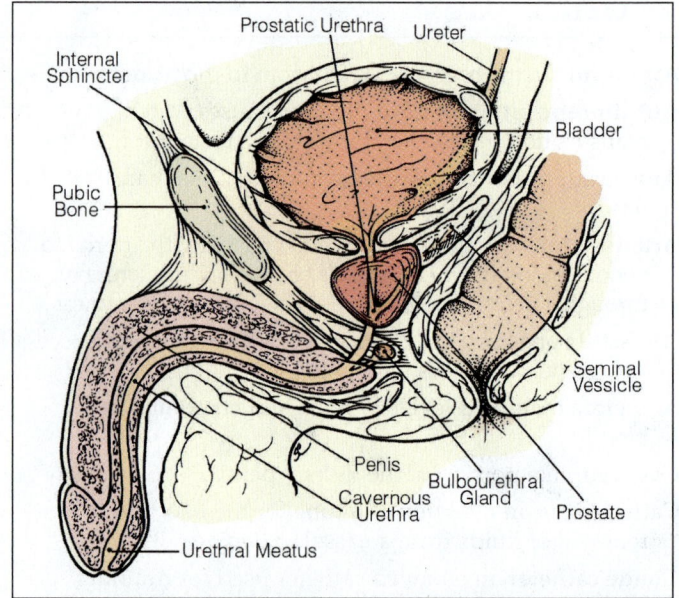

FIGURE 22-2 Male genitourinary system.

Urine Production

Nephrons, the functional units of the kidneys, produce urine. Each nephron consists of a **renal** corpuscle (Bowman's capsule) and a renal tubule, which is surrounded by a capillary bed. Each kidney has approximately a million nephrons.

Urine formed in the renal tubules enters collecting ducts, which empty urine into the kidney **calyx**. As urine collects in the renal pelvis, it flows to the bladder. If movement of urine from the pelvis is interrupted, infection, hydronephrosis, or formation of calculi may occur.

Blood is circulated to kidneys by way of the renal artery. This artery branches into arterioles, which supply a capillary tuft (glomerulus) filter. Under the influence of blood pressure, plasma is forced through the glomerulus and enters renal tubules. Filtered blood then passes from the glomerulus through an efferent arteriole and finally a capillary system that surrounds the renal tubules (**peri**tubular capillaries). Kidneys filter approximately 140 L of blood each day, but only 1,500 mL of urine is produced. As blood pressure falls, urine production decreases.

The plasma that is filtered into the renal tubule contains water, glucose, **electrolytes**, and nitrogenous wastes. This "filtrate" is then modified as it moves through the tubular system (Table 22-1 ■). Substances such as medications are secreted from the peritubular capillaries and into the filtrate for elimination. Most of the plasma fluid is reabsorbed into the bloodstream by way of peritubular capillaries, and excess fluid is removed along with acid waste products (urea, creatinine, hydrogen ion) in the form of urine. Through this process, kidneys maintain fluid and electrolyte and acid–base balance. In addition to urine production, kidneys play an important role in maintenance of blood pressure by secreting renin, activation of vitamin D to facilitate calcium absorption, and stimulation of red blood cell production by erythropoietin. It is easy to appreciate that loss of kidney function has a profound and widespread effect on homeostasis since it influences elimination of waste products, bone metabolism, blood pressure, tissue oxygenation (RBC production), acid–base balance, and fluid and electrolyte balance.

Micturition

Micturition (urination or voiding) is a voluntary response to pressure changes within the bladder. When urine begins to collect, the muscular walls of the bladder are relaxed, with little change in pressure. After about 300 mL of urine accumulates, pressure increases. This rising pressure stimulates receptors in the bladder wall, which send impulses to the spinal cord. After 400–500 mL of urine is collected, the bladder walls contract and the internal sphincter relaxes, causing a sense of needing to void. Under voluntary control, urine enters the urethra, the external sphincter relaxes, and voiding occurs.

Micturition can occur sooner if the tone of the bladder is increased because of such factors as emotional stress or infection. Micturition can be delayed by voluntary contraction of the external sphincter or pelvic floor muscles. Once the volume of urine reaches about 700 mL, however, most individuals lose their ability to delay micturition.

If an individual is unable to void, as much as 1,000 mL of urine can accumulate in the bladder. When a large volume of urine is retained, the bladder's lining and blood vessels can be damaged by the increased stretching and pressure. When this happens, an individual experiences pain, restlessness, chilling, flushing, headache, diaphoresis, and a rise in blood pressure.

Alterations in Urinary Elimination

Alterations in urinary elimination can result from changes in the intake and output of fluids, obstructions to the flow of urine, changes in the secretion of **antidiuretic** hormone (ADH), and changes in blood volume or blood pressure. See Table 22-2 ■ for normal results of a urine exam.

Alterations Related to Fluids

The average individual takes in approximately 2,600 mL of fluid each day: 1,200 mL from drinking, 1,100 mL from the water content of food, and 300 mL from metabolism.

Table 22-1 Tubular Alterations of Filtrate

Proximal tubule and descending limb	Obligatory water reabsorption, which accounts for about 80% of the absorption of water, occurs in the proximal tube and descending limb. Glucose, amino acids, vitamins, and sodium are actively reabsorbed. Chloride, sulfate, phosphate ions, and urea are passively reabsorbed. Bicarbonate is actively reabsorbed in relation to systemic pH. Water is reabsorbed with these substances, leaving the filtrate's osmotic pressure unchanged.
Loop of Henle	Sodium is actively transported from the filtrate in the ascending limb into the medullary interstitial fluid, thus raising its osmotic pressure. This rising pressure causes more water to be reabsorbed from the descending limb and the collecting duct and results in the concentration of the urine.
Distal tubule and collecting ducts	Facultative or optional reabsorption of water, which accounts for about 10–15% of the absorption of water, occurs in the distal tubule and collecting ducts. Sodium is actively reabsorbed in exchange for secreted potassium or hydrogen. As water continues to be reabsorbed, the filtrate becomes more concentrated and its volume is greatly reduced.

Table 22-2 Urine Exam: What to Check

Urine color: pale yellow to amber
Clarity and odor: clear with minimal odor
Urine pH: 4.5–8
Urine **specific gravity**: 1.005–1.020
Protein, glucose, and ketone bodies
Urine **sediment**: abnormal; red and white blood cells, casts, crystals, and bacteria

An increase or decrease in fluid intake results in a parallel increase or decrease in urine output.

Healthy individuals rarely experience decreases in urine output because they take in more fluids whenever they are thirsty. Individuals who are ill, however, may experience decreases in urine output because they are unable to respond to thirst, their intake is limited due to testing that requires NPO preparations, or their IV fluid intake is insufficient to balance fluid losses.

Fluid is lost from the body not only through urine, but also through respiration, perspiration, and feces. On a daily basis, most individuals lose approximately 2,400 mL of fluid: 1,500 mL through urine output, 200 mL through respiration, 600 mL through perspiration, and 100 mL through the elimination of feces. Individuals who are ill may also lose fluids through vomiting, bleeding, wound drainage, and suctioning or decompression of the GI tract.

Alterations Related to Obstructions

A decrease in the output of urine may also be caused by an obstruction (tumor, clot, tissue hypertrophy) to the flow of urine from the bladder. If the obstruction is great enough, the bladder does not empty completely. Instead, it retains fluid and, over time, becomes distended. Individuals who have urinary outlet obstructions experience the need to void more frequently. When they do void, however, they eliminate only very small amounts of urine.

Alterations Related to Aldosterone and Antidiuretic Hormone

Changes in the secretion of ADH and aldosterone also alter urine output since these hormones control the amount of water that is reabsorbed in the distal renal tubules and collecting ducts. Common factors that increase the secretion of ADH and aldosterone and reduce urine output include the physiologic stress response to accidental or surgical trauma, pain, hemorrhage, decreased cardiac output, anesthesia, and drugs, such as morphine and barbiturates. Factors that reduce the secretion of ADH and thus increase urine output include alcohol, caffeine, cold, disease states, and medications such as diuretics.

Alterations Related to Changes in Blood Volume

Because the production of urine is influenced by the volume of blood perfused to the kidneys, decreases in perfusion lead to reduction in the output of urine. Hemorrhage, **dehydration**, and **shock** reduce the flow of blood to the kidneys and cause decreased glomerular filtrate. If the volume of filtrate is reduced substantially, **oliguria**, or even **anuria** and accumulation of nitrogenous wastes (**azotemia**), may occur.

Other factors that may increase or decrease urine production include pathophysiologic states of the kidneys or other body systems, drugs, treatment modalities, diet, and metabolic rate.

Alterations in Disease States

Urinary outlet diversion is required when the bladder is obstructed or has been removed due to disease or trauma. Diversion can be created anywhere along the urinary pathway and is named for the structure involved in the diversion (Box 22-1 ■; Table 22-3 ■). The most common **urinary diversion** is the ileal conduit, named because it uses the ileum of the bowel to form the conduit. A segment of the ileum close to the ileocecal valve is resected with its mesentery intact to create the conduit. The proximal end of this segment is closed and the distal segment is brought out through the lower quadrant of the abdominal wall to form the **stoma**. The ureters are anastomosed to the ileal segment at the proximal end or side of the conduit. This type of diversion is an incontinent urinary diversion. Clients with incontinent diversions must wear a pouch for urine collection.

Ileal reservoirs are continent diversions that do not require the use of a collection device. The ileal reservoir is created with valves that allow it to function as a "bladder," which is regularly emptied by client self-catheterization through the abdominal stoma.

The "neo bladder" is created by connecting the ureters to a segment of ileum that is connected to the urethra. The client has no stoma; therefore, no collection device is required. The "bladder" is emptied by timed voiding or urethral self-catheterization.

Box 22-1 **NEW TRENDS: ROBOTIC SURGERY**

With the advent of robotic surgeries, many of the urinary diversion procedures are now being done robotically. Clients may now have options in certain situations to have robotic-assisted radical cystectomy procedures instead of the open, radical cystectomy previously done when clients who had bladder cancer needed surgery to remove their bladder and create an ileal conduit.

Table 22-3 Types of Urinary Diversion

Type of Diversion	Nursing Considerations
I. Ileal or Colonic Conduit • Urostomy is constructed from portion of bowel—ileum is resected and an internal conduit formed and attached to abdominal wall. • Ureters are connected to internal conduit. • An external pouch collects urine.	• Provide care of urinary pouch. • Monitor peristomal skin for breakdown. • Monitor stoma.
II. Continent Urostomy **A. (Kock's Reservoir)** • Reservoir is constructed from ileum and ascending colon. Two nipple valves are created by pulling ileum back onto itself. • Ureters are implanted near internal nipple valve (valve prevents reflux). • Outlet valve is attached to abdominal wall and stoma. • Reservoir is catheterized to drain urine.	• Instruct in clean intermittent self-catheterization every 2–4 hr.
B. Indiana Pouch • Internal pouch is created from the ascending colon and terminal ileum. • Pouch is larger than Kock's reservoir. • Reservoir is catheterized to drain urine.	• Instruct in clean intermittent self-catheterization every 2–4 hr. • Monitor for electrolyte imbalance; reservoir may absorb urea and electrolytes.
III. Neo Bladder • Created from cecum or ileum with ureters attached. • Has no stoma. • Requires no external appliance. • Urine exits via urethra. • Preserves normal body image.	• Client may eliminate with timed voiding. • Client may require self-urethral catheterization.

Alterations Related to Chronic Renal Failure

A number of disease states and socioeconomic factors place clients at risk for chronic renal failure. Nephron loss is irreversible as it progresses through five stages of deterioration marked by a declining glomerular filtration rate, glomerular leakage of protein into urine, and the retention of nitrogenous wastes in the blood (rise in the serum creatinine).

The presence of micro **albuminuria** (Stage 1) is the initial indicator to manage risk factors (e.g., diabetes and blood pressure control). With stage progression, proteinuria worsens and the glomerular filtration rate is reduced from a normal 120 to below 15 mL/min (Stage 4). Unfortunately, the chronic decline in renal function is often asymptomatic until the client has reached this fourth stage when the kidneys are unable to maintain their homeostatic role and are unable to excrete wastes or excess water. It is at this stage that the client is usually referred to a nephrologist to prepare for lifelong renal replacement therapy (**hemodialysis**, peritoneal dialysis, or transplantation).

In the final, fifth stage, the client has become uremic, having lost 90% of nephrons. The retention of nitrogenous wastes and loss of renal homeostatic processes alters all body system functions and is responsible for a constellation of signs and symptoms. **End-stage renal disease** (ESRD) is a term used for clients treated with dialysis or transplantation (renal replacement therapy), but does not actually define a stage of severity of renal disease.

Nursing Interventions

The primary purpose for performing nursing interventions associated with urinary elimination is to maintain the integrity of the urinary system, which eliminates excess fluid and wastes and thereby promotes homeostasis.

Aseptic technique is essential whenever performing procedures that could introduce bacteria into the urinary tract. Handwashing, using sterile gloves, and maintaining a closed urinary collection system decrease the incidence of ascending bladder contamination and subsequent **urinary tract infection (UTI)** (Box 22-2 ■). Maintaining aseptic technique throughout dialysis procedures is necessary to prevent infection in grafts, fistulae, and catheters.

Indwelling Catheters

Millions of Americans have bladder dysfunction every year. Twenty-five percent of these individuals are older adults in acute care hospitals; 7% of clients are in long-term care facilities. Due to the dysfunction, they require urinary drainage systems to drain and collect urine. The median time of urinary drainage system usage in home care is 3 to 4 years.

Indwelling catheters are invasive devices with significant complications. Infection and **encrustation** are common. Long-term use of catheters provides access for bacteria from a contaminated environment. As a result, catheter-associated urinary tract infections (CAUTIs) occur.

Adaptations for Home Care

Home care clients who require assistance with emptying their bladders are usually placed on intermittent clean **catheterization** protocols rather than having an indwelling catheter. This procedure assists in preventing penoscrotal abscess formation, overwhelming infection, and altered body image. Fluid intake needs to be monitored and restricted to 1,500 mL/day to avoid bladder **distention**. If spontaneous voiding returns, frequency of catheterizations can be extended to every 12 hr and discontinued when the residual urine is consistently less than 100 mL in 24 hr.

When an indwelling catheter is used, it is important to be aware that it may lead to UTI. The nurse must teach the client and family to observe for signs and symptoms of UTIs and **sepsis**. They should note odor, color, and consistency of the urine; burning pain; and flank pain. Catheter changes are the responsibility of the nurse and are usually performed once a month. Encouraging fluids becomes a major role assumed by family members and monitored by the nurse. Urinary antiseptics are adjunctive measures when catheterizations are required.

Home care dialysis is common in many areas of the country. The principles and procedures are similar to those in a hospital or free-standing dialysis unit. The major change is the advent of portable dialysis methods such as continuous ambulatory peritoneal dialysis (CAPD) and continuous cycling peritoneal dialysis (CCPD). These procedures allow individuals to participate in a normal lifestyle. However, use of these methods requires monitoring by the nurse and specific teaching of the essential components to prevent complications and promote health. Peritoneal dialysis (PD) reflects more normal kidney function than hemodialysis. Fluid and electrolytes are removed gradually and, therefore, clients have fewer complications with blood pressure alterations and disequilibrium syndrome. There are fewer dietary and fluid restrictions, allowing clients to lead a more normal life. PD provides the client with a more flexible schedule, allowing him or her to work, travel, and participate in activities. One major restriction, besides ensuring the ordered number of exchanges each day, is the monthly appointment at the dialysis center for lab work and consultation with the healthcare provider or nurse.

The catheter is placed in a dependent position in the peritoneal cavity to minimize the chance of catheter obstruction or erosion into other abdominal organs. The other end of the catheter is placed outside of the abdomen to decrease the likelihood of infections. There are several devices that are placed around the catheter that prevent fluid leak from the peritoneal cavity. These devices impede the migration of bacteria.

CAPD does not require a machine and can be done almost anywhere that is clean and well lit. The client performs four to five exchanges daily that take approximately 30–45 min each. Each exchange allows a prescribed amount of a dextrose solution, termed *dialysate*, 1,500–2,000 mL for adults, to flow into the abdomen. The dialysate remains in the abdomen, called *dwell time*, for approximately 4 hr, and then it is drained out of the abdomen for about 10 min. The last exchange of the day is before bedtime. The dialysate remains in the abdomen overnight.

CCPD requires a portable machine that connects to the catheter and automatically fills and drains the dialysate from the abdomen at night while the client sleeps. This procedure usually takes 10–12 hr every night.

Cultural Awareness

- African Americans have a more rapid decline in glomerular filtration rate than do Caucasians.
- Hypertensive African Americans have decreased renal excretion of sodium, making sodium restriction an important factor in treatment.
- Hypertension, diabetes, and ESRD are three to four times more common in African Americans and American Indians than in Caucasians.

Nursing Diagnoses

The following nursing diagnoses may be appropriate to use on client care plans when the components are related to promoting urine elimination.

NURSING DIAGNOSIS	RELATED TO . . .
Disturbed Body Image	Alteration in body appearance, urinary diversion stoma, use of appliance, catheter presence, fear of rejection, psychosocial factors
Ineffective Coping	Poor adjustment to illness or treatment, chronic disease state
	Inadequate knowledge base, denial of health status, cultural or spiritual beliefs
Deficient Fluid Volume	Increased urine output, decreased fluid intake
Excess Fluid Volume	Decreased urine output, renal system dysfunction, decreased cardiac output
Infection, Risk for	Vascular access site, altered immunity, urine retention, presence of catheter, malnutrition
Noncompliance	Inadequate knowledge base, inability to manage equipment for **irrigation**, denial of health status, cultural or spiritual beliefs
Impaired Urinary Elimination	Inability to retain urine related to stress, surgery, anatomic or functional problems, infection, motor or sensory impairment
Stress Urinary Incontinence	Inability to retain urine related to stress, surgery, anatomic or functional problems, infection, motor or sensory impairment
Urinary Retention	Inability to void, bladder distention or atony, surgical repair

Source: Herdman, T. H. & Kamitsuru, S. (Eds.) *Nursing Diagnoses – Definitions and Classification 2015-2017.* Copyright © 2014, 1994–2014 by NANDA International. Used by arrangement with John Wiley & Sons Limited. Companion website: www.wiley.com/go/nursingdiagnoses. In order to make safe and effective judgments using NANDA-I nursing diagnosis it is essential that nurses refer to the definitions and defining characteristics of the diagnoses listed in this work.

Nursing Process Data

ASSESSMENT Database

- Assess whether strict measurement of intake and output (I&O) is ordered.
- Assess client's ability to assist in keeping intake and output record.
- Assess all potential sources of intake (e.g., IVs, oral fluids, tube feeding) and output (e.g., urine, emesis, diarrhea, drainage from tubes).
- Observe color, clarity, and odor of urine.
- Assess for signs of dehydration or fluid excess.
- Evaluate weight changes (most accurate assessment of fluid balance).

PLANNING Objectives

- To accurately measure all sources of fluid intake
- To accurately measure all sources of fluid output
- To identify alterations in fluid balance
- To record data on appropriate records

IMPLEMENTATION Procedures

DOCUMENTATION AND EVALUATION

Expected Outcomes

- All sources of fluid intake and output are recorded.
- Client's intake and output balance.

Unexpected Outcomes/Alternative Actions

Pearson Nursing Student Resources

Find additional review materials at
nursing.pearsonhighered.com.
Prepare for success with NCLEX®-style practice questions and Skill Checklists.

Skill 22.1.1 | Measuring Intake and Output

Equipment

I&O electronic health record (EHR)

Client's own graduated container

Bedpan, urinal, or underseat basin for toilet ("hat")

Hourly inline urine measurement device for client requiring frequent monitoring

Clean gloves

Preparation

1. Perform hand hygiene.
2. Identify client using two client identifiers. Provide privacy.
3. Explain purpose of keeping I&O record to client.
4. Instruct client to keep record of all fluids taken orally. Keep an I&O record at the bedside for the client to document intake.
5. Instruct client to void into bedpan, urinal, or underseat basin for toilet.
6. Instruct client not to place toilet tissue in bedpan or defecate in bedpan.

Procedure

Fluid Intake

1. Measure all fluid intake (including oral, IV, fluid medications, and tube feedings) according to hospital values (e.g., cup = 150 mL, glass = 240 mL).
2. Record time and amount of fluids in the appropriate space on bedside form or in the EHR. ❶
3. Check bedside I&O record for approximate amounts of fluid containers.
4. Total 8-hr fluid intake on bedside I&O record.
5. Complete 24-hr intake record by adding together all three 8-hr totals.

Fluid Output

1. Don clean gloves to measure output from all sources.
2. Empty urinal, bedpan, or drainage bag into client's graduated container. ❷ ► *Rationale:* Measurement is only approximate from drainage bag or "hat." (Include other sources of output such as drainage, diarrheal stools, draining wounds, or emesis on output record.)

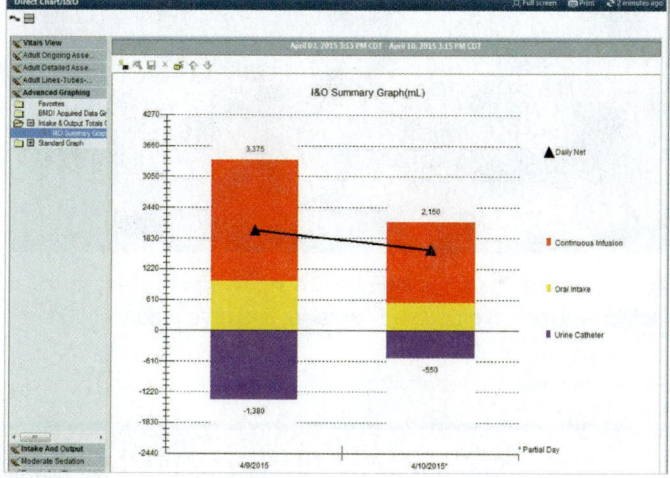

❶ Bedside intake and output EHR.

Source: From Cerner Electronic Health Record. © Cerner Corporation. Pearson has restricted permission to reproduce and distribute this copyrighted work. Further reproduction or distribution is strictly prohibited without written consent of Cerner Corporation.

3. To drain urine collection bag:
   a. Use client's individual (labeled) graduated receptacle.
   b. Slide port opener clockwise to allow urine to drain.
   c. Turn port opener counterclockwise to close.

(continued)

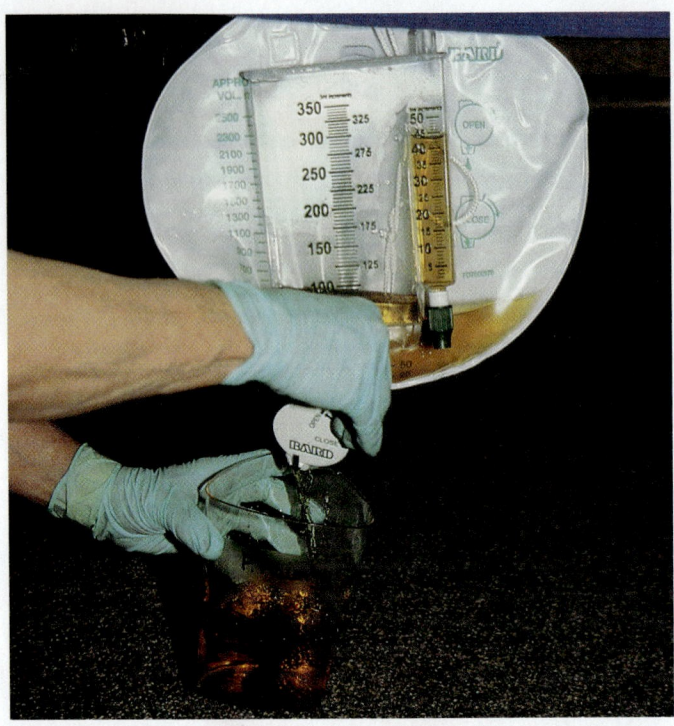

❷ Empty urinal, bedpan, or Foley drainage bag into client's individual (labeled) graduated container and note amount of urine.

If using drainage tube with plastic clips:

a. Raise drainage tube to drain urine into collection bag.

b. Hold bag over receptacle; squeeze plastic pieces together gently. The clips will come out off edge of holder.

c. Slide tube out of holder and point into receptacle.

d. Open metal clamp by pushing down on bottom metal pieces and wait until all urine has drained from bag.

e. Close clamp by pressing metal pieces together. Listen for click sound. ➤ *Rationale:* Click means clamp is now closed.

f. Clip drainage tube back into holder.

4. Remove gloves and perform hand hygiene.

5. Record time and amount of output on bedside I&O record.

6. Complete 24-hr output record by adding together all intermediate output totals during that 24-hr period, and place total on graphic sheet.

7. Notify healthcare provider of any significant imbalance; more intensive monitoring may be indicated.

Unit 22.1 Documentation and Evaluation

DOCUMENTATION for Intake and Output

- Time and amount of all oral fluid intake
- 8-hr total of all IV and enteral fluids
- 24-hr total of all fluid intake
- Time and amount of all urinary output
- Time and amount of all drainage (e.g., nasogastric or NG)
- 8-hr total of all fluid output
- 24-hr total of all fluid output

EVALUATION/Critical Thinking

Expected Outcomes

- All sources of fluid intake and output are recorded.
- Client's intake and output balance.

Unexpected Outcomes

- Client voids in toilet.

Alternative Actions

- Document "voided in toilet" on I&O record.
- Review instructions for accurate I&O monitoring with client.
- Post sign above toilet: "All urine must be measured and recorded."
- Place urine collection container or "hat" receptacle in toilet.

• Family members obtain fluids for client without notifying staff.	• Post sign indicating need to record all fluid intake. • Remind family of importance of I&O monitoring; provide cups with measured increments and paper for them to record fluids given (unless fluids are restricted).
• Fluid intake and output do not balance (intake greater than output).	• Initiate daily weight measurement (weigh before breakfast, after voiding, same scale, same clothing). • Compare losses or gains with client's daily weight measurement. • Fluid intake and output generally are relatively equal (assuming numbers are accurate). Output should be about 500 mL less per 24 hr due to insensible fluid loss. • Determine whether treatment goal is to rehydrate or diurese the client. • Use graduated container to accurately measure output in "hat." • Search for sources of unmeasured output (fever, wound drainage, diarrhea).
• Fluid output is greater than intake.	• Analyze whether treatment goal (rehydration, **diuresis**) has been achieved. • Reposition client cautiously, monitoring for possible orthostatic hypotension. • Identify when "dry weight" has been achieved (intake balances output after therapy received). • Search for sources of unrecorded intake (family offerings, flush solutions, ice chips, full-liquid foods).

Nursing Process Data

ASSESSMENT Database

- Assess that client is able to empty bladder completely and spontaneously.
- Assess the genital area for signs of irritation and **edema** during the use of condom catheter for urine collection.
- Assess activity level of client to determine when a leg bag or a continuous drainage system is necessary.

PLANNING Objectives

- To provide a means for managing incontinence
- To provide a means of collecting urine in a system that allows client ambulation
- To prevent skin breakdown due to incontinence of urine
- To prevent UTIs in clients who are at risk and require a method of urine collection

IMPLEMENTATION Procedures

DOCUMENTATION AND EVALUATION

Expected Outcomes

- Client remains dry with condom catheter for urine collection.
- Skin irritation does not occur with condom catheter use.

Unexpected Outcomes/Alternative Actions

Pearson Nursing Student Resources

Find additional review materials at
nursing.pearsonhighered.com.
Prepare for success with NCLEX®-style practice
questions and Skill Checklists.

Skill 22.2.1 | Applying a Condom Catheter for Urine Collection

Equipment
Soap, water, towel, washcloth
Commercial condom catheter; select appropriate size
Leg bag or bedside drainage system
Skin barrier prep
Clean gloves
Drape
Scissors

Preparation
1. Check healthcare provider's orders and client care plan.
2. Gather equipment.
3. Identify client using two client identifiers and explain procedure.
4. Perform hand hygiene and provide privacy.
5. Raise bed and lower side rail on working side of bed. Place client in flat supine position.
6. Don clean gloves.
7. Drape for privacy.
8. Wash genital area with soap and water, and dry area thoroughly. (If client is uncircumcised, gently attempt to retract foreskin, cleanse shaft beneath it, then replace foreskin to normal position.)
9. Clip hair from base of penis if necessary. ➤ *Rationale:* This is to avoid catching it in adhesive strip.

Procedure
1. When commercial condom catheter is used, apply protective coating to skin on penile shaft and allow to dry completely (60 sec).
2. If adhesive strip is required, peel off paper from one side of the adhesive strip according to product instructions. Spirally wrap the adhesive strip around the penile shaft starting behind the glans, then peel outer paper from adhesive strip.
3. Take the condom catheter and place the prerolled sheath so that funnel is against the glans, but *not* rubbing it.
4. Unroll the condom up the penis until it is completely over the adhesive strip. ❶

❶ After unrolling condom onto penis, apply pressure to ensure smooth fit.

5. Gently squeeze condom against strip to seal it after sheath is completely rolled over the penis. Do not wrinkle as wrinkles cause urine to leak through catheter.
6. Clip rolled portion of condom if necessary to prevent constriction at base of penis.
7. Connect condom to a drainage system. The drainage system can be a leg bag or a bedside drainage system depending on activity level and condition of client.
8. Cover the client. Lower bed, and raise side rail or assist client out of bed if he is to be ambulated.
9. Remove gloves and perform hand hygiene.
10. Assess penis 30 min after condom is applied to check for edema, discoloration, and urine flow. ➤ *Rationale:* This detects complication with application.

> **CLINICAL ALERT**
> Use of an external urine collection system is recommended for incontinent men without urine retention. These devices are comfortable, and there is less chance of a UTI than with indwelling catheters.

Skill 22.2.2 | Attaching Urine Collection Condom Catheter to Leg Bag

Equipment
Leg bag with Velcro straps (or stockinette to secure bag) ❶
Antimicrobial swabs
Clean gloves

Preparation
1. Obtain order for leg bag from healthcare provider.
2. Gather equipment.
3. Identify client using two client identifiers and explain procedure.
4. Provide privacy.
5. Raise bed, and lower side rail on working side of bed.
6. Perform hand hygiene and don clean gloves.

Procedure
1. Remove protective cap from connecting tube on top of leg bag.
2. Disconnect drainage tubing from indwelling or condom catheter.
3. Cap bedside drainage tubing end with protective cap from leg bag. ➤ *Rationale:* This maintains sterility of connecting parts.

(continued)

Skill 22.2.2 | Attaching Urine Collection Condom Catheter to Leg Bag *(continued)*

❶ Leg bag with Velcro straps to secure to leg.

4. Wipe leg bag and catheter connectors with swab, if not already sterile.
5. Connect tip of leg bag into catheter. ❷ ❸
6. Secure leg bag to thigh by placing Velcro strap through bag and around leg. Alternately, secure with stockinette.
7. When removing leg bag, disconnect catheter from leg bag and wipe each connection end with antimicrobial wipes.
8. Take leg bag cap off drainage tubing and replace it onto leg bag.
9. Connect catheter to bedside drainage tubing.
10. Lower bed and raise upper side rails.
11. Rinse leg bag in warm soap and water, and place in bathroom to dry.
12. Remove gloves and perform hand hygiene.

❷ Connect longer tube from leg bag to condom catheter.

❸ Maintain sterility when placing the tip of leg bag into condom catheter.

Unit 22.2 Documentation and Evaluation

DOCUMENTATION for External Urine Collection System

- Type and size of condom catheter applied
- Condition of genital area
- Protective coating (prep) applied to skin

- Type of drainage collection device attached
- Amount, color, and odor of urine obtained
- Client's tolerance of procedure and ability to perform self-care

EVALUATION/Critical Thinking

Expected Outcomes

- Client remains dry with condom catheter for urine collection.
- Skin irritation does not occur with condom catheter use.

Unexpected Outcomes

- Condom catheter leaks.

Alternative Actions

- Use smaller size condom to provide *wrinkle-free* fit.
- Replace adhesive strips for better condom adherence.
- Make sure penis is thoroughly dry before applying condom system.
- Ensure that drainage collection system is dependent of condom tubing to promote gravity flow.
- Consider using a retracted penis pouch.

- Penis becomes reddened with condom catheter use.

- Remove condom.
- Notify wound care specialist or healthcare provider for topical medication order.
- Apply adult brief and change frequently until problem resolves.
- Make sure penis is clean and dry and protective coating is applied before condom application.
- Clip rolled portion of condom to prevent constriction at base of penis.

Nursing Process Data

ASSESSMENT Database

- Assess the client's bladder for distention.
- Assess purpose of catheterization or urine output monitoring.
- Check healthcare provider's orders for method of catheterization to be done.
- Assess urinary meatus for exudate or inflammation.
- Assess character and amount of urine.
- Note client's I&O balance.

PLANNING Objectives

- To prevent or relieve discomfort due to bladder distention
- To promote urinary elimination
- To obtain a sterile urine specimen
- To provide continuous urinary bladder drainage
- To provide bladder irrigation
- To measure the amount of residual urine (postvoid)
- To monitor the output of a critically ill client

IMPLEMENTATION Procedures

DOCUMENTATION AND EVALUATION

Expected Outcomes

- Catheterization is avoided with use of bladder scanner.
- Sterile technique is maintained throughout catheterization procedure.
- Catheter enters bladder as evidenced by urine outflow.
- Client remains free of urine leakage around retention catheter.
- UTI does not occur secondary to catheterization.

Unexpected Outcomes/Alternative Actions

Pearson Nursing Student Resources

Find additional review materials at
nursing.pearsonhighered.com.
Prepare for success with NCLEX®-style practice questions and Skill Checklists.

Skill 22.3.1 | Using a Bladder Scanner

Equipment
Ultrasound bladder scanning device
Ultrasound conducting gel
Tissues

Preparation
1. Check healthcare provider's order to evaluate client's bladder; gather equipment.
2. Identify client using two client identifiers and explain procedure and purpose (Box 22-3 ■).
3. If female, ask client if she has had a hysterectomy or is pregnant. If the client has had a hysterectomy use the appropriate setting or the results may be inaccurate. Follow manufacturer directions. ➤ *Rationale:* Scanner is not indicated for pregnant clients.
4. Provide privacy.
5. Determine time and amount of last void or assist client to empty bladder if residual volume is to be evaluated.
6. Determine that client does not have an indwelling catheter. ➤ *Rationale:* Scanner reflects off the catheter bulb, giving an echo reading.
7. Perform hand hygiene.
8. Place client flat and supine, and palpate client's bladder to locate appropriate site.

Procedure
Note: Refer to manufacturer's directions or agency policy for particular scanner in your facility.
1. Turn the device on and press "SCAN."
2. Apply conducting gel to scanner head.
3. Select MALE or FEMALE mode on scan unit. Select *MALE MODE* if female client has had a hysterectomy.
4. Fanfold linens to expose client's suprapubic area.
5. Place head of scanner 3 cm (1½ in.) above client's symphysis pubis, directed toward the bladder, and align the icon.
6. Press scan head button and hold scanner still until a beep is heard.
7. Scan until bladder image is lined up on cross-hairs.
8. Take several scans at different angles and press DONE when finished.

❶ Handheld portable ultrasound bladder scanner.

9. Press PRINT for a printout of client's bladder volume in milliliters.
10. Wipe gel from client's skin. Cover client.
11. Reposition client for comfort.
12. Wipe ultrasound probe with antiseptic solution.
13. Perform hand hygiene.

Box 22-3 ESTIMATING BLADDER FULLNESS
- The bladder is not normally palpable until it contains more than 150 mL of urine.
- Normally, suprapubic percussion produces a hollow sound. A dull or flat sound indicates bladder distention.
- A bulge may be noted in the suprapubic area when the bladder contains 500 mL.
- Pain is often felt after bladder capacity has been reached, commonly after 400–500 mL.
- Subjective symptoms are not reliable indicators of bladder fullness.

Skill 22.3.2 | Inserting a Straight Catheter (Female)

Equipment
Disposable catheterization tray with straight catheter (14 Fr) and specimen cup. Determine type of catheter to use. See Table 22-4 ■.
Biohazard specimen transport bag
Bath blanket or turn sheet

Additional light source, if needed
If necessary for cleansing, towel, washcloth, basin with warm water and soap
Clean gloves

Note: If bladder scanner is not available, this skill may be indicated after client voids to determine residual volume.

(continued)

Skill 22.3.2 | Inserting a Straight Catheter (Female) *(continued)*

Table 22-4 Types of Catheters*

Latex	Rubber, ideal for forming the core of an indwelling catheter, due to its flexibility. Comfortable for client. Can cause urethral trauma. Latex swells as it absorbs body fluids.
100% Silicone	Larger drainage lumen due to having a coating. Biocompatible with urethra mucosa and is resistant to encrustation. Major advantage is hypoallergenic. Less flexible than latex. Up to 50% water loss from balloon can occur due to gas diffusion. Can stay in place up to 12 weeks. Used for clients with latex hypersensitivity. Discomfort in removal can occur as a result of incomplete cuff deflation of the balloon.
Latex Catheter Coated With Hydrogel	Gel is a polymer that absorbs water and forms a smooth surface on catheter. It is resistant to encrustation and settlement of bacteria, which diminishes risk of infection. Can stay in place up to 12 weeks. Used for clients with latex hypersensitivity.
Silicone–Elastomer	Coated latex catheter that is biocompatible and reduces urethra mucosal irritation. Flexibility provides comfort and can remain in place up to 12 weeks. Useful for clients with latex hypersensitivity.
PTFE-Coated Catheter	Teflon is fixed onto a latex core to form a catheter; used short term. Client is more comfortable, and there is decreased incidence of urethritis and encrustation that with latex catheters. Can stay in place for 28 days. Loss of balloon water occurs. Clients with latex hypersensitivity can use this catheter.
Silver Alloy	Lower incidence of bacteriuria than with silver oxide catheter. Clinically effective in reducing CAUTI if used short term (14 days). Silver is an antiseptic and inhibits growth of gram-positive and gram-negative bacteria. Silver-coated catheters may reduce catheter-related infections and have a low risk for generating antibiotic resistance.
Antiseptic-Impregnated or Antimicrobial-Coated	Significantly prevents or delays onset of CAUTI. Both the outer wall and inner drainage lumen are impregnated with an antibacterial agent that exudes from the catheter over time.

*Catheter tip shapes are either Coudé or Tiemann, and size of lumen is based on French scale (each unit equals 0.33 mm of internal lumen).

CLINICAL ALERT

A silicone-coated **Foley catheter** is not preinflated for testing before insertion because a ridge is present in the balloon when it is deflated, and ridges can lead to irritation of the urethra. Silicone catheters are used for clients with latex allergies. They are also used if a urethral stricture is present, and during radical prostatectomy surgery, as there is less meatus.

Preparation

1. Bring equipment to client's room. **❶**
2. Check lighting source.
3. Identify client, and explain procedure and need for client to keep knees positioned during procedure.
4. Provide privacy (close curtains or door; be sensitive to modesty concerns).
5. Perform hand hygiene.

❶ Disposable kit includes equipment necessary for performing a catheterization. (Retention catheter/Foley is shown here)

6. Place bed in comfortable working position, and lower side rail on working side.
7. Fold linens to foot of bed and cover client's lower body.
8. Provide perineal care, if necessary, with soap and water using clean gloves. Dry perineum thoroughly.
9. Discard towels and water and replace basin.
10. Dispose of gloves and perform hand hygiene.
11. Drape bath blankets around the client's legs if client modesty is a concern.
12. Have client bring knees up and out. May need assistance to keep knees in this position. ➤ *Rationale:* This position provides for good visualization of the urinary meatus.
13. Adjust light source to ensure that meatus is adequately visualized.

EVIDENCE-BASED PRACTICE

Best Practice for Preventing Catheter-Associated Urinary Tract Infections—Follow Your ABCDEs

A simple rubric for avoiding CAUTIs can be used and is based on some solid evidence.

Adherence: Be sure to follow good infection control practices and use hand hygiene and aseptic technique when inserting catheters.

Bladder: Use a bladder scanner to avoid placing indwelling catheters.

Condom catheters or other alternatives such as intermittent catheters should be used when appropriate.

Do not use an indwelling catheter unless it is the only option.

Early removal of the catheter is critical—Use reminder systems or nurse-driven protocols to facilitate this.

Source: Saint et al. (2009)

Procedure

1. Open sterile catheter set package by tearing the package on the lined edge of plastic wrap. Place plastic wrap at foot of bed for waste disposal.
2. Place catheter set on bed between client's legs or on a bedside table near the client.
3. Fold back drape to expose perineum.
4. Open white outer wrap away from sterile package with last turn toward client.
5. Remove sterile absorbent pad, and position plastic side down under client's buttocks. Have client lift buttocks if able. Position pad by holding corners of pad only. ➤ *Rationale:* Pad creates a sterile field.
6. Put on sterile gloves.
7. Place fenestrated drape over client's perineum, exposing meatus.
8. Place tray on sterile field, which may be enlarged by utilizing sterile wrapping, with care not to contaminate sterile field.
9. Open package, and pour antiseptic solution over cotton balls or open package of antiseptic-soaked swabs with stick ends up, according to facility policy.
10. Uncap syringe filled with lubricant, or tear open lubricant package, pick up catheter tip, and lubricate the tip of the catheter generously. ➤ *Rationale:* Removing catheter from sterile container (tray) increases risk of contamination.
11. If specimen is required, uncap sterile specimen container.
12. Move catheter tray close to client on sterile field.
13. Prep client's meatus according to hospital policy.

    a. Separate the client's labia minora with your nondominant hand (maintain separation throughout prep). **2**
    b. With your dominant hand, *use forceps* to pick up an absorbent ball that has been saturated with antiseptic solution. (If Betadine swabs are used, pick up one swab.)
    c. Cleanse client's meatus using the procedure in the above note, or with one downward stroke of forceps or swab.

➤ *Rationale:* Using a downward stroke cleans from least contaminated to most contaminated area.

    d. Discard absorbent ball or swab in the plastic cover at foot of bed. ➤ *Rationale:* Using a new cotton ball or swab with each downward stroke prevents transfer of microorganisms.
    e. Repeat Step c at least three to four times.
    f. Continue to hold client's labia apart until you insert catheter. ➤ *Rationale:* This prevents contamination of the urinary meatus.

14. Using sterile gloved hand, pick up lubricated catheter, keeping drainage end in collection container, and insert 5 cm (2 in.) or until urine begins to flow.
15. Move nondominant hand from holding labia open to hold catheter in place.
16. Instruct client to take a deep breath. While client is exhaling, insert catheter. ➤ *Rationale:* Sphincter will relax, decreasing discomfort and resistance to insertion of catheter.
17. Place sterile specimen container under drainage end of catheter if specimen is needed, and fill container with approximately 30 mL of urine. **3**
18. Replace catheter drainage end into collection container, and allow urine to flow until it ceases.
19. Pinch catheter closed when urine ceases to flow, and remove gently and slowly.
20. Remove drapes and dry the perineum.
21. Cover the client. Position client for comfort; put the bed in LOW position with the upper side rails raised.
22. Measure and record urine output on I&O bedside record.
23. Discard gloves and equipment appropriately.
24. Perform hand hygiene.
25. Label specimen, place in transport bag, and send to lab.
26. Document procedure.

Clitoris
Labia Majora — Urethral Orifice
Labia Minora — Vagina
Anus

2 Anatomic view of female perineal area showing urethral orifice.

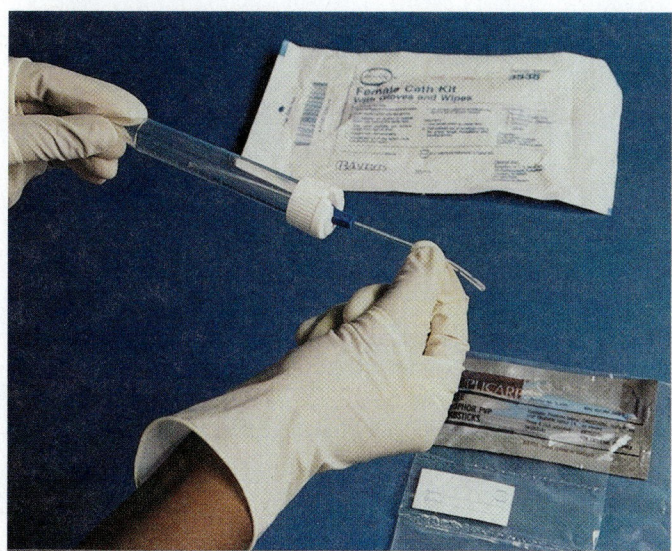

3 Female mini-catheter used to obtain sterile urine specimen.

Skill 22.3.3 | Inserting a Straight Catheter (Male)

Equipment
Same as for Inserting a Straight Catheter (Female)
15–20 mL, 2% lidocaine gel for lubricant, if ordered

Preparation
1. Follow Preparation Steps 1–6 in Skill 22.3.2, Inserting a Straight Catheter (Female). Provide privacy.
2. Place client in a supine position with knees slightly apart. ➤ *Rationale:* This position relaxes abdominal and perineal muscles.
3. Drape client by placing a bath blanket or drawsheet over chest area and fanfold top linen down to cover lower extremities, exposing only genital area.
4. Don clean gloves, and wash genital area if necessary.
5. Remove gloves and perform hand hygiene.

Procedure
1. Open sterile package by tearing the package on the lined edge of plastic wrap. Place plastic wrap at foot of bed for waste disposal.
2. Place sterile kit at client's side near thigh.
3. Open outer wrap away from sterile package.
4. Remove absorbent drape from package and place between the legs under the genitalia.
5. Don sterile gloves.
6. Place fenestrated drape over penis.
7. Open antiseptic package and pour solution over cotton balls or open package of antiseptic-soaked swabs with stick ends up, according to hospital policy.
8. Open lubricant packet or syringe—eject onto prep tray. Lubricate tip of catheter.
9. If specimen is required, uncap the specimen container.
10. Hold penis upright with your nondominant hand.
11. With your dominant hand, use forceps to pick up cotton ball saturated with antiseptic solution or pick up Betadine swab.
12. Cleanse meatus with circular expanding stroke using cotton ball or swab. Discard cotton ball or swab into plastic bag at foot of bed.
13. Repeat circular cleansing motion prep around tip of penis. Cleanse three times using a new cotton ball or swab each time.
14. Continue to hold penis with your nondominant hand.
15. Discard forceps into plastic bag.
16. Lubricate catheter about 8–10 cm (3–4 in.) using generous amount of lubricant.
17. *Alternate Method:* Insert tip of lubricant syringe at urethral opening and instill lubricant (or 2% lidocaine gel if ordered) directly into urethra. (If catheter tray does not have syringe, place sterile syringe on tray before gloving.) ➤ *Rationale:* Lidocaine gel facilitates catheter placement by expanding, anesthetizing, and lubricating the urethra.
18. Pick up catheter with sterile gloved hand about 8–10 cm (3–4 in.) from tip of catheter.
19. Lift penis to a 90-degree angle (perpendicular to body) and exert slight traction by pulling upward. ➤ *Rationale:* This movement straightens the urethra for easier insertion of catheter.
20. Instruct client to take a deep breath and, while client is exhaling, insert catheter. ➤ *Rationale:* Sphincter will relax, decreasing discomfort and resistance to insertion of catheter.
21. Insert catheter about 25–30 cm (10–12 in.) or until urine is obtained.
22. If catheter meets resistance, decrease angle of penis to 45 degrees or less, and ask client to take a deep breath. ➤ *Rationale:* Taking a deep breath helps relax the external sphincter. If persistent resistance is felt and catheter cannot be inserted without difficulty, remove catheter and notify healthcare provider.

> **CLINICAL ALERT**
> A **Coudé catheter** or 12 Fr catheter may be easier to insert if the client has an obstruction.

23. Fill sterile specimen container from drainage end of catheter if specimen is needed.
24. Pinch tubing, and transfer end of catheter into collection container.
25. Allow urine to drain into collection container until flow stops.
26. Remove catheter, and place lid on specimen bottle.
27. Dry penis and remove drapes. Cover the client.
28. Make client comfortable. Place bed in LOW position with upper side rails raised.
29. Discard equipment in appropriate container.
30. Remove gloves and perform hand hygiene.
31. Label specimen, send specimen to lab, and document procedure.

EVIDENCE-BASED PRACTICE
Nurse-Directed Interventions to Reduce CAUTIs
An evidence-based intervention done at the University of Colorado Hospital found that a combination of nurse-driven interventions, product changes, and client/family involvement were key factors in reducing CAUTIs. Some of the key changes that improved client outcomes were:

- Emptying Foley bags when they are two-thirds full, every 8 hr, or before transfers, to avoid putting traction on the bladder that would increase the risk of infection
- Keeping the Foley below the level of the bladder to avoid urine flowing back into the bladder
- Using a device to secure the Foley to the client's leg to avoid catheter movement that can cause irritation and is a risk factor for infection

Source: Oman et al. (2012)

Skill 22.3.4 | Inserting an Indwelling Catheter (Female)

Equipment

Disposable indwelling catheter kit with appropriate size catheter (size 14–16 Fr for adult female, size 16–18 Fr for adult male with 10-mL balloons) and preconnected closed system

2,000-mL drainage bag with MONO-FLO antireflux device

Closed drainage set with or without urimeter or urometer, if indicated

Label for urine specimen if indicated

Biohazard bag for specimen if indicated

Additional lighting if needed

Bath blanket or turn sheet

Towels, washcloth

Clean gloves

Basin with warm water

Soap

Tape or commercial catheter securement (Bard Catheter leg strap, Dale Anchor Strap, StatLock Foley)

Preparation

Check healthcare provider's orders for indwelling catheter (Table 22-5 ■). Preparation is the same as for Skill 22.3.2, Inserting a Straight Catheter (Female).

> **CLINICAL ALERT**
> Chronic irritation and inflammation of bladder mucosa due to long-term (more than 8 months) presence of an indwelling catheter (urethral or suprapubic) is associated with an increased risk for bladder cancer.

Procedure

1. Open sterile package by tearing the package on the lined edge of plastic wrap. Place plastic wrap at foot of bed for waste disposal. Provide privacy. ❶
2. Place catheter kit on bed between client's legs or on a bedside table near the client.
3. Fold back corner of bath blanket or drape to expose perineum.
4. Open white outer wrap away from package with last turn toward client.

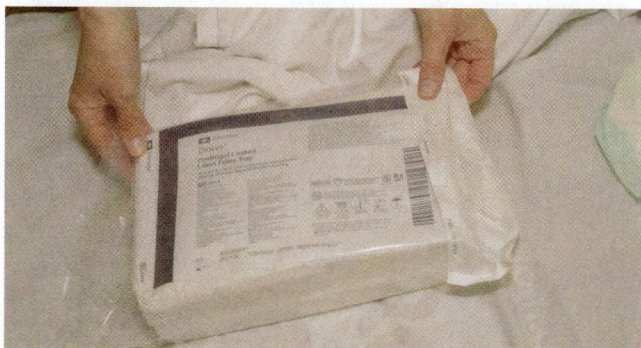

❶ Open the sterile package by tearing it along the lined edge of the plastic wrap.

5. Remove sterile absorbent pad, ❷ and position under client's buttocks plastic side down. Have client lift buttocks if able. Position pad by holding corners of pad only. ➤ *Rationale:* Holding onto the edges keeps the center sterile.
6. Don sterile gloves. ❸

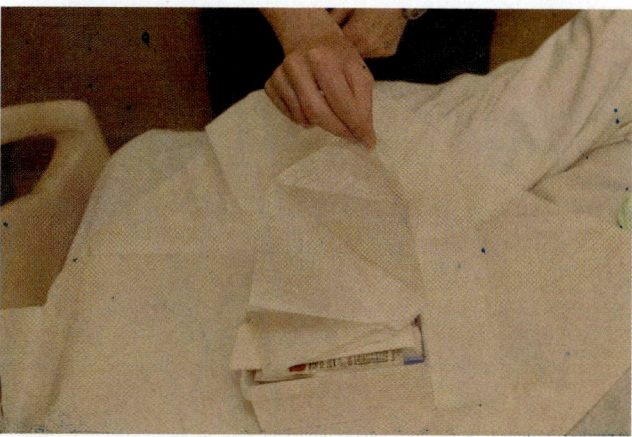

❷ Remove the sterile absorbent pad.

❸ Don sterile gloves, being careful not to contaminate the sterile field.

Table 22-5 Appropriate Indications for Indwelling Urethral Catheter Use to Prevent CAUTI

• Acute urinary retention or bladder outlet obstruction
• Need for accurate measurement of urinary output in clients who are critically ill
• Clients who have open sacral or perineal wounds and are incontinent to assist in healing
• Clients requiring prolonged immobilization
• To improve comfort for clients for end-of-life care (if needed)

Source: Gould (2009)

(continued)

Skill 22.3.4 | Inserting a Straight Catheter (Female) *(continued)*

7. Position fenestrated drape over the client to expose the genitalia. **4**

8. Separate prep tray from container, placing prep tray with cotton balls, antiseptic solution packet or according to hospital policy and lubricant onto sterile field toward client.

> **CLINICAL ALERT**
> It is no longer recommended that nurse preinflate to test the balloon before insertion. Many manufacturers are testing this during the manufacturing process, and there is some concern that it may contribute to CAUTIs.

9. Open package and pour antiseptic solution over cotton balls. **5**

10. Uncap syringe filled with lubricant and eject onto prep tray to lubricate catheter tip at time of catheter insertion, or open lubricant packet, remove catheter from protective sleeve and insert catheter tip into lubricant, keeping catheter in tray. **6 7 8**

11. Remove cap from specimen cup if indicated.

12. Remove rubber protector and insert tip of prefilled sterile water syringe into catheter side arm to inflate balloon after insertion. **9**

13. Prep client's meatus:

a. Separate client's labia minora with your nondominant hand.

b. With your dominant hand, *use forceps* to pick up an absorbent cotton ball that has been saturated with antiseptic solution, according to hospital policy. See Step 13c in Skill 22.3.2, Inserting a Straight Catheter (Female).

c. Cleanse client's meatus with one downward stroke. Discard absorbent cotton ball or swab in plastic bag at foot of bed. **10**

6 Squeeze lubricant onto the tray.

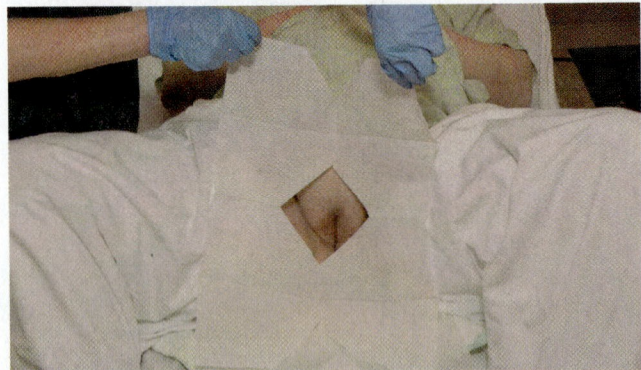

4 Position sterile fenestrated drape over client to expose genitalia.

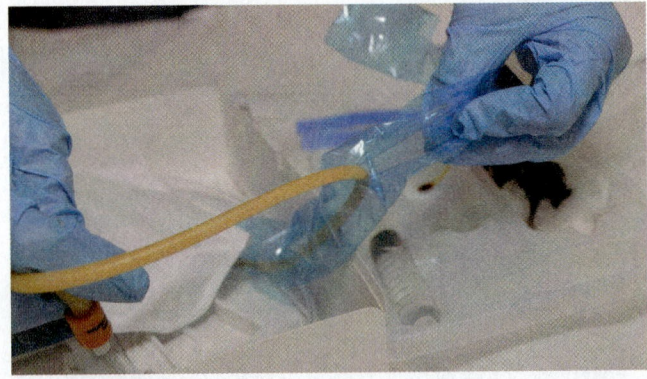

7 Remove Foley from protective sleeve.

5 Pour antiseptic solution completely over cotton balls.

8 Lubricate tip of catheter to facilitate insertion without trauma.

d. Repeat Step c at least three times.

e. Continue to hold the client's labia apart until you insert the catheter. ⑪

14. Discard forceps in plastic bag at foot of bed.

15. With uncontaminated hand, take catheter from container, lubricate tip, and insert gently into meatus 5 cm (2 in.) or until urine starts to flow. ⑫

16. Guide the catheter gently 2.5 to 3.5 cm (1–1.5 in.) just beyond the point at which urine begins to flow.
    ➤ *Rationale:* Inserting catheter further into bladder ensures it is beyond neck of the bladder.

17. Inject entire contents of prefilled (10–30 mL sterile water) syringe into the side arm of the catheter used for balloon inflation. ⑬ ➤ *Rationale:* Underinflation can cause balloon distortion and catheter tip deflection.

18. If client complains of pain on balloon inflation, immediately aspirate the sterile water. ➤ *Rationale:* The catheter may be in the urethra rather than the bladder.

19. Gently retract the catheter until you feel resistance.
    ➤ *Rationale:* This indicates the balloon is resting against the bladder neck and in the correct position.

20. Obtain urine specimen before attaching catheter to drainage tubing, if indicated.

⑨ Insert the tip of the prefilled sterile water syringe into the catheter side arm to inflate the balloon after the catheter is inserted.

⑩ Cleanse meatus by using downward strokes with cotton balls or use single-use lubricant or anesthetic gel.

CLINICAL ALERT

Immediate assessment and documentation of the amount of urine obtained after inserting the retention catheter is important. If the client has urinary retention, it may alter clinical decisions.

CLINICAL ALERT

Do not obtain a urine specimen from the catheter drainage bag. Pathogens in drainage bag do not necessarily represent those present in lower urinary tract.

⑪ With nondominant hand hold the labia open as you approach with the catheter being careful to keep the catheter sterile.

⑫ Insert catheter gently into meatus until urine begins to flow; then advance another 2.5–5 cm (1–2 in.).

⑬ Inject water from prefilled syringe into catheter balloon after inserting catheter.

(continued)

Skill 22.3.4 | Inserting an Indwelling Catheter (Female) *(continued)*

21. Remove protective cap from drainage tubing and attach securely to catheter, if indicated.
22. Apply catheter holder or tape catheter to client's upper thigh. Place one piece of tape on thigh. Take second piece of tape and encircle catheter, leaving two "tails" on tape. Secure "tails" from tape on catheter to tape on leg. ⑭ ⑮ ➤ *Rationale:* This stabilizes the catheter, minimizes urethral trauma, and avoids tension on the bladder neck. This helps prevent CAUTI.

⑭ Tape catheter to side of client's thigh using nonallergenic tape.

⑮ Securement device (StatLock Foley) stabilizes catheter to minimize urethral trauma.

23. Attach drainage bag to bed frame (not side rails); coil tubing to allow free gravity flow of urine. ⑯
24. Remove drapes. Cover the client.
25. Reposition client for comfort; put bed in LOW position with upper side rails up.
26. Remove equipment, including gloves, and discard disposable trash in appropriate container.
27. Perform hand hygiene.
28. Record urine output on I&O.
29. Label specimen and place cup in biohazard transport bag.
30. Send urine specimen to lab and document procedure.

Note: The optimal drainage system is a closed system with a one-way valve between the bag and tubing. ➤ *Rationale:* This system reduces UTIs for clients with a short-term indwelling urinary catheter.

⑯ Attach urine collection bag to nonmovable part of bed. Do not allow tubing to hang below collection bag.

Skill 22.3.5 | Inserting an Indwelling Catheter (Male)

Equipment
Same as for Skill 22.3.4, Inserting an Indwelling Catheter (Female)

Preparation
1. Follow Preparation Steps 1–6 in Skill 22.3.2, Inserting a Straight Catheter (Female).

2. Place client in a supine position with knees slightly apart. ➤ *Rationale:* This position relaxes abdominal and perineal muscles.
3. Drape client by placing a bath blanket or turn sheet over chest area and fanfold top linen down to cover lower extremities, exposing only perineal area.

4. Don clean gloves and wash client's perineal area if necessary.
5. Remove gloves, perform hand hygiene, and prepare for catheterization.

Procedure

1. Open sterile package by tearing package on lined edge of plastic wrap. Place plastic wrap at foot of bed for waste disposal. **1**
2. Place sterile kit on bed at client's side near thigh.
3. Open closed drainage set and place on bed near work area.
4. Open outer white wrap away from sterile package and remove drape. **2**
5. Place sterile drape over thighs and under penis.
6. Don sterile gloves; set fenestrated drape aside on sterile field. **3**
7. Separate prep tray from container, placing prep tray with cotton balls, antiseptic solution packet, and lubricant onto sterile field toward client.
8. Open package and pour antiseptic solution over cotton balls according to facility policy. **4**

9. Remove cap from specimen cup if indicated.
10. Uncap syringe filled with lubricant and eject onto rolling prep tray, or open lubricant package. **5**

3 Don gloves. Be careful not to contaminate the sterile field.

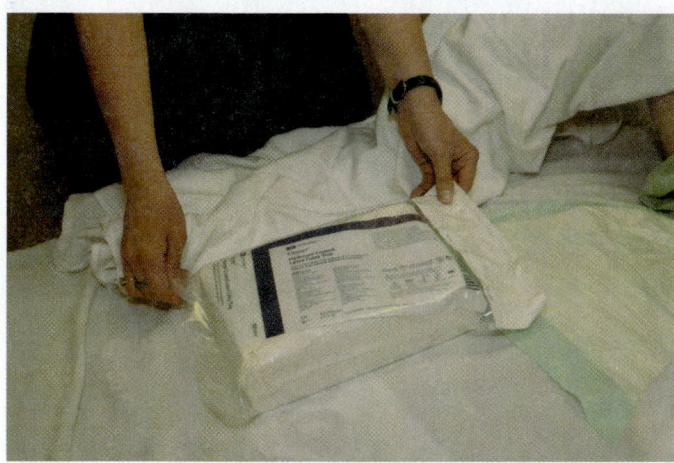

1 Open the sterile package.

4 Pour Betadine over the cotton.

2 Remove the drape.

5 Express lubricant onto the tray.

(continued)

Skill 22.3.5 | Inserting an Indwelling Catheter (Male) *(continued)*

11. Remove catheter from its protective sleeve and lubricate it generously about 8–10 cm (3–4 in.), keeping catheter in tray or, if using alternate method, insert lubricant directly into the urethra using a prefilled syringe. **6** **7**
12. Position fenestrated drape over the penis. **8**
13. Hold penis upright with your nondominant hand. Hold sides of penis to prevent closing of urethra.
14. With your dominant hand, use forceps to pick up cotton ball saturated with antiseptic solution or pick up swab.
15. Cleanse meatus first with expanding circular stroke using the cotton balls held by forceps or Betadine swab. Check facility policy for Betadine use. **9**
16. Discard swab into plastic wrap at foot of bed.
17. Repeat circular prep around head of penis. Cleanse three times using a new cotton ball or Betadine swab each time. ➤ *Rationale:* Using a circular motion around head of penis prevents bacteria from entering urinary meatus.
18. Continue to hold penis with your nondominant hand.

19. Discard forceps into plastic bag.
20. Pick up catheter with sterile hand about 8–10 cm (3–4 in.) from tip of catheter.
21. Lift penis to a 90-degree angle (perpendicular to body) and exert slight traction by pulling upward. ➤ *Rationale:* This movement straightens the urethra for easier insertion of catheter.
22. Insert catheter about 25–30 cm (10–12 in.). **10**
23. If resistance is met, lower angle of penis to 45 degrees and ask client to take a deep breath. ➤ *Rationale:* Taking a deep breath helps relax the external sphincter.
24. Guide catheter gently 2.5–5 cm (1–2 in.) beyond point at which urine begins to flow. ➤ *Rationale:* Inserting catheter further into bladder ensures it is beyond neck of bladder.
25. Inject entire contents of prefilled sterile water syringe into side arm of catheter for balloon inflation.
26. Gently retract catheter until you feel resistance of the balloon at neck of bladder.

6 Remove the Foley catheter from its protective sleeve.

8 Place the fenestrated drape over penis.

7 Lubricate the tip of the catheter to facilitate insertion without trauma.

9 Cleanse the meatus with circular expanding strokes.

27. Obtain urine specimen if indicated.
28. Remove protective cap from drainage tubing and attach securely to catheter if indicated.
29. Tape catheter to abdomen with 2.5-cm (1-in.) tape if client is not ambulatory, or use securement device (Box 22-4 ■) with Velcro strap. ⓫ ➤ *Rationale:* This prevents pressure on the penoscrotal angle and ventral urethral meatus. Tape catheter to upper thigh if client is ambulatory.

30. Attach drainage bag to bed frame (not side rails).
31. Cover the client. Reposition client for comfort; put bed in LOW position with upper side rails raised.
32. Remove all equipment, including gloves, and discard disposable trash in the appropriate container.
33. Measure and record urine output in I&O bedside record.
34. Perform hand hygiene.
35. Label specimen cup, place in biohazard transport bag, and send to lab.
36. Document procedure, including amount of urine obtained.

CLINICAL ALERT

Optimal management of an indwelling catheter includes securing catheter to thigh or abdomen to prevent catheter or balloons from exerting excessive force on bladder neck or urethra. Maintaining a sterile, continuously closed and sealed urinary drainage system is critical to prevent CAUTI.

⓾ Insert the catheter about 25–30 cm (10–12 in.).

⓫ Tape catheter to abdomen to prevent pressure in penoscrotal angle if client is on bed rest.

Box 22-4 TYPES OF SECUREMENT DEVICES

Categories of securement devices for short- and long-term indwelling catheters:

- Improvised devices using adhesive tape, safety pins, and sutures
- Manufactured devices with an adhesive backing and a mechanism for attaching catheter
- Nonadhesive devices that incorporate Velcro and straps to secure the catheter to the upper thigh

Note: Securement products developed specifically to hold indwelling catheters include the nonadhesive products that secure to the upper thigh or abdomen with a soft closure strap. These products are latex-free with hypoallergenic backing and use the Velcro locking system to hold the catheter securely in place. Reusable leg anchors are available from several companies.

EVIDENCE-BASED PRACTICE

Preventing CAUTIs by Providing Appropriate Catheter Care

Providing appropriate care for an indwelling catheter should be based on evidence. The following are guidelines to help prevent infections from occurring when caring for a client with an indwelling catheter:

- Always maintain a closed system when possible.
- Remember that bladder irrigations do not prevent CAUTIs.
- Use computerized reminders; these help staff with early catheter removal.
- Do not clean the urinary meatus with antiseptics for daily catheter care; use soap and water daily or twice a day.

Source: Dailly (2011)

Skill 22.3.6 | Providing Catheter Care

Equipment
Soap and water
Washcloth
Towel
Clean gloves
2.5-cm (1-in.) tape or commercial catheter holder

Preparation
1. Check client care plan.
2. Gather equipment.
3. Identify client using two client identifiers.
4. Provide privacy.
5. Perform hand hygiene.
6. Explain procedure to client.
7. Raise bed, and lower side rail on working side.

Procedure
1. Place client in supine position, and expose perineal area.
2. Remove catheter securing tape.
3. Don clean gloves.

Female
   a. Cleanse urinary meatus using circular motion moving outward with washcloth, soap, and water.
   b. Dry area with towel.
   c. Resecure retention catheter with tape or commercial holder.

Circumcised Male
   a. With mitten washcloth, soap, and water, cleanse around urinary meatus.

> **CLINICAL ALERT**
> Almost all clients will be bacteriuric after 1 month of catheterization. Indwelling urinary catheters promote UTIs by creating a portal of entry for microorganisms, and healthcare-associated UTIs increase mortality rate threefold (Box 22-5 ■). The client should be assisted to urinate by using noninvasive techniques before resorting to catheterization.

   b. Dry area with towel.
   c. Using separate washcloth, clean area between scrotum and rectal area, and then dry.
   d. Place soiled linen in hamper.

Uncircumcised Male
   a. Retract foreskin back away from catheter.
   b. With mitten washcloth, soap, and water, cleanse around urinary meatus.
   c. Dry penis with towel.
   d. After drying, pull foreskin back around the catheter.
   e. Place soiled linen in hamper.

4. Remove gloves and discard. Retape catheter.
5. Cover the client. Position client for comfort.
6. Lower bed and raise upper side rail.
7. Perform hand hygiene.

EVIDENCE-BASED PRACTICE
Cranberry for Urinary Tract Infection Prophylaxis
There is a growing accumulation of evidence-based information in support of use of cranberry in UTI prevention. Its beneficial effect is not by acidifying urine, but by inhibiting adherence of *E. coli* and other gram-negative uropathogens to urinary tract epithelial cells. A recent randomized controlled trial demonstrated that one tablet of concentrated cranberry extract (300–400 mg) twice daily or 8 oz of pure unsweetened cranberry juice three times daily is safe and effective for up to 12 months. Cranberry may increase urinary oxalate levels and so may increase risk of kidney stone formation in clients with a history of oxalate calculi.

Cranberry also seems to inhibit the aggregation of dental plaque bacteria.

Source: Callahan (2015)

Box 22-5 COMPLICATIONS ASSOCIATED WITH LONG-TERM INDWELLING CATHETER PLACEMENT
- UTIs
- Catheter leaks
- Bladder spasms
- Urethral erosion
- Urethritis
- Epididymitis
- Prostatitis
- Scrotal abscess
- Prostatic abscess
- Urinary stones
- Urethral sphincter damage
- Bladder cancer

Skill 22.3.7 | Removing an Indwelling Catheter

Equipment
10-mL syringe without needle
Paper towel

Clean gloves
Client's calibrated graduate

Preparation

1. Check healthcare provider's orders for removing catheter.
2. Perform hand hygiene.
3. Identify client using two client identifiers.
4. Gather equipment.
5. Explain procedure to client.
6. Provide privacy.
7. Don clean gloves.

Procedure

1. Remove tape attaching catheter to client.
2. Insert syringe into balloon port of catheter. Do not cut port with scissors. ➤ *Rationale:* Balloon may not totally deflate if inflation port is cut.
3. Withdraw fluid from balloon (usually 10 mL of water in balloon). ❶

> **CLINICAL ALERT**
> Do not aspirate balloon vigorously. Doing so may collapse inflation lumen and prevent balloon deflation.

4. Pull gently on catheter to ensure balloon is deflated before attempting to remove. ➤ *Rationale:* Damage to urethra can occur if balloon is not totally deflated. ❷
5. Hold paper towel under catheter with your nondominant hand.
6. If resistance is not met, slowly withdraw catheter, allowing it to fall into paper towel.
7. Disconnect urine drainage bag from bed frame.
8. Empty drainage bag into graduate and measure.
9. Record output on I&O bedside record.
10. Dispose of catheter in appropriate receptacle.
11. Cover the client. Position client for comfort.
12. Remove gloves and perform hand hygiene.
13. Instruct client to drink oral fluids as tolerated and observe for symptoms of UTI (burning, frequency, urgency).
14. Offer bedpan or urinal after removing catheter, until voiding occurs. Keep accurate I&O record of time and amount of postcatheterization voidings.
15. Report to healthcare provider if client has not urinated in 8 hr or is uncomfortable.

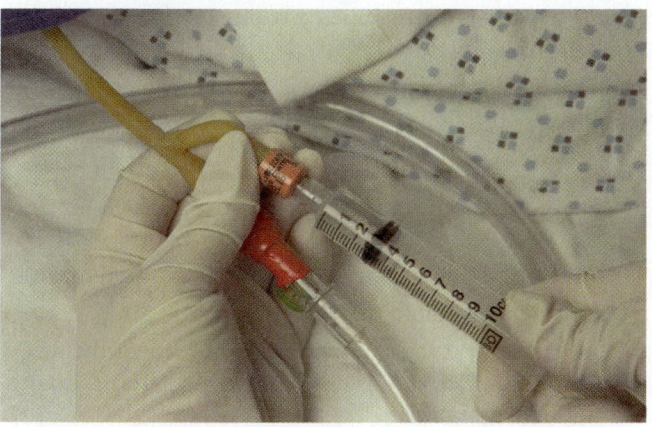

❶ Insert syringe hub into balloon port and withdraw fluid from retention catheter balloon.

❷ Balloon (shown here inflated) must be deflated before removing to prevent damage to urethra.

Unit 22.3 Documentation and Evaluation

DOCUMENTATION for Catheterization

- Time and purpose
- Type and size of catheter
- Amount, color, and odor of urine obtained
- Client's tolerance of procedure
- Specimen sent to lab (if ordered)

- Catheter care provided
- Catheter removed
- Voiding: time and amount after catheter removal
- Intake and output
- Residual volume amount and time since last void

EVALUATION/Critical Thinking

Expected Outcomes

- Catheterization is avoided with use of bladder scanner.
- Sterile technique is maintained throughout catheterization procedure.
- Catheter enters bladder as evidenced by urine outflow.
- Client remains free of urine leakage around retention catheter.
- UTI does not occur secondary to catheterization.

Unexpected Outcomes	Alternative Actions
• Bladder scan does not give reading.	• Make certain adequate conducting gel has been used. • Have obese client bend knees so that feet are flat on the bed. • Have thin client partially sit up to compress abdomen. • Apply more pressure with scan head, depressing 2.5–5 cm (1–2 in.) into client's abdomen.
• Catheter is contaminated during procedure.	• Obtain new kit (or sterile catheter) and repeat procedure. • Keep catheter tip in lubricant packet until ready to catheterize. • If catheter has tearaway sleeve, leave catheter within it while catheterizing client.

• Catheter is inserted into female client's vagina.	• Leave the catheter in place and follow these actions:
	  • Have someone obtain a new sterile catheter and gloves.
	  • Reposition fingers to better visualize urethral meatus.
	  • Obtain an assistant to provide direct lighting.
	  • Insert new catheter pointing upward (toward client's umbilicus), as downward angle insertion tends to follow vaginal inlet.
	  • Place obese client in side-lying position and flex upper leg for catheterization.

• Catheter cannot be inserted into male client.	• Obtain new catheter kit and follow these actions:
	  • Obtain order for intraurethral lidocaine gel.
	  • Hold penis vertical to client's body; insert lidocaine gel.
	  • Insert catheter while applying slight traction by gently pulling upward on the shaft of the penis.
	  • If resistance encountered, rotate catheter, increase traction, and lower angle of penis.
	  • Ask client to cough.
	  • Try using a Coudé or 12-Fr catheter.

- Urine leaks around indwelling catheter.

- Inflate catheter balloon with full amount of sterile water in syringe (10 mL) to fill balloon and catheter inflation lumen as well.
- If client still requires the catheter, replace the catheter.
- Do not increase catheter size, as this increases bladder irritation, spasm, and leakage.
- Obtain urine culture and sensitivity, as leakage may be sign of UTI.
- Obtain order for anticholinergic medication to relieve bladder spasms.

- Client develops UTI while catheterized.

- Remind healthcare provider that client has a catheter; reevaluate need for continued use.
- Keep urine collection system below level of client's bladder—avoid any chance of bacteria entering system caused by retrograde flow from collection bag to bladder.
- Encourage fluid intake of 2–3 L/day unless contraindicated.
- Maintain client and system positioning so that continuous urine drainage is unobstructed.
- Make certain that catheter is secured properly (thigh of female, abdomen of male).
- Maintain/coil drainage tubing to allow straight drainage into urine collection bag.
- Empty the collection bag regularly.
- Provide daily perineal care with soap and water only.
- Don clean gloves to empty urine collection bag; avoid contamination of drain port.
- Suggest external collection system (condom catheter) for male client.

Bladder Irrigation

Nursing Process Data

ASSESSMENT Database

- Determine rationale for irrigation.
- Note rate of urine flow from bladder, color of urine, and presence of clots or debris.
- Assess for distended bladder.
- Assess for bladder discomfort.
- Note client's I&O balance.

PLANNING Objectives

- To remove blood clots from client's bladder
- To ensure patency of drainage system
- To relieve bladder spasm discomfort

IMPLEMENTATION Procedures

- **Skill 22.4.1** Maintaining Continuous

DOCUMENTATION AND EVALUATION

Expected Outcomes

- Continuous bladder irrigation is maintained to prevent clot formation and catheter obstruction.
- Client does not experience discomfort.

Unexpected Outcomes/Alternative Actions

Pearson Nursing Student Resources

Find additional review materials at
nursing.pearsonhighered.com.
Prepare for success with NCLEX®-style practice questions and Skill Checklists.

Skill 22.4.1 | Maintaining Continuous Bladder Irrigation

Equipment

Irrigating solution (2,000 mL of sterile normal saline or less than drainage bag volume) as prescribed
IV tubing with roller clamp
IV pole
Antiseptic swabs
Clean gloves

Procedure

1. Check healthcare provider's orders and client care plan.
2. Note whether client has triple-lumen indwelling catheter and drainage bag. ❶
3. Identify client using two client identifiers.
4. Explain procedure to client and provide privacy.
5. Perform hand hygiene and don clean gloves.
6. Remove protective covering from spike on tubing, and insert spike into insertion port of solution container. Use aseptic technique.
7. Hang irrigating solution container on IV pole and prime tubing. Height of pole is usually 60–90 cm (24–36 in.) above bladder. ❷

   a. Remove protective cover from end of tubing using aseptic technique.
   b. Open roller clamp, and allow irrigating solution to run through tubing until all air is expelled. ➤ *Rationale:* This prevents air from entering the bladder and causing discomfort.
   c. Close roller clamp.

8. Connect tubing to catheter irrigating (indwell) lumen using aseptic technique.
9. Check for **patency** of catheter; ensure there is an absence of clots or foreign bodies that may obstruct catheter.
10. Remove gloves and perform hand hygiene.
11. Adjust drip rate of irrigating solution by adjusting the clamp on the tubing to increase or decrease based on urine outflow color.

    a. Infuse continuously to keep urine drainage pink to clear.
    b. When drainage is dark red or contains tissue or blood clots, irrigate manually, and then increase drip rate.
       ➤ *Rationale:* Increased drip rate will clear the drainage and flush out debris and clots.
    c. Change irrigation solution bottle using aseptic technique.

12. Check for bladder distention or abdominal pain; note urine color.
13. Monitor urine output at least every hour to observe patency of system.
14. Empty drainage bag as needed. Subtract amount of irrigant infused from total output to obtain urine output and record.
15. Maintain catheter traction if taped to thigh. ➤ *Rationale:* This promotes venous hemostasis.
16. Remove gloves and perform hand hygiene.

Note: Procedure is done to flush clots and debris from bladder or obstruction of catheter after prostatic surgery and to prevent catheter obstruction and promote patency. Immediately report bright red urine outflow, as this indicates an arterial bleed.

❶ Maintain continuous bladder irrigation by using a triple-lumen catheter for procedure.

❷ Hang irrigating solution on IV pole at height of 60–90 cm (24–36 in.) above bladder.

Unit 22.4 Documentation and Evaluation

DOCUMENTATION for Bladder Irrigation

- Type and amount of solution administered for irrigation
- Rate of administration of irrigating solution
- Description of urinary output, including color and presence of clots or debris
- Any statements of discomfort or cramping
- Medication given for pain
- Amount of actual urine output (total urine output minus amount of irrigant instilled)

EVALUATION/Critical Thinking

Expected Outcomes

- Continuous bladder irrigation is maintained to prevent clot formation and catheter obstruction.
- Client does not experience discomfort.

Unexpected Outcomes	Alternative Actions
• Irrigation flow is not infusing at prescribed rate.	• Raise or lower IV standard with attached irrigation bag to assist in regulating flow using gravity. • Move flow adjuster clamp to new site on tubing. • Suspect obstruction.

• Irrigation outflow is less than expected.	• Suspect obstruction:
	  a. Check tubing for kinks.
	  b. Have client change position.
	  c. Maintaining sterile technique, disconnect catheter outflow port, and gently aspirate solution from catheter to remove clots.
	  d. Instill 30–50 mL of irrigating solution to free clots.
	  e. Reconnect drainage system and observe for 30 min; bladder spasms may block outflow of urine.
	  f. Notify healthcare provider if problem is not resolved or client develops nausea, hypertension, and bradycardia (client may develop transurethral resection of the prostate (TURP) syndrome due to absorption of hypotonic irrigating solution).
	• Increase irrigation inflow rate; monitor vital signs.
	• Do not allow client to cough.

• Client's urine outflow is dark pink with blood clots.	• Keep client's catheter-taped leg straight to maintain traction on catheter inflation bulb. • Suspect obstruction. • Increase irrigation rate. • Notify healthcare provider if problem continues.
• Client experiences painful bladder spasms during irrigation.	• Notify healthcare provider to obtain order for urinary antispasmodic medication. • Assist client to change position.

Suprapubic Catheter Care

Nursing Process Data

ASSESSMENT Database

- Observe for urine flow through catheter.
- Observe for excessive bleeding through catheter or at insertion site.
- Check that suture site is clean, dry, and intact.
- Check that straight drainage is maintained.
- Assess that fluid intake is at least 2,000 mL daily.
- Assess client for pain, bladder distention, or spasms.
- Assess client's ability to assist with clamping procedure.
- Assess client's ability to tolerate catheter being clamped.

PLANNING Objectives

- To prevent UTI when a suprapubic catheter is inserted
- To maintain a patent suprapubic catheter
- To monitor the catheter clamping procedure
- To prevent infection at catheter insertion site
- To provide discharge teaching if catheter is to remain in place when client is discharged

IMPLEMENTATION Procedures

DOCUMENTATION AND EVALUATION

Expected Outcomes

- Suprapubic catheter remains intact.
- Client remains free of UTI.

Unexpected Outcomes/Alternative Actions

Pearson Nursing Student Resources

Find additional review materials at
nursing.pearsonhighered.com.
Prepare for success with NCLEX®-style practice questions and Skill Checklists.

Skill 22.5.1 | Providing Suprapubic Catheter Care

Equipment

Closed drainage system, including Foley catheter tubing and bag
Catheter clamp and plug
Dry sterile dressing and tape if ordered
Cleansing solution
Clean gloves
Sterile gloves

Preparation

1. Check healthcare provider's orders and client care plan.
2. Identify client using two client identifiers and explain purpose of catheter.
3. Describe procedure for continuous or intermittent urinary drainage.
4. Perform hand hygiene.
5. Provide privacy.

Procedure

1. Observe catheter for patency. ➤ *Rationale:* The most common problem with suprapubic catheters is occlusion with sediment or clots.

   a. First 24 hr: Check the catheter every hour to detect possible obstruction. Urine output should be in excess of 30 mL/hr.
   b. Second day: Check the catheter every 8 hr.
   c. Third day: Check the catheter when the catheter is unclamped.

2. Maintain a closed drainage system. Do not open system to irrigate or obtain urine sample.
3. Observe for signs of UTI (color, odor, presence of sediment).
4. Keep the dressing dry around site of insertion. Apply a new dressing, maintaining sterile technique, every morning and as necessary.

   a. Place bed in high working position.
   b. Perform hand hygiene and don clean gloves.
   c. Remove old dressing, discard gloves, and dispose in appropriate container.
   d. Perform hand hygiene and open sterile supplies.
   e. Open cleansing solution and pour over sterile gauze.
   f. Don sterile gloves.
   g. Assess skin surrounding suprapubic catheter.
   h. Cleanse area with cleansing solution. Allow to dry.
   i. Apply sterile dressing and secure with tape. ❶
   j. Remove gloves and supplies and discard in appropriate container.
   k. Perform hand hygiene.
   l. Replace bed in LOW position.

5. Perform clamping protocol according to healthcare provider orders for intermittent urinary drainage.

   a. Explain the clamping procedure and ask client to help monitor the clamping.
   b. Instruct client to report if he or she feels fullness in the bladder during clamping.
   c. Don clean gloves.
   d. Clamp the catheter.

❶ Tape catheter and connect to a closed system.

6. Empty the drainage bag or remove drainage tubing from catheter, maintaining aseptic technique.

   a. Place drainage tubing in sterile package to maintain sterility.
   b. Place catheter plug in catheter end.
   c. Remove gloves and perform hand hygiene.
   d. Record urine output on I&O record.
   e. Leave the catheter clamped or plugged for 3–4 hr depending on client's level of comfort and healthcare provider's orders.

7. At 3- to 4-hr intervals, or when client feels bladder fullness, ask client to void normally. Don clean gloves to measure the urine and record output on I&O bedside record.
8. Immediately after client voids, unclamp catheter and leave unclamped for 5 min, collecting the residual urine.

   a. Don clean gloves to measure the residual urine after unclamping of the catheter.
   b. Reclamp catheter.
   c. If ordered, send a urine specimen to laboratory after the first clamping. ➤ *Rationale:* This checks for the presence of microorganisms.

9. Repeat clamping protocol every 3–4 hr according to healthcare provider's orders. The catheter may be open to drainage from bedtime until 6 a.m.
10. When the client is voiding normally, clamp the catheter throughout the night in preparation for its removal.
11. When the client's residual urine output is less than 100 mL or retains less than 20% of residual urine on two successive checks, notify the healthcare provider for removal of the catheter.
12. Cleanse insertion area with antimicrobial swab.
13. Deflate balloon and remove catheter, if order written for nurse to remove.
14. Apply a 2 × 2 sterile dressing over insertion site. Cover client.
15. Dispose of the catheter in biohazard bag.
16. If the client is discharged from the hospital with the catheter, provide the following teaching for home care:

    a. Instruct the client to drink one glass of fluid every hour while awake.

b. Instruct client to follow clamping procedure when awake or as instructed by the healthcare provider.

c. Instruct the client to leave the catheter open to the drainage system at night (drainage system may be urinary tubing and bag or leg bag).

d. Tell client to notify healthcare provider if **dysuria** occurs when voiding or if urine becomes cloudy, odorous, or has sediment.

Removing the Suprapubic Catheter

a. Don clean gloves.

b. Prep the catheter and the insertion site with Betadine or antiseptic prep.

c. Deflate balloon: Insert syringe into inflation tube of catheter and withdraw fluid from balloon, which will deflate.

d. Gently withdraw catheter.

e. Place 2×2 sterile dressing over the insertion site.

Reinserting at Established Suprapubic Catheter Site

Note: In selected hospitals, nurses are now allowed to reinsert suprapubic catheters per healthcare provider's orders.

a. Obtain same size suprapubic catheter as used previously (check size at distal end of catheter).

b. Insert new catheter 2.5–5 cm (1.5–2 in.) or add length if large amount of adipose tissue. There may or may not be urinary return with insertion of catheter.

c. Inflate balloon with appropriate volume of sterile water.

Unit 22.5 Documentation and Evaluation

DOCUMENTATION for Suprapubic Catheter Care

- Time catheter clamped
- Length of time clamped
- Client's ability to void spontaneously
- Client's feelings of fullness
- Time specimen sent to laboratory
- Color, amount, and odor of urine obtained
- Color, amount, and odor of residual urine

EVALUATION/Critical Thinking

Expected Outcomes
- Suprapubic catheter remains intact.
- Client remains free of UTI.
- Client is able to void naturally.

Unexpected Outcomes	Alternative Actions
• Suprapubic catheter becomes dislodged.	• Place sterile dressing over catheter insertion site; do not attempt to replace catheter. • Notify healthcare provider. • Obtain new catheter to prepare for insertion by healthcare provider.
• Client develops UTI.	• Note signs and symptoms of UTI: cloudy malodorous urine with sediment, bladder discomfort or spasms, elevated temperature. • Notify healthcare provider to obtain order for urinalysis and antimicrobial therapy. • Increase fluid intake to at least 2–3 L/day (unless contraindicated). • Maintain continuous urine drainage per suprapubic catheter.
• Client is unable to void spontaneously through urethra.	• Maintain suprapubic urine drainage. • Notify healthcare provider.

Specimens from Closed Systems

Nursing Process Data

ASSESSMENT Database

- Assess the type of specimen needed.
  Note: From a closed system, all will be sterile specimens—voided urine is a clean specimen.
- Identify amount of urine needed for specimen.
- Check to see if the closed urinary system has a port for obtaining a specimen.

PLANNING Objectives

- To prevent urinary infection by obtaining a urine specimen without interrupting a closed urinary drainage system
- To determine the specific microorganism causing a UTI
- To obtain a urine specimen for diagnostic purposes

IMPLEMENTATION Procedures

DOCUMENTATION AND EVALUATION

Expected Outcomes

- Urine specimen is obtained from the closed urinary drainage system.
- Urine specimen remains sterile.

Unexpected Outcomes/Alternative Actions

Pearson Nursing Student Resources

Find additional review materials at
nursing.pearsonhighered.com.
Prepare for success with NCLEX®-style practice questions and Skill Checklists.

Skill 22.6.1 | Collecting Specimen From a Closed System

Equipment
Catheter tubing clamp or rubber band
Kova specimen trap syringe *or* syringe with blunt cannula
Sterile specimen container with label if necessary
Label
Biohazard bag
Antimicrobial swab
Clean gloves

Procedure
1. Gather equipment.
2. Identify client using two forms of identification.
3. Explain the procedure and rationale to the client.
4. Clamp (or crimp and bind) retention catheter drainage tubing a few inches distal to sample access port (approximately 15 min to allow urine to collect in tube). ➤ *Rationale:* This ensures the urine specimen is adequate.
5. Perform hand hygiene and don gloves.
6. Wipe the sample access port of the drainage tubing with the antimicrobial swab.
7. Insert cannula of specimen trap syringe into port. Alternately, insert blunt cannula of syringe, or engage uncapped Luer-Lok syringe with port. ❶ ➤ *Rationale:* Different manufacturers recommend using different equipment with their products.
8. Aspirate urine sample (at least 2 mL) by gently pulling back on syringe plunger, and then remove syringe. ❷
9. For Kova specimen syringe, maintain sterility of cap while obtaining specimen; cap syringe, completely retract plunger, snap it off from end of syringe barrel, and discard. ❸

10. Apply identifying label to specimen syringe.
11. For syringe with blunt cannula or Luer-Lok syringe, transfer urine sample into specimen container and apply client label.
12. Remove drainage tubing clamp.
13. Remove gloves and perform hand hygiene.
14. Send specimen syringe or container in biohazard bag to laboratory as soon as possible, or place in unit refrigerator.

❷ Specimen trap syringe: Insert specimen collection syringe cannula into aspiration port and gently pull back on plunger to aspirate urine.

❶ Luer-Lok syringe: Obtain specimen using Luer-Lok syringe and transfer urine to sterile specimen cup.

❸ Kova specimen syringe: Snap off plunger of Kova specimen collection syringe, place in biohazard bag, and send as self-contained unit to lab for urine analysis.

Unit 22.6 Documentation and Evaluation

DOCUMENTATION for Specimens From Closed Systems

- Type and amount of specimen obtained
- Type of specimen container or syringe used to obtain specimen
- Color, consistency, and odor of urine
- Time of urine collection
- Time specimen sent to laboratory

EVALUATION/Critical Thinking

Expected Outcomes

- Urine sample is obtained from closed urinary drainage system.

Unexpected Outcomes

- Insufficient amount of urine is obtained when collection is attempted.

Alternative Actions

- Check that client has had sufficient fluid intake.
- Check for kinking of catheter.
- Clamp catheter tubing for 45 min before specimen collection.
- Reposition client.

Nursing Process Data

ASSESSMENT Database

- Assess location of stoma on client's abdomen (depends on type of diversion).
- Determine type of urinary diversion.
- Observe stoma color (same color as mucous membrane lining the mouth).
- Assess skin for condition.
- Assess presence of ureteral stents for new ileal conduit.
- Assess most appropriate pouching system for client. (System depends on client's age, manual dexterity, size of stoma, stoma location, presence of skin folds, and bony prominences.)
- Assess client's ability to manage self-care.
- Assess urine output (amount and character).

PLANNING Objectives

- To provide a pouching system that prevents skin irritation
- To instruct the client in self-care
- To monitor stoma for viability
- To obtain a sterile urine specimen

IMPLEMENTATION Procedures

DOCUMENTATION AND EVALUATION

Expected Outcomes

- Pouching system does not leak.
- Client demonstrates self-care skills.
- Urine specimen is readily obtained from urinary diversion system.
- Peristomal skin remains intact and healthy.

Unexpected Outcomes/Alternative Actions

Pearson Nursing Student Resources

Find additional review materials at
nursing.pearsonhighered.com.
Prepare for success with NCLEX®-style practice questions and Skill Checklists.

Skill 22.7.1 | Applying a Urinary Diversion Pouch

Equipment

One- or two-piece urinary pouch with skin barrier, flange, and spigot at bottom of pouch to empty urine ❶

Items to clean stoma (e.g., soft cloth or gauze sponges) and warm water

Plastic bag for disposal of used equipment

Gauze for drying skin and for wicking stoma

Underpad to protect bedding

Scissors if indicated

Protective barriers such as skin prep, skin gel, or protective barrier film if necessary

Stoma measuring guide

Clean gloves

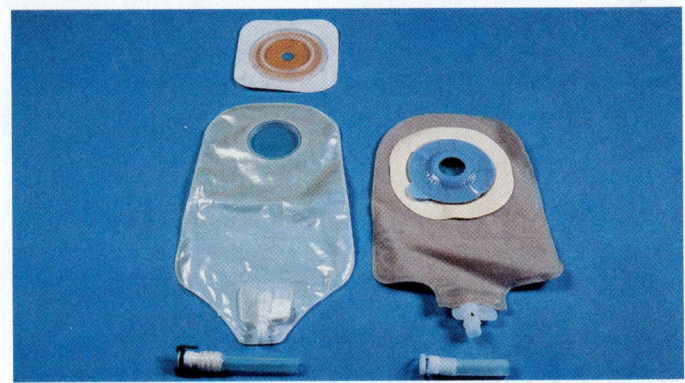

❶ One-piece and two-piece urinary diversion pouches.

Preparation

1. Check healthcare provider's order and client care plan. Pouch should be changed every 3–7 days.
2. Gather equipment.
3. Perform hand hygiene.
4. Identify client using two client identifiers and explain procedure.
5. Provide privacy.
6. Place client in a position that promotes visualization and self-care.
7. Place protective pad under client.
8. Place bath blanket over client's chest and position top covers over lower abdomen without impeding client's visualization of procedure.

❷ Cleanse stoma and periostomal skin; dry thoroughly.

Procedure

1. Don clean gloves.
2. Empty, and then remove entire ostomy appliance by pushing the skin gently away from the appliance and peeling the appliance downward. Discard in plastic bag.
3. Wash stoma and peristomal skin with warm water and soap if needed, rinse well, and pat skin dry. ➤ *Rationale:* Chemical or perfumed wipes can irritate skin or may interfere with pouch seal. ❷

Note: Stoma may bleed slightly when wiped.

CLINICAL ALERT

Thin plastic tubes (stents) may be placed in each ureter during surgery. These exit stoma and remain in place for up to 10 days. They serve to maintain patency until swelling has subsided at ureteroileal anastomosis site (6–10 days). Their presence and length of exposure should be documented. The surgeon should be notified when they wash out into collection pouch.

---

4. Check stoma for healing; it should be bright but not dark red and moist, and raised 0.5–1 in (1.2–2.5 cm). above skin surface (or may be flush). Check for mucocutaneous separation, ulceration, encrustation, and signs of infection, and sensitivities or allergies.

5. Check skin surrounding stoma to ensure urine hasn't been draining under wafer, causing skin irritation.
6. Prepare new urinary pouch. Place gauze over stoma to prevent urine from oozing onto skin. A wick can be placed in stoma, if needed. Measure stoma site with measuring guide, unless pouch has precut opening. ➤ *Rationale:* This is to keep urine from contact with skin during pouch change.
7. Trace size of stoma on wafer and cut ¹⁄₁₆–¹⁄₈ in (0.2–0.3 cm) larger than size. ❸ ➤ *Rationale:* This small opening prevents leakage of effluent onto skin; however, the size is large enough to prevent pressure on the stoma from the wafer rubbing on skin.

❸ Cut wafer opening slightly larger than stoma.

8. Apply protective barrier (only if indicated) to skin surrounding stoma or to wafer. ❹ Do not use lotion. ➤ *Rationale:* Protective barriers contain alcohol and cause burning and may interfere with seal. In addition, barrier must be removed with adhesive remover.
9. Let site dry thoroughly.
10. Remove paper from adhesive on wafer of one- or two-piece appliance.
11. Remove wick and center wafer over stoma; apply to dry skin, starting at bottom, and working up around stoma. Press wafer on skin for 3 min. ❺ ➤ *Rationale:* This promotes adherence to skin. If two-piece pouch, attach pouch to wafer flange.
12. Remove air from clean pouch and close spout. Attach pouch to gravity drainage bag only while client is in bed. Empty pouch when one-third full.
13. Cover client. Discard equipment in appropriate receptacle.

14. Remove gloves and perform hand hygiene.
15. As ordered, provide client teaching for emptying the pouch (Box 22-6 ■).

Box 22-6 CLIENT TEACHING FOR EMPTYING POUCH

Instruct client to:

- Empty pouch when one-third full.
- Use bathroom if possible.
- Place distal end of pouch between thighs or stand over toilet.
- Open drainage port to allow urine to drain.
- Dry drainage port with toilet paper.
- Close drainage port.
- Perform hand hygiene.

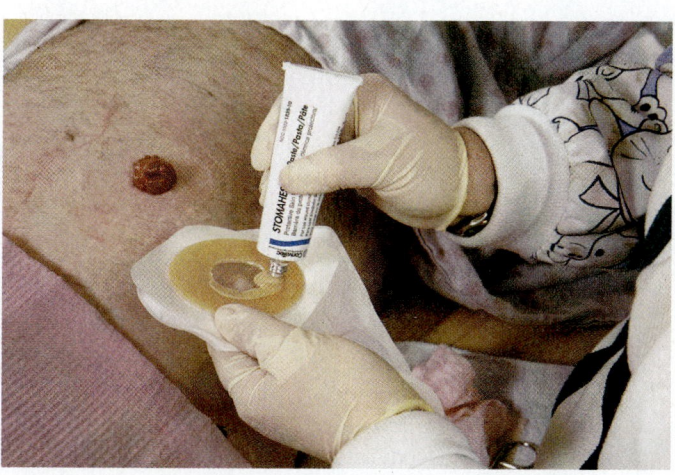

❹ Apply protective paste to wafer, only if indicated.

❺ Apply the wafer and press it to the skin.

Skill 22.7.2 | Obtaining Urine Specimen From an Ileal Conduit

Equipment
Sterile catheter kit
Prep solution
Sterile saline or water
Underpad
New urinary pouch
Supplies necessary to apply new pouch
Bath blanket, towels
Clean gloves
Soap and water
Pitcher of water and glass
Biohazard bag

Preparation
1. Check healthcare provider's orders and client care plan.
2. Gather equipment.
3. Perform hand hygiene.
4. Identity client using two client identifiers.

5. Explain procedure to client.
6. Provide privacy.
7. Place bath blanket over client's chest and position top covers over lower abdomen.
8. Place towels around stoma. ➤ *Rationale:* Urine will leak around catheter.
9. Don clean gloves.

Procedure
1. Open sterile packages.
2. Remove pouch or snap pouch off wafer flange.
   Note: Do not use pouch contents to obtain urine specimen.
3. Remove gloves. Wash hands. Put on sterile gloves.
4. Place sterile drape over stoma.
5. Remove lid from specimen container and place end of catheter into container.
6. Apply lubricant to catheter.

(continued)

Skill 27.7.2 | Obtaining Urine Specimen From an Ileal Conduit (continued)

7. Use forceps to pick up cotton ball and prep stoma with solution using a circular motion from stoma opening outward.
8. Blot stoma dry with sterile gauze.
9. Insert tip of straight catheter into stoma approximately 5–7.5 cm (2–3 in.). 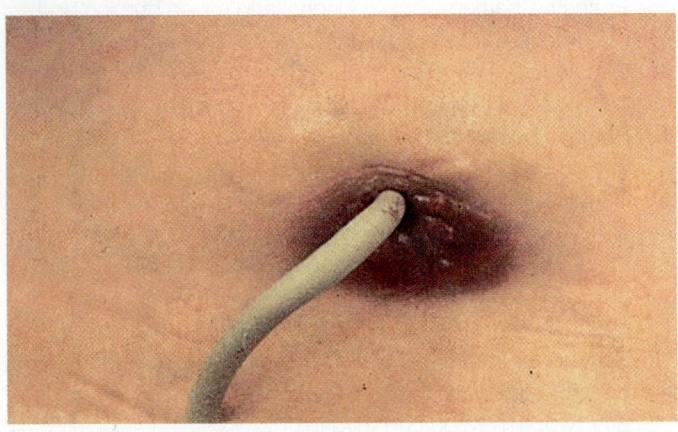 ❶
10. If using a double catheter, insert 2.5–5 cm (1–2 in.).
11. When urine specimen is obtained (usually not more than 5–25 mL), remove catheter. If no urine is obtained, have client drink water.
12. Return lid to specimen container and apply label.
13. If wafer removed, wash and dry peristomal area.
14. Replace pouch or apply new pouch. Cover client.
15. Remove gloves and perform hand hygiene.
16. Place specimen container in biohazard bag and send specimen to lab immediately or refrigerate.

❶ Catheter is used to obtain specimen from ileal conduit.

Skill 22.7.3 | Catheterizing Continent Urinary Reservoir

Equipment
Sterile catheter (if client hospitalized)
Water-soluble lubricant
Clean gloves
Bedpan (if client is unable to use toilet)
Warm water and soap
Washcloth, towel

Preparation
1. Check healthcare provider's orders and client care plan.
2. Gather equipment.
3. Identify client using two client identifiers and explain procedure.
4. Perform hand hygiene and don gloves.
5. Provide privacy.
6. Position client on chair facing toilet or place bedpan next to client if on bed rest.

Procedure
1. Open lubricant packet.
2. Lubricate tip of catheter, maintaining sterility.
3. Insert catheter 2.5–5 cm (1–2 in.) into stoma. Place distal end of catheter over toilet or bedpan.

CLINICAL ALERT
Irrigation: During the immediate postoperative period after formation of a continent reservoir, irrigation of the reservoir must be done. A plug of mucus can block the catheter, leading to overdistention of the reservoir and perforation or disruption of the surgical reconstruction. Teach the client with a continent reservoir to irrigate the reservoir with warm water daily using catheter and bulb or piston syringe to remove collected mucus. ➤ *Rationale:* Mucus produced by the bowel segment will accumulate in the reservoir.

4. Instruct client to take deep breath and gently insert catheter through nipple valve until urine returns. ➤ *Rationale:* When the abdominal muscles are relaxed, it is easier to advance catheter through nipple valve.
5. Hold catheter in place until urine stops draining.
6. Remove catheter.
7. Wash and dry peristomal area with soap and water.
8. Assist client back to bed, or position for comfort.
9. Remove gloves and perform hand hygiene.

Unit 22.7 Documentation and Evaluation

DOCUMENTATION for Urinary Diversion

- Color and amount of urine obtained from catheterizing continent reservoir
- Catheter size used for catheterization
- Status of ureteral stents, if present

- Peristomal skin and stoma condition
- Client's acceptance of stoma, participation in self-care
- Type and method of drainage pouch applied
- Specimen sent to lab

EVALUATION/Critical Thinking

Expected Outcomes

- Pouching system does not leak.
- Client demonstrates self-care skills.
- Urine specimen is readily obtained from urinary diversion system.
- Peristomal skin remains intact and healthy.

Unexpected Outcomes	Alternative Actions
• Pouching system leaks.	• Check area for crease or dip in skin, which allows urine to pool and leak out. • Fill in dip area with skin barrier to prevent pooling. • Apply belt to improve fit. • Apply another type of pouch (e.g., convex). • Change more frequently if leak is due to dissolving of skin barrier—or use different barrier. • Advise client to avoid using soaps or wipes to clean area because they interfere with pouch adhesion.
• Client is unable to manage own urinary diversion.	• Simplify pouch procedure if possible. • Provide detailed instruction in more simplified manner. • Include caregiver in teaching to assist and support client. • Refer client to home health agency for follow-up care.
• Client is offended by odor in urine collection system.	• Recommend urine-acidifying agent (e.g., vitamin C, 500 mg BID to TID); avoid alkaline ash citrus juices (e.g., grapefruit, tomato). • Wash reusable equipment with mild soap and water and rinse in vinegar weekly or use commercial deodorant. • Inform client that certain foods and drugs (asparagus, vitamin B complex) give odor to urine. Empty pouch frequently if these are ingested. • Inform client that cloudy urine and strong odor may indicate a UTI. Advise healthcare provider and collect sterile urine specimen.
• No urine is obtained from conduit.	• Rotate catheter, or position client on side to allow urine to flow into catheter. As little as 1 mL is needed for urine culture and sensitivity testing. • Have client drink water.
• Erythematous vesicular rash appears on peristomal skin.	• Suspect possible allergic reaction; obtain patch test for allergy. • Avoid use of chemical wipes and perfumed soaps. • Suspect yeast infection; report to healthcare provider.

Hemodialysis (Renal Replacement Therapy)

Nursing Process Data

ASSESSMENT Database

- Assess patency of vascular access.

  Femoral vein catheter: dual-lumen vascular device used for immediate vascular access in life-threatening situations

  Central venous dual-lumen catheter (DLC): vascular device placed in internal jugular vein used for temporary access for acute hemodialysis clients

  Permanent dual-lumen catheter (PDLC): vascular device inserted through internal jugular vein and advanced to superior vena cava (SVC)

  ***Arteriovenous** fistula:* surgically created internal anastomosis between an artery and vein; used for clients undergoing chronic hemodialysis

  Arteriovenous graft: surgically implanted synthetic material (GOR-TEX) or biologic material (human umbilical vein) used for anastomosis between an artery and vein for clients undergoing chronic hemodialysis

- Review chart and laboratory reports for factors that may alter management of dialysis (especially potassium, sodium, calcium, and phosphorus levels; albumin; hemoglobin; hematocrit levels; BUN; and creatinine).

- Assess vital signs.

- Assess causes of hypotension: fluid loss, hypoalbuminemia, large interdialytic weight gain.

- Check serum electrolyte levels, BUN, and creatinine before and after dialysis according to healthcare provider's orders.

- Weigh client before and after dialysis to determine fluid loss.

PLANNING Objectives

- To maintain a patent access site for hemodialysis
- To provide care for a client after receiving hemodialysis
- To maintain patent catheters centrally placed

IMPLEMENTATION Procedures

DOCUMENTATION AND EVALUATION

Expected Outcomes

- Dialysis proceeds without complication (excess fluids and wastes removed from blood).
- Vascular access site remains patent.

Unexpected Outcomes/Alternative Actions

Pearson Nursing Student Resources

Find additional review materials at
nursing.pearsonhighered.com.
Prepare for success with NCLEX®-style practice questions and Skill Checklists.

The Hemodialysis Process

Hemodialysis works by removing blood from the client's arterial access site (graft, fistula, or catheter). It travels through a blood pump and an arterial pressure monitor to a **dialyzer** (filter). In the dialyzer, the blood is separated from the dialysate by a synthetic semipermeable membrane. The dialysate (bath) runs against the blood flowing on the opposite side of the semipermeable membrane, leading to osmosis, diffusion, and ultrafiltration. Fluid, electrolytes, and toxins are removed from the blood. The blood then flows from the dialyzer through a tubing system to the client's venous access site (Figure 22-3 ■). Fluid is removed through the use of **hydrostatic pressure** applied to the blood and a negative hydrostatic pressure applied to the dialysate bath. The difference between these two pressures is termed *transmembrane pressure,* and this results in the process of ultrafiltration.

An adequate vascular access should permit blood flow to the dialyzer at 200–400 mL/min. Optimal blood access and blood flow to the dialyzer influences dialysis efficiency.

FIGURE 22.3 Arterial and venous needles placed in graft for hemodialysis.

SAFETY ALERT

Precautions for Fistula or Graft

When a hemodialysis client is hospitalized, place an identifying bracelet on the access arm. Post safety precautions at head of bed (e.g., "Do not use access arm for blood pressure or venipuncture," and "Fluid restriction specified").

- Regularly feel for vibration (thrill) over access site.
- Do not measure blood pressure on the affected extremity.
- Do not perform venipuncture in the affected extremity.
- Counsel the client:
  - Avoid lying on the affected extremity.
  - Avoid carrying heavy loads with access extremity.
  - Do not wear constrictive clothing on the affected extremity.
  - Immediately report swelling, discoloration, drainage, or coldness, numbness, or weakness of hand.

Skill 22.8.1 | Providing Ongoing Care of Hemodialysis Client

Procedure

1. Limit fluid intake to prescribed amount (e.g., 1,500 mL/day).
2. Maintain individualized diet as prescribed: high-quality protein 1.1 g/kg ideal body wt/day; sodium 70 mEq/day; potassium, average 70 mEq/day.
3. Check blood pressure for hypertension or hypotension; check temperature for possible infection.
4. Auscultate heart and lung sounds for signs of fluid overload (pulmonary edema and pericarditis).
5. Assess the **AV fistula** (Box 22-7 ■). Provide access site care.
6. Observe mental status—indicative of fluid and electrolyte imbalance.
7. Administer Epogen, if ordered, to improve hemoglobin level (given at time of dialysis).
8. Encourage regular rest periods.
9. Weigh daily to assess fluid accumulation.
10. Use antibacterial soap and lotion to bathe. ➤ *Rationale:* This decreases risk of staphylococcal infections.

Box 22-7 ASSESSING ARTERIOVENOUS FISTULA

- Perform hand hygiene.
- Position client's arm, so fistula is easily accessed.
- Palpate the area to feel for thrill (vibration). This indicates arterial to venous blood flow and fistula patency.
- Auscultate with a stethoscope to detect a bruit (swishing noise). This indicates a patent fistula.
- Palpate pulses distal to fistula to check circulation.
- Observe capillary refill in extremity digits.
- Assess for numbness, tingling, coldness, pallor, or alteration in sensation in digits of fistula extremity.
- Assess for signs and symptoms of infection: redness, edema, soreness, warmth, or increased temperature.

Note: Vascular access promotes more efficient removal and replacement of blood during dialysis and fewer complications occur. Vascular access should be prepared weeks or months before using it for dialysis. This will stabilize the graft site and ensure adequate blood flow when used for dialysis.

(continued)

Skill 22.8.1 | Providing Ongoing Care of Hemodialysis Client *(continued)*

11. Determine that client understands when and how to take medications.
12. Provide continued emotional support.
    a. Allow for expression of feelings about change in body image and role performance.
    b. Encourage expression of fears.
    c. Encourage caregiver support.
    d. Give support for required change in lifestyle.
13. Instruct client to prevent obstruction to blood flow on fistula arm.
14. Predialysis care
    a. Assess vital signs, including apical pulse and orthostatic blood pressure (provides baseline comparison).
    b. Obtain client weight.
    c. Assess heart and lung sounds.

15. Postdialysis care
    a. Assess vital signs, including apical pulse and orthostatic blood pressure.
    b. Obtain weight.
    c. Assess heart and lung sounds.
    d. Assess fistula site for bleeding.
    e. Assess for dialysis disequilibrium syndrome (headache, nausea and vomiting, altered level of consciousness, hypertension). ➤ *Rationale:* Rapid changes in BUN, pH, and electrolyte levels during dialysis may lead to cerebral edema and increased intracranial pressure.
    f. Assess for other complications of dialysis such as bleeding and transfusion reaction if client received blood.
16. Monitor BUN, serum creatinine, serum electrolyte, and hematocrit levels.

Unit 22.8 Documentation and Evaluation

DOCUMENTATION for Posthemodialysis

- Status of fistula, graft, or catheter access site and distal circulation
- Time dialysis initiated and terminated
- Dialyzer type and dialysate used
- Volume of blood processed

- Any complications during procedure and actions taken
- Client symptoms at 30-min intervals
- Vital signs as ordered
- Postdialysis assessment

EVALUATION/Critical Thinking

Expected Outcomes
- Vascular access site remains patent.
- Client demonstrates self-care after teaching.

Unexpected Outcomes
- Client states hand feels weak; neither thrill nor bruit can be assessed in fistula or graft.

Alternative Actions
- Notify physician of potential clotting of fistula or graft.
- Prepare to possibly send client to radiology for vascular procedure.
- Review safety precautions to prevent constriction of blood flow in access extremity.

• Client gains 7 lb between dialysis sessions; blood pressure is elevated.	• Assess client's understanding of fluid restriction (1,500 mL/day); advise of hidden fluid in certain foods (such as ice cream or watermelon). • Encourage client to control blood sugar (if diabetic) to help relieve thirst; decrease salt intake, but avoid salt substitute (KCl). • Encourage client to weigh daily.
• Client's predialysis phosphorus level is excessively elevated.	• Review foods high in phosphorus (colas, red meat, dairy products, eggs). • Encourage client to continue calcium and vitamin D supplement as prescribed. • Remind client to take phosphorus binder medication with meals; if not taking, inquire if constipation is reason and recommend stool softener.

Nursing Process Data

ASSESSMENT Database

- Assess the client's bladder for distention.
- Assess the client's physical ability to cooperate with positioning.
- Assess urinary meatus and catheter for exudate, edema, inflammation, and general cleanliness.
- Assess need for perineal care before catheterization procedure.
- Assess dialysate solution for clarity.
- Assess dialysis returns for cloudiness.
- Assess family's ability to use gloving technique and maintain asepsis when needed.
- Assess need for suprapubic catheter care.
- Assess need for catheterization procedure.
- Assess for proper function of dialysis machine.

PLANNING Objectives

- To prevent or relieve discomfort due to bladder distention
- To promote urinary elimination
- To identify family's knowledge related to signs and symptoms of dialysis-related infections
- To prevent UTIs through aseptic catheter care
- To prevent infection at peritoneal catheter site
- To use aseptic technique when instituting CAPD
- To identify client's and family's knowledge base regarding CAPD or CCPD

IMPLEMENTATION Procedures

DOCUMENTATION AND EVALUATION

Expected Outcomes

- Catheterization performed using aseptic technique.
- Bladder emptied when client is unable to void.
- UTI prevented through aseptic catheter care.
- Aseptic PD procedure used.
- Catheter site remains free of infection.
- Suprapubic catheter care is completed and client is free of UTIs.

Unexpected Outcomes/Alternative Actions

Pearson Nursing Student Resources

Find additional review materials at
nursing.pearsonhighered.com.
Prepare for success with NCLEX®-style practice questions and Skill Checklists.

Skill 22.9.1 | Teaching Clean Technique for Intermittent Self-Catheterization

Equipment

Straight catheters in clean container, plastic bag, or wrapped in aluminum foil
Washcloth, soap, water
Water-soluble lubricant (K-Y; Surgilube)
Plastic bags
Basin or container
Mirror

Procedure

Note: The nurse will instruct the client in steps to perform self-catheterization.

Female Client

1. Attempt to urinate. If unable to do so, continue to follow these steps.
2. Perform hand hygiene and gather equipment. (Keep equipment in one large container.)
3. Assume sitting position on the bed or commode. (Place plastic under towel if bed is used.)
4. Separate labia with one hand while cleaning with soap and water front to back with other hand.
5. Position mirror to visualize urinary meatus.
6. Remove catheter from container (plastic bag or aluminum foil).
7. Lubricate end of catheter with water-soluble lubricant and place other end in container to catch urine.
8. While holding labia apart with one hand, insert catheter about 8 cm (3 in.) or until urine flows.
9. Press down with abdominal muscles to promote bladder's emptying.
10. Pinch off catheter after all urine has drained and withdraw gently, holding tip of catheter upright.
11. Wash and dry perineal area.

12. Wash catheter in warm, soapy water.
13. Rinse with clear water and dry the outside with paper towel.
14. Place in plastic bag for storage.
15. Perform hand hygiene.
16. Use catheters for 2–4 weeks and then discard.

Male Client

1. Attempt to urinate. If unable to do so, continue to follow these steps.
2. Perform hand hygiene and gather equipment. (Keep equipment in one large container.)
3. Assume sitting position on the bed or commode. (Place plastic under towel if bed is used.)
4. Retract the foreskin, if present, and wash tip of penis with soap and water.
5. Remove catheter from container (plastic bag or aluminum foil).
6. Lubricate the first 18–25 cm (7–10 in.) of catheter with water-soluble lubricant. Place other end in container to catch urine.
7. Hold penis at right angle to body, keeping foreskin retracted. Insert catheter 18–25 cm (7–10 in.) into penis or until urine begins to flow. Then insert catheter 2.5 cm (1 in.) farther.
8. Press down with abdominal muscles to promote bladder's emptying.
9. Pinch off catheter after all urine has drained and gently withdraw, holding tip of catheter upright.
10. Wash and dry area. Replace foreskin, if present.
11. Wash catheter in warm, soapy water.
12. Rinse with clear water and dry the outside with paper towel.
13. Place in plastic bag for storage.
14. Perform hand hygiene
15. Use catheters for 2–4 weeks and then discard.

Skill 22.9.2 | Providing Suprapubic Catheter Care in Home Care

Equipment

Catheter plug and clamp
Closed drainage system
Sterile dressings if necessary
Clean gloves
Receptacle to drain urine from drainage bag
Normal saline solution or mild soap and water
White vinegar
Applicator sticks
4×4 gauze pads
Paper tape

Procedure

1. Instruct client to gather equipment for specific skill to be done.
2. Perform hand hygiene and don gloves.
3. Clean around catheter site with normal saline solution or mild soap and water. Use applicator sticks to remove material from around catheter opening.
4. Ensure catheter is not pulling on exit site. Tape catheter to skin so a gentle curve is present. This prevents tugging on the catheter.

(continued)

Skill 22.9.2 | Providing Suprapubic Catheter Care in Home Care *(continued)*

5. Empty catheter bag. Some clients use leg bags. Empty into container and then dispose of contents in toilet or, if removing bag, empty directly into toilet.

6. Clean drainage bags with warm water and soap every day or two. Place one teaspoon of vinegar in rinse water to reduce odor.

7. Replace catheter bag on catheter.

8. Remove gloves and perform hand hygiene.

9. Instruct client in bladder testing:

   a. Wash hands and catheter connections with soap and water.

   b. Clamp the suprapubic tube so it does not drain. Use catheter plug or clamp.

   c. Have client attempt to void when client feels urge to urinate. Measure the amount of urine.

   d. Unclamp the suprapubic tube immediately after voiding; empty urine into container and measure residual urine amount.

   e. Instruct client to keep a log of each voiding and residual amount.

   f. Call healthcare provider with findings when residual amount is less than 20% of voided amount. Usually, this amount is about 60 mL. Usually, the suprapubic tube is removed when client is able to urinate without complications.

10. Instruct client to monitor carefully for signs of UTI and notify healthcare provider immediately. Check for bladder pain, bleeding, temperature over 100°F (37.8°C), chills, cloudy urine, and drainage or edema around the suprapubic tube.

Skill 22.9.3 | Administering Continuous Ambulatory Peritoneal Dialysis (CAPD)

Equipment

Sterile dialysate solution, 1–2 bags, warmed
Heating pad
Transfer set, either Y tubing or straight, and cap
Hook on wall of room used for dialysis
Clamp
Paper towels
Low stool or table
Intake and output record
Two pairs of sterile gloves
Mask
Antibacterial soap
Cleansing solution for catheter
Medication, if ordered

Preparation

1. Perform hand hygiene thoroughly; dry using paper towel.
2. Obtain container of sterile dialysate.
3. Check that strength and amount of solution are accurate as ordered (Box 22-8 ■).
4. Take equipment to clean area for assembly.

Procedure

Draining Fluid

1. Perform hand hygiene and don gloves. ➤ *Rationale:* Hand washing is an infection control precaution for the caregiver when there is potential contact with blood or body fluids.
2. Don mask.
3. Uncap catheter maintaining aseptic technique.
4. Attach sterile bag and transfer set to catheter for draining dialysate.
5. Place bag on low stool or table below level of client's abdomen. ➤ *Rationale:* This position allows fluid to drain by gravity from client's peritoneal cavity.
6. Unclamp tubing.

7. Allow fluid to drain into bag from abdomen until flow ceases, approximately, 10–20 min.

8. Reclamp tubing.

9. Examine drainage for discoloration or cloudiness.
   ➤ *Rationale:* Change in color may indicate presence of infection, or if white gelatin-like material is present, it indicates shredding of the peritoneal lining's old skin; an increase in this fibrin indicates potential peritonitis.

10. Disconnect tubing from drainage bag while maintaining aseptic technique. Unscrew catheter from tubing and attach Mini Cap, according to clinic's instruction. ➤ *Rationale:* The glucose in the dialysate solution predisposes the client to infections.

11. Weigh drainage bag on scale. Effluent should weigh at least 4.5 lb. This is equal to 2 L of fluid. ➤ *Rationale:* This is to ensure all fluid is drained from abdomen.

12. Dispose of effluent into toilet.

Box 22-8 PRINCIPLES OF PERITONEAL DIALYSIS

- Works on principle of diffusion and osmosis.
- Diffusion—particles move through semipermeable membrane from area of high to low solute concentration.
- Osmosis—fluids move through a semipermeable membrane from an area of low solute concentration to an area of high solute concentration from the blood, creating a high osmotic gradient.
- Peritoneal dialysis—used for chronic states of renal failure. Acute renal failure clients do not benefit because it is not efficient or rapid enough to adequately remove the waste products, such as urea when it accumulates in catabolic acute renal failure clients.

13. Double-bag tubing and drainage bag. Place biohazard label on bag. Discard by placing in biohazardous container. Tubing is usually disposed of after each exchange.
14. Remove and discard gloves and mask.
15. Perform hand hygiene.
16. Check blood pressure and pulse. ➤ *Rationale:* Rapid fluid shift may cause hypotension.

Note: Mini Cap disinfects dialysis tubing between exchanges.

Infusing Dialysate

1. Warm dialysate. The bag can be encased in a heating pad for 1 hr. DO NOT PLACE IN MICROWAVE. ➤ *Rationale:* Microwave heating will produce uneven heating and can cause burning in the client.
2. Perform hand hygiene for 3 min with antibacterial soap. ➤ *Rationale:* This is to prevent contamination.
3. Gather equipment and don gloves.
4. Open plastic wrap on dialysate solution, inspect solution bag for expiration date and color and consistency of dialysate, and assess bag for possible leaks.
5. Add medications as ordered. Maintain sterile technique in this step. ➤ *Rationale:* Some clients add routine drugs to dialysate, such as insulin.
6. Connect tubing to dialysate bag by removing protective cover from port and spiking into dialysate bag. Maintain sterility throughout this step. Each manufacturer has a slightly different mechanism for connecting the tubing and bag. Follow manufacturer's directions. See Box 22-9 ■, Transfer Sets.
7. Hang new dialysate bag on hook, which is positioned above client at shoulder height.
8. Open clamp and adjust height to ensure inflow of solution by gravity over a 10- to 20-min period.
9. Clamp tubing.
10. Discard empty dialysate bag or place in a holding pouch at client's waist, according to type of transfer set being used.
11. Allow fluid to remain in peritoneal cavity for approximately 4 hr.
12. Remove gloves.
13. Perform hand hygiene.

14. Repeat procedure four times daily, the last time at bedtime, allowing fluid to remain in peritoneal cavity overnight.
15. Ensure that client and caregiver are knowledgeable in strict aseptic technique.
16. Instruct client to notify healthcare provider if there is evidence of infection.
17. Document findings and bring to healthcare provider at each visit.

Box 22-9 TRANSFER SETS

A transfer set is tubing that connects the bag of dialysate solution to the catheter. There are two types used for CAPD.

Straight Tubing

Straight tubing stays connected to the catheter. For each exchange, the "free" end is connected to the solution. With this type of transfer set, the empty solution bag is rolled up and worn under clothing. That bag is then unrolled, placed on the floor, and used to drain dialysate from the abdomen. After draining is completed, tubing is disconnected from the straight transfer set and a new solution bag and tubing are connected to the catheter.

Y-Set Tubing

This type of tubing is disconnected between exchanges. The base of the Y is connected to the catheter. One branch of the Y is connected to a new bag of solution and the other to an empty bag. The base of the Y is closed, and a small amount of solution is drained from the full bag into the empty bag. This is done to rid the transfer set of any bacteria that might be in the tubing. The branch that leads to the empty bag is then closed, and the solution flows into the abdomen. Once the solution bag is empty, the Y-set is disconnected from the catheter. This removes the need to wear the bag around the waist while solution is in abdomen. The catheter is then reconnected to the Y-set and solution is drained into an empty bag to discard. A new bag of solution is hung and the process continues. The Y-set is filled with disinfectant when not in use. The disinfectant is flushed out with the used dialysate. The Y-set can be reused for several months.

Skill 22.9.4 | Changing Dressing for CAPD Client

Equipment

Dressing according to facility policy
Antimicrobial swabs or sterile 4×4 dressings and Betadine solution
Tape
Sterile gloves (two pair)
Forceps (optional)
Povidone iodine ointment
4×4 gauze pads and precut drain dressings
Warm soapy water, if needed

Procedure

1. Perform hand hygiene.
2. Don sterile gloves.
3. Remove old dressing with sterile gloves.

4. Remove any dried blood or drainage with warm, soapy water.
5. Saturate 4×4 dressings with Betadine solution, or use swabs, and clean skin around catheter, moving in concentric circles from the catheter site outward. Remove crusted material, if present.
6. Inspect site for infection (erythema, edema, warmth, exudate).
7. Apply povidone iodine ointment to catheter site using sterile dressings.
8. Change gloves.
9. Place two precut drain dressings over catheter site, and tape dressing. ➤ *Rationale:* Secure dressings help to prevent infection at the site.
10. Remove gloves and perform hand hygiene.

Unit 22.9 Documentation and Evaluation

DOCUMENTATION for Home Care

Use Appropriate Home Care Documentation Forms.

- Client's assessment appropriate for skill; suprapubic catheter care and catheterization
- Peritoneal catheter site assessment

- Peritoneal dialysis site fluid assessment
- Complications associated with skill
- Client's response to interventions
- Ability of client and family to participate in skill

EVALUATION/Critical Thinking

Expected Outcomes

- Client's PD is efficient and promotes urinary waste removal.
- Client remains infection-free from catheterizations and catheter changes.
- Peritoneal catheter site remains infection-free.

Unexpected Outcomes	Alternative Actions
• Client's peritoneal catheter becomes occluded.	• Check tubing. • Raise bag to higher level above abdomen to increase the inflow. • Turn client to side-lying position to facilitate drainage. • Notify healthcare provider to check position of catheter, or fibrin can be occluding catheter. • Instruct client and family on specific positions and interventions to increase dialysis outflow.
• Vital signs are increased above normal.	• If BP is elevated, check for retention of dialysate solution in abdomen. • Temperature and pulse increase may be result of peritonitis. • Instruct client and family on how to promote sterile technique when assisting with dialysis.
• Client experiences respiratory distress.	• Increased respirations or distress are a result of increased pressure in peritoneal cavity. • Evaluate dialysate output.
• Client experiences constipation.	• This can be caused by inflow–outflow complications. • Administer stool softener or laxative.
• Client experiences CAUTIs.	• Determine whether client can urinate without catheter. • Promote toileting every 2 hr. • Use external condoms for men instead of indwelling catheters. • Use intermittent catheterization using sterile technique.

Chapter Wrap-Up

GERONTOLOGIC Considerations

Some changes in the urinary system that occur naturally with aging may be difficult to differentiate from pathologic processes.

Changes Seen With Aging

- Reduced activation of vitamin D results in decreased absorption of calcium from the gut.
- Reduction in glomerular filtration rate by 1 mL/min each year after age 40. The diabetic client loses 5 mL/min per year.
- Medications eliminated by the kidneys may require dosage modification; the older adult client should be monitored closely for signs of drug toxicity.
- Lower specific gravity of urine occurs due to decreased ability to concentrate urine; may cause **nocturia**.
- Any acute fluid loss may cause renal insufficiency.
- The bladder has reduced holding capacity, weaker smooth muscle contractility, and decreased sphincter tone, but lack of bladder control is *not* a normal part of aging.
- Urgency as well as urge **incontinence** and nocturia are common among all older adult clients due to decreased bladder capacity.
- In the older adult, postvoiding residual volume increases, but remains within the normal range, usually no more than 50 mL.
- Prostatic enlargement in men causes obstruction with resultant urinary retention, frequency, urgency, and UTIs.
- Reduced estrogen levels in women lead to atrophy of tissues that line and surround the urethra, bladder outlet, and vagina, contributing to urinary incontinence.
- Many older adults have coexistent urge and stress incontinence.
- Women may experience weakening of pelvic muscles, causing urethral shortening and urinary retention.

MANAGEMENT Guidelines

Each state legislates a Nurse Practice Act for RNs and LVN/LPNs. Healthcare facilities are responsible for establishing and implementing policies and procedures that conform to their state's regulations. Verify the regulations and role parameters for each healthcare worker in your facility.

Delegation

- Certified nursing assistants (CNAs) may document intake and output findings on bedside records. Some facilities allow CNAs to chart these findings on flow sheets. Check the facility policies and procedures regarding this.
- Unlicensed assistive personnel (UAP) may apply condom catheters and provide catheter care.
- UAP may perform the same tasks as the CNA. In addition, many states are allowing "clean" catheterization on clients requiring long-term procedures. It is advisable to check the policy and procedure manual to determine the tasks UAP may perform.
- Technicians may be trained to perform certain tasks in hemodialysis units. They may initiate the dialysis treatment and monitor clients while they are on dialysis but may not give medications or make nursing judgments.
- LVNs/LPNs may be assigned to clients with urinary diversion. They may change pouches and empty continent ileostomies.

Interprofessional Communication

- It is very important that all staff be informed about which clients require intake and output recordings. Families can also help out by writing down what their family member drinks while they are visiting.
- Healthcare team members should report any complaints of pain or discomfort from the client, as well as unusual odor, color, or abnormal findings from urinary catheter drainage systems.
- Urinary diversion pouches should be emptied when one-third full. If the facility policy does not allow ancillary personnel to complete this task, the nurse will instruct them to observe the amount of urine in the pouch and report when it needs to be emptied.

CASE STUDY Applications

Scenario 1

Your 55-year-old neighbor confides in you that every time she coughs or sneezes she loses urine. She asks if this is normal since so many of her friends have the same problem.

1. Describe various types and causes of urinary incontinence.

2. What lifestyle changes help to correct stress incontinence?

3. What noninvasive measures help to correct stress incontinence?

Scenario 2

Mrs. Christofferson, a 64-year-old female client, is a first-day postoperative client. She had a bowel resection yesterday.

The healthcare provider ordered her Foley catheter discontinued at 8 a.m. today. His additional order is to check for residual urine after her first voiding.

1. The client has not voided since the Foley catheter was removed 2 hr earlier. What is your priority nursing intervention?

2. The client voids 600 mL of urine 6 hr after the Foley catheter was removed. What further actions should the nurse take at this time?

3. Checking for residual urine, you obtain 120 mL of urine. What is your next intervention? What alternative action might you take if you suspect the client may exceed the normal amount of residual urine?

NCLEX® Review Questions

Unless otherwise specified, choose only one (1) answer.

1. To what is the amount of urine production directly related?
   A. Renal perfusion
   B. Fluid intake
   C. Bladder capacity
   D. Metabolic rate

2. A scanner is useful to reflect the client's bladder volume but is not reliable for assessing which of the following? *Select all that apply.*
   A. Obese clients
   B. Catheterized clients
   C. Clients with hysterectomy
   D. Pregnant clients
   E. Male clients
   F. Children

3. For male catheterization, how far is the catheter inserted?
   A. 5-10 cm (2–4 in.)
   B. 10-15 cm (4–6 in.)
   C. 15-20 cm (6–8 in.)
   D. 25-30 cm (10–12 in.)

4. For female catheterization, how far is the catheter inserted?
   A. 1.25 cm (0.5 in.)
   B. 5 cm (2 in.)
   C. 7.5 cm (3 in.)
   D. 10 cm (4 in.)

5. What does urine leakage in the client with a urinary retention catheter indicate?
   A. The need for a larger-size catheter
   B. The need for an additional 10 mL of water to be added to the indwelling balloon
   C. A possible urinary tract infection
   D. The ability now for the client to urinate normally

6. What are common causes of urinary tract infection associated with indwelling catheters? *Select all that apply.*
   A. Long-term use
   B. Break in aseptic technique
   C. Inadequate catheter stabilization
   D. Overfilled drainage bag
   E. Only using soap and water for perineal care
   F. Urine specimen sampling

7. What does continuous bladder irrigation (CBI) after prostate surgery help to prevent?
   A. Catheter obstruction
   B. Bladder infection
   C. Bladder spasms
   D. Postoperative bleeding

8. When applying a urinary diversion pouch, when should a protective barrier product be used?
   A. Only if absolutely necessary
   B. When the client has sensitive skin
   C. When pouch adherence must be ensured
   D. Only with a two-piece pouch

9. Which of the following is true about a client with end-stage renal disease?

    A. Has no functioning nephrons

    B. Receives renal replacement therapy

    C. Produces no urine

    D. Is uremic

10. The nurse is caring for a client who has a urinary catheter in place. Which of the following indicate that the client meets criteria for continuing with the Foley?

Select all that apply.

A. The client is incontinent and had a hip replacement.

B. The client has a stage III pressure ulcer on her coccyx and is incontinent.

C. The client is terminally ill and has less than 6 months to live and is incontinent.

D. The client had surgery 2 days ago for a knee replacement and is incontinent.

E. The client has acute urinary retention.

QSEN Activity

DOMAIN: Evidence-Based Practice

KSA: Integrate best current evidence with clinical expertise and client/family preferences and values for delivery of optimal health care.

Activity:

Objective: Participate in structuring the work environment to facilitate integration of new evidence into standards of practice.

You are working in a small community-based hospital that has had a problem with high rates of catheter-associated urinary tract infections (CAUTIs). You have been reading about the Centers for Disease Control (CDC) CAUTI Guidelines and prevention toolkits available on its website. You would like to work with your hospital administrators to develop a nurse-driven protocol to help nurses better identify appropriate indications for Foley catheter use and when to remove Foley catheters without needing to obtain healthcare provider orders every time. Put together a proposal using the information from the CDC and other evidence-based practice sites to develop a nurse-driven protocol to reduce CAUTI rates in your hospital.

Bibliography

Callahan, B. (Ed.). (2015). Clinical *nursing skills: A concept-based approach to learning*, Vol 3. (2nd ed.) Hoboken: Pearson.

Carter, N. M., Reitmeier, L., & Goodloe, L. R. (2014). An evidence-based approach to the prevention of catheter-associated urinary tract infections. *Urologic Nursing, 34*(5), 238–245.

Centers for Disease Control and Prevention. (2015). Healthcare-associated infections: Catheter-associated Urinary Tract Infections (CAUTI). Retrieved from http://www.cdc.gov/HAI/ca_uti/uti.html

Dailly, S. (2011). Prevention of indwelling catheter-associated urinary tract infections: Sue Dailly outlines best practice in caring for patients with urethral catheters and how staff can promote their removal. *Nursing Older People, 23*(2), 14–19.

Flasar, C. (2008, Jul.). What is urine specific gravity? *Nursing, 38*(7), 14.

Gould, C. V., Umscheid, C. A., Agarwal, R. K., Kuntz, G., & Pegues, D. A. (2009). Guideline for prevention of catheter-associated urinary tract infections. *Infection Control & Hospital Epidemiology, 31*(4), 319–326.

Johnson, C., Levey, A. S., Coresh, J., Levin, A., Lau, J., & Eknoyan, G. (2004). Clinical practice guidelines for chronic kidney disease in adults. Part I. Definition, disease stages, evaluation, treatment, and risk factors. *American Family Physician, 70*(5), 869–876.

LeMone, P., Burke, K., Dwyer, T., Levett-Jones, T., Moxham, L., Reid-Searl, K., ... & Raymond, D. (2013). *Medical-surgical nursing.* Hoboken, NJ: Pearson.

Linton, A. & Lach, H. (2007). *Matteson & McConnell's gerontological nursing: Concepts and practices* (3rd ed.). Philadelphia, PA: Saunders.

Mahoney, M., Baxter, K., Burgess, J., Bauer, C., Downey, C., Mantel, J., ... & Sheppard, S. (2013). Procedure for obtaining a urine sample from a urostomy, ileal conduit, and colon conduit: A best practice guideline for clinicians. *Journal of Wound Ostomy & Continence Nursing, 40*(3), 277–279.

Oman, K. S., Makic, M. B. F., Fink, R., Schraeder, N., Hulett, T., Keech, T., & Wald, H. (2012). Nurse-directed interventions to reduce catheter-associated urinary tract infections. *American Journal of Infection Control, 40*(6), 548–553.

Pyrek, K. (2010, Apr.). Catheter-related infection prevention: A review of the basics. *Infection Control Today, 14*(4), 30–32.

Recalla, S., English, K., Nazarali, R., Mayo, S., Miller, D., & Gray, M. (2013). Ostomy care and management: A systematic review. *Journal of Wound Ostomy & Continence Nursing, 40*(5), 489–500.

Saint, S., Olmsted, R. N., Fakih, M. G., Kowalski, C. P., Watson, S. R., Sales, A. E., & Krein, S. L. (2009). Translating health care–associated urinary tract infection prevention research into practice via the bladder bundle. *Joint Commission Journal on Quality and Patient Safety/Joint Commission Resources, 35*(9), 449.

Wilson, T. G., Guru, K., Rosen, R. C., Wiklund, P., Annerstedt, M., Bochner, B. H., ... & Catto, J. (2015). Best practices in robot-assisted radical cystectomy and urinary reconstruction: Recommendations of the Pasadena Consensus Panel. *European Urology, 67* (3): 363–375.

Wound Ostomy Nurses Society. (2013). Teen chat: You and your ostomy. Retrieved March 8, 2015 from http://c.ymcdn.com/sites/www.wocn.org/resource/resmgr/Publications/Teen_Chat_You_&_Your_Ostomy_.pdf?hhSearchTerms=%22ileal+and+conduit%22.

Chapter 23
Bowel Elimination

Learning Objectives

23.1 Explain both the mechanical and chemical aspects of digestion.

23.2 Compare and contrast hypermotility with hypomotility.

23.3 Discuss what is meant by obstruction of the bowel.

23.4 Describe the anatomic locations for an ileostomy, cecostomy, or colostomy.

23.5 List the components of a good bowel training program.

23.6 Outline the essential steps in administering a tap water or saline enema to an adult client.

23.7 Describe the precautions necessary when performing digital stimulation to remove a fecal impaction.

23.8 Compare and contrast stoma care of an ileostomy and a colostomy.

23.9 Outline the steps for developing a regular bowel routine.

23.10 Describe at least three interventions used when skin is denuded from leakage.

23.11 Describe at least three precautions necessary when applying a fecal ostomy pouch.

23.12 Discuss the corking and intubation procedure for a client with a continent ileostomy.

23.13 Describe the precautions necessary when using a rectal tube.

23.14 Distinguish clients who should have a rectal tube from those who should have a bowel management system (BMS) in place.

23.15 Compare and contrast nursing interventions for clients with alterations in bowel elimination in home care and hospital.

Chapter Outline

Terminology

Bowel the intestine.

Bowel movement the emptying of the intestinal tract.

Carminative having to do with an agent that removes gases from the gastrointestinal tract.

Cathartic a drug to induce emptying of the intestinal tract; a laxative.

Chyme the viscous, semifluid contents of the stomach present during digestion of a meal. Chyme then passes through the pylorus into the duodenum, where further digestion occurs.

Colitis inflammation of the colon.

Colon the large intestine, which extends from the cecum to the anus.

Colostomy an artificially created opening from the colon to the abdominal surface for the elimination of waste.

Constipation difficulty or straining in defecation and infrequent bowel movements over an extended period of time.

Defecation elimination of waste products of digestion from the body by evacuation of bowel.

Diarrhea the passage of unformed liquid stools.

Digestion the process by which food is broken down, mechanically and chemically, in the gastrointestinal tract.

Diverticulitis inflammation of diverticula in the intestinal tract causing stagnation of feces in the small, distended sacs (diverticula).

Dyssynergic defecation the result of pelvic floor dysfunction in the muscles and nerves within the pelvic floor, resulting in chronic constipation.

Emulsification the breaking down of large fat globules in the intestine to smaller, uniformly distributed particles.

Enema the introduction of fluid through a tube into the lower intestinal tract.

Fecal incontinence involuntary or inappropriate passing of liquid or solid stool.

Feces body wastes such as food residue, bacteria, epithelium, and mucus discharged from the bowels by way of the anus.

Fistula an abnormal tube-like passage from a normal cavity or tube to a free surface or another cavity.

Flaccid relaxed, flabby; having defective or absent muscle tone.

Flatulence excessive gas in the stomach and intestines.

Hemorrhoids abnormally distended rectal veins caused by congestion in the veins of the rectal venous plexus.

Hypermotility unusually quick motility or movement in the gastrointestinal tract.

Hyperreflexia increased action of reflexes.

Hypertonic having a higher osmotic pressure than normal body fluid.

Hypomotility unusually slow motility of the gastrointestinal tract.

Ileostomy an artificially created opening from the ileum to the abdominal surface for the elimination of wastes.

Impaction condition of being tightly wedged into a place, such as tight wedging of feces in the bowel.

Laxative a mild-acting drug to induce emptying of the intestinal tract.

Mucosa mucous membrane.

Necrosis death of areas of tissue or bone caused by enzymatic action or lack of circulation.

Obstipation severe obstruction of the normal flow of feces through the bowel.

Occluded blocked off, obstructed.

Occult blood blood in such minute quantities that it can only be detected by a microscope or chemical means.

Ostomy a surgically formed artificial opening that serves as an exit site for the bowel or intestine.

Parasite an organism that lives within, on, or at the expense of another organism known as the host.

Perforation the act or process of making a hole, such as that caused by an ulcer.

Peristalsis a progressive wave-like movement that occurs involuntarily, as in the gastrointestinal tract.

Reflux a return of or backward flow.

Sphincter circular band of muscle fiber constricting a natural orifice.

Stoma an artificially created opening between two passages or between a passage and the body surface.

Stool waste matter discharged from the bowels.

Suppository semisolid substance for introduction into the rectum, vagina, or urethra, where it dissolves; serves as a vehicle for medicines to be absorbed.

Villi short filamentous processes found on certain membranous surfaces.

Anatomy and Physiology

The gastrointestinal system converts food into products that can be used as nutrients on the cellular level and disposes of wastes incurred in the process. The primary structures in this system include the mouth, esophagus, stomach, small intestine, and large intestine (Figure 23-1 ■).

The mouth, esophagus, and stomach are the structures of the upper gastrointestinal tract, where the process of digestion begins. The small intestine, where digestion is completed and most absorption takes place, is a 12-foot tube composed of the duodenum, jejunum, and ileum. The large intestine is made up of the cecum, **colon**, and rectum. The cecum contains the ileocecal valve and the appendix. The colon is divided into the ascending, transverse, descending, and sigmoid colon. The rectum extends from the sigmoid colon to the anus. The terminal end of the rectum is called the anal canal and is guarded by the internal and external **sphincter** muscles. The chief functions of the colon are to reabsorb water and sodium and to store wastes.

Digestion is accomplished mechanically and chemically. Food is mechanically churned through the intestinal tract by sharp contractions, or peristaltic waves, of the circular and longitudinal muscles of the intestinal wall. Muscular sphincters and valves are located at strategic points throughout the intestinal tract. These structures help propel the food bolus or feces at appropriately timed intervals in a process called rhythmic segmentation. The sphincters and valves, when functioning properly, prevent **reflux** of contents. Peristaltic waves, coupled with rhythmic segmentation, allow maximal contact between food and the bowel wall so that chemical reactions can accomplish digestion and absorption can take place.

The chemical aspects of digestion in the small intestine begin in the duodenum with the introduction of pancreatic juices and bile. Pancreatic juices are rich in enzymes, which work to break down proteins and fats and to complete the transformation of starch to sugar. Bile, secreted from the liver, aids in the **emulsification** and absorption of fats. These substances work in an alkaline medium that combines with the acidity of **chyme** to provide a neutral pH in the duodenum, thereby protecting the duodenal **mucosa**.

In the 20 feet of jejunum and ileum, approximately 3,000 mL of digestive enzymes are secreted. These enzymes, which are secreted by the mucus glands of the **bowel** (intestines), complete the digestive processing of food before absorption. Again, the alkaline nature of these secretions works to protect the mucous membrane of the intestinal tract.

The peristaltic activity of the gastrointestinal tract, as well as its secretory functions, is governed, to a large degree, by parasympathetic and sympathetic nerve fibers. Stimulation of the parasympathetic system increases the activity of the intestinal tract, while stimulation of the sympathetic nervous system inhibits activity in the tract. The internal anal sphincter, however, is activated by sympathetic stimulation, whereas the external anal sphincter is under voluntary control.

Absorption, another primary function of the small bowel, is the passage of prepared materials from the gastrointestinal lumen to the blood and cells. Most absorption in the small intestine results from the churning action of the bowel. Chyme is continually exposed to the circular folds of the mucosal surface, which is lined with thread-like projections called **villi**. Villi serve as the sites of absorption of fluid and nutrients. The duration of contact between chyme and the mucosal surface of the bowel is very important in absorption. **Hypermotility** in the small intestine can result in decreased contact with the mucosal wall and deficient absorption; **hypomotility** can result in increased absorption of fluids, as well as problems with elimination.

The circulatory system delivers nutrients to tissue cells and transports the waste products of metabolism. Arterial circulation to the small bowel and colon is via the superior and inferior mesenteric arteries. Blood that contains absorbed nutrients is carried from the gastrointestinal tract by the superior and inferior mesenteric veins, which become a part of the portal system delivering blood to the liver. Each villus on the intestinal wall contains a network of small capillaries, which absorb sugar and amino acids, and a central lymph channel, which absorbs fatty acids and glycerol. When circulation is compromised, absorption is decreased and cells are lost.

By the time chyme reaches the ileocecal valve—the junction between the small and large intestines—most nutrients have been absorbed. Whereas 3 L of fluid passes through the small bowel, only 500 mL actually passes through the ileocecal valve. The semiliquid material received by the large intestine consists of living and dead bacteria, undigested food and residue, and cell debris. As residue is slowly passed along the colon by peristaltic mass movements, fluid is absorbed. These movements occur relatively infrequently (perhaps two or three times per day) and are stimulated by the entrance of food into the stomach by the gastrocolic reflex.

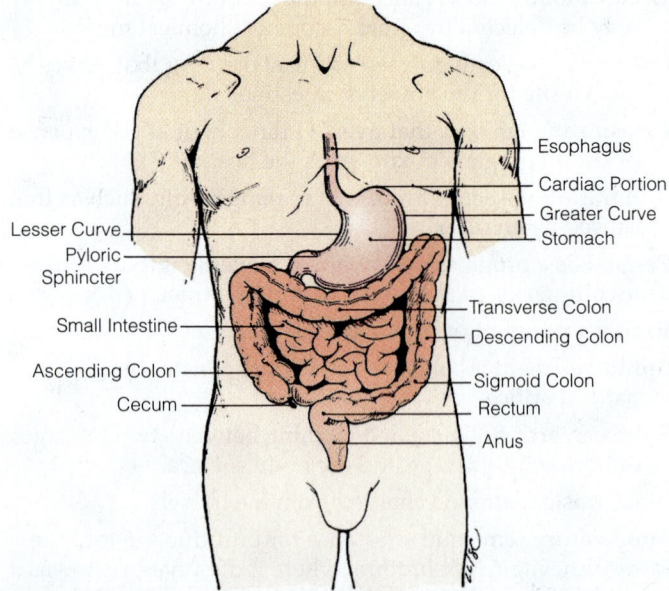

Lesser Curve
Pyloric Sphincter
Small Intestine
Ascending Colon
Cecum

Esophagus
Cardiac Portion
Greater Curve
Stomach
Transverse Colon
Descending Colon
Sigmoid Colon
Rectum
Anus

FIGURE 23-1 Anatomy of the gastrointestinal tract.

Absorption of fluid in the colon takes place primarily in the ascending and transverse colon. Fecal masses are stored in the sigmoid colon and move into the rectum with mass peristaltic movement. When the rectum fills and becomes sufficiently distended, centers in the sacral area of the spinal cord facilitate a defecation reflex, which contracts the rectum and relaxes the internal and external anal sphincters. The resulting urge, facilitated by the autonomic nervous system, leads to contraction of the abdominal, perineal, and diaphragmatic muscles. Willful defecation is a coordinated, learned habit. Voluntary inhibition of the act returns the stool to the sigmoid colon.

Defecation

Defecation is defined as elimination of waste products of digestion from the body by evacuation of the bowel. Excreted waste products are termed **feces** or **stool**. The pattern of defecation varies with each individual. It can occur from several times each day to two or three times each week. The type and amount of stool evacuated is also individualized. It is determined by such factors as diet and normal changes in the intestinal flora. Additional factors that influence bowel patterns include age, fluid intake, exercise, psychological factors, alterations in lifestyle, and medications.

For healthy bowel elimination, the client needs to have sufficient bulk (cellulose and fiber) to produce adequate fecal volume. Daily fluid intake of 2,000–3,000 mL is essential to maintain a soft stool for easy elimination, as well as to promote adequate urine output. Food intake at specified times and food that does not produce **flatulence** are also important for healthy elimination. Daily exercise stimulates peristaltic activity, facilitating **bowel movement**.

Normal feces are composed of about 75% water and 25% solid material. The stool is soft, but formed, and the color ranges from light to dark brown. The color of the stool is due to the presence of stercobilin and urobilin, derived from bilirubin. In the absence of bile pigment, the stool takes on a characteristically clay-colored or white appearance. The action of bacteria in the colon plays a role in the color of the stool. Ingestion of certain foods, drugs, and vitamins can alter the color and consistency of the stool. The nurse must complete an accurate bowel history to determine normal or abnormal findings. Conclusions should not be made on observation alone. Iron supplements, vitamins with iron, beets, red peppers, licorice, grape juice, and spinach affect the color of the stool, which could lead to an incorrect conclusion of blood in the stool. Feces that are red or black in color can be a direct result of ingestion of these foods. Medications can also affect the color and consistency of the stool. In addition to consistency and distinct color of the feces, there is an odor associated with the feces. The odor is a result of the action of microorganisms on the chyme.

Abnormal characteristics of feces include the presence of exudate, a **parasite**, fat, and large amounts of mucus. Large amounts of mucus are generally associated with an inflammatory process of the bowel. The stool appears slimy in this condition. Diseases, such as ulcerative **colitis** or Crohn's disease, produce a stool with large amounts of pus when inflammation is present. Stools with abnormally high fat content are foul-smelling and float to the top of the water. Children with cystic fibrosis commonly produce this type of stool.

Constipation

Constipation is not a well-defined disease entity but rather a general term used to describe the difficulties that clients experience with moving their bowels. The prevalence of constipation increases with age, especially after 65 years of age. Among older adult clients living in the community, the prevalence of constipation is 50%. The number is even higher in nursing home residents, with 74% of these residents using daily laxatives (Toner, 2012). Older women are two to three times more likely to report constipation, and clients taking multiple medications are more affected.

Because many factors influence the development of constipation, it is not well defined. The management of constipation is also individualized according to each client's needs. Loss of mobility, medications, underlying diseases, impaired anorectal sensation, and ignoring the urge to defecate are as important as **dyssynergic defecation** or irritable bowel syndrome in causing constipation.

There are two types of constipation: acute and chronic. Acute constipation is usually managed with a **suppository**, enema, or osmotic **laxative** to clear the rectum. A bowel program is generally indicated after the initial treatment to include modification of the diet and fluid intake, as well as education about bowel habits.

Chronic constipation requires the use of bulk-forming agents if the client has a low dietary fiber and no specific underlying cause for the constipation. Osmotic agents may be effective for immediate results, but the goal of the bowel management is to establish regular bowel habits, using only small doses of laxatives.

In addition to medical conditions, general anesthetics block parasympathetic stimulation to the colon, leading to potential constipation.

Bowel (Fecal) Incontinence

Normal bowel function is based on the client having functioning muscles and nerves, a healthy bowel structure and tissues, normal bowel organisms, proper diet, adequate fluids, and physical activity.

Bowel incontinence can occur when any of these factors are not functioning properly. It can also be caused by disease, injury, stress, poor elimination habits, and side effects of medications. Structure and functional changes as a result of aging can result in bowel incontinence. Structural changes include rectal prolapse, surgical interventions of the bowel, colectomy, and prostate or rectal surgery. Functional causes are often related to an individual's lifestyle or behaviors.

These causes may be related to medication effects or nerve damage. Common causes include severe diarrhea, leakage due to chronic constipation, stress, chronic laxative use, and general functional damage from a stroke or other debilitating condition.

Several medical tests are used to determine the cause of **fecal incontinence**. Before interventions are discussed, it is imperative that the etiology of the condition be determined. Examples of common tests include proctoscopy, ultrasonography, electromyography, and colonoscopy.

An older approach, the placement of a rectal tube, is not encouraged because of major trauma to the anus and surrounding tissue with prolonged use. There are newer treatments available for treating bowel incontinence. A surgical procedure is also available, which inserts an inflatable artificial sphincter in clients who have incontinence caused by a sphincter dysfunction or injury.

The new systems are used for long-term fecal diversion for clients with associated conditions such as skin breakdown, wounds or grafts in danger of contamination, or immobilized clients. The BMS system can be in place up to 29 days without removing and changing the catheter.

Alterations in Elimination

By-products of digestion must be continually eliminated to maintain normal body function. Alterations in normal elimination can result from changes in motility, obstruction of the lumen of the bowel, circulatory deficiencies, disease process, and surgically induced alterations to the structures of the intestinal tract.

Changes in Motility

Normal motility of the bowel provides peristaltic activity that pushes and churns food and chyme through the upper tract and feces through the lower tract at timed intervals.

Hypermotility may be caused by direct stimulation or irritation of the autonomic nervous system, as well as by inflammatory processes in the gastrointestinal tract. Stimulation of parasympathetic nerves promotes **peristalsis** and increases bowel muscle tone. Increased peristalsis speeds the propulsion of chyme through the upper tract, resulting in deficient absorption of nutrients. When increased peristalsis speeds the propulsion of feces through the lower tract, **diarrhea** occurs.

Stimulation of the autonomic nervous system may be psychic in origin. Anxiety, for example, may be mediated through either parasympathetic nerves, with resultant diarrhea, or through sympathetic nerves, with resultant constipation. The action on the parasympathetic nervous system of certain drugs may also cause hypermotility of the intestine. Antihypertensive drugs, such as reserpine, and cholinergic drugs can cause diarrhea by their stimulation of parasympathetic nerves.

Hypermotility caused by the stimulating effect of an irritant on intestinal peristalsis may arise from infectious agents, chemical agents, or inflammatory disease processes. The most common intestinal irritants are the products of certain bacteria that release toxins in the digestive tract. Chemical agents that irritate the intestinal mucosa include cytotoxic drugs, castor oil, and quinidine. Ulcerative and inflammatory disease processes include **diverticulitis**, tuberculous lesions, ulcerative colitis, and Crohn's disease.

Hypomotility may be caused by direct stimulation or blockage of the autonomic nervous system, intestinal muscle weakness, and chemical agents that inhibit peristalsis and induce flaccidity in the intestinal tract. Decreased peristalsis causes chyme to move sluggishly through the upper tract so that fluids are overabsorbed. Decreased peristalsis also slows the propulsion of feces through the lower tract and causes constipation, fecal **impaction**, and obstruction.

Stimulation or blockage of the autonomic nervous system may be congenital in origin, as is the case in Hirschsprung 's disease, where the absence of parasympathetic nerve ganglia results in failure of peristalsis of the affected portion of the bowel. The effects of trauma or toxins on autonomic innervation of the intestine, which occur with paralytic (adynamic) ileus, inhibit motility to the point of obstruction.

Intestinal muscle weakness that results from disease processes, old age, or a lack of essential vitamins (notably the B group) or electrolytes (particularly potassium) may all contribute to hypomotility. Certain drugs, such as codeine and morphine, can also cause hypomotility by relaxing the smooth muscles of the digestive tract and by increasing spasms of the intestinal sphincters.

Obstruction of the Lumen of the Bowel

Obstruction of the lumen of the bowel may be partial or complete. The severity of the obstruction depends on the region of the bowel that is affected, the degree to which the lumen is **occluded**, and the degree to which the circulation in the bowel wall is disturbed.

A small bowel obstruction that occurs as a consequence of persistent vomiting (reverse peristalsis) can cause severe disturbances in the electrolyte balance of the body. Large bowel obstructions, even if complete, are not as dramatic, provided that the blood supply to the colon is not disturbed.

The causes of intestinal obstruction are varied. In rare instances, obstruction may result when a foreign body, such as a large fruit stone or a mass of parasitic worms, becomes lodged in the bowel. Intestinal obstruction is more frequently caused by strictures, adhesions, hernias, volvulus, intussusception, polyps, neoplasms, and fecal impaction.

The physiology of an obstruction in the lumen of the bowel is generally the same, regardless of cause. As the lumen of the bowel is blocked, the body attempts to overcome the obstruction by increasing peristalsis. During this process, liquid feces move past the site of obstruction and cause diarrhea and increased obstruction, which leads to constipation. Within several hours peristalsis is reduced, and the bowel becomes **flaccid**. As intraluminal pressure builds up, fluid is retained, and absorption decreases. The increased intraluminal pressure then leads to the compression of the bowel wall and its capillaries, which causes **necrosis** of the bowel wall.

Circulatory Deficiencies

An adequate circulatory flow is essential for maintaining the structure of the bowel and for carrying on cellular nutrition. Any interruption of the arterial blood supply inhibits the bowel function. An occlusion of the circulatory flow, also called an intestinal infarction, results in gangrene of the bowel unless surgical intervention is carried out. A partial occlusion of the mesenteric arteries due to atherosclerosis can cause intestinal angina, a condition that occurs when the blood supply is increasingly interrupted.

Surgically Induced Alterations in Bowel Elimination

When alterations in bowel elimination become life-threatening and medical management fails, surgical intervention becomes necessary. Potential complications of surgical intervention are described in Box 23-1 ■. Diversionary surgical procedures of the bowel include cecostomy, ileostomy, and colostomy.

An **ostomy** may be temporary or permanent, depending on the etiology (Figure 23-2 ■). The most common indication for a permanent ostomy is low cancer of the rectum or advanced metastatic cancer involving the colon. A temporary ostomy is usually created with the intent of reconnecting it in the future. The anatomy of the GI system is left intact. Many of these ostomies are done as an emergency. The temporary ostomy may be performed because a bowel prep could not be done due to obstruction or **perforation**, or to protect a distal surgery of the colon. Reversal, or reanastomosis, can be done at a later time when infection is unlikely and healing can take place. **Ileostomy** and **colostomy** are the most frequent type of fecal diversion. Today, both of these ostomies can be reversed as long as the anatomy of the GI system is left intact. Children with certain congenital intestinal disorders may require an ostomy. These are

FIGURE 23-2 A sigmoid colostomy. An ileostomy.

usually temporary and reversed once the child reaches a certain weight.

A cecostomy is a surgically created opening from the cecum through the abdominal wall. This procedure is a quick and temporary method to decompress the right side of the colon. This is usually done with the insertion of a catheter into the colon. This catheter requires frequent irrigation to ensure patency. If stool leaks around the site, a pouch should be applied to collect the output.

An ileostomy is a surgically created opening from the terminal ileum through the abdominal wall. The entire large intestine is bypassed or removed. Permanent ileostomies are usually performed on clients with Crohn's disease of the entire large intestine and those clients with a weakened rectal sphincter, which would leak stool if a pull-through procedure was performed. The stoma is smaller than the colostomy stoma as it is formed by the small intestine. The tip of the small intestine is brought to the skin's surface and folded back on itself. The stoma size is about the size of a quarter or half-dollar. The effluent has a pastelike consistency, although it can be more liquid if fluid intake is abnormally high.

In recent years, new surgical procedures have eliminated many permanent ileostomies. Clients with polyposis or ulcerative colitis may choose to have a continent ileostomy or Kock Continent Ileostomy or Kock pouch, an internal reservoir of the ileum constructed at the rectum (Figure 23-3 ■). The Kock reservoir consists of an internal pouch with two limbs of the ileum, one forming an internal valve. Continence occurs as a result of the stool collecting in the internal pouch. The pouch must be intubated four to six times a day to evacuate the stool. The rectal reservoir is created by joining the ileum to the anus after the colon is removed. The client will have 4–10 stools a day and must have good sphincter control. Any of the surgeries that remove or bypass the large intestine produce a soft-to-watery effluent that contains water and many digestive enzymes that have not yet been absorbed by intestinal villi. The daily output varies from 500 to 2,000 mL.

Another type of continent internal reservoir is the Barnett Continent Intestinal Reservoir (BCIR) shown in Figure 23-4 ■. The pouch is made from the ileum, the last segment of the small intestine. A self-sealing valve

Box 23-1 POTENTIAL POSTOPERATIVE COMPLICATIONS

- Hemorrhage
- Shock
- Thrombophlebitis
- Pulmonary embolism
- Sepsis
- Paralytic ileus
- Intestinal obstruction (**obstipation**)
- Impaired intestinal absorptive capability
- Leaky anastomosis
- **Stoma** necrosis

Total Proctocolectomy with Kock Pouch

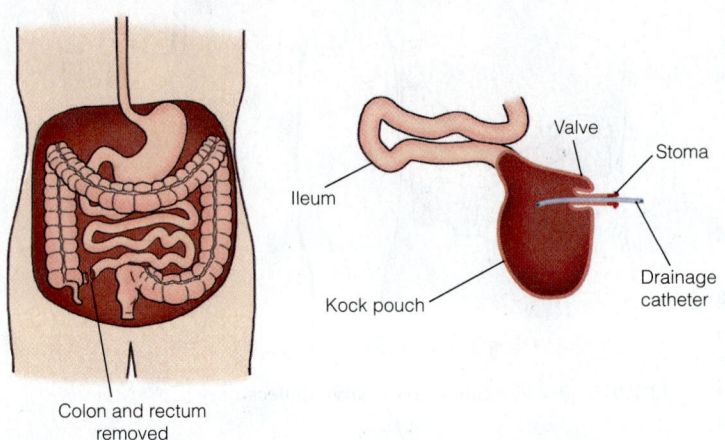

FIGURE 23-3 Kock pouch.
Source: Alila Medical Media

FIGURE 23-4 Barnett Continent Intestinal Reservoir.

mechanism and "living collar" is constructed from the intestine, which prevents leaking from the pouch. The pouch stores liquid waste and is drained several times each day using a small catheter. The catheter is inserted through the opening on the abdomen into the pouch. The pouch holds about 1,000 mL a few months following surgery. The advantage of the Barnett pouch stoma is that, unlike the conventional ileostomy, it does not need to be situated above the skin to form a spout. The stoma is flush with the skin, and no appliance is needed. It is placed just above the pubic hairline to the right of midline. There are no clothing restrictions and there is no bulge. The major problem with the continent ileostomy is the potential need for additional surgery due to a slipped nipple valve or a **fistula**. If a slipped valve occurs, it requires a revision to restore normal pouch function. Other potential problems are difficulty inserting the drainage catheter and leakage of gas or waste out of the stoma opening.

A colostomy is a surgically created opening from the colon through the abdominal wall and can be created using any segment of the large intestine. With a colostomy, the diseased portion of the colon is bypassed or removed and a portion of healthy colon is brought to the outside of the abdomen to form a stoma. The type of stoma is named after the segment of bowel used to form the stoma; most colostomies are sigmoid colostomies. The type of output from the stoma is determined by how far to the right side of the colon the stoma is placed. See Table 23-1 ■ for a comparison of ostomies.

The most common surgery performed for cancer of the colon is a low anterior resection. In this procedure, a wide excision of the tumor and surrounding lymph nodes is made and the remaining colon is reconnected. The client may have a diverting ostomy proximal to the resected area to protect the surgical site from leakage.

Abdominal–perineal resections with permanent *sigmoid colostomy* are usually done only when the tumor is located too low in the rectum for the client to maintain continence. Output from colostomies on the left side of the intestine

will eventually become formed and firm, since most of the water has been absorbed by the time the feces reaches these portions of the colon.

A *descending colostomy* is usually temporary. It is seen frequently in children with congenital disorders. Adults may have a descending colostomy after trauma or severe diverticulitis when perforation is present.

A *transverse colostomy* can be located anywhere along the transverse colon. It is also usually temporary and is done for either a bowel obstruction or perforation.

Colostomies can also be named for the way they are constructed. A *loop colostomy* is a very quick surgical procedure to exteriorize the bowel (Figure 23-5 ■ A and B). A loop of intestine is brought out to the surface of the abdomen and some type of plastic bridge is placed under the loop to prevent it from falling back inside the abdomen. This bridge is left in place for 7–14 days until the abdominal wall has sealed.

A *double-barrel colostomy* is one that has two stomas. One is the proximal or functional stoma. The second is the distal stoma that connects the remaining stoma and rectum. In any of the surgeries that leave the rectum intact, the client can expect to pass any old stool remaining from before surgery, plus mucus produced by the lining of the intestine on an ongoing basis.

An *end colostomy* has only one stoma, which originates from the proximal portion of the bowel. The distal end of the colon is either resected or is closed off with sutures and remains in the abdomen. This can also be called a Hartman's procedure. All of these ostomies can be reversed once the distal site is healed and an adequate bowel prep can be done.

Another type of colostomy is the Pelvic Pouch or Ileo-Anal Pull-through, better known as the *J Pouch, S Pouch,* or *W Pouch,* depending on the stoma location in the intestine.

Table 23-1 Comparison Chart for Ostomies

Colostomy	Ileostomy
Etiologic Factors	
Cancer of colon	Ulcerative colitis
Traumatic or congenital disruption of intestinal tract	Crohn's disease (regional ileitis)
Diverticulitis	Birth defects Trauma Protect distal surgery Distal obstruction
Surgical Procedure	
Portion of colon brought through abdominal wall	Portion of ileum brought through abdominal wall
Bowel Control	
Sigmoid—Sometimes	None
Ascending—No	
Stool Consistency	
Sigmoid—Formed	Liquid to semisoft
Ascending—Semiformed	
Irrigation for Bowel Control	
Sigmoid or descending colon, but rarely used	No
Use of Appliance	
Yes, use nondrainable, but only if evacuation pattern is not achieved	Yes
Nursing Care Priorities	
Maintain skin integrity a. Keep skin clean and dry b. Provide skin barrier c. Ensure proper fit of appliance	Same as colostomy
Fluid Requirement	
Sigmoid—Normal intake	8–10 glasses per day
Transverse—8–10 glasses per day	
Diet Control	
Avoid gas-forming foods	Same as colostomy
Eat odor-forming foods in moderation	
Chew food well	
Medications	
Sigmoid—none	Same as colostomy
Transverse—Avoid enteric-coated meds	B_{12}
May need Na replacement	
Vitamins, especially K, minerals	
Psychosocial	
Promote self-image	Same as colostomy
Refer to an ostomy support group	

In this type of colostomy, there is no external stoma. An internal pouch is constructed from the rectum, allowing waste products to accumulate before being expelled in the normal manner, although bowel movements will be more watery and more frequent than usual. The client is not a candidate for this pouch procedure if the rectum is too diseased and the anal sphincter muscle was removed. The J Pouch is also not recommended for clients with Crohn's disease, as the disease can return and infect the pouch, requiring its removal.

FIGURE 23-5 A. Loop colostomy with rod. A loop of bowel is brought onto the abdomen and is supported by a plastic rod. **B.** Loop colostomy with rod removed 7–14 days after surgery, when the abdominal wall has sealed. Two openings are made in the colostomy. The proximal loop is functional and discharges fecal material. The distal end is nonfunctional and discharges only mucus.

Clients usually reestablish bowel habits similar to those they had before surgery. Colostomy irrigations are *not commonly used* today to establish regularity of bowel elimination. Some clients may perform daily irrigations; however, irrigations are *always contraindicated* in clients with unstable fluid and electrolyte balance and in those clients in whom vagal stimulation is dangerous. Irrigations are *also contraindicated* when clients are receiving radiation therapy or are experiencing chemotherapy-induced diarrhea.

Adaptation for Home Care

The actual care of clients requiring interventions for altered bowel elimination is basically the same for home care clients as hospitalized clients. Equipment may be slightly different, but it is similar enough to make it easy to teach clients and family members to perform the skills.

A major responsibility of the nurse is to provide client and family education in the care and management of the ostomy, bowel elimination interventions (see Box 23-2), and **enema** administration. At the time of discharge from the hospital, most clients and family members need support in the management of an ostomy. The home care nurse will not only need to demonstrate and evaluate the performance and outcome of the ostomy care, but will also need to provide emotional support.

It is important for the nurse to discuss dietary requirements for clients with an ostomy. Some foods are restricted because they are not completely digested and could cause blockage at the stoma opening. This is most common for clients with an ileostomy. Nuts, seeds, popcorn, raisins, dried fruit, and coconut are among the most common. Certain foods also can cause odors and should not be eaten. These include yogurt, bananas, cranberry juice, applesauce, sticky white rice, buttermilk, and white toast. Other foods to be limited in order to make it easier to manage a colostomy include: raw vegetables; dairy products; very high-fiber foods such as wheat bran cereal and breads, beans, peas, lentils, corn, brown and wild rice; sweets such as cakes, pies, and cookies; and high-fat and fried foods such as fried chicken or sausage.

Cultural Awareness

When providing nursing care for clients requiring an intervention for bowel elimination, remember that many cultures are very modest and do not like to talk about elimination issues. Privacy during the procedure and a respectful approach are critical for all clients, in order for them to feel comfortable with the task that needs to be completed. Some cultures have greater concerns than most. For example, Chinese Americans may request to use the toilet and not a bedpan. Arab Americans may prefer to wash rather than use toilet paper after every urination and bowel movement and may insist on using a bidet to wash. Muslims may require additional bathing rituals.

Nursing Diagnoses

The following nursing diagnoses may be appropriate to use on client care plans when the components are related to alterations in bowel elimination.

NURSING DIAGNOSIS	RELATED TO . . .
Disturbed Body Image	Presence of stoma, fear of rejection, psychosocial factors (loss of body contiguity related to operative procedure such as colostomy, ileostomy)
Constipation, Risk for	Inadequate intake of fluid or bulk, decreased exercise, disease states, medication, personal habits
Diarrhea	Nutritional intake, medication, disease state
Deficient Fluid Volume	Effluent from ileostomy is watery to semisoft; excessive use of enemas or laxatives
Ineffective Health Maintenance	Cognitive impairment, depression, immobility, cultural beliefs, lack of social support
Deficient Knowledge	Inability to manage ostomy, constipation
Noncompliance	Inability to manage equipment, impaired manual dexterity, poor vision
Impaired Skin Integrity	Skin irritation or breakdown, poor pouching techniques, incontinence or diarrhea, poor-fitting equipment, economic situation

---

Nursing Process Data

ASSESSMENT Database

- Assess for symptoms indicating presence of impaction: nausea; headache; abdominal pain; malaise, abdominal distention, or bloating.
- Evaluate client's diet:
  Amount of high-bulk foods
  Amount of fluid intake daily
- Evaluate client's physical status:
  Extent of physical exercise performed daily
  Ability to ambulate (i.e., spinal cord injury, CVA)
  Ability to perform bed exercises, abdominal exercises
  Extent of disease process
  Medications routinely taken
- Assess effectiveness of drugs, such as stool softeners, bulk formers, and suppositories.
- Assess time of day client usually evacuates bowels and any changes in normal routine.
- Identify client's ability to adapt and psychological readiness for the above program.
- Identify position most effective for bowel evacuation.
- Assess consistency and amount of stool for abnormal findings (diarrhea, fecal impaction, thin, pencil-like stool, or blood in stool).
- Assess when client had last bowel movement.
- Assess perianal area for tears, ulcerations, or excoriation.
- Assess for fecal contamination of wounds or grafts.
- Assess for postoperative constipation.
- Assess the need for colostomy irrigation for home care client.

PLANNING Objectives

- To promote regular bowel evacuation
- To prevent constipation
- To promote removal of flatulence
- To remove a fecal impaction
- To promote colostomy evacuation at same time each day
- To establish a bowel program to which the client can easily adapt
- To develop a bowel program that the client can perform him- or herself
- To prevent skin breakdown or wound contamination from fecal incontinence
- To manage stool elimination for clients with mobility issues
- To relieve pain and discomfort

IMPLEMENTATION Procedures

DOCUMENTATION AND EVALUATION

Expected Outcomes

- Client establishes regular bowel evacuation program.
- Constipation is prevented.
- Fecal impaction is removed.
- Client is able to evacuate bowel at a convenient and consistent time.
- Client is free of pain, flatus, and discomfort.
- Digital stimulation is performed without cardiac complications.
- Rectal tube insertion relieves flatus.
- Colostomy irrigation promotes routine daily bowel evacuation.

Unexpected Outcomes/Alternative Actions

Pearson Nursing Student Resources

Find additional review materials at
nursing.pearsonhighered.com.
Prepare for success with NCLEX®-style practice questions and Skill Checklists.

Skill 23.1.1 | Providing Assistive Digital Evacuation

Equipment
Clean gloves, 2 or 3 pairs
Water-soluble lubricant
Absorbent pad
Washcloth and towel
Bath blanket
Bedpan
Basin of warm water

Preparation
1. Check physician's order for impaction removal if the client is at risk for possible complications from vagal stimulation (i.e., cardiac or spinal cord–injured client). ➤ *Rationale:* Vagal stimulation can result from manual removal of feces. It should be used only as a last resort and with specific physician's order. It causes a decreased pulse rate by decreasing conductivity at the sinoatrial (S-A) node and decreasing the rate of impulse firing at the node.
2. Gather equipment.
3. Introduce yourself, identify the client using two forms of identification, and explain procedure.
4. Provide privacy.
5. Perform hand hygiene.

Note: An oil retention enema may be used before removing the impaction. ➤ *Rationale:* It helps soften and lubricate stool.

Procedure
1. Obtain baseline pulse and blood pressure.
2. Place client on left side with knees flexed. ➤ *Rationale:* Positioning on left side allows easier access to sigmoid colon.
3. Place absorbent pad on bed. Cover client with bath blanket.
4. Place bedpan next to client's buttocks.
5. Don gloves, and lubricate fingers of dominant hand. You may want to double-glove dominant hand to prevent contamination if glove tears.
6. Ask client to take a slow, deep breath and exhale slowly through the mouth as your index finger is gently inserted into rectum moving toward the umbilicus. ➤ *Rationale:* Encouraging breathing assists in relaxing the sphincter.

> **CLINICAL ALERT**
> Removal of fecal impaction is usually performed in small steps to reduce the risk of injury to the rectal tissue. A series of suppositories may be given between manual removal attempts to assist in clearing the bowel.

> **CLINICAL ALERT**
> Due to risk factors, manual evacuation should be considered an acute intervention, not a regular intervention. Stimulation of rectum could result in excessive stimulation of the vagal nerve in the rectal wall with subsequent autonomic **hyperreflexia.** Other risk factors include rectal trauma or perforation, rectal bleeding, and history of abuse.

7. Gently massage around stool and remove the hardened stool by working the forefinger into and around the mass to break it up. ➤ *Rationale:* Smaller pieces allow for easier expulsion of stool.
8. Allow client to rest between digital removal if any untoward effects, such as palpitations or faintness, are exhibited.
9. Obtain vital signs if client complains of any discomfort.
10. Provide hygienic care, as needed.
11. When stool is removed, change gloves; wash and dry buttocks thoroughly.
12. Dispose of stool in toilet or send stool specimen to laboratory.

> **CLINICAL ALERT**
> Even though manual evacuation of stool is considered within the scope of practice for a registered nurse, nurses receive little or no training to perform the procedure. At a minimum, the practitioner should:
>
> - Be knowledgeable about the anatomy and physiology of the lower rectum.
> - Demonstrate awareness of common perineal and anal conditions.
> - Be able to discuss constipation management options.
> - Utilize critical synthesis of evidence-based practice and relevant literature.
> - Demonstrate professional accountability.

13. Clean bedpan and replace in appropriate area.
14. Remove gloves and perform hand hygiene.
15. Position client for comfort.
16. Perform hand hygiene.
17. Follow physician's orders for administering a cleansing enema or inserting a suppository. ➤ *Rationale:* These procedures will assist in the removal of any remaining feces.
18. Instruct client in management of simple constipation, if appropriate. Include diet, exercise, and laxatives or stool softeners.

Skill 23.1.2 | Providing Digital Stimulation

Equipment
Bath blanket (optional)
Clean gloves, 1 or 2 pairs
Lubricant
Bedpan or commode
Absorbent pad
Washcloth and towel
Medication if ordered
Toilet tissue

Procedure
1. Check physician's orders and client care plan. Determine client's usual bowel habits and time of evacuation.
2. Perform hand hygiene.
3. Gather equipment.
4. Identify client using two identifiers, introduce yourself, and explain the procedure.
5. Provide privacy and place absorbent pad on bed as necessary.
6. Place client in position in the bed for bowel evacuation (bedpan in place). Place client in either left or right lateral position (if on right side, sigmoid is uppermost) and assist with feces removal.
7. Place bath blanket over client if appropriate.
8. Don gloves, and lubricate fingers of nondominant hand. You may want to double-glove to prevent contamination if gloves tear. ➤ *Rationale:* Lubrication reduces resistance by fingers moving through anal sphincter.

9. Insert finger into rectum 3.5–5 cm (1.5–2 in.).
10. Move your finger from side to side in a circular motion to slightly stretch the rectal wall. Move toward the spine and not the bladder to prevent injury to the bladder. ➤ *Rationale:* This stimulates lower bowel and helps relax sphincter.
11. Instruct client to take slow, deep breaths during procedure.
12. Continue stretching the rectal wall for 1–3 min until the internal sphincter muscle relaxes.
13. Work with client to discover an associated stimulus to help establish a good bowel routine. ➤ *Rationale:* Abdominal massage, coughing, deep inhalations, and tightening of abdominal muscles, in conjunction with digital stimulation, assist in bowel evacuation.
14. Repeat digital stimulation for 1–3 min at 5-min intervals up to 20 min if a bowel movement does not occur.
15. Use two fingers if necessary to break up hard stool for evacuation to occur.
16. Place stool in bedpan as it is removed.
17. Assess vital signs if prolonged digital removal is required. ➤ *Rationale:* Vagal nerve stimulation can occur.
18. Assess for bleeding.
19. After bowel evacuation occurs, assist the client with cleaning and drying perineum.
20. Remove equipment from room.
21. Wash equipment and return to storage area.
22. Discard gloves and perform hand hygiene.
23. Position the client for comfort.

Skill 23.1.3 | Developing a Regular Bowel Routine

Equipment
Clean gloves, 1 or 2 pairs
Lubricant
Bedpan or commode
Absorbent pad
Specific enema if ordered
Washcloth and towel

Preparation
1. Check physician's orders and client care plan.
2. Identify the correct client using two forms of identification and explain procedure (Boxes 23-2 and 23-3 ■).
3. Identify time of day client usually evacuates bowels.
4. Evaluate diet, exercise, and former use of medications for bowel evacuation.
5. Administer the following drugs as ordered:
   a. Stool softener (Colace, Dialose, DCS, Coloxyl) daily
   b. Bulk former (Metamucil or FiberCon)—daily to TID
   c. Mild laxative (Senokot, Doxidan, Dulcolax) 8 hr before program
   d. Suppository (glycerin or Dulcolax) just before digital stimulation
6. Perform hand hygiene.

Box 23-2 **BOWEL TRAINING**
Good bowel training programs include:

- Initiation of defecation on demand with digital stimulation and abdominal massage
- Evacuation at same time each day; best time 20–40 min after a meal
- Proper diet, increased fiber and fluids
- Daily physical exercise regimen
- Client and family education

CLINICAL ALERT
A daily routine should be set up for at least 2–3 weeks to establish a pattern.

Procedure

1. Don gloves. You may want to double-glove to prevent contamination if glove tears.
2. Perform digital stimulation ½ hr after dinner or breakfast or according to client's time schedule for evacuation (see Skill 23.1.2). ➤ *Rationale:* Food stimulates bowel activity.
3. Place client on toilet or commode. (Use bedpan if client is on bedrest.) ➤ *Rationale:* Assuming normal posture for bowel movement facilitates evacuation.
4. Encourage client to contract abdominal muscles or bend forward while bearing down. ➤ *Rationale:* Increases abdominal pressure and helps evacuate the bowel.
5. Remove gloves.
6. Perform hand hygiene.
7. Provide privacy and sufficient time for evacuation.

Box 23-3 RECOMMENDATIONS FOR PREVENTING CONSTIPATION IN THE OLDER ADULT POPULATION

- Assess constipation by obtaining the client's history, including information regarding the amount of fluid intake, food ingested, and dietary fiber.
- Review medications associated with an increased risk of developing constipation; screen for polypharmacy.

Teach older adults about home care:

- Identify bowel patterns using a bowel diary.
- Increase fluids to 2.7 L/day for females and 3.7 L/day for males. Minimize both caffeine and alcohol intake.
- Increase fiber to 21 g/day for females and 30 g/day for males ages 51–70.
- Maintain regular consistent toileting.
- Tailor physical activity to their physical abilities.

---

8. Don gloves.
9. Wash and dry perineal area if client is unable to do so.
10. Remove gloves.
11. Place client in wheelchair or bed and position for comfort.
12. Perform hand hygiene.
13. Wean client away from suppositories and laxatives when spontaneous bowel movements occur with digital stimulation.

EVIDENCE-BASED PRACTICE
Management of Constipation in Older Adults

Early studies conducted in Britain and the United States indicated that between 10% and 18% of otherwise healthy adults had frequent straining on defecation. Constipation appeared to be more common in women than men, and about 20% of older adults identified the problem. Constipation is not a physiologic consequence of the aging process, but decreased GI motility is a contributing factor to its prevalence in older adults. Constipation may occur secondary to other conditions, such as colorectal cancer or strictures. It is also associated with contributing factors such as inadequate fluid intake, absence of dietary fiber, caloric intake, and lack of exercise.

Newer studies based on these reports indicate that insufficient amounts of fluid could predispose older adults to constipation. Fluid intake for hydration should be 11 cups (2.7 L) per day for females and 3.7 cups (15 L) for males, with 20% of fluid coming from food and 80% from beverages. Fluids are water, juice, and caffeinated fluids. A diet high in fiber is not recommended for individuals who are immobile or who do not consume at least 1.5 L/day of fluids. The recommended total fiber is 21 g/day for females and 30 g/day for males ages 51–70.

Sources: Gallelli, Pirritano, Palleria, & De Sarro (2012) and McKay, Fravel, & Scanlon (2009)

Skill 23.1.4 | Administering a Suppository

Equipment

Clean gloves
Lubricant
Bedpan or commode
Absorbent pad (optional)
Suppository as ordered
Washcloth and towel
Paper towel

Procedure

1. Check physician's orders and MAR.
2. Perform hand hygiene.
3. Gather equipment.
4. Identify client with two forms of ID and explain procedure.
5. Provide privacy. Place client in Sims position with upper leg flexed.
6. Place bed protector on bed if necessary. Fold back top bed covers.
7. Remove suppository foil; lubricate tip of suppository. ➤ *Rationale:* This prevents tissue damage and promotes easy insertion of suppository.
8. Don gloves; lubricate fingers of nondominant hand.
9. Place small amount of lubricant on paper towel.
10. Lift upper buttock to expose the rectal area.
11. Instruct client to breathe through mouth. ➤ *Rationale:* This relaxes anal sphincter.
12. Gently insert suppository (usually glycerin) with pointed end first, and place high in rectum beyond external and internal sphincters, approximately 8–10 cm (3–4 in.) ❶. ➤ *Rationale:* This prevents expulsion of suppository.
13. Push the suppository against the side of the rectal wall. Ensure it is not placed into fecal mass. ➤ *Rationale:* The suppository is ineffective if placed in feces because it cannot be absorbed.

(continued)

Skill 23.1.4 | Administering a Suppository *(continued)*

Rectum
Suppository
Rectal-Anal Ridge
Anus
Rectal Sphincter

1 Insert rectal suppositories beyond the rectal-anal ridge for retention.

> **CLINICAL ALERT**
>
> If client has a spinal cord injury, observe for signs of autonomic hyperflexia (goose pimples, pounding headache, hypertension, perspiration above level of spinal cord injury).
>
> If signs and symptoms of autonomic hyperflexia occur, discontinue digital stimulation. Apply dibucaine hydrochloride (Nupercainal) and lidocaine (Xylocaine) ointment around anus and rectum as ordered. This anesthetizes the area and decreases the stimulation that caused the response. Wait 10 min for symptoms to decrease, and then gently remove the feces.

14. Withdraw finger and press client's buttocks together for a few minutes. ➤ *Rationale:* To prevent expulsion of suppository.
15. Instruct client to stay in Sims position for at least 5 min. ➤ *Rationale:* This position helps retain the suppository.
16. Remove gloves by turning inside-out and discarding in appropriate receptacle.
17. Perform hand hygiene.
18. Place client on toilet or commode. If bowel movement does not occur in 30 min, perform digital stimulation. A suppository is usually effective within 30 min.
19. Repeat with stronger suppository if ordered (bisacodyl [Dulcolax]) after 30 min if there are no results. Follow steps for inserting the suppository, including donning gloves.
20. Allow client to retain Dulcolax suppository for 30 min. If no results, do digital stimulation again.
21. After bowel evacuation, cleanse and dry perineal area.
22. Remove gloves and perform hand hygiene.
23. Position client in wheelchair or bed.

> **CLINICAL ALERT**
>
> Although widely used, stool softeners have limited clinical efficacy. Suppositories may be used in institutionalized clients with obstructed defecation to help with rectal evacuation.

EVIDENCE-BASED PRACTICE
Incontinence-Associated Dermatitis

In 2010, an international consensus conference was held to review current evidence regarding pathology, prevention, and management of incontinence-associated dermatitis (IAD). A consensus of the panelists at the conference agreed upon the evidence-based guidelines for prevention and management of IAD.

1. IAD is clinically and pathologically distinct from pressure ulcers and intertriginous (skin-fold) dermatitis.
2. A consistently applied, structured, or defined skin care program is effective for prevention and management of IAD.
3. Evidence is lacking concerning which products and protocols provide the best outcomes for IAD prevention and treatment in individual clients.
4. Clinical observation and histopathologic analysis suggest that IAD is the result of "top-down" injury.
5. Major etiology is skin exposure to urine or stool, with liquid stool being the potent irritant.
6. Factors associated with IAD are presence of high levels of *Staphylococcus aureus* or *Candida albicans*.
7. The use of occlusive products is associated with an increased likelihood of IAD. The use of products that provide enhanced water vapor transmission may reduce the risk of IAD.
8. Most studies support the consistent use of a well-defined skin care regimen.
9. The key components of an effective program for IAD prevention is:
   a. Gentle cleansing with a no-rinse cleanser with pH range similar to normal skin.
   b. Moisturization to maintain normal levels of intercellular lipids and the skin's normal barrier function.
   c. Application of moisture barrier product (petrolatum-based, dimethicone-based, zinc oxide-based, or liquid film-forming acrylate).

Source: Doughty et al. (2012)

Skill 23.1.5 | Inserting a Rectal Tube

Equipment

Rectal tube: size 22–24 straight (Fr) for adults and size 12–18 Fr for children
Small plastic bag or stool specimen container
Hypoallergenic paper tape

Water-soluble lubricant
Bed protector
Clean gloves, 2 pairs
Washcloth and towel

CLINICAL ALERT

Rectal tubes should be used only for removal of flatus, not to manage diarrhea. They should not be used routinely because of the risk of injury to rectal tissue.

Procedure

1. Check physician's orders and client care plan.
2. Perform hand hygiene.
3. Gather equipment.
4. Identify the correct client with two forms of identification and explain the procedure.
5. Provide privacy. Place client on left side in a recumbent position and drape. ➤ *Rationale:* This position facilitates insertion of tube following the normal curve of rectum and sigmoid colon.
6. Place bed protector under client.
7. Tape the plastic bag around the distal end of the rectal tube or insert the tube into the stool specimen container.
8. Vent the upper side of the plastic bag to prevent inflation.
9. Don gloves.
10. Lubricate the proximal end of the rectal tube with water-soluble lubricant.
11. Gently separate buttocks and ask client to take a deep breath. Gently insert the tube into the client's rectum, past the external and internal anal sphincters (5–10 cm [2–4 in.] in adults, 2.5–7 cm [1–3 in.] in children) ❶. Do not force the rectal tube.
    ➤ *Rationale:* Taking a deep breath relaxes the anal sphincter and prevents tissue trauma during tube insertion.
12. With adults, gently tape the tube in place, using hypoallergenic paper tape. With children, hold the tube in place manually.
13. Remove gloves and place in appropriate receptacle. Perform hand hygiene.
14. Take client's pulse. ➤ *Rationale:* Alterations in pulse rate can indicate a vagal stimulation and the rectal tube may

❶ Insert rectal tube past the external and internal anal sphincters.

need to be removed. This can occur particularly in a client with a cardiac condition.

15. Leave the tube in place no longer than 20 min.
    ➤ *Rationale:* Prolonged stimulation of the anal sphincter may result in a loss of the neuromuscular response. The prolonged presence of a catheter may cause pressure necrosis of the mucosal surface.
16. Don gloves.
17. Remove the tube and provide perianal care.
18. Help the client assume a comfortable position.
19. Clean the tubing, and replace in bathroom if to be reused. Remove and discard the plastic bag.
20. Instruct client that chewing gum, sucking on candy, drinking liquids through a straw, carbonated beverages, and smoking tend to promote the swallowing of air and increase abdominal distention.
21. Remove gloves and perform hand hygiene.

Skill 23.1.6 | Instructing Client in Colostomy Irrigation

Equipment

Solution container with 1,000 mL warm water 40.5–43°C (105–110°F)
Irrigating tubing with cone
Clean gloves, 3 pairs
Irrigating sleeve cut long enough to reach water level in toilet
Items to clean skin and stoma (e.g., washcloths or gauze)
Plastic bag for disposal of used pouch
Clean pouch and closure device
Skin barriers
Water-soluble lubricant
Hook near toilet

CLINICAL ALERT

Colostomy irrigations are done *only* if normal bowel evacuation cannot be achieved *and if not contraindicated*.

Preparation

1. Identify client using two forms of identifiers.
2. Check client chart for orders to perform irrigation. ➤ *Rationale:* This procedure is contraindicated for many clients.
3. Introduce self and explain the procedure. Provide privacy.

Procedure

1. Fill container with 1,000 mL lukewarm water (500 mL for first irrigation). ➤ *Rationale:* Lukewarm water temperature is 40.5–43°C (105–110°F). This temperature prevents injury from hot solutions and cramping from cold solutions.
2. Suspend container on bathroom hook at same level as client's shoulders (no higher than 46 cm [18 in.] above stoma).
3. Instruct client in benefits of relaxing and taking periodic deep breaths.
4. Perform hand hygiene and don clean gloves.

(continued)

Skill 23.1.6 | Instructing Client in Colostomy Irrigation *(continued)*

5. Remove and dispose of used pouch in plastic bag.
6. Clean stoma and skin with warm water and soft cloth. Assess skin for signs of irritation or breakdown.
7. Apply irrigation sleeve to peristomal skin, and place belt around waist.
8. Open roller clamp and allow solution to run through tubing; close clamp. ➤ *Rationale:* This removes air from tubing and prevents discomfort for client.
9. Assist client to sit on toilet or on chair in front of toilet.
10. Place sleeve between client's thighs and direct end into toilet.
11. Lubricate cone tip with water-soluble lubricant.
12. Position cone in sleeve by placing through top opening. If cone cannot be inserted easily, do not force it.
13. Hold cone snugly against stoma. ➤ *Rationale:* This prevents backflow of solution.
14. Open roller clamp on tubing and allow water to run through cone while inserting cone into stoma.
15. Instill solution (750–1,000 mL) over 5–10 min. ➤ *Rationale:* The container height and rate of water flow affect results obtained. If client complains of feeling light-headed or has vertigo, take pulse and stop instillation. ➤ *Rationale:* These are symptoms of a vagal response.

Skill 23.1.7 | Instructing Home Care Client in Colostomy Care

Procedure

1. Identify client using two forms of ID. Perform hand hygiene.
2. Instruct client and family on ostomy care (Box 23-4 ■).
3. Provide telephone number and address of supply vendors.
4. Refer client to community support groups for psychological support as needed.
5. Review infection control measures when caring for ostomy pouches or dressings. Dispose of used equipment in appropriate receptacle.
6. Review potential skin and infection signs and symptoms and when to report findings to healthcare provider.

Box 23-4 CLIENT TEACHING: CARE OF AN OSTOMY

- Empty pouch when it is one-third full of stool or flatus.
  a. Empty into toilet.
  b. Pouch should last for 3–4 days.
- Rinse pouch using room temperature water and a rubber ear syringe (squirt into pouch).
- Use pouch deodorant if desired.
- Empty each morning and last thing at night, even if not one-third full.
- Check seal on daily basis for tight fit; change if needed.
- Instruct client to always carry a supply of ostomy equipment for emergency use.
- Instruct client on emptying and cleaning pouch, opening and closing clamp, observing and cleaning peristomal area, and changing pouch.
- Have client return demonstration until able to perform activities correctly.

Unit 23.1 Documentation and Evaluation

DOCUMENTATION for Bowel Management

- Type and number of suppositories used
- Digital stimulation used
- Approximate time used for digital stimulation
- Amount, consistency, and characteristics of stool
- Protocol for bowel evacuation for client
- Untoward complications of bowel training program
- Nursing interventions needed to correct complications
- Time rectal tube inserted, size of tube
- Amount, color, and consistency of feces collected
- Time rectal tube removed
- Presence, absence, or change in abdominal distention
- Client's reaction to procedure
- Any unexpected outcomes and measures taken to treat these outcomes
- Take pulse rate before and during procedure
- Colostomy irrigation, amount, color, and concentration of return solution
- Interventions related to stool modification plan
- Irrigation solution; type and amount

EVALUATION/Critical Thinking

Expected Outcomes

- Client establishes regular bowel evacuation program.
- Constipation is prevented.
- Fecal impaction is removed.
- Client is able to evacuate bowel at a convenient and consistent time.
- Client is free of pain, flatus, and discomfort.
- Digital stimulation is performed without cardiac complications.
- Rectal tube insertion relieves flatus.
- Colostomy irrigation is effective in promoting consistency in daily evacuation time.

Unexpected Outcomes	Alternative Actions
• When digital stimulation is performed, client exhibits reflex spasm that prevents stool expulsion.	• Apply local anesthetic around rectum and anus, if ordered. • Wait for spasm to relax, and then proceed with stimulation.
• Client develops diarrhea.	• Identify possible cause of diarrhea. • Observe dietary intake for possible cause. Provide for bulk. • Hold the laxatives and stool softeners temporarily. • Instruct client to eat yogurt and drink milk if not contraindicated by condition. • Inform physician of diarrhea and obtain orders for Kaopectate. Administer 2 teaspoons after each loose stool for 24 hr. • Check with physician if medications should be readjusted for bowel training as needed.
• Client exhibits signs and symptoms of vagal response during removal of fecal impaction.	• Immediately discontinue procedure. • Place client in shock position. • Monitor vital signs every 5–15 min until condition is stable. • Notify physician of findings and request medication order for antispasmodic such as atropine. • Be prepared for "Code" situation, even though it is not likely to occur.
• Effective bowel evacuation program is not established.	• Ask dietitian for altered diet (including more fruits and vegetables). • Check if contraindication exists for increasing fluids to 3,000 mL daily. • Obtain order from the physician to administer a different stool softener and bulk former or increase dosage. • Have client increase physical activity, especially exercise of the abdominal muscles if not contraindicated by condition. • Ensure that client begins bowel training program one half hour after a meal.

(continued)

Unexpected Outcomes	Alternative Actions
• No relief of abdominal distention.	• Reposition client at an angle that raises the lower part of the body (e.g., in a prone position with the foot of the bed raised).
	• Instruct client to circle, raise, and lower his or her legs.
	• Reinsert the tube after 2–3 hr.
	• Remove the tube and check for feces that may be clogging the outlet. Clean tube, and reinsert.
• Fecal impaction lower in rectum prevents insertion of rectal tube.	• Perform digital examination with gloved finger and water-soluble lubricant.
	• Break up impaction if present.
	• Position client on left side in Fowler's position.
	• Reinsert the rectal tube.
• Client is impacted with stool even after stool modification program is instituted.	• Irrigate aggressively to loosen stool.
	• Irrigate every 8–12 hr if necessary to maintain loose stool.
	• Administer enema and/or laxatives.

Enema Administration

Nursing Process Data

ASSESSMENT Database

- Review client's present and past eliminatory status.
- Assess the need for an enema.
- Evaluate amount of solution a client can tolerate.
- Assess if fecal impaction is present.
- Assess the degree of abdominal distention.
- Assess degree of sphincter control.
- Assess current medical regimen.
- Assess dietary history.
- Assess vital signs before and after procedure, as necessary.

PLANNING Objectives

- To relieve constipation
- To relieve fecal impactions
- To cleanse the bowel before surgery or diagnostic examination
- To evacuate the bowel in clients with neurologic dysfunction
- To provide nutrients
- To introduce an exchange resin
- To relieve abdominal distention
- To stimulate peristalsis

IMPLEMENTATION Procedures

DOCUMENTATION AND EVALUATION

Expected Outcomes

- Client experiences increased comfort and relief from abdominal distention.
- Enema administered without difficulty.
- Returns are clear if preparing client for diagnostic examination or surgery.
- Relief is obtained from fecal impaction or constipation.
- Return of solution plus formed, soft feces is complete.

Unexpected Outcomes/Alternative Actions

Pearson Nursing Student Resources

Find additional review materials at
nursing.pearsonhighered.com.
Prepare for success with NCLEX®-style practice questions and Skill Checklists.

Skill 23.2.1 | Administering a Large-Volume Enema

Equipment

Fluid container with attached rectal tube (size 22–30, straight, or Fr, for adults)

Normal saline, tap water, soap (for adult, 750–1,000 mL of solution; Table 23-2 ■ lists fluid volume of enemas for different client ages)

Water-soluble lubricant

Bath blanket, if desired

IV pole

Clean bedpan, commode, or toilet

Bed protector pad

Skin care items (e.g., soap, water, towels)

Clean gloves, 2 pairs

Toilet tissue

Table 23-2 Fluid Volume for Enema Administration

Age	Amount (mL)
Infant	50–150 mL
Toddler	250–350 mL
Child	300–500 mL
Adolescent	500–750 mL
Adult	750–1,000 mL

Preparation

1. Check physician's orders and client care plan. Types of enemas are listed in Box 23-5 ■.
2. Gather equipment.
3. Identify correct client using two client identifiers, introduce yourself, and explain the procedure. Explain the benefits of relaxing and taking periodic deep breaths and that he or she will need to hold solution for specified time.
4. Provide privacy.
5. Perform hand hygiene.

Procedure

1. Fill water container with 750–1,000 mL of lukewarm solution, 40.5–43°C (105–110°F). ❶ ➤ *Rationale:* Solutions that are too hot or too cold or solutions that are instilled too quickly can cause cramping, damage to rectal tissues, and extreme shock.
2. Allow solution to run through tubing until air is removed ❷. Clamp tube. ➤ *Rationale:* If air is instilled during procedure, client experiences discomfort as a result of distension of the colon.
3. Hang container on IV pole next to bed. Solution should hang 30–46 cm (12–18 in.) above buttocks.

Box 23-5 TYPES OF ENEMAS

Cleansing

- Stimulates peristalsis through irritation of colon and rectum and by distention. Agents: Soap suds, tap water, and saline. This type of enema is used to prepare the client for a colonoscopy or x-ray and can be used as a small- or large-volume cleansing enema.
- *Soap suds*: Mild soap solutions stimulate and irritate intestinal mucosa. Strong soap solutions can cause severe irritation of the mucous membrane of the colon. Dilute 3–5 mL of mild soap in 1,000 mL of water.
- *Tap water*: Give with caution to infants or to adults with altered cardiac and renal reserve. Tap water is a hypotonic solution.
- *Saline*: For normal saline enemas, use a smaller volume of solution. **Hypertonic** solutions draw fluid into the colon from the body tissues. These solutions are mildly irritating to the mucous membrane of the colon.

Retention

- Solution or nutrient is retained for specified time. Agents: mineral oil, olive oil, cottonseed oil, liquid petrolatum. Nutrient agent: dextrose solution.
- *Emollient (Oil)*: Lubricates the rectum and colon, protecting the intestinal mucous membrane. Feces absorb oil and become softer and easier to expel. Client retains enema for prescribed time, usually 30–60 min. Mineral oil is used for fecal impaction removal. It should be followed immediately with a sodium phosphate enema or soap suds enema to relieve the fecal impaction and constipation.
- *Nutritive*: Provides nourishment in temporary or emergency situations. Enema is retained.

Distention Reduction

- Provides relief from flatus causing distention. It improves ability to expel flatus. Types: carminative and return flow.
- **Carminative:** Two common types include: 1-2-3 enema (30 g of magnesium sulfate, 60 g of glycerin, and 90 mL warm water) and milk and molasses (180–240 mL of equal amounts).
- *Return flow*: Harris flush is the most common. Mild colonic irrigation using 100–200 mL of enema solution. After instillation, enema container is lowered and solution siphoned back into container.

Medicated

- Enemas containing drugs used for reducing bacteria or removing potassium. Agents: Kayexalate and neomycin.
- *Kayexalate*: A resin is introduced into the large intestine, removing the excess potassium by exchanging it for sodium ions.
- *Neomycin*: Antibiotic solution is used to reduce bacteria before bowel surgery.

1 Fill bag to 750–1,000 mL with tepid solution.

2 Allow solution to run through tubing to expel air.

4. Raise bed to HIGH (comfortable working height), and lower side rails on side where you will be working.
5. Don gloves.
6. Place bed protector under client.
7. Place bedpan within easy reach, or place commode near bed.
8. Place client on left side in Sims position. ➤ *Rationale:* This facilitates flow of solution using contour of bowel. Do this by bringing client's right leg toward the chest.
9. Provide privacy, and drape client with bath blanket.
10. Lubricate tip of tubing 5–10 cm (2–4 in.) with generous amount of water-soluble lubricant **3**.
11. Gently spread buttocks, instruct client to take a slow breath, and insert tubing 7–10 cm (3–4 in.) Observe the client carefully, particularly if the client has a cardiac condition.
    ➤ *Rationale:* The insertion of the tube may stimulate the vagus nerve, which could trigger bradycardia.
12. Raise the solution container to a maximum height of 46 cm (18 in.) above rectum when giving a high enema and 30–46 cm (12–18 in.) when giving a low enema **4**. ➤ *Rationale:* To assist in fluid movement, turn client to supine position midway through procedure, and then to right side.
13. Open regulating clamp and allow solution to flow slowly.
    ➤ *Rationale:* If the flow is slow, client experiences fewer cramps. The client will also be able to tolerate and retain a greater volume of solution. If cramping occurs, lower container to slow influx of solution to decrease cramping. When cramping decreases, raise container to 46 cm (18 in.) above buttocks.

3 Lubricate tip of tubing to prevent rectal injury.

14. Hold tubing in place in client's rectum at all times. Keep a bedpan nearby.
15. Lower solution container or momentarily clamp tubing if client experiences cramping, is unable to retain solution, or exhibits anxiety. Resume infusion of solution after a few minutes.

(continued)

Skill 23.2.1 | Administering a Large-Volume Enema *(continued)*

18 Inches High

❹ Place enema solution container no more than 46 cm (18 in.) above rectum for safety.

16. After you have instilled the solution, gently remove the tubing. Instruct client to hold solution for 10–15 min or as long as tolerated. ➤ *Rationale:* The longer the solution is retained, the more effective the results.
17. Clean and dispose of equipment.
18. Place client on bedpan, elevate the head of the bed so that client can assume a squatting position on bedpan, or assist to commode.
19. Remove gloves and perform hand hygiene.
20. Provide privacy until client has expelled total volume of instilled solution.
21. Don clean gloves before removing bedpan, or assist client to bed.
22. Remove bedpan when client is ready, and immediately empty, clean, and replace in proper storage area.
23. Assist client with perineal care, and help client to assume a comfortable position.
24. Lower bed and raise side rails.
25. If client is on strict I&O, measure returns. ➤ *Rationale:* This is to make sure total volume of the solution is expelled.
26. Remove gloves, dispose in a trash receptacle, and perform hand hygiene.

Skill 23.2.2 | Administering an Enema to a Child

Equipment
Water container with attached rectal tube (size 14–18 straight [Fr] for children, and size 10–12 Fr or infant enema syringe with bulb for infants)
Normal saline, tap water, soap solution
Water-soluble lubricant
Clean potty chair for children
Bed protector
Skin care items (e.g., soap, water, towels)
Clean gloves

Preparation
1. Check physician's orders and identify client using two forms of identification.
2. Gather equipment.
3. Provide privacy for child.
4. Perform hand hygiene.
5. Explain procedure to child or family. Inform an older child he or she will feel like he or she has to go the bathroom while the solution is flowing in. Take time to calm a frightened child and to answer the child's questions.
6. If child is toilet trained, place potty chair next to crib or bed.

Procedure
1. Fill water container with 38°C (100°F) solution, using appropriate volume according to age.
2. Open clamp and allow solution to run through the tubing so that air is removed.
3. Clamp tube and hang solution container on IV pole.
4. Place bed protector under child.
5. Place child on left side or in knee–chest position. ➤ *Rationale:* This facilitates flow of solution using contour of bowel.
6. Don clean gloves.
7. Lubricate tip of tubing or infant enema syringe with bulb.
8. Gently separate buttocks and insert catheter or syringe into child's rectum (2.5–3.8 cm [1–1.5 in.] for infants, 5–7.6 cm [2–3 in.] for children) at an angle pointing toward the navel.
9. If there is resistance when inserting the tip or solution, carefully withdraw the tip and try a different angle.
10. Elevate solution container no more than 30–46 cm (12–18 in.) above the child's hips, according to hospital policy. ➤ *Rationale:* Height increases pressure of solution entering colon—too much pressure may damage colon.
11. Open clamp and allow solution to flow slowly for 10–15 min. If the solution starts to ooze out of rectum, briefly squeeze child's buttocks firmly together around the tube.
12. After you have instilled the solution, close clamp and gently remove the tubing or syringe.
13. Hold child's buttocks together or tape them with hypoallergenic paper tape.
14. Retain solution 10–15 min for cleansing enemas.
15. Place the child on a potty chair or bedpan to expel solution.
16. Remove gloves and place in trash receptacle. Perform hand hygiene.
17. If there are no contraindications, you may gently massage child's abdomen to help child expel returns.

18. If the child wants to be left alone while expelling returns, provide privacy. Child should expel the total volume of the instilled solution.
19. Don gloves.
20. Remove the potty chair or bedpan.

21. Clean the child's perineal area, and help child assume a comfortable position.
22. Estimate returns of solution. ➤ *Rationale:* This determines that the child expelled the total volume of the solution.
23. Clean all equipment, and replace in appropriate area.
24. Remove gloves and perform hand hygiene.

Skill 23.2.3 | Administering a Small-Volume Enema

Equipment
Commercially prepared enema
Water-soluble lubricant
Bedpan, commode, toilet
Clean gloves, 2 pairs
Bed protector
Skin care items (e.g., soap, water, towels)

Preparation
1. Check physician's orders and identify client using two forms of identification.
2. Gather equipment.
3. Perform hand hygiene.
4. Identify correct client and explain the procedure. Explain the benefits of relaxing and taking periodic deep breaths.
5. Place bed protector under client.
6. Place client on left side in a Sims position.
7. Provide privacy.
8. Read directions on enema container.
9. Don clean gloves.

Procedure
1. Fold linen down to expose buttocks.
2. Lubricate with water-soluble lubricant if necessary (usually rectal tube is self-lubricated).
3. Expose the anal opening to assist you in inserting the tube without traumatizing the tissue.
4. After inserting rectal tube, gently squeeze the container, and empty entire 120 mL of hypertonic solution. ❶
5. Keep pressure on container while removing from rectum. ➤ *Rationale:* This prevents solution from being drawn back into container.

6. Instruct client to hold solution 5–7 min.
7. When ready to expel solution, elevate the head of the bed so that the client can assume a squatting position on the bedpan. If able, client may expel solution in toilet.
8. Remove and dispose of gloves.
9. Provide privacy until the client has expelled the total volume of the instilled solution.
10. Don gloves and remove bedpan if client is using bedpan.
11. Assist client with perineal care, and help client to assume a comfortable position.
12. Measure returns if on strict I&O.
13. Dispose of equipment. Remove and dispose of gloves.
14. Perform hand hygiene.

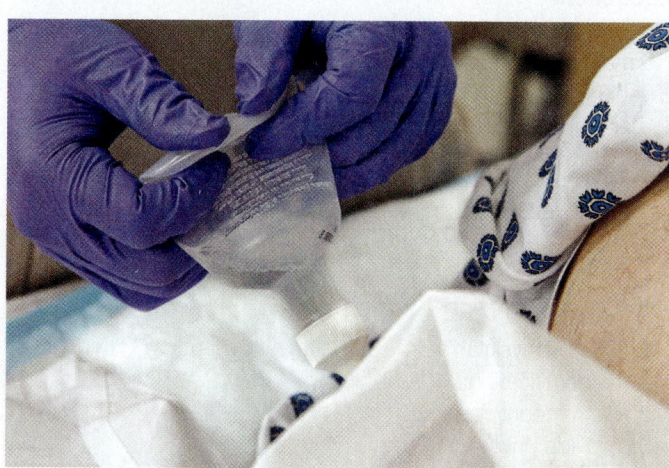

❶ Insert tip of container gently into rectum and expel all fluid.

Skill 23.2.4 | Administering a Retention Enema

Equipment
Commercially prepared disposable oil retention enema

Note: For retention enema, only these types of enemas are used: medication and oil, including nutritive, antibiotics, and anthelmintics.

Oil: Adult 150–200 mL, child 75–100 mL, 32.8°C (91°F)
Water-soluble lubricant
Bedpan or commode

Bed protector
Skin care items (e.g., soap, water, towels)
Clean gloves

Preparation
1. Identify client using two forms of identification and prepare client as for any enema.
2. Provide privacy.

(continued)

Skill 23.2.4 | Administering a Retention Enema *(continued)*

3. Gather equipment—disposable oil retention enema is administered like a small enema. Read directions on enema container.

Procedure

1. Explain steps of procedure to client.
2. Raise bed to HIGH position (comfortable working height).
3. Perform hand hygiene and don gloves.
4. Place bed protector on bed.
5. Expose anal opening, and gently insert rectal tube tip of container 7–10 cm (3–4 in.). Commercially prepared enemas are prelubricated.
6. Squeeze contents slowly, and empty entire amount into rectum.
7. Keep container compressed and remove rectal tube gently. ➤ *Rationale:* This prevents solution from being drawn back into container.

8. Lower bed.
9. Discard equipment and gloves, following Standard Precautions. Perform hand hygiene.
10. Explain to client that oil should be retained for 30–60 min before it is expelled. ➤ *Rationale:* The purpose of the enema is to soften stool.
11. A cleansing enema may need to be given to remove oil and stimulate defecation.
12. Don gloves and provide hygienic care if needed. Discard washcloth and towel in laundry.
13. Remove gloves, discard in appropriate container, and perform hand hygiene.

Skill 23.2.5 | Administering a Return Flow Enema

Equipment

Fluid container with attached rectal tube
Normal saline or tap water at 40.5–43°C (105°–110°F), or enema solution
Water-soluble lubricant
Clean bedpan
Bed protector
Skin care items (e.g., soap, water, towels)
Clean gloves

Preparation

1. Check physician's orders and identify client using two forms of identification.
2. Gather equipment.
3. Provide privacy.
4. Perform hand hygiene.
5. Fill fluid container with 100–200 mL of ordered solution; check that temperature is between 40.5 and 43°C (105–110°F). ➤ *Rationale:* Cool solutions increase cramping.
6. Allow solution to run through tubing so that air is removed. ➤ *Rationale:* If air is instilled during procedure, client experiences discomfort.
7. Hang container on IV pole.

Procedure

1. Explain procedure to client. Explain the benefits of relaxing and taking periodic deep breaths during procedure.
2. Raise bed to HIGH position, and lower side rails.
3. Don gloves.
4. Place bed protector under client.
5. Place client on left side in Sims position with right leg flexed as much as possible. ➤ *Rationale:* This position facilitates instillation of fluid.

6. Lubricate tip of tubing with water-soluble lubricant.
7. Gently spread buttocks, and insert tubing 7–10 cm (3–4 in.) into client's rectum, past external and internal sphincters. Avoid traumatizing **hemorrhoids** during insertion. ➤ *Rationale:* Vagal nerve stimulation from enemas may cause cardiac arrhythmias.
8. Raise water container to a maximum height of 30–46 cm (12–18 in.) above rectum.
9. Open clamp and allow 200 mL of solution to flow slowly into rectum and sigmoid colon. If cramping occurs, clamp tube for a few minutes and then continue infusion.
10. Lower solution container 30–46 cm (12–18 in.) below level of rectum and allow all fluid to flow back into container.
11. Raise container 30–46 cm (12–18 in.) above rectum and allow solution to flow back into rectum.
12. Repeat inflow–outflow process five or six times, changing solution when it becomes thick with feces. ➤ *Rationale:* This assists in stimulating intestinal peristalsis with expulsion of flatus.
13. Provide privacy until client has expelled total volume of instilled solution after last inflow–outflow series.
14. Assist client with perineal care, and help client assume a comfortable position.
15. If client is on strict I&O, measure returns to make sure total volume of solution is expelled.
16. Clean all equipment, and replace in bathroom or appropriate location.
17. Remove gloves and perform hand hygiene.
18. Lower bed and raise side rails.

Unit 23.2 Documentation and Evaluation

DOCUMENTATION for Enema Administration

- Purpose of enema
- Time enema given
- Volume and type of solution used
- Results obtained: amount, consistency, and color
- Any unexpected outcomes and measures taken to remedy problems
- Client's reactions to procedure
- Relief of flatus and distension

EVALUATION/Critical Thinking

Expected Outcomes

- Client experiences increased comfort and relief from abdominal distention.
- Enema administered without difficulty.
- Returns are clear if preparing client for diagnostic examination or surgery.
- Relief obtained from fecal impaction or constipation.
- Return of solution plus formed, soft feces is complete.

Unexpected Outcomes	Alternative Actions
• Client expels solution prematurely.	• Calm and ease client's distress by reassuring him or her as you clean the equipment. • Place bedpan under client. Place client in semi-Fowler's position with knees flexed. • Hold the rectal tube in client's rectum between thighs. Slow the water flow, and continue with the enema.
• Client complains of severe and sudden abdominal pain, nausea, and distention.	• Remove tubing and notify physician immediately of possible perforation (this is an uncommon complication). • Assess vital signs. If you suspect cardiac dysrhythmias, remove bedpan and notify physician immediately. • Be prepared to administer emergency drugs, such as atropine. • If an IV is not in place, start an IV of 5% dextrose in water (D_5W) using a large-bore needle for emergency use.
• The flow of water is impeded or an obstruction is felt.	• Open clamp on tubing. Allow a small amount of solution to flow (the warm solution may help relax the internal sphincter). • Withdraw tube slightly and reinsert. • Gently perform a digital examination for the possibility of fecal impaction. Break up impaction if present. Ask physician for order to give a retention enema, followed by a cleansing enema 2–3 hr later.

Unexpected Outcomes	Alternative Actions
• Client cannot return enema solution.	• Gently massage client's abdomen if not contraindicated. • Replace rectal tube. Lower the enema bag below the level of the bed. • If client is not uncomfortable, do nothing. If client complains of discomfort or pain, notify physician.
• Enema returns are not clear before surgery or diagnostic testing.	• Repeat enema. If, after three enemas, returns are still not clear, notify physician of findings. • May need to give an enema with a stronger solution. • Physician may need to order magnesium citrate or electrolyte solution (e.g., GoLYTELY).
• Fecal impaction is not relieved.	• Check orders for oil retention enema. • Check catheter size needed. • Obtain order for and use digital stimulation and manual extraction of feces if not contraindicated by diagnosis of cardiac or neurologic involvement.

Fecal Ostomy Pouch Application

Nursing Process Data

ASSESSMENT Database

- Assess type and location of stoma (section of bowel used to create stoma).
- Observe stoma color, which should be beefy red and moist.
- Inspect client's abdomen for creasing, firmness, softness, contour, scars, folds, and incisions.
- Inspect client's peristomal skin for signs of erythema, excoriation, ulceration, and fistula formation.
- Assess how far stoma protrudes above skin surface; it should be 1.25–2.5 cm (0.5–1 in.).
- Assess size of stoma.
- Assess output of effluent, including amount, consistency, and odor.
- Assess client's learning abilities, age, manual dexterity, and visual acuity.

PLANNING Objectives

- To assist client to feel more confident that colostomy will not evacuate once appliance is intact
- To collect effluent for accurate assessment of output in the hospital
- To collect effluent for the comfort of the client
- To contain stool and odors to facilitate the client's return to a productive lifestyle, including the resumption of satisfying and meaningful relationships
- To protect peristomal skin from erythema, excoriation, and infection
- To protect the client's clothing

IMPLEMENTATION Procedures

DOCUMENTATION AND EVALUATION

Expected Outcomes

- Pouch remains intact without leakage for 3–5 days.
- Pouching system provides maximal skin protection.
- Pouching system remains odor-proof for 3–5 days.
- Client gradually assumes an active role in applying the pouch.
- Client's skin remains free of erythema or excoriation and infection.

Unexpected Outcomes/Alternative Actions

Pearson Nursing Student Resources

Find additional review materials at
nursing.pearsonhighered.com.
Prepare for success with NCLEX®-style practice questions and Skill Checklists.

Skill 23.3.1 | Applying a Fecal Ostomy Pouch

Equipment

One- or two-piece transparent ostomy pouch with adhesive wafer ❶
Warm water and mild soap
Soft cloths
Bath blanket
Plastic bag for pouch disposal
Tail closure or night adaptor for pouch
Clean gloves
Graduate or bedpan
Measuring guide
Tissues
Ostomy scissors and dark marking pen

Preparation

1. Check client care plan and identify client using two forms of identification.
2. Introduce yourself and explain procedure to client.
3. Determine exact supplies client uses.
4. Gather equipment.
5. Provide privacy.
6. Raise bed to HIGH position (comfortable working height).
7. Perform hand hygiene and don gloves.

(continued)

Skill 23.3.1 | Applying a Fecal Ostomy Pouch *(continued)*

A. Supplies for two-piece pouches.

B. Supplies needed to change one-piece pouches.

C. Two-piece fecal pouches.

D. Fabric pouches, convexity faceplates, pouch with filter.

❶ Supplies needed for ostomy care.

Procedure

1. Place bath blanket over client. Place absorbent pad or towels under client. ➤ *Rationale:* This protects bed from spillage.
2. Observe placement and condition of stoma. **❷**
   ➤ *Rationale:* This determines normal amount of output and consistency (immediately after surgery, all stomas will have very liquid stool and high flatus output).

> ### CLINICAL ALERT
> To promote the client's self-esteem and body image, be aware of your own body language. Even subtle changes in the way you look at the stoma could indicate disgust or disapproval, and an altered self-esteem could result.

3. Empty old pouch into graduate, bedpan, or toilet.
4. Remove old pouch by pushing against skin as you pull backing from skin, and discard in plastic bag. Save tail closure on bottom of pouch. **❸**
5. Measure output, if ordered.

A

B

C

Source: © B. Slaven

❷ A. Viable stoma. **B.** Nonviable parastomal hernia. **C.** Necrotic stoma.

Changing One-Piece Fecal Ostomy Pouch

A. Starting at upper corner, remove old pouch.

B. As you remove old pouch, push against skin while pulling down on pouch.

C. Clean skin with warm water, dry well.

D. Measure stoma size.

E. Remove plastic covering from one-piece pouch.

F. Cut pouch opening to ⅛ in. larger than the size of stoma.

G. Remove paper from inner wafer. Save pattern for future pouch changes.

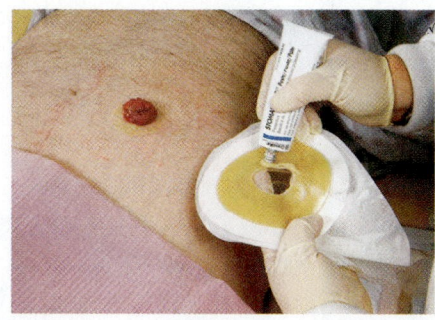

H. Apply ring of paste to opening on pouch.

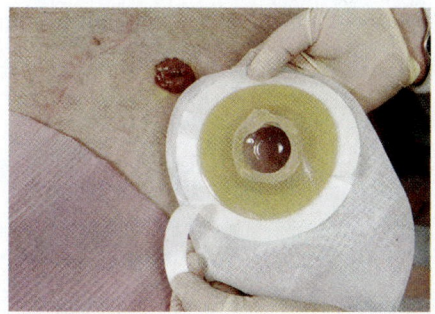

I. Remove paper from outer adhesive ring of pouch.

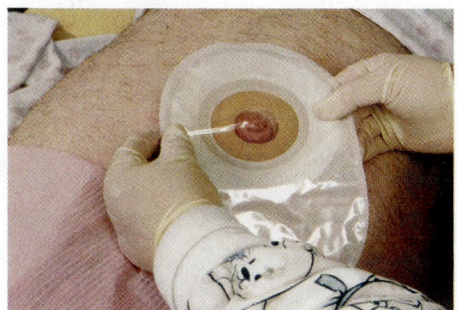

J. Center and apply pouch to clean, dry skin.

K. After applying one-piece pouch, clamp bottom of pouch.

❸ **A.–K.** Changing a one-piece fecal ostomy pouch.

(continued)

Skill 23.3.1 | Applying a Fecal Ostomy Pouch *(continued)*

6. Clean skin and stoma gently with warm water and soft cloth. ➤ *Rationale:* Oily substances can interfere with pouch adhesive. If adhesive doesn't come off, leave it on the skin. If you pick at it, the peristomal skin can be damaged.

7. Dry skin well with soft cloth. Keep tissues available if stoma functions while pouch is off.

8. Observe skin; it should be free of erythema or excoriation. The stoma is assessed for changes in size, ulceration, and color (stoma should be moist, pink, or beefy red). Notify the physician if stoma is black, blue, or purple. This indicates a nonviable stoma.

9. Measure stoma at the base with measuring guide.

10. Trace measured pattern on pouch.

11. Cut pouch to pattern, making sure opening is large enough (at least 0.3 cm [⅛ in.] wider than stoma) to encircle stoma without pushing on edges. ➤ *Rationale:* No skin should appear between the pouch edge and the stoma to ensure the entire stoma is covered.

12. If using a two-piece pouch, snap the wafer and pouch together. ❹

13. Remove paper from skin barrier on pouch and save it. ➤ *Rationale:* This may be used as a pattern for next pouch change.

14. Apply a ring of skin barrier paste to opening on pouch.

15. Apply Stomahesive powder to denuded skin only.

16. Remove paper from outer ring.

17. Center and apply pouch to clean and dry skin. Smooth edges of adhesive to skin. ➤ *Rationale:* If adhesive is wrinkled, it may result in leakage from pouch. To promote optimum wear of the pouch, warm the adhesive by placing your gloved hand over the adhesive and gently hold it over the site for ½–1 min. ➤ *Rationale:* This will activate the adhesive in the skin barrier.

18. Pouches can be applied over an incision. ➤ *Rationale:* Incisions are sealed within 24 hr of surgery.

19. Close and secure end of pouch with tail closure.

    a. Ensure bowed end is next to body. ➤ *Rationale:* This provides a better fit to body, and prevents outpouching of clamp through clothing.

    b. Lay hook on top of bag and fold bag 2.5 cm (1 in.) over end of pouch.

    c. Squeeze clamp together to close.

20. Remove soiled pouch and tissues from bedside.

21. Remove gloves and perform hand hygiene.

22. Position client for comfort. Return bed to LOW position.

23. Put away supplies and reorder as necessary.

Note: Complications of a colostomy skin irritation resulting from stool leaking underneath the pouch can cause a hernia to develop around a colostomy, or the bowel can prolapse or become narrow.

CLINICAL ALERT

Clients with ostomies need a nutritional consult and a written dietary guide. They need to limit the amount of hard-to-digest foods for at least the first 2–3 weeks postop. Also, limiting gas-producing foods will prevent gas-forming odors.

Applying Two-Piece Fecal Ostomy Pouch

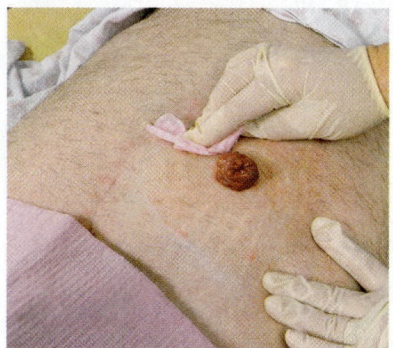

A. Clean and dry skin thoroughly before applying two-piece pouch.

B. Cut opening of a two-piece pouch to exact size of stoma.

C. Check size of opening to ensure proper fit.

D. Snap pouch onto wafer when using a two-piece pouch.

E. Check for secure fit by tugging at bottom of pouch.

F. Remove paper from inner barrier.

G. Apply paste to inner circle of wafer.

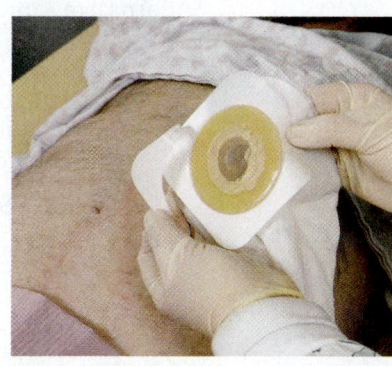

H. Remove paper from outer adhesive ring.

I. Center pouch over stoma and press onto skin.

J. Secure adhesive to skin.

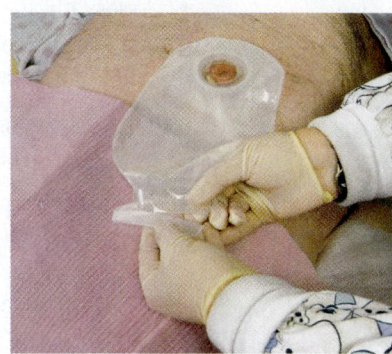

K. Clamp bottom of pouch.

L. Check that clamp is secure.

4 **A.–L.** Applying a two-piece fecal ostomy pouch.

Unit 23.3 Documentation and Evaluation

DOCUMENTATION for Fecal Ostomy Pouch Application

- Type of pouch and skin barrier used
- Time pouch applied
- Time pouch emptied
- Amount, color, and consistency of stool emptied from pouch
- Presence or absence of flatus through the stoma
- Location of stoma
- Client participation in and toleration of pouch application
- Condition of peristomal skin and stoma, including color and size
- Condition of incision line (i.e., any erythema or edema)
- Condition of abdomen (e.g., distention)
- Client teaching, which has been completed

EVALUATION/Critical Thinking

Expected Outcomes

- Pouch remains intact without leakage for 3–5 days.
- Pouching system provides maximal skin protection.
- Pouching system remains odor-proof for 3–5 days.
- Client gradually assumes an active role in applying the pouch.
- Client's skin remains free of erythema, excoriation, and infection.

Unexpected Outcomes	Alternative Actions
• Stoma appears dark, dusky-colored, or black.	• Notify physician of findings, and document in chart (usually indicates stoma is ischemic).
• Stoma becomes ulcerated or cut.	• Examine pouching system to see if opening of pouch may be cutting into stoma. • Recut opening to exact size of stoma.
• Stoma remains a persistent pale pink.	• Request physician to order Hgb, Hct (usually the result of low Hgb). • Instruct client to monitor effluent for constipation if iron preparation ordered.
• Bleeding occurs when stoma is touched.	• Observe and note—usual occurrence postoperatively.
• Erythematous rash at site of pouch.	• Assess for allergic reaction to product being used. • Client may need to change to different type of adhesive on pouch or change to a pouch with no adhesive.
• Papular rash appears on peristomal skin.	• Assess for possible yeast sensitivity. • Be sure skin is clean and dry before applying pouch. • Do not rinse pouch with water because this traps water under wafer. • Client may need to use antifungal powder on skin with each pouch change until skin clears.

(continued)

Unexpected Outcomes	Alternative Actions
• Peristomal skin complications occur.	• Evaluate cause of leakage.
	• Be sure pouch is cut to correct size.
	• Measure stoma at each pouch change for 4–6 weeks. Size will change as edema subsides.
	• Measure stoma at base.
	• Client may need to fill any creases around stoma with skin barrier paste.
	• Apply thin layer of ostomy powder over area and seal with an alcohol-free coating.
	• Client may need to use secondary skin barrier like Eakin seal.
	• Client may need to attach belt to minimize lateral leakage.
	• Change to a product like Durahesive that swells around stoma, preventing leakage, and holds up well to liquid output.
	• Be sure pouch is emptied before it is more than one-third full of stool or flatus, since an overfull pouch can break seal of pouch.
	• Pouches should not be changed more than once daily.
• Ostomy is flush or below the surface.	• Apply convex pouch system to assist ostomy to protrude.
	• Apply ostomy belt.
• Ostomy is in skin fold or crease.	• Apply a one-piece pouch for more flexibility.
	• Fill deep crevices with caulking material.
• Client experiences itching or burning under appliance.	• This may be a sign that stool is undermining seal of pouch.
• Client not coping with altered body image.	• Refer to United Ostomy Associations of America, Inc., the Crohn's and Colitis Foundation of America, American Cancer Society, or the local Enterostomal Therapy nurse.

Chapter Wrap-Up

GERONTOLOGIC Considerations

- Older adult clients frequently have concomitant cardiac problems, which can be affected by vagal stimulation during fecal removal or enema administration. Check with the physician before these skills are performed on older clients. Monitor the pulse carefully during the procedure.
- Fecal impaction is not uncommon with older clients due to decreased mobility and exercise, dietary habits, and tendency to overuse enemas and laxatives.

- Encourage clients to decrease use of laxatives and enemas, increase fluid intake and fiber in diet, and increase exercise. Dehydration resulting from inadequate fluid intake leads to constipation and fecal impaction.
- To select the proper ostomy appliance for an older adult client, the nurse must determine whether the client has any physical limitations that could influence the type of appliance needed. These limitations include poor vision, use of only one hand, arthritis, and inability to perform cleaning and pouching procedure.

MANAGEMENT Guidelines

Each state legislates a Nurse Practice Act for RNs and LVN/LPNs. Healthcare facilities are responsible for establishing and implementing policies and procedures that conform to their state's regulations. Verify the regulations and role parameters for each healthcare worker in your facility.

Delegation

- A CNA or unlicensed assistive personnel (UAP) may be assigned to administer a disposable enema or tap water enema in most facilities. This information is presented in the CNA curriculum. These personnel are not allowed to administer enemas with medications or a Harris flush.
- An LVN/LPN may be assigned to insert a rectal tube, administer enemas, and perform colostomy care.
- In some rehabilitation settings, aides may be instructed to administer glycerine suppositories. This requires additional training. Check facility policy and procedure manuals to determine which healthcare worker may be assigned to this task.
- *A CNA cannot be assigned to perform a fecal impaction removal because of the risk of a vagal response during the procedure.*

Interprofessional Communication

- Information relative to bowel elimination is provided both through report and written information on the Kardex card.
- Before delegating any of the tasks associated with bowel elimination to a CNA or UAP, determine his or her knowledge base to perform the task. Ask him or her to explain the procedure if you are unsure of their ability to perform the task.
- When an LVN/LPN or RN is assigned to perform colostomy care or assist a physician with an intestinal tube insertion, ensure he or she is familiar with the procedure. Review the procedure as needed.
- Clients who require a bowel program need instruction on the process so they may become independent in the skill. If someone else will be assisting them with this procedure, he or she should be included in the teaching process. The RN is responsible for establishing the teaching program. An LVN/LPN may assist in carrying out the plan.
- When special steps or supplies are needed to perform a task (e.g., colostomy care), information should be written on the client care plan or clinical pathway. This allows all staff to perform the procedure the same way. Clients feel more secure when procedures are completed in a uniform method.

CASE STUDY Applications

Scenario 1

You are assigned to a 74-year-old man who had a transverse colostomy for cancer 4 days ago. During the night report, you heard the night nurse say his pouch is leaking and he is very angry with the staff for causing the mess. As you prepare to enter his room, you decide how to approach him.

1. Determine the most appropriate communication technique to use with the client. Provide rationale for your response.
2. As you observe the stoma and pouch, you determine the leak is at the bottom of the pouch.
   a. State two reasons the pouch may be leaking.
   b. Describe your initial nursing action after you assess the leaking pouch.
   c. What steps do you take to ensure the new pouch will not leak?
3. After removing the first pouch, you assess the skin and determine the peristomal skin to be erythematous and the stoma reddened and slightly edematous.
   a. What is your priority nursing intervention? Provide the rationale for your response.
   b. After completing the priority intervention, what is your next action?
4. After the application of the new pouch, you determine that a teaching plan needs to be developed for the client.
   a. Describe the method of developing a teaching plan for this client.

b. After developing a plan, indicate the first step the nurse should incorporate to implement the plan.
c. Describe your rationale for the first step of the teaching plan.
d. List at least three nursing diagnoses that are appropriate for this client's care plan.
e. Identify at least one community resource that is appropriate for a referral.

Scenario 2

You assess Mrs. Jacob, a 65-year-old who had a colostomy performed 6 days ago, for cancer of the descending colon. When you tell her you will be instructing her on how to apply a new pouch, she starts to cry and says, "No, I don't want to know how because all it does is leak everywhere."

1. Identify the initial nursing intervention and discuss additional actions you would take to resolve this problem.
2. Describe the assessment database that should be completed before a plan can be implemented.
3. Outline the steps in designing a client teaching plan for a client with an ostomy.

NCLEX® Review Questions

Unless otherwise specified, choose only one (1) answer.

1. The client is undergoing diagnostic tests for fecal incontinence. You would expect to prepare the client for which of the following tests?
   Select all that apply.
   A. Ultrasonography
   B. Electromyography
   C. MRI
   D. Colonoscopy
   E. CAT scan

2. The client is scheduled for surgery in the morning for an ileostomy. He asks you what to expect when he returns from surgery. What would your best response be?
   A. "You will need to ask the physician. I can't tell you."
   B. "You will have an opening through the abdominal wall where the stool will pass into a bag."
   C. "You will have a drain in place from the abdominal incision until bowel function returns."
   D. "You will have a catheter inserted into the colon until the colon has healed."

3. What is one of the major differences between care of a client with a colostomy and care of a client with an ileostomy?
   A. The stool of the ileostomy is liquid to semisoft, which requires increased fluid intake.

B. Only the client with an colostomy will require the use of an ostomy bag.
C. The ileostomy is usually able to be reversed when the disease process heals.
D. There are usually no dietary restrictions with either client.

4. What would the nurse do just before removing a fecal impaction?
   A. Obtain a consent form for the procedure.
   B. Infuse at least 500 mL of fluid through a rectal tube into the lower colon.
   C. Obtain baseline pulse and blood pressure.
   D. Give the client a laxative to assist with the fecal removal.

5. The client requires a rectal suppository. Which of the following actions is appropriate when inserting the suppository?
   A. Ask the client to bear down when you insert the suppository just beyond the external sphincter.
   B. Place the flat end of the suppository into the external sphincter.
   C. Insert the suppository into the fecal material if at all possible.
   D. Place the pointed end of the suppository 7–10 cm (3–4 in.) beyond the internal sphincter.

6. A client has just come home from the hospital following a colectomy with a colostomy. His wife wants to know what foods he should avoid to minimize odors.

   Select all that apply.
   A. Dairy products
   B. Brown rice
   C. Cookies
   D. Bananas
   E. White toast

7. How much fluid intake do older clients require per day to prevent constipation?
   A. Females 2.7 L/day
   B. Females 2 L/day
   C. Males 2.7 L/day
   D. Males 2 L/day

8. The client has an enema ordered before surgery. Which one of the following nursing actions will you perform when administering a large-volume enema?
   A. Place client on right side in Sims position.
   B. Instruct the client to take in a slow, deep breath and insert tubing 7–10 cm (3–4 in.).
   C. Raise height of enema solution to the level of the client's shoulder.
   D. Instill solution over 5–10 min.

9. The student nurse has been instructed to teach the client and family the application procedure for a fecal ostomy pouch. In reviewing the skill, which of the following actions would be considered inappropriate teaching for applying a pouch?
   A. Remove old pouch by pushing against skin as you pull backing from the skin.
   B. Cleanse skin and stoma with warm water and a generous amount of soap.
   C. Cut new pouch at least 0.12 cm (⅛ in.) larger than the stoma.
   D. Apply ring of skin barrier paste to the opening on the pouch.

10. The student nurse is preparing to begin the leadership component of the nursing program. Which of the following is included in appropriate delegation of nursing skills?
    A. Assigning the nursing assistant to complete a fecal impaction removal on an older adult client.
    B. Determining that the unlicensed assistive personnel cannot be assigned to care for a client requiring a tap water enema.
    C. Asking the RN team leader to administer a carminative enema to the client.
    D. Assigning the LVN to develop an ileostomy teaching plan for the client and family.

QSEN Activity

Teaching Client and Family About Colostomy Care at Home

Domain: Patient Centered Care

KSA: Knowledge and Skills

Activity:

Have students develop a plan of care that includes applying a fecal ostomy pouch, colostomy irrigation (if appropriate), and dietary instructions on foods to eat and avoid based on the client's condition and fluid intake. After the care plan is completed, implement a client scenario with a client and family member.

Bibliography

Anastasi, J., Capill, B., & Chang, M. (2013, Jul.). Managing irritable bowel syndrome. *American Journal of Nursing, 113*(7), 42–51.

Bailes, B. K. & Reeve, K. (2013). Constipation in older adults. *Nurse Practitioner, 38*(8), 21.

Burch, J. (2014). What you need to know about caring for the skin around a stoma. *Journal of Community Nursing, 28*(4), 90–93.

Collins, E., Hibberts, F., Lyons, M., Williams, A. B., & Schizas, A. M. P. (2014). Outcomes in non-surgical management for bowel dysfunction. *British Journal of Nursing, 23*(14), 776.

De Paepe, K., Sieg, A., Le Meur, M., & Rogiers, V. (2014). Silicones as nonocclusive topical agents. *Skin Pharmacology and Physiology, 27*(3), 164–171. doi:10.1159/000354914

Dietz, K., & Gares, J. (2010, Feb. & May). Wound & skin care: Basic ostomy management, part 1. *Nursing, 40*(2), 61–62; part 2 *40*(5), 62–63.

Dixon, S. (2014, Dec. 16). Do I need a special colostomy or colectomy diet after surgery? Retrieved from www.coloncancer.aboutcom/od/nutrition and diet/a/colostomydiet.htm

Doughty, D., Junkin, J., Kurz, P., Selekof, J., Gray, M., Fader, M., ... & Logan, S. (2012, May/Jun.) Incontinence-associated dermatitis: Consensus statements, evidence-based guidelines for prevention and treatment, and current challenges. *Wound, Ostomy, and Continence Nurses Society, 39*(3), 303–315.

Free Ostomy Care Guides. (2014) The phoenix: The official publication of UOAA. Retrieved from http://www.phoenixuoaa.org/free-magazine-for-new-ostomy-patients

Gallagher, P. & O'Mahony, D. (2009). Constipation in old age. *Best Practice & Research, 23*(6), 875–887. doi:10.1016/j.bpg.2009.09.001

Gallelli, L., Pirritano, D., Palleria, C., & De Sarro, G. (2012). Constipation treatment. In Catto-Smith, A. (Ed.). *Neurological disorders, constipation—causes, diagnosis and treatment.* Rijeka, Croatia: InTech. Retrieved from http://www.intechopen.com/books/constipationcauses-diagnosis-and-treatment/constipation-treatment-in-neurological-disorders

Grant, M., Mccorkle, R., Hornbrook, M. C., Wendel, C. S., & Krouse, R. (2013). Development of a chronic care ostomy self-management program. *Journal of Cancer Education, 28*(1), 70–78. doi: 10.1007/s13187-012-0433-1

Guidance on OASIS-C1. (2014). Integumentary items: Best practices for nurses. *Wound, Ostomy and Continence Nurses Society.* 2:28.

Klein, J. & Holowaty, S. (2014). Managing constipation: Implementing a protocol in a geriatric rehabilitation setting. *Journal of Gerontological Nursing, 40*(8), 18–27.

McKay S. L., Fravel M., & Scanlon, C. (2009, Oct.). *Management of constipation.* Iowa City, IA: University of Iowa Gerontological Nursing Interventions Research Center, Research Transition and Dissemination Core.

Massey, R. L. (2012). Return of bowel sounds indicating an end of postoperative ileus: Is it time to cease this long-standing nursing tradition? *Medsurg Nursing, 21*(3), 146–150.

Polk, T. M. & Schwab, C. W. (2012). Metabolic and nutritional support of the enterocutaneous fistula patient: A three-phase approach. *World Journal of Surgery, 36*(3), 524–533. doi:10.1007/s00268-011-1315-0

Rao, S. S. C. & Go, J. T. (2010, Aug. 9). Update on the management of constipation in the elderly: New treatment options. *Clinical Interventions in Aging, 5,* 417–418.

Toner, F. & Claros, E. (2012, Dec.). Preventing, assessing, and managing constipation in older adults. *Nursing, 42*(12), 32–39.

Wierzchowski, P., Dabrowiecki, S., Szczesny, W., & Szmytkowski, J. (2013). Clinical research: Nonvariceal upper gastrointestinal tract bleeding—Risk factors and the value of emergency endoscopy. *Archives of Medical Science, 9*(5), 843. doi:10.5114/aoms.2013.36911

Chapter 24
Heat and Cold Therapies

Learning Objectives

24.1 Describe the mechanisms responsible for the body's heat loss and heat production.

24.2 Discuss the role of the hypothalamus in thermoregulation.

24.3 List at least three adaptive processes that maintain the body temperature within a normal range.

24.4 Discuss how heat transfer occurs.

24.5 Identify various modes of heat therapy.

24.6 Describe the physiologic effects of local heat applications (thermotherapy).

24.7 Identify various modes of cold therapy (local cryotherapy and induced hypothermia).

24.8 Describe the physiologic effects of local cold applications (cryotherapy).

24.9 Identify indications and contraindications for various heat and cold therapies.

24.10 Predict the type of thermal agent that would be most therapeutic for a particular client's condition.

24.11 Discuss the rationale for induced hypothermia for special clients.

24.12 List four safety precautions to consider when applying heat and cold treatments.

24.13 State two nursing diagnoses related to thermal therapies.

Chapter Outline

Terminology

Afterdrop reduction in core temperature upon discontinuation of rewarming therapy.

Ambient temperature temperature of the air surrounding an individual.

Antipyretic an agent that reduces fever.

Compress a pad of cloth applied firmly to a part of the body; compress may be dry or wet, cold or warm.

Conduction heat transfer between materials of different temperatures that are in direct contact with each other (e.g., hot or cold pack).

Convection heat transfer by contact with circulating gas or fluid of a different temperature (e.g., whirlpool, wind).

Core temperature the temperature of internal sites; may be increased in rectum or tympanic membrane.

Cryotherapy transfer of heat from the client by use of a cooling agent.

Cyanosis bluish coloring of the skin and the mucous membrane due to decreased oxygenation.

Erythema reddish color of the skin due to dilation of capillaries.

Evaporation absorption of heat (energy) as a result of conversion of a material from a liquid to a vapor state (e.g., sweating, spraying).

Fever regulated rise in body temperature to a new hypothalamic "set point"; usually mediated by internal stimuli (e.g., pyrogenic cytokines), often caused by infection. Metabolic rate is increased; shivering and diaphoresis occur.

Hyperemia increased blood supply to an area with resultant erythema.

Hyperthermia nonregulated rise in core body temperature exceeding 41.1°C (106°F); due to dysfunction of thermoregulation caused by injury to the hypothalamus (central fever), or failure of the body's ability to eliminate excess heat (e.g., environmental exposure, medications).

Hypothermia a reduction in core body temperature due to environmental exposure or thermoregulatory dysfunction: mild (33°–36°C [91.4°–96.8°F]), moderate (26°–32°C [78.8°–89.6°F]), deep (13°–25°C [55.4°–77°F]), and profound (<12°C [<53.6°F]).

Insulator substance that is a poor conductor or nonconductor of heat; substance that helps prevent the escape or entrance of heat.

Mottling blue-gray to purplish blotches seen peripherally; usually the result of peripheral vasoconstriction.

Overshoot temperature overcompensation due to external temperature management therapy.

Pallor loss of reddish hue due to superficial vasoconstriction.

Radiation exchange of heat through the air without an intervening medium (e.g., heat lamp).

Shivering production of body heat by involuntary muscle activity, which increases metabolic rate and oxygen consumption and possible anaerobic metabolism with resulting acidosis.

Suppuration the process of pus formation.

Thermogenesis heat production by the body.

Thermotherapy transfer of heat to a client by use of a heating agent.

Vasoconstriction narrowing of blood vessels.

Vasodilation expansion of blood vessels.

Temperature Regulation

Body temperature is regulated and maintained by interrelated feedback systems, which can be altered by disease or environmental conditions. Temperature regulation is a homeostatic function that balances heat production and loss to maintain body temperature within a fairly constant range or "set point" (36.4°–37.3°C [97.5°–99°F]), with temperature normally being lowest in the morning and highest in late afternoon. This function is controlled by the body's thermostat, the hypothalamus.

Twenty percent of the body's afferent temperature information reaches the hypothalamus indirectly through superficial thermal receptors in the skin and subcutaneous tissue by way of the spinal cord. Internal organs send **core temperature** information (80% of input) directly by circulating blood. The hypothalamus interprets information from both the superficial and internal (core) sources and triggers vasomotor responses to maintain a normal temperature through processes of conduction, convection, evaporation, and radiation (Figure 24-1 ■).

FIGURE 24-1 The hypothalamus is located in the diencephalon portion of the brain. It controls the body's thermostat.

As heat is gained through metabolism, exercise, or environmental factors, the body loses excess warmth through *convection, conduction, radiation,* or *evaporation.* In contrast, on sensing a loss of heat (cold), the body triggers one or more processes to produce heat (thermogenesis) or conserve it. Although these dynamic processes cannot be observed, their resulting effects, such as **shivering,** are readily evident. In addition, we consciously and unconsciously alter levels of activity in response to the physiologic stimulus from the body's thermostat, the hypothalamus. When we sense cold, we huddle or curl up and add clothing to decrease heat loss from the body surface. When warm, we extend our bodies, separate our limbs, and shed our clothes.

When the hypothalamus perceives cooling, the sympathetic nervous system is activated to conserve and produce heat. Release of norepinephrine causes vessel constriction (a heat-conserving mechanism), which removes warm blood from the skin. This, along with *piloerection* (hair-raising), reduces conductive heat loss to the cooler environment. Increased muscle tension and shivering increase the metabolic rate, and heat is produced (**thermogenesis**). These responses continue until the temperature, as sensed by the hypothalamus, has reached its thermostat "set point." Extreme increases in tissue metabolism may result in metabolic acidosis.

In contrast, when the body perceives excess heat, opposite responses are activated. Peripheral **vasodilation** occurs and blood is brought to the surface, promoting radiation of heat away from the body. Behavioral responses (lighter clothing) expose the body for greater heat radiation into a cooler environment. A fan is used to assist heat convection.

Heat and cold therapies utilize physical principles/processes of conduction, convection, radiation, and evaporation to manipulate *heat transfer.*

Processes of Heat Transfer

Conduction is heat transfer when a warmer object is in direct contact with a cooler object (e.g., hot or cold pack, water-flow cooling blanket). The greater the temperature difference, the faster heat will transfer; however, very hot or very cold applications can cause tissue injury. Different objects have different heat conductivity. Metal conducts heat readily, but air has low conductivity. Therefore, metal objects should be removed from the treated area, and a towel may be placed under a hot or cold pack to trap air (insulate) and limit heat transfer in order to prevent tissue injury. The body's superficial tissues transfer (conduct) heat readily, but cooling or warming the surface has little impact on changing the temperature of deeper tissues. Therefore, surface measures to alter core temperature have limited effectiveness.

Convection is heat transfer by direct contact with a circulating medium (agent in motion) and another material of a different temperature. Therapeutic examples include whirlpool, aquathermic pad, air-flow cooling or warm-air blanket, irrigations, or infusions. Heat transfer by convection is more rapid than heat transfer by conduction, and convection modalities that circulate fluid are more effective than those that circulate air. The body utilizes convection by circulating warm blood away from and cooler blood into an area to stabilize tissue temperature.

Radiation is heat transfer through the air (no intervening medium) from a *warmer* to a *cooler* area. Since the exposed head is responsible for 65% of body heat loss, a head covering will help prevent radiant heat loss. An example is putting a cap on a newborn's or operative client's head.

Evaporation is heat transfer by conversion of a liquid to a vapor. Heat transfer by evaporation is more effective than heat transfer by air current (radiation). Evaporation of sweat serves to cool the body as long as the humidity of the environment is low enough to support evaporation. Another example is a moist open body cavity that evaporates heat to the cooler environment of the surgical suite. Therapeutic examples of evaporation include tepid sponging or cold spraying.

Conditions Affecting Temperature Regulation

Fever

Fever, a temperature over 38.3°C (101°F), is the most commonly encountered alteration of thermoregulation. Exogenous pathogens (viruses, bacteria) trigger the release of endogenous pyrogens or cytokines that cause the hypothalamus to reset its normal range (thermostat) higher. In response, the body perceives that it is cold and seeks to conserve and produce heat by peripheral **vasoconstriction,** piloerection, and shivering until the new set point is reached. Peripheral vasodilation follows as the thermostat is set to a lower temperature in response to a decrease in pyrogen concentration or **antipyretic** medication. This is accompanied by a feeling of warmth as the body cools by vasodilation and sweating until the lower set point is reached. Medications can lower hypothalamic set point as well as affect one's ability to shiver or to exert vasomotor control.

Fever increases metabolic rate, oxygen utilization, and cardiopulmonary load. It also places the client at risk for dehydration. Still, many studies substantiate that fever, as a natural defense, correlates positively with a quicker recovery and improved survival rates. Antipyretic agents do reduce fever, but their benefit has not been established beyond that of making clients feel more comfortable. *External* cooling measures (tepid sponging and the use of cooling blankets) are ineffective antipyretics because they only lower skin temperature. If the hypothalamic set point is high, external cooling can induce adverse counteractive mechanisms (shivering). Shivering imposes a tremendous metabolic burden by increasing metabolic rate and oxygen demand four- to fivefold.

Hyperthermia (Body Temperature Exceeding 41.1°C [106°F])

Hyperthermia, sometimes called *central fever*, is a heat-related emergency that can cause irreversible brain damage. Hyperthermia may be caused by strenuous exercise, environmental exposure (heat stroke), or central nervous system injury. It differs from fever because it is not mediated by pyrogenic cytokines but develops when the body's metabolic heat production or environmental heat load exceeds the body's ability to lose heat. The body's core temperature may exceed 41.1°C (106°F), even though the hypothalamic temperature set point is normal. No diurnal temperature variation, shivering, or sweating is observed.

In contrast to fever, which responds to antipyretic agents, hyperthermia tends to be refractory to treatment, requiring external cooling measures that combine evaporation and convection, such as water spraying and warm air fanning. More aggressive cooling measures (e.g., hypothermia garment) may induce shivering by creating a skin-to-core temperature gradient. The cool skin initiates shivering before the brain temperature cools. Vasoconstriction and risk of resultant shivering can be reduced by insulating the client's extremities and confining external cooling only to the torso. Additionally, the use of various sedating and analgesic medications can inhibit shivering and its resultant metabolic burden.

Hypothermia (Body Temperature Below 36°C [96.8°F])

Unintentional **hypothermia**, a potentially lethal condition, is body temperature below 36°C (96.8°F) measured by bladder catheter, pulmonary artery catheter, or an esophageal or rectal probe. It may be caused by loss of heat due to environmental exposure to cold or vasodilation (general anesthesia, cold IV fluids), decreased heat production (hypothyroidism, neuromuscular blockade), or loss of thermoregulation secondary to CNS pathology, injury, or multiple trauma. Hypothermia decreases respiratory drive; slows peripheral nerve conduction, myocardial repolarization, and GI motility; and impairs coagulation. The skin is colder than core tissues, creating a skin-to-core temperature gradient that results in both vasoconstriction to conserve heat and shivering to generate heat. Changes in cognitive and cardiorespiratory function occur, followed by deterioration of all body functions as body temperature continues to drop.

The Inflammatory Response

Inflammation is the immediate local adaptive response of the body to external or internal tissue injury (Table 24-1 ■). The response is the same regardless of the cause of injury: physical (e.g., burn), metabolic (e.g., ischemia), biological (e.g., bacteria), or chemical (e.g., acid). The purpose of inflammation is to minimize injury, kill offending agents, and dispose of debris so healing can take place. The response may be acute, subacute, or chronic.

Cardinal signs of inflammation are redness, swelling, heat, pain, and loss of function. These are due to the action of chemical mediators (histamine, bradykinin, prostaglandins, and cytokines) activated at the time of the primary injury. Vasodilation, circulatory slowing, and increased vascular permeability allow the passage of protein-rich fluid (exudate) and white blood cells (neutrophils) into the site to initiate the process. These circulatory changes result in localized ischemia. Neutrophils destroy invaders by phagocytosis and enzymatic digestion, but this process results in production of oxygen-free radicals and release of cytokines that may destroy other neutrophils and/or injure healthy adjacent tissue and perpetuate the inflammatory response (secondary injury). WBCs also initiate repair by inducing healthy cell division and new blood vessel growth.

Superficial heat and cold therapies are used to minimize or enhance the inflammatory response that accompanies acute tissue injury (e.g., musculoskeletal sprain, strain, fracture, or surgery). Effects of heat and cold are listed in Table 24-2 ■. Cold (cryo) therapies reduce inflammation; heat (thermo) therapies enhance inflammation and increase circulation. For each degree centigrade increase or decrease in the injured site's temperature, the tissue metabolic rate is increased or decreased by 13%. The magnitude of this response is influenced by the temperature of the modality, duration of therapy, and surface area exposed to the treatment.

Local Heat Therapies (Thermotherapy)

The physiologic effects of heat are generally opposite to those of cold. Heat applications (**thermotherapy**) are inappropriate during the acute inflammatory phase of musculoskeletal injury (with the exception of neck or back muscle strain), but are beneficial for subacute and chronic inflammation. Heat produces analgesia and sedation by promoting release of endorphins and by stimulating nerve endings to block pain transmission by the gate control theory of pain modulation. The benefits of heat therapy last only as long as the heat stimulus is applied. When removed, effects quickly disappear. Indications for heat therapies are listed in Table 24-3 ■.

Heat facilitates soft tissue repair by increasing delivery of nutrients and oxygen and removal of cellular debris. Heat relaxes skeletal muscles, increases elasticity, and decreases viscosity of connective tissue and thereby facilitates other treatments by producing relaxation.

Although tissue conduction of heat is limited to a depth of about 2 cm (about ¾ in.), burns can occur if heat application is too hot or prolonged, or if the tissue is unable to mount the increased metabolic demand imposed. The body tends to acclimate to heat therapies; insulation is recommended with heat applications to prevent tissue injury caused by adaptation to harmful levels. Superficial heating

Table 24-1 Categories of Cold and Heat Injuries

Categories of Hypothermia	Signs and Symptoms	Management
Mild (33°–36°C [91.4°–96.8°F])	Tachycardia, tachypnea, hypertension, shivering	*Note:* Rewarming the unintentionally hypothermic client should not exceed 2°C (3.6°F) per hour. Remove wet clothing, place in supine position, avoid excessive movement, monitor core temperature and cardiac rhythm. *Passive rewarming* (blanket, head covering) *Active external rewarming* (heat pad to torso only, forced air warmer, warmed blankets, radiant light, immersion in 40°C [104°F] bath)
Moderate (26°–32°C [78.8°–89.6°F])	Atrial arrhythmias, slow heart rate, hypotension, decreased reflexes	*Passive rewarming, plus active external rewarming* of torso only *Active internal rewarming* (IV saline warmed to 40°–45°C [104°–113°F], warm humid oxygen, 42°–46°C [107.6°–114.8°F], endovascular warming device, extracorporeal blood warming, warm lavage of body cavities)
Severe (13°–25°C [55.4°–77°F])	Oliguria, pulmonary edema, ventricular arrhythmias, nonreactive pupils coma, apnea Client appears to be dead; has no vital signs	Active rewarming, CPR, defibrillation/resuscitation until core temperature is at least 32°C (0°F)
Hyperthermia		
Dehydration	Sweating, ruddy appearance, signs of volume depletion	Rehydrate with caffeine-free or sugar-free beverages.
Heat cramps	Painful leg or abdominal cramps associated with exercise in hot weather	Cease activity, move to cool location, and rehydrate with cool fluids with electrolytes.
Heat exhaustion (37°–40°C [98.6°–104°F])	Tachycardia, normal- or hypotension, weakness, nausea, flushed skin, headache, concentrated or decreased urine output	Apply cool packs to neck, axilla, groin, or spray skin with cool water with warm fanning to speed evaporation. IV fluids may be necessary for rehydration.
Heatstroke (>40°C [104°F])	Heatstroke is a medical emergency associated with hyperthermia and central nervous system dysfunction. Dizziness, delirium, confusion, seizures, coma, coagulopathies, and multisystem failure may develop.	Seek emergency services. Provide oxygen, IV fluids, monitor core temperature, urine output, place NG tube. Begin immediate evaporative external cooling and internal cooling with chilled saline infusion, ice water lavage of body cavities to reduce body temperature to 38.3°–38.9°C (101°–102.2°F) in 1 hr.

Table 24-2 Physiologic Effects of Heat and Cold Therapies

Thermotherapy	Cryotherapy
Increases superficial temperature	Reduces local tissue temperature
Increases local metabolic rate, oxygen consumption, may cause rewarming acidosis, arrhythmias	Decreases cellular metabolism and oxygen consumption
Dilates arterioles and capillaries, increases capillary permeability; may cause hypotension	Constricts arterioles, capillaries; reduces capillary permeability; may cause hypertension
Decreases blood viscosity; promotes bleeding Enhances blood flow to area (including nutrients and WBCs)	Increases blood viscosity; controls bleeding Decreases blood flow; reduces delivery of phagocytes Decreases secondary metabolic injury
Improves lymphatic and venous drainage of fluid and metabolites	Reduces venous and lymphatic drainage
Promotes inflammation	Blunts inflammatory response
Enhances flexibility of muscles, ligaments	Decreases muscle spasticity
Provides *analgesia* via gating mechanism; stimulates endorphin release	Has extreme *anesthetic* effect; slows nerve conduction via gating mechanism; stimulates endorphin release
Reduces edema *not* associated with acute inflammation	Reduces acute edema formation and accumulation

Table 24-3 Indications for Heat Therapies

Indications	Contraindications
Subacute or chronic inflammation Subacute edema joint stiffness	Acute musculoskeletal injury Acute pain or inflammation Acute edema
Subacute or chronic pain	Impaired circulation (peripheral vascular disease)
Muscle soreness/spasm Postherpetic neuralgia infection (supports **suppuration**) *Consensual vasodilation* (spinal cord reflex that causes vasodilation in distal cutaneous vessels as well as at site of heat application) Chronic ulcer	Sensory impairment Bruising or bleeding Malignancy Open wound

Table 24-4 Indications for Cold Therapies

Indications	Contraindications
Acute inflammation, acute or chronic pain	Impaired circulation (peripheral vascular disease)
Acute swelling or bleeding	Raynaud disease/phenomenon
Muscle spasm	Hypersensitivity to cold or cold intolerance
Strain, sprain, or contusion Joint stiffness	Decreased sensation Open wound

therapies that get cooler during application (e.g., moist packs) are safer than therapies with a constant maintained temperature (e.g., heating pad).

A unique benefit of heat is its ability to inhibit sympathetic nervous system outflow. Heat promotes vasodilation both at the site of application and in distal cutaneous vessels (called *consensual vasodilation*). By way of this spinal cord reflex, heat may be applied proximally (e.g., to low back) to increase peripheral circulation and facilitate healing in an area that lacks sufficient circulation or sensation to tolerate direct application of heat.

Local Cold Therapies (Cryotherapy)

Cold therapies (**cryotherapy**) facilitate heat transfer from the body and are the treatment of choice immediately after local tissue injury and throughout the acute inflammatory phase. Cold applications are usually accompanied by compression and elevation of the affected area (see Orthopedic Interventions, Chapter 27). Indications for cold therapies are provided in Table 24-4 ∎.

The immediate benefits of cryotherapy are inhibition of local enzymatic and metabolic activity and limitation of secondary metabolic injury. Cold constricts vessels, controls bleeding, reduces edema formation, decreases nerve conduction velocity, increases the pain threshold, and decreases muscle spasticity.

> **CLINICAL ALERT**
> Cold-induced vasodilation may occur when applications to distal extremities (fingers, toes) exceed 15 min at temperatures below 1°C (34°F). The amount of vasodilation is usually small but should be avoided in certain situations, and therapy time should be limited to 15 min or less when treating fingers and toes. Longer treatment durations may be used for other areas of the body.

With cold therapy, the area temperature remains lower than normal for 1 or 2 hr after removal of the cooling modality, so cold therapies are usually applied for 30–60 min, and then repeated every 1–2 hr.

While cryotherapy prevents acute edema formation (swelling) during the first 24–48 hr after injury, it cannot remove swelling that has occurred. Swelling only decreases as inflammatory exudate (free protein) is removed from the area by lymph flow. Cryotherapy is beneficial in the rehabilitation period as it produces anesthesia and facilitates exercise, which stimulates lymph flow.

Induced Hypothermia

Hypothermia may be therapeutically induced in certain situations to protect vital organs because it provides metabolic quiescence. Central (internal) cooling, during cardiac or neurosurgery, can also induce postoperative shivering. Rewarming the blood or infusing warmed saline before terminating surgery helps to warm core tissues and a forced warm air blanket (e.g., Bair Hugger) may be used for active external rewarming. Peripheral vasculature, however, remains constricted for some time, unable to receive the warmed blood. Later, peripheral vessels dilate and hypotension may occur. As cool blood from the periphery moves to mix with warmer blood in the core, central temperature drops 2°–5°C (3.5–9°F) (*afterdrop*). Acidosis may also occur as accumulated tissue acids enter the central circulation. Even a combination of measures may fail to promote homogeneous body rewarming; therefore, pharmacologic agents that blunt hypothalamic responses may be necessary adjuncts to suppress shivering in the centrally cooled client postoperatively.

Fever has a negative effect on neurologic outcome in various types of neurologic injury. An increase in core temperature of 1°C (1.8°F) results in a 10% increase in energy expenditure. A growing number of studies demonstrate that induction of mild induced hypothermia (32°–35°C [90°–95°F]) for 24 hr provides neuroprotection. Mild induced hypothermia used early on improves rates of survival with meaningful neurologic recovery to victims of postanoxic brain injury (those with return of spontaneous circulation after cardiac arrest). Controlled hypothermia also shows promise as a treatment for severe traumatic brain injury (Glasgow Coma Score <8), stroke, myocardial infarction, refractory intracranial hypertension, bacterial meningitis, and hepatic encephalopathy.

EVIDENCE-BASED PRACTICE
Mild Hypothermia Improves Stroke Outcomes

In a prospective cohort study at two separate Stroke Centers, clients underwent mild hypothermia after successful reperfusion (thrombolysis). The findings suggest that mild induced hypothermia clients have less cerebral edema, less hemorrhage, and better outcomes.

Source: Hong, Lee, Song, Jeong, & Lee (2014)

For each degree centigrade reduction in core body temperature, the cerebral metabolic rate is decreased by 6%–7%. Additional neuroprotection include decreased neutrophil infiltration with reduced cytokine, leukotriene, and oxygen-free radical production (secondary injury); increased blood–brain barrier stability; and decreased intracranial pressure due to vasoconstriction.

The four modes of heat transfer are utilized in a variety of hypothermia techniques, including the following:

- Surface cooling with ice packs, body wraps (most effective), and an isolated head cooling helmet
- Vascular cooling using chilled crystalloid infusion, endovascular heat exchange via central venous catheter, and hemodialysis
- Intracavitary cooling including chilled lavage (gastric, bladder) and delivery of a nasopharyngeal coolant

Cultural Awareness

Determining the client's perspective about illness and treatment practices may provide a framework for developing a plan of care that is therapeutic and acceptable to both the client and the caregiver.

The application of heat and cold would seem to align with beliefs and practices of several cultures that seek a balance of life forces. However, hot–cold theories of health and disease do not relate to body temperature, but rather to a therapy's symbolic strength. For example, to regain balance, a "cold" disease is treated by eating or exposing oneself to "hot" therapies, such as acupuncture and cupping. For some cultures, an orange ("hot") medication may be more acceptable for a "cold" ailment than a blue ("cold") medication.

The gender and race of an individual affect susceptibility to direct cold injury and hypothermia. Nonwhite older adult men are the most at risk, while young white women are the least at risk. Women have a higher gradient of temperature from the skin to the body core (they are more likely to have cold hands, for instance) and so they are more able to maintain a constant body core temperature in cold conditions. Subcutaneous fat acts as an **insulator**, and women generally have more fat than men to help them stay warm. On the other hand, because of the high temperature gradient from skin to core, women are more likely to sustain surface cold injury such as frostbite.

Nursing Diagnoses

The following nursing diagnoses are appropriate to use on client care plans when the components are related to heat and cold therapies.

NURSING DIAGNOSIS	RELATED TO . . .
Impaired Comfort	Environmental exposure, tissue injury, inflammatory process
Hyperthermia	CNS injury, strenuous exercise, environmental exposure, medications
Hypothermia	CNS injury, diabetes, hypothyroidism, environmental exposure, major trauma, surgery, alcoholism, medications
Deficient Knowledge (Specify)	*Lack of understanding* about inflammatory process; rationale for and hazards of heat and cold therapies
Peripheral Neurovascular Dysfunction, Risk for	Prolonged application of heat or cold therapy to joints or areas with impaired circulation
Impaired Skin Integrity, Risk for	Prolonged use of cold or heat therapy, excessive temperature of therapy, impaired sensation, impaired circulation
Ineffective Thermoregulation	Anesthesia, medications, alcoholism, infection, CNS injury, environmental exposure

Unit 24.1
Local Heat Therapies (Thermotherapy)

Nursing Process Data

ASSESSMENT Database

- Determine rationale for heat therapy.
- Review client's history for possible circulatory problems (peripheral vascular disease, diabetes).
- Assess environmental exposure, induced central cooling.
- Determine site, type, and duration of therapy to be applied.
- Assess area to be treated.
- Determine client's ability to sense temperature at site.
- Assess skin condition before and throughout therapy.

PLANNING Objectives

- To increase circulation to area
- To provide analgesia
- To promote inflammatory process
- To facilitate mobilization of interstitial fluid (noninflammatory edema)

IMPLEMENTATION Procedures

DOCUMENTATION AND EVALUATION

Expected Outcomes

- Circulation is increased to area.
- Client reports decrease in pain.
- Inflammation or suppuration is enhanced.
- Tissue fluid is mobilized and edema reduced.

Unexpected Outcomes / Alternative Actions

Pearson Nursing Student Resources

Find additional review materials at
nursing.pearsonhighered.com.
Prepare for success with NCLEX®-style practice
questions and Skill Checklists.

Skill 24.1.1 | Applying a Commercial Heat Pack

Equipment
Prepackaged heat pack
Tape

Preparation
1. Check healthcare provider's orders for type and duration of heat treatment.
2. Gather equipment.
3. Perform hand hygiene.

Procedure
1. Check two forms of client ID and introduce yourself.
2. Explain procedure to client.
3. Provide privacy.
4. Remove heat pack from outer wrapper.

5. Break inner seal by holding pack tightly in the center and in an upright position.
6. Squeeze firmly to break seal. ➤ **Rationale:** Breaking the seal activates the chemical ingredients and produces the heat.
7. Check for leakage from pack. Remove pack immediately if leakage occurs. ➤ **Rationale:** Chemicals from the pack may burn the skin.
8. Gently shake the pack, and then apply to treatment area. **Note:** Never apply directly to the skin. ➤ **Rationale:** Application directly to skin may cause burns.
9. Remove pack after 5 min and assess skin for **erythema**.
10. Replace pack and secure with tape. Keep in place 15–30 min or as ordered by healthcare provider.
11. Place call bell in client's reach.
12. Remove pack and discard in appropriate container.
13. Perform hand hygiene.

Skill 24.1.2 | Applying an Aquathermic Pad

Equipment
Aquathermic reservoir container with pump
Aquathermic pad (disposable)
Distilled water
Tape

Preparation
1. Review healthcare provider's orders to determine treatment area, type of application, and temperature of treatment.
2. Perform hand hygiene.
3. Gather equipment, and check it for safety factors (e.g., frayed cords, water leaks).
4. Take equipment to client's room.
5. Check two forms of client ID and introduce yourself.
6. Connect aquathermic pad to pump hoses (male and female fittings).
7. Snap locking rings into place to ensure hose fittings are snug, and then open hose clamps.
8. Fill reservoir two-thirds full with *room temperature* distilled water.
9. Place pump on bedside stand or other surface at or above level of the pad. ➤ *Rationale:* If pump is placed below pad level, water will drain back into pump when it is shut off.
10. Use plastic key to set reservoir temperature as ordered, and then remove key. ➤ *Rationale:* Temperature range is 30°–42°C (86°–108°F). Removing key prevents tampering.
11. Plug pump into grounded wall outlet.
12. Turn pump power switch ON. Set temperature is reached in about 20 min.

Procedure
1. Explain procedure to client and provide privacy.
2. Apply aquathermic pad with its coiled surface against client's extremity or over moist pack that has been placed on area to be treated.
3. Secure pad with tape if necessary; *do not use safety pins*. ➤ *Rationale:* Pins can pierce coils in pad.
4. Check client's skin after 2–5 min. ➤ *Rationale:* This is to assess for possible skin reaction caused by a hot pad.
5. Instruct client to notify you if the pad feels too warm. ➤ *Rationale:* This prevents burning of skin.
6. Remove pad after 15–20 min. Observe area for redness, pain, or any untoward reaction.

> **CLINICAL ALERT**
> Heat transfers more quickly than cold. Do not allow the client to lie on a "constant heat source" such as a heating pad or an aquathermic pad.

7. When pad is used to keep dressings or soaks warm, continue treatment longer than 20 min if ordered. Treatment may be continuous when used for clients with subacute lower back or neck pain.

❶ Connect Aqua-K pad to pump hoses.

❷ Aquathermic pad is a form of local heat therapy.

8. Turn pump OFF. Close hose clamps; hold hose with connectors above pump and pad. ➤ *Rationale:* This prevents water spillage.
9. Remove aquathermic pad and join male and female connectors.

> **CLINICAL ALERT**
> Contraindications to heat therapies include acute injury or inflammation, recent or potential hemorrhage, deep-vein thrombophlebitis, impaired circulation, impaired sensation, and impaired mentation.
>
> When treating an area where skin is not intact, cover lesion with sterile gauze and insulating barrier before applying heat (see Wound Care, Chapter 25).

10. Place pad on bedside stand until next treatment or place in appropriate disposal area.
11. Reposition client for comfort.
12. Perform hand hygiene.

Skill 24.1.3 | Applying a Hot Moist Pack

Equipment

Box of 4×4 gauze sponges or other absorbent material necessary for size of area to be treated
Optional large dressing (ABD pad)
Hot tap water or ordered solution and container
Plastic moisture barrier (plastic bag)
   Or
Aquathermic pad (optional)
Tape
Bath thermometer
Gloves

Preparation

1. Check healthcare provider's order for type of hot moist treatment ordered, length of treatment, and time interval between treatments.

CLINICAL ALERT

Do not apply heat to an edematous area until the reason for edema has been determined.

---

2. Gather specific equipment for type of hot moist pack ordered.
3. Place material in a warming solution (usually water).
4. Determine amount of time elapsed since last application.
5. Considering age of client, body part involved, and type of treatment, determine safe temperature of application to prevent burning. ➤ *Rationale:* Water temperature in hospitals is usually controlled at 43.3°C (110°F), but the individual client may require altered temperature.
6. Perform hand hygiene.

Procedure

1. Check two forms of client ID and introduce yourself.
2. Provide privacy.
3. Position client appropriately to expose and assess area to be treated. ➤ *Rationale:* Open wounds are generally *not* treated with heat application because heat increases the area's need for oxygen and may injure granulation tissue. Heat therapy to a recent bruise can restart bleeding.
4. Assess client's ability to sense touch and heat or cold at site to be treated. ➤ *Rationale:* Impaired skin sensation may contraindicate therapy.

5. Remove any jewelry from area to be treated. ➤ *Rationale:* This decreases risk of burn due to conductive potential of metal.
6. Open container of gauze sponges or **compresses**. Open ABD outer wrap if used.
7. Don gloves.
8. Saturate gauze sponges (or other selected material) with warm water (no greater than 43.3°C [110°F]).

Note: Water in hospitals is usually controlled at 43.3°C (110°F) to prevent injury.

9. Pick up soaked sponges and wring out excess solution.
10. Place warm moist pack over area to be treated.
11. Use plastic barrier or aquathermic pad to mold and secure pack to site. ➤ *Rationale:* Barrier helps maintain heat by preventing evaporative cooling.
12. Set aquathermic pad temperature at 41°C (105.8°F). ➤ *Rationale:* While the warm moist pack will cool quickly, the aquathermic pad maintains heat—this also increases the risk of burns.
13. Use tape to secure the barrier. Do not allow client to lie on pack or pad.
14. Ensure that nurse call system is in client's reach. ➤ *Rationale:* Client should summon nurse if discomfort is felt.
15. Assess area in 5 min for signs of redness, **mottling**, or blistering. ➤ *Rationale:* These may be signs of burning. Thermotherapy should be discontinued and a cool pack should be applied.
16. Remove and dispose of pack after 20 min or as prescribed.
17. Assess and dry the treated area. ➤ *Rationale:* Slight redness and warmth are expected responses.
18. Document procedure and client's response to treatment.
19. Discard gloves and perform hand hygiene.

LEGAL ALERT

Salter v. Deaconess Family Medicine Center, 1999
Although this judgment was made many years ago, the case is still relevant. A nurse and hospital were found liable for injuries to an infant's foot after a nurse's application of a wet washcloth that had been heated for 1 full minute in a microwave oven, and then applied to the infant's heel to facilitate drawing blood. Application of the hot cloth was the proximate cause of second-degree burns to the infant's heel.

Skill 24.1.4 | Assisting With a Sitz Bath

Equipment

Disposable sitz bath with tubing and bag ❶
Warm water (40°–43°C [104°–109°F])

Note: Cold temperature may be indicated for client's situation.

Towels for drying
Thermometer
Clean gloves

Preparation

1. Verify healthcare provider's order for sitz bath, and duration and frequency of treatments.
2. Raise toilet seat and place sitz bath basin with FRONT facing the front of the toilet bowl.
3. Fill basin with warm water (40°–43°C [104°–109°F]) one-half to two-thirds full.
4. Close the flow tubing clamp.
5. Open top of plastic bag and fill with hot water (40°–43°C [104°–109°F]).
6. Hang bag at a level higher than the sitz basin so that fluid will flow by gravity.
7. Insert tubing through front or rear entry hole in sitz bath, and then snap or secure tubing into channel or "eye" in bottom of basin.
8. Perform hand hygiene.

Procedure

1. Identify client by checking identification band and asking client to state name.
2. Introduce self.
3. Explain procedure and rationale for sitz bath.
4. Assist client to treatment area with accessible call bell.
5. Provide privacy by placing sign on door.
6. Check to ensure that temperature is 40.5°–43.3°C (105°–110°F).
7. Assist client to sit in sitz bath for 15–20 min.
8. Maintain water temperature by continually adding water of appropriate temperature to bag. ➤ *Rationale:* Overflow will drain into toilet through openings in back of basin.
9. Upon completion, assist client to dry the perineal area and allow client to sit briefly to allow normalization of blood pressure and to prevent hypotension upon standing. ➤ *Rationale:* Orthostatic hypotension may occur with rapid position change after warm sitz bath due to vasodilation.
10. Don clean gloves, empty and rinse client's sitz basin, and store in convenient location for future use.
11. Discard soiled linen.
12. Perform hand hygiene.

❶ Individual disposable sitz bath units are used for infection control purposes.

Unit 24.1 Documentation and Evaluation

DOCUMENTATION for Local Heat Therapies

- Time of application
- Type of heat therapy applied
- Area of body treated
- Status of area pre- and post-treatment
- Positioning of area treated
- Duration of treatment
- Client's response to treatment

EVALUATION/Critical Thinking

Expected Outcomes

- Circulation is increased to area.
- Client reports decrease in pain.
- Inflammation is enhanced.
- Noninflammatory edema is reduced.

Unexpected Outcomes	Alternative Actions
Client experiences pain, asks about alternative measures for relief.	Cold therapy may be an option, or heat–cold alternating therapy as counterirritants; these therapies alter nerve transmission.
	Assess if application is too hot.
	Ensure that temperature is not over 43.3°C (110°F) if heating pad is used.
Swelling is not reduced with heat therapy.	Ensure that acute inflammation is not present, as heat therapy will not reduce swelling (exudate) due to acute tissue injury.
	Support venous return by elevating the part.
Aquathermic pump signals "Over Temp."	Check reservoir water level; it may be low or empty.
	Be sure to use room temperature (not hot) distilled water in reservoir. Check that hoses are not kinked or hose clamps closed.
Pump continues to signal "Over Temp" after previous actions.	Disconnect, label, and send to BioMed department.
	Obtain a different pump.

Local Cold Therapies (Cryotherapy)

Nursing Process Data

ASSESSMENT Database

- Determine purpose for cryotherapy (acute injury, joint stiffness).
- Review client's history for possible circulatory problems (Raynaud phenomenon, diabetes, peripheral vascular disease).
- Assess baseline data (peripheral circulation).
- Determine client's ability to sense temperature at site.
- Assess skin condition before and throughout cryotherapy.
- Assess for adverse responses to cryotherapy.

PLANNING Objectives

- To reduce local tissue metabolic and oxygen demand and prevent secondary metabolic injury
- To promote vasoconstriction and reduce bleeding
- To control the inflammatory response (edema formation)
- To achieve an anesthetic effect
- To reduce muscle spasticity and promote motion
- To facilitate rehabilitation exercise to stimulate lymph flow and reduce inflammatory edema

IMPLEMENTATION Procedures

DOCUMENTATION AND EVALUATION

Expected Outcomes

- Inflammatory response is controlled.
- Bleeding and edema formation are reduced or controlled.
- Local anesthetic response is achieved.
- Cryotherapy promotes rehabilitation exercise to reduce edema.
- Local cryotherapy causes no adverse effects.

Unexpected Outcomes/Alternative Actions

Pearson Nursing Student Resources

Find additional review materials at
nursing.pearsonhighered.com.
Prepare for success with NCLEX®-style practice questions and Skill Checklists.

Skill 24.2.1 | Applying an Ice Pack or Commercial Cold Gel Pack

Equipment

Small plastic bag, ice bag, or glove (consider size to be treated and necessity to mold)

Flaked or crushed ice from an ice machine (−1°C [30°F])

Salt

Or

Reusable silicone gel cold pack that has been in freezer (−5°C [23°F]) for at least 1.5 hr before initial use

Cloth or towel

Elastic bandage or towel

Tape (*do not use pins*)

Pillows

Preparation

1. Verify healthcare provider's order for type of cold pack, duration, and frequency of therapy.
2. Fill ice bag one-half to two-thirds full. ➤ *Rationale:* This facilitates molding of pack to treatment area.
3. Remove excess air from bag. ➤ *Rationale:* Air interferes with cold conduction.
4. Add salt to ice if a colder slush mixture is needed.
5. Take equipment to client's room.
6. Perform hand hygiene.

Procedure

1. Check two forms of client ID and introduce yourself.
2. Provide privacy.
3. Explain procedure and rationale to client. Discuss sensory experiences to expect with cold therapy.

EVIDENCE-BASED PRACTICE
Cold Gel Packs Useful for Analgesia

Clients receiving cold gel application four times a day for 14 days after soft tissue injury had less pain at rest and with movement and had less functional disability than those receiving a room temperature gel application.

Source: Martin, Paulson, & Nichols (2008)

4. Position client to expose area to be treated and remove any jewelry if present.
5. Assess circulation and client's ability to sense touch and heat or cold at site to be treated. ➤ *Rationale:* Inadequate circulation or impaired sensory perception may contraindicate therapy.
6. Use pillows or other item to elevate area to be treated. ➤ *Rationale:* Elevation promotes venous return, reduces swelling and pain.
7. Place towel directly onto skin area. ➤ *Rationale:* Towel provides a barrier to protect the skin from extreme temperature.
8. Place ice or cold gel pack atop towel and mold it to fit the treatment area. Bony areas (knee, ankle, elbow) usually require half the treatment time of fatty areas. Superficial

nerves at these joint sites are especially vulnerable to cold-induced neuropathy, especially if cold is combined with compression. ➤ *Rationale:* Manufacturer's instructions vary among products and must be followed for safe use.

9. Secure pack in place with toweling or elastic wrap using tape. ❶ ➤ *Rationale:* Outer wrap decreases warming effect of environmental air.
10. Place call bell within client's reach.
11. Assess client and treatment site in 5 min. ➤ *Rationale:* If **pallor**, blanching, mottling, or blisters occur, or client reports increased pain, burning, or severe numbness, discontinue pack immediately.

CLINICAL ALERT

- Frozen gel packs and crushed ice packs using ice frozen in a refrigerator or freezer (−16° to −19°C [3° to −2°F]) should not be applied directly to the skin.
- Packs with ice from an ice machine (−1°C [30°F]) do not require insulation and may be applied directly to the skin.
- During cryotherapy, erythema will occur.
- The client will experience four stages of cold progression: cold, stinging, burning, and numbness.
- Discontinue therapy when numbness occurs.

12. Limit treatment time to 10–15 min, or longer as prescribed. ➤ *Rationale:* A reusable cold pack usually loses its effectiveness after 15 min. Application time can be increased if cold is applied over bandages or against a cast. Never apply a fully cooled *reusable cold pack* directly to the skin; also, do not over-insulate the area.
13. Assess treatment area for adverse signs (wheals, **cyanosis**, pallor, pain, and tingling or numbness *distal* to treatment over a superficial nerve such as the radial nerve at the lateral elbow).
14. Discard used towels in linen hamper.
15. Return reusable ice bag or cold pack to freezer for at least 30 min before reusing.

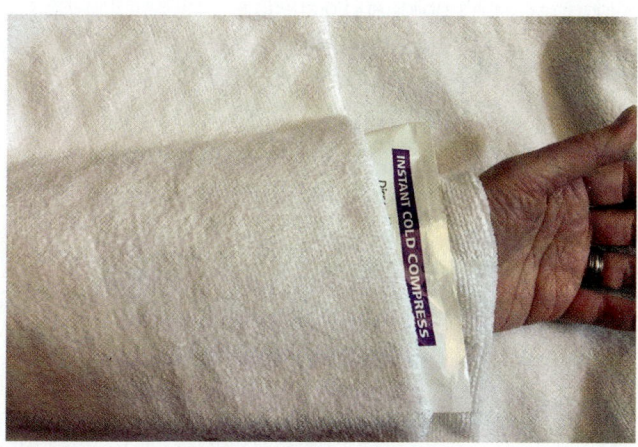

❶ Wrap and tape around pack to secure.

Skill 24.2.2 | Applying a Disposable Instant (Chemical) Cold Pack

Equipment

One-time-only use instant chemical cold pack (kept at room temperature)
Moist cloth or towel (if indicated on pack instructions)
Elastic bandage or towel
Tape
Pillows for elevation of part treated

Preparation

1. Review healthcare provider's order for local cryotherapy.
2. Gather equipment.
3. Perform hand hygiene.
4. Identify client by checking two forms of ID and having client state name and birth date.
5. Introduce self and explain the procedure.
6. Provide privacy and position the client.

❶ Follow manufacturer's instructions to activate chemical cold pack.

Procedure

1. Grasp top of cold pack and shake contents to bottom of bag. ❶
2. Hold package in the middle with both hands and follow manufacturer's directions on package.
3. Locate inner pouch and squeeze the package firmly to break the inner pouch.
4. Shake the package gently to mix the chemicals together.
5. Check that package is not punctured or opened.
   ➤ *Rationale:* If solution touches the skin, the chemicals can burn the skin.
6. Use pillows or other item to elevate part to be treated.
   ➤ *Rationale:* Elevation promotes venous return, reduces swelling and pain.

7. Avoid applying pack directly to skin; place disposable cold pack atop towel (according to instructions).
8. Mold pack to fit area and secure in place with toweling or elastic wrap and tape. ➤ *Rationale:* Outer wrap decreases warming effect of environmental air.
9. Place call bell within client's reach.
10. Assess client and treatment site in 5 min. ➤ *Rationale:* If mottling or blisters occur, or client reports numbness, discontinue pack immediately.
11. Limit treatment time to 30 min or as prescribed.
12. Dispose of one-time-only use pack. ➤ *Rationale:* Product cannot be reused by freezing, as frostbite may result.
13. Perform hand hygiene.

Skill 24.2.3 | Applying a Circulating Cold Therapy Pad

Note: There are many cold therapy systems available. Check with your institution's policy and procedure.

Equipment

Cold therapy system (e.g., EBIce) for single client use (cooler, site-specific disposable pad and straps, hose with connectors, pump with temperature control module)
Ice (4 quarts)
Cold water (2 quarts)
8-ply gauze or towel for insulation

Preparation

1. Review healthcare provider's order for application site.
2. Take cooler to client's room.
3. Check two forms of client ID and introduce yourself.

4. Explain purpose of cold therapy (to reduce pain, swelling).
5. Place 2 quarts cold water into cooler to reach water line marker.
6. Add ice to ice line marker (the pump inside cooler must be completely covered with ice–water).
7. Join short connectors on treatment pad to connectors on end of cooler system hose (disconnect these to discontinue treatment if, for instance, client gets out of bed). ❶
8. Plug DC power cord into jack on side of cooler.
9. Plug wall mount adapter into wall electrical outlet.
10. Turn system to coldest setting to initiate circulating cold water into treatment pad. ❷
11. Place cooler at or slightly *below* the level of the treatment site.
12. Perform hand hygiene.

❶ Join connectors on treatment pad to connectors on end of cooler system hose.

❷ Turn system to coldest setting to initiate treatment.

Procedure

1. Place protective gauze or towel over area to be treated (e.g., knee). ➤ *Rationale:* Pad should not be placed directly on client's skin.
2. Place treatment pad over area to be treated.
3. Secure pad and hose in place with enclosed straps. ➤ *Rationale:* Tight securing may restrict water flow through the pad.
4. Turn temperature control knob to 12:00 midpoint position. ➤ *Rationale:* Cold water will circulate into pad for 30 sec, and then stop for 70 sec. Intermittent cycling helps prevent treatment from being too cold.
5. After 10 min, assess color and sensation of site. ➤ *Rationale:* If site is discolored or numb, discontinue the treatment and notify healthcare provider.
6. Adjust cold water on–off cycling frequency according to client's comfort level. ➤ *Rationale:* Cycling periods may be 9, 30, or 52 sec; off periods may be for 91, 70, or 48 sec.
7. Periodically reassess client's response to cold treatment.
8. To refill ice and water, disconnect power cord from wall mount and cooler. ➤ *Rationale:* Cooler provides approximately 3 hr of treatment.
9. Discontinue treatment by unplugging power cord from wall and cooler, and remove treatment pad; empty ice and water from cooler; and place system in storage carton. ➤ *Rationale:* System belongs to the individual client.
10. Position client for comfort.
11. Perform hand hygiene.

Unit 24.2 Documentation and Evaluation

DOCUMENTATION for Local Cold Therapies

- Specific cold application used
- Area of body treated
- Positioning of area treated

- Duration and frequency of treatment
- Status of area pre- and post-treatment
- Client's response to therapy

EVALUATION/Critical Thinking

Expected Outcomes

- Inflammatory response is controlled.
- Bleeding and edema formation are minimized.
- Local anesthetic response is achieved.
- Local cryotherapy causes no adverse effects.
- Local cryotherapy facilitates rehabilitation therapies.

Unexpected Outcomes	Alternative Actions
• Local edema is increasing.	• Elevate extremity above level of heart. • Ensure that area is sufficiently covered with cold application to cause vasoconstriction. Check that area is not overinsulated.
• Bleeding or bruising continues in spite of local cold applications.	• Reassess area for possible "bleeders," which may require cautery or ligation by the healthcare provider. • Apply pressure to site to stop bleeding. • Assess pulse distal to bleed.
• Area to be treated is near superficial nerve.	• Use caution: Reduce time and duration of cold application. • Ask client to report any itching or tingling and discontinue therapy if these occur.
• Hand develops waxy white sheen, mottling, and numbness during local cold therapy.	• Immerse part in moving water at 40°–42°C (104°–107.6°F) until area flushes (about 30 min). • Do not apply dry heat; keep area uncovered at room temperature. • Do not rub part; keep part elevated.
• Cold cycling pad is not cooling properly.	• Examine if pad or hose is folded or kinked. • Determine whether securing straps are too tight and restricting flow of cold water. • Make sure pump inside cooler is completely covered with ice water. • Check all connections between hose and treatment pad. • If still not cooling properly, disconnect, label, and send to BioMed. • Obtain different machine.

Temperature Management Therapies

Nursing Process Data

ASSESSMENT Database

- Determine purpose for ordered temperature management therapy.
- Assess medications client has received (e.g., sedative).
- Determine desired core temperature target.
- Assess client data: vital signs, neurologic status, cardiovascular status, complete blood count (CBC), serum chemistries, and coagulation studies before and throughout treatment (if indicated).
- Assess ECG tracings throughout treatment (if indicated).
- Assess that temperature management system is functioning properly.
- Assess for early signs of shivering.

PLANNING Objectives

- To maintain or restore normal body temperature
- To reduce body core temperature
- To reduce metabolic process–tissue oxygen demand
- To prevent secondary metabolic injury
- To improve neurologic outcomes after cardiac arrest and traumatic brain injury
- To ensure temperature management system functions properly
- To monitor for therapeutic or adverse responses to therapy

IMPLEMENTATION Procedures

DOCUMENTATION AND EVALUATION

Expected Outcomes

- Target core body temperature is achieved.
- Tissue oxygen demand is reduced.
- Secondary metabolic injury is minimized.
- Neurologic outcomes are optimized.
- Temperature management system functions properly.
- Client has no adverse responses to therapy (arrhythmias, bleeding, shivering, afterdrop, or rebound hyperthermia).

Unexpected Outcomes/Alternative Actions

Pearson Nursing Student Resources

Find additional review materials at
nursing.pearsonhighered.com.
Prepare for success with NCLEX®-style practice questions and Skill Checklists.

Skill 24.3.1 | Using a Warm Air Blanket

Equipment

Means for continuous core body temperature monitoring (rectal, esophageal, bladder, pulmonary artery catheter), cable and module to monitor depending on thermometer used

Cardiac monitor

Automated blood pressure unit

Disposable warm air temperature management blanket with control unit and tubing

Gown or sheet and bath blanket

Preparation

1. Review healthcare provider order or agency protocol for client rewarming.
2. Obtain equipment and take to client's bedside.
3. Perform hand hygiene.
4. Check two forms of client ID and introduce self.

❶ A forced warm air convection blanket provides active rewarming. Client's temperature should increase gradually (2°–3°C/hr [3.5°–5°F/hr]).

5. Provide privacy and explain purpose of rewarming blanket and associated monitoring.
6. Establish continuous core body temperature, cardiac, and blood pressure monitoring.
7. Obtain baseline vital signs.

Procedure

1. Remove seal from warm air blanket port and insert corrugated tubing connected to unit.
2. Remove all client covering and apply light gown or place sheet over client (not both). ➤ *Rationale:* Warm air must have close contact with client's skin.
3. Place warm air blanket (perforated side down) over client.
4. Apply bath blanket over warm air blanket. ➤ *Rationale:* The bath blanket secures the air blanket.
5. Clamp unit's corrugated tubing to sheet or bed. ➤ *Rationale:* Clamping prevents dislodgement and heat loss.
6. Set unit for overheat (rapid warming), high (43°C [110°F]), medium (38°C [100°F]), or low (32°C [90°F]).
7. Turn system ON and reassure client that hum sound is due to air flow.
8. Monitor core temperature, cardiac rhythm, and blood pressure every 15 min. ➤ *Rationale:* Client's temperature should increase gradually (2°–3°C/hr [3.5°–5°F/hr]). Hypotension may occur due to vasodilation with rewarming; arrhythmias may occur.
9. Discontinue procedure when client's core temperature is 37°C (98.6°F), but continue to monitor. ➤ *Rationale:* **Afterdrop** (drop in temperature) or **overshoot** (overcompensation) may occur.
10. Dispose of single-use warm air blanket and return reusable equipment to appropriate area for cleaning and storage.
11. Perform hand hygiene.

Skill 24.3.2 | Providing Tepid Sponging

Equipment

Water or other coolant at prescribed temperature

Basin or tub

Washcloth and towels

Bath blanket

Electric fan

Automated blood pressure unit

Core temperature thermometer, cable and module to monitor

Preparation

1. Review order for cooling method (Box 24-1 ■).
2. Gather equipment and bring to client's room.
3. Check client's identification band and have client state name and birth date.

4. Provide privacy and explain procedure.
5. Perform hand hygiene.
6. Establish continuous core temperature monitoring (rectal, esophageal, bladder, or pulmonary artery), if indicated.
7. Establish ongoing blood pressure and cardiac monitoring.

Box 24-1 RAPID NONINVASIVE COOLING

Indicated for heat stroke or hyperthermia:

- Remove clothing.
- Place client in lateral recumbent position for maximal skin surface exposure.
- Spray entire body with water (20°C [68°F]), and direct a fan onto client to enhance evaporation.

Procedure

1. Remove client's clothing to allow for cooling and observation. Use bath blanket for privacy.
2. Monitor skin color and vital signs every 15–30 min during cooling. Immerse washcloths or material for sponging in ordered solution, generally 21°–27°C (70°–80.6°F). ➤ *Rationale:* Cool applications reduce heat by conduction.

> **CLINICAL ALERT**
> Do not immerse the client in cold or ice slush. Resulting peripheral vasoconstriction will impair body cooling and induce shivering, which produces heat.

3. Wring out excess solution and place cloths on neck, axillae, and groin. ➤ *Rationale:* The vascularity of these areas promotes cooling.
4. Depending on type of bath, change cloths every 5 min. ➤ *Rationale:* This prevents cloths from warming and losing effectiveness.
5. Cool the **ambient temperature** to 20°–22°C (68°–72°F). ➤ *Rationale:* This enhances therapy by convection and evaporation.

6. Direct a warm fan onto client to promote evaporation. ➤ *Rationale:* This enhances cooling by evaporation.
7. Assess client for early signs of shivering (ECG tremor artifact, palpable jaw line "hum" or trapezius muscle tension).
8. Stop treatment if client has early signs of shivering and notify healthcare provider. ➤ *Rationale:* Shivering raises core temperature, defeating the purpose of cooling interventions. The healthcare provider may order a narcotic or benzodiazepine for sedation.
9. Monitor client's temperature frequently. When temperature has decreased to desired level, dry skin and replace light covering over client and reposition for comfort. ➤ *Rationale:* A thin client will cool faster than one with more subcutaneous fat.
10. Continue to monitor vital signs, cardiac rhythm, I&O, and electrolytes.
11. Provide fluids and a high-calorie diet. ➤ *Rationale:* Increased temperatures increase metabolic rate.
12. Place cloths in linen hamper and return equipment to storage area.
13. Perform hand hygiene.

Skill 24.3.3 | Using a Cooling Blanket

Equipment

Thermal (heating–cooling) unit
Sterile or distilled water
Low-reading (below 34.4°C [94°F]) thermometer: rectal probe and lubricant, esophageal probe, urinary retention catheter, or pulmonary artery catheter with cable and module for continuous core temperature monitoring, depending on thermometer used
Clean gloves
Disposable thermal (cooling) blanket
One sheet or thin blanket
Covering for client
Four towels to wrap client's lower arms and legs
Tape
Leg or foot compression wraps
Sphygmomanometer and stethoscope or automated BP monitoring equipment
Continuous ECG monitoring
(see Circulatory Maintenance, Chapter 31)
Supplemental oxygen therapy equipment

Preparation

1. Check healthcare provider's orders for desired client temperature.
2. Identify medications client has received (narcotic, sedative).
3. Gather equipment and take to client's room.
4. Connect power cord to grounded outlet.
5. Ensure that reservoir (sterile or distilled water) level is adequate.

6. Perform hand hygiene.
7. Check client's identification band and have client state name and birth date.
8. Provide privacy and explain procedure.
9. Obtain baseline vital signs.

> **CLINICAL ALERT**
> Cooling with ice packs, cold fluids, and cooling mats may frequently result in overcooling. A more targeted approach is recommended.

Procedure

1. Place the cooling blanket on bed, and connect it to the Temperature Control Unit machine. ❶ ❷ ➤ *Rationale:* The cooling blanket increases heat transfer from client and reduces body temperature by conduction.

   a. Push the tubing tab to insert male tubing connector of the cooling pad into inlet opening. Release the tab.
   b. Repeat connection using the outlet opening.
   c. Turn the unit ON by pushing power switch. ❸
   d. Enter client's target temperature set point. ❹ ❺

2. Place a sheet or a thin bath blanket over the cooling blanket.
3. Place client on the cooling blanket.
4. Apply leg or foot compression wraps. ➤ *Rationale:* This prevents thrombus formation and reduces edema.

(continued)

Skill 24.3.3 | Using a Cooling Blanket (continued)

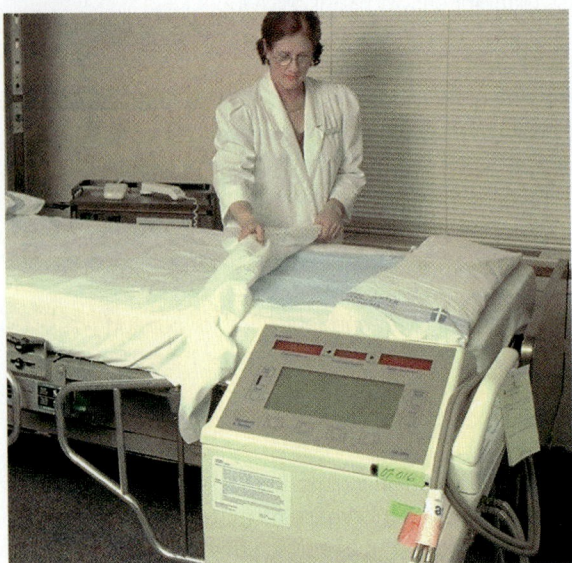

❶ Disposable cooling blanket is covered by sheet to protect the client's skin.

❷ Connect two ends of tubing—one from blanket, the other from machine.

5. Wrap client's lower arms and hands, lower legs, and feet (and scrotum, if indicated) in towels; tape to secure. ➤ *Rationale:* This prevents stimulation of skin thermoreceptors that initiate shivering.

6. Establish continuous core temperature monitoring.

7. Set the master temperature control to either automatic or manual operation. ➤ *Rationale:* There are two separate temperature controls, one for automatic and one for manual operation.

❸ After machine is powered and connected to blanket, push unit ON button.

❹ After checking fluid level, select desired mode: heat, cool, automatic, or monitor.

❺ Set fluid temperature to ordered set point, and press START.

EVIDENCE-BASED PRACTICE

Mild Hypothermia Improves Cardiac Arrest Survival Rates

Evidence has shown that mild therapeutic hypothermia could improve survival and neurologic outcome in clients following cardiac arrest. Healthcare providers do need to be aware that there may be associated adverse events such as bleeding, pneumonia, and bradycardia.

Source: Xiao et al. (2014)

Automatic Control

a. Don clean gloves.

b. If using rectal thermometer probe, digitally examine client's rectum to determine it is empty of stool.
➤ *Rationale:* Rectal temperature probe must make contact with mucosa.

c. Insert lubricated temperature probe into client's rectum 5 cm (2 in.).

d. If using bladder retention catheter with integrated temperature probe, determine that urine output is at least 20 mL/hr. ➤ *Rationale:* Probe actually measures urine temperature.

e. Set temperature control at the desired temperature (fluid temperature set point).

f. Turn automatic mode light on and press "START."
➤ *Rationale:* The pad fluid temperature will adjust automatically to bring client's temperature to a selected set point.

g. Check that the pad temperature limits are set as ordered.

Manual Control

a. Observe that the *manual* mode light is on.

b. Monitor the fluid set point, which indicates temperature of pad. ➤ *Rationale:* This ensures pad temperature is maintained at desired level.

8. Set the temperature control to 37°C (98.6°F), and begin lowering temperature 1°C (1.8°F) every 30 min to 1 hr as tolerated to prevent shivering, until 33° or 34°C (91.4° or 93.2°F) or set temperature is reached. ➤ *Rationale:* Blanket will cool client to set temperature independent of client's temperature. Gradual cooling helps prevent shivering.

9. Monitor client's temperature. ➤ *Rationale:* This will help prevent excessive cooling.

10. Assess client every 15 min for early signs of shivering: ECG muscle tremor artifact, jaw line "hum," trapezius muscle tension.

11. If early signs of shivering occur, discontinue therapy and notify healthcare provider or refer to agency hypothermia protocol. ➤ *Rationale:* Shivering causes an increase in core temperature, thus defeating the purpose of treatment. Shivering imposes a heavy metabolic burden and increases oxygen demand.

Mild	32°–37°C	89.6°–98.6°F
Moderate	28°–32°C	82.4°–89.6°F
Severe	20°–28°C	68.0°–82.4°F

12. Monitor vital signs every 15–30 min during therapy.
➤ *Rationale:* Bradycardia may occur. Blood pressure usually remains elevated due to vasoconstriction.

13. Monitor ECG for possible arrhythmias. ➤ *Rationale:* Potassium shifts into cells with induced hypothermia.

14. Monitor client's serum glucose. ➤ *Rationale:* Insulin levels are decreased with induced hypothermia. Glucose levels may rise with shivering. An *insulin drip* may be necessary to maintain glucose at 70–110 mg/dL.

15. Have client turn, cough, and take a deep breath every 1–2 hr. ➤ *Rationale:* Hypothermia reduces carbon dioxide production with possible resultant hypoventilation.

16. Monitor client's skin condition and bony prominences every 2 hr. ➤ *Rationale:* Client is at risk for pressure ulcers when skin temperature is lowered.

17. Turn off unit when client's temperature is 1°–3°C (1.8–5°F) above desired temperature. ➤ *Rationale:* Cooling will continue upon discontinuation of therapy.

18. Monitor vital signs every 15 min during rewarming.

19. Observe for edema. ➤ *Rationale:* Hypothermia causes fluid shift into the interstitium.

20. Clean and return reusable equipment to appropriate area and dispose of blanket.

21. Monitor client's vital signs frequently after discontinuation of treatment. ➤ *Rationale:* Overshoot hypothermia may occur.

22. Make client comfortable.

23. Perform hand hygiene.

Skill 24.3.4 | Using a Hypothermia Garment (Body Wraps)

Equipment

Water circulating vest and thigh wraps with temperature control console

Distilled water

Low-reading (below 34.4°C [94°F]) thermometer: rectal probe and lubricant, esophageal probe, urinary retention catheter, or pulmonary artery catheter with cable and module for continuous core temperature monitoring depending on thermometer used

Glucometer

Sequential compression devices (calf or foot)

Four towels for hands, feet, scrotum (if indicated)

Tape

Lubricating eye drops

Preparation

1. Review healthcare provider's order for induced hypothermia and target temperature. ❶

(continued)

Skill 24.3.4 | Using a Hypothermia Garment (Body Wraps) *(continued)*

❶ Hyper/Hypo thermia system provides surface warming and cooling to the torso and adjusts automatically to maintain client's target temperature. Medi-Therm MTA7900 and Repround system.
Source: Photo courtesy of Stryker Medical (Gaymar Team).

2. Determine that client has ice packs to axillae, neck, and groin before initiating therapy.
3. Determine that client has infusion of refrigerated normal saline at a rate of 1 L/hr before initiating therapy.
4. Determine client-specific rationale for temperature management (e.g., traumatic brain injury; comatose cardiac arrest client will be intubated and sedated and should be cooled within 4 hr of return of spontaneous circulation).
5. Determine whether client is intubated and receiving moderate sedation (see Chapter 26, Unit 4, Moderate Sedation [Conscious Sedation]).
6. Determine that essential continuous monitoring systems (ECG, arterial BP) have been established. (See Cardiovascular Maintenance, Chapter 31, and Advanced Nursing Skills, Chapter 33.)
7. Identify medications client has received (e.g., insulin drip).
8. Review client's recent lab results, specifically the bleeding profile.
9. Reduce room temperature and remove all sources of heat.
10. Gather equipment. Fill water reservoir of temperature control console per manufacturer's instructions. Perform hand hygiene.

Procedure
For Cooling
1. Identify client, introduce yourself, and briefly explain procedure and rationale, whether or not client is responsive.
2. Apply chest and thigh garments directly to client, fitting securely. ➤ **Rationale:** This is to maximize body surface contact.
3. Connect chest garment tubing to console.
4. Interconnect leg wraps' tubing; connect to single tubing, and then connect to console.

5. Apply towel wraps to client's hands and feet and secure with tape. ➤ **Rationale:** Skin counterwarming prevents stimulation of skin thermoreceptors that initiate shivering and need for sedation.
6. Connect core temperature monitoring thermometer to console. ➤ **Rationale:** A consistent body site must be used for temperature monitoring.
7. Plug console into outlet and turn machine ON.
8. Set target temperature to 33°C (91.4°F). ➤ **Rationale:** Target temperature should be reached in <4 hr. Cool time should be 24 hr from start of cooling.
9. Establish AUTO rapid mode of operation. ➤ **Rationale:** Garment system automatically adjusts to maintain client's target temperature. When client's temperature is within 1°C (1.8°F) of set point, machine will change to a slower mode to reduce overshoot.
10. Obtain basic metabolic panel (BMP) and complete blood count (CBC) every 12 hr during hypothermia. ➤ **Rationale:** Potassium levels decrease as potassium moves into cells with induction; potassium should be repleted to maintain levels >3.5 mEq/L.
11. Monitor client's glucose per agency protocol. ➤ **Rationale:** Insulin levels decrease with hypothermia, and glucose levels may rise with shivering. Every attempt should be made to avoid shivering, which increases basal metabolic rate (BMR).
12. Stop intravenous insulin as soon as glucose levels fall below 200 mg/mL, unless client has type 1 diabetes.
13. Monitor client's BP, ECG, and temperature every 30–60 min for 6 hr or until goal temperature is reached, then hourly. ➤ **Rationale:** BP may remain elevated due to vasoconstriction; bradycardia may occur; and arrhythmias may occur as potassium moves into cells. Overshoot hypothermia may occur with cooling (Box 24-2 ■).
14. Assess client's neurologic status hourly. (For Table 11-2, Glasgow Coma Scale, see Physical Assessment, Chapter 11; for the FOUR SCORE, see Neurologic Management, Chapter 32.)

Box 24-2 HYPOTHERMIA TOXICITY RELATED TO DURATION AND INTENSITY OF THERAPY AND RATE OF REWARMING

Cardiovascular—arrhythmias, bradycardia, reduced left ventricular function
Respiratory—hypoventilation with hypoxemia, atelectasis, and pneumonia
Gastrointestinal—stress ulcer, ileus
Hematologic—platelet dysfunction, coagulopathy (prolonged PT/PTT)
Immunologic—impaired neutrophil function, risk for infection
Metabolic—hypokalemia, hyperglycemia due to decreased insulin release, possible systemic inflammatory response syndrome (SIRS) with rewarming

15. Monitor client every 15 min for early signs of shivering. ➤ *Rationale:* Shivering raises core temperature, interferes with the cooling process, and increases oxygen consumption.
16. Provide additional extremity and face counterwarming to help suppress shivering.
17. If shivering continues, medicate according to protocol (meperidine or benzodiazepine) or notify healthcare provider.
18. Monitor client's skin condition every 2 hr; skin should be kept dry. ➤ *Rationale:* Vasoconstriction increases risk for pressure ulcers.
19. Obtain blood cultures ×2, 12 hr after initiating hypothermia. ➤ *Rationale:* Hypothermia may cause neutropenia and may increase risk for aspiration pneumonia.
20. Provide frequent eye care using lubricating drops.
21. Assess client for signs of bleeding. ➤ *Rationale:* Hypothermia can prolong clotting time and decrease platelet count.
22. Monitor urine output hourly.

For Rewarming

1. Stop all potassium administration 4 hr before rewarming. ➤ *Rationale:* Potassium level will increase with rewarming.
2. Enter target temperature to 36°C (96.8°F) for rewarming.
3. Gradually rewarm client to normothermia over 12–24 hr or remove chest and leg garments and allow client to rewarm passively to normothermia. ➤ *Rationale:* Rewarming should be done slowly, no faster than 0.5°C/hr (1°F/hr) to prevent rewarming acidosis, shivering, or hypotension (due to vasodilation).
4. Continue to monitor client's temperature. ➤ *Rationale:* Rebound hyperthermia may occur with rewarming. Avoid temperature above 37.5°C (99.5°F).

> **CLINICAL ALERT**
> Fever should be controlled during the acute phase of brain injury. Fever is a common occurrence in critically ill neurologic clients and is associated with increased morbidity and mortality after ischemic and hemorrhagic stroke and in subarachnoid hemorrhage. In traumatic brain injury clients, temperature elevation has been linked with increased intracranial pressure.

5. Monitor for hypoglycemia, especially if client has received continuous insulin infusion.
6. Obtain serum potassium level every 6 hr during rewarming. ➤ *Rationale:* Hyperkalemia may occur as potassium shifts out of cells with rewarming.
7. When client is stable, discontinue garment therapy and dispose of single-use body wraps.
8. Return reusable temperature control console to storage area.
9. Perform hand hygiene.

Unit 24.3 Documentation and Evaluation

DOCUMENTATION for Temperature Management Therapies

- Specific type of temperature management therapy used
- Target temperature settings established
- Application of compression wraps
- Application of insulating towel wraps to extremities and scrotum
- Time of initiation and duration of therapy
- Baseline and vital signs trends, including monitored cardiac rhythm
- Serum glucose determinations
- Medications administered
- Client's response to temperature management therapy and any adverse effects
- Healthcare provider notification of client's response (if indicated)

EVALUATION/Critical Thinking

Expected Outcomes

- Target core body temperature is achieved.
- Tissue oxygen demand is reduced.
- Secondary metabolic injury is minimized.
- Neurologic outcomes are optimized.
- Temperature management system functions properly.
- Client has no adverse responses to therapy (arrhythmias, bleeding, shivering, afterdrop or rebound hyperthermia).

Unexpected Outcomes	Alternative Actions
• Client's core temperature decreases rapidly to desired level.	• Turn off cooling blanket or discontinue tepid sponging. • Monitor temperature every 15 min to detect additional temperature decrease.
• Cooling blanket does not function properly.	• Check that plug is connected to the outlet. • Check that the fluid level is sufficient and that unit freezing has not occurred. • Check that the thermistor probe is properly connected. • Check that the cool limit on the pad is not set too high.
• Shows early signs of shivering.	• Adjust rate of cooling every 15 min to detect additional temperature decrease. • Cover client's face for additional counterwarming. • Contact healthcare provider for medication order (narcotic or sedative).
• Hyperthermic client's core temperature is not reduced.	• Discuss need for cold water spray and warm air fan to reduce client's temperature. • Consider that cutaneous vasoconstriction due to external cooling may be conserving core body heat. • Discuss need for more aggressive internal cooling measures (e.g., endovascular cooling).
• Rebound hyperthermia occurs after induced hypothermia cooling and rewarming.	• Provide supplemental oxygen therapy. • Leave the temperature management garment in place for up to 12 additional hr once goal temperature has been achieved. The garment can cool the client if rebound hyperthermia occurs.
• Client shows early signs of skin breakdown with nonblanchable area noted.	• Loosen garment to remove direct cold and compression over area. • Apply a clear adhesive dressing over the area to add a layer of protection and help prevent shearing.

Chapter Wrap-Up

GERONTOLOGIC Considerations

Older Adult Clients Are More Susceptible to Injury From Heat and Cold Therapy as a Result of Physiologic Changes or Medical Conditions

- The epidermal cells are replaced more slowly in older adults.
- Skin in older adults is thin and contains less moisture.
- Older adults have a reduced sensitivity to pain and therefore may not feel untoward effects of heat and cold treatment.
- Temperature should be reduced when using heat therapy because the older adult client's skin burns more easily.

Vital Signs and Frequent Assessment May Be Necessary During Heat and Cold Therapy, as Vasodilation From Heat or Vasoconstriction From Cold Can Cause Changes in Cardiac Function and Blood Pressure

- Peripheral circulation may be compromised due to chronic volume depletion, atherosclerosis, or microvascular disease.
- Sensation in distal extremities may be impaired in older adult clients with neuropathy due to diabetes.
- Older adults may take medications that decrease sweating (anticholinergics for Parkinson) or increase heat production (CNS stimulants or lithium).

- Serious infections may not elicit a febrile response.
- Temperature threshold for sweating is higher in the older client and ability to mount a metabolic response to temperature loss is limited.

- Living conditions and financial limitations may not afford adequate environmental control.
- Hemodynamic responses to heat–cold therapies may be more unpredictable.

MANAGEMENT Guidelines

Each state legislates a Nurse Practice Act for RNs and LPNs/LVNs. Healthcare facilities are responsible for establishing and implementing policies and procedures that conform to their state's regulations. Verify the regulations and role parameters for each healthcare worker in your facility.

Delegation

- RNs may assign LPNs/LVNs to perform most of the skills covered in this chapter. For example, they may apply heat or ice to an extremity, set up a hypothermia blanket, or give a sitz bath.
- Assessment before delegation and evaluation of the client's response during and after therapy is required of licensed delegate.
- Systemic cooling or heating therapies are indicated for critically ill clients in special care settings who may be

sedated. These clients are generally monitored and cared for exclusively by licensed personnel.

- Unlicensed assistive personnel (UAP) may be assigned to do many of the skills with supervision. They should not be assigned to use infant radiant warmers or cooling blankets without special guidance and supervision.

Interprofessional Communication

- Because many of the procedures in this chapter are performed by UAP, there must be excellent reporting to the nurse responsible for client care. The treatment effect of these measures will influence client health, so outcomes of the procedures must be charted as well as orally reported to the nurse.
- Any adverse responses (local or systemic) should be reported to prescribing healthcare provider so that corrective measures can be provided.

CASE STUDY Applications

Scenario 1

Mrs. Moore is a 52-year-old client who has been admitted to your unit after a laparoscopic cholecystectomy. She has a peripheral IV infusion of 5% dextrose in 0.45% NS infusing at 120 mL/hr in the cephalic vein at the left wrist. She receives intermittent antibiotic therapy by IV piggyback.

One hour after the evening IV antibiotic administration, she calls the nurse and reports a discomfort in her left arm. Assessment findings include discomfort in the area, slight pallor, swelling (lower arm circumference 3.8 cm [1½ in.] greater than contralateral arm), and coolness to touch.

1. Based on assessment findings, what is the probable complication and what are possible causes?
2. What should the nurse's first action be?
3. How should the area be treated?
4. When are heat or cold therapies indicated to manage IV complications?

Scenario 2

Mr. X, age 78, lives alone in a small urban dwelling. He has a history of heart failure and COPD, and was found unresponsive in his back yard by his neighbor at 2:00 p.m.

He has been admitted to the ED with a temperature of 40°C (104°F). Additional findings include confusion, lack of perspiration, dizziness, blurred vision, tachycardia, and hyperventilation. His laboratory tests reflect dehydration; insertion of a Foley catheter reveals minimal urine output.

His diagnosis is heatstroke.

1. What causes hyperthermia, and how does it differ from fever?
2. Why are the older adults at great risk for developing heat-related illness?
3. What is the immediate goal of treatment for Mr. X?
4. Why are external cooling measures the treatment of choice rather than the use of antipyretics?
5. What are the principles involved with application of external cooling measures?
6. Why should cooling therapy be discontinued if shivering occurs?
7. What other ongoing assessments are essential during the cooling process?
8. How can heat-related injuries be prevented?

NCLEX® Review Questions

Unless otherwise specified, choose only one (1) answer.

1. What causes the elevation of body temperature in a fever?
   A. Cytokine influence on the hypothalamus
   B. Injury to the hypothalamus
   C. Dehydration
   D. Environmental extremes

2. What is the most effective method to reduce fever?
   A. Tepid sponging
   B. A cooling blanket
   C. Antipyretic medication
   D. Cool packs to axillae and groin

3. What effect does shivering in response to external cryo-therapy have on the febrile client?
   A. Enhances body temperature cooling
   B. Reduces metabolic rate
   C. Increases heat production
   D. Increases pyrogen production

4. To what maximum temperature do most hospitals control facility water?
   A. 30°C (95°F)
   B. 37.8°C (100°F)
   C. 43.3°C (110°F)
   D. 49°C (120°F)

5. When the surgical client wears a head covering, what kind of heat loss is prevented?
   A. Radiation
   B. Evaporation
   C. Convection
   D. Conduction

6. Which of the following fluids is preferred to rehydrate an overheated, dehydrated client?
   A. Water
   B. Intravenous dextrose in water
   C. Sport drink
   D. Sugared cola

7. Expected effects of local cold (cryo) therapy include which of the following?
   Select all that apply.
   A. Pallor
   B. Flushing
   C. Blister formation
   D. Anesthesia
   E. Burning
   F. Numbness

8. After a sitz bath, the nurse should monitor the client for which possible complication?
   A. Orthostatic hypotension
   B. Perineal fungal infection
   C. Increased vaginal bleeding
   D. Exacerbation of hemorrhoid discomfort

9. Why should cold applications to injured joints be of short duration?
   A. Reactive vasodilation may occur.
   B. Joints become less flexible with cold application.
   C. Bleeding may be induced.
   D. Injury to superficial nerves can occur.

10. Why are heat therapies contraindicated for areas with circulatory insufficiency?
    A. It increases tissue need for oxygen.
    B. It decreases metabolic rate, thereby increasing ischemia.
    C. It promotes inflammation.
    D. It decreases sensation and increases risk for injury.

QSEN Activity

Domain: Safety

KSA: Skill

Activity:

You are the licensed nurse on the medical-surgical floor, and you have a UAP working with you. You have just been informed by the UAP that your client's IV has infiltrated.

Upon inspection, you note edema, erythema, and warmth midway from the antecubital fossa to the distal humerus. You discontinue the IV and ask the UAP to apply a warm compress. You instruct the UAP to monitor and report back on the client's condition.

After delegating the task to the UAP, what pieces of information are important to follow up on?

Bibliography

Eliopoulos, C. (2009). *Gerontological nursing* (7th ed.). Philadelphia: Lippincott Williams & Wilkins.

Finkelstein, R., & Alam, H. (2010). Induced hypothermia for trauma: Current research and practice. *Journal of Intensive Care Medicine, 25*(4), 205–226.

Hong, J. M., Lee, J. S., Song, H. J., Jeong, H. S., & Lee, K. (2014). Therapeutic hypothermia after recanalization in patients with acute ischemic stroke. *Stroke, 45*(1), 134–140.

Koran, Z. (2008). Therapeutic hypothermia in the postresuscitation patient: The development and implementation of an evidence based protocol for the emergency department. *Advanced Emergency Nursing Journal, 30*(4), 319–330.

Martin, S., Paulson, C.P., & Nichols, W. (2008). Does heat or cold work better for acute muscle strain? *The Journal of Family Practice, 57*(12), 820–821.

Scirica, B. M. (2013). Therapeutic hypothermia after cardiac arrest. *Circulation, 127*, 244–250. doi:10.1161/CIRCULATIONAHA.111.076851

Smith, J., Stevens, J., Taylor, M., & Tibbey J. (2002, Feb.). A randomized, controlled trial comparing compression bandaging and cold therapy in postoperative total knee replacement surgery. *Orthopaedic Nursing, 21*(2), 61–66.

Xiao, G., Guo, Q., Shu, M., Xie, X., Deng, J., Zhu, Y., & Wan, C. (2014). Safety profile and outcome of mild therapeutic hypothermia in patients following cardiac arrest: Systematic review and analysis. *Emergency Medicine Journal, 13*(30), 91–100. doi:10.1136/emermed-2012-201120

Chapter 25
Wound Care and Dressings

Learning Objectives

25.1 Describe the three phases of wound healing.

25.2 Define the three types of wound healing.

25.3 Discuss three factors that affect wound healing.

25.4 State three complications associated with wound healing.

25.5 State criteria used to assess a wound.

25.6 Compare and contrast the four stages of pressure ulcers.

25.7 Write three nursing diagnoses for a client requiring wound care.

25.8 State three goals of wound care.

25.9 Discuss the effect of topical agents in wound healing.

25.10 Differentiate between clean, contaminated, and infected wounds.

25.11 Compare and contrast clean and sterile technique.

25.12 Describe dressing classification and indication for each type of dressing: gauze, transparent film, hydrogel, calcium alginate, foam, composite, hydrocolloid, and impregnated gauze.

25.13 Explain appropriate use of dressings: gauze, transparent adhesive film, hydrocolloid, and hydrogel.

25.14 Describe two methods to manage bacterial bioburden.

25.15 Outline the steps in irrigating a wound.

25.16 Describe the steps to obtain a wound specimen for culture.

25.17 Perform the steps of a surgical hand scrub.

25.18 Prepare a sterile field for a dressing change.

25.19 Demonstrate the steps of putting on sterile gloves.

25.20 Describe the procedure for cleaning around a drain site.

25.21 List steps used to maintain a Hemovac or Jackson–Pratt suction drain.

25.22 Demonstrate changing a sterile dressing.

25.23 Outline the steps for removal of staples and sutures.

25.24 Outline the procedure for changing a wet-to-moist dressing.

25.25 Compare and contrast the three adjunctive wound care therapies.

25.26 Complete documentation on a wound assessment and wound care.

25.27 State five debridement methods.

25.28 Describe the term *surgical site infection*.

Chapter Outline

Terminology

Adhesions fibrous scar tissue that binds anatomic surfaces that normally are separate from each other, most commonly in the abdomen.

Anemia a condition in which the number of circulating red blood cells, or hemoglobin, is reduced.

Antimicrobial referring to an agent that prevents the multiplication of microorganisms.

Asepsis prevention of contact with microorganisms.

Bacterial bioburden the number of contaminating bacteria present on an object.

Collagen formation build-up or creation of the protein substance of the white fibers of skin, bone, and cartilage.

Debridement removal of damaged tissue and cellular debris from a wound or burn to prevent infection and promote healing.

Debris remains of damaged or broken-down tissue or cells.

Dehiscence a bursting open, as a graafian follicle or wound (especially an abdominal wound).

Dermis synonym for *corium*, the skin layer beneath the epidermis; part of the skin that contains vascular connective tissue.

Edematous having abnormally large amounts of fluid in the intercellular tissue spaces of the body, causing swelling.

Electrical stimulation (of a wound) transfer of electrical current through contact with moist wound bed to promote healing.

Epidermis superficial, avascular layers of skin.

Epithelial having to do with the top layer of skin.

Erythema redness of the skin due to congestion of capillaries.

Eschar scabs or dry crust resulting from trauma such as a thermal or chemical burn, infection, or excoriating skin disease.

Evisceration protrusion of the viscera; removal of the viscera.

Exudate fluid that filters from the circulatory system into areas of the body that are inflamed.

Friable easily shattered, crumbled, or pulverized, such as tissues of the liver.

Gangrene death and putrefaction of body tissue precipitated by poor or absent blood supply to the tissue; occurs as a result of infection, injury, or disease processes.

Granulation formation of granules, fleshy projections formed on the surface of a gaping wound that is not healing by the normal joining together of skin edges.

Hyperbaric oxygen therapy 100% oxygen administered at greater than 1 atmosphere pressure absolute.

Incision a cut made with a knife.

Infection morbid state caused by multiplication of pathogenic microorganisms within the body.

Inflammatory process localized response when injury or destruction of tissue has occurred; destroys, wards off, or dilutes the causative agent or the injured tissue.

Irrigated rinsed or washed out with a fluid.

Ischemia restriction in blood supply (generally due to factors related to blood vessels, such as stenosis and/or occlusions) leading to damage or dysfunction of tissue.

Isolation limitation of movement and social contacts of a client, especially of those having communicable diseases.

Keloid scar-like growth of collagen that results in a rounded, hard, shiny, white benign tumor.

Macrophages large monocytes that have left the circulation and settled and matured in tissue, serving as scavengers of the blood, cleaning it of old cells and cellular debris.

Maceration the softening and whitening of skin that is kept constantly wet.

Microorganisms minute living bodies not perceptible to the naked eye.

Monocytes phagocytic white blood cells that mature into macrophages.

Monokines chemical mediators released by monocytes and macrophages during the immune response, which affect growth and activity of other white blood cells.

Myofibroblasts atypical fibroblasts with features of both fibroblasts and smooth muscle cells.

Necrotic pertaining to the death of tissue in response to disease or injury.

Negative pressure wound therapy negative pressure applied to a wound to promote healing, using an electrical pump.

Neutrophils white blood cells responsible for the body's protection against infection and playing a large role in the inflammatory process.

Organism an individual animal, plant, or single-celled life form.

Pathogenic related to disease-producing organisms.

Periwound area surrounding wound; healthy tissue around wound.

Phagocytosis process by which certain cells engulf and destroy microorganisms and cellular debris.

Pressure ulcer a break in the skin caused by pressure and restricted blood flow to the area; generally occurs over bony prominences of the heels, sacrum, hip, and shoulder; decubitus ulcer.

Primary intention for wounds, closure by approximation of wound edges or by placement of a graft or skin flap.

Purulent containing pus, or caused by pus.

Pus an inflammation containing leukocytes and exudate.

Sanguineous containing blood (used to describe wound drainage); bright red

Secondary intention second stage in wound healing in which granulation occurs.

Semiocclusive dressings materials that create and maintain a moist environment by holding liquid drainage from wound and moisture vapor at the wound surface.

Serosanguineous containing both blood and serous fluid (used to describe wound drainage)

Serous containing clear or watery fluid (used to describe wound drainage)

Slough to shed or cast off dead tissue; the name for dead, cast-off tissue.

Surgical site infection (SSI) an infection related to an operative procedure.

Tertiary intention open method of wound healing, allowing granulation to occur.

Wound dehiscence the separation of layers of a surgical wound.

Wound healing three phases of wound resolution: inflammation, proliferation, and maturation (or remodeling).

Wound Healing

The three major phases of **wound healing** are inflammation (or reaction), proliferation (or regeneration), and maturation (or wound remodeling).

Note: Refer to Chapter 8 for information on prevention of wounds.

Inflammatory Phase (Reaction)

The onset of the first phase of wound healing occurs immediately after an injury and lasts 2–5 days. After the injury, small blood vessels dilate and become more permeable, and serous fluid leaks into the traumatized tissue as a result of histamine and prostaglandin release. Plasma and electrolytes leak into the interstitial spaces, causing edema. The edema leads to a reddened, swollen, and tender wound. **Neutrophils** reach the site in about 6 hr. Through the process of **phagocytosis**, they assist in preventing **infection** by ingesting and digesting bacteria. Oxygen is necessary for the neutrophils to destroy the bacteria. They survive only several hours after ingesting bacteria and **necrotic** tissue before releasing their intracellular contents that form part of the wound **exudate**. By the fourth day, **monocytes** enter the wound and differentiate into **macrophages**, which digest necrotic tissue, remove **debris**, and inhibit microbial growth. Macrophages and monocytes play a role in collagen synthesis. If macrophages are depleted, deposition of wound collagen decreases significantly. Macrophages direct healing through the release of **monokines** (substances that affect the function of other cells and have an effect on the immune system).

Proliferative, or Granulation, Phase (Regeneration)

This phase begins between about 2 days to 3 weeks after the injury and ends 14–24 days later. During **granulation**, rapid growth of **epithelial** cells produces a protective covering for the wound. The granulation tissue is formed by rebuilding the vascular capillary network and collagen tissue. The collagen fibers increase the tensile strength of the wound and provide wound integrity. Collagen fibers fill in the gaps and form a scar. Wound scar tissue is very fragile and susceptible to reinjury. After 6 weeks, the scar has only 10% of the tensile strength of normal skin. Large wounds may take months to build enough granulation tissue to close the wound. Healthy granulation tissue has a reddish-pink color. This color results from the increased blood flow that delivers oxygen and nutrients to the newly formed tissue.

Maturation, or Wound-Remodeling, Phase

Wound contraction begins between 14 and 21 days after the injury and can last up to 2 years. During this phase, the scar shrinks and thins. It becomes less red as the capillaries regress. Contraction of the wound occurs as a result of **myofibroblasts**, which assist in moving the wound edges toward the center of the wound. The skin and fascia of the healed wound achieve only about 70%–80% of the tensile strength of normal skin. Scar tissue has fewer melanocytes and thus has a lighter color than normal skin.

Wound Classification

There are different wound classification systems used to describe wounds. These are useful when the nurse is planning for wound care management. The classification systems include categorizing the wound by cause (intentional or unintentional), cleanliness (clean, contaminated, or infected), depth (superficial, partial thickness, or full thickness), and color.

The RYB (red-yellow-black) classification system has been used in wound care classification since the late 1980s. This system classifies open wounds that are healing by secondary or delayed **primary intention** in both acute and chronic wounds. It is used as an adjunct to other classification systems. It does not provide an in-depth, comprehensive evaluation. It can be used to determine the state of healing. This system identifies what phase a wound is in on the continuum of the wound healing process. Red wounds (R) can be in the inflammatory, proliferative, or maturation phase of wound healing. Yellow wounds (Y) are infected or contain fibrinous **slough** and are not ready to heal. Black wounds (B) contain necrotic tissue and are not ready to heal. Treatment options are based on the color of the wound. Red wounds need to be kept clean and moist. Yellow wounds require the removal of slough or fibrinous tissue. Black wounds must have the **eschar** removed for healing to take place. If the wound has a combination of colors, the rule is that the most severe color treatment is completed.

Wounds are also classified into six main categories, which may overlap: surgical, traumatic, diabetic, venous, arterial, and pressure.

Types of Wound Healing

Primary Intention

This is the simplest form of healing. The skin is cleanly incised through a surgical **incision** or a traumatic laceration. The wound can be closed with sutures or staples that approximate (pull together) the wound edges. These wounds close rapidly because there are no gaps in the tissue. The top layer of cells migrates, or epithelizes, within 72 hr. The wound surface is "sealed," thus preventing bacteria from entering and fluid from escaping. The tensile strength of the wound is very weak at this stage of healing.

Secondary Intention

These wounds heal by granulation. As granulation tissue builds, it fills the gap under the skin and cells epithelize from the edge of the wound to create the closure. Burns, pressure ulcers, and wounds with large pieces of skin missing heal by **secondary intention**. In these wounds, no edges are available to be approximated and sutured. These wounds are at risk for local and systemic infection due to the destruction of the **dermis** and the increased time necessary for healing to occur.

Tertiary Intention

Healing by **tertiary intention** is a method that leaves the wound open to heal. Reasons for this method are that wounds cannot be sutured, **dehiscence** has occurred, or the wound is infected and needs frequent irrigations and dressing changes to facilitate healing. Clients with peritonitis, a ruptured appendix, or diverticula frequently require this type of wound healing. After irrigations and dressing changes have been done for about 10 days, the wound is sutured and allowed to heal by primary and secondary intention.

Major Factors Affecting Wound Healing

In addition to proper wound care and generally good physical health, nutrition plays a major role in wound healing. Calories need to be increased to 30–35 cal/kg/day. Fluid intake should be at least 2500 mL/day unless contraindicated. Medications may interfere with wound healing.

Note: Positioning to help wounds heal and to prevent contamination of wounds is discussed in Chapter 8.

Nutrition

Low serum albumin levels slow the diffusion of oxygen and diminish the ability of neutrophils to kill bacteria. Low oxygen at the capillary level diminishes the proliferation of healthy granulation tissue. Zinc deficiency can slow the rate of epithelization and decrease wound and collagen strength. Adequate amounts of vitamins A, B1, B5, and C and of iron and copper are necessary for effective **collagen formation**. Collagen synthesis also depends on appropriate intake of protein, carbohydrates, and fats. Wound healing requires almost double the usual protein and carbohydrate requirements for age. For the scar to develop adequate tensile strength, the client's intake of vitamin C, iron, and zinc must be increased (Table 25-1 ■).

General Physical Health

The major obstacle to wound healing is infection. Infected wounds have **friable** tissue, bleed easily, and have delayed healing. Immunosuppressed clients have more difficulty healing wounds because the inflammatory phase is impaired. When the blood glucose level is consistently over

Table 25-1 Nutritional Support for Wound Healing

Nutrient	Food Sources
Protein	Meat, fish, poultry, milk, cheese, eggs, dried beans, peas, peanut butter
Carbohydrates	Legumes, fruits, vegetables, whole-grain cereal, bread, pasta
Vitamins	
Vitamin A	Dark green leafy vegetables, milk, eggs, carrots, liver, sweet potatoes
Vitamin C	Citrus fruits, vegetables, potatoes, tomatoes
Minerals	
Iron	Meat, eggs, cereal, vegetables
Copper	Seafood, nuts, seeds, organ meats
Zinc	Meat, liver, seafood, eggs, legumes
Calories	30–35 cal/kg/day

200 mg/dL or the hemoglobin is below 10 g/dL, wounds do not follow the usual phases of healing. Any condition that reduces the formation of adequate white blood cells, especially macrophages, adversely affects healing. Such conditions include diabetes mellitus, **anemia**, uremia, cancer, atherosclerosis, infection, and malnutrition. Older clients, clients who smoke or are obese, and those undergoing radiation or steroid therapy are also prone to delayed wound healing. Laboratory values should be monitored frequently for lymphocytes, protein (albumin), and hemoglobin.

Medications

Any medication that reduces the inflammatory response, such as steroids and nonsteroidal medications used to treat arthritis or respiratory conditions, also impairs wound healing. Anti-inflammatories decrease epithelization and wound contraction and may also affect fibroblast proliferation and collagen synthesis. Steroids decrease the tensile strength of a closed wound and cause inadequate deposits of collagen, but administration of vitamin A can reverse the processes associated with steroid use.

Goals of Wound Care

Wound assessment and measures to treat wounds have changed dramatically in recent years. The major trend is to treat wounds with moisture-retentive dressings rather than by drying them. Wound care specialists diverge on the use of sterile versus clean technique during dressing changes.

Note: Presurgical skin prep is discussed in Chapter 26.

Whatever plan is used in treating a wound, the goals remain the same:

- Remove necrotic tissue to promote wound healing.
- Prevent, eliminate, or control infection.

- Absorb drainage (exudate).
- Maintain a moist wound environment.
- Protect the wound from further injury.
- Protect the surrounding skin from infection and trauma.

To accomplish these goals, a moist wound environment must be maintained to allow tissue to granulate. A wound bed that is too moist or too dry kills healthy tissue and impairs healing. Drainage from the wound site needs to be contained to protect adjacent healthy skin from **maceration**. All wounds require a dressing that is dry on the air-exposed side; this prevents bacterial invasion by downward capillary mobility of contaminants. The dressing should be secured over the wound and taped in place using the "window paning" method of taping if there is no adhesive backing on the dressing. Using this method, the edges remain taped down and the dressing stays intact.

There are many types of wound care products available (Table 25-2 ■), including skin cleansers, skin barriers, irrigants, various types of dressings, gauze dressings, and enzymes. Physician and wound care specialist preferences, as well as type and extent of wound, determine products and methods of wound care.

Complications Associated With Wound Healing

Chronic wounds are wounds that do not heal completely in 6 weeks. Examples of this type of wound include deep ulcers, large burns, and infected cuts. Conditions that lead to slow healing are poor blood supply or low oxygen (caused by low blood pressure or blocked or narrow blood vessels), infection where bacteria is found in the wound due to dead tissue, a weak immune system, and tissue swelling. Diabetes can increase the risk for wound infections.

Adhesions are a complication that may occur after wound healing has seemed to progress satisfactorily. Adhesions frequently form in the peritoneal cavity after abdominal surgery and can either constrict or fold around the intestines.

Incisional strangulated internal hernias, which may even be gangrenous, cause frequent admissions to the hospital. Other complications are surgical or incisional hernias that occur when the intraperitoneal pressure pushes against scar tissue, causing a hernia (or outpouching) through the incision.

Contractures, formed as a result of a shortening of scar tissue, can decrease mobility and joint movement. Contractures caused by incisional scars are far less common than those caused by scar tissue from burns.

Excessive collagen formation results in the formation of a **keloid**, a complication that does not present a serious problem with body function but that generally causes an altered self-image if the keloid is large or in a prominent place on the body.

Wound Infections

Open wounds of any type provide an environment for bacterial invasion. All wounds may be considered contaminated but not necessarily infected. The risk of surgical site infection (SSI) is approximately 1%–3% for elective clean surgeries. Healthcare-associated infections (HAIs) vary depending on the length of hospital stay and present the highest burden on clients and hospitals in terms of morbidity, mortality, prolonged length of hospital stay, and additional costs. Surgical site infections may be the most frequent HAIs after asymptomatic bacteriuria (Johns Hopkins Medicine, n.d.).

Wound care must include regular wound cleansing, use of **semiocclusive dressings**, use of Standard Precautions when providing care to the client, proper hand hygiene technique, and adherence to dressing change protocols. Semiocclusive dressings in wound care have reduced the incidence of wound infections dramatically compared with gauze dressings. These dressings promote a moist environment, provide a mechanical barrier for bacterial invasion, and reduce airborne dispersal of bacteria during dressing changes.

The clinical symptoms of wound infection generally begin 3–5 days postoperatively or after injury. When the client's temperature and pulse rate increase, an associated tachypnea occurs. As the **inflammatory process** occurs, the wound becomes progressively more tender, painful, and **edematous**. **Erythema** surrounds the edges of the wound unless the infection is in the deeper tissues. Abnormal firmness of the wound edge may be present. Usually, a persistent

Table 25-2 RYB Wound Dressing Guidelines*

Dressings Most Commonly Used to Treat RYB Wounds			
Red Wounds	Yellow Wounds (fibrinous slough)	Yellow wounds (infected)	Black wounds
Biologicals	Alginate	Alginates	Alginate
Foams	Exudate absorbers	Impregnated dressings	Hydrocolloid
Gauze	Foams	Exudate absorbers	Hydrogel
Hydrocolloids	Hypertonic gauze	Foams	Gauze
Hydrogels	Hydrocolloid	Hypertonic gauze	Transparent film
Moist gauze	Hydrogel	Wound pouches	
Nonadherent gauze	Transparent film		
Transparent film			

*See Skill 25.3.2, Assessing a Wound.

WBC count of 12,000/mm³ or greater, lasting longer than 72 hr, accompanies the infection. Foul-smelling, **purulent** drainage may occur. An absence of local signs of infection does not necessarily mean that deep wound infections are absent.

Several **microorganisms** are responsible for the majority of wound infections. *Staphylococcus aureus* is still a major cause of postoperative infection. *Escherichia coli, Streptococcus faecalis, Proteus vulgaris, Klebsiella, Enterobacter,* and *Pseudomonas aeruginosa* are also closely associated with wound infection. **Antimicrobial** agents themselves can promote infection by increasing the susceptibility of clients to colonization with nosocomial microflora; these agents also select and concentrate antibiotic-resistant **organisms** on or in the host.

Maintaining **asepsis** during dressing changes assists in preventing wound infections. Using sterile equipment, including gloves, is the first barrier against infection. A mask and gown should be worn during dressing changes to prevent the spread of microorganisms to other clients and to the healthcare worker.

When wounds become grossly infected or are extensive in nature, the physician may order wound irrigations. Normal saline or Ringer's solution are the usual irrigating solutions used for wounds. Most of the agents used in the past have been identified as toxic to the cells generated in the inflammatory phase of healing. Each hospital has its own protocol for wound irrigation, and nurses should become familiar with their institution's procedure. This chapter presents one method of wound irrigation that is helpful in most clinical situations.

Wound Specimens for Culture

Purulent exudate from infected wounds can contain a variety of aerobic and anaerobic microorganisms. In the majority of wound infections, the causative agent is usually found in the upper respiratory tract, gastrointestinal tract, and genitourinary tract. When these organisms invade other body parts, they can cause severe infections and sometimes death.

Before a wound can be cultured, it should be **irrigated** with normal saline to remove the surface bacteria. The best method of obtaining a culture specimen is to rotate a swab along the granulation tissue. Refer to Chapter 20, Unit 20.5, Swab Specimens, for these skills. For the most accurate results, the physician should take a biopsy of the tissue.

Surgical Site Infections

Surgical site infections (SSIs) are best described as infections related to the operative procedure that occur at or near the surgical incision within 30 days of a procedure or within 1 year of an implant left in place.

At the time of the incision, every surgical site becomes contaminated with bacteria inward from the skin or outward from the organs undergoing surgical intervention. The client's endogenous flora at the incisional site leads to the contamination. In addition to the skin, the mucosal membrane or viscera is also involved in the contamination process. The contamination does not cause the infection itself; the virulence of the bacteria and local blood flow and nutritional components lead to the infection. The amount of bacteria in the wound at the end of the surgery is the major cause of the SSI.

SSIs account for more than 20% of all HAIs among surgical clients and 2%–5% of all HAIs. Each client with an SSI is associated with approximately 7–11 additional postoperative hospital days and a risk of death that is 2–11 times higher than operative clients without an SSI. Seventy-seven percent of surgical client deaths are related to a wound infection. Since October 2008, these SSI costs are not reimbursable by Medicare and Medicaid (Yokoe et al., 2014)

Wounds Caused by Vascular Insufficiency

There are three types of wounds caused by vascular insufficiency. These include arterial insufficiency ulcers, venous insufficiency ulcers, and pressure ulcers (capillary insufficiency ulcers). See Table 25-3 ■ for comparison of arterial and venous ulcers.

Table 25-3 Comparison of Arterial and Venous Ulcers

Differentiation	Arterial	Venous
Predisposing factors	Peripheral vascular disease Atherosclerosis Diabetes mellitus Advanced age Raynaud syndrome	Valve incompetence in vein History of deep vein thrombosis (DVT) Obesity Advanced age
Anatomic location	Between toes or tips of toes Over phalangeal heads Around lateral malleolus Area subjected to trauma	Medial distal lower leg and ankle Malleolar area
Wound characteristics	Even around margins **Gangrene** or necrosis Black eschar Deep, pale wound bed Blanched or purpuric **periwound** tissue Severe pain Cellulitis Minimal exudate	Irregular wound margins Superficial to deep wounds "Ruddy" granular tissue Minimal to moderate pain Minimal to moderate pain Moderate to heavy exudate

Five major factors contribute to ulcer formation in vascular insufficiency:

- Poor nutrition and a lack of blood flow causing inability of nutrients to diffuse through the interstitial spaces
- Continuous pressure on certain areas of the body, such as bony prominences
- Mechanical, thermal, or chemical insults to limbs, resulting in lack of nutrients reaching the lower limbs
- Decreased sensation in the lower extremities
- Excess moisture from incontinence

Venous Ulcers

Venous ulcers are sometimes mistakenly termed venous stasis ulcers; however, they are not caused by a lack of venous blood flow, but rather by a diminished ability of nutrients to diffuse through the interstitial space from the capillaries. The usual etiology of this condition includes calf pump failure as a result of outflow tract obstruction, associated with pregnancy, obesity, tumor, or deep vein thrombosis. Insufficient valves, either deep venous valve incompetence or superficial vein incompetence (varicose veins), are causes as well. Peripheral neuropathy and musculoskeletal disorders may lead to venous ulcers as a result of calf muscle disuse.

Compression therapy is used to treat venous ulcers. This therapy includes the use of compression stockings, Unna boot, or a compression dressing when wound care is included in the treatment. Compression therapy is contraindicated in clients with phlebitis, diminished sensation, and arterial insufficiency, as it will exacerbate the insufficiency.

Arterial Ulcers

Arterial ulcers are often seen in clients with diabetes mellitus and atherosclerosis. Clients with a history of smoking and clients who sustain mechanical trauma to the extremity are prone to arterial ulcers. In these situations, there is diminished oxygenation and nutrients to the periphery. Drug therapy with vasodilators, anticoagulants, or thrombolytic agents is part of the treatment plan for these clients. If drug therapy is insufficient, surgical treatment (smpathectomy, endarterectomy, or bypass surgery) may be necessary to treat the ulcer.

Pressure Ulcers

Pressure ulcers are defined by the National Pressure Ulcer Advisory Panel as any lesion caused by unrelieved pressure resulting in damage to underlying tissue. Four mechanical factors contribute to the development of pressure ulcers: pressure, friction, shearing, and moisture. Pressure ulcers are usually located over a bony prominence, where normal tissue is squeezed between the bone and pressure or friction caused by the bed or chair. External pressure that lasts long enough to result in decreased blood flow causes altered oxygenation and nutrition to the tissue, resulting in a pressure ulcer. Immobility, especially associated with the older adult, is the primary cause of pressure ulcer formation. In addition to mechanical factors and immobility, aging skin and malnutrition increase the risk of skin breakdown.

Each year 2.5 million hospitalized clients develop pressure ulcers, resulting in 60,000 deaths. Data suggest that 25% of these clients develop the pressure ulcer in the operating room, especially when the surgery is prolonged beyond 3 hr. Surgical clients experience periods of prolonged immobility, resulting in unrelieved pressure and decreased blood flow to the skin. Pressure ulcer rates vary by clinical setting: from 0.4%–38% in acute care, to 2.2%–23.9% in long-term care, and 0–17% in home care. Older clients are affected most often and account for the highest number of cases. A large percentage of the clients who develop pressure ulcers while in a nursing home die as a result. These statistics are appalling when one considers that ulcers are usually preventable and treatable (Institute for Clinical Systems Improvement, 2014). Pressure ulcers are classified in stages by the degree of tissue damage observed. See Unit 5 of this chapter for illustration and description.

Management of pressure ulcers is best accomplished using a team of healthcare providers, including physicians, nurses, an enterostomal therapist, dietitian, physical therapist, family members, and the client.

Client education should include the following:

- Discussion of options for pressure ulcer treatment
- Discussion of client's active participation in his or her own care
- Developing a plan of care that is consistent with the client's goals and desires

Client treatment plan should include these points:

- Assessment of the pressure ulcer
- Managing tissue loads
- Ulcer care
- Managing **bacterial bioburden** and infection
- Operative repair of the pressure ulcer

Management and prevention of pressure ulcers begins on hospital admission with a thorough assessment of the client's skin, especially over bony prominences. Preventive steps for high-risk clients include the following:

- Ensure that skin is kept clean, and prevent it from getting too dry by using moisturizing lotions.
- Provide a balanced diet high in protein, vitamins, and minerals for tissue repair.
- Ensure a fluid intake of at least 2,000 mL/day for adequate hydration (unless there are fluid restrictions).
- Place clients on a pressure-reducing mattress or chair cushion.
- Use turning sheets to reposition.
- Avoid massaging over bony prominences.
- Do not elevate head of the bed more than 30 degrees.
- Positioning is the basic standard of ulcer prevention.
- Reposition a bedridden client at least every 2 hr; reposition a chair-bound client every hour.
- Complete a risk assessment for the client, evaluating factors for developing pressure ulcers.

Adjunctive Wound Care Therapy

Three of the more common types of adjunctive wound therapy include **electrical stimulation**, noncontact normothermic wound therapy, and the vacuum-assisted closure system (Table 25-4 ■).

Electrical stimulation uses transfer of an electric current through a surface electrode pad that is in contact with external skin surface or the wound bed itself. It influences wound healing by attracting cells of repair, changing cell membrane permeability, enhancing cellular secretion through cell membranes, and orienting cell structure. A moist wound environment must be maintained for this therapy to be successful in healing. Electrical stimulation increases blood flow, oxygen uptake, and DNA and protein synthesis. It can be used in a variety of wound problems, including burns, pressure ulcers, vascular ulcers, and surgical wounds.

Ultrasonic debridement utilizes low-frequency pulsed ultrasound directed to the wound surface via an ultrasound probe. A wound irrigation fluid (0.9% normal saline) is directed through an opening in the probe's tip as a coupling medium, coolant, wound lavage, or flush.

Negative pressure wound therapy uses a foam dressing applied directly to the wound. This system stimulates growth of granulation tissue while promoting a moist environment. Negative pressure is applied to the foam, and tubing connects the foam to a canister where exudate and wound fluids are collected. This system is used with infected wounds, as well as chronic wounds, acute and traumatic wounds, and dehiscence. Since its introduction in the mid-1990s, negative pressure wound therapy has become a leading technology in the care and management of acute, chronic, dehisced, and traumatic wounds, and of pressure ulcers, diabetic ulcers, orthopedic trauma, skin flaps, and grafts. There are many risk factors associated with the use of this system. (Guidelines for safe negative pressure wound therapy are provided in Unit 25.6.)

Hyperbaric oxygen therapy has been approved by Medicare and Medicaid for treatment of clients who have diabetes with leg ulcers and has proven to be very effective in healing. In this therapy, 100% oxygen is delivered and is administered at greater than 1 atmospheric pressure absolute (ATA). This can only be accomplished in an environment of elevated atmospheric pressure, which is in the chamber.

Oxygen has pivotal roles in wound healing. Disruption of microcirculation is the initial event that leads to wound hypoxia, and hypoxia continues in chronic wound conditions. Cellular energy metabolism requires oxygen to produce adenosine triphosphate (ATP). Without tissue oxygen at sufficient levels, acidosis occurs. Furthermore, oxygen consumption and potential for hypoxia of the wound increase as leukocytes migrate to the wound area. An oxygen level of 40 mm Hg is needed to sustain the fibroblast activity that leads to collagen deposits for healing.

Home Care

Before discharge from the hospital, a multidisciplinary team meeting should be held with the client to review home care. The team should include the following: home care RN, dietician, wound care specialist, and mental health CNS, if appropriate. A home care plan needs to include a discussion of the wound care and dressing change; mobility and exercise routine, if appropriate; diet to promote wound healing; and discussions with healthcare workers and family regarding wound care techniques, signs and symptoms of infection, and when to notify the physician or healthcare provider (Box 25-1 ■).

Table 25-4 Adjunctive Therapies in Wound Care

Therapy	Outcomes
Hydrotherapy	Promotes **debridement** and cleans wound
Electrical stimulation	Increases oxygen and nutrients to tissues, reduces pain and edema, and improves scar tissue elasticity
Ultrasound	Increases collagen elasticity, and decreases pain and muscle spasms. Increases oxygen, decreases edema, and accelerates wound recovery
Hyperbaric oxygen	Increases tissue oxygenation and promotes wound healing
Compression	Promotes venous blood return, and prevents pooling of blood and edema formation
Nutritional support	Decreases susceptibility of soft tissue breakdown
Support surfaces	Distributes body weight and reduces tissue pressure; controls shear forces on skin surfaces and provides stability for client's torso
Biological products	Increases wound healing by increasing wound strength, increasing cellular content, and controlling collagen deposition

---

Box 25-1 CLIENT TEACHING FOR DISCHARGE

- Instruct client to eat foods high in protein, carbohydrates, vitamins, and minerals to promote wound healing.
- Teach client to splint wound when coughing or moving from chair or bed to prevent separation of wound edges.
- Provide list of signs and symptoms of wound infection or delayed healing. Include when to notify healthcare provider.
- Encourage use of daily showers; water may run over wound if approved by physician.
- Instruct not to use soap, lotions, or vitamin creams on incision.
- Instruct in dressing change procedure.
- Instruct not to lift heavy objects (anything over 10 lb or 4.5 kg).
- Instruct in measures to promote elimination.

Wound assessments and dressing changes are the same as those in the hospital. The more advanced adjunctive wound therapy modalities are usually not done in the home. If a complicated dressing change is required, a wound care specialist should be assigned to the home care client.

LEGAL ALERT

Wound care practitioners are at risk for litigation. Frequently, clients who experience wounds believe it is because of neglect by healthcare workers. Wound care practitioners may face liability for:

- Negligence
- Violations of Medicare and Medicaid fraud and abuse prohibitions
- Abandonment for terminating services to clients

To prove negligence, a client must show that the provider owed the client a duty and breached the duty owed the client, and the breach of duty must result in injury or damage to the client. Owing a duty of reasonable care to a client incorporates the standards of wound care. Breaching a duty occurs when the healthcare practitioner does something that should not have been done. To be charged with causing injury, the client would need to prove that injuries occurred as a result of practitioner error.

Nursing Diagnoses

The following nursing diagnoses may be appropriate to use on client care plans when the components are related to the client requiring wound care.

NURSING DIAGNOSIS	RELATED TO . . .
Infection, Risk for	Altered circulation, invasive procedures, trauma Exposure to nosocomial agents, surgical incision, open wound
Impaired Physical Mobility	Bed rest, wounds, or pressure ulcers
Chronic Pain	Tissue injury, extensive dressing changes, recent surgery, vascular ulcers
Pressure Ulcer, Risk for	Alteration in cognition or sensation, extremes of age or weight, impaired circulation, inadequate nutrition, physical immobilization
Impaired Skin Integrity	Mechanical factors (shearing force, pressure), altered circulation due to pressure on a bony prominence, immobility, poor nutritional intake
Impaired Tissue Integrity	Interrupted blood supply to site, depleting oxygen and nutrients

Source: Herdman, T. H. & Kamitsuru, S. (Eds.) *Nursing Diagnoses – Definitions and Classification 2015-2017.* Copyright © 2014, 1994–2014 by NANDA International. Used by arrangement with John Wiley & Sons Limited. Companion website: www.wiley.com/go/nursingdiagnoses. In order to make safe and effective judgments using NANDA-I nursing diagnosis it is essential that nurses refer to the definitions and defining characteristics of the diagnoses listed in this work.

Unit 25.1
Measures to Prevent Infection

Nursing Process Data

ASSESSMENT Database

- Identify clients at risk for infection (e.g., clients with diabetes, older adults, malnourished, obese, smokers, immunosuppressed).
- Identify length of time client remained in surgery (the more hours in surgery, the greater the risk for infection).
- Assess incision three times a day.
- Identify the components necessary to prevent infection for individual clients.
- Assess need for sterile technique compliance in client care.
- Assess lab results for abnormal values (i.e., WBC, Hgb, Hct).

PLANNING Objectives

- To remove transient microorganisms from nails, hands, and forearms
- To prevent clients with impaired resistance from becoming infected
- To prevent microorganisms from entering the wound
- To provide a sterile working field for dressing changes

IMPLEMENTATION Procedures

DOCUMENTATION AND EVALUATION

Expected Outcomes

- Infection is prevented in clients with impaired resistance.
- Sterile field is maintained when preparing for dressing changes.
- Sterile technique is maintained throughout wound care.

Unexpected Outcomes/Alternative Actions

Pearson Nursing Student Resources

Find additional review materials at **nursing.pearsonhighered.com.**
Prepare for success with NCLEX®-style practice questions and Skill Checklists.

Skill 25.1.1 | Completing Surgical Hand Antisepsis

Equipment
Plastic or orangewood stick
Antimicrobial solution (soap)
Sterile towel

Procedure
1. Remove all jewelry: rings, watch, bracelets.
2. Turn on water using foot or knee pedal or hand lever. Water should be tepid. ➤ *Rationale:* Hot water dries skin and is uncomfortable. Cold water prevents soap from lathering, and bacteria are not rinsed away.
3. Wet hands first with warm water. Apply 3–5 mL of antimicrobial soap to hands. Rub together for at least 20 sec. ❶ Cover all surfaces of hands and fingers and 3 in. above wrists, keeping fingers pointing upward.
4. Scrub your hands for 10 strokes and nails for 15 strokes with an antimicrobial solution (time based on facility policy). Scrub each side of each finger and all surfaces of the hand for 2 min.
5. Scrub your hands using soap or alcohol-based hand rubs. When using antimicrobial soap, scrub hands and forearms up to 3 in. above elbows. This is done for length of time recommended by manufacturer (2–6 min) for each hand and arm. Most studies indicate this should be done for first OR scrub.
6. Rinse hands and arms by passing them through the water in one direction only, from finger tips to elbows. Do not move the hands and arms back and forth through the water.
7. When using alcohol solution, prewash hands and forearms with nonantimicrobial soap. Completely dry hands and forearms. Then use alcohol-based product according to manufacturer's directions, usually a vigorous 1-min rub. Apply product to palm of one hand and rub hands together covering all surfaces of hands and fingers until surfaces are dry.

> **CLINICAL ALERT**
> Chlorhexidine added to alcohol-based preparations results in greater residual activity than alcohol alone. Minimal absorption, if any, occurs through the skin. Care should be taken to avoid contact with the eyes when using more than 1% chlorhexidine, because it causes conjunctivitis and severe corneal damage.

8. Proceed to operating room and dry hands and arms thoroughly on sterile towel.
9. After drying hands and forearms thoroughly, don sterile gloves.

EVIDENCE-BASED PRACTICE
Hospitals' High-Tech Tools Track Who Is Washing Their Hands
Health professionals' rate of compliance with hand-hygiene guidelines, indicated by the Centers for Disease Control and Prevention and the World Health Organization, has been between 40% and 50% nationally. The CDC states that poor hand hygiene contributes to the country's 1.7 million annual HAIs. About 99,000 clients die of these infections each year. The Joint Commission requires hospitals to follow CDC or WHO guidelines and measure their compliance rates. The measurement method relies on individuals observing hand washing as they roam the hallways. A new hand-hygiene sensing device detects the alcohol in the gel that staff use to wash their hands and sends an infrared signal to the staff's badge to record the washing event. When they enter a 7-foot zone near a client's monitor without washing their hands, the badge will vibrate as a reminder. The badge will vibrate after an additional 6–10 sec if the staff member did not step out of the zone to wash hands. After a third buzz, the instance is recorded as a noncompliant event and sent to the system's database. Email reports of each professional's compliance go to the hospital's infection control department. After the sensing device system was installed, one hospital's compliance with hand washing rose from 67% to 90%.

A second hospital achieved a hand-hygiene compliance rate above 90%, which resulted in an 89% drop in HAIs. Several technologies are being developed throughout the country to track hand hygiene by staff.

Source: O'Reilly, 2011.

❶ Scrub hands with an antimicrobial solution.

Skill 25.1.2 | Donning Sterile Gloves

Equipment
Packaged sterile gloves

Procedure
1. Perform hand hygiene.
2. Place glove package on a clean, dry, firm surface that is at waist height (usually an overbed table). ➤ *Rationale:* Objects below waist level are considered to be out of the sterile field.
3. Remove outside wrapper of glove package by peeling the tabs apart where indicated on the wrapper. ❶ Pull edges laterally to expose glove package. Ensure that this step is accomplished over a firm surface. ➤ *Rationale:* This prevents the glove package from accidentally falling onto a contaminated surface.
4. Place the glove package on the firm surface, maintaining sterility of gloves by touching only outside of wrapper. ❷
5. Grasp two edges of wrapper and lift wrapper edges up and away from gloves, being careful to not touch gloves as you open the package. ➤ *Rationale:* Lifting the edges up and away as you open the package will prevent touching the gloves accidentally and causing contamination.
6. With your nondominant hand, pick up the opposite glove by grasping the section that has a folded edge (inside edge of the cuff). Lift the glove up and away from the wrapper. ❸

➤ *Rationale:* This prevents accidental contamination of the glove or inside of glove package.
7. Holding your hands above waist level, insert your dominant hand into the glove opening. ❹ Gently pull the glove into place with your nondominant hand, touching only the inside of the cuff. Do not attempt to straighten out gloved fingers until both gloves have been put on. ➤ *Rationale:* It is easy to contaminate the glove when attempting to adjust the fingers in the glove.
8. With your dominant, gloved hand, remove the other glove from the package, making sure you touch only the inside of the folded cuff. ❺ Lift this glove up and away from the wrapper. ➤ *Rationale:* This prevents gloves from inadvertently touching wrapper and contaminating gloves.
9. Hold your gloved thumb away from your body to prevent touching your skin.
10. Place your ungloved fingers into the new glove opening. Gently pull the glove over your hand as before. ❻
11. Keeping your hands above waist level, adjust both gloves by touching only your fingers, remembering to touch sterile surfaces with sterile surfaces. ➤ *Rationale:* Fingers of gloves are considered sterile; cuff area is considered contaminated.
12. Keep both sterile gloves in front of you above your waist level. ➤ *Rationale:* Being able to see gloves at all times helps prevent potential contamination.

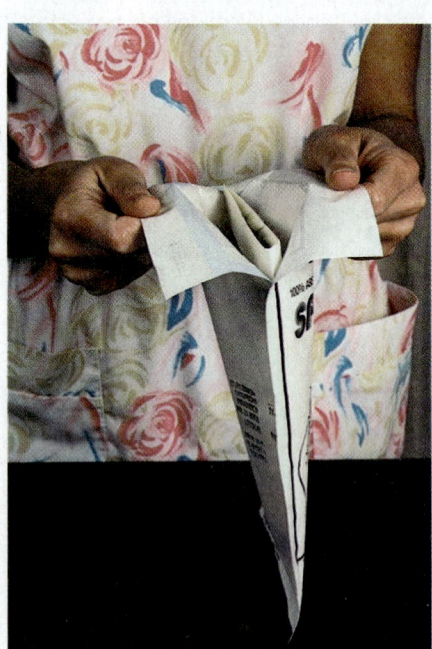

❶ Grasp two upper edges of the glove package and pull laterally to open package.

❷ Place sterile glove wrapper on clean, flat surface and lift wrapper edges away from gloves.

❸ Grasp folded edge of glove with nondominant hand and lift glove away from wrapper.

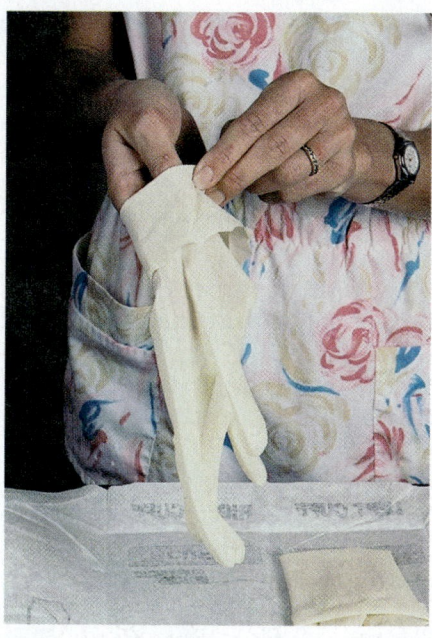

❹ Slip dominant hand into glove opening without contaminating glove.

❺ Remove second glove from wrapper by placing gloved fingers under cuff.

❻ Continue to keep fingers under cuff of glove as the glove is pulled on.

Skill 25.1.3 | Pouring From a Sterile Container

Equipment
Sterile container
Nonsterile container
Sterile solution

Procedure
1. Perform hand hygiene.
2. Gather equipment.
3. Open sterile container according to procedure.
4. Place container on firm surface.
5. Take cap off the bottle and invert the cap before laying on firm surface. ➤ *Rationale:* This keeps the cap sterile.
6. Hold the bottle with the label facing up.
7. Pour a small amount of liquid into a nonsterile container. ❶ ➤ *Rationale:* This action cleans the lip of the bottle.
8. Pour the liquid into the sterile container while keeping the label facing up and not touching the container with the bottle. ❷ Do not reach over a sterile field if the container has been placed on one. ➤ *Rationale:* Crossing over a sterile field can lead to contamination of the field.
9. Replace the cap if liquid remains in the bottle. If total contents have been used, dispose of bottle in trash.
10. Date and initial bottle if reusing.
11. Replace partially filled bottle to storage area if it is to be reused.

❶ First pour a small amount of liquid into nonsterile container.

❷ Pour liquid by placing container close to edge of sterile area.

Skill 25.1.4 | Preparing a Sterile Field

Equipment
Antiseptic cleansing solution, as ordered
Two packages of sterile towels (optional)
Sterile drape package
Number and type of dressings required for dressing change
Tape
Container for antiseptic solution
Paper bag for disposal of soiled dressings
Mask
Sterile gloves

Preparation
1. Check physician's orders and client care plan.

> **CLINICAL ALERT**
> A sterile field is commonly prepared for burn dressings or large wound dressings. It is not used routinely for other dressings.

2. Gather equipment from supply area.
3. Identify client using two forms of identification.
4. Introduce yourself and explain procedure.
5. Clean off overbed table.

Procedure
1. Perform hand hygiene, using aseptic technique.
2. Place sterile drape on overbed table or on another surface close to the table.

Commercially Prepared Packages
   a. Open package at designated end by pulling edges apart and downward to expose contents.
   b. Grasp the edges of the two sides of the package and invert the package over the edge of the sterile field. Allow the contents to drop onto the sterile field.
   c. Repeat procedure for each item to be placed on the sterile field.

Hospital-Wrapped Packages
   a. Hold package in your hand and securely grasp one edge.
   b. Open package wrapper by allowing edges to drop down, away from package.
   c. Grasp the edges of the wrapper with your free hand and pull them toward your wrist, thus exposing the sterile contents.
   d. Gently drop the contents on the sterile field.
   ➤ *Rationale:* Touching the sterile field with the wrapper contaminates it.

   e. Repeat procedure for each item to be placed on the sterile field.

3. If sterile supplies are not to be used immediately, cover with sterile towels.
   a. Open sterile towel package by opening wrapper away from you so that you do not cross over a sterile field (Box 25-2 ■).
   b. Pick up one towel at the edge and open towel by moving yourself away from the sterile field and allowing the towel to fall open.
   c. Grasp the corner of towel opposite the one you are holding. Keep the towel from touching contaminated areas.
   d. Place the towel over the sterile field starting at edge nearest you. Lay the towel down without touching the tray with your hand. Move the towel across the tray toward the opposite edge.
   e. Repeat the procedure with the second sterile towel.

4. If solutions for cleansing the skin are required, place sterile medicine cups near one side of the sterile drape.
   Note: It is best to add the solution to the container after the towels have been removed and just prior to the dressing change. ➤ *Rationale:* This prevents the solution from spilling over the sterile supplies.

   a. Take the cap off the antiseptic bottle.
   b. Pour a small amount of solution into a container, not on the sterile field, keeping the label in uppermost position.
   ➤ *Rationale:* This action rinses contaminated particles from the lip of the bottle.
   c. Pour the antiseptic solution, from the side of the sterile field, directly into the medicine cup. ➤ *Rationale:* Pouring solution from the side prevents crossing over the sterile field.

Box 25-2 GUIDELINES FOR STERILE FIELD
- Never turn your back on a sterile field.
- Avoid talking, coughing, sneezing, or reaching across a sterile field.
- Keep sterile objects above waist level.
- Do not spill solutions on the sterile field.
- Open all sterile packages away from the sterile field to prevent crossover and contamination.
- Consider 2.5 cm (1 in.) around the edges to be contaminated.

Skill 25.1.5 | Preparing a Sterile Field Using Prepackaged Supplies

Equipment
Packaged supplies

Procedure
1. Perform hand hygiene.
2. Ensure working surface is clean and dry. Client's overbed table is frequently used as preparation area. ➤ *Rationale:* This prevents contamination of sterile package.
3. Remove outer plastic wrap.
4. Place package in center of work area and position so that you first open package flap away from you. ➤ *Rationale:* This prevents reaching across the sterile field as you continue to open package.
5. Grasp edge of the first flap of the wrapper, move it away from you, and place it on the working surface. ❶
6. Grasp the first side flap, lift it up, grasp the second side flap, and together move both hands out toward the sides. Place the flaps down on the working surface.
7. Grasp the last flap of the wrapper and open it toward you, taking care not to touch the inside of the flap or any of the contents of the package. ❷ ➤ *Rationale:* This prevents contamination of the supplies.

❶ Grasp edge of top flap of wrapper and lift it away from you.

❷ Open last flap toward you—do not cross over sterile field.

Skill 25.1.6 | Preparing for Dressing Change With Individual Supplies

Equipment
Antiseptic cleaner or cleaning solution
Number and type of dressings needed (e.g., 4×4 gauze pads, ABD pads, application sticks, transparent dressings)
Tape
Clean gloves
Sterile gloves
Disposal receptacle
Mask, if needed

Procedure
1. Perform hand hygiene.
2. Clear bedside stand and wash it thoroughly with antiseptic solution. Dry thoroughly.
3. Place supply packages on table in configuration that allows you to open packages without reaching over sterile field. ➤ *Rationale:* Reaching over sterile field will contaminate supplies.
4. Grasp cover of 4×4 pad plastic container and pull flap back and away from sterile area. ❶ Place cover in disposal bag.
5. Grasp edge of transparent dressing's package, and peel back top covering. ❷ Place open package on work surface. Do not cross over any open supply packages.
6. Continue to open all supplies using steps above.
7. Pour solution over pads in plastic container, if ordered. ❸
8. Open sterile gloves. ❹ Place in position on table where you do not pass over a sterile field.

❶ Open sterile 4×4 pads container by pulling back on flap.

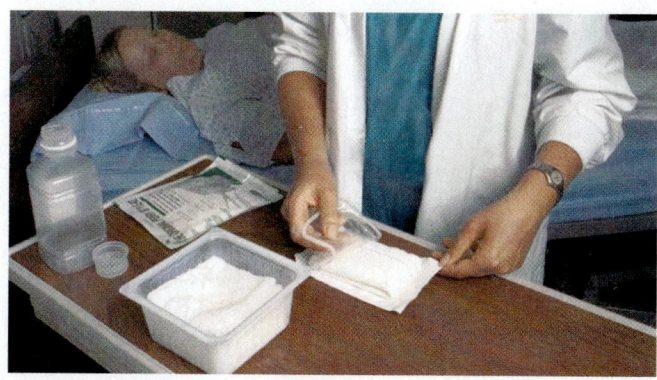

❷ Open transparent dressing packet.

(continued)

Skill 25.1.6 | Preparing for Dressing Change With Individual Supplies *(continued)*

❸ Pour cleaning solution over 4×4 pads.

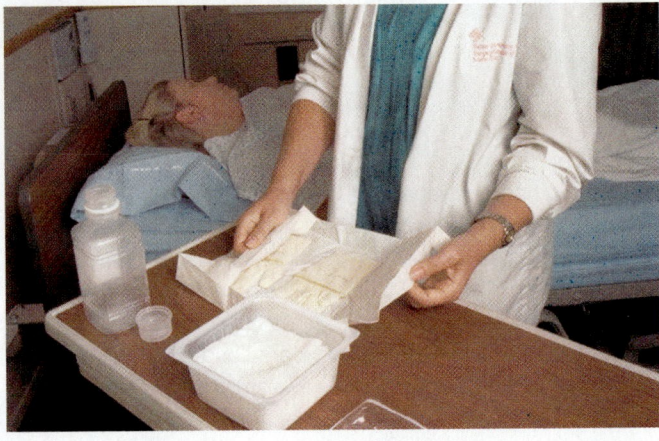

❹ Open sterile glove packet on overbed table.

Unit 25.1 Documentation and Evaluation

DOCUMENTATION for Measures to Prevent Infection

- Type and number of sterile dressings used
- Antiseptic solution used

EVALUATION/Critical Thinking

Expected Outcomes
- Infection is prevented in clients with impaired resistance.
- Sterile field is maintained when preparing for dressing change.
- Sterile field is maintained throughout wound care.

Unexpected Outcomes	Alternative Actions
• Hole develops in glove while performing sterile technique.	• Discard gloves and replace with sterile gloves. • Examine hands for cuts if hole is caused by sharp object. • If hands are cut, scrub hands and replace sterile gloves.
• Sterile field becomes wet or damp.	• Discard supplies on sterile field. • Set up new sterile field.

Unit 25.2
Dressing Change

Nursing Process Data

ASSESSMENT Database

- Identify type of dressing required.
- Determine if sutures or staples need to be removed.
- Assess incision for infection.
- Assess extent of healing.
- Assess nutritional status.

PLANNING Objectives

- To promote incision healing
- To prevent wound infection
- To maintain sterility during dressing change
- To remove sutures or staples using appropriate technique

IMPLEMENTATION Procedures

DOCUMENTATION AND EVALUATION

Expected Outcomes

- Client's wounds do not become infected.
- Client's sutures and staples are removed intact.
- Client's wound remains intact after staple or suture removal.

Unexpected Outcomes/Alternative Actions

Pearson Nursing Student Resources

Find additional review materials at
nursing.pearsonhighered.com.
Prepare for success with NCLEX®-style practice questions and Skill Checklists.

| **Skill 25.2.1** | Changing a Dry Sterile Dressing |

Equipment

Sterile gloves
Clean gloves
Mask
Gown
Disposal receptacle for used dressings
Dressing supplies, as needed
Micropore tape
Sterile normal saline, optional
Package sterile cotton swabs, or 4×4 pads
Bath blanket or sheet

Preparation

1. Check physician's orders and client care plan.
2. Perform hand hygiene.
3. Gather equipment.
4. Identify the client using two forms of identifiers. Introduce yourself and explain procedure. Assess for pain.
5. Provide privacy.
6. Clean off overbed table.
7. Place sterile supplies on overbed table.
8. Raise bed to HIGH position (comfortable working height) and lower side rails, if appropriate.
9. Place bag for soiled dressings near incision site.
10. Fanfold linen to expose incision area.
11. Cover client with bath blanket or sheet, leaving incision area exposed.
12. Open sterile packages and place on overbed table. Arrange packages to ensure you do not cross over the sterile field when reaching for dressings. ➤ *Rationale:* Commercially prepared sterile packages can be opened and used for the sterile field because the inside of the package is sterile.
13. Cut tape into appropriate length strips.

Procedure

1. Don clean gloves.
2. Remove tape slowly by pulling tape toward the wound. ❶
   ➤ *Rationale:* Pulling toward the wound decreases the pain of tape removal by not putting pressure on the incision line.
3. Remove soiled dressings and dispose of them in the proper receptacle. ❷ ❸ Wet dressing with sterile normal saline if it adheres to the suture line.
4. Assess incision area for erythema, edema, or drainage.
   ➤ *Rationale:* Persistent drainage, edema, or temperature above 38°C (100.4°F) 2 days postop indicates a complication is occurring.
5. Assess color of incision. (A healing incision looks pink or red.) ➤ *Rationale:* Redness that does not fade 48 hr after surgery may indicate impaired healing.
6. Remove clean gloves, and discard.
7. Move overbed table next to working area.
8. Don sterile gloves.
9. Cleanse incision area with sterile swabs or 4×4 pads soaked in normal saline, according to facility policy. Cleanse from incision line outward, cleaning from top to bottom, using each swab only once. Discard swabs or 4×4 pads in disposal bag. ➤ *Rationale:* Cleaning outward from incision cleans from least to most contaminated area. Cleaning from top to bottom prevents contamination from secretions that accumulate at the bottom of the wound.
10. Place 4×4 gauze pads over incision area, being careful not to touch incision or client with your gloves. ❹ ➤ *Rationale:* Touching the incision or client contaminates the gloves. You need to reglove if this occurs.
11. Place abdominal pad over incision, being careful not to contaminate the gloves. ❺
12. Remove gloves and discard.
13. Tape dressing securely. ❻
14. Discard trash in appropriate receptacle.
15. Lower bed and raise side rails. Position client for comfort.
16. Perform hand hygiene.

❶ Remove tape by gently lifting toward wound.

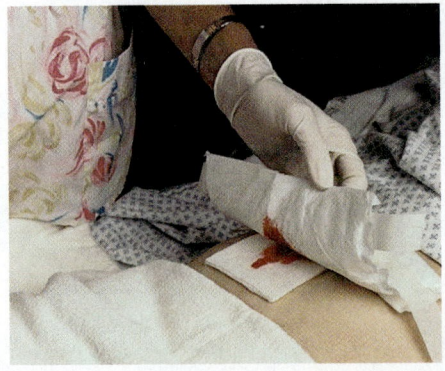

❷ Remove soiled dressing carefully.

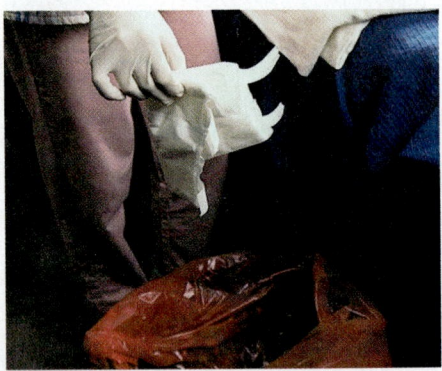

❸ Dispose of dressing in appropriate container.

❹ Do not touch incision with dominant hand when applying dressing.

❺ Place abdominal pad over center of incision.

❻ Tape dressing securely to prevent slipping.

Skill 25.2.2 | Removing Sutures

Equipment
Sterile suture removal set (Box 25-3 ■)
Antiseptic solution
Tape
Butterfly tape
Paper bag for disposal of dressings
Two pairs clean gloves (one pair optional)

Procedure
1. Gather equipment.
2. Perform hand hygiene and don clean gloves.
3. Remove dressing and discard in disposal bag. (Discard gloves only if soiled.)
4. Open suture removal set, and don gloves if second pair needed.
5. Pick up forceps with nondominant hand.
6. Grasp suture at the knot with forceps and lift away from skin. ❶
7. Pick up suture scissors with dominant hand.
8. Place curved tip of suture scissors under suture, next to knot.
9. Cut suture, and with forceps, pull suture through skin with one movement. ❷
10. Discard suture into disposal bag.
11. Check that entire suture is removed.
12. Continue to remove remaining sutures according to hospital policy. Some policies state that every other suture is removed and then remaining sutures are removed at a later time. ➤ *Rationale:* This prevents **wound dehiscence**.

Box 25-3 TOPICAL GLUE FOR WOUND CLOSURE
Dermabond Advanced Glue is now being used to replace sutures and staples. It is used for wounds in areas where skin is not being stretched or pulled and for exterior, hair-free areas of the skin and areas of the face, but not close to the eyes. Dermabond Advanced is used extensively for OB/GYN procedures; general surgery of the abdomen, back, arms, and legs; cosmetic surgery such as breast and abdominoplasty procedures; sports injuries, including lacerations; and some neurological surgeries such as discectomy and laminectomy procedures. Dermabond was approved by the U.S. Food and Drug Administration. It is a synthetic, noninvasive glue that mitigates trauma and postprocedure inflammation while providing a waterproof seal and protecting underlying tissue without the need for bandages. It is also painless, is fast and simple to apply, and naturally sloughs off in 7–10 days.

13. Cleanse suture site with antiseptic solution.
14. Remove gloves and place in disposal bag.
15. Place dressing or butterfly tape over incision area, if ordered.
16. Discard disposal bag into contaminated waste container.
17. Perform hand hygiene.

(continued)

Skill 25.2.2 | Removing Sutures *(continued)*

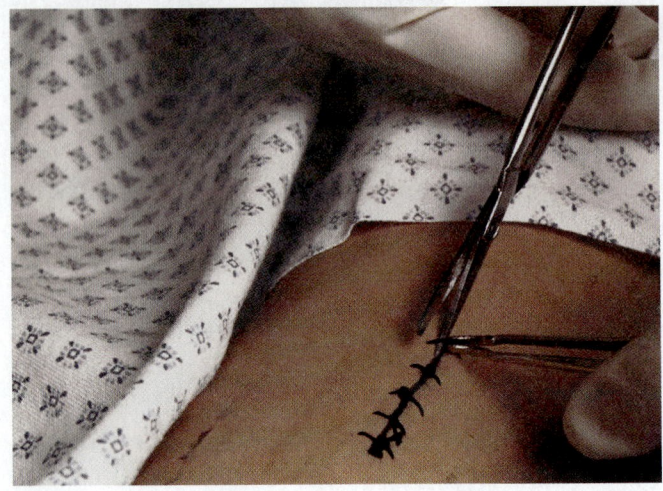

❶ Grasp suture at the knot with forceps and lift away from skin.

❷ After cutting suture, grasp suture at knot and pull through skin.

Skill 25.2.3 | Removing Staples

Equipment

Sterile staple remover
Disposal receptacle
Two pairs clean gloves (one pair optional)
Dressings
Tape or butterfly tape
Antiseptic solution

Preparation

1. Check physician's orders and client care plan.
2. Identify client using two forms of identification.
3. Introduce yourself and explain the procedure to client.

Procedure

1. Gather equipment and open sterile staple remover.
2. Perform hand hygiene and don clean gloves.
3. Remove dressing and discard in disposal bag. ❶ (Discard gloves only if soiled.)
4. Don gloves if necessary.
5. Place lower tip of staple remover under staple. ❷
6. Press handles together to depress center of staple. ❸
7. Lift staple remover upward, away from incision site, when both ends of staple are visible. ❹

❶ Large abdominal wound with staples closing incision.

❷ Place lower tip of staple removal device under staple.

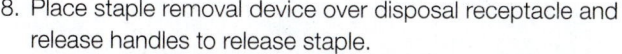

❸ Press handle together to depress center of staple.

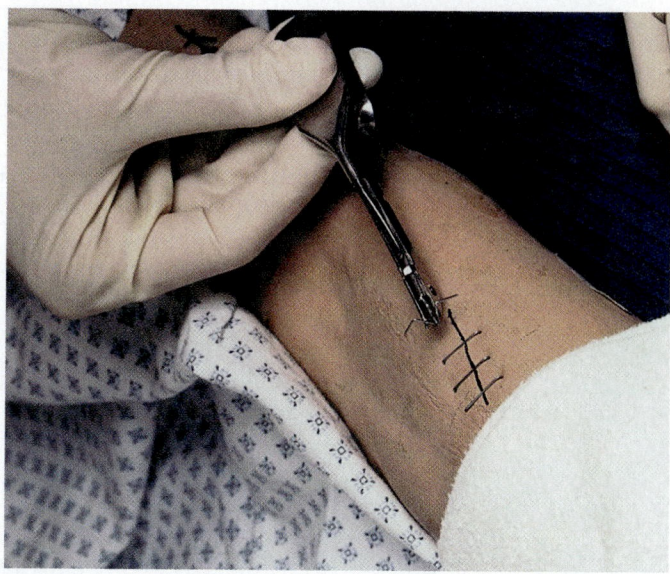

❹ Lift staple removal device upward and away from incision.

8. Place staple removal device over disposal receptacle and release handles to release staple.
9. Remove all staples or as directed by facility policy. Some policies indicate every other staple is removed with remaining staples done at a later time. ➤ *Rationale:* This is to prevent wound dehiscence.
10. Cleanse incision area with antiseptic solution if ordered.
11. Remove gloves and place in disposal receptacle.

12. Place dressing over incision and secure with tape, or place butterfly tape over incision.

> **CLINICAL ALERT**
> Steri-strips may be applied over incision to protect incision after staples are removed.

13. Perform hand hygiene.

Unit 25.2 Documentation and Evaluation

DOCUMENTATION for Dressing Change, Removal of Sutures and Staples

- Conditions of suture line
- Presence of exudate or erythema
- Sutures removed
- Staples removed
- Dressing applied, if appropriate

EVALUATION/Critical Thinking

Expected Outcomes
- Client's wounds do not become infected.
- Client's staples or sutures are removed intact.
- Client's wound remains intact after staple or suture removal.

(continued)

Unexpected Outcomes	Alternative Actions
• Wound appears to be infected.	• Obtain order for wound culture. • Obtain order for different type of dressing. • Document observations.
• Client complains of fever and pain in incisional area.	• Check incision for edema, erythema, or drainage; wound could be infected.
• Wound edges separate when suture or staple is removed.	• Do not continue to remove sutures or staples. • Place Steri-strip over edges. • Notify physician.
• Client complains of pain with dressing change.	• Lift small edge of tape or dressing. • Use alcohol pad, and wipe area next to dressing with pad. • Remove dressing by wiping, with pad, each time the dressing is lifted up until entire dressing is removed.

Nursing Process Data

ASSESSMENT Database

- Identify type of dressing needed.
- Assess level of pain associated with wound care and dressing change.
- Assess wound for color, odor, and drainage.
- Assess extent of wound.
- Assess type of wound.
- Assess for function of wound suction devices, such as Hemovac or Jackson–Pratt suction.
- Assess for extent of wound healing.
- Assess wound.
- Assess for arterial insufficiency, claudication, pain, ischemic tissue loss, and functional limitations.
- Assess for suture site infections.

PLANNING Objectives

- To assess wound appropriately
- To assess for arterial sufficiency
- To promote wound healing by first or second intention
- To prevent microorganisms from entering the wound
- To decrease the presence of purulent wound drainage
- To maintain sterility during a dressing change
- To maintain patency of wound suction devices, that is, Hemovac or Jackson–Pratt suction
- To immobilize and support a wound
- To assist in removal of necrotic tissue
- To apply medication to wound
- To pack a wound to promote granulation of tissue
- To identify potential surgical site infections

IMPLEMENTATION Procedures

DOCUMENTATION AND EVALUATION

Expected Outcomes

- Wound care is provided for contaminated wound, and healing occurs.
- Wound suction devices function without obstruction.
- Wound irrigation is completed using sufficient pressure to cleanse wound bed.
- Abdominal binder supports client's abdominal wound.
- Compression dressing applied to vascular ulcer site.

Unexpected Outcomes/Alternative Actions

Pearson Nursing Student Resources

Find additional review materials at **nursing.pearsonhighered.com.**
Prepare for success with NCLEX®-style practice questions and Skill Checklists.

Skill 25.3.1 | Determining Surgical Site Infections (SSIs)

Preparation

1. Review physician's orders and client care plan.
2. Identify client using two identifiers.
3. Introduce yourself and explain what information is necessary to obtain.
4. Wash hands and obtain necessary information, chart, lab work, and medication list.

Procedure

1. Before surgery, assess client for risk factors associated with surgical site infections (SSIs) (Box 25-4 ■).

   a. Complete health history and physical assessment.
   b. Obtain information on all medications currently taking.
   c. Determine whether client is allergic to specific medications.
   d. Review lab values.

2. Determine whether client has a preexisting viral or bacterial infection. ➤ *Rationale:* If the answer is yes, the client is at an increased risk for SSI.

   a. Clients who must undergo surgery even with existing infections must be monitored closely postoperatively.
   b. Clients scheduled for routine surgery should be treated first and then rescheduled for surgery once the infection is cleared.

3. Check that client does not have nasal bacterial colonization. ➤ *Rationale:* Clients with positive anterior nares cultures of *S. aureus* should receive the topical antibiotic ointment mupirocin before surgical intervention.

4. Complete a nutritional assessment and review lab findings for serum albumin, prealbumin, serum transferrin, and total lymphocyte levels. ➤ *Rationale:* Malnutrition in hospitalized adults is common and can prolong postoperative wound healing, increasing the risk of SSI. The client may need enteral or parenteral nutrition postoperatively.

5. Clients who have diabetes with an elevated fasting serum glucose are at higher risk for SSIs than other clients with diabetes, due to the high glucose levels. ➤ *Rationale:* High glucose levels impair phagocytosis, which affects the body's

Box 25-4 CLIENTS AT RISK FOR SSIs

Advancing age does increase the risk of SSI. One study showed that older clients who developed SSIs after orthopedic surgery were at increased risk for death within the first year postoperatively. Clients with COPD and obesity were at higher risk for SSIs after cardiothoracic and neurologic surgery. Clients who used (or use) nicotine exhibit slow wound healing, leading to SSIs. Obese clients are at higher risk for SSIs due to their inability to ambulate, move in bed, and complete postoperative exercises. Obesity can also lead to a disruption of sutures due to increased stress on the adipose tissue.

It is imperative that high-risk clients be monitored closely for signs and symptoms indicating an SSI could be occurring.

normal defense mechanisms. The client's serum glucose level must be kept below 200 mg/dL during and after surgery to prevent an SSI.

6. Clients with chronic illnesses such as hypertension and other uncontrolled conditions are at high risk for SSIs and must be monitored carefully after surgery. It is preferable to get the conditions under control before surgery is considered.

7. Determine whether client was instructed to perform a preoperative skin cleansing at home. ➤ *Rationale:* The CDC strongly recommends a preventative home cleansing be done for high-risk clients for SSIs. Chlorhexidine gluconate is the most effective cleaning agent in decreasing the microbial count.

8. Check that client has not shaved the surgical site. The CDC recommends that hair be left on client's skin unless it interferes with the surgical procedure. If clipping of the hair is required, the OR staff will complete the clipping. ➤ *Rationale:* Shaving can lead to nicks in the surgical site, predisposing it to an SSI.

9. Check that the client has an antibiotic order for 1 hr before surgery or, if vancomycin is ordered, for 2 hr before surgery.

Skill 25.3.2 | Assessing a Wound

Equipment

Pliable, disposable measuring device or grid
Cotton-tipped applicator sticks
Saline-filled syringe
Plastic disposal bag or receptacle
Clean gloves
Sterile gloves if necessary

Preparation

1. Obtain health history, medical diagnosis, and physical examination data from chart or obtain missing information. The health history must include information on the following:

   a. Initial event and duration of wound
   b. Previous treatments, if any, and the outcome of treatments

c. Current medical diagnosis, including all disease processes. ➤ *Rationale:* Diseases that affect circulation and perfusion of blood can interfere with nutrition and oxygenation of cells and can lead to infection and wounds.

d. Medications, both past and current, including anticoagulants, corticosteroids, immunosuppressives, and antineoplastics. ➤ *Rationale:* These drugs may adversely affect wound healing.

CLINICAL ALERT

Cephalosporins are the drug of choice as prophylaxis for most wound infections. First or second generation drugs such as cefazolin or cefoxitin are used for colon surgery clients. Cephalosporins have a broad spectrum of activity against both gram-positive (gram +) and gram-negative (gram –) bacteria and a wide ratio of therapeutic to toxic dosages. Allergic reactions to these drugs are rare.

---

e. Nutrition and hydration status: Check for signs of malnutrition and assess hydration status of client. ➤ *Rationale:* Malnutrition leads to poor cell growth and repair (Box 25-5 ■). Both dehydration and overhydration lead to impaired oxygen and nutrient transportation.

f. Laboratory data evaluation: albumin, serum total protein, serum transferrin, and total lymphocyte count. ➤ *Rationale:* These lab values are used to determine nutritional status and potential for wound healing.

2. Determine type of wound (acute or chronic) and cause of wound. ➤ *Rationale:* This information is used to evaluate the healing process.

3. Evaluate severity of pain.

4. Perform hand hygiene and don gloves.

Note: Acute wounds progress through the normal process of wound healing in about 1 month. Chronic wounds are wounds that do not go through normal wound healing phases and that do not heal within 1 month.

Procedure

1. Assess location of the wound. ➤ *Rationale:* Location influences rate of healing; the lower body heals more slowly.

2. Assess size of wound: length, width, and depth.

3. Observe color of wound if using this classification.

   a. *Black:* necrotic tissue or black eschar (inhibits formation of granulation tissue)

Box 25-5 **NUTRIENTS FOR WOUND HEALING**

- Protein
- Carbohydrates
- Fats
- Iron
- Zinc
- Copper
- Arginine
- Vitamin A
- Vitamin C
- Vitamin K
- Pyridoxine
- Riboflavin
- Thiamine
- Glutamine

---

b. *Yellow:* presence of exudate or slough; **pus**, fibrin, debris (will advance to eschar), requires cleaning

c. *Red:* indicates wound ready to heal (granulation tissue present)

4. Assess odor of wound.

   a. *Foul:* infected (necrotic tissue has an odor even if not infected)

   b. *Sweet: Pseudomonas* infection

5. Assess level of moisture in wound. (A moist environment allows wound to heal without forming a scab.)

CLINICAL ALERT

Moist wound environment is essential for healing without a scab. Epithelial tissue will not migrate into wounds with necrotic tissue or if deprived of oxygen.

---

6. Assess wound exudate.

   a. Type: dry or moist

   b. Amount: minimum, moderate, maximum (copious)

   c. Color of drainage: clear (**serous**), brown–brown/yellow (slough), bright red (**sanguineous**), containing blood and clear fluid (**serosanguineous**), yellow–yellow/green (**purulent** from *Streptococcus* or *Staphylococcus* infection), blue-green (*Pseudomonas*)

7. Assess tissue viability.

   a. Presence of granulation tissue; red, moist, beefy appearance

   b. Presence of epithelialized tissue; new pink, shiny **epidermis**

   c. Absence of necrotic tissue; slough of yellow, gray. Green and brown color or eschar of hard, black, leathery tissue

8. Assess periwound condition.

   a. Skin nutrition: loss of hair, thickening of nails, atrophy

   b. Edema of skin or scaly skin

   c. Skin hydration: skin turgor indicates hydration or dehydration

   d. Areas of inflammation surrounding wound

   e. Skin integrity: maceration, induration, crepitus, hematoma, blisters

   f. Color: red (inflammation), white (arterial insufficiency), blue (cyanosis, severe arterial insufficiency), black (necrosis), brown (venous insufficiency)

   g. Skin temperature: cool, cold, warm, normal temperature

9. Assess extent of pain, if present.

   a. Determine whether pain is present during dressing change only or constantly.

   b. Use pain scale to determine severity of pain.

   c. Observe for signs of infection.

   d. Arterial insufficiency wounds are very painful.

   e. Venous insufficiency wounds are relatively pain-free.

10. Measure the length and width of wound using a disposable measuring device or grid. Measure in centimeters (cm).

11. Measure depth of wound by placing a sterile cotton-tipped applicator stick into wound in several areas. Measure depth of each area using measuring device or grid. Measure in centimeters (cm).

(continued)

Skill 25.3.2 | Assessing a Wound (continued)

12. Check for undermining or tunneling or sinus tracts by placing a sterile cotton-tipped applicator stick into suspected areas. Gently probe margins of lesion for extensions into surrounding tissue (*undermining*) and beyond wound base (*sinus tract*).

13. Evaluate laboratory values.

   a. Increased white blood cell count indicates infection, usually before other signs and symptoms are evident.

   b. Low hemoglobin and hematocrit indicate **anemia**, which can decrease oxygen transport to the wound.

   c. Altered serum glucose levels may indicate presence of diabetes mellitus, which interferes with normal wound healing.

14. Evaluate client's stress level. Increased stress leads to hypermetabolic states, which use up oxygen and nutrients and affect wound healing.

15. Complete skill by following appropriate steps described in Skill 25.3.3, Changing a Wound Dressing. See moisture-retentive dressings in Table 25-5 ■.

16. Document findings and notify physician of any changes or unusual findings in the assessment.

Table 25-5 Moisture-Retentive Dressings

	Advantages	Disadvantages	Clinical Use
Transparent Adhesive Film	• Transparency allows wound visualization but is nonabsorptive • Conforms to area of application • Can reduce friction of area • Promotes autolysis of dry eschar • Semipermeable: Vapor can escape and environmental oxygen can enter to reduce chance of anaerobic bacterial growth. • Barrier to bacterial invasion; can aspirate fluid and patch • Does not require secondary dressing	• Does *not* absorb exudate • Exudate may macerate skin around wound • Edges will roll in friction area • May be difficult to apply • May be too tightly applied • Removal may tear underlying skin • May increase bacterial growth in infected wounds	• Pressure ulcers, stage I and II • Donor sites • Abrasions • Partial-thickness wound with little or no exudate • Wound without necrotic tissue or slough • Extend edge to minimum 3.2 cm (1¼ in.) beyond wound; skin around wound must be dry for adhesion; apply without tension. • Change when fluid buildup and leaking occurs and when edges are loosening to potentially expose wound.
Hydrogel	• Comes in sheets or gel to conform to the wound • May have soothing and coating effect • Absorbs some exudate • Softens slough or eschar in necrotic wounds • Can be used when infection is present • Provides moist wound healing • Rehydrates dry wound beds	• Expensive • Held in place with gauze dressing or transparent film • May have transparent film on both sides (Film next to wound must be removed.)	• Wounds with necrosis and slough • Partial thickness (use sheets) • Gel can be used to fill wound cavity. • Change every day or twice a day, based on wound exudate.
Hydrocolloid	• Used on acute and chronic wounds • Absorbs exudate in limited capacity • Conforms to area • Prevents bacterial invasion • May be occlusive or semiocclusive	• Not transparent • Melts down with exudate • Characteristic drainage and odor • Edges may need to be taped to prevent rolling. • Most do *not* allow environmental oxygen, so growth of anaerobic bacteria may be a problem. • Cannot be used for infected wounds	• Noninfected dermal ulcers • May leave in place up to 7 days • Change if leaking. • Change if clinical signs of infection present. • Cleanse wound before application. • Roll dressing over wound. • Do *not* stretch; press securely.

Skill 25.3.3 | Changing a Wound Dressing

Equipment

Sterile, prepackaged dressing(s) as needed
Tape; micropore, paper, or Montgomery tie tapes
Clean gloves

Sterile gloves
Sterile normal saline irrigation solution or commercially prepared cleansing spray
Wound culture media, as needed

Plastic bag
Bath blanket or sheet
Emesis basin

Preparation

1. Complete steps in Skill 25.3.2, Assessing a Wound.
2. Check physician's orders and client care plan.
3. Perform hand hygiene.
4. Gather equipment. ❶
5. Identify the client, using two forms of identification, introduce yourself, and explain procedure. Assess for pain.
6. Provide privacy.
7. Clear overbed table.
8. Place sterile supplies on the overbed table.
9. Raise bed to HIGH position (comfortable working height), and lower side rails on working side of bed, if necessary.
10. Place bag for soiled dressings near wound site.
11. Open sterile packages and place on overbed table. Arrange packages to ensure that you do not cross over the sterile field when using dressings. ➤ *Rationale:* Commercially prepared sterile packages can be opened and used for the sterile field; the inside of the package is sterile.
12. Fanfold linens to expose wound site.
13. Cover client with bath blanket or sheet, leaving wound area exposed.
14. Cut tape into appropriate strips.

❶ PYXIS supply station provides easy access for dressing supplies.

Procedure

1. Remove tape slowly by pulling tape toward the wound.
   ➤ *Rationale:* Pulling toward the wound decreases the pain of tape removal by not putting pressure on the incision line.
2. Don clean gloves.
3. Remove soiled dressings, and dispose of in bag. Soaking dressings that are dried to skin or incision with sterile normal saline prevents tissue damage and pain when dressings are removed.
4. Obtain wound specimen for culture if ordered (Box 25-6 ■).
5. Remove clean gloves and discard into plastic bag.
6. Bring overbed table close to working area.
7. Open sterile saline solution or commercially prepared cleansing spray and pour over wound. Place emesis basin next to skin surface to catch overflow.
8. Don sterile gloves.
9. Form a ball with gauze pads by tucking all four corners together. Use the center of gauze pads to cleanse the wound. ➤ *Rationale:* This action prevents contamination of your hands during cleansing.
10. Cleanse wound. Always start at the cleanest area and work away from it. Never return to a previously cleaned area. Usually start at top of wound and work toward bottom.
    ➤ *Rationale:* This prevents contamination of area.
11. Assess the wound, measure, identify type, and determine whether signs of infection are present. ➤ *Rationale:* This allows nurse to determine most effective treatment and type of dressing to be used (Box 25-7 ■).

Box 25-6 **HOW TO OBTAIN A WOUND CULTURE**

- Rinse wound thoroughly with sterile saline.
- Use non–cotton-tipped swab.
- Rotate swab while obtaining specimen.
- Swab edges starting at top, crisscross wound to bottom.
- Do not take specimen from exudate or eschar.
- Place swab in culture medium and take to laboratory immediately.

Box 25-7 **USE OF ANTIMICROBIAL AGENTS IN WOUND CARE**

Antiseptics and antibiotics are two types of antimicrobial agents used in wound care management. Antiseptics, unlike antibiotics, cannot be used exclusively to kill bacteria. Systemic antibiotics only should be used to treat wound infections; however, wounds that have impaired blood flow will not receive the systemic antibiotics. Topical antibiotics are used only for a limited time when infection is present. These agents are not used preventively.

Antiseptics return the wound back to bacterial balance, promoting wound healing. Cadexomer iodine gel is used to absorb wound exudates and assists in autolytic debridement. Silver nitrate and sulfadiazine are used against many antibiotic-resistant strains of bacteria, as they reduce the number of viable bacteria.

(continued)

Skill 25.3.3 | Changing a Wound Dressing (continued)

12. Cleanse under the drain and around the site with a 4×4 gauze pad and cleansing solution if a drain is present. Do not use a cytotoxic or dangerous chemical. ➤ *Rationale:* These agents may harm granulating tissue.
13. Place several gauze pads under the drain.
14. Place several 4×4 gauze pads at wound center, extending at least 2.5 cm (1 in.) beyond the wound. Loosely pack a tunneling area of wound, if present, before filling the base of the wound. Cover with an ABD pad if necessary; remove gloves, and tape securely. Montgomery straps (tie tapes) may be used if frequent dressing changes are required or the client has sensitive skin. ❷ ➤ *Rationale:* Once a dressing has been placed over the wound, it is not to be moved or readjusted, as microorganisms from the skin could be introduced into the wound. The type of dressing used depends on the type of wound, the presence of infection or debris, the amount of exudate, the cost, and client comfort.
15. Use skin sealants or moisture barrier ointments on intact skin and moisture-retentive dressing over 4×4 gauze pad and even over ABD, if used. ➤ *Rationale:* Moisture-retentive dressings are flexible and water resistant, which allows clients to move freely and take showers without disturbing the dressing.

> **CLINICAL ALERT**
> Gauze dressings alone do not support healing or prevent entry of exogenous bacteria.

❷ Montgomery straps are used to prevent skin irritation when frequent dressing changes are required.

16. Cover client.
17. Close the plastic bag and dispose of bag as **isolation** material.
18. Remove gloves and perform hand hygiene thoroughly.
19. Check with client to see that he or she is comfortable before leaving room.
20. Lower the bed and raise the side rail, according to facility policy.

Skill 25.3.4 | Packing a Wound

Equipment
Dressing pack, optional
Sterile narrow packing gauze or 4×4 gauze pads
Normal saline solution
Alcohol wipe
Dressings
Forceps, optional
Sterile scissors
Paper tape
Montgomery tapes
Plastic bag or receptacle
Clean gloves
Sterile gloves

Procedure
1. Follow steps in Preparation for Skill 25.3.3, Changing a Wound Dressing.
2. Determine client's need for pain medication before beginning procedure. ➤ *Rationale:* Pain can be present, particularly when removing old packing that may have become attached to the tissue.
3. Perform hand hygiene, don clean gloves, and place plastic bag near wound site.
4. Remove tape slowly by pulling tape toward wound.
5. Remove soiled dressings and dispose of dressings and packing into plastic bag. Moisten packing with sterile saline solution if dry.
6. Assess wound site.
   a. Identify location of wound.
   b. Observe wound bed and appearance.
   c. Check wound size, shape, depth, and margins.
   d. Observe exudates or drainage.
   e. Evaluate presence of pain.
7. Remove clean gloves and discard.
8. Don sterile gloves.
9. Clean inside of the wound by pouring saline solution over the wound and pat wound dry with 4×4 gauze pads. If the wound is deep, wet several pieces of gauze with sterile saline, and swipe the gauze across the sides of the wound.

> **CLINICAL ALERT**
> Normal saline or Ringer's solution are widely advocated as fluids of choice for cleansing and irrigating wounds. Iodine and chlorhexidine are cytotoxic, particularly to fibroblasts. In severely infected wounds, antimicrobial irrigations may be used.
>
> Povidone iodine, hydrogen peroxide, Dakin's solution, and other agents are not used on acute wounds. These agents dry the wound bed and remove the exudate and all its beneficial cells from the area. Wounds maintained in a moist environment have a lower infection rate than dry wounds.

10. Moisten the packing gauze with sterile saline. Place packing material in wound by pushing a corner of the gauze into the wound, and then pack the rest of the gauze on top of it. Pack lightly, filling tunneling or undermined areas. Forceps can be used to place packing material into corners and wound areas hard to reach. ➤ *Rationale:* Pack lightly to prevent wound margins from contracting. Wound packing is used to facilitate healing by secondary intention. Type of packing material is dependent on type of wound and material available. Gauze pads should be moistened before packing.

11. Cut ribbon gauze with sterile scissors and leave small wick exposed, if used for packing.

12. Cover packing with gauze dressing and tape securely.

13. Dispose of used packing and gloves.

14. Perform hand hygiene.

15. Position client for comfort.

❶ Pack wound dressing in all tunneled and undermined areas.

Skill 25.3.5 | Assessing a Venous Ulcer

Equipment
Blood pressure cuff and stethoscope
Dressings
Chux
Clean gloves (two pairs)
Sterile normal saline
Scissors, if needed

Procedure
1. Perform hand hygiene.
2. Don clean gloves.
3. Identify client using two forms of identification, introduce yourself, and explain the procedure.
4. Place absorbent pad (Chux) under leg.
5. Remove dressings and discard into trash bag.
6. Cleanse site with normal saline as needed.
7. Remove gloves and don new gloves.
8. Observe lower leg. ➤ *Rationale:* The medial malleolus is the usual site for ulcer area.
9. Observe surrounding area of ulcer for any of the following:
   a. Dilated veins
   b. Edema
   c. Maceration
   d. Hyperpigmentation
   e. Eczematous skin change: scaling, pruritic, erythema, and vesicle
   f. *Atrophic blanch* (white plaques with dot-like capillaries)
   g. Scarring from prior healed ulcers (*lipodermatosclerosis*)
10. Complete a pain assessment. ➤ *Rationale:* Deep ulcers are most painful.
11. Check wound bed for "ruddy" or "beefy-red" granular appearance.
12. Observe for flat, irregular wound margins without undermining.
13. Assess amount of drainage and exudate (may be heavy to moderate).
14. Complete an ankle–brachial index (ABI) to check for arterial insufficiency. See Skill 25.3.7. Refer back to Table 25-3 for comparison of arterial and venous ulcers. For information on assessment and treatment of an arterial ulcer, see Box 25-8 ■.

Box 25-8 ARTERIAL ULCERS

Assessment
- Assess arterial flow; dorsalis pedis, femoral, popliteal, or posterior tibial.
- Use Doppler to assess pulses if necessary.
- Assess ankle–brachial index; below 0.5 indicates severe arterial insufficiency.
- Assess temperature of skin.
- Observe color of extremities.
- Assess for presence of pain when client resting.

Treatment
- Debridement
- Pain control
- Occlusive dressings: reduce pain, protect the wound from infection, control exudates, enhance autolytic debridement, maintain moist wound environment
- Secure dressing with gauze; do not use tape as skin is fragile and tears easily
- Management of disease process, that is, BP, eliminate smoking, control blood glucose
- Surgical intervention to improve circulation
- Vacuum compression therapy
- Hyperbaric oxygen therapy

Skill 25.3.6 | Changing a Dressing—Venous Ulcer

Equipment

Cleansing solution
Normal saline solution
Sterile 4×4 dressings
Moisture-retentive dressings (hydrocolloid, transparent film or
    foam for light-to-moderate drainage)
Absorbent dressings (foams, alginates, and absorptive dressings)
    for moderate to heavy exudate
Compression dressing
Clean gloves
Sterile gloves
Biohazard bag
Scissors
Absorbent pad

Preparation

1. Perform hand hygiene.
2. Gather equipment. ❶
3. Identify client using two forms of identification, introduce
   yourself and explain procedure to client.

4. Provide privacy for client.
5. Raise bed to HIGH working height position and lower side rails.
6. Open sterile packages and arrange on overbed table.
7. Place absorbent pad under wound.

Procedure

1. Don clean gloves.
2. Remove compression bandage and old dressing and place
   in biohazard bag. ❷ Compression dressings may be left in
   place for 3–7 days depending on amount of drainage and
   type of dressing.
3. Assess and measure wound. ❸ ❹ ➤ *Rationale:* This
   determines effectiveness of treatment.
4. Clean off debris by pouring cleansing solution over wound. ❺
5. Rinse wound with sterile normal saline.
6. Debride wound, if ordered (Box 25-9 ■), using one of the
   following methods:

   a. Autolytic: Apply occlusive dressings that assist in
      maintaining a moist wound environment, therefore
      promoting reepithelialization. ➤ *Rationale:* Autolytic

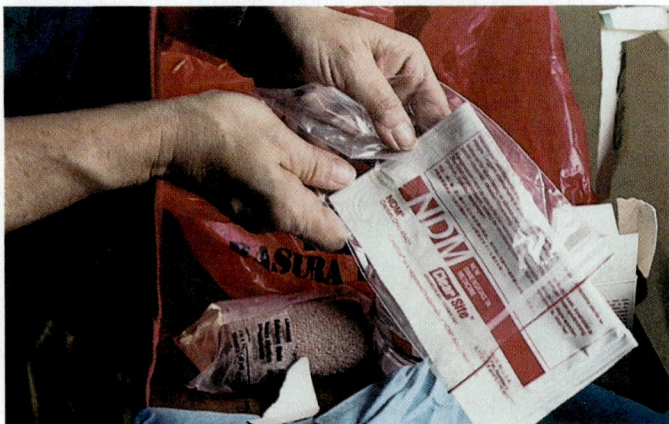

❶ Obtain appropriate wound dressing kit, if available.

❸ Assess wound healing and evaluate progress (stage II).

❷ Remove compression dressing, being careful not to cut skin.

❹ Measure wound to evaluate effectiveness of treatment.

debridement uses the body's own enzymes and moisture to rehydrate, moisten, and slough tissue.

   b. Chemical: Apply enzyme-debriding agents (accuzyme, collagenase, papain, etc.). *Note:* The major disadvantage of the chemical method is that viable tissue is removed with necrotic tissue.

   c. Mechanical: Apply wet-to-dry dressings, use hydrotherapy, irrigation.

7. Dry the wound using sterile 4×4 dressings. Place waste in biohazard bag. **6 7**

8. Remove gloves, and don sterile gloves.

9. Apply medicated moisturizer over wound, if ordered. **8**

   ➤ *Rationale:* This keeps wound area moist.

CLINICAL ALERT

Moisture promotes granulation and reepithelialization and reduces pain. Ointments provide the most occlusive moisturizer because they contain oil and water.

EVIDENCE-BASED PRACTICE
Medieval Remedies Make a Comeback

Medieval remedies, like maggots for bedsores, are enjoying a renaissance to debride or eliminate necrotic tissue and remove **pathogenic** bacteria. There is evidence from recent studies that they may accelerate wound healing by promoting the formation of granulation tissue. Maggots feed on dead tissue, cellular debris, and exudates from necrotic wounds. Maggot treatment has proven to be effective in clients with venous ulcer, diabetic ulcers, and arterial ulcers.

In a 2011 study of people with nonhealing wounds, maggot therapy was more effective in debriding than conventional surgical wound cleaning during the first week, but there was no significant added benefit by day 15. Wounds debrided by maggots showed significantly increased wound surface compared to surgical debridement. However, the second week of treatment could be deleterious because a significant increase in wound surface area was observed by day 15 in the maggot group.

Source: Opletalova et al. (2012)

5 Pour normal saline solution over wound to clean off debris.

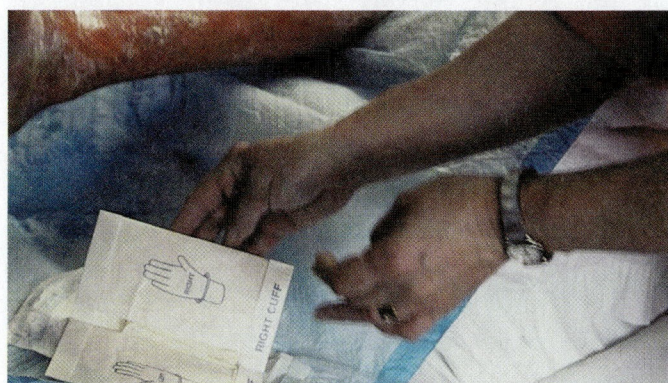

6 Don sterile gloves before cleaning wound with 4×4 gauze pads.

7 Dry with 4×4 gauze pad after cleansing.

Box 25-9 DEBRIDEMENT

Physical removal of affected tissue by debridement is the most effective method of cleaning the wound. Infected tissue is best removed by surgical debridement. Other common methods of debridement include chemical (enzymatic), mechanical, or autolytic. Stage II ulcers can be debrided by gentle mechanical debridement using mesh gauze moistened with saline, hydrocolloid dressings, or enzymatic debriding. Stage IV and large stage III ulcers require surgical debridement. Surgical debridement uses sterile instruments and requires local anesthesia. Only a qualified clinician can use this technique.

Chemical debridement is slower than surgical debridement but is able to be used in home care and long-term care settings. Proteolytic enzymes such as collagenase or papain-urea are commonly used chemical agents. Mechanical debridement is accomplished through whirlpool treatments. Autolytic debridement uses moisture-retentive or moisture-donating dressings to facilitate digestion of tissue by the client's own enzymes and phagocytes.

Biological or larval debridement is uncommon but is finding increased use for wounds that are difficult to heal.

(continued)

Skill 25.3.6 | Changing a Dressing—Venous Ulcer *(continued)*

8 Apply medicated moisturizer on wound, if ordered.

10 Apply compression dressing for venous or lymphatic conditions.

9 Apply moisture-retentive dressing over wound site.

11 Cover entire area with compression dressing.

10. Remove backing on moisture-retentive dressing and place over open wound site. These dressings prevent entry of bacteria from surface of dressing. **9**

CLINICAL ALERT
Use of semiocclusive dressings reduces incidence of wound infections by maintaining a moist environment, reducing airborne bacteria, and providing a mechanical barrier for bacterial entry.

11. Palpate arterial system: dorsalis pedis, posterior, or tibial pulse. If pulses are nonpalpable, obtain an ankle-brachial index (ABI).

12. Apply compression dressing if ABI is greater than 0.6. **10**
11 ➤ *Rationale:* If arterial insufficiency is present, another ulcer can occur. Effective compression bandages generate 40–70 mm Hg of pressure.

CLINICAL ALERT
Compression Therapy
Elastic Therapy
Graduated compression and multilayer compression stockings and compression pumps are effective in increasing venous return. Both mobile and immobile clients can use these stockings, although it is more difficult for the client who is mobile. The stockings are available in different pressures.

Intermittent Pneumatic Compression
Therapy comprises a pump that delivers air to inflatable and deflatable sleeves that embrace extremities, providing intermittent compression. It is used for bedridden clients who cannot tolerate continuous compression therapy. The benefits of this type of therapy are less clear than for the elastic therapy.

13. Reposition leg in elevated position. Leg should be elevated 18–20 cm (7–8 in.) above heart for 2–4 hr during the day and night. ➤ *Rationale:* This prevents edema and venous stasis and promotes healing.
14. Remove gloves and place in biohazard bag. Place all used supplies in bag.
15. Place biohazard bag in appropriate receptacle.
16. Perform hand hygiene.
17. Lower bed and raise side rails.
18. Assess peripheral circulation every 4 hr. ➤ *Rationale:* This ensures compression dressing is not too tight.

EVIDENCE-BASED PRACTICE
Algorithm for Treating Venous Leg Ulcers Utilizing the Cochrane Database of Systematic Reviews

A literature review was done to develop an evidence-based algorithm for the treatment of venous leg ulcers that may improve outcomes, restore function of the affected limb, and reduce healthcare costs. Based on the data obtained, an algorithm was established outlining the use of compression therapy in venous leg ulcers for less than 4 weeks. If a wound is present after 4 weeks of therapy and has not reduced in size by 40%, bilayered living skin equivalents may be indicated. The algorithm recommendations were based on an analysis of wound characteristics and healing rates in 29,189 clients with 56,488 venous leg ulcers. The median wound size was 189 mm^2 and the median wound duration was 3 months. By the 12th week of care, 45.2% of clients had healed. Those who healed had smaller wounds at baseline and wounds of shorter duration than those who did not heal.

Source: Kimmel & Robin (2013)

Skill 25.3.7 | Assessing Ankle–Brachial Index (ABI)

Equipment
Sphygmomanometer (two cuffs, one arm and one leg)
Stethoscope
Doppler, handheld

Procedure
1. Review chart to determine whether client has diabetes.
   ➤ *Rationale:* The ABI may not be reliable in these clients because arterial calcification causes false readings (high). The ABI is used to indirectly assess lower-extremity peripheral blood flow.
2. Identify client using two forms of identification, introduce yourself, and explain procedure to client.
3. Place client in supine position. Instruct to lie quietly for 5 min.
4. Place cuff above right or left elbow, and apply ultrasound gel to brachial pulse area.
5. Hold ultrasound probe at 90-degree angle on top of gel.
   ➤ *Rationale:* This position opposes direction of brachial artery blood flow.
6. Inflate cuff pressure to the point that the "whooshing" sound of the brachial pulse stops, and continue inflating at least 20 mm Hg above that point.
7. Slowly deflate pressure until systolic pulse sound is heard (when "whooshing" sound restarts).
8. Obtain blood pressure readings in both arms. Use the higher systolic pressure as the brachial pressure for the ABI calculations.
9. Wrap leg cuff around leg 5 cm (2 in.) above ankle's medial malleolus. Place conductivity gel over posterior tibial or dorsalis pedis artery.
10. Place Doppler probe at a 90-degree angle to dorsalis pedis or posterior tibial artery.
11. Inflate cuff until Doppler sound stops.
12. Deflate cuff slowly while maintaining Doppler probe in place over artery.
13. Obtain two readings of posterior tibial or dorsalis pedis measurements and select highest value to be used in ABI calculation.
14. Divide ankle systolic pressure by brachial systolic pressure to obtain ankle–brachial index (ABI). Normally, ankle pressure is equal to or slightly higher than brachial pressure.
15. Review ABI guidelines to determine severity of arterial insufficiency (Box 25-10 ■).
16. Document findings in nurses' notes and place note on chart for physician.

Box 25-10 ANKLE-BRACHIAL INDEX (ABI) GUIDELINES

1.0–1.2 ABI	Normal—No arterial insufficiency
0.8–1.0 ABI	Mild insufficiency
0.5–0.8 ABI	Moderate insufficiency
<0.5 ABI	Severe insufficiency
<0.3 ABI	Limb threatening

Skill 25.3.8 | Caring for a Wound With a Drain

Equipment
Same items as for Skill 25.3.3, Changing a Wound Dressing
Sterile cotton applicators
Sterile safety pin
ABD dressings
Gauze pads
Sterile scissors
Sterile gloves
Clean gloves
Cleansing solution

Preparation
1. Check physician's orders (Box 25-11 ■).
2. Perform hand hygiene.
3. Gather equipment.
4. Provide privacy.
5. Identify client using two forms of identification, introduce yourself, and explain procedure. Assess for pain.
6. Clear off overbed table.
7. Raise bed to HIGH position (comfortable working height) and lower side rails on working side of bed.
8. Place plastic bag for soiled dressings on bed near wound site.
9. Open sterile packages and place on overbed table.

Procedure
1. Remove tape from client's skin by pulling *toward* the incision. ➤ *Rationale:* This decreases pain and prevents damage to wound site by preventing a "pull" on the incision.
2. Don clean gloves.
3. Remove soiled dressing.
4. Discard gloves and dressings into plastic bag.
5. Observe wound closely for signs of infection or healing. Don sterile gloves.
6. If pin on the Penrose drain is crusted, replace it with a sterile pin. Be careful not to dislodge drain or suction tubing.
7. Using cotton applicators or gauze pads, cleanse drain site with cleansing solution and then saline.
8. Start cleansing at drain site, moving in a circular motion toward the periphery, unless using chlorhexidine swab; with chlorhexidine, use back-and-forth motion. ❶ ❷

❶ Use drainage pouches for wounds with drains.

❷ Clean the drain site, using a circular motion (unless using chlorhexidine) from the inside to the periphery of the wound. With chlorhexidine, use a back-and-forth motion.

❸ Place a precut sterile 4×4 gauze dressing around the drain site to prevent skin excoriation.

Box 25-11 DRAINAGE POUCHES AND DRAINAGE SYSTEMS

Drainage Pouches

Apply a pouch to:

- Collect drainage
- Measure drainage
- Protect skin from drainage
- Contain drainage
- Contain microorganisms so spread is decreased
- Lessen frequency of care; dressing change is every 24–48 hr

Drainage Systems

Open drains: Discharge flows freely into an absorbent dressing or a drainage bag.

Closed systems: Remove fluid and debris into a closed container (i.e., Hemovac or Jackson–Pratt). Fewer wound infections occur with this drainage system.

Hold drain erect while cleaning around it. ➤ *Rationale:* This prevents contamination of drain site area.

9. Dry the surrounding skin with gauze swab.
10. Discard applicators in plastic bag.
11. Advance drain if ordered:

  a. Using sterile forceps, pull drain out of wound the ordered number of centimeters. ➤ *Rationale:* To facilitate tissue healing.

  b. Reposition the safety pin so that it is at the level of the skin. ➤ *Rationale:* The pin prevents the drain from slipping back into the wound.

  c. Cut off the excess tubing with sterile scissors. Leave at least 5 cm (2 in.) of tubing on the outside. ➤ *Rationale:* This prevents drain from being drawn up into the wound opening.

Note: Drains vary in length (25–35 cm [10–14 in.]) and width (1.2–4 cm [0.5–1.5 in.]).

12. Place several 4×4 dressings around the drain. ❸
13. Apply gauze pad with a precut slit under the drain site.
14. Apply dry, sterile gauze pads over drain.
15. Apply ABD pads over sterile gauze.
16. Remove gloves and dispose of them in refuse bag.
17. Tape dressing or retie Montgomery straps (tie tapes).
18. Remove bag with soiled dressing from room.
19. Perform hand hygiene.
20. Position client for comfort.
21. Lower bed and raise side rail.

Skill 25.3.9 | Applying an Abdominal Binder

Equipment

Abdominal binder: woven-cotton, synthetic, or elasticized material. Most facilities use commercial Velcro binders.
Safety pins for binders without Velcro closure

Procedure

1. Perform hand hygiene.
2. Identify client, introduce yourself, and explain use of binder to client. Assess for pain.
3. Place client in supine position.
4. Ask client to raise hips, and then slide the binder under client's hips at level of gluteal fold. Place top of binder at client's waist.
5. Bring ends of binder around client, and secure by pressing Velcro surfaces together. ❶ If using non-Velcro binder, secure binder with safety pins placed vertically along edges from bottom of binder and toward waist. ➤ *Rationale:* Pinning binder from bottom to waist provides uplifting support for abdominal muscles.

6. Observe for wrinkles in binder. ➤ *Rationale:* Wrinkles can cause pressure areas, especially over iliac crest.
7. Assess client's ability to move freely, breathe deeply, and feel secure pressure over abdominal incision. ➤ *Rationale:* A binder that is too tight may compromise breathing or place pressure on the incisional area.
8. Assess effectiveness of binder every 4 hr, and rewrap every 8 hr if non-Velcro binder is used. ❷ Many clients use this binder only when ambulating.

❶ Bring end of binder around client and secure Velcro surfaces.

❷ Assess effectiveness of binder every 4 hr.

Skill 25.3.10 | Maintaining Wound Drainage System

Equipment
Specimen cup for measuring drainage
I&O bedside record
Absorbent pad
Clean gloves
Hemovac suction or Jackson–Pratt suction drainage system ❶

❶ Jackson–Pratt drainage system in place.

Preparation
1. Check physician's order and client care plan.
2. Bring specimen cup to bedside.
3. Identify client using two forms of identification, introduce yourself, and explain the procedure, giving the client time to ask questions.
4. Provide for comfort and privacy.
5. Perform hand hygiene and don gloves.
6. Elevate bed to workable height.

Procedure
1. Expose catheter insertion site while keeping client draped. Place drainage system on absorbent pad.
2. Examine pump and catheter for patency, seal, and stability. If catheter is occluded, notify physician.
3. Remove Hemovac plug, which is labeled "Pouring Spout," or disconnect tubing from Jackson–Pratt system.
4. Pour drainage into specimen cup. ❷
5. Compress bulb on Jackson–Pratt or compress the Hemovac by pushing the top and bottom together with your hands. ❸

A

B

❷ **A.** Empty, measure, and record drainage every shift. **B.** Remove Hemovac plug from "Pouring Spout" for emptying.

A

B

❸ **A.** Squeeze bulb and reconnect to drainage tubing after emptying. **B.** Compress Hemovac by pushing top and bottom together.

6. Hold pump or bulb tightly compressed, and reinsert plug or connect tubing to Jackson–Pratt system. ➤ *Rationale:* This will reestablish closed drainage system.
7. Position suction devices on bed.
8. Measure and record amount of drainage.
9. Examine drainage for color, consistency, and odor.
10. Discard drainage and container; remove gloves, and wash hands.
11. Send culture specimen to laboratory if ordered.
12. Make client comfortable, and lower bed.
13. Compress evacuator at least every 4 hr to provide suction. Measure drainage at least every 8 hr.

Skill 25.3.11 | Irrigating Wounds

Equipment

Sterile irrigation solution, preferably saline or Ringer's solution
Commercial wound cleaner container with nozzle
   Or
Sterile irrigating set with 35-mL syringe and 19-gauge
Angiocath tip or 19-gauge needle
Absorbent pad
Clean gloves
Sterile gloves
Equipment for dressing change
Mask, goggles, and gown
Plastic bag to dispose of soiled dressings

Preparation

1. Check physician's orders and client care plan.
2. Identify client using two forms of identification and introduce yourself to the client. Assess for pain.
3. Gather irrigation equipment and dressing material. Put on mask, goggles, and gown. ➤ *Rationale:* These are part of Standard Precautions. The gown protects clothes from contamination should splashing occur. Goggles protect the eyes from contact with irrigating fluid or wound drainage, and the mask prevents splashing into the mouth.
4. Assemble equipment. Place the plastic bag in a convenient place for waste disposal.
5. Explain procedure to client and answer any questions.
6. Raise bed and lower side rails.
7. Perform hand hygiene.
8. Open sterile packages on the overbed table as with dressing change.
9. Pour sterile irrigating solution into container.

Procedure

1. Place absorbent pads under the client. Place a bath blanket under absorbent pads when irrigating a large wound.
   ➤ *Rationale:* This will absorb any spilled irrigation solution.
2. Position client so that solution flows from wound to basin.
3. Don clean gloves.
4. Remove and discard used dressing.
5. Remove gloves and discard into plastic bag.
6. Place overbed table near working area with all packages open.
7. Don sterile gloves.
8. Inspect area surrounding wound for redness, tissue integrity, and signs of granulating tissue.
9. Place sterile basin under wound area.

10. Draw solution from sterile container into 35-mL syringe with syringe or Angiocath tip. Increasing syringe size decreases pressure of stream or increasing bore of catheter tip increases pressure.

Note: The goal of irrigation is to remove bacteria and debris without injury to normal tissue (see Box 25-9). Irrigation pressure of 5–15 pounds per square inch (psi) is required to accomplish the goal.

> ### CLINICAL ALERT
> If wound has moderate to heavy drainage, alginate dressings should be used. Alginate forms a gel when it comes in contact with wound fluid. It absorbs up to 20 times its weight in fluid. It can be used in infected and noninfected wounds. It is not to be used in dry wounds, because it can dehydrate the wound.

11. Cleanse wound in the direction from least contaminated to most contaminated areas.
12. Open commercial cleaning solution package if using for irrigation.
    a. Read directions on commercial wound cleaner container to determine appropriate distance nozzle is positioned from wound during irrigation.
    b. If nozzle is too close to the wound, force may be higher than expected.
    c. If nozzle is too far from the wound, force may be lower than needed.
    d. If saline solution is used, deliver irrigant with 8 psi pressure. The 35-mL syringe and 19-gauge Angiocath tip delivers this pressure. ➤ *Rationale:* Pressures effective in wound cleansing should be between 4 psi and 15 psi in order to effectively clean the wound surface by forcefully loosening foreign materials and nonattached bacteria.
    e. Repeat until all irrigation solution has been used.
13. After the irrigation, cleanse client's skin around wound and dry.
14. Apply sterile dressing.
15. Dispose of equipment properly.
16. Remove gloves. Check to see that client is comfortable before leaving the room.
17. Lower bed and raise side rails.
18. Perform hand hygiene.

| **Skill 25.3.12** | Teaching Wound Care to Clients |

Procedure

1. Begin client teaching as soon as client is able to participate in activity. ➤ *Rationale:* Client will need to care for wound at home for a period of time before sutures are removed and wound is healed.
2. Assess wound daily for any changes in color, odor, or drainage. Assess for pain.
3. Keep wound dry and clean.
4. Instruct client that he or she can take a shower, unless contraindicated by wound condition (i.e., dressing on wound, splint, or other contraindication).
5. Do not remove dressing unless it is wet or soiled. If soiled or wet, change dressing according to directions. Wound or dressing can be covered by plastic when taking shower.
6. Report any signs of infection to healthcare provider: erythema, edema around incision site, warmth or tenderness surrounding incision site, discharge or foul odor from site, streaks on the skin running from wound, and chills or temperature above 37.8°C (100°F). ➤ *Rationale:* These are signs and symptoms of SSIs.
7. After sutures are removed, instruct client to:
   a. Follow instructions from healthcare provider regarding activity level. ➤ *Rationale:* Even though sutures are removed, wound is not completely healed and will continue to strengthen over the next weeks.
   b. Keep suture line clean, cleansing it using soft strokes, and pat dry.
   c. Observe wound edges, they will appear red and slightly raised; this is normal.
   d. Observe suture site; if site continues to be reddened and painful to pressure beyond 8 weeks, notify healthcare provider. ➤ *Rationale:* This could indicate excessive collagen formation.

Unit 25.3 Documentation and Evaluation

DOCUMENTATION for Wound Care

- Observation of wound site, including amount, color, and odor of drainage, as well as appearance of suture site
- Color of wound drainage: *serous*—clear, watery plasma; *serosanguineous*—plasma and red blood cells; *sanguineous*—blood; *purulent*—thick drainage suggestive of infection
- Observation of granulating necrotic or epithelial tissue
- Observations pertinent to client's tolerance of procedure
- Observation of skin condition around incision site; erythema, maceration, induration, edema
- Changes in vital signs that indicate possible infection
- Client's activity level, any incontinence
- Compliance with prescribed treatment

- Type of dressing applied
- Material used in wound packing
- Observations on wound irrigation
- Type and amount of irrigation solutions used
- Unusual tension on sutures if present
- Amount and color of Hemovac or Jackson–Pratt drainage
- Document undermining using clock orientation (e.g., 2 to 5 o'clock); measure in centimeters
- Tissue viability; percent healthy and necrotic tissue relative to entire wound
- Signs and symptoms indicating potential SSI
- Teaching information provided to client

EVALUATION/Critical Thinking

Expected Outcomes

- Wound care is provided for contaminated wound and healing occurs.
- Drainage system functions without obstructions.
- Wound irrigation is completed using sufficient pressure to cleanse wound bed.
- Abdominal binder supports client's abdominal wound.
- Compression dressing applied to vascular ulcer site.

Unexpected Outcomes	Alternative Actions
• Wound becomes infected with multiple microorganisms.	• Notify physician about changes in color or odor of drainage. • Obtain culture and sensitivity if physician orders one. • Wash your hands thoroughly after caring for client to prevent the spread of infection. • Pay strict attention to changing dressings.
• Wound does not heal.	• Evaluate use of dressing and perhaps choose a different type of dressing. • Assess nutritional status. Increase protein and carbohydrates if not contraindicated. • Determine availability of a vacuum-assisted closure machine.
• Edges of wound split open (wound dehiscence).	• Place client in supine position. Apply butterfly tape to wound edges. Cover opening with sterile dressings. • Apply binder for abdominal incisions after obtaining order. • Notify physician if signs of infection are present. • Obtain culture of drainage if physician orders one. • Observe client for signs of shock. If client is in shock, notify physician immediately. • Encourage high-protein diet.
• **Evisceration** occurs (protrusion of bowel contents).	• Institute emergency measures. Place the client in supine position. Cover bowel with sterile gauze moistened with sterile saline. Have IV-certified nurse insert IV catheter and infuse normal saline. Reassure client. Obtain vital signs, and treat for shock if present. • After above measures are completed, notify physician, and prepare client for return to surgery. • After surgical repair, notify dietician for diet change to increase protein and vitamin C in diet. • Apply abdominal binder if ordered.
• Wound hemorrhages.	• Outline area of blood on dressing with a pen and observe outline to see how quickly the bleeding spreads. • If bleeding is excessive, notify the physician immediately. • Apply pressure dressing to site if there is excessive bleeding.
• Skin appears red and broken.	• Clean area with sterile saline and dry thoroughly with sterile 4×4 pads. • Apply moisture-retentive dressing.
• Wound is too extensive for application of drainage.	• Obtain Stomahesive or Hollihesive 8×8 sheets and cut on diagonal 0.3–0.6 cm (⅛–¼ in.) larger than wound.
• ABD pads cannot contain drainage.	• If larger barrier needed, Stomahesive may be pieced together to form larger barrier, reinforcing juncture points with Karaya paste. • A superadhesive pouch may then be app lied. • If dressings are used, they may be secured with Montgomery straps (tie tapes).

(continued)

Unexpected Outcomes	Alternative Actions
• Abdominal binder is not effective in supporting incisional area.	• Evaluate the effectiveness of the abdominal binder. • Assess if the binder is properly positioned at the hip level and waist level to provide support. • Assess if the binder is too loose.
• Client is too large for the abdominal binder.	• Fold a drawsheet in half lengthwise and place under client. Position the edges at the waist and pubic area. • Pull tightly on the drawsheet, and secure the edges with safety pins.
• Drainage system expands quickly after being reconnected. • Client is too large for bed. • Client's assessment indicates that he or she is at high risk for SSI.	• Check all connections for an air leak because properly functioning reservoirs expand slowly. • Request use of BariCare bed. • Administer appropriate antibiotic 1 hr before surgery. • If client has a chronic illness, monitor carefully for signs and symptoms of SSIs postoperatively. • If client's surgery is not urgent, treat condition and then reschedule surgical intervention.

Promoting a Moist Environment

Nursing Process Data

ASSESSMENT Database

- Assess wound edges for presence of granulation tissue.
- Assess for changes in amount of drainage.
- Assess whether necrotic tissue is decreasing in amount.
- Identify whether appropriate dressing is used for wound care.

PLANNING Objectives

- To promote wound healing by secondary intention
- To maintain a moist environment conducive to wound healing
- To provide the most appropriate treatment for wound care
- To enhance local healing
- To maintain sterile technique throughout procedure
- To remove trapped exudate from wounds

IMPLEMENTATION Procedures

DOCUMENTATION AND EVALUATION

Expected Outcomes

- Wound heals without complications.
- Sterile technique is maintained throughout procedure.

Unexpected Outcomes/Alternative Actions

Pearson Nursing Student Resources

Find additional review materials at
nursing.pearsonhighered.com.
Prepare for success with NCLEX®-style practice questions and Skill Checklists.

Skill 25.4.1 | Applying Wet-to-Moist Dressings

Equipment

Sterile 4×8 noncotton gauze dressings
Semiocclusive dressing, optional
Sterile gloves
Clean gloves
Tape
Plastic bag or receptacle for contaminated dressings
Sterile normal saline solution
Sterile receptacle (round basin or emesis basin) if dressing not in commercial pack
Montgomery straps, if desired

> **CLINICAL ALERT**
>
> Wet-to-dry dressings are used only to debride wounds, as they cause tissue damage. Maceration of healthy tissue can occur with dressings that are always wet. Dry dressings cause damage to granulating tissue if removed without first soaking the gauze.

Preparation

1. Check physician's orders and client care plan.
2. Perform hand hygiene and gather equipment.
3. Identify client using two forms of identification, and introduce yourself.
4. Explain procedure to client. Assess for pain.
5. Provide privacy.
6. Raise bed to HIGH working height; lower side rail near you.
7. Remove tape by pulling it toward the wound. ➤ **Rationale:** This action prevents injury to newly formed tissue.
8. Don clean gloves.
9. Remove wound packing by gently grasping the gauze without touching the wound and tear it away at a right angle from the wound surface. ➤ **Rationale:** Touching only the gauze prevents contamination of the wound.
10. Place soiled dressings in disposable bag.
11. Remove gloves, and dispose of them in bag.
12. Perform hand hygiene.

Procedure

1. Open packages of dressings making sure sterility is maintained. ❶
2. Pour normal saline solution over dressings. ❷
3. Don sterile gloves.
4. Pick up sterile gauze dressings one at a time.
5. Fluff each dressing, and place over wound. ❸ ➤ **Rationale:** If packed tightly, dressing can prevent wound edges from contact with capillaries.
6. Place gauze in the wound, covering all exposed surfaces and tunneling. Press gauze lightly into depressions or cracks. ➤ **Rationale:** Necrotic tissue is more prevalent in these areas.
7. Unfold a moist, sterile, 4×8 ABD pad dressing into a single layer and place it on top of wet dressings covering the wound area (not on skin). ❹
8. Place a dry 4×8 pad over the dressing to hold it in place. Some protocols call for semiocclusive dressing in place of pad.
9. Remove gloves, and place in plastic bag.
10. Tape only the edges of the dressing. Montgomery tapes may be used to prevent excessive skin irritation and damage due to frequent dressing changes.
11. Position client for comfort. Lower bed and raise side rail to UP position, if appropriate.
12. Discard soiled material in appropriate container.
13. Perform hand hygiene.
14. Observe wound for excessive drainage or drying out of dressing between dressing changes. Remoisten dressing if dry. ➤ **Rationale:** Unless excessive drainage occurs, or dressing dries out, dressings are usually changed every 8 hr. See list of additional dressings in Table 25-6 ■.
15. Provide client or family teaching regarding wound care, if appropriate.

Note: These dressings function as osmotic dressings. Normal saline is isotonic. As water evaporates from saline dressing, it becomes hypertonic and fluid from wound tissue is drained into dressing.

❶ Open sterile packages before beginning dressing change.

❷ Pour sterile saline solution over dressings to moisten.

❸ Fluff dressings and apply over wound, covering all exposed surfaces.

❹ Place moist ABD pad over dressings; then cover with dry pad.

Table 25-6 Additional Moist Wound Dressings

Type of Alternative	Use	Outcome of Treatment	Considerations
Hydrogel Sheet	• Interacts with aqueous solutions • Used with minor wounds with light to moderate drainage • Absorbs minimal to heavy exudates • Cannot be used with infected wound • Nonadherent	Softens necrotic tissue Creates moist environment	Use outer dressing to prevent wound from drying out. Change dressing every 1–2 days.
Impregnated Gauze Dressing	• Absorbs minimal to moderate exudates • Nonadherent	Conforms to irregular surfaces Eliminates dead space Creates moist environment	Requires outer dressing Change daily. Nonabsorptive
Alginate*	• Absorbs heavy exudates • Converts to gel when comes in contact with wound drainage • Easily removed from wound • Nonadherent • Absorbs up to 20 times its weight in fluid • Can be used in infected and noninfected wounds	Maintains moist environment Promotes fast healing of wound	Not to be used on dry wounds Dehydrates wound, delaying healing of eschar-covered wounds, third-degree burns, or surgical wounds
Foams	• Absorbs minimal to heavy exudates • Highly absorbent • Used for deep cavity wounds	Maintains moist environment Decreases tissue trauma when removed Increases time between dressing changes (3–4 days)	Requires external dressing Can cause drying effect on wound
Hydrophilic	• Type of foam dressing • Nonadherent • Very absorbent	Cushions wound Traps exudate	Used in wounds with moderate to heavy drainage
Hydrophobic	• Nonadherent flexible dressing • Minimal or no necrotic tissue • Used with lightly to moderately exudating wounds	Resists fluid penetration into wound Provides cushion to irritated skin	Use on lightly draining wounds
Medical hydrolysate of collagen	• Soluble, and degrades in wound site • Absorbs wound exudates • Is interactive with wound site to provide mechanical protection against physical and bacterial insult	Absorbs up to 30 times own weight Used in stages I–IV pressure ulcers Accelerates tissue remodeling and reduces scarring	Cover with nonstick dressing Soak dressing in warm water before removing

*Alginates are made from acids obtained from brown seaweed. The calcium salts of alginic, mannuronic, and guluronic acids are processed into nonwoven, biodegradable fibers. When the fibers come into contact with fluids, sodium, and calcium ions, they form soluble sodium gel.

(continued)

Skill 25.4.1 | Applying Wet-to-Moist Dressings (continued)

Table 25-6 Additional Moist Wound Dressings (continued)

Type of Alternative	Use	Outcome of Treatment	Considerations
Anticoat 7 Silver-coated contact dressing	• Used for wounds with moderate to heavy exudates • Has an antimicrobial barrier to protect against bacterial contamination and infection • Calcium in the dressing provides antimicrobial to protect against bacterial contamination and infection. • Kills bacteria faster than any other form of silver dressing	Used for leg ulcers, pressure ulcers, diabetic foot ulcers, and burns	Stays in place for up to 3 days to provide moist environment

Skill 25.4.2 | Using a Hydrocolloid Dressing

Equipment

Sterile normal saline

Hydrocolloid dressing (e.g., DuoDERM, Restore, Ultec, Comfeel Plus) (Table 25-7 ■)

Hydrogel if needed (ClearSite, Aquasorb)

Sterile 4×4 gauze pads

Hypoallergenic tape

Clean gloves

Skin prep, optional

Note: These dressings are a combination of adhesive and gelling polymers that are impermeable to oxygen, water, and water vapor. They promote a moist wound environment, aid in autolytic debridement, and have no toxic components. They are waterproof and bacteria proof. These dressings are best used in clients who have partial- to full-thickness wounds with minimal to moderate exudates such as for pressure ulcers, skin tears, surgical wounds, and burns.

Procedure

1. Select dressing size to ensure coverage 3.2 cm (1¼ in.) beyond ulcer margin. (Dressing available in 4×4 to 8×8 sizes.) ➤ **Rationale:** This ensures complete covering of wound. Use for small ulcers and in stages II and III ulcers.

Note: These dressings can be used for dry wounds, as they contain 95% water. They are occlusive and do not allow water or bacteria into the wound. Hydrocolloid causes the pH of the wound surface to drop, and this acidic environment can inhibit bacterial growth.

CLINICAL ALERT

Hydrocolloids cannot be used if wound or surrounding skin is infected. The dressings are not used on wounds with heavy drainage or wounds with deep tunnels.

---

2. Perform hand hygiene and don clean gloves. Assess for pain.
3. Cleanse skin with gauze pad moistened with sterile normal saline and pat dry with gauze pad.
4. Measure wound using pliable device.
5. Apply skin prep to surrounding skin to protect, if ordered.

Table 25-7 Hydrocolloid Dressings

Dressing	Uses
Hydrocolloid dressing (2 mm thick) Exterior surface protects wound from contamination	On partial- and full-thickness wounds with exudate
Thin hydrocolloid dressing (less than 1-mm thick)	On superfluid wounds with minimal exudate and to protect areas at risk for skin breakdown
Hydrocolloid paste	To manage dermal wounds with light drainage
Hydrocolloid gel	On partial- and full-thickness wounds Fills dry wound cavities Promotes autolytes debridement

6. Fill ulcer area with hydrogel if ordered—usually used with stage III or IV pressure ulcer of the hip when exudate is present (Box 25-12 ■). Do not overfill with gel. ➤ **Rationale:** This facilitates autolytic debridement of devitalized tissue.

Box 25-12 **HYDROGEL DRESSINGS**

• Hydrogel dressings contain 95% water; they are very absorbent and dehydrate easily when not covered with a secondary dressing.

• Dressings cannot absorb much exudate; they should be used for dry wounds such as skin tears, surgical wounds, and radiation therapy burns.

• Dressings are nonadhesive, can be transparent, and conform to wound surfaces.

• Sterile aqueous hydrogen fiber is used to fill cavity with gel; it is also used to fill dead space in large wounds. Do not overfill wounds to prevent tissue damage.

• Hydrogel sheets are placed in direct contact with wound bed and margins; air bubbles and plastic covering on sheet must be removed. The unique cooling properties soothe painful wounds.

7. Warm dressing by holding in hands. ➤ *Rationale:* This increases activity of adhesive, and it makes dressing more pliable.

8. Remove silicone release paper backing from dressing. Minimize finger contact with adhesive surface. ➤ *Rationale:* Dressing is sterile, and contamination should be avoided.

9. Center dressing over affected area and extend at least 2.5 cm (1 in.) onto periwound skin. Gently roll dressing over pressure ulcer—do not stretch dressing. ❶ ➤ *Rationale:* Stretching the dressing may cause wrinkling of dressing, which allows air to enter wound.

10. Placing dressing one-third above wound and two-thirds below wound maximizes time between dressing changes. ➤ *Rationale:* This increases absorption capacity of dressing.

❶ Hydrocolloid dressing.

11. Mold the dressing gently to skin and hold down with hand for approximately 1 min.

12. Apply skin prep to area that is to be covered by tape if ordered. Allow to dry. Do not apply skin prep under hydrocolloid dressing. ➤ *Rationale:* Hydrocolloid dressings are placed over broken skin; skin prep may cause damage to skin.

13. Picture-frame sides of hydrocolloid dressing with silk or hypoallergenic tape.

14. Check dressing each shift for impaired integrity.

15. Change dressing at first sign of impaired integrity. Dressings should not be left on longer than 7 days; usually left in place for 3–4 days.

Note: DuoDERM is removed when exudate seeps from edges of dressing or white blister appears under dressing. Comfeel Plus is changed when dressing becomes transparent or there is leakage.

16. Remove dressing by pressing hand down on adjacent skin surface while carefully lifting edge of dressing from skin. Continue lifting dressing around periphery until all edges are released, and then lift dressing carefully away from wound.

17. Remove gloves and perform hand hygiene.

18. Record stage, size, and appearance of ulcer; date; and reason for removal of hydrocolloid dressing.

Note: Although frequently listed as wound care alternatives, topical disinfectant agents such as iodine and silver sulfadiazine are very controversial in wound care. Iodine is cytotoxic to fibroblasts and can impair wound healing. Silver solutions are sometimes used to prevent bacterial colonization in infection-prone areas. They do not eliminate existing infections.

Skill 25.4.3 | Using a Hydrocolloid Wafer Dressing

Procedure

1. Warm hydrocolloid sheet wafer between hands.
2. Apply wafer 2.5–5 cm (1–2 in.) larger than wound.
3. Monitor for periwound maceration.
4. Monitor dressing, as moisture from wound causes wafer to form a gel over wound.
5. Change every 3–7 days or as needed.
6. Secure edges with tape.
7. Remove dressing carefully. Residual may be noted on wound. Do not remove residual.

EVIDENCE-BASED PRACTICE

Silver-Eluting Antimicrobial Dressings Do Not Help Leg Ulcers

Silver-eluting antimicrobial dressings have not been found to help heal leg ulcers to any greater extent than other dressings. A study conducted in the United Kingdom compared these dressings with standard low-adhesive bandages in 213 older adult clients. The results in 6 months indicated the wounds of the clients in the control group had healed 77% and those of the clients in the pilot group had healed 85%. By 1 year, the wounds of clients in both groups had healed by 96%. The silver dressing cost five times as much as the standard dressing. The cost of treating the client with the silver dressing was 30% more than the standard dressing. The study found there was little to support the use of silver or any other antimicrobial dressings in the treatment of venous leg ulcers.

Source: Kennedy, S. (2010)

Skill 25.4.4 | Applying a Foam Dressing

Equipment
Adhesive foam dressing
Receptacle for soiled dressing

Preparation
1. Identify client using two identifiers.
2. Perform hand hygiene.
3. Remove old dressing and discard in appropriate receptacle.
4. Clean wound according to policy.
5. Complete skin assessment and identify wounds that need dressings. Assess for pain.
6. Measure wound and obtain dressing 2.5–5 cm (1–2 in.) larger than wound.

Note: Foam dressings are particularly useful for wounds with moderate to heavy exudate (Box 25-13 ■). The absorptive ability of the foam dressing must match the amount of the exudate the wound is producing. Dry wounds with a scab or eschar are not candidates for foam dressing. They do not benefit from the foam dressing, and the wound may dry out.

Procedure
1. Using foam dressing as primary dressing, measure wound and cut 2.5–5 cm (1–2 in.) larger than wound. ➤ *Rationale:* This is to protect periwound areas.

Box 25-13 **FOAM DRESSINGS IN WOUND CARE**
Foam dressings are useful in the following wounds:

- Wounds requiring negative pressure
- Minor burns
- Skin grafts and donor sites
- Pressure ulcers
- Arterial and venous leg ulcers
- Sutured wounds

Foam can also be used around tracheostomy and gastrostomy tubes to absorb drainage and manage heavy exudate in wounds.

2. If wound is irregular, cut foam dressing to match shape of wound or specific part of body, such as toes.
3. If using foam under compression stockings, place foam in cavity of the wound. Leave space in cavity for expansion of dressing as exudates are absorbed.
4. Press down adhesive border to secure dressing.
5. Apply barrier cream to surrounding skin according to policy.
6. Perform hand hygiene.
7. Assess wound frequently if large volume of exudates in wound.
8. Change dressing every 3–5 days unless wet or soiled, and then change as necessary

Skill 25.4.5 | Applying a Transparent Film

Equipment
Sterile normal saline
Transparent dressing (e.g., Op-Site, Tegaderm, Bioclusive); see moisture retentive dressings in Table 25-8 ■.
Sterile 4×4 gauze pads
Scissors
Hypoallergenic tape
Clean gloves
Plasticizing agent (e.g., skin prep [optional])
Syringe with 26-gauge needle, if needed

Preparation
1. Check physician's orders and client care plan.
2. Check type of dressing ordered. ➤ *Rationale:* These dressings are very important in preventing pressure ulcers; they prevent friction and shear over bony prominences when moving clients.
3. Gather supplies. ❶
4. Obtain appropriately sized transparent dressing. Dressing can be applied to flat surface. (Coccyx area cannot be treated with this type of dressing.) ❷

❶ Dressing carts may be used to keep supplies closer to client area.

Table 25-8   Comparisons of Moisture-Retentive Dressings

	Transparent	Hydrocolloid
Common Brands	Tegaderm Op-Site Bioclusive	Tegasorb DuoDERM Comfeel Restore
Characteristics	Sterile Semipermeable membranes with hypoallergenic adhesive Permeable to oxygen and moisture vapor Allows oxygen exchange Impermeable to bacteria, prevents contamination	Impermeable to oxygen Dressing gel maintains moist environment that promotes autolysis. Impermeable to external bacteria and contamination Minimally to moderately absorptive
Function	Provides moist environment Promotes autolysis and protects newly formed tissue Assists with debridement	Dressing contains hydroactive particles that absorb exudate to form a hydrated gel over wound. When dressing is removed, gel separates from dressing, which protects newly formed tissue.
Use	Easy assessment of wound; dressing is transparent. Nondraining or minimally draining wounds only, nonabsorbable Pressure ulcers, stage I and some stage II Minor burns, lacerations	Absorbs exudate while preserving moist environment needed for autolysis of slough Irrigate gel with saline to allow for assessing wound. Pressure ulcers, some stage III and some clean stage IV Wounds with mild or moderate exudate Wounds with necrosis or slough
Contraindications	Infected wounds Wounds with fragile surrounding skin	Wounds that need frequent assessment, not transparent Wounds with heavy exudate

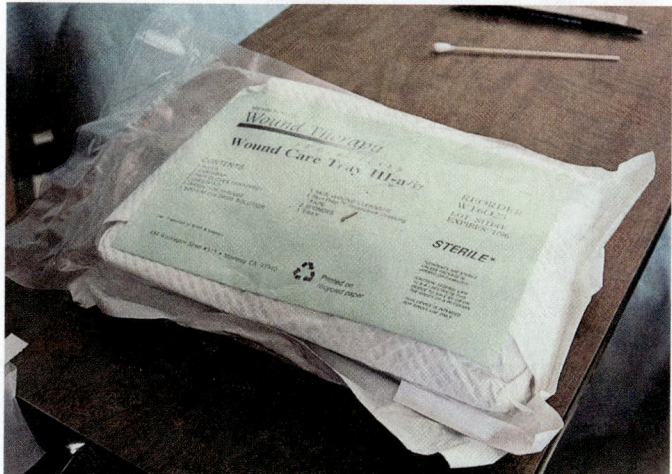

❷ Obtain specific dressing tray for ordered treatment.

❸ Assess size of wound to determine appropriate size of transparent dressing.

5. Perform hand hygiene.
6. Identify client using two types of identification, introduce yourself, and explain procedure to client. Assess for pain.
7. Provide privacy.

Procedure

1. Raise bed to HIGH position (comfortable working height), and lower side rail on working side of bed.
2. Don clean gloves.
3. Remove old dressing, "walk off" dressing from one edge to the other, and discard in appropriate receptacle.

4. Wash pressure ulcer with sterile gauze pads moistened with sterile normal saline.
5. Dry thoroughly with sterile gauze pad.
6. Measure wound using pliable device. ➤ *Rationale:* Comparison of measurement assists in determining effectiveness of treatment. ❸
7. Apply plasticizing agent (skin prep, skin gel) over surrounding tissue if ordered. ➤ *Rationale:* Do not apply directly on ulcer area because the agent contains alcohol, which burns the ulcer area. *Alternate Treatment*: If skin is irritated, apply No Sting Barrier Film Spray to area surrounding tissue.
   ➤ *Rationale:* This protects and prevents skin breakdown.

(continued)

Skill 25.4.5 | Applying a Transparent Film (continued)

8. Loosen transparent dressing from backing paper. **4**
9. "Walk on" dressing: Start at one edge of site and gently lay the dressing down, keeping it free of wrinkles. Allow at least a 3-cm (1.5-in.) margin of dressing beyond ulcer margin. **5** ➤ *Rationale:* This ensures coverage of entire wound area.
10. If using Op-Site, cut off tabs after wound is completely covered.
11. Tape edges with hypoallergenic tape. ➤ *Rationale:* This assists in preventing frequent dressing changes due to loose dressings. These dressings can remain in place for 1 week.

CLINICAL ALERT

Transparent film dressings remain in place for 5–7 days. These dressings are adhesive, permeable to moisture, vapor, and atmospheric gases. They are bacteria-proof and waterproof. It is imperative to observe the ulcer area daily to determine whether a large amount of secretions or serous fluid has accumulated under dressing. If fluid has increased, aspirate with a 26-gauge needle. These dressings are not used for infected areas.

12. Remove gloves and discard in appropriate receptacle.
13. Position client for comfort.
14. Lower bed and raise side rails.
15. Remove and discard equipment.
16. Perform hand hygiene.

4 Remove backing from Op-Site dressing before applying.

5 Apply transparent adhesive dressing over wound.

Unit 25.4 Documentation and Evaluation

DOCUMENTATION for Promoting a Moist Environment

- Condition of wound, location, size of wound
- Solution used
- Number and type of dressings used
- Signs and symptoms indicative of wound infection

- Color, consistency, presence of odor, amount of drainage on soiled dressings
- Presence of granular, necrotic, or epithelial tissue
- Condition of skin surrounding wound
- Client's reaction to procedure

EVALUATION/Critical Thinking

Expected Outcomes

- Wound heals without complications.
- Sterile technique is maintained throughout procedure.

Unexpected Outcomes	Alternative Actions
• Wound drainage increases.	• Decrease time between dressing changes. Change every 4 hr. • Obtain order for culture and sensitivity to determine whether different microorganisms are present or antibiotic medication is not sensitive to microorganism.
• Dressings dry between dressing changes.	• Moisten dressing with sterile normal saline before removing to prevent debridement of granulation tissue. • Ensure that dressing is moist when applied to wound and cover with moist dressing. • Moisten and change dressing more frequently. • Semiocclusive dressing should be considered.

Nursing Process Data

ASSESSMENT Database

- Assess stage of ulcer.
- Assess size and depth of pressure ulcer.
- Assess presence and location of undermining, tunneling, and sinus tracts.
- Identify if infection is associated with pressure ulcer.
- Assess wound exudate.
- Evaluate effectiveness of ulcer treatment.
- Assess healing process of the ulcer.
- Assess other bony prominences for potential formation of pressure ulcers.
- Assess for presence of conditions that inhibit wound healing.
- Assess wound size for changes.

PLANNING Objectives

- To identify the stage of the ulcer
- To provide appropriate treatment for specific ulcer stage
- To promote healing of established ulcer
- To prevent new ulcer formation
- To prevent spread of pathogens from ulcerated area

IMPLEMENTATION Procedures

DOCUMENTATION AND EVALUATION

Expected Outcomes

- Stage of pressure ulcer is accurately assessed.
- Pressure ulcer is treated effectively according to stage of ulcer formation.
- Pressure ulcer is healing within usual time frame.
- Skin remains free of breakdown in surrounding areas of pressure ulcer.
- Absence of additional pressure ulcer formation.

Unexpected Outcomes/Alternative Actions

Pearson Nursing Student Resources

Find additional review materials at **nursing. pearsonhighered.com.**
Prepare for success with NCLEX®-style practice questions and Skill Checklists.

Pressure ulcers are preventable. Nurses must understand the mechanisms and staging of pressure ulcers (Box 25-14 ▪; Table 25-9 ▪).

Box 25-14 NURSING GUIDE FOR ASSESSMENT OF CLIENTS AT RISK FOR PRESSURE ULCERS

Four main factors contribute to development of pressure ulcers:

- Pressure
- Friction
- Shearing
- Moisture

It is a nursing priority to identify at-risk individuals needing preventative measures:

- Bed- and chair-bound individuals
- Clients with impaired ability to reposition themselves
- Clients who are immobilized
- Clients who are incontinent
- Clients with nutritional deficits, such as inadequate dietary intake and malnutrition
- Clients with altered level of consciousness

- Identification of stage I pressure ulcer may be difficult in a dark-skinned client.

A risk assessment tool should be used for all clients admitted to a long-term care facility, an acute care setting, or receiving home care (Braden scale or Norton scale). Systematic reassessments should be done at designated intervals.

- Nursing homes: Assess on admission and every week for 1 month, and then every 3 months. Clients may develop pressure ulcers within the first month in a nursing home.
- Home: Assess at first visit and every visit. Instruct family to notify nurse if skin condition changes.
- Acute care: Assess on admission and every shift for at-risk clients in critical care units or daily to every other day for stable clients.

Table 25-9 Pressure Ulcer Staging

Category/Stage I: Nonblanchable Erythema

Intact skin with nonblanchable redness of a localized area usually over a bony prominence. Darkly pigmented skin may not have visible blanching; its color may differ from the surrounding area. The area may be painful, firm, soft, warmer or cooler as compared to adjacent tissue. This may be difficult to detect in client with dark skin tones (Box 25-15 ▪). It may indicate "at-risk" clients.

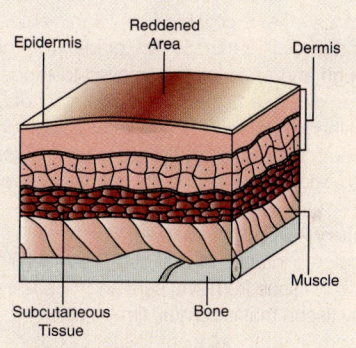

Stage I pressure ulcer.

Category/Stage II: Partial-Thickness Skin Loss

Partial thickness loss of dermis presenting as a shallow, open ulcer with a red-pink wound bed, without slough. May also present as an intact or open/ruptured serum-filled blister or serosangineous-filled blister. It presents as a shiny or dry shallow ulcer without slough or bruising. Bruising indicates suspected deep tissue injury. This stage should not be used to describe skin tears, tape burns, perineal dermatitis, maceration, or excoriation.

Stage II pressure ulcer.

(continued)

Table 25-9 Pressure Ulcer Staging *(continued)*

Category/Stage III: **Full-Thickness Skin Loss**

Full-thickness tissue loss: Subcutaneous fat may be visible, but bone, tendon, or muscle is not exposed. Slough may be present but does not obscure the depth of tissue loss. It may include undermining and tunneling. The depth of this stage varies by the anatomical location. The bridge of the nose, ear, occiput, and malleolus do not have subcutaneous tissue and therefore the ulcers can be shallow. In contrast, areas of significant adipose tissue can develop extremely deep Stage III pressure ulcers. Bone or tendon is not visible or directly palpable.

Stage III pressure ulcer.

Category/Stage IV: **Full-Thickness Tissue Loss**

Full-thickness tissue loss with exposed bone, tendon, or muscle: Slough or eschar may be present on some parts of the wound bed. It often includes undermining and tunneling. The depth of this stage ulcer varies by anatomical location. The bridge of the nose, ear, occiput, and malleolus do not have subcutaneous tissue and these ulcers can be shallow. This stage can extend into muscle or supporting structures (fascia, tendon, or joint capsule) making osteomyelitis possible. Exposed bone or tendon is visible or directly palpable.

Stage IV pressure ulcer.

Unstageable–Unclassified. Full-thickness skin or tissue loss—depth unknown in which the base of the ulcer is covered by slough (yellow, tan, gray, green, or brown) and/or eschar (tan, brown, or black) in the wound bed. Until enough slough and/or eschar is removed to expose the base of the wound, the true depth, and therefore stage, cannot be determined, but it will be either Category/Stage III or IV. Stable (dry, adherent, intact without erythema or fluctuance) eschar on the heels serves as the body's natural (biological) cover and should be removed.

Suspected Deep Tissue Injury—Depth Unknown. Purple or maroon localized area of discolored intact skin or blood-filled blister due to damage of underlying soft tissue from pressure and/or shear. The area may be preceded by tissue that is painful, firm, mushy, boggy, warmer or cooler as compared to adjacent tissue. Deep tissue injury may be difficult to detect in individuals with dark skin tones. Evolution may include a think blister over a dark wound bed. The wound may further evolve and become covered by think eschar. Evolution may be rapid exposing additional layers of tissue even with optimal treatment.

Source: National Pressure Ulcer Advisory Panel, European Pressure Ulcer Advisory Panel, & Pan Pacific Pressure Injury Alliance (2014)

Box 25-15 **ASSESSMENT FOR DARK-SKIN-TONE CLIENTS**

Stage I. Ulcers appear with persistent red, blue, or purple hues. To assess darker skin tones that do not show erythema, shine a light at skin level to check for color change. Palpate area for induration or edema.

Stage II. Ulcers appear as solid, smooth, dark pink tissue exposing basal membrane; there is exposed dermis epithelization.

Skill 25.5.1 | Preventing Pressure Ulcers

Procedure

1. Inspect skin at least on admission and once a shift, particularly over bony prominences. Heels and sacrum are most common areas for skin breakdown. Use Braden or Norton scale for assessment (Table 25-10 ■). Document assessment findings. **①–⑥** ➤ *Rationale:* If skin is red or skin breakdown is evident on admission, Medicare and other payers will reimburse for treatment. If not evident on admission, treatment costs will not be reimbursed.

2. Individualize client's bathing schedule. Daily baths are not essential. ➤ *Rationale:* Daily cleansing can destroy the skin's natural barrier, making it more susceptible to external irritants.

   a. Avoid hot bath water. ➤ *Rationale:* Tepid water prevents injury to skin.

   b. Use mild cleansing agents to minimize dryness.

   c. Cleanse skin immediately if urine, fecal incontinence, or wound drainage seeps onto skin.

   d. Provide humidity to prevent drying of skin.

   e. Use cream or thin layer of cornstarch to protect skin.

3. Avoid massaging bony prominences. ➤ *Rationale:* Massaging can lead to deep tissue trauma.

   a. Keep bony prominences from direct contact with one another.

   b. Use pillow, foam wedges, or other positioning devices.

   c. Use elbow pads and heel elevators.

4. Promote adequate dietary intake of protein, calories, and nutrients. Protein should be approximately 1.2–1.5 g/kg body weight daily. ➤ *Rationale:* Adequate protein intake in addition to vitamins and minerals help prevent pressure ulcer formation.

> **CLINICAL ALERT**
> Heat lamps should not be used to treat pressure ulcers. Preferred wound care is to promote a clean, moist environment.

5. Ensure adequate fluid intake. ➤ *Rationale:* This prevents dehydration, which is a risk factor for pressure ulcer formation.

Table 25-10 Pressure Ulcer Risk Assessment Scales

Norton Scale									
Physical Condition		**Mental Condition**		**Activity**		**Mobility**		**Continence**	
Good	4	Alert	4	Walks	4	Full	4	Good	4
Fair	3	Apathetic	3	Walks with help	3	Slightly limited	3	Occasional incontinence	3
Poor	2	Confused	2	Sits in chair	2	Very limited	2	Frequent incontinence	2
Very poor	1	Stuporous	1	Remains in bed	1	Immobile	1	Urine and fecal incontinence	1
Total ____		Total ____		Total ____		Total ____		Total ____	
Grand total = _____									

A score of 14 or less indicates risk of pressure ulcer; a score under 12 indicates high risk.

Braden Scale											
Sensory Perception		**Moisture**		**Activity**		**Mobility**		**Nutrition**		**Friction and Shear**	
No impairment	4	Rarely moist	4	Walks frequently	4	No limitations	4	Excellent	4		
Slightly limited	3	Occasionally moist	3	Walks occasionally	3	Slightly limited	3	Adequate	3	No apparent problems	3
Very limited	2	Very moist	2	Chairfast	2	Very limited	2	Probably inadequate	2	Potential problem	2
Completely limited	1	Constantly moist	1	Bedfast	1	Completely immobile	1	Very poor	1	Problem	1
Total ____		Total ____		Total ____		Total ____		Total ____		Total ____	
Grand total = _____											

Assign a score of 1–4 in each category. Total the score; Low risk 15–16, Moderate risk 13–14, High risk 12 or less.
Norton and Braden Scales adapted from AHCRP (1992, May)
Note: Refer to actual scales for detailed information about both scales.

(continued)

Skill 25.5.1 | Preventing Pressure Ulcers (continued)

6. Reposition bedridden client every 1–2 hr.

   a. Do not position directly on trochanter.

   b. Do not turn the client more than 30 degrees in one position change.

   c. Raise heels off bed by placing pillows under legs; allow heels to hang over edges.

   d. Use trapeze or turning sheet to reposition client.

> **CLINICAL ALERT**
> Be alert to altered skin integrity when pressure is reduced in one anatomical area by turning and repositioning, as the newer location may be placed at risk for pressure ulcer formation.

❶ Stage I pressure ulcer.

❷ Stage II pressure ulcer.

❸ Stage III pressure ulcer.

❹ Stage IV pressure ulcer.

❺ Eschar must be removed by debridement before staging is done.

❻ Clinical signs of infection.

7. Encourage mobility or range-of-motion exercises.
   ➤ *Rationale:* Range-of-motion exercises promote activity and reduce effects of pressure on tissue.

8. Minimize force and friction on skin when turning or moving client. Use turning sheets or Hoyer lift.

9. Maintain head of bed at lowest degree of elevation consistent with medical problem; below 30 degrees if possible.

10. Place at-risk clients on pressure-reducing devices in both bed and chair. Devices include foam, alternating gel, water mattress, or air-fluidized mattress.

11. Place client on specialty bed or mattress if highly at risk for pressure ulcer formation or has an ulcer.

12. Encourage chair-fast clients to shift position every 15 min.

CLINICAL ALERT

Air-fluidized beds and low-air-loss beds are recommended to manage pressure ulcers, especially in clients with large or multiple ulcers.

Air-Fluidized

Warm, pressurized air circulates through beads in the bed and creates support surface. Polyester sheet allows for moisture and air to pass through, keeping skin dry.

Treatment can take several months. Use of this bed is very expensive.

Low-Air-Loss

Head and foot of bed can be elevated. Bed is a modified standard bed frame, lighter and more portable than air-fluidized bed. Bed circulates cool air. Urine and feces do not pass through fabric on the bed.

See also Box 8-3, Support Surfaces and Specialty Beds and Table 8-2, Therapeutic Beds.

EVIDENCE-BASED PRACTICE

Pressure Ulcer Formation and At-Risk Clients

Evidence shows that there is a need for hospitals to increase documentation, prediction, and prevention strategies for clients at risk for pressure ulcers. Use of a risk scale can provide triggers to plan care to decrease risk factors. As a predictive measure, individuals should be assessed for risk of pressure ulcer development upon admission to acute care and rehabilitation hospitals, nursing homes, home care programs, and other healthcare facilities.

Source: Agency for Healthcare Research and Quality (2014)

Skill 25.5.2	Providing Care for Clients With Pressure Ulcers

Procedure

1. Monitor client's overall condition daily. ➤ *Rationale:* Clients who are dying will have the tendency to develop new skin breakdown (skin failure) as other organs fail. Existing pressure ulcers of lesser staging (I and II) almost always worsen over time and become at least stage III.
2. Differentiate type of ulcer, pressure versus nonpressure.
3. Determine stage of ulcer.
4. Monitor and assess ulcer characteristics daily:

   a. Observe dressing to determine whether dry, intact, and not leaking.

   b. Observe ulcer bed, if appropriate, and document findings.

5. Assess pain level of client and provide adequate pain relief.
6. Photograph ulcer according to facility policy.

   ➤ *Rationale:* This is to determine progress of ulcer healing.

7. Monitor progress toward healing and for potential complications.

   a. Measure pressure ulcer size weekly using a Pressure Ulcer Scale. Usual healing time is 2–4 weeks.

   b. If healing is not progressing or ulcer has not healed in usual time frame, reevaluate treatment plan and client's condition.

8. Maintain turning and positioning schedule to promote healing and prevent additional ulcer formation.
9. Complete a nutritional assessment. ❶ ❷ Positive nitrogen balance and protein intake are necessary for healing.

❶ Nutritional assessment of client with pressure ulcer(s).
Source: From Cerner Electronic Health Record. © Cerner Corporation. Pearson has restricted permission to reproduce and distribute this copyrighted work. Further reproduction or distribution is strictly prohibited without written consent of Cerner Corporation.

(continued)

10. Complete a psychosocial assessment to determine client's adherence to pressure ulcer treatment regimens.

> **CLINICAL ALERT**
>
> Clients near the end of life have the right to refuse ulcer care. However, "Do Not Resuscitate" orders do not relieve the staff from providing quality pressure ulcer prevention or treatment.

11. Complete dressing change according to facility policy and type of dressing used. Follow manufacturer's guidelines for dressing change.
    ➤ *Rationale:* Dressing changes are based on a combination of factors, such as manufacturer suggested use, pressure ulcer characteristics, and goals for healing.

> **CLINICAL ALERT**
>
> Centers for Medicare and Medicaid Services have indicated that long-term care facilities must implement evidence-based protocols of prevention and care for pressure ulcers.

Incision/Wound Detailed

Routine Wound Assessment

	Type	Location	Description/ Assessment	Length (cm)	Width (cm)	Depth (cm)	Surrounding Tissue	Drainage	Cleansing/ Irrigation	Dressing	Comment
Incision/Wound #1	<Alpha>		<MultiAlpha>				<MultiAlpha>	<MultiAlpha>	<MultiAlpha>	<MultiAlpha>	
Incision/Wound #2	<Alpha>		<MultiAlpha>				<MultiAlpha>	<MultiAlpha>	<MultiAlpha>	<MultiAlpha>	
Incision/Wound #3	<Alpha>		<MultiAlpha>				<MultiAlpha>	<MultiAlph>	<MultiAlpha>	<MultiAlpha>	
Incision/Wound #4	<Alpha>		<MultiAlpha>				<MultiAlpha>	<MultiAlph>	<MultiAlpha>	<MultiAlpha>	
Incision/Wound #5	<Alpha>		<MultiAlpha>				<MultiAlpha>	<MultiAlpha>	<MultiAlpha>	<MultiAlpha>	
Incision/Wound #6	<Alpha>		<MultiAlpha>				<MultiAlpha>	<MultiAlpha>	<MultiAlpha>	<MultiAlpha>	
Incision/Wound #7	<Alpha>		<MultiAlpha>				<MultiAlpha>	<MultiAlph>	<MultiAlpha>	<MultiAlpha>	

Detail for Complicated Wounds

	% Pink	% Red	% White	% Yellow	% Black	Pressure Ulcer Stage	Tunneling/Undermining Location/Depth	Tunneling/Undermining % Wound Involvement	Comment
Incision/Wound #1						<Alpha>			
Incision/Wound #2						<Alpha>			
Incision/Wound #3						<Alpha>			
Incision/Wound #4						<Alpha>			
Incision/Wound #5						<Alpha>			
Incision/Wound #6						<Alpha>			
Incision/Wound #7						<Alpha>			

Stage I: Observable pressure related alteration of intact skin whose indicators as compared to the adjacent or opposite area on the body may include changes in one or more of the following: skin temperature (warmth or coolness), tissue consistency (firm or boggy feel), and/or sensation (pain, itching). The ulcer appears as a defined area of persistent redness in lightly pigmented skin, whereas in darker skin tones, persistent red, blue or purple hues.

Stage II: Partial thickness skin loss involving epidermis, dermis, or both. The ulcer is superficial and presents clinically as an abrasion, blister, or shallow crater.

Stage III: Full thickness skin loss involving damage to or necrosis of subcutaneous tissue that may extend down to, but not through, underlying fascia. The ulcer presents clinically as a deep crater with or without undermining of adjacent tissue.

Stage IV: Full thickness skin loss with extensive destruction, tissue necrosis, or damage to muscle, bone, or supporting structures (e.g., tendon, joint capsule). Undermining and sinus tracts also may be associated with Stage IV pressure ulcers.

❷ Incision wound detail. From Cerner Electronic Health Record. © Cerner Corporation. Pearson has restricted permission to reproduce and distribute this copyrighted work. Further reproduction or distribution is strictly prohibited without written consent of Cerner Corporation.

Unit 25.5 Documentation and Evaluation

DOCUMENTATION for Pressure Ulcers

- Client's general skin condition
- Periwound assessment
- Assessment of wound (i.e., size, presence of tunneling drainage, evidence of tissue granulation)
- Color, volume, and type of exudate
- Type of ulcer care provided
- Type of pressure-reducing or relieving device used
- Results of Braden or Norton pressure ulcer assessment scale
- Pressure ulcer record completed
- State the exact location of pressure ulcer; if bony prominence involved, use an anatomic name. Indicate turning surface involved (i.e., RI, LI, post., ant., medial, lateral).
- Size: Indicate size in centimeters.
- Identify ulcers by number; use chart.
- Measure depth of ulcer.
- Identify and measure undermining and tunneling location.
- Stage: Write the number of the stage that corresponds to the description of the pressure ulcer (stage I–IV).
- Treatment: Chart treatment used (e.g., hydrocolloid dressing applied, transparent adhesive film applied, and so on).
- Position: Indicate time client's position was changed.

EVALUATION/Critical Thinking

Expected Outcomes

- Stage of pressure ulcer is accurately assessed.
- Pressure ulcer is treated effectively according to stage of ulcer formation.
- Pressure ulcer is healing within usual time frame.
- Skin remains free of breakdown in areas surrounding pressure ulcer.
- Absence of additional pressure ulcer formation.

Unexpected Outcomes	Alternative Actions
• Client does not have sufficient exercise; appetite decreased.	• Encourage small, frequent feedings. • Offer high-calorie drinks like eggnog or Isocal.

• Client's wound does not heal with traditional types of treatments.	• In client care conference discuss the following:
	  • Is everyone following same treatment?
	  • Are causative agents preventing healing?
	  • Should treatment be adjusted or changed?
	  • Would use of a support surface be effective?
	  • Is surgical debridement and grafting necessary for healing?

• Skin is exposed to moisture.	• Establish bowel or bladder program and select absorbent products for wound care that wick the moisture from skin. • Cleanse skin with pH-balanced cleansers, avoiding friction, and thoroughly dry skin after each incontinence. • Apply skin barrier product. • Consider use of fecal management system or urinary catheter.
• Nutritional or hydration deficit occurs.	• Monitor nutritional and fluid intake accurately. • Obtain order for vitamin supplements if client is not already on vitamins. • Increase protein intake by supplementing with high-protein drinks.
• Shearing and friction secondarily related to immobility or reduced activity.	• Keep head of bed in lowest position possible to prevent client from sliding down in bed. • Use lifting devices to move client up in bed or out of bed to prevent friction on skin. • Instruct client on use of trapeze to assist in repositioning.

Nursing Process Data

ASSESSMENT Database

- Identify why usual wound therapy treatments are ineffective.
- Identify most effective adjunctive treatment for client.
- Assess wound for baseline data before initiating treatment.
- Determine if wound is healing using adjunctive therapy.
- Assess if client is good candidate for adjunctive therapy.
- Assess client's nutritional status to ensure best results from V.A.C. therapy.
- Determine if wound is maintaining a moist environment with adjunctive therapy.
- Assess periwound area for signs of maceration.
- Assess for adverse reactions during hyperbaric oxygenation therapy (HBO).

PLANNING Objectives

- To assess if adjunctive therapy is providing adequate wound healing
- To place client on pressure relief surface if wound is over bony prominence
- To determine if client is able to participate in specific therapy
- To select appropriate type of dressing for adjunctive therapy
- To determine if client is a good candidate for HBO

IMPLEMENTATION Procedures

DOCUMENTATION AND EVALUATION

Expected Outcomes

- Granulation tissue is evident using adjunctive therapy.
- Periwound area remains healthy without evidence of maceration.
- Moist wound environment is maintained.
- Pain is reduced with adjunctive therapy.
- Wound progresses through usual phases with electrical stimulation.
- Exudate is removed and wound healing occurs with negative pressure wound therapy.
- Hyperbaric oxygen therapy is effective in treating diabetic leg ulcers.

Unexpected Outcomes/Alternative Actions

Pearson Nursing Student Resources

Find additional review materials at
nursing.pearsonhighered.com.
Prepare for success with NCLEX®-style practice questions and Skill Checklists.

Skill 25.6.1 | Using Electrical Stimulation

Equipment
Normal saline solution
Bag for soiled dressings
Gauze pads
Two sterile basins
Hydrogel sheets
Electrode
Bandage tape
Alligator clip
Stimulator
Clean gloves (two pairs)
Sterile gloves

Preparation
1. Determine whether client is a candidate for electrical stimulation (Box 25-16 ■).
2. Determine phase of wound healing. ➤ **Rationale:** This determines the correct treatment protocol.
3. Set the stimulator settings according to manufacturer's directions, based on client's phase in wound healing. The settings include polarity, pulse rate, intensity, duration, and frequency.
4. Identify client using two forms of ID. Explain procedure. Assess for pain.
5. Gather equipment.
6. Perform hand hygiene.
7. Provide privacy.

Procedure
1. Raise bed to HIGH working height; lower near side rail.
2. Place client in position to enable staff to work with wound area and equipment. (Placement depends on wound site.)
3. Place supplies on overbed table, near working area.
4. Open all supply packages, maintaining sterility.
5. Pour sterile normal saline into one basin.
6. Don clean gloves.
7. Place disposal bag near wound. ➤ **Rationale:** This is for ease in disposing of soiled dressings.

Box 25-16 CANDIDATES FOR ELECTRICAL STIMULATION

- Pressure ulcers, stages I–IV
- Diabetic ulcers
- Venous ulcers, ischemic ulcers
- Traumatic wounds
- Surgical wounds
- Wound flaps
- Donor sites, burn wounds

---

8. Remove dressing carefully to avoid interfering with granulation tissue.
9. Remove clean gloves; place in disposal bag. Don sterile gloves.
10. Place sterile basin next to wound to catch irrigation solution as wound is cleansed.
11. Pour sterile normal saline into wound to cleanse wound. ➤ **Rationale:** This is to remove exudates, slough, and petrolatum products. Current will not be conducted into wound tissue if petrolatum products remain in the wound.
12. Remove excess irrigation solution using sterile gauze pads.
13. Place fluffed gauze pads into normal saline solution; squeeze out excess liquid.
14. Fill wound cavity with gauze, including any undermined or tunneled spaces. Pack gently.
15. Place surface (active) electrode in wound bed, over gauze packing. ➤ **Rationale:** This transfers electrical energy into wound bed, producing positive effects on necessary components for wound healing (i.e., blood flow, oxygen uptake, DNA, and protein synthesis).
16. Cover with dry gauze pad.
17. Tape dry pad securely.
18. Connect alligator clip to foil.
19. Connect to stimulator lead.
20. Place a wet washcloth over area where dispersive electrode will be placed.
21. Select a dispersive pad that is larger than the sum of areas of active electrodes and wound packing.
22. Place dispersive electrode proximal to wound, over soft tissue, avoiding bony prominences.

Note: The greater the separation between two electrodes, the deeper the current path. Larger separation space is used to treat deep and undermined wounds. Closer separation space is used for shallow or partial-thickness wounds. Ensure electrodes do not touch.

23. Ensure all edges of electrode are in good contact with skin. Hold electrode in place with nylon elasticized strap.
24. Place client in position of comfort. Electrical stimulation treatments usually last 60 min.
25. Remove gloves and discard.
26. Perform hand hygiene.
27. Don clean gloves.
28. Remove electrode from wound after treatment.
29. Remove saline-soaked gauze and cover wound with occlusive dressing.

Note: Hydrogel sheets or amorphous hydrogel-impregnated gauze can be used to conduct current. If hydrogel gauze is the conductor, it is changed BID.

Skill 25.6.2 | Using Negative Pressure Wound Therapy

Equipment

Foam, Black or White V.A.C. kit
Gauze pads
Sterile normal saline
Irrigating syringe
Moisture proof pad or sterile basin
Skin prep agent, optional
Razor, optional
Clean gloves
Sterile gloves
V.A.C. device
Disposal bag
Sterile scissor

❶ V.A.C. unit.

Box 25-17 GUIDELINES FOR SAFE NEGATIVE PRESSURE WOUND THERAPY

To prevent complications when using the system, follow these guidelines:

1. Understand the equipment and its use. Read manufacturer's directions for use.
2. Assess clients thoroughly. Confirm they are candidates for the treatment.
3. Assess the order. ➤ *Rationale:* You are responsible if complications occur.
4. Ensure there is a proper written order, which should specify the following:
   a. Wound filling material
   b. Negative pressure setting (20–200 mm Hg)
   c. Therapy setting (continuous, intermittent, or variable)
   d. Frequency of dressing changes
5. Assess the wound. Develop a systematic approach to ensure the treatment is appropriate.
6. Complete ongoing client assessment and monitoring.
7. Evaluate client understanding of teaching.

Source: Rock (2014)

Preparation

1. Evaluate whether client is candidate for V.A.C. therapy (Boxes 25-17 and 25-18 ■): nutritionally stable, able to use device 22 hr each day, uses a pressure support surface if wound is over a bony prominence. ➤ *Rationale:* If therapy is turned off longer than 2 hr/day, dressing must be removed and replaced with traditional dressing.
   a. Wound open enough to insert foam dressing that touches all edges.
   b. Wound debrided
   c. Sufficient circulation to assist in healing process
   d. Does not have bleeding tendencies or infections.
      ➤ *Rationale:* These are major complications associated with the use of wound therapy.
2. Select correct foam dressing according to size and type of wound. ❶ Black foam has larger pores and is used to stimulate granulation tissue and wound contraction. White (soft) foam is used when granulation tissue needs to be restricted or client cannot tolerate pain associated with black foam. White foam is used with superficial wounds, shallow chronic ulcers, and tunneling or undermining wounds.
3. Gather equipment and supplies.
4. Provide privacy.
5. Identify client using two forms of identification. Introduce yourself and explain procedure to client and determine his or her willingness to use this therapy. Assess for pain.
6. Perform hand hygiene.

Procedure

1. Place disposal bag near wound.
2. Open supplies and place on overbed table. Open kit, maintaining sterility.

Box 25-18 NEGATIVE PRESSURE WOUND THERAPY

Uses	Contraindications
Acute and chronic wounds	Malignancy in wound
Trauma	Untreated osteomyelitis
Partial-thickness burns	Nonenteric and unexplored fistula
Dehisced wounds	Necrotic tissue with presence of diabetic ulcers
	Eschar
Pressure ulcers	Directly over exposed blood flaps, vessel, or organ
Grafts	When using hydrogen peroxide and alcohol-based solutions
	Clients who cannot tolerate temperature of fluid

3. Draw up normal saline irrigating solution in syringe.
4. Don clean gloves.
5. Place moisture-proof pad or sterile basin under wound. ➤ *Rationale:* This protects skin and bed during irrigation.
6. Clean wound using aggressive irrigation. If debridement is to be done, only a trained professional can perform the skill. Notify the appropriate individual. ➤ *Rationale:* Devitalized tissue should be removed because areas of soft or stringy slough delay the healing process.
7. Remove gloves and place in disposal bag.
8. Don sterile gloves.
9. Dry wound and prepare periwound tissue with skin preparation agent if necessary. ➤ *Rationale:* This is to promote an airtight seal.
10. Cut the V.A.C. foam to fit the shape and entire wound cavity, including tunneling or undermined areas. White foam is used for tunneled wounds. ❷
11. Size and trim drape to cover foam dressing, leaving a 3.5-cm (1.4 in.) border around the wound area.
12. Gently place the foam into the wound, ensuring the entire wound is covered.

> **CLINICAL ALERT**
> Do not pack foam into any areas of the wound. Forcing foam dressings into any wound may lead to risk of adverse health issues.

13. Apply tubing to foam. Tubing can be laid on top of foam or placed inside foam dressing. Keep tubing away from bony prominences.
14. Cover foam and 3.5 cm (1.4 in.) of the periwound area with drape (Box 25-19 ■). Do not stretch drape or compress foam with drape. ➤ *Rationale:* This ensures a tight seal without causing tension or a shearing force on periwound tissue.
15. Lift tubing and place on drape that has been bunched up to protect skin from pressure of tube.

❷ V.A.C. foam cut to fit shape and wound cavity, with tubing attached to vacuum pump.

> **CLINICAL ALERT**
> For deep wound, reposition tubing to minimize pressure on wound edges every 2 hr. Excess foam can be used to cushion skin under tubing.

16. Secure tubing with additional piece of drape or tape several centimeters away from dressing. ➤ *Rationale:* This prevents pulling on the dressing, leading to a leak.
17. Remove gloves and discard.
18. Remove canister from sterile package and push it into the V.A.C. unit until you hear it click in place. Alarm will sound if canister is not properly inserted into unit.
19. Connect dressing tubing to canister tubing.
20. Open both clamps, one on dressing tubing and one on canister tubing.
21. Place V.A.C. unit on level surface or hang from footboard.
22. Press power button ON.
23. Adjust V.A.C. unit settings according to physician's orders or guidelines for treating wound types in the manufacturer's manual. Target pressure should be set for 5 min on and 2 min off (intermittent therapies on machine). Intensity of setting sets the negative pressure.
24. Assess dressing in 1 min. ➤ *Rationale:* The dressing should collapse unless air leak is present.
25. Dressing changes must be completed every 48 hr unless wound is infected, and then change every 12 hr.

Removing Dressing

1. Perform hand hygiene.
2. Don clean gloves.
3. Raise tube connector above level of pump unit.
4. Tighten clamp on dressing tube.
5. Separate canister tube and dressing tubes by disconnecting the connector.
6. Allow pump unit to pull exudates in canister tube into canister; then tighten clamps on canister tube.
7. Press Therapy ON/OFF to deactivate pump.
8. Stretch drape horizontally and slowly pull up from skin. Gently remove it from skin. Do not peel it off skin. ❸
9. Discard disposable equipment including gloves in appropriate bag or container.
10. Perform hand hygiene.

Note: Dressing changes are completed every 48 hr; if infected, every 12 hr.

Box 25-19 **V.A.C. GRANUFOAM SILVER**

- Provides continuous delivery of silver directly to wound bed
- Provides a protective barrier to reduce aerobic, gram-negative, and gram-positive bacteria, yeast, and fungi, and may reduce infections in wounds
- Indicated for client with chronic, acute, traumatic, and dehisced wounds, partial-thickness burns, and pressure ulcers

---

(continued)

Skill 25.6.2 | Using Negative Pressure Wound Therapy *(continued)*

❸ Remove adhesive drape by gently pulling away from skin.

EVIDENCE-BASED PRACTICE
Use of Negative Pressure Wound Therapy for Chronic Wounds

Evidence-based recommendations were obtained by a systematic review of the literature with 422 independent healthcare professionals who were able to agree or disagree with the recommendations. They were graded with evidence presented in the literature. The criterion for agreement was set at 80% agree. Evidence and recommendations were graded according to the Scottish Intercollegiate Guidance Network Classification System. The primary treatment goal for Negative Pressure Wound Therapy in most chronic wounds is to achieve wound closure (secondary intention or preparing the wound for surgical closure). The evidence base was strongest for the use of negative pressure wound therapy in nonischemic diabetic foot ulcers and weakest in venous leg ulcers.

Source: Vigs et al. (2011)

Disconnecting V.A.C. Unit
1. Turn the unit to OFF.
2. Clamp both clamps on tubing.
3. Press quick-release connector to separate dressing tubing from canister tubing.
4. Cover ends of tubing with gauze and secure.

Reconnecting V.A.C. Unit
1. Remove gauze from ends of tubing.
2. Connect tubing.
3. Unclamp clamps.
4. Press V.A.C. green power button to ON.
5. Select NO at new client prompt. Unit will resume previous settings.
6. Press therapy to ON.

SAFETY ALERT
Tips for Negative Pressure Therapy
- Maintain therapy 22 hr/day.
- Perform wound cleansing and dressing changes every 48 hr unless wound infected, and then change to every 12 hr.
- Monitor wound and dressing at least every 4 hr to ensure foam is collapsed and for signs of infection or other complications.
- Change type of wound system or medicate if client complains of pain or discomfort during treatment.
- Use continuous therapy (24 hr) to minimize movement and help stabilize wound bed over unstable body structures such as chest wall.
- Change canister when full, or at least weekly. Use Standard Precautions.

Changing Canister
1. Don clean gloves.
2. Assess that canister unit is full. Unit will alarm when full.
3. Tighten clamps on canister tubing from dressing tubing.
4. Pull back on release knob on V.A.C. unit at same time as you pull canister from slot.
5. Put canister in biohazard disposable bag and place in designated area for disposal.
6. Dispose of gloves.
7. Perform hand hygiene.

Note: Average length of treatment is 4–6 weeks. Home systems are available as well.

Skill 25.6.3 | Using Hyperbaric Oxygenation for Diabetic Ulcers

Equipment
Hyperbaric chamber (Box 25-20 ■)
Compressed air mask (optional)

Preparation
1. Identify client using two forms of identification. Introduce yourself.
2. Explain the procedure to client.

Procedure
1. Perform hand hygiene.
2. Ensure client is wearing 100% cotton fabrics only.
   ➤ *Rationale:* This prevents spark potential.
3. Ensure client does not have petroleum- or alcohol-based products or cosmetics on hair or skin. ➤ *Rationale:* Vapors from sprays, cosmetics, and Vaseline can spontaneously combust in an increased atmospheric environment of 100% oxygen.

Box 25-20 **HYPERBARIC OXYGEN (HBO) THERAPY CHAMBERS**

Two types of chambers are used in HBO therapy: multiplace chamber and monoplace chamber.

Multiplace chamber

- Compressed with 100% oxygen administered through direct piped-in gas.
- As many as 12 clients can be treated at one time.
- Nurse is in chamber to provide care.
- Critically ill clients can be more readily treated.

Monoplace chamber

- Single client therapy
- Uses 100% O_2 to compress chamber
- Client can breathe compressed air by mask during treatment
- For clients with claustrophobia or who cannot tolerate mask, alterations in treatment protocols may be required.

Risk to nurse is minimized by strict adherence to diving protocols that allow for period of decompression of the nerve. See also Box 30-7, New Trends: Hyperbaric Oxygen Therapy (HBOT).

---

4. Check that topical wound and skin care products with petroleum base are not present on client.
5. Take client to treatment area.
6. Once client is placed in chamber, the following observations must be made constantly during compression and during entire treatment (Box 25-21 ■). ❶
   a. Assess client for ability to equalize pressure changes in ear. Client will complain of ear pain. Instruct client to yawn, swallow, or perform Valsalva maneuver.
   b. Determine if client has sensation of warmth as the pressure and temperature increase and the rate of compression of the chamber decreases.

c. Check for confinement anxiety. Minimize this potential adverse effect through orientation to the process of decompression. Anxiolytic therapy using benzodiazepines may be ordered.
   d. Determine potential for hypoglycemia with client who has diabetes. Assess client during decompression for loss of consciousness, disorientation, and seizures. Preventive measures include maintaining blood glucose levels by adequate nutrition and timing of insulin injections in relationship to treatment. Peak insulin levels should not occur during treatment.
7. Observe client continuously while in chamber and when decompression is reversed.
8. Evaluate client for signs of oxygen toxicity or other potential adverse reactions. Report adverse findings to physician.

Box 25-21 **USES OF HYPERBARIC CHAMBERS**

Hyperbaric clinics are used to treat many client conditions, including:

Autism	Traumatic brain injuries
Arthritis	Stroke
Fibromyalgia	Migraines
Heart issues	Inflammation
Cancer	Cerebral palsy
Lyme disease	Parkinson's
Surgery	

The Monoplace chamber can be used at home as well as in clinics.

❶ Hyperbaric chamber.

Unit 25.6 Documentation and Evaluation

DOCUMENTATION for Adjunctive Wound Care Therapy

- Wound assessment, including location, measurement of wound, and presence of tunneling or undermining
- Color of wound, presence of exudates, color, and odor
- Wound stage, if appropriate
- Eschar description if present

- Presence of pain in periwound area
- Type, frequency, and duration of adjunctive therapy
- Client's response to therapy
- Length of time negative pressure therapy treatment is off
- Client's reaction to HBO and any adverse effects

EVALUATION/Critical Thinking

Expected Outcomes

- Granulation tissue is evident using adjunctive therapy.
- Periwound area remains healthy without evidence of maceration.
- Moist wound environment is maintained.
- Pain is reduced with adjunctive therapy.
- Wound progresses through usual phases with electrical stimulation.
- Wound healing occurs faster with radiant heat dressing.
- Exudate is removed and wound healing occurs using negative pressure wound therapy.
- Client's diabetic wound heals with hyperbaric oxygen therapy.

Unexpected Outcomes	Alternative Actions
• Wound is too large for V.A.C. kit.	• Use more than one foam piece. • Place pieces so they touch each other. • Use only one tubing to one of the pieces.
• Periwound skin is fragile.	• Use skin prep before applying drape. • Frame wound with skin barrier or DuoDERM. • Cut drape large enough to enclose foam dressing and skin barrier layer.
• Dressing does not collapse following V.A.C. application.	• Listen for whistling sound indicating a leak in the system. • Gently press around tubing; check for wrinkles or drape not covering correctly. • Most leaks occur around tubing. • Use excess drape to patch over leak.
• Foam is not collapsed in wound bed.	• Ensure therapy is ON. Ensure clamps are open and tubing is not kinked. • Check for leaks and patch.
• Audible alarm sounds on V.A.C. system, and therapy is stopped.	• Check for blockage in tubing and replace as needed. • If problem continues after tubing is replaced, notify company that produces the system.
• Dressing adheres to wound with negative pressure system.	• Instill sterile water or normal saline into dressing, let sit for 15–20 min, and then gently remove dressing from wound.
• Client exhibits signs of anxiety when providing education regarding use of hyperbaric chamber.	• Place client in multichamber where a nurse is present to assist client with anxiety-reducing interventions.

Chapter Wrap-Up

GERONTOLOGIC Considerations

As Clients Grow Older, the Usual Function of the Skin Declines, Leading to Major Complications; Nearly 40% of Clients Aged 65–75 Have at Least One Significant Problem Related to the Skin

- Dry skin present in 77% of clients over 64
- Vitamin D deficiency
- Decrease in sebum production
- Decrease in sweat production
- Decrease in thermoregulation
- Basal cell carcinoma most common skin malignancy
- Decrease in sensory perception
- Decrease in adequate oxygen or nutrition when tissue is subjected to excessive pressure

The Inflammatory and Proliferation Phases of Wound Healing Are Often Defective With Older Clients Who Have Chronic Diseases

- A hemoglobin below 10 g/dL increases susceptibility.
- Uncontrolled diabetes mellitus or a blood glucose level that exceeds 200 mg/dL presents a risk.
- Hyperglycemia retards neutrophil production.
- T and B cells diminish in function and number, indicating a reduced inflammatory response. Older clients are at risk for cutaneous viral and fungal infections.
- Clients with rheumatoid arthritis who take steroids or nonsteroidal anti-inflammatory medications are at risk for decreased wound healing. There is a slower rate of epithelialization and severely inhibited contraction.
- **Ischemia**, anemia, and edema from vascular insufficiency or pressure leads to lack of blood flow to a wound area. Lower oxygen-carrying capacity results from anemia. Edema makes it difficult to transport oxygen and cellular wastes to and from cells. Ischemia leads to diminished oxygen necessary for wound healing.

Nursing Actions to Counteract Risks Against Wound Healing

- All at-risk older clients should have a pressure ulcer risk assessment completed at the time of admission and at regular intervals thereafter.
- Use of compression stockings assists in treating both the edema and ultimately the ischemia, therefore increasing blood flow to wound area.
- Turning frequently, at least every 2 hr, for clients free of pressure ulcers and every 1 hr for those at high risk, should be a priority.
- Use of pressure-relieving mattresses decreases risk potential.
- Wound care, including irrigation, use of appropriate dressings, and maintaining aseptic technique with dressing changes, should be priority care for clients with any type of wound.

MANAGEMENT Guidelines

Each state legislates a Nurse Practice Act for RNs and LVNs/LPNs. Healthcare facilities are responsible for establishing and implementing policies and procedures that conform to their state's regulations. Verify the regulations and role parameters for each healthcare worker in your facility. Nurses working in a hyperbaric chamber must be trained in how to work with the clients and how to protect themselves when in the chamber. Before assigning nurses to this activity, ensure they have had the education necessary to work in this environment.

Delegation

- Assessment and evaluation of wounds and their management modalities are only RN functions and may not be delegated to other healthcare workers. The RN in collaboration with the physician develops a plan of care for clients requiring wound management.
- An LVN/LPN may be assigned to complete a sterile dressing change following instructions from the RN and in accordance with the wound care protocol established for the individual client.
- An LVN/LPN may remove staples and sutures after instruction and return demonstrations have been documented. (Most nursing programs include this information in the curriculum.)
- A CNA may apply a dry dressing, but may not perform a sterile procedure.

Interprofessional Communication

- Information regarding assessment of the wound should be reported to all staff caring for the client. This can be accomplished during report or documented on the nurses' notes and on client care plans or clinical (critical) pathway documents, or electronic forms.
- Wound care procedures (e.g., dressing changes) should be outlined or special wound care steps inserted into computer record. Specific instructions regarding type and amount of dressing material needed and specific directions in the application of the dressings must be written clearly, so all nurses may follow appropriate directions.

- Specific directions for wound management and use of specialized equipment must be given to the nurse during report from the RN team leader or manager.
- Reports outlining specifics of the wound, such as color, odor, and amount of drainage, must be provided to the RN manager after the dressing change has been completed.
- Any change in wound appearance must be immediately reported to the RN team leader or manager before the dressing change has been completed.

CASE Study Applications

Scenario 1

Mrs. Johnson is an 84-year-old retired school teacher who was widowed 10 years ago and now lives alone. She developed diabetes mellitus at the age of 58. She has been in failing health for the last 3 years and has been at home with the assistance of home health aides and weekly visits by the RN. Her coccyx area has had frequent skin breakdown. The homecare RN determined she now has a stage III pressure ulcer as a result of being on bed rest the past week. She is being admitted to the hospital for treatment of the ulcer.

1. Identify risk factors for Mrs. Johnson developing pressure ulcers.
2. Describe the stage III pressure ulcer.
3. Identify the most effective treatment for the stage III pressure ulcer.
4. Compare and contrast the two Pressure Ulcer Assessment Scales and identify the score indicating that Mrs. Johnson is a high risk for pressure ulcer formation on one of the scales.
5. In addition to dressing changes, identify a preventative therapy that should be used for clients at high risk for pressure ulcers.
6. Explain why massaging bony prominences should be avoided for clients at risk for pressure ulcer formation.

7. Briefly describe the application of a hydrocolloid dressing.
8. Identify and briefly explain the use of one new advance in the treatment of pressure ulcers.

Scenario 2

A young client was in a motor vehicle crash and has numerous wounds on his buttocks, back, and both legs. He is in extreme pain and is on a PCA pump with morphine sulfate for pain control. He is able to respond to questions. His vital signs are BP 140/88, P. 110, R. 26, O2 Sat 96% on room air.

1. When assessing the client's wounds, what questions will you need to ask to determine the client's history and physical findings that contribute to his treatment?
2. Describe how you would determine the extent of the wounds.
3. The physician has determined that the negative pressure wound therapy protocol would be the most beneficial treatment for the leg wounds. This decision is based on what criteria?
4. Compare and contrast the use of white foam and black foam for the leg wounds.
5. Describe the method you will use to prepare the wound for the V.A.C. system.
6. Provide the rationale for using GranuFoam silver dressings for wound care.

NCLEX® Review Questions

Unless otherwise specified, choose only one (1) answer.

1. What phase of wound healing begins about 2 days to 3 weeks after injury?
   A. Maturation
   B. Inflammatory
   C. Regeneration
   D. Wound remodeling

2. Which of the following is a description of tertiary intention in wound healing?
   A. A wound that heals by granulation
   B. The simplest form of wound healing
   C. A clean skin incision through a surgical incision
   D. A wound that heals by leaving it open

3. When instructing clients in measures to increase wound healing, which of the following should the nurse include as the increased daily intake of calories?
   A. 20–25 Cal/kg/day
   B. 30–35 Cal/kg/day
   C. 35–45 Cal/kg/day
   D. 45–50 Cal/kg/day

4. What should be included in instructions to student nurses about the use of antimicrobial soap to decontaminate hands for surgical asepsis?
   A. Apply 3-5 mL of antimicrobial soap in palm of hand and rub hands together.
   B. Vigorously rub hands for 10 sec, covering all hand surfaces.
   C. Scrub hands for 3 min.
   D. Move arms forward and back to rinse, and dry using a single-use towel.

5. What does the nurse need to do to maintain a sterile field?
   A. Place the sterile package near the edge of the overbed table on the opposite side of the bed.
   B. Open the package by holding it directly in front of you and grasping the wrapper.
   C. Open the last flap of the wrapper toward you.
   D. Move the sterile dressing tray toward you after opening the last flap of the wrapper.

6. The physician asks you to remove the sutures on a client with an abdominal incision. Which one of the following steps is appropriate to carry out?
   A. Don sterile gloves before removing sutures.
   B. Grasp suture at knot with forceps and lift away from skin.
   C. Place straight tip of suture scissors over knot and cut knot.
   D. Begin to remove sutures in the middle of the incision to ensure it is healed.

7. What are advantages of using transparent adhesive film dressing for wound care?
   Select all that apply.
   A. Transparent adhesive film allows visualization of wound.
   B. It promotes autolysis of dry eschar.

   C. It does not require a secondary dressing.
   D. It may have a soothing, cooling effect.
   E. It may warm up the wound.

8. A wound culture has been ordered for a client with a leg wound. What is the appropriate method for obtaining the culture?
   A. Clean the wound area with hydrogen peroxide before swabbing the wound.
   B. Swab the wound using a single straight motion with the swab down the middle of the wound.
   C. Swab the edges of the wound starting at the top and crisscrossing the wound to the bottom.
   D. Clean the edge of the wound with saline and then swab the inner aspects of wound.

9. The client requires a wet-to-moist dressing change daily. What is the most appropriate method when placing the dressing in the wound?
   A. Pack several flat sterile 4×4 dressings into the wound bed.
   B. Fluff each sterile dressing and place it over the wound.
   C. Place a moist dressing on top of the sterile dry dressings in the wound.
   D. Unfold a dry dressing and place it on top of moistened dressings in the wound.

10. The physician has ordered negative pressure wound therapy. The nurse needs to evaluate the wound before this therapy can be initiated to ensure it can be effective. What assessments indicate that the wound can accommodate this type of therapy?
    Select all that apply.
    A. It is surrounded by at least 2 cm (¾ in.) of intact periwound tissue.
    B. It is open enough to insert the foam dressing that must touch all edges.
    C. It is debrided.
    D. It must be on the extremities.
    E. It must be able to accommodate the therapy for at least 2 hr.

QSEN Activity

Domain: Patient Centered Care

KSA: Knowledge and Skills

Activity:

Identify Pressure Ulcer stages using photos. Select one stage and discuss how you will assess the ulcer area using the Braden and Norton Scales. Document the assessment and determine a plan of care.

Bibliography

Agency for Health Care Policy and Research. (1992, May). Pressure ulcers in adults: Prediction and prevention. Quick reference guide for clinicians. *Decubitus, 5*(3), 26–30.

Agency for Healthcare Research and Quality. (2014). Preventing pressure ulcers in hospitals. Retrieved from http://www.ahrq.gov/professionals/systems/hospital/pressureulcertoolkit/putool3.html#33

Best Practice. (2008, Feb.). Pressure ulcers: Prevention of pressure related damage. *Evidence Based Information Sheets for Health Professionals, 12*(2), 1–4.

Blaney, W. (2010, Mar.). Taking steps to prevent pressure ulcers. *Nursing, 40*(3), 44–47.

Braden Scale: Adapted from *Pressure Ulcers in Adults: Predictions and Prevention*. (1992, May). AHCRP Publication No. 92-0047, pp. 16–17.

Chettle, C. (2008, Apr.). Shockingly high rates of surgical site infections remain a constant threat. *NurseWeek, CA, 4*, 24–27.

Cleveland Clinic. (2011). Venous insufficiency. Retrieved from http://my.clevelandclinic.org/services/heart/disorders/hic_Venous_Insufficiency

Collins, L., & Seraj, S. (2010). Diagnosis and treatment of venous ulcers. *American Family Physician,, 81*(8), 989–996.

Halperin, E., Engel, T., Sherman, S., & Justo, D. (2012). Low admission Norton scale scores are associated with falls long after rehabilitation in the elderly with hip fractures. *Clinical Intervention in Aging, 7*:431–436. Retrieved from http://www.ncbi.nlm.nih.gov/pmc/articles/PMC3479894/

How wound dressings affect wound healing times. (2014). Retrieved from http://www.advancedtissue.com/wound-dressings-affect-wound-healing-times/

Iker, U., Harbarth, S., Peter, R., Lew, D., Hoffmeyer, P., & Pittet, D. (2010). Preventing surgical site infections. *Expert Review of Anti-Infective Therapy, 8*(6), 657–670. Retrieved from www.medscape.com/viewarticle/723601

Institute for Clinical Systems Improvement. (2014, Mar.). Pressure ulcer prevention and treatment protocol (3rd ed.). Retrieved from https://www.icsi.org/_asset/6t7kxy/PressureUlcer.pdf

Johns Hopkins Medicine. (n.d.). Surgical site infections. Retrieved from http://www.hopkinsmedicine.org/healthlibrary/conditions/surgical_care/surgical_site_infections_134,144/

Jolly, J. (2008). Laceration repair with tissue adhesives: A solution for simple wounds. *Advance for Nurse Practitioners, 16*(3), 63–64.

Kennedy, S. (ed.). (2010, Jan.) NewsCap: Silver-eluting antimicrobial dressings don't help leg ulcers. *The American Journal of Nursing, 110*(1), 20.

Kimmel, H., & Robin, A. (2013). An evidence-based algorithm for treating venous leg ulcers utilizing the Cochrane database of systematic reviews. Disclosures. *Wounds, 25*(9):242–250.

Kirman, C. (2014). Pressure ulcers and wound care treatment and management. Retrieved from http://emedicine.medscape.com/article/190115-treatment

Livingston, M., & Wolvos, T. (2009). *Scottsdale wound management guide*. Malvern, PA: HMP Communications, LLC.

Martindell, D. (2012, Jun.) The safe use of negative-pressure wound therapy. *American Journal of Nursing, 112*(6), 59–61.

Meehan, M. (2009, Oct.). Pressure ulcers: The stakes just got higher. *Nursing, 39*(10), 45–47.

Mercandetti, M., & Cohen, A. (2008, Mar.). Wound healing, healing and repair: eMedicine plastic surgery. Retrieved from http://emedicine.medscape.com/article/1298129-overview

Murphy, P., & Evans, G. (2012). Advances in wound healing: A review of current wound healing products. *Plastic Surgery*

International. Retrieved from http://www.hindawi.com/journals/psi/2012/190436/ref/

National Pressure Ulcer Advisory Panel, European Pressure Ulcer Advisory Panel, and Pan Pacific Pressure Injury Alliance. Prevention of pressure ulcers: Quick reference guide. (2014). Emily Haesler (ed.). Perth, Australia: Cambridge Media. Retrieved from http://www.npuap.org/wp-content/uploads/2014/08/Updated-10-16-14-Quick-Reference-Guide-DIGITAL-NPUAP-EPUAP-PPPIA-16Oct2014.pdf

National Pressure Ulcer Advisory Panel. (2014). NPUAP pressure ulcer stages/categories. Retrieved from http://www.npuap.org/resources/educational-and-clinical-resources/npuap-pressure-ulcer-stagescategories/2014

Opletalova, K., Blaizot, X., Mourgeon, B., Chêne, Y., Creveuil, C., Combemale, P., … & Dompmartin, A. (2012, Apr.). Maggot therapy for wound debridement. A randomized multicenter trial. *JAMA Dermatology, 148*(4), 432–438.

O'Reilly, K. (2011). Hospital's high-tech tools track who's washing their hands. *American Medical News*. Retrieved from http://www.amednews.com/article/20110425/profession/304259947/4/

Orgill, D., & Bayer, L. (2011). Negative pressure wound therapy: Past, present and future. Retrieved from http://onlinelibrary.wiley.com/doi/10.1111/iwj.12170/abstract

Rock, R. (2014, Mar.). Guidelines for safe negative-pressure wound therapy. *Wound Care Advisor, 3*(2), 29–33. Retrieved from http://woundcareadvisor.com/guidelines-for-safe-negative-pressure-wound-therapy-vol3-no2/

Snyder, L. (2008, Aug.). Wound basics: Types, treatment, and care. *RN, 71*(8), 32–36.

Surgical Care Improvement Project (SCIP). (2014). CMS core measures. Retrieved from https://www.bannerhealth.com/NR/rdonlyres/B0DB7AEE-6141-4C56-808E-23DE26B07B02/68540/SCIPInpatientmeasuresfor2014.pdf

Surgical Site Infection (SSI) Event. (2015). Retrieved from www.cdc.gov/nhsn/pdf's/pscmanual/9pscDDICurrent.pdf

Sweetland, S. & Gerts, W. (2010). FDA warning about negative pressure wound therapy. *American Journal of Nursing, 110*(3), 16–19.

The Joint Commission. (2014). Surgical care improvement project (SCIP). Retrieved from http://www.jointcommission.org/surgical_care_improvement_project/.

Toth, P., Stricker, L., & Rijswijk, L. (2010, Feb.). Wound wise: Peristomal skin complications. *American Journal of Nursing, 110*(2), 43–48.

U.S. Department of Health and Human Services, AHCPR. (n.d.). Pressure ulcer treatment: Quick reference guide for clinicians, no. 15. Retrieved from http://www.ncbi.nlm.nih.gov/books/NBK63851/?report=reader

Vigs, S., Dowsett, C., Berg, L., Caravaggi, C., Rome, P., Birke-Sorensen, H., … & Smith, J. (2011, Dec.). Evidence-based recommendations for use of negative-pressure-wound therapy in chronic wounds: Steps toward and international consensus. *Journal of Tissue Viability, 20*(1), S1–S18.

Weir, G., Smart, H., van Marle, J., & Cronje, F. J. (2014). Arterial disease ulcers, part 1: Clinical diagnosis and investigation. *Advances in Skin and Wound Care: The Journal for Prevention and Healing, 27*(9), 421–428.

Yokoe, D. S., Anderson, D. J., Berenhdzsm, S. M., Calfee, D. P., Dubberke, E. R., Ellingson, K., … & Maragakis, L. L. (2014). Introduction to "A Compendium of Strategies to Prevent Healthcare-Associated Infections in Acute Care Hospitals: 2014 Update." *Infection Control and Hospital Epidemiology, 35*(5): 455–459.

Chapter 26
Perioperative Care

Learning Objectives

26.1 Define the word *perioperative*.

26.2 Discuss the nursing care focus in each of the three stages of the perioperative period.

26.3 Identify at least three factors that influence the surgical client's degree of stress.

26.4 Explain why postoperative complications are reduced by decreasing the stress level.

26.5 Describe at least one potential problem and the suggested solution for clients demonstrating high stress levels in the preoperative period.

26.6 State the primary purpose of providing preoperative care for clients.

26.7 Discuss how preoperative teaching can reduce the surgical client's stress.

26.8 Describe the information contained in the surgical permit.

26.9 Outline the essential steps in physically preparing a client for surgery.

26.10 Describe information contained in the surgical safety checklist.

26.11 Explain the purpose for administering the three classifications of drugs used for preoperative medications.

26.12 Describe the nurses' role in caring for a client with moderate sedation (conscious sedation).

26.13 Outline the essential postoperative nursing interventions completed in the surgical unit.

26.14 Summarize the major categories of postoperative pain medications and describe the general side effects of each category.

26.15 Discuss at least three major postoperative complications and the nursing interventions to prevent and treat the complications.

26.16 Describe the process of Hand-off communication.

26.17 Discuss the differences in procedure when a client is discharged to home after outpatient surgery.

Chapter Outline

Terminology

Adaptation ability of an organism to adjust to a change in the environment.

Analgesia absence of the sense of pain.

Analgesic a drug that relieves pain without altering the conscious state.

Anesthesia partial or complete loss of sensation by administration of a drug or gas.

Anxiety a vague, uneasy feeling, the source of which is often nonspecific or unknown to the individual.

Arthrogram a diagnostic radiological test involving use of dye, which is injected into a joint to visualize tears in ligaments and surrounding tissue.

Arthroscopy the examination of the interior of a joint by inserting a specially designed endoscope through a small incision.

Asepsis sterility; a condition free from germs.

Atelectasis collapse of a section of the lungs.

Bronchitis inflammation of the bronchial mucous membrane.

Bronchoscopy examination of the bronchi with a magnifying device.

Capnography measure of $ETCO_2$ (end-tidal carbon dioxide); a means of identifying respiratory depression.

Contamination the introduction of disease, germs, or infectious materials into or onto normally clean or sterile objects.

Dehydration loss of water from the body or tissues due to low intake or high output of fluid.

Emesis vomiting.

Emphysema a condition in which the alveoli of the lungs become distended or ruptured.

Enema injection of water or fluid into rectum and colon to empty the lower intestine or to introduce medicine or food for therapeutic purposes.

Euphoria an exaggerated feeling of well-being.

Exudate fluid, cells, or other substances that have been slowly discharged from cells or blood vessels through small pores or breaks in cell membranes.

Hand-off method of reporting between one nurse and another or between nursing units.

Hernia the protrusion or projection of an organ or part of an organ through the wall of the cavity that normally contains it.

Hypertension higher than normal blood pressure, usually above 140/90 mm Hg.

Hypnotic causing insensibility to pain or partial to complete unconsciousness; hypnotic drugs include sedatives, analgesics, anesthetics, and intoxicants.

Hypothermia state of low body temperature.

Hypovolemia diminished intravascular volume.

Immunosuppressive acting to suppress the body's natural immune response to an antigen.

Induction the process of causing or producing; in anesthesia, the period from the initial inhalation or injection until optimum level of anesthesia is reached, including airway competency intubation.

Laparoscopy a magnifying device inserted into the abdominal cavity to perform diagnostic or surgical procedures.

Laser therapy procedure using laser beams to divide or cause adhesions or to destroy or fix tissues in place.

Lethargy a condition of sluggishness; stupor.

Lithotripsy procedure for eliminating a calculus (stone) in the renal pelvis, ureter, bladder, or gall bladder.

Maladaptive poorly adjusted; unable to adapt.

Mesentery a peritoneal fold connecting the intestine with the back of the abdominal (postabdominal) wall.

Moderate sedation (conscious sedation) a medically controlled state of depressed consciousness that allows protective reflexes to be maintained.

Narcotic producing stupor or sleep; a drug that depresses the central nervous system.

Neurohormonal concerning the interaction between nerves and hormones.

Orthopedic concerning the prevention or correction of deformities of the musculoskeletal system, especially bones, tendons, and ligaments.

Palpitations rapid, violent, or throbbing pulsations, as an abnormally rapid, throbbing, or fluttering heart.

Perioperative having to do with the three phases of the surgical experience: preoperative, intraoperative, and postoperative.

Peritonitis inflammation of the peritoneum.

Pneumonia inflammation of the lungs caused primarily by bacteria, viruses, and chemical agents; can be characterized by chills, high fever, pain in the chest, cough, and purulent or bloody sputum.

Stress a mentally or emotionally disruptive or disquieting influence; distress.

Surgical site infection (SSI) infection that results from the surgical procedure.

Therapeutic having medicinal or healing properties.

Thrombophlebitis inflammation of a vein associated with thrombus (clot).

Topical pertinent to the surface of a particular area of the body; local.

Trauma a physical injury or wound caused by external force or violence; an emotional or psychological shock that may produce disordered feelings or behavior.

Vasoconstriction tightening of a blood vessel.

The Surgical Experience

Surgery used to involve 3–10 days in a hospital setting, but increasingly it is now a short hospital stay or an outpatient experience. Many same-day surgical procedures last only a few hours. The short-stay procedure involves an observation period during an overnight stay in the facility, usually less than 24 hr, and much of the postoperative period is managed at home. Depending on the protocol, a home health nurse may visit, or there may be a postoperative follow-up visit by the nursing staff. In all cases, where outpatient procedures are performed, the nurse does phone follow-up within the first to third postoperative day.

Surgical procedures are classified as either emergency or elective procedures. *Elective procedures* can be scheduled in advance. This allows the client time to plan for child care arrangements and employment responsibilities, as well as to prepare psychologically for the experience. *Emergency procedures* usually are a result of a life-threatening situation such as hemorrhage, obstruction, malignancy, or body system disruption. Procedures are also termed major or minor according to the degree of risk to the client. *Major surgical procedures* involve a risk of bleeding and loss of organs or bodily parts. *Minor surgical procedures* usually involve less risk of bleeding and fewer complications. Examples of these procedures include arthroscopic procedures of the knee, rhinoplasty, and eye surgeries.

One in ten general surgery clients returns to the hospital due to postoperative complications (Cheung-Larivee, 2012). Researchers reviewed the data from the American College of Surgeons National Surgical Quality Improvement program. Of the nearly 1,500 general surgery clients, 11.3% were readmitted within 30 days of discharge. The major causes for readmission were gastrointestinal problems (27.6%), surgical infection (22.1%), and failure to thrive or malnutrition (10.4%). Clients with pancreatectomy, colectomy, and liver resection procedures were more likely to be readmitted. Clients with no complications following surgery had a median length of stay of 5 days; clients with three or more complications stayed in the hospital for an average of 24 days.

According to the CDC, of the 27 million surgeries performed each year, about 1% result in infection and approximately 1 in 8,000 deaths occur each year. Common surgical complications include: pain, infection, blood clots, **atelectasis**, muscle atrophy, fatigue and lack of energy, and **anesthesia** effect (nausea, sore throat, sleepiness, and confusion or delirium).

Perioperative nurses are well-acquainted with the movement to reduce surgical complications. The Surgical Care Improvement Project (SCIP) is a national quality partnership of many organizations with a goal of reducing surgical complications by focusing on high-quality client care. SCIP measures are evidence-based interventions, performance processes, and outcomes that were developed after in-depth assessment by a panel of experts.

Nurses' Role   Nurses take an active role in the psychological and physiologic preparation of the surgical client. Nurses instruct the preoperative client in stress-reduction techniques, explanations of the operating room experience, expectations for the postoperative period, and use of special postoperative equipment. In fact, some hospitals provide time for the operating room nurse to make postoperative visits to clients to assess the client's evaluation of the surgical intervention.

Perioperative Care

Perioperative Areas   There are specific physical areas of the hospital where client care takes place during the operative experience.

Personnel working in these areas must adhere to regulations regarding appropriate attire with personal protective equipment identified for each specific area. Personnel must also follow Standard Precautions and are not permitted to work if they have open lesions on the hands or arms, eye infections, diarrhea, or respiratory infections.

Preoperative Area   Preoperative care can take place in a holding area for invasive procedures or the preoperative area of the operating room. Care can also take place in a central testing area, an inpatient room, or a clinic's examination or treatment room. During this stage, the client must be identified by at least two identifiers (e.g., name, birth date, medical record number). This phase is used to perform tests, attempt to limit preoperative **anxiety**, provide preoperative teaching, and complete client assessments.

The operative site needs to be verified, both to site and side, and then marked by two parties (ideally the client and the physician).

If a female client is of childbearing age, a pregnancy test is usually done. The potassium levels are checked if the client is on diuretics.

Intraoperative Area   This includes the operating room suite or a procedure room where invasive surgical procedures occur. The intraoperative area of the operating room suite includes the area surrounding the operating room and the actual operating room suite. Intraoperative care begins when the client enters the invasive procedure area or the operating room suite and ends when the client is transferred to the PACU (postanesthesia care unit). During the intraoperative period, the client is placed on the operating table, anesthetized, monitored, prepped, and draped, and the surgical procedure is completed. Nursing activities include the focus on client safety, infection prevention, and physiological response to anesthesia.

Postoperative Area   Care can commence in the operating room suite, the procedure room, a recovery room or postoperative area, a client room (ICU), or a treatment room. The postoperative care begins immediately after the completion of the surgical procedure.

Perioperative Stages

Preoperative Stage   The first stage of the perioperative period is the *preoperative stage*. During this stage, a health history, including identification of all allergies (including latex allergies and Betadine or prep solutions), medical concerns in other systems, identification of side and site of procedure, and verification of a client's understanding of the procedure including side and site, a thorough physical assessment, and review of all laboratory tests ordered is completed. Some clients will require an ECG, chest x-ray, pregnancy test, or blood type and screen. The registered nurse completes the operative check list and notifies the surgeon and anesthesiologist of any abnormal findings according to facility policy and procedures. Infections such as urinary tract infections must be treated before any surgical procedure is done. Not all infections such as urinary tract or respiratory are obliterated before surgery, but they must be identified and reported to the surgeon and anesthesiologist to determine whether surgery can proceed. Some clients receive preoperative IV antibiotic therapy before surgery. The nurse must ensure that these orders have been completed before surgery. If clients are to receive preoperative antibiotics, they should be administered before the beginning of surgery to maximize the effects. The antibiotics are frequently administered in the holding area.

Admission to the hospital or outpatient surgery facility and anticipation of surgery result in some degree of anxiety and **stress**. Stress is a physiologic and psychological response to a stressor. Anxiety is one of the manifestations of stress. The degree of anxiety and stress depends on many factors:

- The client's likelihood of reacting to anticipated stressors with high anxiety
- The number of stress-producing events that have occurred recently in the client's life or within the client's family
- The client's perceptions of the hospitalization and surgical experience
- The significance of the surgery to the client and how life will be altered

- The number of unknowns that confront the client on admission
- The client's degree of self-esteem and self-image and perception of how surgery will impact body image
- The client's belief system and religious conviction

The body responds physiologically to an actual or perceived threat. The hypothalamus controls a **neurohormonal** response. The heart rate is increased, and the heart contracts more forcefully. Blood volume is redistributed by **vasoconstriction** of the vessels in the skin, stomach, **mesentery**, and kidneys. Increased blood volume increases cardiac output. Increased blood flow to the skeletal muscles results in the muscles becoming tensed for action. The bronchi dilate, and the increased respiratory rate increases oxygenation. Mechanisms that provide energy include increased glucose release and decreased insulin production. The effects of these mechanisms make it important to know the blood glucose status of a client with diabetes; a higher blood glucose level immediately preceding the procedure is better than one that is too low.

Behavioral responses to stress or anxiety can be adaptive or **maladaptive** (Table 26-1 ■). Adaptive behaviors are purposeful. The client adapts to a stressful situation by preparing to face it or by removing the threat. Maladaptive behaviors result from the inability to adapt to a stressful situation.

One of the objectives of providing preoperative care is to identify the level of stress present in the client. If nursing interventions can be planned that reduce high anxiety levels, the result is a safer intraoperative period (Table 26-2 ■).

High levels of anxiety can prevent successful preoperative **adaptation** and can negatively influence postoperative recovery. Mild anxiety, on the other hand, increases alertness, increases the ability to learn, and increases the ability to assess and to adjust to the environment. Mild anxiety also increases the ability to adjust to several simultaneous stressors. In the preoperative client mild anxiety is adaptive, while a high level is maladaptive. When levels of anxiety or stress become intolerably high, defense mechanisms are unconsciously implemented to reduce the distress by concealing, falsifying, or distorting reality.

Preoperative anxiety is increased by ambiguity, conflicting perceptions, misconceptions, fears of the unknown, and bombardment by many simultaneous stressors. Ambiguity occurs from uncertainty or vagueness concerning the hospital environment, preoperative procedures, intraoperative procedures, or postoperative events.

Conflicting perceptions occur when preconceived notions about the operative experience are different from those actually encountered. A client may not have comprehended the pertinent facts about the procedure (e.g., incision site and how the procedure is going to be done). The client who thought that a herniorrhaphy would be a quick, safe cure can become quite anxious after the anesthesiologist informs him or her of potential complications.

Misconceptions arise when inaccurate information is given, or accurate information is misinterpreted, when terminology is not understood, and when events are not explained clearly. A client who is scheduled for a **bronchoscopy** in the morning, and whose nurse silently

Table 26-1 Responses to Anxiety States

Low Anxiety	High Anxiety
Less likely to react with high anxiety to stressors	Likely to react with high anxiety to stressors
Few changes in personal situation in recent past	Many changes in personal situation in recent past
Perceives hospital and surgical experience as beneficial	Perceives hospital and surgical experience as threatening
Believes surgery will end chronic problem	Fears that surgery may lead to pain, disability, and possibly death
Regards admission procedures as friendly and supportive	Regards admission procedures as strange and frightening
Finds hospital conditions comfortable and the nursing staff supportive and informative	Finds hospital conditions unbearable and the nursing staff nonsupportive

Table 26-2 Managing Surgical Clients

Conscientious Preoperative Care of Clients Prevents Postoperative Complications
- Preparing the client psychologically reduces the client's stress level and helps to prevent postoperative complications.
- Teaching coughing and deep breathing exercises, procedures for getting out of bed, and uses of specialized equipment enhances the client's cooperation and prevents postoperative complications.

Scrupulous Asepsis Throughout the Perioperative Period Reduces Complications
- Maintaining strict **asepsis** reduces cross-contamination.
- Completing the surgical scrub reduces microorganisms on the body surface and the possibility of wound infections postoperatively.
- Identifying breaks in sterile technique and taking appropriate actions are ways to decrease the risk of postoperative complications.

Accurate Identification of Client and Surgical Site Prevents Surgical Errors
- Marking of correct site and side by client, nurse, and surgeon reduces errors.
- Reconfirmation of client identifiers and correct procedure should involve the entire surgical team.

places an NPO sign over the bed, may believe that he is destined for the same hospital regimen as his roommate who had a gastrectomy.

Stress responses are cumulative. An increasing number of stressors can eventually drain adaptive energy. The newly admitted surgical client who has been confronted with many stressors before admission is more likely to respond with a higher level of stress as each new stressor is encountered.

Preoperative teaching is essential for clients undergoing any surgical procedure. Research studies have repeatedly identified the positive outcomes of client teaching as decreased perception of pain, increased compliance with treatments, decreased postoperative complications, and decreased duration of hospitalization. Of course, fear and anxiety are greatly reduced when explanations are complete and time is allowed during the teaching session to answer questions by both the client and family. The client has the right to know what to expect during the surgical procedure and the postoperative period as set forth in The Client's Bill of Rights.

Postoperative cooperation is promoted by informing the client, before anesthesia, about what he or she can expect postoperatively, such as presence of a urinary catheter, drainage tubes, central or arterial IV lines, cast, and so on.

The teaching plan needs to include the preoperative preparation, time of surgery, and postoperative activities. A tour of the postoperative unit is also an important aspect of the teaching, particularly if the client will be going to a critical care or special care unit. Clients should also know what to expect about invasive tubes (e.g., Foley catheter, drain, chest tube) and monitoring lines (i.e., arterial and central venous pressure), which will help to decrease their postoperative anxiety. A demonstration of specific equipment such as incentive spirometer, PCA pump, cardiac monitor, and immobilizer should be presented to increase compliance with the equipment postoperatively. Information regarding time of arrival to the hospital and fluid and food restrictions should be provided before hospitalization, whether it is for outpatient or inpatient surgery.

Other topics covered in the preoperative stage are the type of anesthesia (usually described by the anesthesiologist) and the physical preparation of the client, which includes preoperative skin preparation, identifying the correct client in the operating room, and in some cases, the preoperative scrub. This may include the surgical cleansing prep and hair removal. Cutting or clipping excessive hair has replaced shaving, which produces minute dermal cuts and increased risk of infection. If it must be completed in the intraoperative area, a method that controls aerosolization of hair and epithelium is utilized.

Intraoperative Stage This stage includes the time the client arrives in the preinduction or holding room until he or she arrives in the recovery room. The client may well complain of being cold. The operating room is kept cool, so offering a warm blanket will make the client more comfortable. The Bair Paws Warming System provides heat more effectively than a blanket. Nurses complete an assessment, and may insert IVs and Foley catheters.

Once the client is moved to the operating room itself, a "Time Out" is called before anything transpires. The Time Out is a formal verbalization and checking of "Correct Client, Correct Procedure, Correct Site." (Box 26-1 ■). All members of the OR team must participate in the process, including surgeon, anesthesiologist, surgical assistant, circulating RN, and surgical scrub nurse or technician. The process includes verification of antibiotic administration, allergies, presence of appropriate prosthesis or implant, and correct client positioning. The process is an Association of Perioperative Registered Nurses (AORN) Standard of Practice and a mandate of The Joint Commission. The anesthesiologist prepares the client for and administers the anesthesia while monitoring the client throughout the procedure. The operating room nurses, circulating and scrub, prepare the operating room and provide for client safety. Operating room technicians are used in many facilities in place of scrub nurses.

In 2004, AORN developed a position statement regarding the role of the scrub nurse to achieve optimal client outcomes ("Perioperative Patient-focused Model: Standards Recommendations, Practices, and Guidelines"). An RN must be assigned to the operating room when an OR technician is used as a member of the team. In this case, the OR nurse functions as the circulating nurse. The circulating nurse must always be an RN. The nurse assists in the preparation of the client, positions the client on the operating room

---

Box 26-1 UNIVERSAL PROTOCOL FOR PREVENTING WRONG SITE, WRONG PROCEDURE, WRONG PERSON SURGERY

The implementation of the universal protocol is required by all hospitals accredited by The Joint Commission. The protocol is based on the consensus of experts from clinical specialties and professional disciplines and more than 40 professional medical associations and organizations (The Joint Commission, 2013b).

The protocol identifies the principles necessary to eliminate a surgical client's injury from a wrong procedure, wrong site, or wrong person. It includes the method of marking the operative site and active communication among all surgical team members to ensure that procedures are carried out to prevent these tragedies.

Markings are required whenever there is a procedure involving right–left distinction, multiple structures such as toes and fingers, or levels such as spinal procedures. These markings are placed at the operative site indicating the exact surgical site. This is critical when it involves limbs to ensure the surgical procedure is performed on the correct limb. The individual performing the surgical procedure should do the marking. If the surgeon is unable to perform the markings, a surgical team member can be designated to mark the site. In most states, nurses on the surgical team may be delegated to mark the surgical site.

Source: The Joint Commission (2012c)

table, and ensures that a grounding pad (if electrocautery is used) is securely attached to the client. The role of the circulating nurse in maintaining client safety is highly complex due to the mandates, technical innovations, client advocacy issues, interactions with physicians, operating room personnel, and scheduling or timing of cases. Critical responsibilities of the circulating RN include ensuring sterile technique, correct counts of instruments and sponges, and availability of correct instrumentation. The circulating nurse must be an RN as he or she supports the anesthesiologist during the procedure. The assistance includes starting and monitoring venous lines, administering IV medications when necessary, verifying and hanging blood, and assisting in monitoring the condition of the client. The circulating nurse also assists the team in gowning and gloving for the procedure.

MODERATE SEDATION (CONSCIOUS SEDATION) **Moderate sedation** is used for some surgical procedures and for invasive procedures or tests. Procedures once performed only in an operating room can now be safely done in outpatient settings and special procedures rooms. Moderate sedation may be used in critical care units in clients whose restlessness and anxiety prove detrimental to treatment. Moderate sedation, like general anesthesia, requires a signed permit. Moderate sedation is the administration of an IV sedative, opioid, or **hypnotic** drug that produces sedation, **analgesia**, and amnesia. Clients receiving moderate sedation can respond to commands and maintain their own airway. Clients under light sedation are able to maintain normal respiration, eye movements, and protective reflexes. They usually do not remember the procedure or even the environment. After moderate sedation, the client may have slurred speech and nystagmus at the end point of the sedation.

Moderate sedation (conscious sedation) occurs on a continuum from alertness to deep sedation. In a minimum sedation state, the client can still be anxious. In deep sedation, the client is in a controlled state of depressed consciousness or unconsciousness, is not easily aroused, and does not respond to command. Moderate sedation is considered to be safer than general anesthesia; however, there are risks involved with its use. As the level of sedation increases, the risk of complications increases as well. Clients can become too deeply sedated and require intervention to maintain a patent airway and breathing. Unlike general anesthesia, moderate sedation (conscious sedation) allows clients to maintain a patent airway and respond appropriately to physical stimulation and verbal commands. Another benefit of moderate sedation (conscious sedation) is a quicker return to baseline neurologic status.

A qualified anesthesia provider must give orders for administration of moderate sedation. Some states and institutional guidelines allow qualified registered nurses to administer sedating drugs. The American Nurses Association (ANA) and other nursing organizations have written position papers relative to the practice of administering and monitoring clients undergoing moderate sedation. Nurses must be familiar with the state Nurse Practice

Act as well as the institutional policies regarding their role in this procedure. Nurses allowed to administer moderate sedation (conscious sedation) must meet additional criteria and demonstrate proficiency in the skill. The nurses are working under *standard procedures* in this situation. Nursing students are not allowed to administer moderate sedation or monitor clients while they are receiving moderate sedation.

During the entire procedure, the safety of the client is the priority goal for the entire staff assigned to the procedure (Box 26-2 ■). All staff assist in monitoring the client, ensure that sterile technique is maintained throughout the procedure, and maintain accurate and complete documentation, including sponge and instrument counts. OSHA guidelines are followed by the staff to protect both the client and the staff from exposure to bloodborne pathogens.

After the procedure the client is transferred to the postanesthesia room by the anesthesiologist and/or surgeon and, in some facilities, the circulating nurse. A complete report of the client's status is provided to the postanesthesia staff.

EVIDENCE-BASED PRACTICE

Effect of Using a Safety Checklist on Patient Complications After Surgery: A Systematic Review and Meta-Analysis

The systematic review explored the evidence and found that checklist implementation was linked to a reduction in overall surgical complications. The authors recommend the checklists be used with other interventions to augment safety.

Results of the 207 intervention studies, representing 37,339 clients, indicated seven studies were included in a meta-analysis, and all were cohort studies. Results showed that the use of checklists in surgery, compared with standard practice, led to a reduction in complications. There was no significant reduction in mortality, pneumonia, or unplanned return to the OR.

Source: Gillespie et al. (2014)

Postoperative Stage The *postoperative stage* can be divided into three segments. The immediate postoperative period includes the care given to the client in the postanesthesia room and in the first few hours on the surgical floor. The intermediate period usually involves the care given during the course of surgical convalescence to the time of discharge. The third segment in the postoperative stage is discharge planning, teaching, and referral. Discharge planning and teaching begin during the preoperative period and are reinforced and continued in the postoperative period.

Besides nursing care, nursing management during the postoperative period centers on assessing the client's postoperative condition and monitoring for complications. It also includes client teaching, pain control, and psychological support of both the client and family.

When the client is deemed stable, he or she is transferred to the nursing unit, critical care unit, and in the case of an outpatient client, to home. The nursing care provided in the postoperative period is described in this chapter.

Box 26-2 **SURGICAL SAFETY CHECKLIST**

The surgical safety checklist was established in 2008 as a result of the World Health Organization (WHO) published guidelines, with recommended practices to ensure the safety of surgical clients worldwide. The guidelines were developed to reduce the rate of major surgical complications. A worldwide study was completed to determine whether complications could be reduced by following the surgical checklist before each surgical procedure.

Before Induction of Anesthesia*
(Involves at least nurse and anesthetist)

Has the patient confirmed his or her identity, site, procedure, and consent?
[ ] Yes

Is the site marked?
[ ] Yes
[ ] Not applicable

Is the anesthesia machine and medication check complete?
[ ] Yes

Is the pulse oximeter on the patient and functioning?
[ ] Yes

Does the patient have a:
Known allergy?
[ ] No
[ ] Yes

Difficult airway or aspiration risk?
[ ] No
[ ] Yes, and equipment and assistance available

Risk of >500 mL blood loss (7 mL/kg in children)?
[ ] No
[ ] Yes, and two IVs/central access and fluids planned

Risk of hypothermia (operation >1 hr)?
[ ] No
[ ] Yes, and warmer in place

* **BEFORE INDUCTION,** check these are complete.

Before Skin Incision**
(Involves nurse, anesthetist, and surgeon)

Confirm all team members have introduced themselves by name and role.
[ ] Yes

To surgeon, anesthetist, and nurse:
[ ] What is this patient's name?
[ ] What procedure is planned?
[ ] Where will the incision be made?

Has the antibiotic prophylaxis been given within the last 60 min?
[ ] Yes
[ ] Not applicable

Is venous thromboembolism prophylaxis needed?
[ ] Yes, and boots/ anticoagulants in place
[ ] Not applicable

Anticipated Critical Events to Surgeon:
[ ] What are the critical or nonroutine steps?
[ ] How long will the case take?
[ ] What is the anticipated blood loss?
[ ] What implants/equipment issues or any concerns?

To Anesthetist:
[ ] Are there any patient-specific concerns?

To Nursing Team:
[ ] Has sterility (including indicator results) been confirmed?
[ ] Are there equipment issues or any concerns?

Is essential imaging displayed?
[ ] Yes
[ ] Not applicable

** **BEFORE SKIN INCISION,** check these are complete.

Before Patient Leaves Operating Room†
(Nurse or anesthetist reads out loud.)

Nurse verbally requests from the team:
[ ] How shall I record the name of the procedure?
[ ] Are the instrument, sponge, and needle counts complete?
[ ] How shall I label the specimens (including patient name)?
[ ] Are there any equipment problems to be addressed?

To Surgeon, Anesthetist, and Nurse:
[ ] What are the key concerns for recovery and management of this patient?

† **BEFORE LEAVING ROOM,** check this is complete.

Source: World Alliance for Patient Safety (2008–2009)

Cultural Awareness

Most religions and cultures allow the administration of blood and blood products. The main exception is Jehovah's Witnesses, who forbid the use of blood and blood products. Christian Science followers ordinarily do not allow blood and blood products either. Surgical procedures are accepted by all religions and cultures with some modification. Buddhists permit surgery, but will avoid extremes in surgical procedures. Roman Catholics do not allow abortion or sterilization procedures.

Nursing Diagnoses

The following nursing diagnoses are appropriate to include in a client care plan when the components are related to a surgical experience.

NURSING DIAGNOSIS	RELATED TO . . .
Ineffective Airway Clearance	Pulmonary secretions, allergic response, medications, suppressed cough reflex, decreased oxygen intake, pain, mechanical obstruction
Anxiety	Actual or perceived threat to body image, ability to maintain independence, long-term effects of surgical procedure
Ineffective Coping	Inadequate support system, change in body integrity, unrealistic expectations regarding surgical outcome, stress from surgery
Infection, Risk for	Impaired wound healing, nutritional deficits, inadequate acquired immunity
Deficient Knowledge	Inadequate understanding of surgical procedure, language barrier, incomplete client teaching, lack of motivation, cognitive limitation
Latex Allergy Response, Risk for	Clients with allergies to bananas, tropical fruit, and poinsettia plants at risk; also clients with multiple surgical procedures who have repeated contact with natural latex rubber
Acute Pain	Tissue damage resulting from surgical intervention, ineffective pain relief, psychological factors
Perioperative Positioning Injury, Risk for	Joints and extremities malpositioned or maintained in one position for long period of time
Impaired Skin Integrity, Risk for	Excessive hours on operating table, operative table drapes wrinkled, excessive fluid accumulation on drapes
Delayed Surgical Recovery	Evidence of interrupted healing of surgical area; difficulty in ambulation, pain, fatigue

Source: Herdman, T. H. & Kamitsuru, S. (Eds.) *Nursing Diagnoses – Definitions and Classification 2015-2017.* Copyright © 2014, 1994–2014 by NANDA International. Used by arrangement with John Wiley & Sons Limited. Companion website: www.wiley.com/go/nursingdiagnoses. In order to make safe and effective judgments using NANDA-I nursing diagnosis it is essential that nurses refer to the definitions and defining characteristics of the diagnoses listed in this work.

Nursing Process Data

ASSESSMENT Database

- Identify if high level of stress exists.
- Assess exaggerated anxiety or stress behaviors.
- Assess client's use of defensive behaviors.
- Assess client's vulnerability to number and significance of changes in life before admission.
- Assess client's level of knowledge and perceptions of the impending surgery and perioperative period.

PLANNING Objectives

- To identify the level of stress and anxiety present in preoperative clients
- To provide interventions that decrease stress levels and promote optimal preoperative behavioral and physiologic responses
- To observe for use of defensive behaviors that mask a failure to adapt appropriately in stressful situations
- To prepare the client for a smooth preoperative and postoperative period
- To prevent postoperative complications

IMPLEMENTATION Procedures

DOCUMENTATION AND EVALUATION

Expected Outcomes

- Client's level of stress and anxiety is identified.
- Nursing interventions are provided that decrease stress levels and promote optimal preoperative responses.
- Denial, as a defense mechanism, is identified in the client and therapeutic interventions are made.
- Client identifies stressors and own stress response.
- Client demonstrates coping strategies to control stress and anxiety.
- Client and family state expectations for perioperative experience.
- Client demonstrates activities that will be performed postoperatively.

Unexpected Outcomes/Alternative Actions

Pearson Nursing Student Resources

Find additional review materials at
nursing.pearsonhighered.com.
Prepare for success with NCLEX®-style practice questions and Skill Checklists.

Skill 26.1.1 | Preventing Anxiety and Stress

Preparation

1. Identify client using two identifiers.
2. Introduce yourself and explain what you will be discussing.
3. Complete hand hygiene and provide privacy.

Procedure

1. Establish a trusting relationship.
2. Encourage verbalization of feelings.
3. Listen attentively.
4. Communicate acceptance of the client as an individual.
5. Identify the client's needs (Table 26-3 ■) and keep the charge nurse informed of them.
6. Give adequate information regarding hospital procedures.

   a. Hospital environment, including sights, sounds, and equipment

   b. Hospital personnel and routine procedures: mealtimes, telephone usage, call light
   c. Ordered preoperative procedures: lab tests, diagnostic procedures (Explain the sensory experiences that will be encountered.)
   d. Scheduled time of surgery
   e. Hospital regulations: visiting hours, children's age for visiting
   f. Preoperative procedures: skin preparation, NPO, medications, side rails, dentures, nail polish
   g. Anticipated intraoperative events: monitors, oxygen mask, intravenous line, and others.
   h. Anticipated postoperative events: recovery room, pain and pain medications, coughing and deep breathing exercises, dressings, IVs, Foley catheter

Table 26-3 Preoperative Stress Assessment

Physiologic Responses	Emotional and Defensive Responses	Anxiety and Activity Responses
Heart rate: rate increases 10 beats/ min over baseline during three observations	Withdrawal: daydreaming, increased time in sleep, unwillingness to talk, disinterest	Hyperactivity: pacing, hand-wringing, lip or nail biting, finger-tapping, impatience, irritability, insomnia
Presence of **palpitations**	Anger: resentment, aggressiveness, noncompliance, swearing, boasting, attempts to gain control, and independence	Disorganization of thought: repetitive speech, constant conversation, difficulty concentrating
Blood pressure: increases more than 10 mm Hg over baseline during three observations		
Respiratory rate: increases more than 5 per minute over baseline during three observations	Denial: joking, carefree attitude, inappropriate laughter, refusal to discuss impending surgery	Increased sensitivity to environmental noise, light, temperature, activity
Vasoconstriction of blood vessels near the skin: cool, pale fingers and toes; increased capillary filling time of more than 3 sec		Increased muscle tensing: furrowed eyebrows, facial tics, clenched jaws, loud or high-pitched voice, stammering, rapid speech, elevated shoulders, clenched fists, urinary frequency, tension, or inability to relax
Vasoconstriction of renal vessels: decreased urine output compared with baseline and fluid intake		Increased energy and preparedness: restlessness, easily startled, increased activity level
Vasoconstriction of gastric and mesenteric vessels: anorexia, nausea, vomiting, abdominal distention with flatus, decreased bowel sounds, hyperactivity, diarrhea		

Skill 26.1.2 | Reducing Client Anxiety and Stress

Equipment
Portable audio device (CD player or iPod)
Appropriate relaxation tape

Preparation
1. Identify client using two identifiers.
2. Introduce yourself and explain what you will be discussing.
3. Complete hand hygiene and provide privacy.

(continued)

Skill 26.1.2 | Reducing Client Anxiety and Stress *(continued)*

Procedure

1. Establish a trusting relationship.
2. Encourage verbalization of feelings.
3. Use touch to communicate caring and genuine interest, if culturally appropriate.
4. Avoid false reassurance.
5. Use realistic outcomes.
6. Assist client in exploring effective coping methods to reduce anxiety and stress.

   a. Ask the client or the family what method the client normally uses to successfully reduce stress.
   b. Provide activity: walking, range of motion.
   c. Provide a back rub to loosen tense muscles.
      ➤ *Rationale:* Physical relaxation will often lead to mental relaxation.

   d. Teach client relaxation techniques. One technique is to ask the client to picture a blue sky that is clear except for one white, fluffy cloud. Tell client to concentrate on this scene for 10 min. This often relaxes the mind and body.
   e. An alternative is to ask the client to picture a favorite place (e.g., a warm, sunny beach with sand and a clear, blue lake).

7. As the client begins to relax, reinforce success. Assist client in recognizing his or her strengths.
8. Encourage self-awareness of increasing tension and immediate reversal of escalation.

Note: Some hospitals allow one family member to stay with the child while in the PACU. Not many facilities permit adult clients to have family members in the PACU.

Skill 26.1.3 | Assisting the Client Who Uses Denial

Procedure

1. Establish a trusting relationship.
2. Encourage verbalization of feelings and use an interpreter if necessary.
3. Use touch to communicate caring and genuine interest if acceptable to client (i.e., some cultures prefer not to be touched).
4. Do not attempt to enforce reality. The client is denying reality to prevent outright panic. Allow use of this defense.
5. Use techniques to reduce anxiety and stress to manageable proportions.
6. Attempt to determine the cause of the need for denial.
7. Listen for cues that indicate readiness to discuss the stressors causing the need for denial.
8. Notify physician of your findings.

Unit 26.1 Documentation and Evaluation

DOCUMENTATION for Preoperative Stress

- Objective and subjective indications of anxiety or stress levels
- Nursing interventions used to decrease stress and the results of the intervention
- Changes that occurred as a result of the nursing interventions
- Specific fears verbalized by the client
- Nonverbal indications of stress or anxiety

Expected Outcomes

- Client's level of stress and anxiety is identified.
- Nursing interventions are provided that decrease stress levels and promote optimal preoperative responses.
- Denial, as a defense mechanism, is identified in the client and **therapeutic** interventions are made.
- Client identifies stressors and own stress response.
- Client demonstrates coping strategies to control stress anxiety.
- Client and family state expectations for perioperative experience.
- Client demonstrates activities that will be performed postoperatively.

Unexpected Outcomes	Alternative Actions
• Anxiety level increases rapidly.	• Maintain calm composure and speak in a soft, caring manner. • Use touch to communicate caring and peacefulness, if culturally appropriate. • Reinforce client self-acceptance as an individual. • If unable to achieve success with stress-reducing techniques, notify physician.
• Client becomes angry or hostile.	• Maintain calm composure. • Accept anger, but place limits on how it may be expressed (e.g., no destructive behavior). Understand that anger is usually the result of feeling helpless and powerless to change an intolerable situation. • Do not reward this behavior, but explore other means of meeting client's needs. • Do not isolate client, but continue to respond to needs. • Notify physician of client's behaviors and the actions you used to decrease anger or hostility.
• Client becomes depressed because of overwhelming anxiety and feelings of helplessness or hopelessness.	• Convey respect and belief that the client is worthwhile. Question the client's appraisal of reality and provide support while the client works through his or her feelings. • Provide positive feedback and recognition of strengths, progress, and improved self-esteem. • Spend additional time with the client to allow time to verbalize fears.

Nursing Process Data

ASSESSMENT Database

- Identify type of surgical procedure planned.
- Determine whether client understands type of anesthesia planned.
- Assess client's sociocultural needs.
- Assess client's learning needs.
- Determine most appropriate method of client teaching.
- Assess client's willingness and ability to learn.
- Determine availability of prepared audiovisual material or printed information regarding surgical procedure.

PLANNING Objectives

- To reinforce physician's explanation of surgical procedure and answer questions regarding treatment
- To identify client's readiness to learn about surgical treatment
- To select appropriate time and place for client instruction regarding surgery
- To provide instruction in measures to prevent postoperative complications
- To provide a time for client to ask questions regarding surgical procedure
- To instruct client in use of special equipment required during the postoperative period
- To provide tour of specialty units, such as critical care unit, lithotripsy, or laser rooms

IMPLEMENTATION Procedures

DOCUMENTATION AND EVALUATION

Expected Outcomes

- Client is psychologically and physically prepared for surgery.
- Client demonstrates deep breathing, coughing, turning, and leg exercises accurately.
- Client verbalizes knowledge of operative procedure, potential problems, and expected nursing actions postoperatively.
- Client's family states what they expect during perioperative period.
- Client uses appropriate audio-visual and written materials to increase understanding of perioperative experience.
- Client reports decreased fear regarding special equipment used during perioperative experience.
- Client states safety precautions used with laser and lithotripsy surgery.

Unexpected Outcomes/Alternative Actions

Pearson Nursing Student Resources

Find additional review materials at
nursing.pearsonhighered.com.
Prepare for success with NCLEX®-style practice questions and Skill Checklists.

Skill 26.2.1 | Providing Surgical Information

Equipment

Quiet room for client and family where there will be no interruptions during the teaching program

Equipment that may be used postoperatively by the client (e.g., IV solution, drainage tubes, nasogastric tube, suction equipment, cardiac monitor, and electrodes)

Preparation

1. Identify client using two forms of identification.
2. Introduce yourself and explain what you will be discussing.
3. Complete hand hygiene and provide privacy.

Procedure

Preoperative Client in the Hospital

1. Explain necessity for blood work, ECG, urinalysis, and chest x-ray.
2. Describe preoperative skin preparation.
3. Discuss placement of nasogastric tube and Foley catheter, as indicated.
4. Describe **enema** or special bowel preparation as ordered.
5. Explain use of ongoing medications preoperatively and postoperatively.
6. Demonstrate deep breathing and coughing exercises (use of incentive spirometer if indicated).
7. Assess alcohol use and smoking habits. Emphasize smoking cessation techniques.
8. Assess and document medications used at home, including prescribed, OTC, and herbal remedies; verify that medications related to clotting have been discontinued for an adequate amount of time, usually 1 week before surgery.

> **CLINICAL ALERT**
>
> All herbal medications must be stopped at least 2 weeks before surgery. Side effects vary depending on type of herbal remedy, ranging from sympathomimetic effects, tachycardia, and **hypertension** to inhibition of platelet activity.

9. Demonstrate leg exercises, antiembolic stockings, and sequential compression device.
10. Demonstrate turning and moving in bed.
11. Explain use of postoperative medications for pain control; PCA.
12. Discuss reason for NPO, when it begins, and medication schedule.
13. Explain alterations in diet preoperatively or postoperatively.
14. Describe activities and preparation the morning of surgery, including their participation in the "Time Out" process.
15. State need for quiet environment after medications have been given.
16. State time of surgery to client and family.
17. Describe and reinforce information usually provided by anesthesiologist and surgeon.
18. Offer tour of procedure room, PACU, or ICU that would be used with client and explain monitoring devices and special equipment used there.

Preoperative Client in an Outpatient Setting

1. Check two forms of client ID.
2. Verify accurate consent form has been signed by the client.
3. Call the client several days in advance if long-duration surgical preparations need to be completed before the procedure. If short-duration preparations are required, call the client in the afternoon before the procedure. It is best if the nurse who will care for the client during the surgery calls the client. ➤ *Rationale:* The call begins the nurse–client relationship and helps decrease anxiety.
4. Assess client's ability to understand instructions. If necessary, ask to speak to someone else in the home. ➤ *Rationale:* If instructions are not followed, it could result in unsafe or canceled surgery.
5. Review any lab work that needs to be completed before the scheduled surgery. Explain where the lab work is to be done.
6. Answer the client's questions regarding the surgery and the procedures carried out by the staff during the surgery, including "Time Out" process.
7. Arrange for preadmission as needed.
8. Discuss the procedure for admission to the facility; when to check in at the facility (usually 1.5–2 hr before the scheduled surgery), and what documents need to be available at the time of registration (e.g., insurance card and possibly deductible payment).
9. Determine whether client has an advance directive available or explain what it is and how to obtain a temporary advance directive.
10. Discuss procedure-appropriate clothing to be worn to the setting. For example, clients having knee surgery should wear loose-fitting sweatpants or shorts.
11. Explain that all jewelry and valuables should be left at home for safekeeping.
12. Explain that someone needs to be with the client to take him or her home.
13. Instruct client to not shave surgical site at home. ➤ *Rationale:* Skin nicks increase the risk of infection.

Intraoperative Client

1. Describe mode of transportation to operating room.
2. Discuss procedure in preinduction room or operating room suite in relationship to anesthesia.
3. Reinforce physician's explanation of surgery.
4. Describe dressings, tubes, or equipment that will be used postoperatively.
5. Verify side of body and site involved. See Clinical Alert on page 980 for "Time Out" process.
6. Describe postanesthesia room physical environment and procedures.
7. Explain administration of oxygen.
8. Explain administration of medications.

Postoperative Client

1. Describe assessment procedures.
2. Provide overview of routine procedures of vital signs.

(continued)

Skill 26.2.1 | Providing Surgical Information *(continued)*

3. Demonstrate deep breathing, turning, and coughing exercises.
4. Describe IV therapy if indicated.
5. Explain irrigation of tubes when indicated.
6. Discuss Foley catheter care if indicated.
7. Review dietary alterations.
8. Describe observation and changes of dressing.
9. State ambulation or restrictions in ambulation.
10. Define type of medications used postoperatively.
11. Provide anticipated discharge and plans for assisted care if needed.

Skill 26.2.2 | Providing Client Teaching

Equipment

Prepared teaching aids when available: audio-visual, videos, interactive computer programs, pamphlets, pictures, posters, programmed learning modules, cassette tapes, overhead transparencies, equipment used with client.

Note: Ask client about the best way he or she learns (auditory, kinesthetic, visual). This will determine the best method for teaching.

Preparation

1. Identify client using two forms of identification.
2. Introduce yourself and describe what you will be discussing.
3. Perform hand hygiene and provide privacy.

Procedure

1. Assess client's knowledge base and readiness to learn.
   ➤ *Rationale:* This provides framework for client education at the level client can understand.

   a. Determine the information provided to client by the physician by reading the physician's progress notes and asking client-specific questions.
   b. Identify client's psychosocial and cultural background and ability to listen to teaching by communicating with client and asking direct questions.
   c. Be alert for cultural or religious beliefs that may influence client's surgical experience.
   d. Identify client's perceptions of expected surgical experience and preferences for learning.

2. Develop individualized teaching plan based on client's needs.

   a. Choose appropriate equipment for teaching ❶, based on client's level of understanding, knowledge base, learning style, and language of preference.
   b. Review information previously provided. ➤ *Rationale:* This is to determine retention of information and prevent needless repetition of information already mastered.

❶ Demonstrate use of special equipment in prospective teaching plan.

   c. Choose a quiet environment, and provide for sufficient time to allow client to ask questions. ➤ *Rationale:* This is to ensure client understands planned surgical experience.
   d. Be alert for clues indicating client confusion or misunderstanding of information. Clients may be nodding "yes" even though they do not understand, especially non–English-speaking clients. ➤ *Rationale:* Misunderstanding information can be detrimental to the client's sense of well-being.

3. Select appropriate audio-visual materials to assist with teaching.
4. Demonstrate use of special equipment or devices (e.g., incentive spirometer, chest tubes, suction equipment).
5. Evaluate client teaching by assessing client's ability to return demonstration of exercises and verbally answer specific questions. Reinforce information or provide additional data as needed.

Skill 26.2.3 | Providing Family Teaching

Procedure

1. Include family in teaching provided to client.
2. Instructions to family members should include:

   a. Visiting hours
   b. Where to wait during surgery
   c. Where the surgeon will meet with them and when
   d. Where they can find bathrooms, telephones, and food and beverage service

e. When they can see the client after surgery

f. How to contact a spiritual or religious resource individual

g. How they can best get information regarding the client's condition while they are at home or at the hospital

h. Whether they will be called if there is a change in the client's condition

i. What to expect: client's behavior, which may be regressive; attitude, which may be depressed or angry; physical condition, which may appear worse than

it is; and postrecovery period. ➤ *Rationale:* Some medications may impair client's memory of events.

j. If parents are allowed in recovery room, remind them that the child will still be under effects of anesthesia. Child may cry, be combative, or agitated. Child may be held down by nurses to prevent injury.

k. Instruct parents that they should touch and speak to child to promote reassurance until medications and anesthesia effects are diminished.

Skill 26.2.4 | Teaching For Laser Therapy

Procedure

1. Determine type of laser (Table 26-4 ■) to be used for surgery. There are several types of lasers. However, the three primarily used in client care are: gas, dye, and solid state.

2. Check two forms of client identification and introduce yourself.

3. Determine client's willingness to accept instruction.

4. Determine most appropriate time and place for instruction.

5. Identify client's level of understanding of surgical procedure and what information the physician has provided (Table 26-5 ■).

6. Reinforce explanation of surgical procedure by physician as needed.

7. Describe operating room setting or outpatient setting, including the environment.

8. Explain that client and operating room staff will wear goggles. ➤ *Rationale:* Goggles protect eyes from the laser beam.

9. Explain the use of wet drapes placed over client's skin if required. ➤ *Rationale:* Wet drapes protect skin from burns when some types of **laser therapy** are used.

10. Describe that laser machine may be very noisy.

11. Describe physician's actions during laser therapy. Physician will discharge laser by using a foot pedal while at the same time issuing instructions to nurses, using terms such as *fire, watt seconds,* and *stand by.* ➤ *Rationale:* Describing these words to client allays fear of unfamiliar terms or actual fire. It also describes nurses' role of regulating power and duration of laser beam use.

12. Caution client, if under local anesthesia, he or she may feel heat and smell smoke and a burning odor from tissue being lased.

13. Instruct client to tell physician if pain occurs. ➤ *Rationale:* Additional anesthetic may need to be administered, as client should not feel pain.

14. Instruct client to maintain NPO status 6–8 hr before surgery.

15. Instruct client in postoperative care specific to procedure performed.

16. Instruct client to notify if temperature is above 37.8°C (100°F) for more than 24 hr after laser therapy.
➤ *Rationale:* Infections are unlikely but can occur; therefore, client needs to monitor for presence of symptoms.

Table 26-4 Types of Laser*

Types	Uses
Carbon dioxide (gas)	High-precision cutting instrument used in areas where function must be preserved (e.g., vocal cords, brain, GYN procedures). Also used to treat snoring and for dermatology procedures (e.g., removal of scars and skin cancers).
Holmium (solid state)	Combines the cutting properties of the CO_2 laser with the coagulation properties of the YAG laser. It is used in targeted tissue affecting adjacent, healthy tissue. Can be used with dense or hard tissue. Used in urology procedures (e.g., laser ablation of the prostate [TLAP, HOLAP], stone fragmentation [**lithotripsy**], strictures, obstructions, condylomata, bladder and ureteral tumors and contractures)
Nd:YAG (solid state)	Laser made of a neodymium alloy, yttrium, aluminum, and garnet crystals; deep penetration of beam; can be passed through flexible fibers for cardiovascular laser therapy and scopes (e.g., cystoscope, bronchoscope, and endoscope to treat bladder, prostate, and lung tumors and to coagulate esophageal varices; also used for eye surgery)
Argon (gas)	Used for ophthalmic and dermatologic procedures (e.g., treating glaucoma, cataract, retinal detachment, and removing birthmarks, hemangiomas)
Liquid dye	Used for diagnostic procedures and in conjunction with drugs for photodynamic treatment (e.g., lithotripsy)

*Laser is an acronym for *light amplification by the stimulated emission of radiation.* Choice of laser type is determined by procedure required for treatment.

(continued)

Skill 26.2.4 | Teaching for Laser Therapy (continued)

Table 26-5 Common Types of Laser Surgical Procedures and Complications

Procedure	Client Teaching	Assessment Findings for Potential Complications
Pulmonary	Gag reflex returns in 2–4 hr. Begin taking fluids when gag reflex returns. Expect hoarseness, dyspnea, sore throat, difficulty swallowing for 48–72 hr.	Bright red blood expectorated related to hemorrhage Fever, shortness of breath Use of accessory muscles for breathing related to tracheal edema Wheezing related to airway obstruction **Pneumonia** and respiratory insufficiency related to aspiration of secretions Altered arterial blood gases and sudden pain causing altered vital signs related to pneumothorax
Upper GI	May experience burning sensation in esophagus May experience difficulty swallowing Heartburn present for 3 days.	Poor skin turgor and decreased urine output related to **dehydration** that may be caused by dysphagia Vomiting bright red blood related to perforation Abdominal pain related to perforated bowel Vomiting and abdominal distention related to obstruction of GI tract due to edema
Urology	May experience traces of blood, small blood clots, or traces of tissue in urine for 24 hr Catheter, or more frequently a stent, may be left in place temporarily for up to 1 week. Urinary frequency and urgency may occur for 1 week.	Bright red urine related to hemorrhage Abdominal pain related to perforated bladder Fever, increased pulse, malaise related to infection Inability to void related to blood clots
Cardiovascular	May experience slight burning or chest pain over coronary vessels	Arrhythmias related to hypoxia or laser treatment Bleeding at site of percutaneous laser angioplasty; related to catheter insertion Intake and output values altered related to osmotic contrast media used for laser treatment Changes in vital signs (i.e., may become hypotensive with cardiac tamponade)
Eye	Most clients feel no pain because local or **topical** anesthesia is used. Need to remain quiet during procedure	Corneal injury can occur if eye is rubbed or bumped. Increased intraocular pressure is unusual but can occur.

Skill 26.2.5 | Teaching for Lithotripsy

Preparation

1. Identify type of extracorporeal shock wave lithotripsy (ESWL) used for kidney stones and occasionally for gallstones.
2. Identify type of anesthesia that will be used: local, epidural, spinal, or general. General anesthesia may be used to prevent pain as stones are fragmented.
3. Identify whether client will have a ureteral stent or Foley catheter inserted after the procedure. A string may be visible at the end of the penis and is attached to a stent; this will aid in the removal of the stent at a later time.

Procedure

1. Check two forms of client ID and introduce yourself.
2. Determine client's knowledge base and information provided by physician.
3. Reinforce physician's description of procedure, as needed.
4. Answer client's questions regarding procedure.
5. Explain that lithotriptor discharges a series of shock waves through water-filled cushion.

6. Describe to client that he or she may feel fluttering or mild blows where shock waves are beamed. From 500–2,400 shocks are required to disintegrate stones.
7. Discuss specialized equipment that will be used. Client may lie with water-filled cushion pressed against area of back or abdomen where stones are present.
8. Describe use of monitoring equipment throughout procedure. ▶ *Rationale:* The heart rate and rhythm are monitored throughout procedure and shocks may be synchronized with the rhythm to prevent arrhythmias.
9. Explain that the procedure takes 20 min to 2 hr, depending on type of procedure.
10. Describe postlithotripsy care.

    a. After procedure, client is covered with a warm blanket and taken to recovery or treatment room.
    b. Vital signs are monitored as with any surgical client.
    c. Urine output is monitored for hematuria.

       ▶ *Rationale:* This is to determine kidney damage from procedure.

d. Strain all urine at the facility and at home. ➤ *Rationale:* This is to obtain fragments of the stones in order to send them for analysis. In some cases, knowing the composition of the stone is essential for altering dietary habits.

e. Liver function studies are performed after lithotripsy for gallstones. ➤ *Rationale:* This is to assess whether shock waves have damaged liver.

f. Pain management is monitored and maintained as gravel is passed after disintegration of stones.

g. Medication is provided for nausea and vomiting.
➤ *Rationale:* Nausea and vomiting often accompany pain and postanesthesia.

h. Intake and output measurements are taken.
➤ *Rationale:* Fluids are encouraged to hydrate clients with kidney stones to assist in the excretion of gravel.

i. Catheter care is provided for clients having kidney procedure requiring indwelling catheters. If a stent is used, it may cause urgency, dysuria, frequency, and bleeding.
➤ *Rationale:* Indwelling catheters and ureteral stents, if used, are left in place for 24 hr to assist with passage of gravel or if second lithotripsy treatment is required.

j. Exercise is encouraged to assist with passing of gravel.

k. Ecchymoses and discomfort may be felt over area of the body that experienced shock waves.

11. Provide tour of lithotriptor room, if possible.

Skill 26.2.6 | Teaching for Laparoscopy

Preparation

1. Identify purpose of **laparoscopy** (Box 26-3 ■).
2. Identify type of anesthesia that will be used. Usually, it is done under general anesthesia.
3. Determine whether ultrasound, CT scan, or MRI was done; if so, have results available for physician.
4. Obtain results of standard blood tests and urine tests, if done.

Procedure

1. Check two forms of client identification and introduce yourself.
2. Determine client's knowledge base and information provided by physician.
3. Reinforce physician's description of procedure, as needed.
4. Describe equipment used for procedure: Instrument used in procedure is a medical telescope with a light and high-resolution television camera so that physician can see what is in the abdomen.
5. Describe procedure to client: Incision is made into umbilicus; CO_2 gas is infused into abdomen to insert a small air pocket; a small camera and instruments are inserted through incision.
6. Instruct client that procedure is usually done in a same-day surgery setting. Client will go home the same day. Major procedures require overnight stay for observation and pain management.
7. Instruct client to not eat or drink for 6–8 hr before procedure.
8. Explain that client should shower evening before or day of surgery with chlorhexidine or agent prescribed by physician. The umbilicus is cleaned with soap, water, and a cotton-tipped swab (e.g., Q-tip). ➤ *Rationale:* Chlorhexidine is well tolerated and does not leave discoloration on skin as a povidone–iodine preparation does.
9. Instruct client to be at the hospital 1–2 hr before the scheduled surgery, according to hospital policy. Tell client to bring someone to drive home.

Box 26-3 THERAPEUTIC AND DIAGNOSTIC USES OF LAPAROSCOPY

Therapeutic Uses of Laparoscopy

Therapeutic procedures commonly include:

- Cholecystectomy
- Bowel resection
- Nephrectomy
- Adrenalectomy
- Radical prostatectomy
- Tubal ligation
- Hysterectomy
- Repair of pelvic prolapse
- Appendectomy
- **Hernia** repair
- Pulmonary resection
- Nissen procedure
- Urethral repair

Diagnostic Uses of Laparoscopy

Diagnostic laparoscopy is used for the following purposes:

- Diagnosis of cause of abdominal pain
- Obtaining tissue from an abdominal mass to determine diagnosis
- Determining cause of ascites
- Obtaining liver tissue for diagnosis
- Assisting in cancer staging or a "second look" procedure
- Treatment of endometriosis and pelvic inflammatory disease

10. Have client discuss with the surgeon whether to take routine medications the morning of surgery. If medications are taken, only a sip of water is used to swallow pills. Medications causing increased risk for bleeding need to be discontinued before surgery, such as those prescribed for arthritis, anticoagulants, OTC (e.g., aspirin), or certain alternative herbal medications, according to physician's orders.

(continued)

Skill 26.2.6 | Teaching for Laparoscopy *(continued)*

11. Instruct client to follow specific orders from physician's office regarding other preoperative directions.
12. Explain setting where surgery will be performed. If possible, allow client to visit the area if he or she is anxious.
13. Describe postlaparoscopy care to client:

   a. After surgery, client will go to the recovery room.
   b. Vital signs are monitored, dressing will be observed for signs of bleeding, and medication for pain may be administered. IV fluids will be infused and monitored until effects of anesthesia have dissipated.
   c. Client is discharged home as soon as he or she is fully awake and able to get out of bed unassisted. Many facilities require the client to urinate and manage nausea without **emesis** after light intake of crackers and soda or juice before discharge. Client must be accompanied by someone who can drive him or her home. ➤ *Rationale:* The effects of anesthesia may persist for several hours or as long as a day, even if the client feels fully awake.
   d. Instruct client that some soreness around incision is normal. Take pain medications as prescribed by physician. It is important to take pain medication on time or at the beginning of pain cycle for first 24–48 hr.
   e. Notify physician if chills, vomiting, redness at incision site, or worsening pain is not controlled by medication, or if unable to urinate. ➤ *Rationale:* These are signs of infection.
   f. Instruct client there may be a sharp pain under the scapula up to 24–48 hr postop and that changing positions may relocate "gas" bubble. ➤ *Rationale:* Retained carbon dioxide irritates the phrenic nerve in the diaphragm, causing referred pain. Carbon dioxide is used to distend the abdominal cavity to aid in visualization and provide working space during a laparoscopy.
   g. Instruct client to schedule a follow-up appointment with physician within 2 weeks.

Skill 26.2.7 | Teaching for Arthroscopy

Preparation

1. Determine joint on which **arthroscopy** will be performed. Most common joints: knee, shoulder, elbow, ankle, hip, and wrist (Box 26-4 ■).
2. Identify type of anesthesia that will be used. General, spinal, or local anesthetic is used, depending on specific joint involved and suspected problem.
3. Determine whether diagnostic tests were done, that is, MRI, x-rays, or **arthrogram**. Obtain results for physician.

Procedure

1. Check two forms of client ID and introduce yourself. Perform hand hygiene.
2. Determine client's knowledge base and information provided by physician.
3. Reinforce physician's description of procedure, as needed.
4. Describe equipment used for the procedure: pencil-sized instruments (arthroscope) that contain small lens and lighting system to magnify and illuminate structures inside the joint are inserted through incision.
5. Describe procedure to client: A small incision is made in client's skin to allow instruments to be inserted into the joint so that physician can see the interior of the joint. Several small incisions may be made to see other parts of the joint if needed. The image is projected on a television screen. The surgeon can then determine the amount or type of injury and repair or correct the problem.
6. Instruct client that procedure is usually done in an outpatient setting and he or she will go home the same day.
7. Explain preoperative preparation that is completed before the day of surgery:

   a. Diagnostic tests completed
   b. Operative permit signed
   c. Physical examination and health history completed
   d. Physician informed of routine medications and any allergies
   e. Procedure discussed with physician and anesthesiologist
   f. Client meets with physical therapist to be fitted with crutches and/or knee brace, if lower extremity is affected.
8. Instruct client to not eat or drink anything after midnight unless otherwise instructed by physician.
9. Explain skin prep that is to be completed the night before surgery. A 5-min scrub with an antiseptic is usually ordered. Follow facility policy for specifics—some physicians order a full shower and some concentrate on the surgical site.

Box 26-4 CONDITIONS FOUND AND CORRECTED BY ARTHROSCOPY

- **Inflammation:** synovitis
- **Injury:** acute and chronic:
   Shoulder—rotator cuff tendon tears, dislocation, and impingement syndrome
   Knee—meniscal tears, chondromalacia, and anterior cruciate ligament (ACL) tears and instability
   Wrist—carpal tunnel syndrome
- **Loose bodies of bone and/or cartilage:** knee, shoulder, elbow, ankle, or wrist

10. Instruct client to follow surgeon or anesthesiologist instructions regarding taking routine medications.
11. Instructions to client before admission:

    a. Remove all nail polish and make-up according to hospital policy. (This may not be necessary as newer oxygen saturation monitors that use laser light are not affected by nail polish.) ➤ *Rationale:* Capillary refill and skin coloration are assessed on all clients receiving anesthesia.

    b. Do not bring jewelry, money, or other valuables to facility. ➤ *Rationale:* Facility is not responsible for client's valuables.

    c. Wear comfortable, loose-fitting clothes such as loose-fitting button-down shirts or blouses, drawstring shorts, sweatpants, and boxer-style shorts. ➤ *Rationale:* This is to make it easier to dress after surgery, especially if a brace or sling has been applied.

    d. Bring crutches, brace, sling, or immobilizer to facility, if available.

    e. An adult must accompany client to facility to provide transportation home. ➤ *Rationale:* Even if client feels alert and awake, effects of anesthesia can last up to a day or two.

    f. Arrive at the facility 1.5–2 hr before scheduled surgery, according to facility policy.

12. Describe postarthroscopy care to client:

    a. After surgery he or she will go to recovery room.

    b. Vital signs, circulatory assessments, pain management, and IV fluid infusion will continue until client is fully awake and ready for discharge.

    c. A pressure dressing, brace, and/or ice may be applied to joint.

    d. Discharge instructions are based on joint involved with arthroscopy. Most common joint is knee. Client is to use crutches for short time. Weight bearing is allowed according to physician orders. Brace is worn when walking. Physical therapy will begin within a day or two of surgery.

13. Repeat instructions for home care.

    a. Explain to client that wound and dressing is to be kept clean and dry and changed if it becomes soiled.

    b. Instruct client to place a plastic bag over brace and tape it securely when showering.

    c. Instruct client to apply ice to joint for 24–48 hr after surgery. ➤ *Rationale:* Ice reduces pain and edema.

    d. Demonstrate how to elevate joint (leg, ankle, wrist) to reduce pain and edema.

    e. Explain how pain medication is to be taken: 30 min before exercises; tell client to not drink alcohol when on medications.

    f. Discuss symptoms that indicate complications and should be reported immediately to physician: swelling; tingling; pain or numbness in extremities; drainage that is yellow, green, or foul-smelling; chills or temperature above 38.5°C (101.3°F).

Skill 26.2.8 | Instructing in Deep Breathing Exercises

1. Check two forms of client ID and introduce yourself. Perform hand hygiene and provide privacy.
2. Explain procedure and purpose of exercises. ➤ *Rationale:* Deep breathing and coughing exercises promote lung expansion; lower the risk of pneumonia, atelectasis, and pulmonary emboli.
3. Instruct and have client demonstrate deep breathing exercises. ➤ *Rationale:* Encouraging the client to practice and return the demonstration before surgery assists him or her to deep breathe more effectively after surgery.
4. Have client sit in upright position.
5. Place client's hands along lower borders of rib cage. Client should feel rib cage expand when breathing in. ➤ *Rationale:* This assists client to feel adequate chest movement.
6. Instruct client to breathe through nose slowly, take a deep breath, hold 1–3 sec, and then exhale through mouth. ➤ *Rationale:* This expands alveoli and prevents hyperventilation if client is breathing too quickly.
7. Repeat exercise sequence three to four times, at least every 2 hr when awake.

Note: Incentive spirometry is preferred by most facilities. Refer to Skill 30.1.4 for incentive spirometry instructions.

Skill 26.2.9 | Instructing in Coughing Exercises

Procedure

1. Check two forms of client ID and introduce yourself. Complete hand hygiene.
2. Explain procedure and purpose of exercises. Provide privacy for client.
3. Instruct and have client demonstrate coughing exercises.
4. Have client sit in upright position.
5. Instruct client to splint incision when deep breathing and coughing.
6. Demonstrate placement of hands on either side of incision. Instruct client to press hands firmly toward incision during exercises. ➤ *Rationale:* This prevents tension on the suture line and diminishes pain.

(continued)

Skill 26.2.9 | Instructing in Coughing Exercises *(continued)*

1 Instruct client in coughing exercises using cough pillow or demonstrate placement of hands on either side of incision for support during coughing.

7. Instruct in use of cough pillow. **1** Place folded bath towel in pillowcase. Hold pillow directly over incision and press on pillow when performing exercises. ➤ *Rationale:* This prevents pain and discomfort by splinting the incision and reducing stress on suture line.
8. Demonstrate technique for inhaling deeply and holding breath for 1–2 sec.
9. Instruct client to take 2–3 breaths slowly and exhale passively; on third breath, hold for 2–3 sec.
10. Encourage client to cough forcefully two to three times by using abdominal and other respiratory muscles to assist with coughing. ➤ *Rationale:* This extra force provides a more effective cough.
11. Have client cough a second time.
12. Instruct client to do coughing exercises after deep breathing exercises at least every 2 hr when awake.
13. Have tissue available for secretions if client has a productive cough.

Skill 26.2.10 | Providing Instruction to Turn in Bed

Procedure

1. Check two forms of client ID and introduce yourself. Complete hand hygiene and provide privacy.
2. Explain turning procedure and purpose. ➤ *Rationale:* Turning assists in the prevention of **thrombophlebitis**, pressure ulcer formation, and respiratory complications.
3. Instruct and demonstrate turning procedure.
4. Instruct client to splint incision whenever turning.
5. Have client move to far side of bed with side rails up.
   ➤ *Rationale:* This position allows client to turn without rolling to edge of bed.

6. Instruct client to splint incision with hand on side toward which he or she will be turning. ➤ *Rationale:* This leaves the uppermost hand available to grasp side rail or trapeze to assist with turning.
7. Instruct client to keep leg straight on side to which he or she will turn.
8. Flex other leg over straight lower leg. ➤ *Rationale:* Flexing the leg assists in shifting the weight when turning to opposite side.
9. Instruct client to turn on side and grasp side rail.
10. Instruct client to move pillow into comfortable position under head or place pillow under top leg and place arm into comfortable position.

Skill 26.2.11 | Instructing in Leg Exercises

Procedure

1. Check two forms of client ID and introduce yourself. Complete hand hygiene and provide privacy.
2. Explain exercise and purpose. ➤ *Rationale:* These exercises assist in preventing stasis of blood in lower extremities and thus thrombophlebitis.
3. Place client in supine or semi-Fowler's position.
4. Instruct client to bend knee, raise foot in air, and hold this position for 2–3 sec.
5. Have client extend the leg and lower it to bed.
6. Repeat procedure with other leg.

Note: Inhale when extending leg and exhale slowly when lowering leg. This prevents back strain and strengthens abdominal muscles.

7. Complete sequence 5–10 times each hour while awake.
8. Have client extend toes (plantar flexion) toward bottom of bed, and then flex (dorsiflexion) toward head of bed.
9. Repeat foot extension and flexion with other side.
10. Repeat sequence five times each hour while awake.
11. Instruct client to make circles with the ankle moving first to the left and then to the right.
12. Repeat sequence five times each hour while awake.

Note: Sequential compression devices are more commonly used during the postoperative period. See Skill 31.2.2, Applying Sequential Devices.

Unit 26.2 Documentation and Evaluation

DOCUMENTATION for Preoperative Teaching

- Type of instruction provided
- Amount of time provided for instruction
- Type of audio-visual materials or written information used
- Client's response to teaching
- Accuracy and participation in return demonstration exercises
- Areas of instruction that need to be reinforced
- Psychological response to preoperative teaching and impending surgery
- Preop teaching form if available

EVALUATION/Critical Thinking

Expected Outcomes

- Client is psychologically and physically prepared for surgery.
- Client demonstrates deep breathing, coughing, turning, and leg exercises accurately.
- Client verbalizes knowledge of operative procedure, potential problems, and expected nursing actions postoperatively.
- Client's family states what they expect during perioperative period.
- Client uses appropriate audio-visual and written materials to increase understanding of perioperative experience.
- Client reports decreased fear regarding special equipment used during perioperative experience.
- Client states safety precautions used with laser and lithotripsy surgery.

Unexpected Outcomes

- Client refuses to participate in preoperative teaching.

Alternative Actions

- Encourage client to state reasons for refusal.
- Encourage client to discuss knowledge of surgery.
- Assess whether client is experiencing fear or denial regarding impending surgery.
- Ask client to provide a time frame more acceptable for teaching.
- Notify physician of client's refusal if facility policy.

(continued)

Unexpected Outcomes	Alternative Actions
• Client unable to understand directions.	• Identify client's learning capabilities. • Determine whether a language barrier exists. If so, find an individual who speaks client's primary language and ask for assistance with teaching. • Use different words to explain information. • Determine a different teaching strategy that the client can understand, or involve family members who can assist with explanations to client. • Evaluate client's stress level to determine whether it is interfering with learning. • Establish a new time for teaching when client may be able to concentrate on teaching. • Develop a slower pace for instruction and present less information at one time.
• Client not adequately prepared for surgery.	• Ascertain where data are insufficient or unclear and provide additional instruction in that area. • Use a different approach or teaching style to provide information. • Select different teaching materials that may explain information in a more useful way.
• Client becomes angry or hostile.	• Maintain calm composure. • Acknowledge anger, but place limits on how it may be expressed (e.g., no destructive behavior). Understand that anger is usually the result of feeling helpless and powerless to change an intolerable situation. • Do not reward this behavior, but explore other means of meeting client's needs. • Do not isolate client; continue to respond to needs. • Try to defuse anger, but if safety is threatened, call for assistance.
• Client becomes depressed because of overwhelming anxiety and feelings of helplessness or hopelessness.	• Convey respect and belief that client is worthwhile. Question client's current appraisal of reality; provide support while client works through feelings. • Provide positive feedback and recognition of strengths, progress, and improved self-esteem. • Spend additional time with the client to allow time to verbalize fears.

Preoperative Care

Nursing Process Data

ASSESSMENT Database

- Assess type of surgical procedure to be carried out and extent of database needed.
- Evaluate the client's ability to provide accurate information.
- Assess level of anxiety present that may interfere in the transmission of information at that moment.
- Identify the appropriate physical care needed for the specific surgical intervention.
- Assess special needs for the surgical clipping.
- Check hospital protocol for shaving surgical site or if a special permit is needed for shaving, such as the head for neurosurgical clients, extremities for orthopedic clients, or children.
- Check for need for special soap or antiseptic scrub before shave.
- Check if a policy exists in the hospital for disposing or handling of scalp hair.
- Assess surgical site before preparing; observe for unusual cuts, abrasions, or markings, and report findings to charge nurse.
- Assess client's knowledge of side and site of surgical procedure.

PLANNING Objectives

- To assist with monitoring the client's progress through the operative experience
- To assist in identifying deviations from the client's baseline data that may occur as a result of anxiety or stress of admission, preoperative events, diagnostic procedures, the surgical trauma, postoperative complications, and responses to and side effects of drugs

- To provide appropriate preoperative physical care to enable the client to have a safe intraoperative and postoperative period
- To report client's statements about allergies or chronic problems that could affect postoperative nursing care
- To complete a surgical prep correctly

IMPLEMENTATION Procedures

DOCUMENTATION AND EVALUATION

Expected Outcomes

- Client's physical or emotional deviations from normal are identified preoperatively.
- Preoperative baseline data are obtained.
- Surgical site is marked and prepared correctly.
- Client states expectations regarding intraoperative and postoperative course.

Unexpected Outcomes/Alternative Actions

Pearson Nursing Student Resources

Find additional review materials at **nursing.pearsonhighered.com.**
Prepare for success with NCLEX®-style practice questions and Skill Checklists.

Skill 26.3.1 | Obtaining Baseline Data

Equipment
Thermometer
Sphygmomanometer and stethoscope
O_2 saturation probe
Chart or computer for documenting findings

Procedure
1. Check two forms of client ID and introduce yourself. Perform hand hygiene. Provide privacy.
2. Ask about allergies to drugs, food, or latex.
3. Assess for surgical risk: nutritional status, fluid and electrolyte balance, use of prescribed medications, over-the-counter complementary medications (i.e., herbs), and illicit drugs. ➤ *Rationale:* Medications such as anticoagulants, tranquilizers, or CNS depressants can adversely affect surgical experience.
4. Assess for alcohol use and smoking habits. ➤ *Rationale:* Complications can arise in clients using these substances, particularly with anesthesia.
5. Take and record vital signs and weight of client. Obtain oxygen saturation levels.
6. Check if client wears dentures, hearing aid, glasses, has an artificial eye, or body piercing jewelry. Check for toe rings. If body piercing jewelry cannot be removed, cover with tape to protect skin from electrical arcing from the electrical surgical unit, which could cause skin burns.
7. Assess mental attitude; record any unusual stress or anxiety exhibited by the client.
8. Complete a physical assessment and health history. Report unusual findings to physician, OR staff, and anesthesiologist if client has history of methicillin-resistant *Staphylococcus aureus* (MRSA), vancomycin-resistant enterococci (VRE), hepatitis B or C, or tuberculosis (TBC).

> **CLINICAL ALERT**
> It is imperative that nurses on the surgical floor check documentation carefully to find any abnormalities in the history and physical, lab results, or assessment indicating potential complications during procedure. This information must be reported to the anesthesiologist and OR staff.

9. Evaluate lab values for abnormalities (ECG, x-rays, blood work, urinalysis) and pregnancy test on age-appropriate client if she has an intact uterus. ➤ *Rationale:* This is to detect potential sources for complications (e.g., low Hct, Hgb, urine glucose, lung or cardiac abnormalities).
10. Determine whether skin preparation was completed either evening before or morning of surgery. Check if shower or bath with designated antiseptic was completed.
11. Assess for fall potential (unsteady gait, use of assistive devices).
12. Identify topics requiring client teaching.
13. Identify discharge plans.
14. Determine religious or cultural beliefs that may affect surgical experience.

Skill 26.3.2 | Preparing the Surgical Site

Equipment
Washcloth and towels
Absorbent pad
Bath blanket or drape
Scissors or electric clippers
Two sterile bowls
4×4 gauze pads
Emesis basin
Applicator sticks
Cleansing solution
Sterile water
Clean gloves
Depilatory
Antiseptic solution
Tongue blade

Procedure
1. Refer to physician's orders for specific operative site or area to be prepared. If orders do not state preference for site, refer to procedure manual for appropriate area to be prepared, based on surgical procedure.
2. Determine type of preparation to be done: clipping of hair or hair removal using depilatory. ➤ *Rationale:* The older process of shaving hair was determined to cause **surgical site infection (SSI)**; therefore, it has been eliminated in most surgical hair removal.
3. Gather equipment.
4. Check two forms of client ID and introduce yourself.
5. Explain procedure to client and provide privacy.
6. Adjust light to ensure good visualization.
7. Perform hand hygiene.
8. Position client for maximum comfort and site exposure.
9. Drape client for comfort and to prevent undue exposure.

10. Protect bed with absorbent pad.
11. Arrange equipment for your convenience.
12. Put on clean gloves.
13. Assess surgical site before skin preparation for moles, warts, rash, and other skin conditions. ➤ *Rationale:* Inadvertent removal of lesions traumatizes skin and may contribute to infection.

Note: CDC standards indicate that clients are to shower or bathe with an antiseptic agent at least the night before surgery. The FDA has also shown that antimicrobial activity of the antiseptic agent prevents skin infections.

EVIDENCE-BASED PRACTICE
Preparing the Skin for Surgery
The science of preoperative skin preparation has grown more sophisticated, but it continues to be the cornerstone of evidence-based practice to prevent SSIs and to promote positive surgical outcomes.

Procedures for skin preparation vary based on client and surgical procedure factors. Of the 21,000 SSIs reported to the National Healthcare Safety Network in 2009–2010, 30.4% were attributed to *S. aureus*, a type of bacteria commonly found on the skin. Close to half of the infections were MRSA. The AORN Practice Committee recommended the following goals of preoperative skin preparation:

a. The removal of soil and transient microbes from the skin.
b. The rapid reduction of resident microbes without tissue irritation.
c. The inhibition or rapid, rebound growth of these microbes.

Because most planned procedures have clients who begin the skin preparation at home, the AORN recommends two showers using 4% chlorhexidine gluconate before surgery to decrease the number of microorganisms on the skin. The contact with the skin prep should last 2 min, followed by a thorough rinsing to remove the residual chlorhexidine and drying with a clean towel. The CDC supports clients showering with an antiseptic agent at least once the night before surgery.

Source: Barzoloski-O'Connor (2014)

14. Prepare site using scissors or clippers according to facility policy/procedures.
    a. Use scissors or electric clippers and cut hair 1 cm (about ⅜ in.) above surgical site or according to facility policies.
    b. Clip small amount of hair each time.
    c. Cut in direction hair grows.
15. Clipping should be completed close to the time of surgery. The prep is completed close to the time of surgery and not the night before. ➤ *Rationale:* The risk of SSI is greater if done the night before.
16. Remove all hair from site and discard.

CLINICAL ALERT
Electric or battery-powered clippers are preferred to razors to prevent skin irritation and microscopic cuts to the skin. Clippers must have a disposable head that is changed between clients. Handles should be disinfected.

---

17. Prepare site using depilatory (if ordered by physician).
    a. Clip hair before applying cream.
    b. Apply cream to designated area using tongue blade or gloved hand.
    c. Leave on skin for designated time, according to directions on package, usually 10 min.
    d. Remove cream by rubbing off with tongue blade or moistened 4×4 gauze pads.
    e. Wash skin with antiseptic soap; dry area thoroughly. Remove all hair with washing. ➤ *Rationale:* This provides clean, smooth skin, free of abrasions and cut.
18. After removing hair, apply antiseptic solution with 4×4 pads or use disposable prep kit.
19. Begin at incision site and, with light friction, make ever-widening circles, moving outward from the center to the most distant line of area. ➤ *Rationale:* Working from most clean to least clean area prevents **contamination**. Scrub area for 2–3 min.
20. Rinse area with warm water and blot dry with 4×4 gauze pads.
21. Remove and dispose of equipment; scissors and razors are disposed of in sharps container.
22. Remove gloves and discard.
23. Perform hand hygiene.
24. Assist client to put on clean gown.
25. Position the client for comfort.

EVIDENCE-BASED PRACTICE
Infection Control: Recognizing Surgical Site Infections
SSIs are the most common healthcare-associated infections in clients undergoing surgery in the United States. They have contributed significantly to increased morbidity, mortality, and healthcare costs. An estimated 27 million surgical procedures are performed each year, and the rate of SSIs in surgical clients ranges from 2% to 5%. That is 540,000 to 1.3 million SSIs annually. Infection is the cause of death in 77% of surgical clients who have SSIs at the time of death. SSIs develop within 30 days after a surgical procedure, or within 1 year if an implant was placed. A thorough assessment can help recognize an SSI early in the process. The way to ensure early detection and diagnosis of SSIs is for clinicians to provide direct client care and teach clients to assess their surgical wounds at home. Close tracking of postoperative assessment data, noting trends that suggest possible infection, and confirmation from lab tests, may prove to be the most reliable indicators of SSIs.

Source: Alexander-Magalee (2012)

Skill 26.3.3 | Preparing the Client for Surgery

Equipment

Preoperative checklist ❶

Operative permit

Specific equipment needed to provide physical care as ordered, such as enema equipment, nasogastric tube, Foley catheter

Antiseptic agent for shower

Procedure

1. Check two forms of client ID and introduce yourself. Perform hand hygiene and provide privacy.
2. Obtain client's signature on surgical consent form ❷ and check agency policy. Ensure all preoperative forms are complete, with no blank areas.

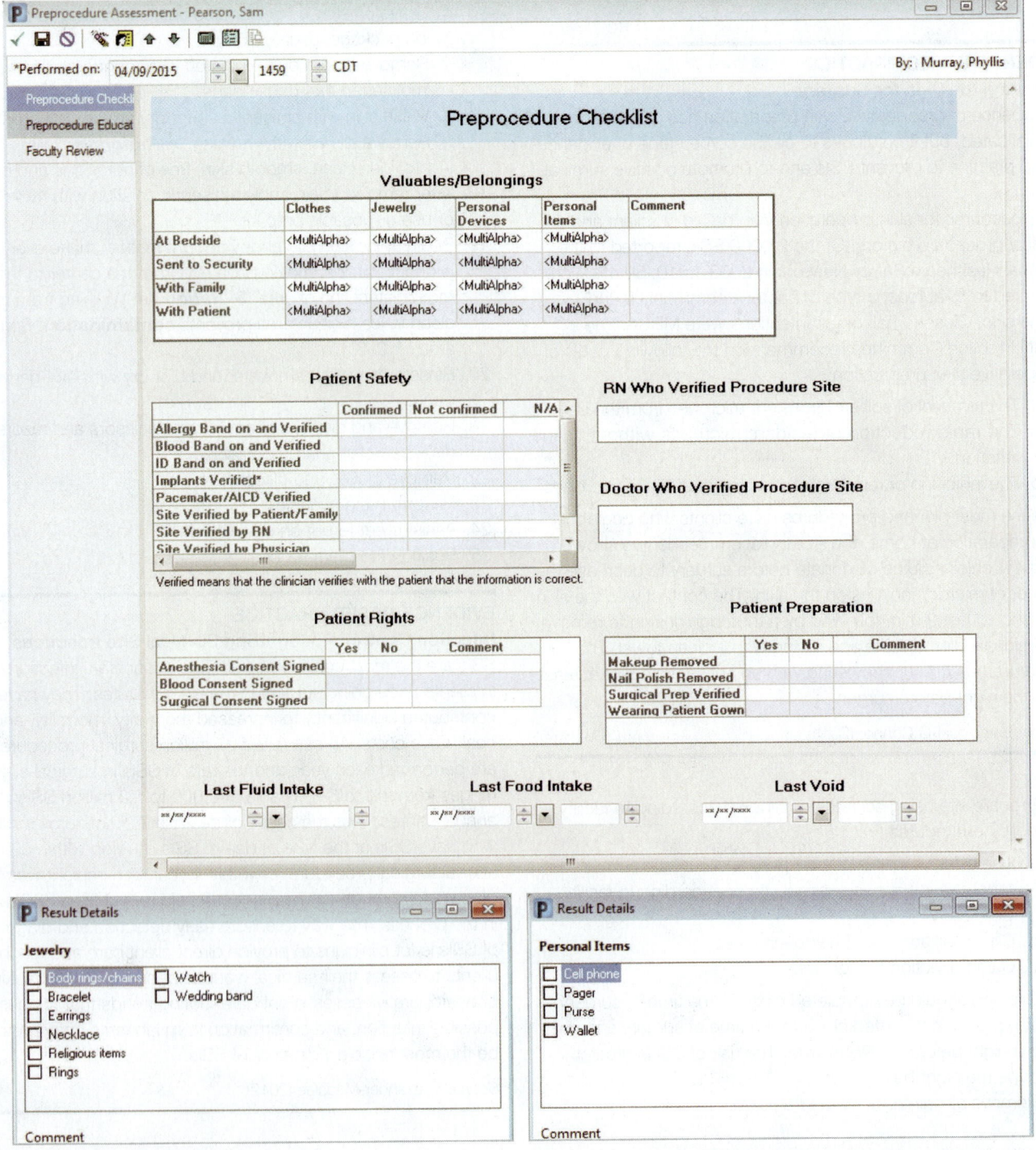

❶ Preoperative checklist. *Source:* From Cerner Electronic Health Record. © Cerner Corporation. Pearson has restricted permission to reproduce and distribute this copyrighted work. Further reproduction or distribution is strictly prohibited without written consent of Cerner Corporation.

Note: Informed consent means that the client has not only consented to the procedure, but is fully knowledgeable about all the possible risks and consequences. A physician having the client sign a general consent form only gives permission for the physician to perform a procedure. No further information is provided. To be able to sign an informed consent, clients must be in full control of their faculties and be legally capable of giving such consent.

❷ Surgical consent form.

❸ Preanesthesia evaluation form. *Source:* From Cerner Electronic Health Record. © Cerner Corporation. Pearson has restricted permission to reproduce and distribute this copyrighted work. Further reproduction or distribution is strictly prohibited without written consent of Cerner Corporation.

3. Assist client to complete anesthesia questionnaire ❸ if required.
4. Assess whether bowel prep was completed at home.
   ➤ *Rationale:* Most clients complete bowel prep before admission to facility. Administer an enema if ordered.
5. Assist client to shower if not completed at home. Instruct on how to shower and specific time guidelines according to facility guidelines.
6. Complete skin prep, if ordered. Follow facility guidelines for skin prep.

CLINICAL ALERT

The AORN recommends preoperative skin prep should be with an antimicrobial agent that has a broad germicidal range and is nontoxic.

The most common antiseptic agents used for preoperative skin preparation and surgical scrubs include alcohol, chlorhexidine, iodine/iodophor, and Triclosan.

Alcohol has the most rapid microbial action, which denatures proteins and is effective against both gram-positive (gram +) and gram-negative (gram –) bacteria, viruses, and fungi.

Chlorhexidine has an intermediate rapidity of action, disrupting the cell membrane. It should not be used on mucous membranes, eyes, or brain tissue (neurotoxic). It works well against gram-positive bacteria, and less well against gram-negative bacteria.

Iodine or **iodophor** has an intermediate action and is acceptable for use against a wide range of bacteria, fungi, and viruses.

Triclosan disrupts the cell wall and has an acceptable kill rate against bacteria. Even though alcohol has microbial action, it is not often used as a surgical skin prep because it does not stay on the skin.

---

7. Assess for latex allergy. If present, ensure allergy band is applied, physician is notified, and OR staff are notified.
   ➤ *Rationale:* All latex products must be removed from OR and client must be scheduled for first case in morning.
8. Assess for symptoms and observe for signs of cold or upper respiratory infection.
9. Explain need for client to be NPO for 8–10 hr preoperatively.
10. Remove lipstick and nail polish if required by hospital policy.
11. Insert Foley catheter if ordered.
12. Take and record vital signs.
13. Remove earrings, necklaces, medals, watch, rings (ring may be taped to finger or toe in some facilities). If possible, remove body piercing jewelry. Cover with tape if not possible to remove. ➤ *Rationale:* This protects skin from possible burns from electrical arcing generated by electrical cautery machines.
14. Remove contact lenses, glasses, hairpieces, and dentures. Some hospitals or anesthesiologists allow full dentures to remain if using a mask.
15. Assist client to void if catheter not inserted, and record time and amount.
16. Check identification band, blood band, and allergy bracelet. During this stage, the client must be identified by at least two identifiers (i.e., name, birth date, medical record number).

(continued)

Skill 26.3.3 | Preparing The Client For Surgery *(continued)*

17. Put antiembolic stockings on client as ordered.
18. Administer preoperative medications.
19. The operative site needs to be verified and marked, both site and side, by the physician while the client is awake.
20. Place side rails in UP position and bed in low position after administration of medications.
21. Darken room and provide quiet environment after administration of medications.
22. Check client 15 min after medication administered to observe for possible side effects.

CLINICAL ALERT

Universal Protocol for Preventing Wrong Site, Wrong Procedure, and Wrong Person Surgery

- Preoperative validation of the right client, procedure, and site should occur when the client is awake, aware, and before he or she leaves the preoperative area or enters the surgical suite.
- Individual performing the procedure must do the marking.
- Incision site must be marked, using a marker that is not easily removed, at or near the incision site.
- DO NOT MARK any nonoperative site(s) unless necessary for some other aspect of care.
- Use initials, word "yes," or a line indicating proposed incision site to prevent ambiguous marks.
- Mark must be visible after client is prepped and draped.
- Final verification of site mark must take place in the location where the procedure will take place. This time is identified as the "Time Out" period. Nothing happens until this has occurred. The entire team must be present during this check.

- Verification must include the following:
  a. Correct client identity
  b. Correct site and side
  c. Agreement on procedure to be done
  d. Correct client position
  e. Availability of any special equipment or implants needed for procedure

Exemptions From the Marking Procedure

Single organ cases (e.g., C-section, cardiac surgery)
Interventional cases: insertion site of instrument or catheter not predetermined
Premature infants: for whom the ink may cause a permanent mark

Source: The Joint Commission (2013)

Note: The Universal Protocol is now accessible as part of the National Patient Safety Goals.

LEGAL ALERT

In 2001, The Joint Commission reported surgical mistakes were on the rise. After this report, a study was completed. The study analyzed 126 cases involving surgical mistakes and found that 76% of the cases involved operating on the wrong body part, 13% involved the wrong client, and 11% involved the wrong surgical procedure.

Reviewing medical liability settlements and judgments from 1990 to 2010, the federal repository of medical liability claims published a report in the December 2012 issue of *Surgery*. Approximately 80 times each week, U.S. clients undergoing surgery experience mistakes that safety advocates say never should happen. Errors consist of surgical instruments or sponges left in the client, wrong procedure performed, wrong surgical site operated on, and surgery done on the wrong client. They indicate a surgical "never" event occurs about once every 12,000 procedures. Even though this does not seem like a high number, it translates to 80 times a week.

Source: O'Reilly (2013)

EVIDENCE-BASED PRACTICE

Surgical Checklist May Improve Outcomes for Noncardiac Surgery

Surgical procedures are estimated at 234 million operations performed yearly throughout the world. A longitudinal study over 1 year utilized eight participating hospitals representing a diverse group of socioeconomic environments within the WHO regions from Amman, Jordan, to Seattle, Washington, and Toronto, Canada. The study included more than 3,700 consecutive inpatient noncardiac surgery clients 16 years or older. The objective of the study was to evaluate the effect on rates of mortality and major complications with implementing the surgical checklist in inpatient surgical units. Data were first prospectively collected regarding clinical processes and outcomes. After implementing the Surgical Safety Checklist, data were collected from the cohort of consecutive inpatient noncardiac surgery clients.

Death rates during hospitalization decreased from 1.5% in the initial cohort to 0.8% after implementing the checklist. This represents a decline in the rate of inpatient complications from 11.0% to 7.0%.

Source: Barclay (2009)

Skill 26.3.4 | Administering Preoperative Medications

Equipment
Preoperative checklist
Preoperative medications

Procedure

1. Check two forms of client identification and introduce yourself. Perform hand hygiene and provide privacy.
2. Complete preoperative checklist.
3. Check orders for medication, dosage, route, and time (Box 26-5 ■).
4. Verify that surgical consent is accurate, understood by client, and properly signed before giving any pre-op sedation.
5. Check history for allergy to ordered medication.
6. Explain purpose of medication to client.
7. Warn client that injection may sting or burn.
8. Follow procedure for administration of injections.
9. Administer medications 30 min before beginning of surgery.
10. Raise side rails to UP position and put bed in low position.
11. Explain why client should not get out of bed after medications have been given. ➤ *Rationale:* Medication makes client drowsy and affects equilibrium.

Box 26-5 PREOPERATIVE MEDICATIONS: TYPE AND ACTION

Hypnotic or Antianxiolytic—Given Night Before Surgery
Decreases anxiety
Promotes good night's sleep

Hypnotic or Opiate—Preoperative Medication
Decreases anxiety
Allows smooth anesthetic **induction**
Provides amnesia for immediate perioperative period

Anticholinergic—Preoperative Medication
Decreases secretions
Counteracts vagal effects during anesthesia

12. Place call light within reach and encourage client to use it.
13. Ask if there are any questions or assistance you can offer before leaving the room. Darken room or close curtains.
14. Inform client of the estimated time he or she will be going to surgery.

EVIDENCE-BASED PRACTICE

Antibiotic Prophylaxis to Prevent Surgical Site Infections

SSIs are the most common healthcare-associated infections in surgical clients. These infections occur at or near a surgical incision within 30 days of the procedure, or within 1 year if an implant is left in place. The Centers for Disease Control and Prevention (CDC) estimates that about half a million SSIs occur annually in the United States. They are the leading cause of healthcare-associated infections after surgery. They account for nearly 4 million excess hospital days annually and nearly $2 billion in increased health care costs. The Surgical Care Improvement Project (SCIP)—created by the CDC and the Centers for Medicare and Medicaid Services (CMS)—developed six infection prevention measures. Of these, three measures contain recommendations regarding selection of a prophylactic antibiotic, timing of administration, and duration of therapy. A cephalosporin was selected as the recommended prophylactic antibiotic for clients undergoing clean-contaminated surgeries (cardiothoracic, gastrointestinal, **orthopedic**, vascular, gynecologic).

The SCIP developed the core infection prevention measures:

1. Prophylactic antibiotics should be initiated within 1 hr before surgical incision, or within 2 hr if the client is receiving vancomycin or fluoroquinolones.

2. Prophylactic antibiotics should be appropriate for their specific procedure.

3. Prophylactic antibiotics should be discontinued within 24 hr after surgery completion (within 48 hr for cardiothoracic surgery).

4. Postoperative 6 a.m. blood glucose levels should be controlled at 200 mg/dL (11.10 mmol/L) or less in clients undergoing cardiac surgery.

5. Surgical site hair removal should be appropriate for the location and procedure (e.g., clippers, depilation, no hair removal).

6. Clients undergoing colorectal surgery should be normothermic (96.8°F [36°C]) within the first 15 min after leaving the operating room.

A recent survey of U.S. hospitals found that the recommendations are not routinely followed. Fewer than 10% of surgical clients received prophylactic antibiotics within 1 hr of incision and they were discontinued within the 24 hr after surgery in fewer than half the clients. Other studies show approximately 80–90% of the clients received antibiotic prophylaxis, but the choice of regimen, timing of administration, or duration of prophylaxis were inappropriate in approximately one-quarter to half those clients. As an incentive, the CMS reduced reimbursement to hospitals for some of these infections.

Source: Salkind & Kavitha (2011)

Unit 26.3 Documentation and Evaluation

DOCUMENTATION for Preoperative Care

- Safety measures carried out preoperatively
- Completion of preoperative site preparation and area involved
- Antiseptic solution used and length of time of scrub
- Operative checklist completed
- Review of physician's explanation of potential surgical complications
- Physical care completed before surgery

- Surgical site marking procedure (site, individual who marked site, individuals present during "Time Out" step in procedure)
- Preoperative medications given and effects of medications
- Time and method of transportation to operating room
- Preoperative teaching completed

EVALUATION/Critical Thinking

Expected Outcomes

- Client's physical or emotional deviations from normal are identified preoperatively.
- Preoperative baseline data are obtained.
- Surgical site is marked and prepared correctly.
- Client states expectations regarding intraoperative and postoperative course.

Unexpected Outcomes	Alternative Actions
• Factors that can affect the postoperative course are identified during the preoperative care (e.g., arthritic changes in client's back, history of thrombophlebitis).	• Place information in client's care plan and inform charge nurse and surgeon about findings. • Write a note in client's chart and alert the operating room and recovery room staff of the findings so that they can assess for the problems.
• Client refuses to go to operating room without dentures.	• Explain to client that dentures are likely to be lost, broken, or inadvertently pushed to back of mouth if not removed. • If client refuses to remove dentures, alert anesthesiologist that dentures are in place.
• Client unable to void before surgery.	• Run water so client can hear trickling sound to stimulate voiding. • Run warm water over perineum. • Place ammonia or oil of wintergreen on a cotton ball in urinal or bedpan. • Help male to stand or sit at edge of bed with urinal positioned. • Help female to commode if urinating into bedpan is difficult. • Notify MD and OR staff. Record in chart.

Unexpected Outcomes	Alternative Actions
• Client appears to be abnormally stressed.	• Explore feelings and reasons for client's or family's stressed behaviors. • Explore more effective methods to reduce stress for client and family. • Provide additional stress reduction exercises. • Clarify misconceptions and inappropriate perceptions. • Introduce client to another client who has had similar surgery. • Have physician speak to client and answer questions.
• Client's preoperative laboratory findings are abnormal.	• Check with laboratory to have them reevaluate if lab results are accurate. • Have laboratory redo tests if extremely abnormal. • Notify physician of abnormal findings. • Notify surgeon and anesthesiologist.
• Client is unable to participate in marking surgical site.	• If client is comatose, non–English speaking, or incompetent, follow protocol as with informed consent. • Guardian or individual with power of attorney should be involved with marking, if possible.
• Client refuses site marking.	• Client has right to refuse; document client refusal on appropriate forms. • Procedure may be performed without marking. • Provide client with information regarding safety aspects for marking procedure. • Discuss rationale for client's refusal to determine whether insufficient information was provided regarding marking procedure.

Moderate Sedation (Conscious Sedation)

Nursing Process Data

ASSESSMENT Database

- Assess type of procedure to be done and determine whether moderate sedation (conscious sedation) is appropriate.
- Assess type of sedation to be used for procedure.
- Determine whether medication can be administered by nurse or only by physician.
- Check whether physician has ordered medication for moderate sedation (conscious sedation) and whether nurse is approved to administer medication.
- Determine whether history and physical is in client's chart.
- Check that signed consent form is in chart.
- Assess client according to American Society of Anesthesiologists (ASA) Classification of Physical Status.

PLANNING Objectives

- To determine whether client is to receive moderate sedation (conscious sedation) from nurse or physician
- To establish venous access before sedation administration
- To monitor vital signs throughout procedure
- To continuously assess for changes in client's condition or untoward responses or effects of medication
- To immediately notify physician of changes in client's condition

IMPLEMENTATION Procedures

DOCUMENTATION AND EVALUATION

Expected Outcomes

- Client maintains airway and respiratory status throughout procedure.
- Client does not experience anxiety or pain during procedure.

Unexpected Outcomes/Nursing Actions

Pearson Nursing Student Resources

Find additional review materials at **nursing.pearsonhighered.com.**
Prepare for success with NCLEX®-style practice questions and Skill Checklists.

Skill 26.4.1 | Preparing Client for Moderate Sedation (Conscious Sedation)

Equipment
Consent form
History and physical
Lab test results, if necessary
Sedation scale ❶

Procedure

1. Ensure that client is candidate for moderate sedation (conscious sedation). Use ASA Classification of Physical Status (Box 26-6 ■). ➤ **Rationale:** Clients in ASA categories 1 and 2 may receive moderate sedation by qualified physicians and nurses. Clients in category 3 or 4 are referred to anesthesia provider for further evaluation because their condition puts them at risk for complications. Further evaluation of older adult, pregnant, or obese clients, and those with a history of substance abuse, sleep apnea, or severe cardiac, respiratory, hepatic, renal, or central nervous system (CNS) diseases is necessary because these clients are placed at higher risk during the use of moderate sedation.

2. Determine whether client has any contraindications for moderate sedation (conscious sedation):

   a. Recent ingestion of large food or fluid volumes (in past 2 hr)

   b. Physical status IV or greater

   c. Lack of support staff or monitoring equipment

   d. Lack of experience on part of clinician

3. Determine whether nurse or physician will administer medication.

4. Check that qualified anesthesia provider has written order for moderate sedation.

5. Check two forms of client ID and introduce yourself. Perform hand hygiene.

6. Check that client has been informed about procedure and use of moderate sedation.

7. Ensure that history and physical has been completed and on client's chart.

8. Obtain height and weight. ➤ **Rationale:** These are needed for drug calculation when administering moderate sedation.

9. Ask about allergies, particularly sedatives.

10. Ensure client has been NPO for at least 2 hr.

11. Explain that the medication will relax him or her during procedure, client will feel sleepy but will not be asleep, and will be able to communicate during procedure.
    ➤ **Rationale:** This is necessary to determine comfort and level of sedation during procedure.

12. Discuss the possibility of unpleasant sensations of pain, nausea, and vertigo.

13. Determine gestures that will be used during procedure to indicate whether client is having pain.

14. Ensure that someone is with the client to take him or her home if discharge is anticipated after the procedure.
    ➤ **Rationale:** Residual effects of sedation can last for several hours. Driving can be impaired and thus it is unsafe for the client to drive home.

Note: The American Nurses Association and other nursing organizations allow nurses to administer sedating drugs, assess client responses, and monitor vital signs during the use of conscious sedation. Nurses who administer conscious sedation must function within the standard of practice and be allowed to administer conscious sedation according to the Nurse Practice Act in the state in which they are practicing. They must also administer conscious sedation according to policies and procedures of the facility in which they are working. At no time are student nurses allowed to administer conscious sedation.

❶ Moderate (conscious) sedation record samples. *Source:* From Cerner Electronic Health Record. © Cerner Corporation. Pearson has restricted permission to reproduce and distribute this copyrighted work. Further reproduction or distribution is strictly prohibited without written consent of Cerner Corporation.

Box 26-6 ASA CLASSIFICATION OF PHYSICAL STATUS

Class	Definition
P1	A normal, healthy client
P2	A client with mild systemic disease
P3	A client with severe systemic disease
P4	A client with severe systemic disease that is a constant threat to life
P5	A moribund client who is not expected to survive without surgery
P6	A declared brain-dead client whose organs are being removed for donation

Source: Adapted from the American Society of Anesthesiologists (2010)

Skill 26.4.2 | Monitoring Client During Procedure

Equipment

Crash cart or following list of equipment:

Suction equipment; machine, tubing, and suction catheter (tonsil tip)

Oxygen supply and appropriate delivery system

Laryngoscope handle and blades of appropriate size

Endotracheal tubes and stylets in various sizes

Oral and nasal cannulas

3-mL and 10-mL syringes

Needles, if not using needless system

IV solution bags

Reversal drug agents (i.e., naloxone [Narcan], flumazenil [Romazicon])

Pulse oximeter (optional with capnography)

ECG machine and defibrillator, cardiac monitor

Intubation tray and bag–valve–mask device

Vital sign portable machine

Client's chart

Procedural sedation record

Conscious sedation medications; usually benzodiazepines and opioids

Emergency cardiac drugs, reversal agents: naloxone, flumazenil

Procedure

1. Ensure that backup personnel skilled in advanced cardiac life support (ACLS) are available if needed.
2. Verify correct client by using two identifiers.
3. Evaluate ASA Classification of Physical Status again.
4. Check that chart contains appropriate documents.
5. Check that preprocedural assessment is completed on sedation record.
6. Check that consent form was signed.
7. Gather emergency equipment, including reversal drugs, and place near client.
8. Determine whether premedication was ordered and given.
9. Obtain vital signs and document findings on procedural sedation record.
10. Start peripheral IV with ordered solution.
11. Determine gesture to be used for communication regarding pain and sedation.
12. Place ECG leads on, if appropriate.
13. Administer oxygen via nasal cannula at 2 L/min.
14. Monitor end-tidal CO_2 with capnography (Box 26-7 ■).

15. Begin administration of medication as ordered.
16. Monitor for signs of drug reactions.
17. Monitor vital signs, oxygen saturation, sedation level, pain level, ECG rate, and rhythm every 1–5 min according to facility policy and client condition (Table 26-6 ■).
    ➤ *Rationale:* Close monitoring of these values identifies potential complications such as respiratory depression, oversedation, hypoxia, and hypotension.

> **CLINICAL ALERT**
>
> The sedation assessment parameters that need to be observed during the procedure include responsiveness, speech, facial expressions, and eyes. Scales available that provide a scoring system are the Ramsay Sedation Scale and the Riker Sedation–Agitation Scale.

18. Continue to monitor client every 15 min until stable after completion of procedure using conscious sedation.

> **LEGAL ALERT**
> **Operating Room Negligence**
>
> A common litigation against operating room nurses involves sponges or instruments left in a client after a surgical procedure. It is the nurse's responsibility to accurately count and monitor the sponges and equipment.

Box 26-7 CAPNOGRAPHY

Capnography has been shown to be effective in detecting hypoventilation during procedural sedation. The traditional PCA pump now has built in sensors that monitor ventilation and oxygenation. It is also used to monitor clients on PCA pumps using **narcotics**.

A capnography monitor is a device that measures carbon dioxide. The monitor is attached to tubing at the end of the tracheostomy or endotracheal tube. The Alaris PCA pump with capnography/pulse oximetry has a module that measures CO_2. CO_2 can also be measured by attaching a tube to an oxygen mask or nasal cannula. The mask or nasal cannula contains a sensor that measures CO_2. The results are reported on a handheld device rather than the monitor.

Table 26-6 Levels of Sedation/Analgesia

Level of Sedation	Client Response
Minimal (Anxiolysis)	Client is relaxed but able to respond to verbal commands. Cognitive function and coordination may be impaired; ventilator and cardiovascular functions are not affected.
Moderate (conscious)	Client has depression of consciousness that is drug induced but still responds purposefully to verbal commands. Airway remains patent with spontaneous ventilation and cardiovascular status maintained.
Deep	Client will sleep through procedure with little or no memory of the procedure. Airway intervention may be required (supplemental oxygen or ventilator support); cardiovascular status is maintained

Source: Orlewicz (2014)

Equipment
Electronic vital sign machine
Oxygen supply
Oxygen nasal cannula
Procedural sedation record
Aldrete scale
Pulse oximeter
ECG monitor and leads
Emergency equipment
Naloxone

Procedure
1. Check two forms of client ID and introduce yourself. Perform hand hygiene.
2. Observe vital signs, oxygen saturation, respiratory rate and rhythm, and ECG rate and rhythm every 15 min unless more frequent monitoring is required according to client condition. ➤ *Rationale:* Major complications during and immediately after the use of moderate (conscious) sedation include respiratory depression, oversedation, hypoxia, and hypotension (Table 26-7 ■). Assess need for naloxone, an antagonist of the opioids, to reverse a narcotic **analgesic** (rarely needed).
3. Observe client for patent airway if he or she was intubated during procedure and ensure oxygen cannula is in place immediately after extubation. Place oxygen cannula on client if using pulse oximeter.
4. Assess client for pain, and medicate accordingly.
5. Monitor client and obtain sedation scale score in preparation for discharge. Client must attain specified score within 1 hr of completion of procedure. ➤ *Rationale:* If using Aldrete Scale, client must attain Aldrete score of ±1 point of preprocedure score before discharge. This score should be achieved within 1 hr of the procedure. A potential complication is occurring if this score is not attained within the specified time.
6. Provide instructions as needed before client is discharged.
7. Ensure client has someone with him or her if discharged to home.
8. Complete documentation on Procedural Sedation Record.

Note: Monitor ECG continuously if client is at high risk or has had a prolonged procedure.

Table 26-7 Moderate Sedation (Conscious) Sedation Medications

	Benzodiazepines	Opioids
Drugs	Midazolam (Versed), diazepam, lorazepam*	Fentanyl, morphine, meperidine; ketamine is used for pediatric clients.
Action	Produce anxiolysis and amnesia	Produce sedation, **euphoria**, pain relief
Disadvantages	Lack of analgesic properties	Can cause respiratory depression and decreased level of consciousness
Side Effects	Decreased blood pressure, increased heart rate	Apnea, hypotension, vertigo, nausea
Reversal Agent	Flumazenil	Naloxone

Note: The most common drugs used for conscious sedation are the benzodiazepines and opioids.

*Frequently administered with narcotics; Versed and Fentanyl are the most commonly used drugs in these classifications.

Unit 26.4 Documentation and Evaluation

DOCUMENTATION for Moderate Sedation (Conscious Sedation)

- Preprocedural assessment: past medical history, drug allergies, anesthetic history
- Consent form signed
- Baseline vital signs, particularly respiratory and cardiac findings, ECG findings
- Height and weight
- Teaching provided regarding medication and procedure
- ASA rating
- Continuous documentation of level of consciousness, speech, facial expression, agitation level, pupils, respiratory rate and rhythm, ECG findings if appropriate during procedure
- Score on a sedation scale (Aldrete, Ramsay, or Riker)
- Oxygen saturation levels during and after procedure

- Amount and type of medication administered
- Supplemental oxygen, liter flow, and system used
- Aldrete score before discharge

- Complications that occurred during the procedure and actions taken
- Complete Procedural Sedation Record

EVALUATION/Critical Thinking

Expected Outcomes

- Client maintains airway and respiratory status throughout procedure.
- Client does not experience anxiety or pain during procedure.

Unexpected Outcomes

Alternative Actions

- Client is scheduled to have conscious sedation for procedure but scores above P2 on ASA scale.

- Notify anesthesiologist and physician; nurses may not administer conscious sedation if the client scores above P2 on the scale.
- Client is physically compromised and could be unstable during use of conscious sedation medications.

- Client does not respond to verbal commands during procedure when using minimal or moderate sedation.

- Notify physician of change in client's status.
- Notify anesthesiologist immediately and prepare for intubation.
- Have reversal drug available to administer if directed by physician.
- Continue to monitor client every 1 min for changes in status.
- Administer oxygen via nasal cannula if not already in place.

- Client experiences airway obstruction or respiratory depression.

- Reposition client's head, lifting jaw and tipping back the head.
- Suction client or insert oral airway.
- Be prepared to bag client with bag–valve–mask device.

- Client experiences hypoxemia.

- Ensure pulse oximeter is on client.
- Check respiratory rate, pattern, and effort.
- Increase amount of oxygen delivered. May need to change delivery system to oxygen mask.
- Use capnography to evaluate CO_2 level.

- Client experiences a 20% drop in blood pressure during procedure.

- Inform physician.
- Assess client for potential complications leading to decrease in blood pressure.
- Check for presence of hypovolemia. Administer 200 mL bolus of fluid and monitor for response.

- Client experiences pain during procedure.

- Dosage of amnesia or analgesic agents needs to be reviewed.
- Ensure client's weight was calculated correctly.
- Allow sufficient time for agents to work.
- Allow time to titrate effect of medication.

Postanesthesia Care Unit (PACU) and Discharge

Nursing Process Data

ASSESSMENT Database

- Assess for patent airway.
- Assess for order and type of oxygen administration set.
- Check gag reflex and remove endotracheal tube as ordered.
- Assess vital signs and appropriate pulses.
- Assess body temperature.
- Check all IVs for type, amount of fluid, and infusion rate.
- Observe all dressings, tubes, and drains.
- Monitor urine output, color, and consistency.
- Assess color, skin temperature, and condition.
- Assess monitor findings if ordered.
- Assess neurologic status if necessary.
- Assess heart and lung sounds.
- Assess bowel sounds.
- Assess residual anesthetic effect.
- Assess for postoperative bleeding.

PLANNING Objectives

- To provide safe, effective nursing care during the immediate postoperative period for clients in the recovery room
- To promote and maintain adequate airway function
- To monitor and maintain adequate circulatory status
- To identify potential postanesthesia complications and initiate nursing interventions to prevent complications
- To evaluate pain control
- To identify client's readiness to return to nursing unit or to be discharged if an outpatient
- To use Hand-off communication process when discharging client to surgical unit

IMPLEMENTATION Procedures

DOCUMENTATION AND EVALUATION

Expected Outcomes

- Client has an uneventful experience in the recovery period.
- Potential postoperative complications are identified early, and corrective interventions prevent occurrence of complications.
- Client is discharged to home or nursing unit within prescribed time frame.
- Client reports pain: <4 on a scale of 0–10.
- Client does not experience nausea or vomiting.

Unexpected Outcomes/Alternative Actions

Pearson Nursing Student Resources

Find additional review materials at **nursing.pearsonhighered.com.**
Prepare for success with NCLEX®-style practice questions and Skill Checklists.

EVIDENCE-BASED PRACTICE
Effects of Poor Hand-Offs

Incomplete **Hand-offs** and insufficient communication regarding key clinical information may lead to adverse events or missed or delayed diagnoses. This analysis of data from the AHRQ Hospital Survey of Patient Safety Culture sought to determine how perceptions of organizational factors that affect safety can contribute to optimal Hand-offs. Although client Hand-offs have been studied extensively, they continue to be problematic. Studies have shown poor Hand-offs are associated with increased costs, morbidity, and mortality. No prior research had compared perception of management and

clinical staff regarding Hand-offs. The purpose of the study was to determine whether perceptions of organizational factors that can influence client safety are positively associated with perceptions of successful client Hand-offs. Perceived teamwork across units was a significant predictor for successful Hand-offs. Perceptions of staffing adequacy and management support for client safety efforts were also related to good Hand-offs. Open communication was associated with optimal Hand-offs. The authors of this study advocate for hospital leadership to promote teamwork and open communication to improve Hand-offs.

Source: Richter, McAlearney, & Pennell (2014)

Skill 26.5.1 | Providing Postanesthesia Care

Equipment
Blood pressure cuff and stethoscope
Pulse oximeter
Oxygen administration device: nasal cannula or mask
Cardiac monitor and leads
IV pole
Suction catheters
Gloves
Special equipment needed—based on surgical procedure

Procedure
1. Check two forms of client identification, introduce yourself, and determine surgical procedure performed.
2. Complete Hand-off communication process (Box 26-8 ■).

> **CLINICAL ALERT**
> - Ineffective communication is the most frequently cited root cause of sentinel events.
> - Adverse events occur more often for surgical clients than clients in other clinical specialties.

3. Connect client to monitoring systems.
4. Assess for patent airway. Leave airway in place until gag reflex returns and client attempts to remove it. ➤ *Rationale:* This promotes adequate airway exchange and prevents tongue from falling back and occluding airway.
5. Administer humidified SpO$_2$ by mask or nasal cannula at 6 L/min or as ordered. ➤ *Rationale:* Humidified oxygen prevents drying of the tracheobronchial tree and liquefies secretions to facilitate expectoration.
6. Monitor oxygen saturation using pulse oximetry (SpO$_2$).
7. Monitor carbon dioxide levels in client's expiration, using capnography.
8. Encourage client to cough and deep breathe when awake.
9. Suction client as needed.
10. Position client to ensure adequate ventilation. Side-lying position is best if not contraindicated. Turn every hour if not contraindicated. ➤ *Rationale:* This prevents pooling of secretions in lungs and assists with ventilation.

Box 26-8 HAND-OFF COMMUNICATION
- Report focuses on client safety.
- Report is coordinated effort among healthcare professionals involved in changeover of client.
- Communication must be accurate, clear, specific, and allow time for questions and concerns.
- Communication occurs in all areas of surgical care.

SBAR Approach to Hand-off Communication
S – Situation—Identify yourself and the client. State what is happening with the client.
B – Background—Review chart. Provide the client's background. Anticipate other caregiver's questions.
A – Assessment—Provide your observations and evaluation of client's current state. Be accurate and complete.
R – Recommendations—Make informal suggestions based on correct information for continued care of client.

Note: Standardized approach to Hand-off communications is part of National Patient Safety Goals from The Joint Commission.

---

11. Monitor vital signs every 5–15 min as condition warrants. Vital signs are sometimes difficult to obtain due to **hypothermia** and movement from operating room to postanesthesia care unit. ❶
    a. Check pulse rate, quality, and rhythm; include pulse distal to surgical site. ❷
    b. Check blood pressure, pulse pressure, and quality.
    c. Check respiratory rate, rhythm, depth, and pattern.
    d. Assess pain level, determine cause, and medicate as needed.
12. Maintain body temperature by applying warm blankets or use Bair Paws Warming System. This same system can be used throughout the perioperative process, PACU, and nursing unit.
13. Observe for adverse signs of general or spinal anesthesia:
    a. Level of consciousness
    b. Movement of extremities

1 Recovery room is usually an open space for easy observation of all clients.

2 Clients are connected to a monitoring system for cardiac surveillance.

14. Monitor IV fluids.

    a. Verify correct type and amount of solution being administered.

    b. Set appropriate flow rate using IV pump or controller if needed.

    c. Observe IV site for signs of infiltration.

    d. Maintain accurate IV intake record.

15. Monitor blood or blood component infusions.

    a. Identify appropriate replacement fluid.

    b. Check client's name and identification number with fluid.

    c. Check blood type, blood bank number, and expiration date.

    d. Check time infusion initiated.

    e. Observe and record amount of fluid remaining in bag when admitted to recovery room.

    f. Determine time frame for completion of fluid.

16. Monitor and measure urine output hourly if indwelling catheter is in place or before client leaves recovery room.

17. Observe surgical dressings and drains hourly.

    a. Follow hospital policy for marking drainage on dressings.

    b. Note color and amount of drainage on dressings and from drains or tubes.

    c. Check that dressings are secure.

    d. Reinforce dressings as needed.

    e. Empty drainage collection device as needed.

    f. Report unusual amount or type of drainage to physician before client leaves recovery room.

18. Monitor skin for warmth, color, and moisture.

19. Check nail beds and mucous membranes for color and blanching. Immediately report unusual findings or signs of cyanosis to physician.

20. Orient client to surroundings and relieve anxiety and fear.

21. Observe for return of movement, especially if client received spinal or epidural anesthesia.

22. Monitor for muscle strength and movement.

23. Administer all STAT drugs.

24. Provide pain medication as needed.

25. Complete PAR record.

26. Assess parameters for discharge from postanesthesia room.

Skill 26.5.2 | Discharging Client From Postanesthesia Unit to Nursing Unit

Procedure

1. Assess that lung sounds are clear to auscultation and airway is maintained without artificial measures (unless client is to remain on mechanical assistance).

2. Assess that vital signs are within normal range for at least 1 hr and appropriate for client's condition.

3. Observe that client is awake, alert, and responds to commands.

4. Assess that reflexes are present (including gag, swallowing) and that client can move all extremities.

5. Assess skin color and nail beds for signs of cyanosis.

6. Ensure IVs are patent, infusing with correct solution and at prescribed rate. Record total amount of IV fluid infused and amount remaining in bags. Ensure all IVs and irrigating solutions are in sufficient quantity for transfer and immediate continuity of care.

7. Check that all dressings are intact, and there is no excessive drainage from drains or tubes. Reinforce dressings if needed and empty all drainage collection receptacles before returning to nursing unit.

8. Ensure urinary output is adequate. Record all urine output and empty drainage bag before transporting to nursing unit.

(continued)

Skill 26.5.2 | Discharging Client From Postanesthesia Unit to Nursing Unit *(continued)*

9. Record all medications administered in recovery room.
10. Medicate client ½ hr before transport if vital signs are stable and client requires pain medication. ➤ **Rationale:** Transporting clients from postanesthesia room can increase pain due to moving and transfer from gurney to bed.
11. Call anesthesiologist for discharge orders or use Aldrete Postanesthesia Recovery Scoring System if used by facility (Table 26-8 ■).
12. Call for transport assistance if available. Postanesthesia room nurse accompanies client to nursing unit.

13. Call nursing unit and provide information on equipment needs for client (e.g., oxygen, IVs).
14. Document all findings in computer or in chart before discharge.
15. Prepare data for Hand-off communication with surgical floor RN (Box 26-9 ■).

Table 26-8 Aldrete Postanesthesia Recovery Scoring System

Activity
2 = moves all four extremities voluntarily or on command
1 = moves two extremities voluntarily or on command
0 = unable to move any extremity voluntarily or on command
Respiration
2 = able to breathe, cough freely
1 = requires assistance, shallow or limited breathing
0 = apneic
Circulation
2 = BP +20 mm Hg of preanesthetic level
1 = BP +20 to +50 mm Hg of preanesthetic level
0 = BP +50 mm Hg of preanesthetic level
Consciousness
2 = fully awake
1 = arousable on calling
0 = not responding
Oxygen saturation
2 = SpO$_2$ greater than 92% on room air
1 = Supplemental O$_2$ required to maintain SpO$_2$ greater than 90%
0 = SpO$_2$ supplementation
10 = Total score higher than 9 for PACU discharge

Note: This is one method for determining whether postanesthesia room discharge criteria have been met. In addition to stable vital signs, a total score of 10 for the five assessed areas must be achieved for nurses to discharge clients without a physician's order.

Box 26-9 SBAR DATA TO INCLUDE IN HAND-OFF COMMUNICATION PROCESS

Situation
1. Client's name and date of birth
2. Procedure completed with site identified

Background
1. Type of anesthesia and name of anesthesia care provider
2. Intraoperative PACU medications; dose and time
3. IV fluids administered in OR and PACU
4. Estimated blood loss
5. Data regarding dressings, tubes, drains, or packing
6. Significant OR events and PACU events

Assessment
1. Hemodynamic stability
2. Airway and oxygenation status
3. Temperature
4. Urine output
5. Surgical complications if present
6. Pain level
7. Type of pain management

Recommendations
1. Ensure PACU MD orders were completed.
2. Ensure surgeon's plan of care has been implemented.
3. Identify educational needs for client and family.
4. Provide discharge instructions.
5. Discharge within 2 hr or when stable.

Source: Amato-Vealey, Barba, & Vealey (2008)

Skill 26.5.3 | Discharging Client From Phase II Unit to Home

Procedure

1. Follow all actions for Skill 26.5.2, Discharging a Client From Postanesthesia Unit to Nursing Unit.
2. Assess for nausea or light-headedness. ➤ **Rationale:** These symptoms may be a result of anesthesia or **hypovolemia**. The client is not discharged until these symptoms have abated or are medically treated.

3. Provide discharge teaching regarding medications, activity, dressing changes, healthcare provider office visit, etc. (Box 26-10 ■). If client is unable to understand instructions, provide information to the individual taking the client home. Send written instructions home with the client as well.

4. Assist client to side of bed, feet on floor, and allow client to sit for a few minutes. ➤ *Rationale:* This is to prevent a fall as a result of postural hypotension when standing.
5. Assess client's ability to dress self or identify what assistance is needed.
6. Ensure client has urinated, ambulated to bathroom, and is not vomiting before discharge.
7. Obtain prescriptions from pharmacy if needed.
8. Place client's equipment, supplies, and medications in a plastic bag and hand to the individual taking the client home.
9. Transfer client to wheelchair.
10. Take client to car and assist with transfer.
11. Document all activity related to discharge, including individual taking the client home and method of transport.

Box 26-10 SURGICAL SITE INFECTION (SSI) SIGNS AND SYMPTOMS

Hot incision: The incision may feel hot to the touch, resulting from the body sending infection-fighting blood cells to the site of infection.

Edema or hardening of the incision: The tissue underneath the incision is inflamed. The incision itself may appear edematous or puffy.

Redness: Some redness is normal at the incision site, but it should dissipate over time, rather than becoming more red.

Drainage from the incision: Foul-smelling or purulent drainage on the infected incision. The color ranges from blood-tinged to green, white, or yellow. It can be thick.

Pain: If pain level increases for no apparent reason over time at the surgical site, an infection may be developing.

Unit 26.5 Documentation and Evaluation

DOCUMENTATION for Postanesthesia Care

For Nursing Unit

- Assessment findings—follow SBAR
- Effects of anesthesia
- Status of airway management
- Need for oxygen administration
- Status of neurologic signs and reflexes
- Fluid replacement—type and amount
- Blood and blood product replacement
- Medications administered
- Condition of dressings, drains, and tubes
- Intake and output from all sources: urine, drains, tubes, IVs
- Vital signs: T, P, R, BP, and pain
- Description of pain and interventions for relief of pain
- Response to postanesthesia room activities
- Discharged to room (number) and transporter
- Hand-off communication data

For Discharge Home

- Additional charting includes ability to stand or transfer to wheelchair and having urinated
- Discharge teaching completed
- Signs or symptoms of nausea, light-headedness
- Discharged to care at home
- Discharged via automobile or other means of transportation

EVALUATION/Critical Thinking

Expected Outcomes

- Client experiences no untoward effects during recovery period.
- Potential postanesthesia complications are identified early, and appropriate nursing actions are taken to prevent occurrence of complications.
- Client is discharged from postanesthesia unit at appropriate time.

(continued)

Unexpected Outcomes	Alternative Actions
• Client experiences untoward effects in postanesthesia room.	• Contact physician for additional orders. • Complete physical assessment. • Identify and initiate appropriate nursing interventions within allowed guidelines and parameters of the facility.
• Client does not awaken easily.	• Retain client in postanesthesia room; check Glasgow scale. • Continue to provide oxygen. • Arouse every 15 min. • Check pain medication (may need Narcan).
• Client has postoperative hemorrhage.	• Apply direct pressure. • Notify physician immediately. • Assess for signs of hypovolemia. • Assess for signs of overt bleeding (i.e., saturated dressings, large amount of drainage in drainage collection devices, increase in girth of affected surgical area). • Check lab values for hematocrit, hemoglobin, and coagulation levels. • Check records for estimated blood loss during surgery.

Unit 26.6
Postoperative Care

Nursing Process Data

ASSESSMENT Database

- Assess for patent airway.
- Check if oxygen is ordered.
- Check pulse oximetry.
- Auscultate lungs.
- Assess heart sounds and peripheral pulses.
- Observe for adverse signs of general anesthesia or spinal anesthesia.
- Assess pain level using pain scale assessment.
- Take vital signs (T, P, R, BP).
- Check client's temperature for heat control.
- Observe dressings and surgical drains.
- Check IVs for type and amount of fluid to be infused.
- Assess I&O, skin turgor, and hydration.
- Observe color and amount of urine.
- Auscultate bowel sounds, and verify bowel movement and flatus.
- Observe client's overall condition.

PLANNING Objectives

- To ensure that the client experiences an uneventful postoperative course
- To provide safe, effective nursing care in the immediate postoperative period
- To ensure that postoperative pain is relieved promptly
- To be aware of the common postoperative drugs for pain control

IMPLEMENTATION Procedures

DOCUMENTATION AND EVALUATION

Expected Outcomes

- Client experiences an uneventful postoperative course.
- Postoperative nursing interventions are carried out effectively and in a timely manner.
- Client reports pain levels: less than 4 on scale of 0–10.
- Client is free of nausea and vomiting.

Unexpected Outcomes/Alternative Actions

Pearson Nursing Student Resources

Find additional review materials at
nursing.pearsonhighered.com.
Prepare for success with NCLEX®-style practice questions and Skill Checklists.

Skill 26.6.1 | Providing Postoperative Care

Equipment

Absorbent pads
Warm blankets or Bair Paws Warming System
IV pole
Oxygen source, tubing, and equipment
Emesis basin and tissues
Sphygmomanometer and stethoscope
Thermometer (tympanic, oral, or rectal)
Nurses' notes
Intake and output record
Special equipment depending on type of surgery
Pulse oximeter
Sterile dressings

Procedure

1. Perform hand hygiene before each client contact.
2. Check two forms of client identification and introduce self to client.
3. Orient client to time, person, and place. Reorient as needed.
4. Complete a focused assessment.
5. Assess for patent airway and level of consciousness; administer oxygen if ordered. Attach pulse oximeter.
6. Assess for effects of anesthesia including general, regional, or local. ❶
7. Take vital signs, including pain assessment: usual orders are every 15 min until stable; then every half hour for 2 hr; every hour for 4 hr; then every 4 hr for 24–48 hr, or according to hospital policy. ❷

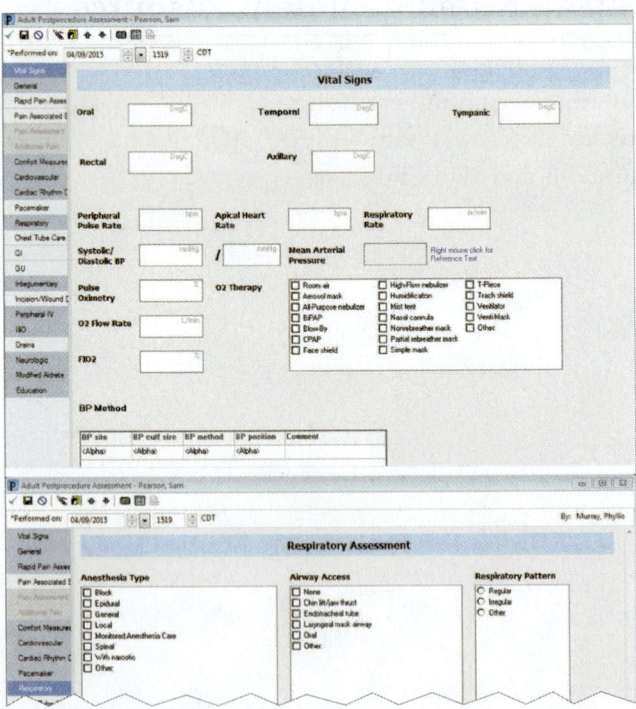

❶ PAR record. *Source:* From Cerner Electronic Health Record. © Cerner Corporation. Pearson has restricted permission to reproduce and distribute this copyrighted work. Further reproduction or distribution is strictly prohibited without written consent of Cerner Corporation.

❷ Recovery room monitoring is accomplished using computerized systems.

8. Check pulse oximetry every hour for 4 hr, then every 4 hr. ➤ *Rationale:* This is to detect early signs of hypoxemia.
9. Check $ETCO_2$ using capnography monitoring, if available.
10. Check for nausea and vomiting.
11. Check IV site and patency frequently.
12. Observe and record urine output, amount, and color.
13. Measure intake and output.
14. Observe skin color and moisture and nail beds. ➤ *Rationale:* This is to determine adequacy of tissue perfusion.
15. Position client for comfort and maximum airway ventilation according to orders.
16. Turn every 2 hr and PRN.
17. Give back care at least every 4 hr.
18. Encourage coughing and deep breathing every 2 hr (may use spirometer or Tri-flow if ordered).
19. Keep client comfortable with medications.
20. Monitor for side effects of medications.
21. Check dressings and drainage tubes every 2–4 hr; if abnormal amount of drainage, check more frequently. Empty drainage system when needed
22. Assess for signs and symptoms of SSIs. Preventive measures and types of SSIs are listed in Box 26-11 ■ and conditions that contribute to risk for SSIs are listed in Box 26-12 ■.

    a. Superficial incisional:
    - Purulent drainage with or without elevated white blood cell count
    - Pain or tenderness at the site
    - Localized swelling, heat, or redness
    - Positive wound culture

    b. Deep incisional:
    - Purulent drainage
    - Temperature above 100.4°F (38°C)
    - Leukocytosis
    - Localized pain or tenderness

    c. Organ or space:
    - Purulent drainage from a drain placed in an organ or space
    - Positive culture from fluid or tissue in the organ or space
    - Temperature above 100.4°F (38°C)

- Leukocytosis
- Pain
- Abscess formation or other evidence of infection in the organ or space

Note: See Wound Care, Chapter 25, for further information.

23. Provide oral hygiene at least every 4 hr; if nasogastric tube or nasal oxygen is inserted, give oral hygiene every 2 hr. ➤ *Rationale:* This decreases risk of infection from presence of oral bacteria.
24. Bathe client when temperature can be maintained. ➤ *Rationale:* Bathing removes the antiseptic solution and stimulates circulation.
25. Keep client warm and avoid chilling, but do not increase temperature above normal. Use of Bair Paws Warming System allows client to maintain warmth and provides comfort. ➤ *Rationale:* Increased temperature increases metabolic rate and need for oxygen. Excessive perspiration causes fluid and electrolyte loss.

26. Irrigate nasogastric tube every 4 hr and PRN, as ordered, with normal saline to keep patent and to prevent electrolyte imbalance.
27. Maintain dietary intake: Type of diet depends on type and extent of surgical procedure.
    a. Minor surgical conditions: Client may drink or eat as soon as he or she is awake, desires food or drink, and has gag reflex present.
    b. Major surgical conditions: NPO until bowel sounds return. Clear liquid advanced to full diet as tolerated.
28. Place client on bedpan 2–4 hr postoperatively if catheter not inserted.
29. Check physician's orders when to begin the client's postoperative activity. Most clients are ambulated within first 24 hr.
30. Observe for signs and symptoms of possible postoperative complications (Table 26-9 ■), particularly postoperative bleeding and infection.
31. Dangle or position client in chair as ordered.

Box 26-11   SURGICAL SITE INFECTIONS

Prevention
- Appropriate use of prophylactic antibiotics
- Appropriate hair removal
- Maintenance of perioperative glucose control
- Maintenance of perioperative normothermia

Bacterial Causes of SSIs

Common battery of infections
- *Staphylococcus*
- *Enterococcus*
- *Pseudomonas*
- *Streptococcus*

Newer causes (due to antibiotic resistance)
- *Escherichia coli*
- MRSA
- *Candida*

Box 26-12   CONDITIONS THAT PLACE CLIENTS AT RISK FOR POSTOPERATIVE INFECTION

- Uncontrolled diabetes
- Renal failure
- Obesity; advanced age
- Receiving corticosteroids
- Receiving **immunosuppressive** agents or are immunosuppressed
- Prolonged antibiotic therapy
- Protein or ascorbic acid deficiencies
- Marked dehydration and hypovolemia
- Decreased cardiac output
- Edema and fluid and electrolyte imbalances
- Anemia
- Preoperative infection

Skill 26.6.2 | Administering Postoperative Medications

Equipment

Medication as ordered (see Chapter 16, Pain Management)
Appropriate syringe and needle for parenteral medications
PCA pump and IV tubing, if appropriate

Procedure

1. Check two forms of client ID and introduce self to client. Perform hand hygiene.
2. Evaluate client's need for pain relief.
3. Provide nonmedication measures for relief of pain, such as relaxation techniques, back care, and positioning.
4. Identify the pharmacologic action of the ordered medication.
5. Review the general side effects of the medication.
    a. Drowsiness
    b. Euphoria

    c. Sleep
    d. Respiratory depression
    e. Nausea and vomiting
6. Administer medications as ordered, usually at 3- to 4-hr intervals for first 24–48 hr for better action and pain relief. Assess for pain relief.
7. Instruct in use of PCA pump, if ordered.
8. Know the action of the following drugs:
    a. Opiates
    b. Synthetic opiate-like drugs
    c. Nonnarcotic pain relievers
    d. Narcotic antagonists
    e. Antiemetics

Table 26-9 Postoperative Complications

Potential Complication	Clients at Risk	Indicative Findings	Prevention	Intervention	Drug Therapy
Atelectasis: Collapse of alveoli; may be diffuse and involve a segment, lobe, or entire lung *Potential Onset:* First 48 hr	All with general anesthesia *Special risk clients:* Smokers Chronic **bronchitis** **Emphysema** Obesity Elderly Upper abdominal surgery Chest surgery Abdominal distention	Fever to 39°C (102°F) Tachycardia Restlessness Tachypnea 24–30 min *Altered breath sounds:* Dullness to percussion Diminished or absent breath sounds Crackles ABGs: decreased PaO_2	*Preoperative:* Have client practice turning, coughing, and deep breathing. Discuss importance of exercises. *Postoperative clients at risk:* Turn every 30 min. Deep breathe and cough. *Other clients:* Initiate turning and deep breathing exercises every 1–2 hr. Ambulate as soon as possible. Medicate to reduce pain, splinting, and resistance to treatment.	Encourage deep breathing and incentive spirometry. Administer supplemental oxygen as ordered. Monitor response to treatment. Monitor for onset of pneumonia. If entire lobe of lung is involved, prepare for bronchoscopy to remove plug. Change position every 2 hr.	Analgesics: pain control Bronchodilators (nebulizer through IPPB); liquefy secretions Water or saline (nebulizer through IPPB); to liquefy secretions
Pneumonia: Inflammatory process in which alveoli are filled with **exudate** *Potential onset:* First 36–48 hr	Clients with unresolved atelectasis Following aspiration Smokers Older adult Chronic bronchitis Emphysema Heart failure Debilitated Alcoholic Immobile Cough suppressant medications Respiratory depressant medications	Client complains of dyspnea, tachycardia, increasing temperature, productive cough, and increasing amount of sputum becoming tenacious, rusty, or purulent. Tactile fremitus Dullness to percussion Bronchial breath sounds Increased crackles or rhonchi Voice sounds present ABGs: decreased PaO_2	Provide vigorous treatment of atelectasis. Prevent aspiration. Ambulate as soon as possible.	Turn, cough, and deep breathe every 1 hr. As needed, stimulate cough with nasotracheal suctioning. Send sputum for culture and sensitivity. Provide frequent mouth care for comfort. Administer oxygen as ordered. Increase fluid intake. Monitor for response to treatment.	Antibiotics: Cephalosporin or ampicillin prophylactically for 48 hr for high-risk clients Cephalosporin IV or parenteral for infections Antipyretics to decrease temperature
Pulmonary embolism: Foreign object has migrated to branch of pulmonary artery *Potential onset:* Seventh to tenth day	Superficial vein thrombosis: rare Deep vein thrombosis: 40–60% Air emboli: intraperitoneal surgery Fat emboli: long bone fracture, split sternum	Only 10% recognized clinically Pain, sharp and stabbing, occurs with breathing; localized (right lower lobe most frequent). Marked shortness of breath Increased heart rate—tachycardia Restlessness and other symptoms of hypoxia (severe anxiety)	Provide range of motion. Encourage early ambulation. Prevent thrombophlebitis. Do not massage an area with potential for or suspected thrombus. Provide elastic stockings or leg compression devices.	Administer oxygen to relieve hypoxia. Reduce anxiety. Position client on left side with head dependent to prevent air embolus. Prevent recurrent embolization; prepare for fibrinolysis; prepare for anticoagulation.	Anticoagulation therapy: IV heparin to maintain therapeutic APTT Sodium prophylactically for high-risk clients Urokinase; t-PA; streptokinase: thrombolytic effect (24 hr) Analgesics: pleuritic pain control X-ray or scan Adequate hydration

	Causes	Signs and Symptoms	Prevention	Treatment	Medications/Therapy
Thrombophlebitis: Inflammation of vein with clot formation *Potential onset:* Seventh to fourteenth day	*Abnormal vein walls:* Varicose veins Previous thrombophlebitis **Trauma** to vein wall Tight strap on operating room table Surgery on hips or in pelvis Age over 60 years (arteriosclerosis) *Venous stasis:* Immobility, long duration surgery Casts, restrictive dressings Constant Fowler's position Prolonged dependent lower extremities Knee gatch elevated Pillows under knees, calves Obesity Abdominal distention Shock Heart failure *Hypercoagulability:* Surgical stress response Anesthesia Decreased circulation Hypovolemia, dehydration Malignant neoplasms Postpartum Oral contraceptives Insert rectal tube	*Superficial vein thrombophlebitis:* Pain, redness, tenderness, and induration along course of vein Palpable "cord" corresponding to course of vein History of trauma, including IV site *Deep small vein thrombophlebitis:* Increased muscle turgor and tenderness over affected vein Deep muscle tenderness Most frequent site: vessels at calf Affected limb warm to touch with occasional swelling Client complains of tightness or stiffness in affected leg Positive Homan's sign (dorsiflexion of foot leads to calf pain) Fever rarely more than 38.3°C (101°F) *Major deep vein thrombophlebitis:* No superficial signs of inflammation Homan's sign unreliable *Femoral vein thrombosis:* Pain and tenderness in distal thigh and popliteal region Swelling extends to level of knee	*Avoid injury to vein wall:* Use care when strapping to operating room table. Avoid IVs in lower extremities. Pad siderails for restless, convulsive, or combative client. Avoid restraints. *Avoid venous stasis:* Encourage early ambulation. Provide feet and leg exercises. Provide elastic stockings; sequential-compression devices. Increase frequency of exercise for client at risk. Prevent client's sitting with legs in dependent position. Place pillow between legs while client is lying on side to prevent pressure from upper leg on lower. Provide deep breathing exercises. Provide range of motion. Increase velocity of blood flow: No standing Steady IV flow Antiembolic stockings (controversial) Decrease hypercoagulability: Provide adequate hydration. Prevent infections. Maintain circulation. Decrease stress/anxiety.	*Superficial vein thrombophlebitis:* Treat symptoms. Continue ambulation unless accompanied by deep venous involvement. Monitor for progression toward saphenofemoral junction (may need ligation). *Deep vein thrombophlebitis:* Provide adequate bed rest. Provide elastic stockings, sequential-compression devices. Elevate foot of bed with 6- to 8-in. blocks Administer warm, moist compresses to relieve venospasm and help resolve inflammation. Monitor for pulmonary embolism.	Streptokinase: thrombolytic effect (24 hr) Heparin IV or subcutaneous: decrease clotting time (short-term) Nonorthopedic surgery—low-dose subcutaneous heparin (or low molecular-weight heparin) Coumadin PO: decreased clotting time (long term) Analgesics: pain control Low-molecular-weight dextran IV on operative day and 2 days postoperative Aspirin 1.2 g/day in divided doses
Ileus: Failure of peristalsis *Potential onset:* First 24–36 hr	All surgical clients Stress response to surgical trauma	No bowel sounds or fewer than 5/min (normal: 5–35 clicks or gurgles/min) Vomiting Abdominal distention	Do not feed until bowel sounds return. Offer only sips of water until return of bowel sounds. Maintain normal serum potassium level.	Monitor for return of normal bowel sounds (enteral feeding following non-GI surgeries will resolve ileus faster). Monitor for distention. Monitor for passage of flatus signaling return of peristalsis. Monitor signs of hypokalemia.	Switch to nonopioid analgesic (opioids slow GI motility), NSAIDs, or acetaminophen.

(continued)

Table 26-9 Postoperative Complications *(continued)*

Potential Complication	Clients at Risk	Indicative Findings	Prevention	Intervention	Drug Therapy
Paralytic ileus: Paralysis of intestinal peristalsis *Potential onset:* First 3–4 days	Intraperitoneal surgery **Peritonitis** Kidney surgery Decreased cardiac output Pneumonia Electrolyte imbalance Wound infection	No bowel sounds Abdominal distention No passage of flatus or feces Nasogastric drainage green to yellow, 1–2 L in 24 hr Anorexia, nausea Complaints of fullness and diffuse pain	Maintain electrolyte balance, especially potassium. Maintain cardiac output. Prevent pneumonia. Provide early ambulation.	Treat the cause. Maintain nasogastric suction until peristalsis returns. Monitor for intestinal obstruction.	Potassium chloride if serum level is low Dexpanthenol (Ilopan) to stimulate return of peristalsis; total parenteral nutrition (TPN) if indicated
Urinary tract infection *Potential onset:* Third to fifth day or 48 hr after removal of catheter	*Decreased resistance:* History of bladder distention History of urinary retention Previous urinary tract infection History of prostatic hypertrophy History of catheterization Client has diabetes Debilitated Immobile	Dysuria Frequency Urgency High fever: up to 40°C (104°F) with fewer systemic toxic symptoms than would be expected Change in urine odor Pus in urine Sediment May be asymptomatic	Maintain sterile technique with catheterization and catheter removal. Provide competent indwelling catheter care. Encourage early ambulation to decrease retention and stasis.	Encourage fluid intake; cranberry juice to decrease urine pH. Increase activity to enhance bladder emptying. Encourage voiding every 2 hr while awake. Send specimen for culture and sensitivity. Monitor for residual urine of more than 100 mL.	Urinary antiseptics (sulfonamides); bacterial suppression Antibiotics (ampicillin, tetracycline); bacterial suppression Anticholinergics; antispasmodic Topical urinary analgesic; pain relief
Wound infection *Potential onset* : Streptococcal: 24–48 hr after contamination *Staphylococcus* gram-negative rods and other signs: 5–7 days postoperatively	*Slow to heal:* Obese Client has diabetes *Poor nutrition:* Debilitated Older adult Ulcerative colitis *Poor circulation:* Older adult Hypovolemic Heart failure *Lack of oxygen to wound:* Vasoconstriction Severe anemia Depressed immunity Cancer Renal failure Preoperative steroid therapy Prolonged complex surgery (stress response leading to increased ACTH) Malnutrition Older adult *At risk for transmission* Proximity of another client with infection Transmission by hands of personnel	Initial inflammation: 36–48 hr Wound tender, swollen, warm, increased redness Increasing heart rate Increasing temperature 38°C (100.4°F or more) Increasing or recurring serous drainage; drainage becomes purulent, foul odor There may be no local signs if infection is deep. Elevated WBC Malaise	Practice meticulous hand hygiene and gloving. Practice aseptic technique in wound care. Separate from infected clients. Use special caution for a new wound, which is easily contaminated. Maintain nutrition. Provide frequent turning. Ambulate as soon as possible. Maintain PaO$_2$. Increase attention to prevention for clients with depressed immunity. Operative site: Clip excess hair and cleanse with chlorhexidine (reduces bacterial counts).	Maintain nutrition. Maintain oxygenation. Maintain circulation and blood volume. Maintain pulmonary toilet. Cleanse wound or irrigate as ordered. Apply wet-to-moist dressings. Monitor for systemic response to infection, fever, malaise, headache, anorexia, nausea. Treat symptoms.	Administer antibiotics as ordered. New cyanoacrylate adhesives (Dermabond, Indermil) close wounds and promote healing. Send wound drainage specimen for culture and sensitivity.

Source: Smith (2016)

Unit 26.6 Documentation and Evaluation

DOCUMENTATION for Postoperative Care

- Postoperative nursing interventions
- Focused assessment findings
- Fluid replacement—type and amount of solution
- Condition of dressings and drains
- Urine output, fluid intake
- Orientation to place, individual, time
- Vital signs
- Signs and symptoms of potential complications

- Preventive nursing measures
- Client's activity level
- Clinical manifestations indicating pain
- Type, time, and amount of pain medication administered
- Site of injection
- Any side effects of medications observed
- Effectiveness of pain medication

EVALUATION/Critical Thinking

Expected Outcomes

- Client has an uneventful experience in the recovery period.
- Potential postoperative complications are identified early and corrective interventions prevent occurrence of complications.
- Client is discharged to home or nursing unit within prescribed time frame.
- Client reports pain: less than 4 on scale of 0–10.
- Client does not experience nausea or vomiting.

Unexpected Outcomes	Alternative Actions
Client develops abnormal breath sounds.	Increase deep breathing and coughing exercises to every 2 hr.
	Medicate for pain before coughing or ambulating.
	Encourage use of incentive spirometer.
	Turn every 1–2 hr and ambulate if allowed.
	Place client in Fowler's position to expand lungs.
	Increase fluid intake to liquefy secretions if not contraindicated.
	Obtain physician's order for nebulizer treatments if indicated.
Bowel sounds are absent.	Do not give ice chips or fluids; keep on NPO status until discussed with physician.
	Notify physician if client is experiencing nausea and vomiting or if abdomen is distended and bowel sounds remain absent. It may be necessary to insert an NG tube.
	Auscultate bowel sounds every 4 hr.
	Encourage frequent turning and ambulation, if allowed.

(continued)

Unexpected Outcomes	Alternative Actions
• Deep vein thrombosis (DVT) occurs.	• Place on bed rest. • Remove antiembolic stockings or compression devices on affected leg. • Check for calf pain, discoloration, or Homan's sign. • Do not massage legs. • Monitor clotting times and titrate anticoagulants if using heparin, according to physician's orders. • Measure circumference of both legs each shift to determine effectiveness of treatment. • Encourage leg exercises on unaffected leg.
• Temperature increases.	• Day of surgery—check for dehydration. • Days 1 and 2—check breath sounds for potential atelectasis. • Fever in first 24 hr is most commonly from atelectasis. • Days 2—check for urinary tract infection. • Days 3–10—check for possible wound infection or pneumonia. • Check breath sounds for adventitious sounds or diminished breath sounds. • Increase fluids if not contraindicated. • Monitor temperature frequently until it returns to normal.
• Blood pressure decreases; pulse and respirations increase.	• Check for IV access. • Check skin turgor and urine output and hypovolemia. • Observe dressings and drains for signs of bleeding. • Check intake and output values to determine hydration status.
• Urinary retention occurs.	• Check bladder using bladder scanner. • Assist to commode or bathroom if possible. • Increase fluid intake if appropriate. • Review I&O record to determine findings. • Assess for signs and symptoms of dehydration. • Obtain order for catheter if necessary.

Chapter Wrap-Up

GERONTOLOGIC Considerations

Statistics for Older Adult Clients Requiring Surgery Are Important to Consider When Providing Care

- Fifty percent of clients over 60 years of age require surgery before they die.
- Forty percent of older clients admitted to hospitals undergo a surgical procedure before discharge.
- The most common surgical procedures for older clients involve tissue biopsy and pacemaker insertion. Fractures comprise a large percentage of surgical interventions, particularly hip fractures.

Older Adult Clients Are More Prone to Fluid and Electrolyte Imbalance

- Dehydration is the most common cause of fluid and electrolyte imbalance.
- Check IV fluid type and amount to ensure adequate hydration.
- Older adult clients require 1.5–2.5 L of fluid every 24 hr.
- Monitor intake and output carefully to ensure adequate hydration.
- Monitor neurologic status for possible electrolyte imbalance.
- Fluid loss occurs with nasogastric tube placement and pre-op bowel preparation; clients requiring either of these interventions should be observed for dehydration.
- Evaluate electrolyte lab values for abnormal levels. (Hyperkalemia is common as a response to age-related alterations in the renin–aldosterone system.)

Older Adult Clients Are at Risk for Complications Associated With Immobility After Surgical Interventions

- Turn client frequently, at least every 2 hr.
- Ambulate as soon as possible postoperatively.
- Evaluate skin for early signs of breakdown (nonblanching erythema).
- Encourage deep breathing and coughing exercises every 1–2 hr. Instruct in use of incentive spirometer if ordered.
- Encourage leg exercises every hour when awake.

Preoperative Teaching Should Be Individualized, Keeping in Mind the Following:

- Older clients may have chronic conditions that make movement difficult, altering preventative measures such as turning.

- Clients may have visual or auditory alterations requiring a quiet environment for teaching.
- Larger print or brochures with photos and large print should be used when teaching older clients.

Chronic Conditions May Alter Normal Vital Signs, Which May Be Misinterpreted During the Perioperative Phases

- Document abnormalities in vital signs on client care plan so that all healthcare workers are alerted to client's usual values. Blood pressure and pulse alterations can be different for this age group.
- Monitor peripheral pulses to ensure adequate circulation.

Altered Physiologic States Need to Be Communicated to All Healthcare Workers

- Document if client has an artificial eye or other prosthesis.
- Document client's visual or auditory alterations. If hearing aid is necessary for client to hear, indicate clearly on care plan.
- Identify if client has any condition that can interfere with postoperative care.

Older Adult Clients May Not Be Candidates for Conscious Sedation

- Many older clients have an ASA reading above 3. This would be considered a contraindication for this sedation.
- Anesthesiologists would most likely have to administer the medication.

Consent Forms Must Be Signed by Legally Competent Client

- Signing of consent form can only be done if client is considered competent to understand directions given and explanation of procedure.
- Signing of consent form must be voluntary.
- Client must be informed about procedure and must understand what he or she is signing.
- A court-appointed conservator may need to be obtained for clients not considered mentally competent to sign for themselves.
- Family members may not sign for client unless they are legally considered the client's guardian or advance directive provides instructions.

- In emergency situations, permission may be obtained from family members, but not for routine procedures.

- Two physicians can sign for emergency surgery; however, the surgeon performing the surgery should not sign the permit.

MANAGEMENT Guidelines

Each state legislates a Nurse Practice Act for RNs and LVN/LPNs. Healthcare facilities are responsible for establishing and implementing policies and procedures that conform to their state's regulations. Verify the regulations and role parameters for each healthcare worker in your facility.

Delegation

- RNs and LVN/LPNs can complete routine preoperative teaching and care. Anything out of the ordinary would be the responsibility of the RN.
- Postanesthesia room staff are usually RNs because they need to make quick decisions and use nursing judgment in times of crisis.
- Postoperative care of clients may be provided by both RNs and LVN/LPNs.
- Clients undergoing conscious sedation may be monitored by RNs if their state's Nurse Practice Act and hospital policy allows it and the clients are in ASA categories 1 and 2 (see section on conscious sedation).
- CNAs can be delegated to take vital signs and do routine hygienic care for clients once they are stable.
- Many facilities use "scrub techs" or OR techs to perform routine duties such as the preoperative scrub. OR techs are also assigned to assist the physician during surgery.

Interpersonal Communication

- It is very important that all preoperative forms be completed in a timely manner. If data are missing, the client's surgery may be delayed while laboratory tests are taken, history and physical examination reports are found and placed in the chart, or chest x-ray results are placed in the chart. History and physical provide information to ensure continuity of care.
- Notify OR staff and physician if client indicates that he or she has a known latex allergy or does not know of a latex allergy. All latex supplies and equipment must be removed from the OR suite before surgery can commence.
- When the phone call is received from the operating room indicating the nurse should give the preoperative medications or that the OR is ready for the client, ensure the message is relayed immediately to the staff caring for the client. This will allow the nurse to give the medication or complete any last-minute charting and have the client ready for the transporter.
- If there are any client issues or problems that directly affect the surgical procedure, contact the operating room or physician immediately. Surgery may need to be delayed or canceled. Examples of issues that could impact the surgery include an overly anxious client, if the client has a temperature, symptoms indicating an upper respiratory or urinary tract infection, labs that are abnormal (bleeding time, cardiac enzymes, electrolytes), or new abnormal ECG changes.
- Specific report regarding the client's condition will be completed upon admission to the postanesthesia room and again when the client is returned to the nursing unit. The report is given by the RN in the operating room to the RN in the postanesthesia room. The postanesthesia room nurse accompanies the client to the nursing unit and gives report to the RN. The report is outlined in Box 26-9.

CASE STUDY Applications

Scenario 1

You are assigned to the postanesthesia room on the day shift. You have just arrived on the unit to begin the shift. There are two clients assigned to your care:

- Mrs. Cohen, a 54-year-old client, had an exploratory laparoscopy with general anesthesia and is just arriving in the recovery room.
- Mr. Brewer is a 24-year-old client who had local anesthesia for an arthroscopy of the right knee. He has been in the recovery room for 1 hr.

1. Which client will you see first? Provide a rationale for your response.
2. Identify the first action you will take when first seeing each of the two clients. Provide a rationale for your response.

3. Identify the priority assessment for Mrs. Cohen and state your rationale.
4. Identify the priority assessment for Mr. Brewer and state your rationale.
5. State nursing interventions that will be provided for all clients in the postanesthesia room.
6. Before discharge from the recovery room, you assess Mr. Brewer on the Aldrete Recovery Scoring System and his score is 7. What is your next action?
7. Mr. Brewer is being discharged home. He tells you he is concerned about going home because he has a dry mouth and is thirsty. What would be an appropriate response to him?
8. Write the SBAR Hand-off communication you will prepare for transfer of Mr. Brown to the surgical floor.

Scenario 2

You assess that Mr. Marconi is very anxious while you are admitting him for a surgical procedure.

1. List four priority components of baseline data you need to obtain before surgery. Provide a rationale to support this data.

2. What factors might contribute to preoperative stress?

3. Identify a priority intervention to use after assessing that Mr. Marconi is in high-level stress.

4. Mr. Marconi becomes angry and hostile when you attempt to provide preoperative teaching. Describe three possible actions you could take, and state the priority intervention and the rationale for selecting this intervention.

NCLEX® Review Questions

Unless otherwise specified, choose only one (1) answer.

1. Which client activity is not completed during the preoperative stage?
   A. Obtaining a health history
   B. Identifying a client's allergies
   C. Beginning the infusion of a moderate sedative drug
   D. Identifying the side and site of the surgical procedure

2. What is the role of the circulating nurse in the operating room?
   A. To identify the correct side and site
   B. To insert the IV and begin infusing fluids
   C. To assist the physician during the operative procedure
   D. To position the client on the operative table and attach grounding pad

3. What is the most common malpractice action against operating room nurses?
   A. Sponges and instruments accidentally left in the surgical site
   B. Surgical procedure performed on wrong site or side
   C. Burns from electrical grounding pad not placed correctly on client
   D. Infection at surgical site after surgical procedure

4. The student's client assignment includes a preoperative client scheduled for surgery in 3 hr. The initial intervention is to reduce anxiety and stress for this client. How can this best be accomplished?
   Select all that apply.
   A. Discussing realistic outcomes with the client
   B. Reassuring the client that everything will be fine
   C. Using touch to communicate caring
   D. Encouraging range of motion and walking activities
   E. Avoiding misconceptions about the procedure.

5. As a student nurse working in the outpatient setting, you are asked to provide postoperative instructions to a client after a laparoscopy. What would the most appropriate instructions be?
   A. Instruct the client that he or she may experience a sharp pain under the scapula up to 24–48 hr after surgery.

B. Inform the client he or she will be hospitalized for a minimum of 24 hr to monitor for pain.
   C. Inform the client that this type of surgery usually requires very little pain medication; Tylenol is sufficient to control the pain.
   D. Explain that the client can return to work the next day, as long as he or she does not lift anything over 50 pounds.

6. While you are working on a surgical unit, you are preparing the client for a surgical procedure. What do your responsibilities in this preparation include?
   A. Asking the client if he or she has made arrangements for home care after discharge
   B. Instructing the client to sign the surgical consent form at the time the OR transporter arrives in the room
   C. Administering the preoperative medication at least 2 hr before the surgery is scheduled
   D. Checking for allergies to latex, food, and medications

7. What do The Joint Commission standards regarding Universal Protocols for preventing wrong site, wrong procedure, and wrong person surgery include?
   Select all that apply.
   A. Marking the surgical site by the preoperative nurse
   B. Validating the correct surgical site by the surgeon before beginning the procedure
   C. Writing the word *yes* on the surgical checklist line indicating the correct incision site
   D. Completing a final verification of the site in the location where the procedure takes place
   E. Not marking single organ surgeries

8. You are caring for a client after a procedure where moderate sedation analgesia (conscious sedation) was used. What must occur in order for the client to be discharged?
   A. Ramsay Sedation Scale is normal.
   B. Riker Sedation-Agitation Scale is −1 to +1.
   C. Aldrete score is within 1 point of the preprocedure score.
   D. Glasgow Coma scale is more than 9.

9. A client is returning to the nursing unit after an abdominal surgical procedure. What is the priority nursing intervention?

   A. Take and record vital signs.

   B. Assess type of IV solution and amount of IV solution remaining in bag.

   C. Check pulse oximeter reading.

   D. Assess for patent airway.

10. Pneumonia is a major postoperative complication related to inactivity and decreased pulmonary ventilation. When postoperatively does the onset of signs and symptoms of pneumonia usually occur?

    A. Within 24 hr

    B. 24–36 hr

    C. 36–48 hr

    D. More than 72 hr

QSEN Activity

Domain: Client-Centered Care

KSA: Knowledge

Activity:

Preparing a preoperative plan of care for a surgical client scheduled for a colon resection.

1. Outline the necessary information that is included in the preoperative preparation for this client such as the blood work.

2. Describe the equipment that will be utilized before and after the procedure.

3. Explain the skin preparation, preoperative medications, bowel preparation, and NPO status.

4. Identify the client's health information and usual activities that will be essential for the physician's knowledge.

5. Discuss the postoperative nursing interventions that all be carried out immediately after surgery.

Bibliography

Allen, G. (2014, May). Contact precautions in the perioperative setting. *OR Nurse 2014, 8*(3), 14–16.

Alexander-Magalee, M. (2012, Nov.). Infection control: Recognizing surgical site infections. *OR Nurse 2012 6*(6), 13–14.

Amato-Vealey, E. J., Barba, M. P., & Vealey, R. J. (2008, Nov.). Hand-off communication: A requisite for perioperative patient safety. *AORN Journal, 88*(5), 763–770. Retrieved from http://www.aorn-greaterhouston.org/files/Nov_08_handoff.pdf

American Association of Nurse Anesthetists. (2011). Moderate (conscious) sedation. Retrieved from http://www.aana.com/practice/conscious.asp

American Society of Anesthesiologists. (2009). Continuum of depth of sedation; Definition of general anesthesia and levels of sedation/analgesia. Retrieved from http://www.asahq.org/publications and serivices/standards/20pdf

American Society of Anesthesiologists. (2010). ASA physical classification system. Retrieved from http://www.asahq.org/clinical/physicalstatus.htm

Antibiotic prophylaxis to prevent surgical site infections. (2011). (EB CME). Retrieved from http://www.allevents24.com/e/cf012-antibiotic-prophylaxis-eb-tickets-7415075691

Association of Operating Room Nurses (AORN). (2004). Proposed AORN position statement on the role of the scrub person. Retrieved from site.blueskybroadcast.com/client/aorn/scrub.pdf

Association of Operating Room Nurses (AORN). (2014). *Perioperative standards, recommended practices, and guideline 2014*. Denver, CO: Author.

Association of Perioperative Registered Nurses. (2015). Guidelines for perioperative practice. Retrieved from http://www.aorn.org/guidelines/#NewIn2015

Barclay, L. (2009, Jan.). Surgical checklist may improve outcomes for noncardiac surgery. *New England Journal of Medicine, 360*, 491–499.

Barletta, J. F. & Senagore, A. J. (2014). Reducing the burden of postoperative ileus: Evaluating and implementing an evidence-based strategy. *World Journal of Surgery, 38*(8), 1966–1977. doi: http://dx.doi.org/10.1007/s00268-014-2506-2

Barzoloski-O'Connor, B. (2014, Mar.). Preparing the Skin for Surgery. *Plastic Surgical Nursing, 34*(1), 12–14.

Cheung-Larivee, K. (2012). One in 10 surgical patients readmitted with post-op complications. Retrieved from http://www.fiercehealthcare.com/story/surgical-patients-bounce-back-post-op-complications/2012-08-29

Criscitelli, T. (2013). Safe patient hand-off strategies. *AORN Journal, 97*(5), 582–585. doi: http://dx.doi.org/10.1016/j.aorn.2013.02.007

Gillespie, B. M., Chaboyer, W., Thalb, L., John, M., Fairweather, N., & Slater, K. (2014, Jun.). Effect of using a safety checklist on patient complications after surgery: A systematic review and meta-analysis. *Anesthesiology, 120*(6), 1380–1390.

Guglielmi, C. L., Stratton, M., Healy, G. B., Shapiro, D., Duffy, W. J., Dean, B. L., & Groah, L. K. (2014). The growing role of patient engagement: Relationship-based care in a changing health care system. *AORN Journal, 99*(4), 517–528.

Hallingbye, T., Martin, J., & Viscomi, C. (2011). Acute postoperative pain management in the older patient. *Aging Health, 7*(6), 813–828. doi: http://dx.doi.org/10.2217/ahe.11.73

Jose, B. & Dignon, A. (2013). Is there a relationship between preoperative shaving (hair removal) and surgical site infection? *The Journal of Perioperative Practice, 23*(1), 22–25. Retrieved from http://search.proquest.com/docview/1272294382?accountid=3588

Joshi, G. P., Beck, D. E., Emerson, R., Hill, J. R., Halaszynski, T. M., Jahr, J. S., Lipman, A. G., & Sinatra, R. S. (2014). Defining new directions for more effective management of surgical pain in the United States: Highlights of the inaugural surgical pain congress (TM). *The American Surgeon, 80*(3), 219–28. Retrieved from http://search.proquest.com/docview/1518527898?accountid=3588

Journeaux, M. (2013). Peri-operative hypothermia: Implications for practice. *Nursing Standard, 27*(45), 33–38. Retrieved from http://search.proquest.com/docview/1413087391?accountid=3588

LaMance, K. (2015). Informed consent for surgery lawyers. Retrieved from http://www.legalmatch.com/law-library/article/informed=consent-for-surgery.html

LegalMatch.com. (2014). What is the difference between "consent" and "informed consent?" Retrieved from http://www.legalmatch.com/law-library/article/informed-consent-for-surgery.html

McCarron, K. (2014). Don't skip the SCIP. *Nursing Made Incredibly Easy, 12*(5), 15–19.

MedlinePlus: U.S. National Library of Medicine NIH National Institutes of Health. (2013). Conscious sedation for surgical procedures. Retrieved from http://www.nlm.nih.gov/medlineplus/ency/article/007409.htm

McMillen, M. (2010). 8 common surgery complications: What to do to reduce your risk of these post-surgery complications. Retrieved from http://www.webmd.com/healthy-aging/features/common-surgery-complications

Nowinski, G. (2008, May). Don't shave unless you have to! *American Academy of Orthopaedic Surgeons.* Retrieved from http://www.aaos.org/news/aaosnow/mayof/clinical9.asp

O'Reilly, K. (2013, Jan.) Surgical errors: In ORs, "never events" occur 80 times a week. *American Medical News.* Retrieved from http://www.amednews.com/article/20130121/profession/130129976/2/

Orlewicz, M. (2014, Dec. 11). Procedural sedation. Retrieved from http://emedicine.medscape.com/article/109695-overview#aw2aab6to3

Reinberg, S. (2015, Feb. 3). Infection most likely cause of hospital readmission after surgery. *Health Day News for Healthier Living.* Retrieved from Consumer.healthday.com/general-health-information-16/doctor-news-206/infection

Richter, J. P., Mc Alearney, A. S., & Pennell, M. L. (2014). The influence of organizational factors on patient safety: Examining successful handoffs in health care. *Health Care Management Review,* Jul. 15, 2014 [epub ahead of print].

Salkind, A. & Kavitha, C. R. (2011, Mar.). Antibiotic prophylaxis to prevent surgical site infections. *American Family Physician.* Retrieved from http//www.aafp.org/afp/2011/0301/p585.html

Smith, S. F. (2016). *Sandra Smith's review for NCLEX-RN* (13th ed.). Burlington, MA: Jones & Bartlett Learning, LLC.

Society of Gastroenterology Nurses and Associates, Inc. (SGNA). (2015). Sedation administration: Levels & definitions. Retrieved from http://www.sgna.org/issues/sedationfactsorg/sedationadministration/sedationlevels.aspx

Starling, J. (2012). Turn the other cheek. Agency for Healthcare Research and Quality web site. Retrieved from http://webmm.ahrq.gov/case.aspx?caseID=265

The Joint Commission. (2012a). Joint Commission Center for Transforming Healthcare releases tool to tackle miscommunication among caregivers. Retrieved from http://www.pwrnewmedia.com/2012/joint_commission/hand_off_communications/index.html

The Joint Commission. (2012b). Safe surgery checklist. Retrieved from http://www.thejointcommission.org/ safe_surgery_checklist/

The Joint Commission. (2012c). The universal protocol for preventing wrong site, wrong procedure, and wrong person surgery™: Guidance for health care professionals. Retrieved from http://www.jointcommission.org/assets/1/18/UP_Poster1.PDF

The Joint Commission (2013a). Ambulatory buzz: Successful time-out solutions for ASCs. Retrieved from http://www.jointcommission.org/musingsambulatory_patient_safety/successful_time-out_solutions_for_ascs/

The Joint Commission. (2013b). Universal protocol for preventing wrong site, wrong procedure, wrong person surgery. Retrieved from http://www.jcaho.org/accredited+organizations/patient+safety/html

The Joint Commission. (2014). Surgical Care Improvement Project core measure set: Effective for discharges January 1, 2014. Retrieved from http://www.jointcommission.org/assets/1/6/SCIP-Measures-012014.pdf

Vitale, M. G. , Riedel, M. D., Glotzbecker, M. P., Matsumoto, H., Roye, D. P., Akbarnia B.A., … & Saiman, L. (2013). Building consensus: Development of a best practice guideline (BPG) for surgical site infection (SSI) prevention in high-risk pediatric spine surgery. *Journal of Pediatric Orthopaedics, 33*(5): 471–478. http://dx.doi.org/10.1097/BPO.0b013e3182840de2

Vogel, T. R., Dombrovskiy, V. Y., & Lowry, S. F. (2009). Trends in postoperative sepsis: Are we improving outcomes? *Surgical Infections, 10*(1): 71–78. http://dx.doi.org/10.1089/sur.2008.046

Walker, I. A., Reshamwalla, S., & Wilson, I. H. (2012) Surgical safety checklists: Do they improve outcomes? *British Journal of Anesthesia, 109*(1), 47–54.

Wang, Y., Xue, S., & Zhu, H. (2013). Risk factors for postoperative hypoxemia in patients undergoing Stanford Aortic dissection surgery. *Journal of Cardiothoracic Surgery, 8*(1), 118. http://dx.doi.org/10.1186/1749-8090-8-118

Whitlock, J. (2014). Signs and symptoms of an infection after surgery. Retrieved from http://surgery.about.com/od/aftersurgery/qt/Signsinfections.htm

World Alliance for Patient Safety. (2008). WHO surgical safety checklist. Geneva, Switzerland: World Health Organization. Retrieved from http://www.who.int/patientsafety/safesurgery/tools_resources/SSSL_Checklist_finalJun08.pdf?ua=1

Chapter 27
Orthopedic Interventions

 ## Learning Objectives

27.1 Identify nursing diagnoses that apply to care of clients with orthopedic conditions.

27.2 Outline emergency measures for an injured extremity.

27.3 Describe different ways to classify fractures.

27.4 Assess circulation, motion, and sensation in an injured limb.

27.5 Recognize indicators of circulatory compromise in an injured or immobilized extremity.

27.6 Apply a variety of immobilizing devices (sling, bandage, splint, brace).

27.7 Describe differences between plaster of Paris and synthetic casts.

27.8 Explain the purpose for skin versus skeletal traction.

27.9 Identify types of skin and skeletal traction.

27.10 Develop a teaching plan for the client with a cast.

27.11 Outline the nursing care needs of the client in traction.

27.12 Outline the teaching needs of a client with an amputation.

27.13 Develop a teaching plan for a client undergoing joint replacement (arthroplasty).

27.14 Discuss the advantages of autologous reinfusion after joint replacement surgery.

Chapter Outline

Terminology

Abduction movement away from the midline of the body or body part, as in raising the arm or spreading the fingers.

Adduction movement toward the midline of the body.

AKA above-the-knee amputation.

Alignment arranged in a straight line.

Amputation traumatic or surgical removal of a diseased limb or part.

Autologous reinfusion collection of shed blood through suction into a reservoir and reinfusion through the client's venous access.

Balanced suspension use of a sling or splint to elevate and support an extremity that is in traction.

BKA below-the-knee amputation.

Bryant's traction a type of skin traction used to treat fracture of the femur in a small child.

Buck's traction a type of skin traction applied to the lower leg to reduce muscle spasm and immobilize hip fracture.

Callus fibrous matrix of protein that bonds a fracture site but has not ossified and cannot support weight bearing.

Cast circumferential immobilizer generally reserved for short-term fracture management.

CMS circulation, motion, and sensation; parameters that provide information on neurovascular status; common assessment for orthopedic clients.

Comminuted broken in pieces; usually occurs in spongy bone areas.

Diaphysis the part of the long bone between the ends, also known as the shaft.

Edema excess fluid in the interstitial space.

Epiphysis the wide spongy end of a long bone.

Extension a movement that increases the angle between two bones, straightening a joint.

External fixation device a metal frame of telescoping rods with attached metal percutaneous pins inserted into or through a bone to maintain alignment.

External rotation turning an extremity away from the midline.

Flexion a movement that decreases a joint angle.

Internal rotation turning an extremity toward the midline.

Intracapsular within the joint capsule (e.g., head and neck of the femur).

Metaphysis wide part of bone at end of shaft adjacent to the epiphysis.

Mobility state or quality of being mobile; facility of movement.

Musculoskeletal pertaining to the muscles and bones.

Osteoblast immature cell, which on maturation plays a role in bone production.

Osteoclast cell that resorbs bone.

Paresthesia abnormal sensation of tingling or numbness.

Pearson attachment attachment to a Thomas splint that supports the lower leg. Used in balanced suspension traction. Allows continuous traction in line with the femur by the use of cords and weights.

Periosteum connective tissue that covers the bone; contains proliferating cells.

Prosthesis artificial replacement for a body part.

Prosthetist specialist who provides preoperative training, prosthetic fabrication, prosthetic training, and follow-up assessments of fit, alignment, and appearance of prostheses.

Restorative promoting a return to health.

Shrinker a rigid or sock device suspended by a strap; worn to reduce edema and protect the stump of an amputated extremity.

Spica figure-eight bandage with one of the two loops larger than the other (used for ankle or stump).

Spiral bandage used to cover a cylindrical part.

Splint noncircumferential immobilizer used for management of a variety of musculoskeletal conditions in which swelling is anticipated (sprain, acute fracture period).

Sprain injury caused by wrenching or twisting of a joint, which results in tearing or stretching of the associated ligaments.

Strain injury caused by excessive force or stretching of muscles or tendons around the joint.

Thomas splint used for balanced suspension along with skeletal traction for fracture of the femur.

Torque a rotary force.

Traction application of a mechanical pulling force applied to soft tissue.

Restoring Function

Orthopedic nursing involves the prevention and correction of alterations in the **musculoskeletal** system. To help clients achieve and maintain optimal **mobility**, nurses use preventative, **restorative,** and rehabilitative methods. Preventative and restorative measures include the use of bandages, positioning, **splints**, casts, and **traction**.

The most common cause of injury to the musculoskeletal system is trauma, which results in soft tissue injuries, fractures, and dislocations. Injuries occurring from falls in the home account for many admissions to healthcare facilities.

Sprains and **strains** are common musculoskeletal injuries. The usual initial treatment is "RICE." "R" stands for resting the injured part, "I" refers to application of ice, "C" stands for compression, such as with a bandage, and "E" stands for elevating the affected part 15 cm (6 in.) above the heart. These early interventions help to minimize pain, muscle spasm, **edema** formation, and secondary injury (review Inflammatory Response in Chapter 24).

Bandages are used for applying pressure over an area, immobilizing a body part, preventing or reducing edema formation, correcting a deformity, and securing splints in place. Several types of material are used as bandages: woven cotton, elastic webbing, gauze, and synthetics.

Fractures

A fracture is a break in the continuity of a bone that occurs when the bone is subjected to stress forces greater than ordinary. No two fractures are alike since forces occur from different directions and in different amounts and muscle pulls differ in response to injury (Figure 27-1 ■).

Long bones, most commonly involved in fractures, are composed of the shaft, or **diaphysis,** and the flared end of the bone, termed the **metaphysis**. In children, the metaphysis consists of two segments: the growth plate and the **epiphysis,** which is directly adjacent to joints. The epiphysis fuses to the metaphysis when long bone growth has ceased. Midshaft injuries to long bones in childhood can result in excessive growth of the extremity, while intra-articular fractures involving the growth plate can cause retardation or arrest in the longitudinal growth of the limb.

Bone healing is similar to soft tissue healing except that bones heal by limited regeneration rather than by scar formation. When a bone is fractured, a specific repair process takes place, beginning with formation of a blood clot at the fracture site. **Osteoblasts** and fibroblasts then converge on the site and start laying down an organic matrix or "**callus**," which bonds the fracture site and is similar to cartilage. Immobilization is an important factor during these critical phases. This callus is then mineralized by calcium deposition and thus converted into bone. In the final stage of the repair, osteoblasts and **osteoclasts** remodel the bone so that it is suited to perform its intended function (Wolff's law).

When a fracture occurs, deformity is noted because bone fragments override due to spasm of surrounding muscles. In order to align ("reduce") fracture components,

Intracapsular
Extracapsular
Spiral
Transverse
Oblique
Greenstick
Comminuted
Compound (open)

FIGURE 27-1 Types of fractures.

muscle spasm must be overcome. Clients may require a sedative to allow them to relax in order to decrease spasms. Fracture reduction can be achieved in various ways. In certain instances, physical manipulation of bone can result in realignment. This can also be accomplished by closed reduction (without surgery) or by open reduction (with surgery). Open reduction with internal fixation (ORIF) incorporates a form of internal fixation of fracture fragments with screws, plates, nails, etc. External immobilization with a **cast** or splint may be used along with either method of fracture reduction. An external fixator apparatus is used to reduce and immobilize fractures often associated with soft tissue injury. The fixator stabilizes fractured parts by the use of percutaneous pins. Recent advances for short-stature and leg-length discrepancy include an internal medullary nail system such as PRECICE, which is a magnetic system that lengthens the bone gradually using a remote control. Recent studies suggest that there are far fewer complications, and less pain than previous implantable systems. Fractures are classified in a variety of ways (Box 27-1 ■). One classification is by fracture configuration. Examples include a transverse fracture, which breaks directly across the bone; an oblique fracture, which breaks at an angle across the bone; and a **comminuted** fracture, which results in more than two fragments of bone. Fractures can also be classified as open or closed. A closed fracture occurs with no break in the skin and is usually reduced without surgery, and then immobilized with a cast. An open fracture is one in which the skin has been broken due to penetration of a bone fragment or external trauma. An open fracture requires additional treatment to prevent infection as a result of tissue exposure to the external environment. Surgical debridement and irrigation must be completed within hours of the fracture.

Casts and Splints

Casts are rigid cylinders applied to maintain the reduced (realigned) fracture in proper **alignment** and usually include the joint adjacent to the fracture. Casts are made from plaster of Paris or synthetic materials, such as polyester, polyurethane, fiberglass, or plastic. Synthetic casts dry faster, weigh less, and can get wet without fear of cracking or disintegration. Splints are not circumferential or as constrictive as casts and may be applied temporarily until swelling in the injured extremity has resolved. Frequent ongoing assessment of circulation, motion, and sensation **(CMS)** in parts distal to the cast is essential for early recognition of neurovascular complications. Splitting or windowing the cast may be necessary to release pressure over a specific area, particularly a bony prominence.

Traction

Skin Traction Traction is the application of a mechanical pulling force. Skin traction can be applied to immobilize an injured site and to relieve pain. A rope, pulley, and weight system (5–10 lb) is attached to the device to provide pulling force to skin and soft tissues.

There are many types of skin traction. **Buck's traction** consists of a foam boot with Velcro straps applied to the lower leg to help immobilize and may relieve pain in clients with fractured hip before surgery. Superficial peroneal nerve compression can result if the straps are too tight. Frequent release of the straps prevents this complication. **Bryant's traction**, another type of skin traction, is used primarily for children under 3 years of age who have sustained a fractured femur. The cervical halter and pelvic girdle are also used in skin traction.

Box 27-1 **CLASSIFICATION OF FRACTURES**

Greenstick

- A crack; the bending of a bone with incomplete fracture; only affects one side of the **periosteum**
- Common in children when bones are pliable

Comminuted

- Bone broken into several fragments
- Common in long bone ends (spongy bone)

Open (Compound)

- Bone exposed to the external environment through a break in the skin
- Can be associated with soft tissue injury
- Infection a common complication

Closed (Simple)

- Intact skin
- Reduced risk for infection

Compression

- Frequently seen with vertebral fractures
- Fractured bone compressed by other bones

Impacted

- One part of fractured bone driven into another

Depressed

- Usually seen in skull or facial fractures
- Bone or fragments of bone driven inward

Pathologic

- Break associated with a disease process (e.g., osteoporosis, cancer)

Skin traction for acute muscle spasm should be continuous, but skin traction for chronic problems such as muscle strain is *intermittent*, removed and reapplied as specified by the healthcare provider. Complications of skin traction relate to skin integrity and neurovascular impairment.

Skeletal Traction Skeletal traction is applied directly to bone to reduce a fracture or to maintain a surgically manipulated bone alignment. Significantly greater weight is used with this mode of traction. Pins or wires are inserted through the skin and soft tissue and into bone, and then the desired weight is applied to maintain bone alignment. This type of traction is *continuous*; removing or lifting weights displaces fragments and can cause neurovascular damage. **Balanced suspension** uses splints and slings to support the extremity and weights applied for countertraction (e.g., **Thomas splint** with **Pearson attachment**). Suspended support allows greater mobility for the client with skeletal traction.

External Fixation Device **External fixation devices** have a rigid metal frame of telescoping rods with attached percutaneous pins or wires. They are used to align and immobilize complex fractures with extensive soft tissue injury or may be used to stabilize a closed fracture that will not remain in position otherwise. These self-contained devices provide traction without the use of ropes and weights and therefore allow client mobility. Similarly, a client with fracture or dislocation of cervical or high thoracic vertebrae can mobilize with a halo ring and vest.

Complications include neurovascular compromise, inadequate bone alignment, skin or soft tissue injury, pin tract infection, and osteomyelitis. Neurovascular function must be assessed every 4 hr because clients requiring these devices usually have extensive soft tissue, nerve, and vessel damage. Extensive client teaching is necessary since these clients go home with the devices in place.

To be effective, any mode of traction must include *countertraction*. This might be provided by the client's body weight, by the pull of weights in the opposite direction, or by elevating the bed under the part in traction. The line of pull must be maintained, weights must hang freely, ropes must be intact and glide freely in the pulley, and knots must be secure. Weights and knots should hang far from the pulleys. The system should be free of any impingement such as linens. It is essential that the nurse have a clear understanding of the traction type and purpose, prescribed amount of weight, and client positioning.

Acute Compartment Syndrome

Since muscle groups are bound in a nonyielding fascia and injury causes swelling due to bleeding, edema, and the like, increased pressure within the "compartment" can compromise circulation to involved tissues. Similarly, external pressure (e.g., a cast) can compromise circulation and cause muscle ischemia and necrosis. As pressure increases within the site, venous return is compressed, leading to increased

---

Box 27-2 MANIFESTATIONS OF ACUTE COMPARTMENT SYNDROME

- Pain on *passive* stretching of the muscle (or distal digits)
- Pain out of proportion to the injury
- Pain that is unrelieved by pain medication
- Pain that increases with *elevation* of the part
- Pain when pressure is applied over the compartment
- Weak active movement of distal digits

---

interstitial fluid (edema), then compression of arterioles and eventually ischemic myositis (necrosis) and contracture formation. The client can nevertheless have intact distal pulses.

To prevent this complication and ultimate loss of limb, immediate fasciotomy is necessary to release the unyielding fascial boundaries. The nurse must be vigilant to early signs and symptoms of acute compartment syndrome (Box 27-2 ■).

Diminished or absent pulses, coolness, and pallor are late signs and unreliable indicators of acute compartment syndrome. In addition to the 5 Ps mentioned above, another very important P is limb pressure. Nurses should include this in their assessment. There are numerous devices on the market and various techniques that can be used to measure compartment pressures. Pressures near 30 mm Hg are generally considered the critical threshold when fasciotomy is considered, but this can vary. Recent technology such as infrared imaging is used to measure the surface skin temperature of the affected extremity for the diagnosis of compartment syndrome; the rationale is based on the known correlation between skin temperature and limb blood flow.

> **CLINICAL ALERT**
> When assessing children for compartment syndrome, use the 3 As: anxiety, agitation, and analgesia (the need for increased pain medication). Nurses must have a high index of suspicion.

Joint Replacement (Arthroplasty)

Degenerative joint disease of the hip and knee is the number one cause of disability among older adults. This chronic disease, sometimes called osteoarthritis, has an insidious onset that may progress to pain and stiffness, which impact the client's activities of daily living (ADLs) and role functioning. Elective total joint replacement (arthroplasty) has become increasingly popular because it restores mobility and relieves pain for clients who cannot be managed by medication or physical therapy.

Total hip arthroplasty includes replacement of both the femoral and acetabular components of the hip joint. The components are usually implanted with cement. Cementless components are also available and are preferred for younger clients who may require implant revision over time. These are textured prostheses that "cement" themselves by bony ingrowth.

After total hip arthroplasty or hemiarthroplasty (femoral **prosthesis** only), the client must adhere to precautions.

Precautions are in place to prevent both prosthesis dislocation and infection in remote sites that may spread by blood to the implanted component's site. Additionally, clients may be on long-term anticoagulant therapy and must understand the need for follow-up laboratory appointments.

Discharge planning begins before admission for elective joint arthroplasty. The client receives education about the perioperative process and "clinical path" expectations, including essentials of self-care rehabilitation. The home is typically equipped with adaptive and safety features before the planned surgery. Prepared clients experience less anxiety, fewer postoperative complications, shorter length of hospital stay, and reduced incidence of hospital readmissions.

Hip Fracture

Hip surgery for the fracture client presents a different challenge. The fracture client is not undergoing *elective* surgery, has had no preoperative preparation, and is frequently ill prepared for hospitalization. The emergent hip fracture client may not have the physical health enjoyed by the elective client. The trauma client is more apt to experience serious adverse consequences of emergent hospitalization and surgery, including delirium, and requires vigilant monitoring. Care and teaching for the client with prosthetic replacement for **intracapsular** hip fracture is identical to care and teaching for the client with total hip replacement.

Hip fracture involving the head or neck of the femur is classified as *intracapsular* (within the joint capsule). Since intracapsular bone lacks periosteum, fracture healing is limited. A hemiarthroplasty is performed whereby the head and neck of the femur are surgically removed and replaced with a *prosthesis*. The client is weight bearing with an assistive device soon after surgery. Because the joint capsule has been surgically disrupted, the hip prosthesis is at risk for dislocation until healing is complete. Specific rehabilitative adherence promotes healing and prevents dislocation of the prosthesis. If the fracture is *extracapsular* (involving the intertrochanteric region), internal fixation with nail, plate, and screws is performed. There is no disruption of the joint capsule, no prosthetic implant, and therefore no risk of femoral head dislocation, and dislocation precautions are not necessary. On the other hand, a repaired fracture site must heal, so total weight bearing is usually delayed.

Amputation

Amputation of a limb may be due to trauma, in which case the psychological ramifications can be very complex, or it can be a planned reconstructive procedure and a welcome source of relief for the client who has sustained painful vascular insufficiency and tissue necrosis (80% of cases). Regardless, the client who has lost a limb must regain psychological equilibrium and learn new skills. A supportive nurse–client relationship can assist the client to cope with grieving and body image reintegration. A rehabilitation team approach addresses goals to reduce stump edema, promote healing, prevent contractures, increase strength, and facilitate adjustment to loss by maximizing functional independence.

It is normal for amputees to experience *phantom sensation*, a feeling that the amputated part is still there. This occurs early postamputation and goes away over time. Clients should be informed of this before amputation, if possible. *Phantom pain*, however, appears later (after 2–3 months) and is more likely to occur in above-the-knee amputees. The client experiences knife-like pain, squeezing, or burning sensations triggered by a number of stimuli (urination, defecation, cigarette smoking, and others). This complication is thought to be due to signals generated by intact nerves previously associated with the amputated part and relayed to the cerebral cortex as originating in the phantom limb, or there may be a response by the central nervous system to a stimulus that seems to come from an intact body or a response to stored pain sensations from the previously intact limb. Analgesics are effective in managing postoperative stump pain, but have no effect on phantom pain. Unfortunately, there is no treatment that is consistently effective. Interventions to reduce phantom pain include:

- Intense preoperative pain management
- Use of opioids, ketamine
- Use of anticonvulsants, antidepressants, and TENS
- Stump desensitization with massage and transdermal anesthetics
- Early prosthetic use

Orthopedic Assessment

All orthopedic clients must be vigilantly monitored for skin and neurovascular status (CMS) of the affected part (Table 27-1 ■). Assessments should be conducted before, during, and frequently after application of any immobilizing modality. The contralateral extremity and documented baseline findings should be used for comparison.

Table 27-1 Neurologic Assessment

	Motion	Sensation
Upper Extremity		
Radial nerve	Hyperextends wrist Hyperextends thumb and four fingers	Web space between thumb and index finger
Ulnar nerve	Abducts (spreads) fingers	Lateral aspect of hand and distal end of little finger
Median nerve	Flexes wrist Opposes thumb and little finger	Distal end of index finger
Lower Extremity		
Peroneal nerve	Dorsiflexes ankle Flexes toes	Web space between great and second toe
Tibial nerve	Plantar flexes ankle and toes	Medial and lateral surfaces on sole of foot

Nursing Diagnoses

The following nursing diagnoses may be appropriate to include in a client care plan when the components are related to a client who requires special orthopedic procedures.

NURSING DIAGNOSIS	RELATED TO . . .
Disturbed Body Image	Trauma or injury, illness, chronic pain, situational crisis, treatments
Acute Confusion	Delirium
Ineffective Health Maintenance	Motor impairment
Injury, Risk for	Altered mobility, risk for falls or trauma, physical environmental factors, impaired balance, gait difficulties
Impaired Physical Mobility	Loss of integrity of bone structures, musculoskeletal impairment, neuromuscular impairment, pain, prescribed movement restrictions
Acute Pain	Physical injury
Chronic Pain	Arthritis, neurologic injury
Impaired Tissue Integrity	Altered circulation, impaired physical mobility, mechanical factors
Ineffective Peripheral Tissue Perfusion	Interruption of arterial flow, interruption of venous flow, mechanical reduction of venous or arterial blood flow

Application of Immobilizing Devices

Nursing Process Data

ASSESSMENT Database

- Recognize need for site immobilization.
- Determine type of immobilization required.
- Select appropriate immobilizing equipment.
- Assess status of surrounding tissue.
- Assess affected extremity for CMS before and after applying modality.

PLANNING Objectives

- To immobilize an extremity or body part
- To maintain functional alignment
- To limit harmful movement
- To reduce or prevent pain
- To prevent further soft tissue injury and complications
- To preserve neurovascular function
- To promote healing

IMPLEMENTATION Procedures

DOCUMENTATION AND EVALUATION

Expected Outcomes

- Treated part is effectively immobilized.
- Pain is reduced.
- Edema and bleeding are controlled.
- Further injury is prevented.

Unexpected Outcomes/Alternative Actions

Pearson Nursing Student Resources

Find additional review materials at
nursing.pearsonhighered.com.
Prepare for success with NCLEX®-style practice questions and Skill Checklists.

Skill 27.1.1 | Applying a Sling

Equipment
Commercial sling *or*
Triangular cloth or bandage
Safety pins

Preparation
1. Check healthcare provider's orders for a sling.
2. Wash hands.
3. Introduce self and identify client with two identifiers.
4. Assess injured extremity CMS before sling application.

> **CLINICAL ALERT**
> Never move an extremity to see if it is fractured. Ask if the client is able to move the limb instead. Always splint the extremity as found.

5. Explain procedure and purpose of immobilization.
6. Remove any circumferential jewelry (ring, bracelet).
7. Have client sit or stand with forearm across chest.

Procedure
1. Place one end of triangular cloth against the chest on the affected side and over the shoulder of the unaffected arm.
2. Place the apex (point) of the triangle toward the elbow of the affected extremity.
3. Bring the opposite end of the triangle over the affected arm and over the affected shoulder.
4. Tie the sling at the side of the neck.
5. Fold the apex of the triangle over the elbow in the front, and secure with a safety pin or twist end and tie a square knot.
6. Assess client for comfort and for support of the affected arm.
7. Assess for neck pressure and peripheral CMS after 30 min and then every 2–4 hr.

Note: If using commercial sling, check directions on package for proper application. ❶ ❷

> **CLINICAL ALERT**
> If greater immobilization is indicated (e.g., for shoulder dislocation or fracture), a swath can be applied over the sling, circling and securing the upper arm to the torso.

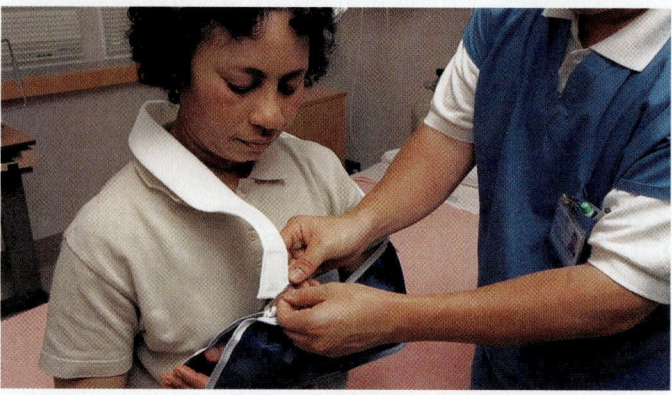

❶ Bring strap over shoulder and pull strap through metal hoops on sling.

❷ Hand should be supported at a level slightly higher than the elbow to prevent edema.

8. Check that hand is supported at a level higher than elbow to prevent dependent edema.
9. Teach client to support the arm higher than heart level and to perform **external rotation** shoulder exercises to prevent shoulder joint stiffness.

Skill 27.1.2 | Applying a Spiral Bandage

Equipment
Elastic or gauze roller bandages (width and number required to treat site)
Safety pins or tape
Supplies for wound care if indicated

Preparation
1. Check healthcare provider's orders, introduce self, identify client with two identifiers, and explain procedure and purpose of immobilization.
2. Wash hands.

3. Assess CMS of extremity before bandage application.
4. Remove any circumferential jewelry (ring, bracelet).
5. Have client sit or lie with part elevated.

Procedure

1. Remove existing elastic bandage or use bandage scissors to remove previously applied gauze bandage. ➤ *Rationale:* This is to prevent further injury and allow direct observation of site and wound care if indicated.
2. Remove dressing and redress wound if indicated (see Chapter 25).
3. Place part to be bandaged in an elevated position. ➤ *Rationale:* This promotes venous return and facilitates bandage compression to control edema and bleeding.
4. If area is functional or to be exercised, apply bandage with muscle in full contraction. ➤ *Rationale:* This prevents bandage constriction with future muscle activity.
5. Hold gauze or elastic roll with loose end of outer part of bandage facing client's skin several inches below the site of injury.
6. Unroll bandage twice around extremity to anchor bandage. ❶

❶ Spiral bandage may be used to secure a wound dressing.

7. Continue wrapping extremity upward, using a moderate amount of tension to stretch and apply bandage uniformly. ➤ *Rationale:* Unequal pressure can adversely affect circulation.
8. Wrap the extremity *proximally* with spiral or angled turns. ➤ *Rationale:* Circular turns create a tourniquet effect. Proximal wrapping promotes venous return.
9. Make bandage turns that overlap by at least one half the previous wrap to prevent bandage separation. ➤ *Rationale:* Bandage turn separation tends to pinch the skin.

CLINICAL ALERT

Cryotherapy Limits Injury

Application of ice (cryotherapy) causes vasoconstriction, reduces capillary permeability, and decreases tissue metabolism. The decreased metabolism results in decreased secondary metabolic injury and thus less tissue debris (free tissue protein). Cryotherapy used as soon as possible limits the extent of the injury, but once secondary metabolic injury has occurred, cryotherapy has no value in removing edema that has formed. The only way to relieve the edema is by removing excess free protein in the tissue by way of the lymphatic system. This generally requires intermittent compression as occurs with active exercise. (See Chapter 24, Heat and Cold Therapies.)

---

10. Finish wrap with a couple of wraps directly overlying each other.
11. Secure the **spiral bandage** by tying or using tape or safety pin.
12. Observe that bandage is snug but not tight, is free of wrinkles, and is not occluding distal circulation.
13. Assess distal digits for CMS in 30 min and every 2–4 hr initially.
14. Maintain elevation of involved extremity and encourage active motion of digits. ➤ *Rationale:* This helps reduce edema and maintain function.
15. Rewrap bandage at least every 8 hr.

| **Skill 27.1.3** | Applying a Figure-Eight Bandage to the Ankle |

Equipment

Roller bandage
Safety pin or tape

Preparation

1. Introduce self, identify client, and explain procedure and rationale.
2. Wash hands and provide privacy.
3. Position ankle in neutral alignment, neither overflexed nor overextended.

Procedure

1. Gather necessary bandages. The number and width of the bandage depends on the extent and area of the extremity to be bandaged.
2. Hold roll with outer part next to client's skin over instep. ❶
3. Anchor bandage by making an angled turn around instep.
4. Make a circular turn around heel and return to starting point.
5. Make a spiral turn down over the ankle and around the foot.

(continued)

Skill 27.1.3 | Applying a Figure-Eight Bandage to the Ankle (continued)

❶ Make an angled turn around instep.

❷ A figure-eight turn is used to support and limit joint movement.

6. Continue to make alternate turns around the ankle and foot. Overlap the preceding turn by at least two-thirds over the preceding layer.
7. Wrap the entire area below and above the involved joint. **❷**
   ➤ *Rationale:* This immobilizes the affected area.
8. Assess extremity (exposed digits) for CMS and evenness of pressure as well as comfort of client.

9. Assess extremity after 20 min and then every 2–4 hr, and rewrap every 8 hr.
10. Maintain elevation of extremity.

Note: Edema can result if the heel is not enclosed within bandage.

Skill 27.1.4 | Applying a Splint in the Emergent Setting

Equipment
Splint materials: commercial splint
Padding materials: swath, gauze wrap
Wrapping materials: tape, elastic bandage

Preparation
1. Introduce self and identify client using two identifiers. Wash hands. Check orders.
2. Assess involved extremity for deformity or soft tissue injury.
3. Do not remove clothing or shoes (except with scissors).
   ➤ *Rationale:* This prevents excessive manipulation of the injured part.
4. Remove any jewelry from extremity to prevent circulatory compromise with swelling.
5. Assess neurovascular status of distal digits.
6. Explain need for and purpose of splint to client.

Procedure
1. Gather needed supplies.
2. Control bleeding by applying direct pressure and by using pressure dressings; apply clean covering to any wound.

3. Explain the rationale for the intervention to client.
4. Move injured extremity as little as possible and splint as it lies.

> **CLINICAL ALERT**
> Never straighten an injured extremity or push bone or tissue back into place. Splint a deformed extremity in its deformed shape using a soft support such as a pillow.

5. Pad joints, bony prominences, and between digits.
   ➤ *Rationale:* This prevents skin damage. Also make sure that the padding does not affect the client's circulation (e.g., do not put padding in axilla).
6. Use a spiral (not circular) technique to wrap splint.
7. Strap the splint and extremity together securely so that the extremity is immobile. Try to include the proximal and distal points in the splint.
8. Check the client's distal circulation by assessing pulse, capillary refill, color, and temperature.
9. Elevate part to reduce edema formation.
10. Assess extremity after 20 min and then every 2–4 hr, and rewrap every 8 hr.

Skill 27.1.5 | Applying a Cervical Collar

Equipment
Sizing chart
Two collars of appropriate size (a spare for alternate use), each with an additional removable pad
Assistant, if client has known or suspected cervical injury

Preparation
1. Check the healthcare provider's order.
2. Introduce self, identify the client with two identifiers.
3. Explain procedure to the client.
4. Place client flat supine.
5. Select appropriate size collar based on length of neck from client's mandible to the clavicle (the longer the neck, the larger the collar).

Note: Some collars allow for anterior and posterior vertical height adjustment.

6. Select appropriate size collar.

Procedure
1. Perform hand hygiene.
2. Obtain assistance if client has known or suspected cervical injury. One maintains neck alignment while the collar is applied.
3. Follow manufacturer's instructions to apply collar. Save instructions and container for later use.
4. Place back half of collar on client's neck, centering with the spine, arrow pointing up.
5. Center front half of collar on front of client's neck, using a scooping motion upward from the chest so that chin fits into the indentation. ➤ *Rationale:* This ensures neutral alignment.
6. Lap back half over front half of collar.

7. Adjust Velcro straps to ensure a secure fit. ➤ *Rationale:* Collar should be snug enough to prevent movement, but not interfere with client's ability to breathe, swallow, or speak. ❶
8. Inspect skin under collar regularly, and cleanse with soap and water.
9. Assess neurovascular status of upper and lower extremities immediately after application of collar and every 4–8 hr, if indicated.
10. Clean collar and removable pads as needed with soap and water and allow to dry naturally; do not use a hair dryer.
11. Maintain collar use 24 hr/day or as ordered, using alternate collar when necessary.
12. Caution the ambulatory client that without neck **flexion,** visibility of stairs or objects on the floor is limited.

❶ Ensure side straps of collar are properly adjusted for a secure fit.

Skill 27.1.6 | Applying a Jewett–Taylor Back Brace

Equipment
Front and back brace with Velcro straps ❶
T-shirt

Preparation
1. Check healthcare provider's order and determine rationale for brace application.
2. Determine that client's brace has been fitted by an orthotist (brace fitter).
3. Introduce self, identify client, explain procedure, or supervise client's application and reinforce previous teaching.
4. Provide privacy.
5. Change wound dressing, if indicated, before applying brace.

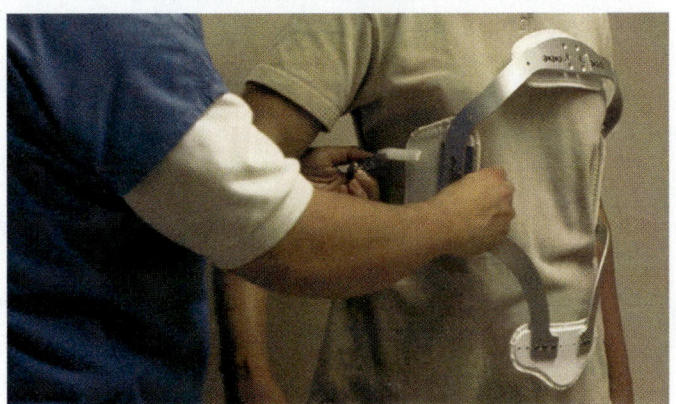

❶ Jewett–Taylor brace being adjusted after application.

(continued)

Skill 27.1.6 | Applying a Jewett–Taylor Back Brace *(continued)*

Procedure

1. Perform hand hygiene.
2. Put T-shirt on client. ➤ *Rationale:* This protects the skin from the brace rubbing on bare skin.
3. Place bed in a flat position. Keep side rail in UP position on side of bed opposite from you.
4. Log-roll or ask client to roll to side away from you.
   ➤ *Rationale:* This position prevents **torque** on the spine.
5. Position brace on back so that struts fit on either side of spine and it fits the natural contour of the back.
   ➤ *Rationale:* Struts provide an open space along the spine, so pressure is not exerted on a surgical site or on vertebrae.
6. Log-roll the client back onto brace to a supine position.

> **CLINICAL ALERT**
>
> In certain nonacute instances, the brace may be applied with the client in the upright position.

7. Place front section of brace over the iliac crest and position iliac wings (made of plastic material). Adjust triangular sternum piece; metal struts will fall into place.
8. Secure brace with Velcro straps.
9. Check under brace for pressure areas. If pressure areas are present, report to orthotist.
10. Provide client with adaptive aids (i.e., reacher).
    ➤ *Rationale:* Client cannot bend forward while wearing brace.

Unit 27.1 Documentation and Evaluation

DOCUMENTATION for Applying Immobilizing Modalities

- Time of application
- Site involved
- Skin integrity or wound status
- Type of immobilizing modality applied

- Circulatory and neurologic status of distal parts before and after modality application
- Site positioning or alignment
- Subjective statements of client

EVALUATION/Critical Thinking

Expected Outcomes

- Treated part is effectively immobilized.
- Pain is reduced.
- Edema and bleeding are controlled.
- Further injury is prevented.

Unexpected Outcomes	**Alternative Actions**
• Bandage securing wound dressing continues to fall off.	• Avoid tape if skin is fragile or area has impaired circulation. An expanding wrap can be used to secure dressings and IV sites. • Consult wound care specialist for alternative suggestions.
• Client with back brace refuses to eat.	• Loosen brace before and for a while after meals. • Encourage small, frequent meals. • Reduce intake of gas-forming foods (cabbage, beans, corn). • Suggest intake of liquid nutritional supplement.
• Client with brace expresses feelings of "being trapped."	• Allow client to voice concerns and explore options for self-control, such as access to telephone, call bell, and so on.

• Elevation of extremity and passive stretching of digits increase pain, pain medications are ineffective, and pressure applied to injured site produces severe pain.	• Suspect acute compartment syndrome and notify healthcare provider immediately. Fasciotomy may be indicated if tissue swelling compromises circulation within a muscle compartment. • Loosen external immobilizing device. • Maintain extremity in *dependent* position.
• Client experiences pain while wearing back brace.	• Encourage the client to not sit for longer than 30 min after back surgery. This increases pain due to spinal alignment in this position.
• Distal edema is noted in bandaged extremity and client is unable to move digits and states sensation is altered.	• Remove bandage and check distal CMS. • Keep extremity elevated. • Rewrap bandage with extremity in elevated position. • If edema persists, notify healthcare provider for possible anti-inflammatory medication, or further evaluation.
• Toes become edematous after ankle bandaging.	• Do *not* apply ice to extremity since this reduces blood flow to area. • Elevate extremity and encourage active exercise of toes to promote venous return. • If area feels warm to touch, consider application of ice to help reduce inflammation. • Loosen bandage.
• Client with neck brace expresses fear of falling.	• Suggest removal of scatter rugs and other obstacles that might cause tripping. • Have client view environment from a distance before advancing into it. • Suggest use of a "blind" cane to scan or tap the area in front of client to warn of potential obstacles or steps.

Nursing Process Data

ASSESSMENT Database

- Identify type of cast applied and rationale for application.
- Note condition for which the cast was applied.
- Observe condition of the cast.
- Assess neurovascular status of involved extremity.
- Assess client's understanding of and adherence to care instructions.

PLANNING Objectives

- To immobilize a fracture site
- To maintain normal sensation, movement, and circulation in a casted extremity
- To improve muscle tone and joint flexibility
- To promote bone healing
- To facilitate self-care after cast application and removal

IMPLEMENTATION Procedures

DOCUMENTATION AND EVALUATION

Expected Outcomes

- Cast integrity is maintained to provide adequate site immobilization.
- Client experiences minimal swelling.
- Neurovascular complications do not occur.

Unexpected Outcomes / Alternative Actions

Pearson Nursing Student Resources

Find additional review materials at
nursing.pearsonhighered.com.
Prepare for success with NCLEX®-style practice questions and Skill Checklists.

Skill 27.2.1 | Caring for a Wet Cast

Equipment
Pillows for support
Pen to mark drainage

Preparation
1. Note healthcare provider's orders for any client-specific instructions about casting, positioning, or cast handling. A cast (Table 27-2 ■) may be applied as long as 48–72 hr after injury. ➤ *Rationale:* This allows the swelling to go down and reduces the risk of compartment syndrome.
2. Introduce self, identify client with two client identifiers, and explain all procedures. Wash hands.
3. Recruit assistant(s) to help turn client.
4. Consider client's need for an analgesic.

Procedure
1. Explain that the cast feels warm as plaster dries, but urge client to report undue warmth or a burning sensation. ➤ *Rationale:* Cast burns can cause serious tissue injury.
2. Until the cast is dry, use *only* the palms of your hands to handle cast when turning and positioning. ➤ *Rationale:* Fingers can indent cast and create pressure areas on underlying tissue.
3. Avoid handling over joints where nerves and blood vessels are superficial.
4. Support cast with pillows, with extremity elevated above heart level. ➤ *Rationale:* This promotes venous return and reduces edema formation. ❶ ❷
5. Maintain contours built into the cast; support leg so that heel is free of pressure. ➤ *Rationale:* This prevents flattening.
6. Keep wet cast uncovered and turn client to both sides, prone, and supine to expose all surfaces, allowing cast to dry by natural evaporation from the inside out.

Note: The wet plaster of Paris cast is dry when musty odor is gone, the cast is white and shiny, and it sounds resonant when tapped.

7. Do not try to hasten drying by using artificial measures such as a hair dryer. ➤ *Rationale:* Outer layer may dry before inner aspect, resulting in cast weakening.
8. If ice pack is ordered to reduce edema, place it alongside of cast, not on cast. ➤ *Rationale:* Placing ice pack on the cast can cause flattening.
9. If cast edges are rough or crumbly, pull inner stockinette out and over the edge and secure with tape.

> **CLINICAL ALERT**
> Injured tissues swell, but encircling therapies do not expand. For any encircling modality, assess distal digits for CMS. Assessment is ongoing and continues after discharge.

Table 27-2 Comparison of Cast Types

	Plaster	Synthetic
Material	Plaster of Paris, comprised of powdered calcium sulfate crystals impregnated into bandages	Polyester and cotton, fiberglass, or plastic. Polyester and cotton are impregnated with water-activated polyurethane resin.
Drying time	24–48 hr No weight bearing until dry	7–15 min for setting 60 min for weight bearing
Advantages	Less costly More effective for immobilizing fracture site Smooth surface Does not require expensive equipment for application	Less likely to indent into skin Lighter in weight Less restrictive Does not crumble Nonabsorbent

❶ Position extremity above heart level to reduce edema formation. Check cast for tightness. The nurse should be able to insert one or two fingers between cast and skin.

❷ Plaster casts are still being used, especially in disaster situations. Position casted extremity above level of heart to reduce edema formation.

Skill 27.2.2 | Assessing a Casted Extremity

Equipment
Pen to mark drainage on cast

Procedure
1. Introduce self, identify client with two client identifiers, and wash hands.
2. Explain rationale for the procedure to client.
3. Encourage client to notify you of any change in sensation, mobility, or color/temperature in the casted extremity.
   a. Circulation ❶
   • Report if digits are swollen despite elevation and active exercise.
   • Report if digits are pale, blue, or cold to touch.
   • Report delayed (>2 sec) capillary refill (pinch finger to blanch and determine length of time required for color to return)
   b. Motion
   • *Immediately* report pain on passive movement of digits.
   • Report inability to actively move digits (see Table 27-1).
   • Compare strength of action with uninvolved extremity.
   c. Sensation
   • *Immediately* report increasing or unrelieved pain, pain with passive motion of digits, or pain that increases when the extremity is elevated.
   • Report numbness or **paresthesia** (pins-and-needles feeling).
   • Assess involved nerve sites for sensation (see Table 27-1).

> **CLINICAL ALERT**
> Always assess active **extension**, flexion, **adduction**, and **abduction** of the fingers; flexion and extension of the toes; and inversion and dorsiflexion of the foot. Pain on passive stretching of the muscle or distal digits is an *early* indicator of circulatory compromise. Diminished or absent pulses, coolness, and pallor are *late* signs and unreliable indicators of acute compartment syndrome.

4. Emphasize that a fine margin exists between reversible and irreversible damage to neurovascular structures.

> **CLINICAL ALERT**
> Do not use abductor bars (incorporated into cast) for moving the client. Move the client as a unit instead.

5. Assess for capillary refill by applying pressure to one of the client's digits. After you stop the pressure, observe the area to see how rapidly the color returns.

> **CLINICAL ALERT**
> When casting material inhibits palpation of peripheral pulses, assess capillary refill, assess for edema, comfort level, and other parameters of CMS as an indication of neurovascular status. Casted extremity should be assessed every half hour for 4 hr, then every 4 hr.

6. Ask the client to move the fingers or toes distal to the cast. The client should be able to move them without difficulty.
7. Check for any drainage on cast. Note color and size of drainage and mark cast with time. ❷

> **CLINICAL ALERT**
> If the client has had open reduction, wound drainage will be absorbed and spread rapidly or seep down to the back of the cast. The visible drainage does not necessarily indicate the amount of actual drainage.
>
> Inspect all cast surfaces and mark drainage regularly if it is increasing. Bleeding should not persist after 24 hr.

❶ Check fingers or toes for color, temperature, capillary refill, sensation, and motion.

❷ Observe casted extremity frequently to monitor and mark drainage. Assess dependent area for drainage as well.

8. Report any unusual odor or increase in drainage.
   ➤ *Rationale:* Active bleeding should cease. Stain should turn brown after 24 hr.
9. Check for redness around casted area.
10. Cover rough edges of cast with stockinette or smooth tape "petals." ➤ *Rationale:* This is to prevent skin irritation, which can lead to skin breakdown.

11. Massage area under cast, but avoid lotions and powders.
12. Remind client to not stick objects inside the cast to scratch skin. ➤ *Rationale:* Skin breakdown can occur, leading to infection.
13. Suggest use of an aseptic syringe or hair dryer (cool setting) to blow under cast to relieve itching or to apply pressure over the area.

Skill 27.2.3 | Instructing Client in Self-Care

Equipment
Instructions pamphlet
Relevant telephone numbers

Preparation
1. Review client's chart for type of reduction performed (open or closed).
2. Introduce self, identify client, wash hands, and explain importance of self-care to prevent complications.
3. Provide written instructions that reinforce teaching.
4. Provide resources for client if relevant for follow-up concerns.

Procedure
1. Demonstrate and teach importance of regular neurovascular checks, comparing with contralateral extremity. (See Skill 27.2.2, Assessing a Casted Extremity.)
2. Teach client to keep casted extremity elevated and to actively exercise digits. ➤ *Rationale:* This reduces edema formation, pain, and stiffness; stimulates lymph flow; and reduces risk of thrombus formation.
3. Report any unusual odor, new drainage, or fever.
   ➤ *Rationale:* These are signs of possible infection, especially if client has had open reduction or an object has been placed or fallen into the cast.
4. Remind client to not stick objects into the cast to scratch the skin. Encourage client to blow cool air (hair dryer on cool setting or Asepto bulb syringe) or to apply pressure over the area to relieve itching. ➤ *Rationale:* Scratching the area abrades the skin and can cause infection.
5. Teach cast protection.

   a. Remove stains with nonabrasive powder cleanser and damp cloth.
   b. Do not shellac or varnish to waterproof the cast. It must "breathe."
   c. Use plastic covering (garbage bag) for showering. Do not cover for prolonged periods as this will cause condensation and weaken the cast.
   d. Report any cracking or softening of cast and redness of skin at cast edges.
   e. Protect cast from urine or stool by covering edge with plastic wrap, as odor cannot be removed.
   f. Sleep with casted lower extremity next to wall, if possible.
      ➤ *Rationale:* If the casted extremity falls off the bed, the client will go with it.

6. Cast removal.

   a. Inform client that cast saw blade is safe. It does not cut through material, but vibrates. ❶
   b. Prepare client that muscle will have atrophied with disuse, joints will be stiff, and bone is vulnerable to refracture. Skin may appear pale and ashen.
   c. Teach client to continue to protect, support, and elevate the extremity after cast removal.
   d. Teach client that skin will be caked with adherent exudate and not to forcibly remove this. Soften exudate with olive oil or use full-strength coldwater wash (e.g., Woolite®), leave on 20 min, and then rinse in warm water. ➤ *Rationale:* Aggressive removal of exudate can cause bleeding. Enzymes in special cleansers will loosen dead cells and fatty or crusty lesions without injuring underlying cells.

❶ Cast is split with a vibrating blade. Underlying padding is cut with bandage scissors.

(continued)

Skill 27.2.3 | Instructing Client in Self-Care (continued)

LEGAL CONSIDERATIONS

***Collins v. Westlake Community Hospital* (1974)**
In this still-relevant case, a client treated for a fractured leg developed ischemia within 3 days, necessitating amputation. The healthcare provider had written an order for the nurses to monitor peripheral CMS, and although the standard of nursing care required frequent monitoring of the client's circulation, the nurses' notes failed to show that the client's circulation had been monitored at any time during the crucial 7-hr period when the client's condition became critical. Nursing negligence was upheld by the court.

Source: Bernzweig (1996)

Standard nursing practice dictates that clients with casts be monitored frequently to detect and prevent complications. Additionally, clients discharged after cast application must receive discharge instructions including self-care, cast care, and adverse signs and symptoms to report.

Note: Monitoring the client's condition and reporting changes are primary nursing responsibilities. Nurses who fail to record their observations run the risk of being unable to convince a jury that such observations actually were made. Failure to report the client's worsening condition is also another source of litigation.

Unit 27.2 Documentation and Evaluation

DOCUMENTATION for Cast Care

- Type of cast applied (see Table 27-2)
- Positioning of cast, repadding
- Client's complaints and nursing responses
- Color, warmth, movement, and sensation in casted extremity

- Presence, location, and amount of drainage from wound
- Client's acceptance of the cast
- Skin assessment
- Actions related to splitting of cast (if needed)

EVALUATION/Critical Thinking

Expected Outcomes
- Cast integrity is maintained to provide adequate site immobilization.
- Client experiences minimal swelling.
- Neurovascular complications do not occur.

Unexpected Outcomes	**Alternative Actions**
• Cast cracks from improper drying or stress.	• Notify healthcare provider immediately. • Reassure client. • Do not reposition client until healthcare provider assesses.
• Synthetic cast has rough edges.	• Smooth edges by filing with nail file if necessary. • Make sure furniture and clothing are protected from scratches and snags by covering cast with stockinette.

• Cast edges begin to crumble.	• "Petal" edges of cast with 2.5- to 5-cm (1- to 2-in.) strips of tape:
	  • Place half of tape inside cast, pull tape over cast, and anchor on outside of cast.
	  • Continue to petal cast until all edges are covered.

• Client develops itching and burning under synthetic cast after swimming.	• Immersion should be avoided. • Flush skin under cast with plain water if it has been exposed to chlorine. • Dry skin under cast thoroughly with hair dryer on LOW. This may require several hours!
• Fingers swell after application of arm cast.	• Assess that there is room for two fingers to be slipped under cast. • Apply ice alongside of cast and maintain elevation after cast application. • Maintain arm positioning with hand higher than elbow. • Encourage client to exercise fingers to help reduce edema. • Monitor neurovascular status frequently.
• Client develops pain not relieved by analgesics, pain that worsens with extremity elevation and passive stretching of digits.	• Maintain extremity in dependent position. • Notify orthopedic technician immediately: Windowing or bivalving cast may be indicated. • Suspect acute compartment syndrome and notify healthcare provider immediately to obtain measurement of compartment pressure. • Fasciotomy may be indicated if tissue swelling or external device compromises circulation within a muscle compartment.

Traction

Nursing Process Data

ASSESSMENT Database

- Determine type and purpose of traction used.
- Note the amount of weight ordered.
- Note any conditions requiring special treatment (i.e., continuous or intermittent traction).
- Assess circulation, motion, and sensation (CMS) of affected extremity.
- Assess pin site for drainage and signs of infection.
- Assess neurovascular status of clients with external fixation devices.
- Assess skin for signs of breakdown due to immobility.

PLANNING Objectives

- To relieve muscle spasm
- To maintain alignment of fracture site
- To prevent unnecessary injury to soft tissue
- To prevent neurovascular complications
- To use for temporary management of fractures in adults
- To maintain pin site free of infection

IMPLEMENTATION Procedures

DOCUMENTATION AND EVALUATION

Expected Outcomes

- Extremity is maintained in correct alignment.
- Neurovascular status is within normal limits.
- Pin site remains free of infection.

Unexpected Outcomes/Alternative Actions

Pearson Nursing Student Resources

Find additional review materials at
nursing.pearsonhighered.com.
Prepare for success with NCLEX®-style practice questions and Skill Checklists.

Skill 27.3.1 | Maintaining Skin Traction

Preparation

1. Determine whether client is preoperative. If so, do not manipulate the extremity.
2. Determine whether client has condition (diabetes, peripheral vascular disease) that predisposes to skin damage with traction.
3. Determine whether traction is continuous or intermittent.
4. Recruit an assistant to apply manual traction when removing and replacing traction. Wash hands.
5. Explain purpose of traction to client and family (Table 27-3 ■).

Procedure

1. Examine type of traction used that attaches weights to the extremity.

    a. Material should be held firmly in place.
    b. Material should fit comfortably, neither too loose nor too tight.
    c. Client should be in functional alignment.

> **CLINICAL ALERT**
> Unless otherwise ordered, the client with Buck's extension should have the knee gatch of the bed elevated 20–30 degrees to flex the hip in a neutral position.

2. Examine all bony prominences of the involved extremity for abrasions or pressure areas.

    a. Traction should be released at least every 8 hr for skin inspection. ❶

❶ Remove straps on Buck's traction every 8 hr to maintain function and allow inspection.

    b. Have an assistant apply manual traction when discontinuing for assessment.
    c. Check for redness, which, if present, indicates excessive pressure on site.

3. Examine extremity distal to the traction.

    a. Note any presence of edema.
    b. Palpate peripheral pulses.

> **CLINICAL ALERT**
> Do not apply Buck's traction over or under a calf compression device. Foot pumps (only around the foot) are acceptable for deep-vein thrombosis prophylaxis.

    c. Check temperature and color contralaterally to see if both extremities are normal.
    d. Check capillary refill time.

4. Assess for possible neurologic impediment from traction slings encroaching on popliteal space, peroneal nerve, or axilla. ❷ ► *Rationale:* Numbness or tingling, if present, indicates possible neurologic involvement.
5. Examine traction system to see that the pull aligns with the long axis of the fractured bone (Box 27-3 ■).

Table 27-3 Skin Traction

Type	Purpose	Bed Position
Buck's extension	Short-term immobilization of a hip fracture before surgical intervention	Head elevated 10–20 degrees for ADLs, knee flexed 20–30 degrees
Cervical	Degenerative or arthritic conditions of cervical vertebrae, neck strain	Flat in bed or head can be elevated 15–20 degrees
Dunlop	Either skin or skeletal, used for fractured humerus	Flat in bed; arm suspended and flexed
Pelvic girdle	Low back pain, muscle spasm, or herniated disc	Head of bed and knee gatch raised, so hips flexed 45-degree angle (William's position)
Russell's	Used for fractured shaft of femur or lower leg and some knee injuries	Head of bed elevated 30–45 degrees
Bryant's	Used specifically for child weighing less than 30 lb for fractured femur or hip dysplasia	Flat in bed with both hips flexed at 45–90 degrees, legs extended and buttocks raised 2.5 cm (1 in.) from mattress

❷ Maintain traction by ensuring that weights hang freely.

(continued)

Skill 27.3.1 | Maintaining Skin Traction (continued)

6. Check the traction mechanism. ❸
   a. Weights should hang freely, off the floor and bed.
   b. Weights are 5–10 lb for adult clients.
   c. Knots should be secure in all ropes.
   d. Ropes should move freely through pulleys.
   e. Pulleys should not be constrained by knots.

7. Position correctly in bed. ❹ The client should be positioned in the center of the bed. Affected leg or arm should be aligned with trunk of body. ➤ *Rationale:* Misalignment is the leading cause of pain for traction clients. The client should not migrate or be pulled down to the end of the bed because this negates the traction.

❸ Bryant's traction is used to reduce fractured femur or treat hip dislocation in a small child.

❹ Ensure client is positioned correctly in bed.

Box 27-3 PRINCIPLES OF TRACTION MAINTENANCE

- Maintain traction pull by ensuring weights are hanging freely, off the floor or bed frame.
- Ensure knots are secure in all ropes.
- Maintain ropes in pulley system and ensure rope moves freely through system and knots do not interfere with movement.
- Maintain prescribed amount of traction (5–10 lb for adult clients).
- Maintain countertraction, with client aligned in center of bed.
- Maintain traction, either continuous or intermittent, according to healthcare provider's orders.

EVIDENCE-BASED PRACTICE
Pin Care

According to the Cochrane Database, there is no strong evidence to support one method of pin care over another. However, there is consensus to support the following: (1) use of chlorhexidine (if there is no skin sensitivity), (2) covering pin sites with a dressing that keeps the exudate away from site, (3) ensuring the dressing is held *in situ*, and (4) cleansing pin sites every 7 days unless there is evidence of infection.

Sources: Cochrane (2013) and Timms & Pugh (2012)

Skill 27.3.2 | Maintaining Skeletal Traction

Equipment
Sterile cotton-tipped applicators
Prescribed cleansing agent such as *chlorhexidine*
Sterile cup for solution
Sterile gloves
Sterile gauze sponges (as ordered)

Preparation
1. Check healthcare provider's orders regarding pin site care and client positioning.
2. Check client using two forms of identification.

3. Gather necessary equipment.
4. Perform hand hygiene.
5. Provide privacy and explain procedure to client (Table 27-4 ■).

Procedure
1. Check pin and site surrounding the pin.
   a. Pin should be immobile.
   b. Pin site should be clean and dry.
2. Assess for infection at the pin site. Note any local pain, redness, heat, or drainage.

Table 27-4 Skeletal Traction

Type	Purpose	Bed Position
External fixation devices Hoffman Synthes	Manage complex fractures with soft tissue damage; provide stability for severe comminuted fractures	Allows client mobility and active exercise of uninvolved joints
Cervical tongs Crutchfield Gardner–Wells Vinke	Used to immobilize and reduce cervical fractures. Tongs maintain alignment of cervical spine	Bed rest, supine position; may be log-rolled
Balanced suspension with Thomas splint and Pearson attachment	Align bone and promote effective line of pull	Bed rest in supine position; may turn side to side for care; knee is flexed

❶ A Thomas splint supports the thigh. It is used for balanced suspension along with skeletal traction for fracture of the femur. A Pearson attachment supports the lower leg.

EVIDENCE-BASED PRACTICE

Pin Site Infections

To date, there are several assessment tools used to examine the clinical state of pin sites and to categorize pin site infections. However, researchers found that these instruments have not been empirically tested for reliability and validity. When assessing pin sites for potential wound infections, it is more important to assess the clinical signs and symptoms of infection than the expected signs and symptoms of an inflammatory response. Clients present with individual findings that must be correlated clinically.

Source: Santy-Tomlinson, Vincent, Glossop, Jomeen, & Pearcey (2011)

3. Provide pin site care if ordered.

   a. Open applicator sticks and gauze package (nonshedding materials).

   b. Open prescribed cleansing agent and pour into cup.

   c. Don sterile gloves.

   d. Clean area with prescribed cleansing agent. Soak cotton-tipped applicators. Dip stick into solution bottle, or pour solution over sticks.

   e. Clean pin site starting at insertion area and working outward (away from pin site). ➤ *Rationale:* This method cleanses the site from cleanest to dirtiest area.

   f. Use new applicator stick for cleaning each pin site.
   ➤ *Rationale:* This prevents cross-contamination of sites.

   g. Loosely dress site with separate gauze sponge (nonshedding materials).

   h. Remove gloves and discard sticks.

   i. Perform hand hygiene.

4. Examine all bony prominences for signs of pressure areas or abrasions.

5. Check for CMS in the affected extremity.

6. Assess distal extremity for color and edema.

7. Check ropes and weights to make sure pull goes directly through long axis of the fractured bone (if applicable).
➤ *Rationale:* This pull maintains fracture in alignment.

8. Check traction mechanism. ❶

   a. Weights should hang freely, off the floor and bed.

   b. Knots should be secure in all ropes.

   c. Rope should move freely through pulleys.

   d. Pulleys should not be constrained by knots.

9. Instruct client to use trapeze correctly to assist in moving in bed and during linen change and back care. ❷
➤ *Rationale:* Use of the heel of the unaffected foot for repositioning can cause pressure ulceration. The foot should be placed flat on the bed for assistance in using the trapeze.

10. Make sure client is positioned correctly in bed.
➤ *Rationale:* If the client is pulled down to the foot of bed, the traction is negated.

11. Check placement of the foot rest. The client's foot should be correctly positioned to prevent footdrop.

12. Check if client has migrated to foot of bed. Pull client up using turn sheet. Do *not* release traction during repositioning.

> **CLINICAL ALERT**
> Skeletal traction is never released without a healthcare provider's order.

13. Change bed linen in a top-to-bottom manner while client uses trapeze to lift buttocks.

❷ A trapeze attached to an overhead frame facilitates client mobility and nursing care. Client uses both hands for repositioning to avoid twisting and back strain.

| **Skill 27.3.3** | Maintaining an External Fixator Device |

Equipment

Sterile cotton-tipped applicators
Prescribed cleansing solution
Sterile gloves
Sterile gauze sponges (as ordered)

Procedure

1. Follow Preparation and Steps 1–5 of Skill 27.3.2.
2. Assess neurovascular status of affected part every 4 hr. ❶
   ➤ *Rationale:* Clients with external fixation devices usually have extensive soft tissue, nerve, and vessel damage.
3. Provide client teaching before discharge.

> **CLINICAL ALERT**
> The fixator–fat-tissue interface may show fatty drainage that appears with movement of the tissue at the pin site. This should not be confused with purulent drainage.

   a. Instruct client on the importance of, and how to perform, neurovascular checks and when to call the healthcare provider.
   b. Demonstrate pin site care. ❷ Have client return the demonstration. ➤ *Rationale:* This is to ensure that he or she is using appropriate technique.

Note: Clean technique is used after discharge.

   c. Reinforce healthcare provider's instructions regarding activity level. Discuss weight bearing on affected limb, if appropriate.
   d. Explain that fixator device is not to be used as a handle.

> **CLINICAL ALERT**
> The extremity and the external fixator should be moved as a unit, supporting the joint above and below the frame. Repeated lifting and manipulation of the frame itself can lead to pin loosening and fracture malalignment.

4. Demonstrate range-of-motion exercises, if appropriate, and have client perform return demonstration. ➤ *Rationale:* This ensures that appropriate exercises are being performed correctly.
5. Instruct client to continue to elevate extremity if edema occurs in affected limb.
6. Teach appropriate use of assistive devices as necessary.
   ➤ *Rationale:* This prevents falls or inappropriate use of the device which could cause injuries. Lower-extremity fixators particularly alter the client's balance.

❶ Hoffman frame, external fixator is used for complex fractures and to allow early mobility.

❷ Pin site care for external fixator.

Skill 27.3.4 | Maintaining Halo Traction

Equipment
Allen wrench
Emergency tracheostomy set (available)
Bag–valve–mask (available)
Bright nail polish
Equipment for pin site care, as ordered
Prescribed cleansing solution, as ordered
Sterile cup for solution
Sterile cotton-tipped applicators
Clean gloves

Preparation
1. Review client's history to determine level and type of spinal injury and purpose of halo brace immobilization.
2. Determine specific assessment required for the particular client (depends on the level of client's spinal injury). ❶ ❷ Cervical injury at C3–C5 may compromise ventilation.
3. Gather necessary equipment.
4. Perform hand hygiene.

Procedure
1. Introduce self and identify client using two identifiers.
2. Evaluate client's understanding of halo traction and its purpose.
3. Assess client's respiratory status regularly.
4. Perform complete neurologic assessment (peripheral nerves, motion, and sensation). ➤ **Rationale:** Because of their location, these nerves are prone to injury or excessive stretching with halo traction.
5. Check alignment of traction–brace system. Client's neck should not be flexed or extended.

> **CLINICAL ALERT**
> Never use the bars of a halo brace to move the client.

❶ Halo brace traction provides immobilization after cervical or upper thoracic vertebral injury.

❷ The halo ring is attached to the vest by vertical bars (two in front and two in back). The ring is attached to the skull by two anterior and two posterior pins. Wrench on vest is for emergency release.

6. Discuss safety issues. Halo alters client's center of gravity and balance.
   a. Client has a limited view of the surrounding environment. Pathways for walking must be clear of obstacles.
   b. Consult PT and OT for adaptive aids and tips for ADLs. ➤ **Rationale:** Client should anticipate situations and problems that may occur at home such as sleeping position, bathing, and getting in and out of a car.
   c. Keep Allen wrench taped to front of vest. Mark anterior screws that attach vertical bars to brace with bright nail polish. ➤ **Rationale:** When marked, they are easy to locate. The anterior vest is removed for emergency measures such as CPR.

> **CLINICAL ALERT**
> If skull pins are loose, apply manual traction and keep client immobilized. Notify healthcare provider immediately.

7. Have emergency equipment available for establishing an airway and maintaining ventilation.
8. Suggest that client cover bolts and screws with moleskin or tape to protect clothing.

(continued)

Skill 27.3.4 | Maintaining Halo Traction *(continued)*

9. Inspect anterior (above eyebrows) and posterior (above and behind ears) pin sites for signs of drainage, crusting, or inflammation.
10. Provide skin care under vest:
    a. Open vest at both sides during bath.
    b. Check skin at vest edges and where vest overlaps.

c. Wash and dry skin thoroughly.
d. Do not use lotion or powder under brace. ➤ *Rationale:* They combine with perspiration and irritate the skin.
e. Replace vest liner if it becomes wet or dirty.
11. Provide pin site care as prescribed. See steps in Skill 27.3.3 for skeletal traction.

Unit 27.3 Documentation and Evaluation

DOCUMENTATION for Traction

- Type and location of traction, intermittent or continuous
- Alignment of traction, client's positioning
- Integrity of the skin
- CMS in extremity
- Specific client concerns and nursing actions taken to solve problems

- Client's comfort and overall feelings
- Pin site, assessment, and care
- Client and family teaching including written materials provided
- Client's progress in self-care

EVALUATION/Critical Thinking

Expected Outcomes
- Extremity is maintained in correct alignment.
- Neurovascular status is within normal limits.
- Pin site remains free of infection.

Unexpected Outcomes	Alternative Actions
• Client in skeletal traction keeps migrating to foot of bed.	• Without releasing traction, use pull sheet and an assistant to reposition client up in bed. • Elevate lower part of bed to provide countertraction. • Increase weight of countertraction at head of bed.
• Bone in skeletal traction has migrated to end of Kirschner wire.	• Notify orthopedic surgeon. • Pin will be sterilized and moved so that bone centers on wire. • Review ordered mobility restrictions with client.
• Client experiences "tightness" in thigh after fracture of the femur.	• Measure thigh circumference and compare with contralateral thigh. • Assess for presence of ecchymosis. • Monitor vital signs closely for hypovolemia (several units of blood may be sequestered in the thigh after fracture of the femur) • Notify healthcare provider for significant changes.

• Client in Buck's traction is unable to dorsiflex the foot.	• Release proximal strap as it may be compressing peroneal nerve over head of fibula. • Assess sensation over dorsum of foot and between big and second toes. • Notify healthcare provider.
• Halo pin site appears to be infected.	• Notify healthcare provider. • Obtain culture of drainage for antibiotic sensitivity studies. • Cleanse pin site as prescribed, using aseptic technique, separate applicator for each site. • Remove crusts to allow drainage. • Monitor for systemic signs of infection.

Client With Joint Replacement

Nursing Process Data

ASSESSMENT Database

- Determine type of joint replacement performed (hemiarthroplasty, total joint arthroplasty).
- Determine surgical approach to total hip arthroplasty (anterolateral or posterolateral).
- Determine whether client has had elective surgery with preoperative preparation.
- Review client's understanding of protective and preventive self-care measures.
- Assess client's progress with clinical path (pain management, activity, client's understanding of expected progress toward discharge).
- Assess that leg position is abducted with pillows or splint.
- Determine whether client uses assistive devices appropriately.

PLANNING Objectives

- To assist the client to progress with self-care after elective joint replacement surgery
- To promote activities that prevent hip dislocation
- To determine that client understands joint motions that could cause joint dislocation
- To encourage use of safety and assistive devices in performing activities of daily living

IMPLEMENTATION Procedures

DOCUMENTATION AND EVALUATION

Expected Outcomes

- Client benefits from autologous reinfusion of wound drainage.
- Client actively participates in elective arthroplasty experience.
- Client describes positions and activities to avoid in order to prevent hip prosthesis dislocation.
- Client voices understanding and demonstrates correct use of assistive devices for ADLs.

Unexpected Outcomes/Alternative Actions

Pearson Nursing Student Resources

Find additional review materials at
nursing.pearsonhighered.com.
Prepare for success with NCLEX®-style practice questions and Skill Checklists.

Skill 27.4.1 | Providing Wound Suction/Autologous Reinfusion

Equipment

Autotransfusion reservoir ready for second collection or reinfusion

Standard blood transfusion tube set with 40- or 20-micron filter

200 mL of normal saline for IV tubing and filter prime and flush postreinfusion

Blood (IV therapy) transfusion documentation form

Clean gloves

Note: A complete collection reinfusion and wound drainage system accompanies the client from PACU, consisting of a drain tube leading from the client's wound to a suction system (e.g., Hemovac). The suction collection unit is attached to the wound drainage evacuator to produce a vacuum.

Preparation

Upon client's return from PACU

1. Review healthcare provider's order for reinfusion.
2. Identify time reinfusion system was activated in the OR.
3. Mark time reinfusion should be completed.
4. Introduce self and identify client using two forms of identification.
5. Ensure that collection reservoir is connected to the wound tubing (done in OR).
6. Ensure that evacuator suction tubing is connected to drainage reservoir and evacuator is compressed for suction.
7. Monitor drainage collection, allowing 4 hr to drain, and then 2 hr for reinfusion. ➤ *Rationale:* Total reinfusion of blood should be completed within 6 hr of system activation in the OR.

Procedure

Reinfusion/Establishing New Collection System

Note: If healthcare provider has ordered to reinfuse a second time, check the reservoir 4 hr after the first reinfusion was started. If more than 100 mL has been collected, repeat the above Preparation.

1. Wash hands and don clean gloves.
2. Place new (empty) collection system in a convenient location.
3. Detach the Hemovac evacuator (secured by clip or Velcro) and remove it from the wound drainage collection reservoir.
4. Close both drain clamps on the evacuator tubing.
5. Unscrew the wound drainage tubing clamps on the evacuator tube.
6. Cap the full wound drainage collection reservoir and set it aside.
7. Connect the evacuator tube to new (empty) reinfusion reservoir.
8. Unscrew tubing connecting Hemovac evacuator to full reservoir to be reinfused.

9. Connect Hemovac evacuator tube onto new (empty) collection reservoir.
10. Uncap the Hemovac attachment spout and activate the evacuator, and then open the client's wound drain clamp.
11. Mark start time on new collection system.
12. Hang new collection unit on client's bed frame.

Reinfusion

1. Remove the spike port cap on full reservoir.
2. Insert the filter spike and begin reinfusion.
3. Gravity-reinfuse autologous blood within 6 hr of system activation (in OR).
4. Dispose of equipment in biohazard receptacle.
5. Remove gloves and perform hand hygiene.

Continued Wound Drainage

1. Connect client's wound drainage tubing to Hemovac evacuator and activate to initiate suction. ❶
2. Empty evacuator every 8 hr.
3. Remove gloves and perform hand hygiene.

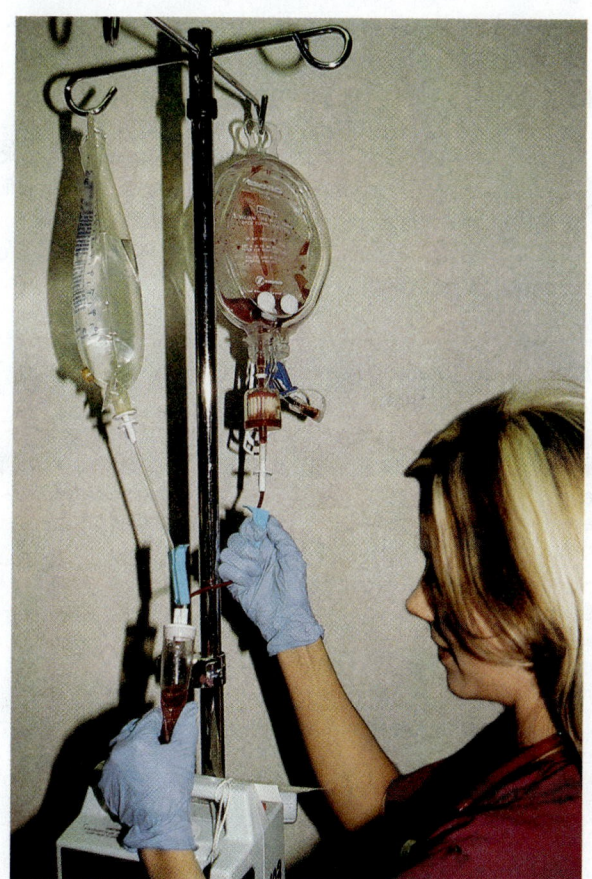

❶ Autoreinfusion system with filter provides gravity infusion of autologous blood obtained within 6 hr of wound suction activation in the OR.

Skill 27.4.2	Caring For a Client With Posterolateral Approach Hip Arthroplasty

Equipment

Abductor pillow ("wedge") or pillows (posterolateral approach)
Nonrotation boot (if ordered)
Bath blanket
Poster reminder for exercises
Walker
Toilet seat extender
Adaptive aids

Preparation

1. Introduce self, identify client, and assess client's understanding of postoperative expectations (Table 27-5 ■).
2. Determine what instructions client has received.
   ➤ *Rationale:* This is to reinforce and not contradict previous teaching. The client may be included in an acute care group exercise program.
3. Wash hands.

Procedure

Bed Positioning

1. Maintain body in alignment using abductor pillow or wedge.
   ❶ ➤ *Rationale:* The abductor serves as a reminder to keep legs in abduction to prevent dislocation of the prosthesis.
   a. Place narrow end of wedge between the thighs, above the knees, as high as possible.
   b. Place legs flush with sides of wedge and strap into place above the knee and above the ankle. ➤ *Rationale:* Avoid pressure over joints where nerves and vessels are superficial.
   c. If abductor has separate leg straps, the *unoperated* side may be loosened for comfort and to allow range of motion while client is supine.

❶ The abduction wedge or pillow prevents hip adduction and internal rotation to prevent dislocation after hemiarthroplasty or posterolateral approach total hip arthroplasty.

Table 27-5 Total Hip Arthroplasty Precautions Differ With Surgical Approach

Posterolateral Approach	Anterolateral Approach
Keep leg in abduction and extension (pillow or wedge often used).	Sitting at 90 degrees is allowed. Avoid active abduction.
Avoid flexion of the hip beyond a 90-degree angle. If while sitting client can put hands on legs below knees, that is too much flexion.	Keep legs side by side without a wedge or pillow between them.
Do not bend at the waist to put on shoes.	Avoid turning toes and knee outward. Do not extend the leg backward.
Keep needed items on the nonoperative side. Use a toilet elevator 53 cm (21 in.) and shower chair. Do not cross the operative leg past the body's midline. Do not inwardly rotate the operative leg.	Place needed items on operative side.
To turn while standing, turn away from the operative side.	To turn while standing, turn toward the operative side.

2. Place rolled soft blanket or towel under ankles to free heels from the mattress. ➤ *Rationale:* This is to prevent skin breakdown.
3. Turn client every 2 hr, keeping legs abducted with both legs strapped. *Although not generally contraindicated, review surgeon's orders before turning client to operated side.*
4. Maintain nonrotation boot (if indicated) while client is supine, but remove when client is turned. ➤ *Rationale:* This boot with bar prevents hip rotation.
5. Encourage standard postoperative preventive measures such as deep breathing, foot pumps, and ankle rotations.
6. Encourage strengthening exercises such as gluteal sets and quadriceps sets.
7. Assess CMS and skin integrity at least every 4 hr.

Strengthening Exercises

1. Place an exercise reminder sign at foot of bed. Have client hold muscle contraction for a count of 5 and repeat 10 times, and then increase hold and number of repetitions each day (may do during commercials if watching TV).

2. Quadriceps strengthening:
   Have client push back of the knee into bed. ➤ *Rationale:* This contracts muscle on top of the thigh. The quadriceps muscle is used to rise to a standing position, to climb stairs, and to walk.
3. Gluteal strengthening:

   a. Have client squeeze buttocks together tightly and hold for a count of 5 and repeat 10 times. ➤ *Rationale:* These exercises help strengthen muscles surrounding the hip.
   b. While standing, move operated leg backward, placing one hand on lower back to prevent arching, and then return leg to starting position.
   c. While standing, move operated leg laterally (out to the side), keeping foot and knee pointing straight forward, and then return to starting position.

EVIDENCE-BASED PRACTICE

Predictors of Mobility Post Hemiarthroplasty

A study conducted in Denmark demonstrated that clients who do not engage in physiotherapy on postoperative day 1 are at greater risk of not regaining basic mobility during hospitalization (OR = 3.3) ($p \leq 0.0001$). Other significant predictors of poor mobility include advanced age (>80 years), prefracture functional status, and Hgb 6 mmol/L. Recommendations to enhance mobility include conducting early discharge planning and attempting to modify other factors.

Source: Hulsbaek, Larsen, & Troelsen (2014)

Mobility and Dislocation Prevention

1. Assist client to get out of bed.

Note: A physical therapist (PT) usually supervises and assists with the first time out of bed.

   a. Raise bed to high position. ➤ *Rationale:* This allows client to exit bed without acute hip flexion.
   b. Elevate head of bed and instruct client to exit bed from unoperated side. ➤ *Rationale:* The stronger side should lead a transfer.
   c. Have client pivot on hips, while keeping legs abducted, and sit on edge of bed with operated leg out in front. Do not allow client to bend forward and push down to stand. ➤ *Rationale:* Bending forward may cause prosthesis dislocation.
   d. Assist client by supporting operative leg.
   e. Have client push down with hands on mattress to rise to a standing position. Walker should not be used for support when rising to a standing position.
   f. Walk client first postoperative day (as ordered) with an assistant and a walker with weight bearing as tolerated.
2. Instruct client about positions to avoid.

Note: Gluteal isometrics strengthen muscles that surround the joint capsule and decrease the risk of dislocation.

   a. Do not cross the legs at ankle or knee. Keep knees apart at all times. ➤ *Rationale:* Adduction can cause prosthesis dislocation.
   b. Do not stand with toes turned in. ➤ *Rationale:* **Internal rotation** can cause prosthesis dislocation.
   c. Do not flex hips greater than 90 degrees. Always sit with knees lower than hips. Avoid low chairs and do not bend over. Use toilet seat extender (elevator). ➤ *Rationale:* Flexion beyond 90 degrees can cause prosthesis dislocation.
   d. Do not sit in bathtub. Use a standing shower or shower/tub chair.
   e. When standing and turning is necessary, turn toward unoperated side. ➤ *Rationale:* Turning toward operated hip can cause hip dislocation due to internal rotation.

> **CLINICAL ALERT**
>
> Hip prosthesis dislocation usually requires a simultaneous combination of contraindicated hip positions, such as crossing the legs and acutely flexing at the same time. Dislocation precautions are continued until the joint capsule has healed. Only the orthopedic surgeon should advise clients when and if precautions are no longer necessary.

Assistive Devices and Adaptive Aids

1. Consult physical therapy and occupational therapist (OT) to obtain a walker, client instruction, and supervised ambulation and activity precautions. ❷

> **CLINICAL ALERT**
>
> The client undergoing hemiarthroplasty (replacement of the femoral head and neck) for fracture of the femur must adhere to the same precautions as client with elective total hip replacement to prevent prosthesis dislocation.

❷ Adaptive aids, such as a reacher, facilitate independence in ADLs.

(continued)

Skill 27.4.2 | Caring For a Client With Posterolateral Approach Hip Arthroplasty *(continued)*

2. Consult occupational therapy for provision and instruction in use of adaptive aids such as toilet seat extender, reachers, sock aid, long-handled sponge, and shoehorn. Instruct client to avoid wearing shoes with laces that must be tied.

3. Discuss home safety adaptations that client may have already installed in preparation for *elective* surgery: toilet extender 53 cm (21 in.), elevated chair seats, shower or tub chair, safety rails, removal of loose rugs and electrical cords, placement of frequently used items within easy reach.

> **CLINICAL ALERT**
> Because of changes in the skin that occur with aging, older clients are at increased risk for blistering and accidental removal of the epidermis by mechanical means such as tape removal. Tape should be applied vertically only, and without tension.

Skill 27.4.3 | Caring for a Client With Knee Arthroplasty

Equipment
Knee splint immobilizer
Continuous Passive Motion (CPM) device ❶ or rocking glider chair

Preparation
See previous skill.

Procedure
Continuous Passive Motion (CPM)

1. Assist client to comfortable position. Client may turn from side to side and may have head of bed up or down. There is little risk of dislocation of knee prosthesis.

2. Place pillows lengthwise under lower leg, but not under knee.

3. Apply soft foam knee immobilizer or brace (if ordered).

   a. Place wide strap over knee.
   b. Allow client to direct tightness of fit.
   c. Monitor surgical wound drainage output frequently for the first 48 hr postoperatively.

❶ CPM (continuous passive motion) device may be used to increase joint mobility after knee surgery.

Postoperative Exercises

1. Maintain accurate positioning of continuous *passive* motion device, if ordered, to gently flex knee by adjusted increments. Settings start at 10–30 degrees and are gradually increased until 90 degrees of flexion is achieved. ➤ *Rationale:* CPM may prevent adhesion formation and improve range of joint motion during early postoperative period.

2. *Alternate:* Client may use a rocking glider chair.
   ➤ *Rationale:* This encourages independent *active knee flexion and extension,* which has added benefit of getting the client out of bed, improving venous return, reducing edema formation, and preventing clot formation and other complications of bed rest.

> **CLINICAL ALERT**
> Infection is a grave complication with joint replacement surgery. It may occur during the first 3 months postoperatively or even after a year. Late infection is usually due to hematogenous spread from a distant site (teeth, GI, or urinary tract).
>
>   Clients should remind their healthcare providers and dentists about their prosthesis; antibiotics may be prescribed before dental work or other invasive procedures to prevent infection.

> **CLINICAL ALERT**
> There may be an increase in wound bleeding when initiating knee flexion exercises (CPM or mobilizing client).

   d. Assess CMS and skin integrity at least every 4 hr while splint is in place.

3. Encourage foot pumps, straight leg raising, ankle rotations, quadriceps, and gluteal sets as for client with a total hip replacement.

Getting Out of Bed

1. Assist client to pivot and sit on side of the bed, supporting the leg.
2. Unless brace is worn, encourage client to alternate bending and straightening the knee. Flex unaffected leg to support weight to a standing position while keeping operative leg extended.
3. Weight bearing as tolerated with an assistant and use of a walker is usually allowed first postoperative day.
4. A raised seat will assist client to get in and out of a chair.

EVIDENCE-BASED PRACTICE
Autologous Retransfusion Drain Compared With No Drain in Total Knee Arthroplasty (TKA)

In a prospective randomized controlled trial ($N = 115$) of clients undergoing total knee arthroplasty, there was evidence to suggest that clients who received **autologous reinfusion** (their own blood returned) after surgery had higher postoperative Hgb levels and less blood loss. In addition, reinfusion resulted in a cost savings for clients when compared to allogeneic blood transfusion.

Source: Horstmann, Kuipers, Ohanis, Slappendel, Kollen, & Verheyen (2014)

Unit 27.4 Documentation and Evaluation

DOCUMENTATION for Client With Joint Replacement

- Character and amount of wound drainage
- Autoreinfusion times and amounts on I&O record as output from a drainage system and intake as a blood product
- Wound assessment findings
- Character and amount of wound drainage
- Client positioning and frequency of turning
- Neurovascular and skin status of involved extremity

- Placement of abductor splint or brace
- Use of continuous passive motion or rocking glider chair
- Exercises performed: type, duration, and client's tolerance
- Client and family teaching; including teaching materials
- Client's understanding of teaching (return demonstration of preventive measures); use of assistive devices and other aids

EVALUATION/Critical Thinking

Expected Outcomes

- Client benefits from autologous reinfusion of wound drainage.
- Client actively participates in elective arthroplasty experience.
- Client describes positions and activities to avoid in order to prevent hip prosthesis dislocation.
- Client voices understanding and demonstrates correct use of assistive devices for ADLs.

Unexpected Outcomes

- Client's hemoglobin lab result remains less than 10 g/dL after reinfusion.

Alternative Actions

- Notify healthcare provider of lab results.
- Obtain order for type and cross and type for possible allogenic blood transfusion.

- Client with knee arthroplasty is fearful of dislocation.

- Assure client that, in contrast to hip arthroplasty, knee dislocation rarely occurs.
- Encourage client to continue quadriceps and gluteal setting and knee flexion and extension exercises.
- Consult with PT regarding client's concerns and need for reassurance and encouragement.

Unexpected Outcomes	Alternative Actions
• Client is unable to remember instructions for hip precautions.	• Provide written instructions with pictures of positions to avoid. • Request OT to work with client and caregiver to reinforce instructions/precautions. • Request Social Service consult for postoperative rehabilitation living needs. • Request OT consult for individualized assessment and recommendations and teaching.
• Client with hip arthroplasty asks about adapting ADLs to accommodate hip precautions.	• Suggest purchasing a raised toilet seat before leaving hospital (many agencies sell these). • Use a standing shower or tub with shower chair for bathing. • Wear lace-up shoes with elastic laces, so tying is not required and the foot can be slipped in with a long-handled shoe horn. • Purchase reachers or long barbecue tongs to retrieve things from the floor. • Place frequently used items at arm level, so bending is not required. • Remove scatter rugs, electric cords, and small objects from the floor. • Move car seat back as far as possible. Keep operated leg out in front, slide back into seat, and then semirecline and pivot to face front of car.

Client With an Amputation

Nursing Process Data

ASSESSMENT Database

- Determine whether amputation was therapeutic or traumatic.
- Determine rationale for therapeutic amputation (tumor, peripheral vascular disease, diabetes).
- Assess status of stump wound.
- Assess stump positioning.
- Inspect stump for presence of edema.
- Assess for phantom sensation or phantom pain.
- Assess client's acceptance of amputation.

PLANNING Objectives

- To promote wound healing
- To reduce edema and discomfort
- To prevent contracture development
- To mold and prepare stump for prosthesis use
- To assist the client in acceptance and self-care

IMPLEMENTATION Procedures

DOCUMENTATION AND EVALUATION

Expected Outcomes

- Stump wound heals without complication.
- Stump maintains functional alignment.
- Stump is prepared for prosthesis use.

Unexpected Outcomes/Alternative Actions

Pearson Nursing Student Resources

Find additional review materials at
nursing.pearsonhighered.com.
Prepare for success with NCLEX®-style practice questions and Skill Checklists.

Skill 27.5.1 | Positioning and Exercising the Stump

Equipment
Pillows

Preparation
1. Check chart for healthcare provider's orders.
2. Introduce self, identify client with two identifiers, and explain purpose of positioning and exercising.
3. Provide privacy.
4. Perform hand hygiene.

Procedure
Preoperative Care
1. Evaluate nutritional status and request nutritional consult if indicated. ➤ *Rationale:* Adequate protein is necessary to promote wound healing.
2. Recruit assistance of OT, PT, and social worker for early multidisciplinary care planning. A **prosthetist** explains future prosthetic care to the client and possibly organizes amputee peer visit, as this helps lessen anxiety about living with an amputation.
3. Explain importance of exercises to client. Tell client that because flexor muscles are stronger than extensors, stump will be permanently flexed and abducted unless the client practices extension and adduction exercises. ➤ *Rationale:* Exercises increase muscle strength and improve mobility of amputated extremity. Both are necessary for optimal ambulation with a prosthesis.
4. Teach client quadriceps-setting exercises with a below-the-knee amputation.
   a. Extend leg and try to push back of knee into bed; try to move patella proximally.
   b. Contract quadriceps and hold contraction for 10 sec.
   c. Repeat this procedure four or five times.
   d. Repeat the exercise at least four times a day.
5. Teach use of ambulatory aids. ➤ *Rationale:* This prepares client for postsurgery mobility.
6. Explain phantom limb sensation; the client may continue to "feel" the lost limb after surgery.

CLINICAL ALERT
Adequate pain management in the preoperative period can reduce the occurrence of phantom limb pain postoperatively.

7. Counsel families, for they also mourn the loss of a visible body part. ➤ *Rationale:* They too need psychological support and education about rehabilitation and necessary skills for self-care.

EVIDENCE-BASED PRACTICE
Mirror Visual Feedback (MVF) and Phantom Limb Pain
Following limb amputation, clients may develop phantom limb pain. This phenomenon is a result of a mismatch between sensory and motor feedback. Mirror visual feedback is a well-established technique that forces the client to view his limb while straddling a mirror, thereby giving the impression of having two "normal limbs." In essence, this is an optical trick that has been cited as effective in modulating pain and making the affected limb "smaller."

Source: McCabe (2011)

Postoperative Care
1. Monitor for complications: hemorrhage, infection, unrelieved pain, wound that will not heal.
2. Assess for excessive wound drainage. Keep tourniquet at bedside. ➤ *Rationale:* If excessive bleeding occurs, tourniquet must be applied, as hemorrhage is a potentially life-threatening complication.

CLINICAL ALERT
Keep a tourniquet nearby in the event of excessive stump incision bleeding.

3. Administer ordered pain medication and continually assess to determine whether pain is controlled.
4. Do not place stump on pillow, but elevate foot of bed for first 24 hr ONLY to reduce stump edema and pain. ➤ *Rationale:* Elevation on a pillow can promote flexion contracture of stump.
5. Turn client to prone or supine position for at least 1 hr every 4 hr. ➤ *Rationale:* This promotes hip extension and helps counteract possible flexion contracture formation.
6. Avoid dependent positioning of stump. ➤ *Rationale:* This is to prevent edema and discomfort. Edema may be present for up to 4 months after amputation.
7. While washing the stump, tap and massage the stump skin toward the incision line. ➤ *Rationale:* This is to prevent development of painful adhesions.
8. Teach stump extension exercises.
   a. Lie in a prone position with foot hanging over the end of the bed.
   b. Keep stump next to intact leg to extend stump and to contract gluteal muscles.
   c. Hold the contraction for 10 sec.
   d. Repeat this exercise at least four times a day.

9. Teach adduction exercise.

   a. Place a pillow between the client's thighs.

   b. Squeeze the pillow for 10 sec and then relax for 10 sec.

   c. Repeat this exercise at least four times a day.

10. Have the client keep track of time spent with the stump flexed and then spend an equal amount of time with the stump extended.

11. Encourage appropriate use of trapeze: Use both hands to pull up with trapeze; place foot flat on mattress to lift body. Do not use heel to push in the mattress. ➤ *Rationale:* Pushing with the heel can lead to pressure ulcers.

12. After stump incision heals, have client begin to bear weight on stump, initially pressing into padded surface (pillow on chair seat). ➤ *Rationale:* This is to reduce pain and help prepare the stump for prosthesis.

Skill 27.5.2 | Shrinking/Molding the Stump

Equipment

Two elastic bandages: 10 cm (4 in.) for below-the-knee amputation (**BKA**), 15 cm (6 in.) for above-the-knee amputation (**AKA**)

Tape or safety pins

Commercial stump **shrinker** (sheath)

Preparation

1. Review client's chart to determine date and type of amputation.
2. Gather equipment.
3. Identify client using two forms of identification. Introduce self and explain rationale for procedure.
4. Perform hand hygiene.
5. Provide privacy.

Procedure

1. Wash stump with soap and water and allow to dry for at least 10 min before bandaging. Do not use lotions, powders, or alcohol.
2. Inspect and encourage client to assess stump for circulatory status, pressure areas, wound healing, and edema.
3. Explain that purpose of wrap is to form a conical AKA stump to prepare for prosthesis use. ❶ ❷
4. Explain that wrap is to be worn at all times except during bathing or when wearing a prosthesis.

5. Start by placing bandage end outer surface on distal stump. ➤ *Rationale:* The pressure gradient of the bandage should be greatest at the distal stump.
6. Wrap bandage medially and diagonally around stump. Have client assist by holding turns. Stretch bandages to two-thirds of the limit of the elastic.
7. Continue to wrap smoothly up the stump with medially directed spirals or figure eight turns (not circular). Progress up the stump and well into groin area. ➤ *Rationale:* Circular turns constrict circulation. Medial turns help correct stump tendency toward abduction.
8. Finish bandaging with a "**spica**" turn over and around the client's pelvis, and then back down to stump. ➤ *Rationale:* Large "spica" turn prevents bandage slipping.
9. Secure the bandage with tape or (*cautiously*) with safety pins. Do not use bandage clips. ➤ *Rationale:* Clips can pierce the skin or easily come loose.
10. Reapply elastic bandage every 4–6 hr or when loose. ➤ *Rationale:* It must never be in place for more than 12 hr without being rewrapped.

❶ Compression bandage may be used after amputation to mold and shrink stump in preparation for prosthesis.

❷ "Commercial shrinkers" may be used for AKA.

(continued)

Skill 27.5.2 | Shrinking/Molding the Stump *(continued)*

11. If client has a stump "shrinker sheath," roll down and stretch the sheath using plastic ring. Fit onto stump end and apply, making sure there are no wrinkles.
12. Teach client home care of residual limb and prosthesis (washing; assessing for redness, pressure points, irritation, swelling, skin breakdown; socket, stump, socks, liners, mechanical parts, etc.).

> **CLINICAL ALERT**
> Amputees use more energy in ambulation than nonamputees. The older adult with an AKA must put forth an effort 100% above normal to walk at a slow rate. The longer the residual limb, the less energy the client must expend for ambulation.

Unit 27.5 Documentation and Evaluation

DOCUMENTATION for Client With an Amputation

- Time, type, and site of bandage application
- Stump positioning
- Stump and wound assessment

- Exercises performed
- Client teaching
- Client's response to stump and participation in self-care

EVALUATION/Critical Thinking

Expected Outcomes
- Stump wound heals without complications.
- Stump maintains functional alignment.
- Stump is prepared for prosthesis use.

Unexpected Problems	Alternative Actions
• Client sits in chair most of the day and keeps stump elevated on a pillow while in bed.	• Discuss hip and knee contracture complications that occur with prolonged flexion positioning of the stump. • Review and reinforce exercises that promote stump adduction and extension to prevent contractures and facilitate prosthesis use.
• Stump edema occurs in spite of compression bandage application.	• Evaluate wrapping procedure. • Ensure that wraps are applied with pressure greater at distal stump and reapplied several times a day. • Instruct client to avoid prolonged dependent positioning of stump. • Consult prosthetist for possible rigid shrinker use. • Apply shrinker before client gets out of bed.
• Client expresses fear of losing other leg.	• Teach client to care for the remaining extremity. • Inspect for lesions; wash and dry daily; use lotion for dry skin (not between toes); keep nails trimmed straight across; avoid mechanical, chemical, or thermal injury; wear shoes that are wide and deep enough for toes. • Teach client to avoid smoking; exercise daily. • Consult podiatrist for individual foot care or shoe orthotic adaptations, especially if client has diabetes. • Consult healthcare provider for management of diabetes or atherosclerosis.

Chapter Wrap-Up

GERONTOLOGIC Considerations

Musculoskeletal integrity can be enhanced and therapeutic goals reached if the aging effect on the musculoskeletal system is appreciated and incorporated into individualized care planning.

Older Adult Clients Generally Experience the Following

- Decreased height
- More brittle bones, decreased density
- Reduced muscle mass
- Diminished strength
- Joint stiffening
- Weakness and slowed movement
- Thinning of the dermis and structures supporting the junction of the epidermis and dermis weaken.
- Increased risk for blistering and epidermal stripping
- Slower and less effective healing, which may result in greater incidence of malunion and nonunion after fracture

Older Adult Clients Are at High Risk for Falls and Musculoskeletal Injury due to the Following Factors

- Weakness and being easily fatigued
- Unsteady balance, gait, and alterations in posture
- Poor eyesight
- Altered mobility resulting from medications or use of assistive device
- Increased time on bed rest, leading to muscle weakness
- Presence of chronic disease

Active Older Clients May Seek Joint Replacement Surgery for Several Reasons

- Decreased pain
- Increased mobility
- Continuation of an active life

MANAGEMENT Guidelines

Each state legislates a Nurse Practice Act for RNs and LPNs/LVNs. Healthcare facilities are responsible for establishing and implementing policies and procedures that conform to their state's regulations. Verify the regulations and role parameters for each healthcare worker in your facility.

Delegation

- All healthcare workers can be assigned to clients with orthopedic conditions for nursing tasks associated with activities of daily living. OTs and PTs are assigned to the more complex tasks of ambulating and teaching clients with joint replacements and clients requiring assistive devices to ambulate.
- Some facilities employ orthopedic technicians who set up and monitor traction; assist with cast application, bivalve, or removal; and help with transfer.

Interpersonal Communication

- The RN needs to assess the skill level of all staff assigned to clients requiring assistive devices or special equipment. Documentation of the skill level for the staff should

be available on the unit. This is a major safety factor for all staff assigned to orthopedic clients.

- When new equipment is purchased, and before it is put into service, the manufacturer should provide in-service education to all staff to prevent damage to the equipment and promote safety in client care.
- Most orthopedic clients are followed by a multidisciplinary care team, which includes healthcare providers, nurses, PTs and OTs, and social workers. The team use the client's DRG-related "clinical path" as an action plan for coordinating hospital, discharge, and subacute setting or home care services. Variances can be identified as the client moves through the sequences of specific interventions that promote timely discharge. Such collaboration requires open and ongoing communication among all members of the team. Special documentation forms may be used to facilitate this process.
- The nurse "Patient Care Coordinator" oversees the client's progress and brings multidisciplinary issues to the healthcare provider's attention so that the "path" can be individualized to reflect the client's unique needs.

- Assistive personnel (aides, orthopedic technicians) must be informed of any restriction in client positioning or mobility. They should report any noted changes in the client's condition or problem with any immobilizing device or equipment to the RN so that further assessment and problem solving can be conducted.

- Oncoming staff should receive information about the client's progress toward satisfaction of expected outcomes, any unexpected variance that impedes the client's progress toward discharge, and any change in the medical plan of care.

CASE STUDY Applications

Scenario 1

Your orthopedic unit has just admitted an 84-year-old female, Nora James. She was brought to the ED after a fall in the grocery store. Her admitting diagnosis is "intertrochanteric fracture of the left hip." She is scheduled for hip "nailing" surgery as soon as she is cleared by her primary healthcare provider, cardiologist, and anesthesiologist.

1. What behaviors would you expect to see upon initial assessment of Miss James?
2. What are the priorities of care in the preoperative period?
3. How will this client's care plan differ from that of the client with hemiarthroplasty replacement of the femoral head and neck?

Scenario 2

Mrs. Jacobson, a 73-year-old retired school teacher, has been admitted to the hospital for a right total hip replacement as a result of osteoarthritis. She has been very active her entire life, playing golf three times a week, bowling on a team, hiking, and gardening. She is very concerned that she will be unable to continue with these activities if she does not have surgery. Her lab work was completed before her admission. She gave 2 units of autologous blood in case she needs it for surgery. Her vital signs are: BP 148/80, P 88, R 26. She uses a cane, which she says is "for balance."

1. Identify the priority preoperative intervention for Mrs. Jacobson. Provide a rationale for your choice.
2. Develop a client care plan: Identify short- and long-term goals, state three nursing diagnoses in priority order, and provide the rationale for your choices. Describe at least two priority nursing interventions for each nursing diagnosis.
3. Identify two safety issues related to Mrs. Jacobson's care.
4. Describe at least three procedures that need to be discussed before her discharge.

NCLEX® Review Questions

Unless otherwise specified, choose only one (1) answer.

1. Which of the following does appropriate application of a sling to the upper arm include?
   A. Positioning so that hand is higher than elbow
   B. Positioning so that hand is lower than elbow
   C. Teaching client to avoid any shoulder joint motion
   D. Teaching client to avoid any movement of distal digits

2. What is the best method of drying wet plaster casts?
   A. Using a hair dryer
   B. Covering with blankets
   C. Using a heat lamp
   D. Natural evaporation

3. Which of the following are true about a synthetic cast compared with a plaster cast?
   Select all that apply.
   A. The synthetic cast is more expensive.
   B. It dries more quickly than plaster.
   C. The synthetic cast is heavier.
   D. It provides greater stability than plaster.
   E. The synthetic cast will not cause skin burns.
   F. The synthetic cast is nonabsorbent.

4. Which of following are early indications of acute compartment syndrome in a casted extremity?
   Select all that apply.
   A. Weak or absent distal pulses
   B. Pain with passive extension of distal digits
   C. Pain relieved with extremity elevation
   D. Pain worsening with extremity elevation
   E. Pain worsening when extremity is dependent
   F. Pain unrelieved by analgesics

5. Injury to the peroneal nerve can result in which permanent condition?
   A. Urinary incontinence
   B. Inability to plantarflex the foot
   C. Inability to dorsiflex the foot
   D. Anesthesia on the sole of the foot

6. In which position should the client with posterolateral approach total hip replacement surgery be kept postoperatively?
   A. Legs adducted
   B. Legs abducted
   C. Operative leg in external rotation
   D. Operative leg in internal rotation

7. What do adaptive aids for the client with total hip replacement primarily help the client to avoid?

   A. Hip flexion

   B. Falls

   C. Hip extension

   D. Pain

8. Studies show which result in clients who do not receive CPM (continuous passive motion) after total knee replacement surgery?

   A. Less joint range of motion

   B. Less venous thrombosis

   C. Less edema

   D. Less wound drainage

9. Phantom pain in the amputated extremity is most apt to occur in clients with which condition?

   A. Drug dependency

   B. Inadequate stump shrinkage or shaping

   C. Traumatic limb amputation

   D. Limb pain preoperatively

10. The client with above-the-knee amputation should be encouraged to perform exercises. What will these stump exercises promote?

   A. Adduction and hip flexion

   B. Abduction and hip flexion

   C. Adduction and hip extension

   D. Abduction and hip extension

QSEN Activity

Domain: Client-Centered Care

KSA: Skill

Activity:

Your client is a 35-year-old male who was involved in a traumatic motorcycle crash, resulting in an AKA of the right leg.

The client is severely depressed and refuses to engage in any of the recommended activities to reduce stump swelling or prevent flexion of the hip. In planning his care, consider the necessary skills and develop a care plan that reflects the QSEN competency of Client-Centered Care.

Bibliography

Bernzweig, E. (1996). *The nurse's liability for malpractice* (6th ed.). St. Louis, MO: Mosby.

Cochrane. (2013). Methods of pin site care for reducing infection and complications associated with external bone fixators and pins. Retrieved from http://summaries.cochrane.org/CD004551/WOUNDS_methods-of-pin-site-care-for-reducing-infection-and-complications-associated-with-external-bone-fixators-and-pins

DelPozo, J. & Patel, R. (2009). Infection associated with prosthetic joints. *New England Journal of Medicine, 361*(8), 787–794.

Eliopoulos, C. (2009). *Gerontological nursing* (7th ed.). Philadelphia, PA: Lippincott Williams & Wilkins.

Horstmann, W., Kuipers, B., Ohanis, D., Slappendel, R., Kollen, B., & Verheyen, C. (2014, Jan. 12). Autologous re-transfusion drain compared with no drain in total knee arthroplasty: A randomized controlled trial. *Journal of Blood Transfusion, Suppl 1*: s176–s181. doi:10.2450/2013.0072-13

Hulsbaek, S., Larsen, R. F., & Troelsen, A. (2014, Oct.). Predictors of not regaining basic mobility after hip fracture surgery. *Journal of Disability and Rehabilitation, 37*(19), 1739–1744. doi:10.3109/09638288.2014.974836

Johnston-Walker, E. & Hardcastle, J. (2011). Neurovascular assessment in the critically ill patient. *Nursing in Critical Care, 16*(4), 170–177.

Lagerquist, D., Dabrowski, M., Dock, C., Fox, A., Daymond, M., Sandau, K. E., & Halm, M. (2012). Care of external fixator pin sites. *American Journal of Critical Care, 21*(4), 288–292. doi:10.4037/ajcc2012600

Lethaby, A., Temple, J., & Santy, J. (2008, Oct 8). Pin site care for preventing infec tions associated with external bone fixators and pins. *Cochrane Database of Systematic Reviews*, (4), CD004551 doi:10.1002/14651858.CD004551.pub2.

McCabe, C. (2011, Apr.–Jun.). Mirror visual feedback therapy: A practical approach. *Journal of Hand Therapy, 24*(2), 170–178.

Metules, T. (2007). Hot and cold packs. *RN, 70*(1), 45–48.

Santy-Tomlinson, J., Vincent, M., Glossop, N., Jomeen, J., & Pearcey, P. (2011). Calm, irritated or infected? The experiences of the inflammatory states and symptoms of pin site infection and irritation during external fixation: A grounded theory study. *Journal of Clinical Nursing, 20*, 3163–3173. doi:10.1111/j.1365-2702.2011.03805.x

Timms, A. & Pugh, H. (2012). Pin site care: Guidance and key recommendations. *Nursing Standard, 27*(1), 50–55.

Chapter 28
Intravenous Therapy

 Learning Objectives

28.1 Describe the role the kidneys play in maintaining fluid and electrolyte balance.

28.2 Discuss the two hormonal regulatory systems that influence urinary excretion by the kidneys.

28.3 Identify the role of the major cations and anions in the body.

28.4 Identify the assessment data to determine a client's fluid status.

28.5 Compare and contrast the client assessment data associated with fluid volume excess or deficit.

28.6 Describe the steps for performing venipuncture using a winged needle or over-the-needle catheter.

28.7 State at least two potential problems that can occur with venipuncture and one suggested solution for each problem.

28.8 Describe the steps for performing vein cannulation.

28.9 Outline the steps in preparing the IV bag for fluid administration.

28.10 Describe the steps for hanging a secondary IV bag.

28.11 Calculate an IV flow rate using a standard formula.

28.12 Describe the procedure for administering an intravenous push medication.

28.13 Discuss client safety and the use of infusion control pumps.

28.14 Describe the proper use of chlorhexidine gluconate or alcohol as a skin preparation for intravenous access.

28.15 Discuss the nursing interventions required for each type of venous access connector.

28.16 Describe safety checks utilized to ensure proper blood administration.

28.17 Differentiate signs and symptoms of hemolytic and allergic blood transfusion reactions.

Chapter Outline

Terminology

Antidiuretic hormone that decreases urine production.

Antimicrobial an agent that prevents the development or pathogenic action of microbes.

Ascites the excessive accumulation of serous fluid in the peritoneal cavity.

Aspirate to remove material by suction.

Autologous blood transfusion use of the client's own blood, collected before a surgical procedure, for the client's future transfusion needs.

Bolus direct injection of a medication intravenously in order to achieve rapid serum concentrations.

BSI bloodstream infection.

Cardiovascular pertaining to the heart and blood vessels.

Central line-associated bloodstream infection (CLABSI) infectious organism that is found in the blood and catheter segment with clinical symptoms of BSI and no other sources of infection present.

Central line bundle a collection of interventions delivered as a group to improve outcomes for catheter-related bloodstream infections.

Colonization presence of bacteria on a body surface (i.e., skin, mouth, airway) without causing disease in the client.

Cyanosis slightly bluish, grayish, slate-like, or dark purple discoloration of the skin or mucous membranes.

Diarrhea frequent passage of watery stool.

Diffusion passive movement of molecules from an area of high concentration to one of lower concentration.

Diuretic a chemical agent that increases the production of urine.

Dyspnea a subjective feeling of difficulty breathing.

Edema an excessive amount of extracellular fluid.

Electrolyte substance that develops an electrical charge when dissolved in water.

Evaporation change from liquid to vapor.

Extracellular outside the cell.

Girth the distance around something; circumference, as in measuring abdominal circumference.

Granulocytes a granular leukocyte (e.g., neutrophil).

Hematoma a collection of blood confined in a space.

Hematuria blood in the urine.

Hemolytic relating to the breakdown of red blood cells.

Homeostasis state of equilibrium of the internal environment.

Homologous blood transfusion blood from another individual used for transfusion.

Hydration the chemical combination of a substance with water.

Hydrostatic pressure the pressure of liquids during equilibrium.

Hypertonic having greater than 340 mOsm, an increased amount of solutes in relationship to plasma.

Hypotonic having less than 240 mOsm, a decreased amount of solutes in relationship to plasma.

Hypovolemia diminished circulating blood volume.

Infiltration inadvertent leakage of blood into surrounding tissue when IV fluids are infusing.

Infusion-related bloodstream infection infectious organism that is found in the infusion and separate percutaneous blood cultures without an identified source of infection.

Infusion introduction of a liquid into a vein or other body part.

Interstitial extracellular fluid found between the cells.

Intracellular inside the cell.

Intravascular within blood vessels.

Isotonic having the same tonicity as plasma, 240–340 mOsm.

Local-catheter-related infection growth of an organism from the proximal or distal catheter or lumen with accompanying signs of inflammation at the catheter site.

Metabolism the sum of all physical and chemical changes that take place within an organism.

Nephrotoxic damaging to renal cells.

Osmolality concentration of osmotically active particles per kg of body water (tonicity).

Osmosis transmission of water across a semipermeable membrane from an area of low solute concentration to one of higher solute concentration.

Osmotic pressure pressure exerted on a semipermeable membrane separating a solution from a solvent, the membrane being impermeable to solutes in solution and permeable only to solvent.

Palpate to examine by touch; to feel.

Pruritus severe itching.

Purulent containing pus.

Skin turgor elastic property of the skin reflecting body fluid status.

Smart pumps computerized IV pumps.

Specific gravity weight of a substance compared with an equal volume of water.

Transfusion administration of whole blood or a component such as packed red cells, to replace blood lost through trauma, surgery, or disease.

Urticaria a vascular reaction of the skin characterized by the eruption of pale raised wheals, which are associated with severe itching.

Venipuncture puncture of a vein with a needle.

Vesicant causing or forming blisters, irritating to blood vessels; a substance that causes blistering.

Viscosity resistance offered by a fluid; property of a substance that is dependent on the friction of its component molecules as they slide by each other.

Fluid and Electrolyte Balance

The body's internal environment is made up of fluids and dissolved substances including electrolytes. Fluids and electrolytes are in a constant state of dynamic equilibrium in order to maintain the delicate balance essential for all the physiologic processes that support life.

Fluids

Body fluid is primarily water. Depending on the amount of body fat, an individual's total body weight is usually 50–70% water. Since fat is essentially water-free, an obese adult's body weight is 50% water. In a leaner individual, the percentage of body weight due to body water is closer to 70%. With aging, there is a decrease in lean body mass; therefore, the older adult may have only 46–52% of body weight as water.

Body water is divided into two main compartments: **intracellular** and **extracellular**. The majority of body water (64%) is located inside the cells. The remaining 36% of body fluid is extracellular. Three fourths of this extracellular fluid is **interstitial** (surrounding cells), and the remaining one fourth is **intravascular** plasma.

Communication between these fluid compartments varies. Intracellular water does not move readily out of the cell. In contrast, in the capillary beds there is constant movement of extracellular fluids between the interstitial and intravascular compartments. The movement of body fluid between the intravascular and interstitial space is controlled by two opposing forces: **osmotic pressure** (holding fluid in the vessels) and **hydrostatic pressure** (forcing fluid out of vessels into tissue spaces). Interstitial and intravascular fluid are similar in composition except for the presence of plasma proteins (which provide osmotic pressure in the intravascular space).

Body water balance is the result of physiologic **homeostasis** responses to the fluid gains (intake) and losses (output) that occur on a daily basis. The major sources of intake and output are shown in Table 28-1 ■.

The primary organ of fluid balance is the kidney. The kidneys excrete the end products of cellular **metabolism**, as well as eliminate excess fluids. In order to clear the blood of wastes, they must produce a minimum of 500 to 600 mL

Table 28-1 Average Daily Fluid Gain and Loss

Intake (mL)		Output (mL)	
Oral intake (liquid and food)	2,300	Urine	1,500
Cellular catabolism of proteins, carbohydrates, and fats }	300	Skin	600 (insensible loss by **evaporation**)
		Lung	300 (insensible loss by vapor)
		Feces	200
	2,600		2,600

Table 28-2 Major Electrolytes

Cations		Anions	
Na^+	Sodium	Cl^-	Chloride
K^+	Potassium	HCO_3^-	Bicarbonate
Ca^{2+}	Calcium	HPO_4^{2-}	Phosphate
Mg^{2+}	Magnesium		

of urine every 24 hr. To balance a typical amount of fluid intake, however, the usual amount of urine produced on a daily basis varies from 1 to 2 L.

Regulation of the volume, composition, and **osmolality** of body fluid is controlled by homeostatic mechanisms. A major regulator of intake is thirst. Thirst is stimulated by receptors in the central nervous system. Under normal circumstances, an individual ingests fluids when these receptors are activated. During illness or an altered level of consciousness, and in the aged, the thirst response may be depressed, resulting in **hypovolemia** and increased tonicity or concentration of the extracellular fluids (Deficient Fluid Volume).

Urine production by the kidneys is influenced by two hormonal regulatory systems: **antidiuretic** hormone (ADH) and aldosterone. When extracellular body fluids become concentrated, osmoreceptors located in the hypothalamus initiates the release of ADH, which stimulates the kidneys to retain more water. As this retained water circulates through the extracellular fluid compartment, the concentration of body fluid is reduced. The osmoreceptors sense this change and slow the secretion of ADH, and the kidneys stop retaining water (negative feedback).

Other conditions that can stimulate the secretion of ADH and lead to increased water retention by the kidneys include hemorrhage, decreased cardiac output, trauma, pain, fear, surgery, and dehydration. Drugs such as morphine, barbiturates, nicotine, and some anesthetics and tranquilizers also increase the secretion of ADH. Secretion of ADH can be inhibited by alcohol, decreased concentration of body fluids, and hypervolemic states.

The other major regulatory hormone is aldosterone, which is secreted by the adrenal cortex. Aldosterone regulates fluid volume by stimulating the kidneys to reabsorb sodium and water (an **isotonic** gain). During this process, sodium is exchanged for potassium or hydrogen; therefore, aldosterone also affects levels of these electrolytes. Secretion of aldosterone is increased in response to several stimuli, which include decreased sodium and increased extracellular potassium, hypovolemia, and stress states.

When blood flow to the kidneys is decreased, a receptor-like area in the glomerulus of the nephron releases an enzyme called renin. As renin circulates in the body, it converts a plasma protein in the liver into a vasoconstrictor substance called angiotensin I. When this substance enters the lungs, it is converted into angiotensin II. Angiotensin II acts directly on the adrenal cortex to increase aldosterone secretion. This then leads to extracellular volume expansion and even possible fluid volume excess if the cause of decreased renal blood flow was due to heart or liver failure.

Electrolytes

In partnership with body fluids are substances called electrolytes. These substances, mostly minerals, contribute to bodily function in many ways and are essential to life (Table 28-2 ■). Electrolytes are important components of intracellular and extracellular fluids. The major intracellular electrolytes are potassium, magnesium, phosphate, and sulfate. Major extracellular electrolytes are sodium, chloride, and bicarbonate.

Electrolytes are distributed throughout the body, both intracellularly and extracellularly. In the extracellular compartment, the main electrolytes are sodium, chloride, and bicarbonate. Intracellular electrolytes are potassium, magnesium, phosphate, and sulfate.

Electrolytes develop an electric charge when dissolved in water. Electrolytes with a positive charge are called cations. Negatively charged electrolytes are called anions. Positive cations and negative anions are attracted to each other because of their opposite electric charges. When they combine with each other, they form neutral compounds that either remain in body fluids or dissociate and regain their electric charges. When they dissociate, or ionize, they are referred to as ions.

Fluid and Electrolyte Imbalance

Alterations in fluid and electrolytes may occur as a primary event or as a secondary response to a preexisting disease state or to a sudden, unexpected traumatic event. When alterations of fluid and electrolytes exceed the narrow limits consistent with health, the body needs to adjust quickly.

Changes in the composition of body fluid and electrolytes may be relative or absolute. Relative losses or gains can occur when fluids or electrolytes shift from one body space to another. Absolute losses or gains occur when fluids and electrolytes are lost outside the body or added to the overall body stores by IV fluid.

The kidney has an obligatory urine output, and the body has an insensible water loss. A daily minimum fluid intake of 1,500 mL is essential to balance these losses. If the loss of body water is greater than fluid intake (fluid volume deficit), weight loss results. If the gain of body water is greater than output, weight gain results. One kilogram of body weight gain or loss is equal to 1,000 mL (1 L) of fluid.

In addition to methods of assessing fluid balance, this chapter discusses interventions for providing fluid and electrolytes to clients who have experienced alterations in their homeostasis. The rationale for interventions associated with alterations in either fluids or electrolytes is to maintain homeostasis.

Clients undergoing major surgery or trauma may be subjected to blood loss necessitating fluid replacement therapy. Clients requiring prolonged intravenous therapy may have associated nutritional losses. Support for these clients must be considered.

IV Administration

Initiating, monitoring, and providing care for clients with IV therapy consumes a large portion of the nurses' time each shift, and requires safe nursing practice to protect the client from complications. Most hospitalized clients require some form of IV therapy.

Administering IV drugs can lead to medication errors, even if the nurse does not mix the medication, but hangs and monitors the IV. Whenever the nurse administers an IV, both the hospital and federal guidelines must be followed. Guidelines include being properly educated in the use of IV equipment, understanding venous anatomy to ensure proper IV selection sites, and knowing the appropriate catheter gauge and length for the vein selected. In addition, it is imperative that the nurse is knowledgeable about drugs and solutions being administered, the side effects, and treatment if a side effect occurs.

Frequent monitoring of IV **infusions** is a requisite for safe nursing practice. Knowing the solution infusing, medications added to the solution, and rate of infusion promotes safe care. Maintaining the IV site and following guidelines established by the Intravenous Nurses Society, The Joint Commission, and the CDC are critical to prevent complications associated with the IV site and cannula.

The CDC Guidelines for Prevention of Catheter-Related Infections state that skin should be disinfected before catheter placement and that chlorhexidine gluconate is preferred. Use of chlorhexidine gluconate has demonstrated superiority to povidone–iodine in decreasing infections at the site of IV catheter insertion. (Some facilities use alcohol swabs.) In addition to the use of chlorhexidine gluconate, the CDC recommends the use of a sterile catheter securement device such as the Statlock. This device protects the client's skin from damage and prevents movement of the IV catheter.

Movement can damage the vessel and lead to infection. Another recommendation is the use of semipermeable transparent film dressings to prevent the passage of liquids, bacteria, and viruses to the IV site. The use of this type of dressing allows easy observation and monitoring of the IV site without removing the dressing. It is recommended that tape not be used to secure the IV site. Tape used to stabilize IVs has historically been unsterile, leading to infections at the IV site. In addition, tape not only allows movement of the catheter, but also has been shown to be the cause of **infiltration**, phlebitis, occlusion/thrombosis, and other device-related complications. If the tape is necessary, it is highly recommended that sterile tape be utilized to prevent infection.

Intravenous devices are an important part of hospital practice for the administration of fluid, nutrients, medications, blood products, and to hemodynamically monitor unstable clients. Providing intravenous therapy for clients is one of the main skills performed by nurses.

These devices are not without problems. **Central line-associated bloodstream infections** can be linked to increased hospital stays, even life-threatening events or death. Central vascular devices are most problematic; peripheral venous catheters are usually not associated with these infections. Phlebitis and infiltration are the most common complications associated with peripheral vein catheters. The risk of phlebitis differs between sites. It is much higher if the lower limb is used as the IV site. Catheters inserted in the hand carry a lower risk of phlebitis than those inserted higher up on the wrist and arm.

Most medication errors resulting in client deaths occur with IV infusions. To meet the need for improved medication safety at the point of care, "smart technology" has been developed to standardize IV infusion administration, reduce IV programming errors, and streamline IV administration processes. The infusion pumps are programmed with a database of information about medications and parameters for correct dosage and infusion rate. The pump can alert the nurse if it is not programmed correctly for a given drug. The pharmacy alters the provided database from the manufacturer to meet the specifications of the hospital and formulary that go into the pump. There are two levels of alerts in the pump: a soft stop and a hard stop. When a minor error is detected, the pump warns the user, but allows the user to override the alert. When a more serious problem occurs, the pump shuts down and does not allow an override.

A point-of-care **smart pump** consists of the computer (brain) that programs the infusions and contains the safety software. Lightweight, large-volume infusion modules, as well as a syringe, client-controlled analgesia (PCA), capnography (ETCO$_2$), and pulse oximetry (SpO$_2$) modules, can be attached to or removed from the smart pump as needed for each client.

The safety software can also be added to some traditional infusion pumps. The hospital can configure up to 10 profiles for specific client care areas such as ICU and Medical–Surgical units. These profiles include customized operating parameters and drug libraries. Each drug library contains institution-specific parameters for up to 1,000 drugs, all of which can be customized. The drug library provides the best-practice guidelines for each medication. If programmed parameters are outside of pre-established limits, the software provides an alert that must be addressed before the infusion can begin.

An IV Medication Harm Index monitors the number of potential errors that were avoided through the use of the system. Potential errors that can be detected are overdose of drugs and adverse events. Having these data available allows the hospital to identify practice issues that were difficult to identify with earlier IV pumps. Several studies have been conducted to determine the extent of the error prevention when using this technology. This chapter presents skills for providing fluids and electrolytes, blood, and blood components, as well as pharmacologic therapy through the intravenous route. Methods for assessing baseline data and evaluating fluid and electrolyte gains or losses are included in this chapter.

Cultural Awareness

Religion and Use of Blood and Blood Products

It is important to know clients' religious beliefs about the use of blood and blood products in order to understand their preferences in choosing to allow or not allow **transfusions**.

- Clients who practice Christian Science (Church of Christ, Scientist) usually do not accept use of blood or blood products in their medical care.
- Clients who are Jehovah's Witnesses believe that blood in any form and agents in which blood is an ingredient are not acceptable. Blood volume expanders are acceptable if they are not derived from blood. Mechanical devices for circulating blood are acceptable as long as they are not primed with blood initially. Their religious belief is based on scripture references and precedents in the history of Christianity. There are times when court orders are obtained for children in life-threatening situations so they may receive blood or blood products.

Nursing Diagnoses

The following nursing diagnoses are appropriate to include in a client care plan when the components are related to intravenous therapy.

NURSING DIAGNOSIS	RELATED TO . . .
Deficient Fluid Volume	Excess fluid loss secondary to vomiting, increased temperature, blood loss, drainage sites or tubes, diarrhea, and diuretics
Excess Fluid Volume	Excessive fluid accumulation secondary to excess sodium intake, medications, renal or cardiac failure; inaccurate IV infusion rate
Infection, Risk for	Chronic diseases, invasive procedures, immunodeficiency, tissue destruction, and increased environmental exposure
Noncompliance	Inaccurate I&O records, denial, lack of instruction regarding I&O, fluid restriction, care of IV site
Impaired Skin Integrity	Alterations in skin turgor, edema, tissue damage, IV infiltration, infection, immobilization
Ineffective Peripheral Tissue Perfusion	Loss of blood related to hemorrhage or loss related to hemodialysis

Source: Herdman, T. H. & Kamitsuru, S. (Eds.) *Nursing Diagnoses – Definitions and Classification 2015-2017*. Copyright © 2014, 1994–2014 by NANDA International. Used by arrangement with John Wiley & Sons Limited. Companion website: www.wiley.com/go/nursingdiagnoses. In order to make safe and effective judgments using NANDA-I nursing diagnosis it is essential that nurses refer to the definitions and defining characteristics of the diagnoses listed in this work.

Nursing Process Data

ASSESSMENT Database

- Validate physician's order for IV therapy.
- Assess need for client teaching about IV therapy.
- Evaluate client for IV site selection.
- Select appropriate vessel for venipuncture.
- Determine appropriate type and size of cannulation device for client.
- Determine IV equipment needed.

PLANNING Objectives

- To maintain fluid and electrolyte balance
- To aseptically prepare infusion system
- To identify and prepare the appropriate site for venipuncture
- To perform successful venipuncture using appropriate equipment

IMPLEMENTATION Procedures

DOCUMENTATION AND EVALUATION

Expected Outcomes

- Fluid and electrolyte needs are met.
- Appropriate IV site is selected and IV inserted without difficulty.
- IV fluids infuse at prescribed rate without complications.
- IV equipment is appropriate for client.
- IV site is maintained using sterile technique.

Unexpected Outcomes/Alternative Actions

Pearson Nursing Student Resources

Find additional review materials at
nursing.pearsonhighered.com.
Prepare for success with NCLEX®-style practice questions and Skill Checklists.

Skill 28.1.1 | Preparing the Infusion System

Equipment

IV solution in bag

Note: The only glass bottles used today are for infusions of certain medications (e.g., nitroglycerin amiodarone and lipids). Check facility procedures for correct infusion of these medications using the glass bottle.

Primary administration tubing set (compatible with infusion pump)

Add-on particulate filter (according to agency policy) compatible with infusion pump psi

Electronic infusion device or free pole for bag suspension and gravity infusion

> **CLINICAL ALERT**
>
> Take IV solutions out of refrigerator (if stored there) and allow to warm to room temperature. This will reduce the number of air bubbles in the IV solution.
>
> It is difficult to detect air bubbles because gas is well assimilated into liquid at low temperatures; thus air bubbles are fully assimilated into the IV solution when kept in refrigerator. Once solution warms to room temperature, air bubbles appear.

Preparation

1. Verify the type and amount of solution with physician's order.
2. Introduce self and identify client using two client identifiers.
3. Perform hand hygiene.
4. Check pharmacy label for client's identification, solution type, additives, and expiration date. ❶
5. Select IV tubing appropriate for infusion device.
6. Select add-on filter if indicated (Box 28-1 ■).

Box 28-1 IN-LINE FILTERS

Except when infusing TPN, TPN with lipids, certain IV medications, PCAs, continuous epidurals, and blood products, in-line filters are not recommended. There is no evidence to suggest that in-line filters prevent infections associated with intravascular devices and infusion systems. Some studies do suggest that they may reduce the incidence of infusion-related phlebitis; however, it has not been proven. Because studies do not justify the cost of the in-line filters, the CDC does not recommend them for infection-control purposes. Before hanging drugs, check the drug formulary to determine the need for an in-line filter.

Procedure

1. Remove outer wrap around IV bag if necessary. (It may be wet due to condensation.)
2. Inspect bag carefully for tears or leaks by applying gentle pressure to bag.
3. Hold bag up against both a dark and light background to examine for discoloration, cloudiness, or particulate matter. ➤ ***Rationale:*** Any evidence of change may indicate contamination, and the bag should be discarded.
4. Hang the IV bag on the IV pole. Close tubing roller clamp. ❷ (Affix time strip on bag according to facility policy.) ***Note***: After checking the client's identification band against the pharmacy label on the bag, place black tape over the client's name. ➤ ***Rationale:*** It is a HIPAA violation for the name to be seen on the IV bag.
5. Remove plastic protector from tubing spike (end of tubing with drip chamber). ❸

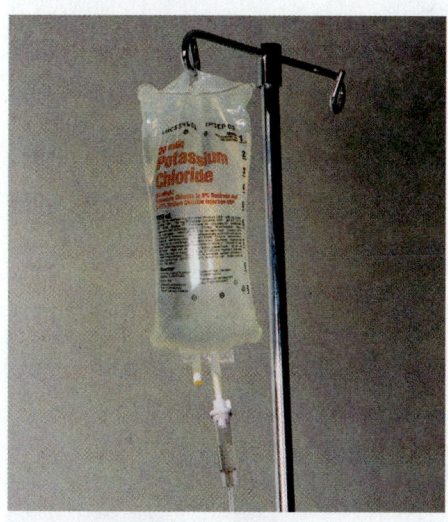

❶ Most hospitals require a "Red Label" if potassium or other drugs are pre-added to the solution.

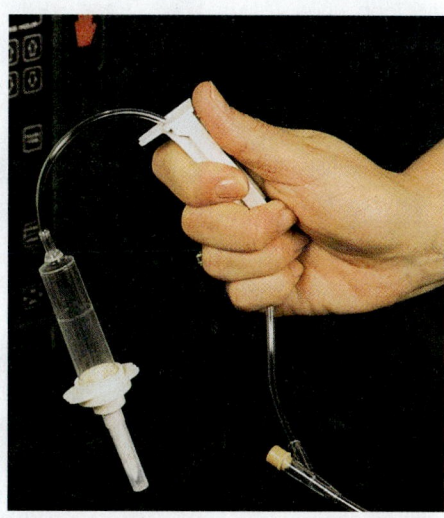

❷ Clamp tubing before spiking IV fluid bag.

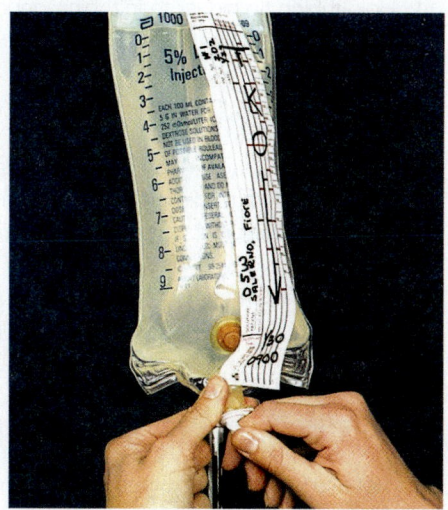

❸ Pull to remove port cap on IV bag.

(continued)

Skill 28.1.1 | Preparing the Infusion System *(continued)*

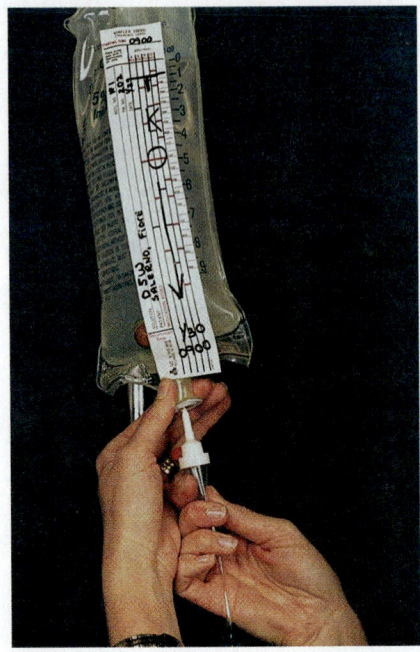

④ Squeeze drip chamber while spiking bag port, maintaining sterility.

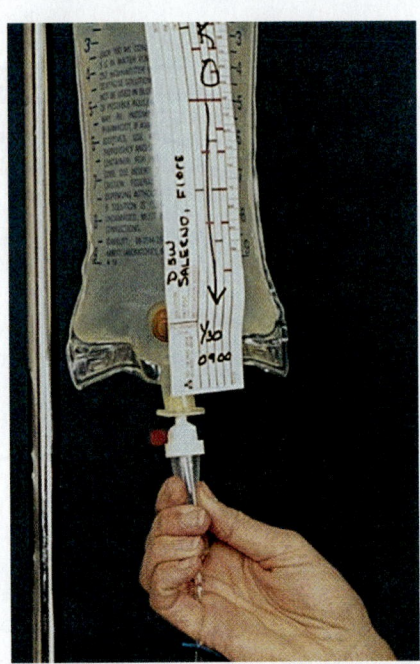

⑤ Squeeze and release drip chamber to fill.

⑥ Fill drip chamber one-half full of fluid.

6. Squeeze drip chamber while inserting tubing spike into bag port, holding port securely to prevent contamination. **④**
   ➤ *Rationale:* Squeezing chamber during insertion prevents air entry into bag.
7. Release pressure on the drip chamber until chamber is partially full. **⑤**
8. Attach add-on terminal filter (if indicated).
9. Remove protective cap at end of tubing.
10. Open clamp on line to prime tubing and filter. (Some IV pumps require that the priming of the tubing be done through the infusion pump, particularly if the tubing comes with an antisyphon valve at the end of the tube).
11. Hold tubing tip higher than tubing-dependent loop while priming. ➤ *Rationale:* Air rises and passes out as fluid primes tubing.
12. Invert and tap Y injection sites to remove air as tubing primes.
13. Hold filter (if attached) pointing downward so proximal half of filter (closest to client) fills with fluid first, then invert to complete filter priming, tapping air out as filter primes. **⑥**
14. Close tubing clamp when primed. **⑦**
15. Load administration set into electronic pump according to manufacturer's instructions. Most pumps require dedicated tubing and a specific loading format.

> **CLINICAL ALERT**
> Do not use felt-tip pens to mark directly on IV plastic bag.
> ➤ *Rationale:* The ink may leach through the plastic and contaminate the solution.

⑦ Close tubing clamp when priming is complete.

Skill 28.1.2 | Adding Extension Tubing

Equipment

Extension tubing

2% Chlorhexidine gluconate or alcohol swab

Injection cap with Luer-Lok adapter, if necessary

Syringe cannula

Two syringes of 0.9% preservative-free normal saline (NS) in volume at least twice the volume capacity of the catheter and any add-on devices

Procedure

1. Gather equipment and determine type of cap, if needed. Extension tubing may be attached directly to IV catheter.
2. Introduce self and identify client using two identifiers.
3. Perform hand hygiene and then swab tubing's terminal injection cap and insert syringe cannula. ❶

> **CLINICAL ALERT**
> Peripheral IVs should be started using aseptic technique. IVs started without proper asepsis, for example, in an emergency or outside the hospital, should be replaced at the earliest opportunity, and within 24 hr.

4. Remove protector at opposite end and prime extension tubing with 1 mL of NS solution.
5. Add needleless IV access device to tubing or use Luer-Lok with attached extension tubing.

❶ Swab injection cap and insert syringe cannula.

6. Swab client's established IV cannula resealable cap and connect extension tubing or insert primed extension tubing directly into client's IV catheter.
7. Flush with 0.9% NS at twice the volume (capacity) of the catheter and any add-on devices.

Note: INS standards discourage the use of additional routine extension tubing. ➤ **Rationale:** This adds additional potential source of IV contamination.

Skill 28.1.3 | Preparing the Venipuncture Site

Equipment

Prepared IV administration setup or sterile needleless access device

Single-use, latex-free tourniquet (constricting band)

Chlorhexidine gluconate swab (not used on infants under 1,000 grams) or alcohol swab

Sterile needle or catheter for venipuncture

Half-inch wide sterile tape

Transparent semipermeable dressing

Securement device per facility policy

Gloves (clean or sterile depending on facility policy)

Electronic infusion pump

Small extension tubing per facility policy (single or double lumen)

Preparation

1. Check physician's orders and MAR.
2. Introduce self and identify client using two forms of identification.
3. Assemble equipment. ❶
4. Flush the extension tubing with saline.

Procedure

1. Explain procedure. ❷
2. Provide privacy.
3. Hang solution bag and primed administration set within easy reach. ❸
4. Position client and adjust lighting as necessary.
5. Perform hand hygiene and don gloves.
6. Select appropriate IV device. Catheter gauge should be smallest size that allows greatest flow, without occluding vessel lumen.

Note: Over-the-needle catheters are used most commonly for IV fluid/blood administration. A smaller catheter (22 gauge) may be used for routine antibiotics or maintenance fluids, but a larger catheter (20 gauge) is needed for blood products. For irritating medications, a small-bore catheter is preferable.

7. If possible, select a vein on client's nondominant arm. ❹ Also consider client's activity level and expected duration of IV therapy. For the client with chronic kidney disease, use the arm opposite the one that has been identified for potential dialysis catheter access (Box 28-2 ■).

(continued)

Skill 28.1.3 | Preparing the Venipuncture Site *(continued)*

❶ Equipment for IV start for over-the-needle.

❷ Explain procedure to client.

❸ Hang IV bag and primed administration set within easy reach.

❹ Anatomical sites used for venipuncture.

a. Inspect both of client's arms, palpating and visualizing the course of the veins.

b. Vein should be superficial, easily **palpated**, and large enough for needle insertion and advancement.

c. Area should be free of lesions or scars and away from joints and areas of frequent motion. ➤ *Rationale:* Motion frequency increases the risk of mechanical phlebitis.

d. Do not use the antecubital fossa except in atypical circumstances.

e. Do not use the same vein below a site where infiltration or phlebitis has occurred.

f. Select shortest and smallest cannula that will be sufficient to deliver fluids/medications. ➤ *Rationale:* The longer the catheter, the greater the risk of infiltration, infection, and thrombus formation. A catheter that is too large does not allow for adequate blood flow around the catheter, and this can lead to phlebitis.

g. Distal end of the vein should be selected first, reserving more proximal sites for future IV therapy.

h. Select larger veins for **hypertonic** solutions, blood, and viscous fluids.

CLINICAL ALERT

Do not shave the **venipuncture** site. Shaving can facilitate the development of infection in resulting microabrasions. Hairy sites can be clipped with scissors.

Box 28-2 IV INSERTION SITES

Select	Avoid
Use vein in nondominant arm.	Antecubital fossa
Use smallest catheter for site.	Lower extremities
Use most distal sites first. Save antecubital site for emergencies.	Previously used veins and injured or sclerotic veins
Assess client's condition; vein condition, size, location; type and duration of therapy.	Veins in affected arm with dialysis fistula, or axillary dissection

i. Avoid using veins in affected arm after mastectomy.

j. Lower extremity sites are associated with complications (e.g., thrombosis) and should be used ONLY if necessary. The legs and feet of clients with diabetes or peripheral vascular disease should never be used. Check facility policies to determine if a physician's order is needed when using a lower extremity for the IV site.

8. Apply tourniquet 15 cm (6 in.) above the selected site to distend vein. ❺ Overlap ends of tourniquet, lift and stretch, then tuck top end under bottom; keep ends pointing away from puncture site. ➤ *Rationale:* Tourniquet traps blood and engorges the vein for better visibility.

> **CLINICAL ALERT**
> Latex-free tourniquets should be used and disposed of after each use.

9. Prepare vein for venipuncture.

> **CLINICAL ALERT**
> Some agencies allow only certified IV therapists to perform venipuncture.

a. Place arm in dependent position. ➤ *Rationale:* This position increases capillary refill and venous distension to increase chance of successful venipuncture.

b. Lightly tap the vein. ➤ *Rationale:* Tapping distends the vein in preparation for venipuncture.

c. Ask client to open and close the fist several times to help distend the selected vein.

d. If vein is difficult to palpate, release tourniquet and apply warm, moist compresses to the arm for 10–20 min before reapplying the tourniquet.

10. Prep site with chlorhexidine gluconate or alcohol swab. ❻ Cleanse area using back-and-forth motion, 5 to 10 cm (2–4 in.) across. ➤ *Rationale:* Vigorous skin preparation decreases organisms at the venipuncture site.

11. Let prep solution air dry for 30 sec or until skin is dry. Do not fan or blow. ➤ *Rationale:* Area must be dry for **antimicrobial** action before continuing with venipuncture.

12. Do not touch selected insertion site after prepping.

13. Proceed to appropriate procedure for inserting the needle.

> **CLINICAL ALERT**
> When repetitive peripheral IV access fails, IV medication doses and fluids are missed. For this reason, many facilities are now inserting PICC lines or implantable ports. Use of PICC lines decreases incidence of phlebitis.

❺ Apply tourniquet 15 cm (6 in.) above insertion site.

❻ Use back-and forth-movement to cleanse the site with chlorhexidine gluconate or alcohol swab.

Skill 28.1.4 | Using a Vascular Imaging Device

Equipment

Infrared or transillumination device
Specific type of IV equipment

Note: The infrared device will project invisible infrared or near-infrared light waves onto the client's skin. The light is reflected off tissue surrounding the vein, but not off blood inside the veins, so it can differentiate between tissue and veins. The transillumination device is applied to the client's skin by focusing bright visible light onto the skin; it illuminates the tissue under the skin and helps locate superficial veins.

(continued)

Skill 28.1.4 | Using a Vascular Imaging Device *(continued)*

Procedure

1. Obtain all IV equipment necessary for specific type of infusion and IV infrared machine.
2. Introduce self and identify client using two identifiers. Wash hands.
3. Explain procedure to client. The vascular imaging device can highlight vein location. It determines sites for placement of IV. Identifying sites can minimize pain and provide more options where sites may be secured. It will not come in contact with the client, nor will they experience heat at the site.
4. Instruct client to take off all jewelry in the area that will be assessed. ➤ *Rationale:* Metal reflects light and can interfere with the projected image, causing blank or distorted images in some instances.
5. Plug in device and lock wheels.
6. Turn on device and calibrate. Place the calibration card on a horizontal surface and position the device head perpendicular over it, approximately 60 cm (2 feet) away. Check the card, which will indicate when the device is successfully calibrated.

7. Place the device head perpendicular to the area and 60 cm (2 feet) from where the IV is to be inserted. ➤ *Rationale:* An inaccurate focus can cause a shift from the projected image away from the vein location, cast shadows, and decrease image quality.
8. Check the focus by making sure the text around the image border is clean and legible.
9. Using the projected image, identify a vein site suitable for IV access.
10. Move the imaging modes and contrast levels to determine the view that is most useful to assist with the venipuncture.

Note: If the site has excessive hair, select the Hair Reduction Mode. ➤ *Rationale:* This mode highlights the veins and minimizes the shadowing caused by the hair.

11. Perform the venipuncture. Insert the needle just outside the lighted area to prevent reflection from the metal of the light. Another option is to turn off the light after marking the IV site with a surgical skin marker and access the vein at the mark.

Skill 28.1.5 | Inserting an Over-the-Needle Catheter

Equipment

Tourniquet (constrictive band)

2% Chlorhexidine swab or alcohol swab

Sterile over-the-needle catheter sizes 12- to 24-gauge, ½- to 2-in. long

Optional: EMLA cream (lidocaine and prilocaine) cream or syringe with local anesthetic (lidocaine) and 25- to 26-gauge needle (check agency policy or physician's orders and client sensitivity before using)

Prepared administration set and infusion solution if ordered

Electronic infusion device

Protective needleless cap if required

Syringe with at least 2 to 3 times the volume capacity of the catheter and add-on devices with preservative-free normal saline for lock (if indicated)

Sterile half-inch tape

Sterile gloves

Sterile transparent dressing

Procedure

1. Introduce self, identify client with two client identifiers, and perform hand hygiene.
2. Prepare IV system and follow steps in Skill 28.1.3, Preparing the Venipuncture Site.
3. Select appropriate size over-the-needle catheter.
4. Perform hand hygiene and don gloves.
5. Position extremity for venipuncture.

Note: Apply EMLA cream or inject site (intradermally) with small wheal of local anesthetic, according to hospital policy. (Allow 60 min for cream and 90 seconds for anesthetic to take effect.)

6. Place extremity flat on bed or place in a dependent position. ➤ *Rationale:* Gravity will slow venous return and thus dilate the vein. If vein is not distended sufficiently for easy venipuncture, ask client to make a fist or lightly tap on the vein with your fingertips.

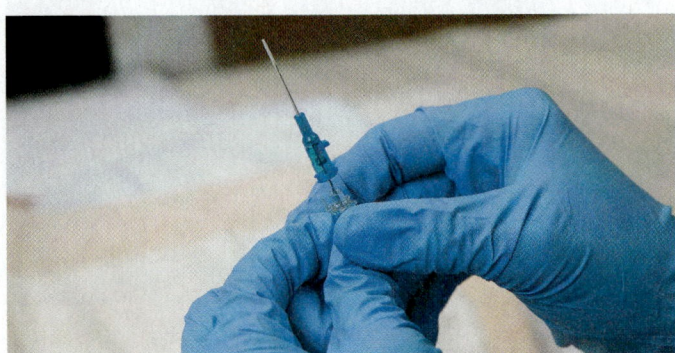

❶ Inspect integrity of needle tip.

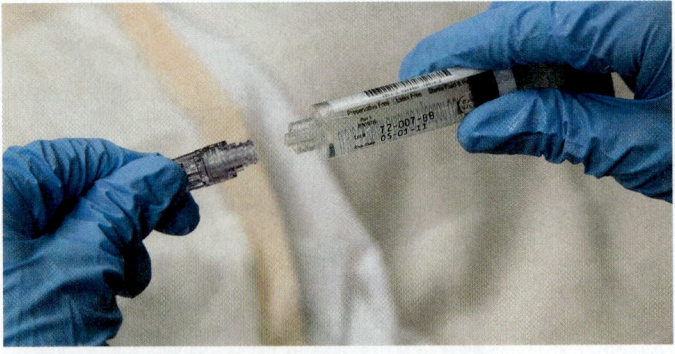

❷ Attach saline-filled syringe to extension tubing.

7. Hold catheter with bevel up and examine the integrity of end of catheter. ❶ ❷
8. Apply traction to stabilize the vein.
9. With bevel of needle up, insert the needle/catheter unit at a 30-degree angle into the client's skin either:

   a. Alongside the vein, or
   b. About a half-inch distal to the selected puncture site.

10. Revisualize vein; reduce angle of cannula to 15 degrees, pierce vein. ❸ A "pop" will frequently be felt. Observe for backflow of blood in the plastic hub. ❹ Slide needle into vein about half a centimeter (¼ in.) after backflow is observed. Continue to apply traction. ➤ *Rationale:* This indicates you are in the vein. If vein is hard to find, use the vascular imaging device if the facility has one.

CLINICAL ALERT

If no blood is observed and you did not feel the catheter enter the vein, pull back on entire catheter apparatus without exiting the skin. Reassess vein position, then reattempt venipuncture. If you are not successful, remove the catheter and look for a different site. Remember, the catheter is now contaminated and cannot be used again. Most facilities allow the nurse to attempt two venipunctures; if unsuccessful, they must notify another professional to attempt venipuncture.

---

11. Hold needle and gently advance plastic catheter hub over the needle and up the vein no more than halfway. ❺

Note: Maintain aseptic technique throughout the procedure and prevent trauma to site and vein. These catheters are associated with a very high rate of phlebitis.

12. Stop and separate, but do not completely remove, the stylet from the catheter. ❻
13. Advance only the catheter until the catheter hub meets the skin. The catheter moves over the stylet. If the hub is against the vein valve, you will need to initiate the infusion of IV fluids in order to float the catheter to the middle of the vein.
14. Release the tourniquet. Leave the stylet in the catheter while you tape the catheter to the skin. When removing the stylet, follow the IV catheter manufacturer's procedure for securing the stylet to prevent needle stick. ➤ *Rationale:* The stylet acts like a plug. Leaving it partially in place allows more time to tape the catheter to the skin.
15. Tape catheter under hub of needle, without touching the puncture site, and without touching the hub–catheter juncture. A securement device may be used in place of the taping procedure.
16. Place digital pressure above the distal end of the catheter and carefully remove the stylet. Maintaining aseptic technique, connect catheter to IV tubing or place a saline lock on the catheter. ❼

❸ Insert needle, with bevel up, at 30-degree angle.

❺ Advance hub over needle.

❹ Slide needle into vein.

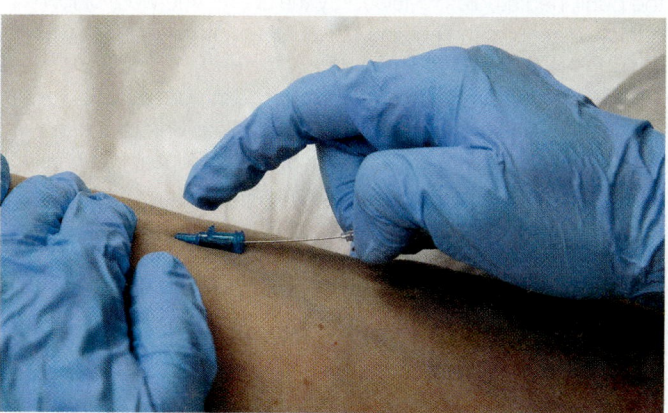

❻ Separate, but do not completely remove, the stylette.

(continued)

Skill 28.1.5 | Inserting an Over-the-Needle Catheter *(continued)*

17. Connect catheter to needleless cap or insert IV tubing into the catheter.

EVIDENCE-BASED PRACTICE

Heparin Versus Saline Solution Flushing for Prevention of Occlusion in Central Venous Catheters in Adults

Central venous catheters (CVCs) can cause blood clots, which can block the line, increase the risk of infection, and travel elsewhere in the body such as the lungs. Heparin is a drug that helps to prevent blood clots and may prevent unwanted consequences. However, heparin can also cause serious adverse effects such as bleeding, allergic reactions, or fall in platelet counts. Normal saline solution, a sterile solution of salt in water at a concentration suitable for the blood, is typically used for IV infusions This study wanted to determine whether heparin helps prevent the effects of blood clots in CVCs, and if the benefit outweighed the risk of harm. Six studies with a combined total of 1,433 participants were included in the study. The review found no compelling evidence of a decrease in the rate of blocking of CVCs flushed with heparin compared with CVCs flushed with sterile saline solution. It found no difference in the number of days the catheter lasted nor in the rates of thrombosis, infection, mortality, bleeding, or heparin-induced fall in platelet count. The conclusion was that there was no good evidence that heparin flushing of CVCs is better than flushing with sterile saline solution. The study suggested that use of heparin, which is more expensive than normal saline, should be challenged for CVC flushing.

Source: Lopez-Briz et al. (2014, Oct. 8)

Heparin Flush Versus Saline Flush for Maintaining CVC

Two studies completed at the University of Pennsylvania and Seattle's Children's Hospital suggested there was insufficient evidence to conclude that a heparin flush is more effective than a saline flush. Flushing CVCs with heparin poses a risk of heparin-induced thrombophlebitis. In the University of Pennsylvania study, the evidence for using heparin to flush CVCs is small, and the published studies reviewed by the committee were of low quality; therefore, the nursing policy for maintaining CVCs was changed to flushing catheters with saline only.

In the first 18 months after the change in policy, there was a reduction in catheter-associated bloodstream infections, no increase in catheter or vein occlusion, and a reduction in nursing workload without compromising client safety.

In a study conducted at Seattle's Children Hospital and reported in *Nursing Times*, there was no evidence to support a difference between normal saline and heparin for patency of locked peripheral IVs. Seattle elected to conform to the Infusion Nurses Society (INS) standards published in late 2008. It recommends the use of NS for flushing peripheral IVs.

Source: Anderson (2010)

18. Open clamp and observe drip chamber for fluid flow (or preserve patency of system by injecting 2–3 times the amount of volume of the catheter and connecting devices using 0.9% preservative free normal saline through access site). ❽ There should not be any sudden swelling at IV site.
19. Observe for signs of infiltration.
20. Reduce flow and proceed with stabilizing the catheter.
    ➤ *Rationale:* Stabilizing the catheter reduces the need for unscheduled restarts and risks for health workers from unnecessary exposure to needles.
21. Prep site with skin protectant and place catheter in the securement device. ❾ ❿ ⓫
22. If using sterile tape, do not tape over connectors. ⓬ ⓭
    ➤ *Rationale:* Taping impedes access to the IV site in emergencies. Cover the insertion site with a sterile transparent dressing.
23. Loop IV tubing only once to prevent decreasing the length of tubing. ➤ *Rationale:* Loops in tubing reduce distance from the IV solution container to client's IV site. This can put excess pressure on the IV site and potentially cause the catheter to dislodge from the vein or infiltration to occur.
24. Loop and tape tubing to client's arm a short distance from the site.
25. Set drip rate according to physician's order.
26. Label IV site with date, time, initials, and size of catheter. ⓮ ⓯
27. Remove gloves and perform hand hygiene.
28. Change cannula and infusion site per hospital policy, unless site shows evidence of phlebitis or cannula was compromised.

The 2011 Infusion Nursing Standards of Practice address the equivalence of two systems: the Statlock system and Nexiva combined with 3M Tegaderm Securement dressing system. There is no evidence for using any other combinations such as a securement dressing on a round hub catheter or a catheter with an integrated stabilization platform and some other type of dressing.

CLINICAL ALERT

If using needleless Angiocath system, once the "flash" is noted and catheter is advanced, the retract button is pushed and the needle is automatically shielded.

❼ Attach extension tubing.

8 Backflush and instill 3 mL of normal saline. Observe for swelling at IV site.

11 Remove cover carefully and press down on the skin.

9 Prep site with skin protectant for securement device.

12 Anchor tubing with tape.

10 Place securement device under cannula with arrows pointing up.

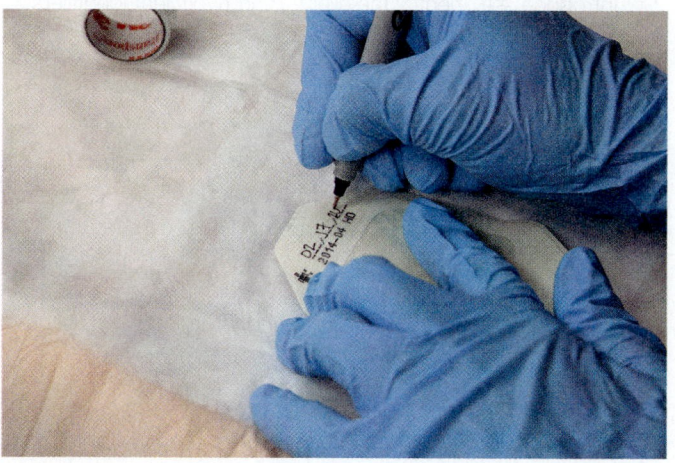

13 Place date, initials, and size of catheter on the dressing tab.

(continued)

Skill 28.1.5 | Inserting an Over-the-Needle Catheter *(continued)*

⑭ Place transparent dressing over the site.

⑮ Secure dressing and place tab on the dressing.

Skill 28.1.6 | Using a NovaCath Integrated IV System

Equipment
Tourniquet
Chlorhexidine 2% or alcohol swab
Sterile gloves
NovaCath tray

Note: The NovaCath integrated IV catheter system is a closed system, since it limits exposure to blood during the catheter insertion process. The needle is withdrawn through a septum that reseals once the needle has been removed, and the female Luer is closed with a vent cap, so blood is contained in the Nova Cath during the catheter insertion process.

Preparation
1. Introduce self, identify the client using two client identifiers.
2. Perform hand hygiene.
3. Follow steps for Skill 28.1.3, Preparing the Venipuncture Site.

Procedure
1. Place the tray on the overbed table. Pull the tray lid all the way back.
2. Remove NovaCath from the tray and turn it over to the upright position. Remove the needle cap by pulling it straight off the needle. Break the seal by sliding the wings and finger tab forward away from the grips and returning them all the way back to the original position.
3. Hold the device gently by the grips, stabilize the blood vessel, and begin insertion. Use the proper position for insertion of the needle,
4. Once the needle is in the vein, look for blood return in the flash chamber, which is located between the grips and behind the needle.
5. Lower the angle of insertion and slightly advance the catheter and needle into the vein.

6. Hold the device in place with one finger on the finger tab and pull back about a quarter inch on the grips.
   ➤ *Rationale:* This ensures the catheter tip moves into the blood vessel ahead of the needle point.
7. Advance the device into the blood vessel as a unit. Remove the tourniquet.
8. Holding the finger tab in place, pull grips all the way back to lock the needle into place. A click can be heard.
   ➤ *Rationale:* Click indicates the safety lock is fully engaged.
9. Check to see if blood is travelling through the extension tubing. ➤ *Rationale:* This indicates the catheter is still in the blood vessel.
10. Hold the grips in place with the dominant hand, and push the finger tab forward with the thumb of the opposite hand.
    ➤ *Rationale:* This advances the catheter into the vein.
11. Advance the catheter off the needle. You should see blood travel through the extension tubing, indicating the catheter is still in the blood vessel.
12. Keep your thumb in place on the finger tab, pull the grips all the way back to click the needle into place. ➤ *Rationale:* A clicking sound indicates the safety lock is fully engaged.
13. Anchor the wings and unfold the stabilization frame.
14. Disconnect the safety needle from the catheter hub. Apply forward pressure to the finger tab while pulling back on the grips.
15. Remove the needle by pulling back on the grips to detach the needle.
16. Cover the insertion site, wings, and septum with a sterile transparent dressing. Ensure the insertion site is clearly visible. Secure the stabilization platform with tape.
17. Engage the multi-access clamp to control blood flow, remove the vent cap, and collect the blood specimen. Flush or begin the infusion.

Unit 28.1 Documentation and Evaluation

DOCUMENTATION for IV Therapy

- Time and date of insertion
- Location of insertion site, name of vein cannulated
- Gauge length and type of needle/catheter inserted or NovaCath inserted
- Number of attempts (if more than one)

- Type of dressing applied
- Flush administered for cannula patency
- Type, amount, and rate of solution infused
- Status of IV site
- Client response to procedure

EVALUATION/Critical Thinking

Expected Outcomes

- Fluid and electrolyte needs are met.
- Appropriate IV site is selected, and IV inserted without difficulty.

- IV fluids infuse at prescribed rate without complications.
- Appropriate IV equipment for client is used.
- IV site is maintained using sterile technique.

Unexpected Outcomes

- Venipuncture is unsuccessful for needle/catheter insertion.

Alternative Actions

- Remove needle/catheter, apply pressure at insertion site until bleeding stops. (This prevents ecchymosis at site.) Apply Band-Aid.
- Apply small pressure dressing if client is on anticoagulant therapy.
- Select another site more proximal in vein or use another extremity.
- Avoid the one-step entry method since this frequently results in a through-and-through vein puncture.
- After two failed attempts, seek a more experienced individual to perform venipuncture.
- Place extremity in dependent position before placing tourniquet. This allows vein to fill.
- Place warm compress on extremity to increase vasodilation before placing tourniquet.
- Use the AccuVein viewing system to identify an appropriate vessel.

- Vein rolls and is difficult to enter.

- Apply traction with thumb and index finger to stabilize skin and vein; maintain traction until venipuncture complete.
- Select a smaller gauge catheter.
- Advance catheter slowly.

- Vein is fragile and "balloons" around needle on vein entry.

- Release tourniquet as soon as vein entry is evident.
- Avoid use of tourniquet if veins are very fragile or client is taking an anticoagulant.
- Enter vein with needle bevel down.

- Infiltration occurs.

- Place warm moist pack; using warm towel, enclose area from fingertips to elbow. Place extremity in plastic bag with open end at elbow. Leave in place no more than 10 min.

- Vesicant drug infuses into tissue.

- Clamp IV tubing.
- Infuse antidote for specific medication, according to physician orders.

Intravenous Management

Nursing Process Data

ASSESSMENT Database

- Assess site for erythema, swelling, or pain.
- Assess infusion for correct solution, amount, and flow rate.
- Assess need to change IV to saline lock.
- Assess need to change client's gown while IV is infusing.
- Assess need to change IV solution/administration set and infusion site.

PLANNING Objectives

- To maintain the IV site free from erythema, swelling, or pain
- To monitor the IV infusion rate accurately
- To change a gown while maintaining the IV site
- To discontinue IV therapy without complication
- To convert IV to saline lock

IMPLEMENTATION Procedures

DOCUMENTATION AND EVALUATION

Expected Outcomes

- Fluids are administered without adverse effects.
- IV site remains clean without signs of infection or filtration.
- IV is converted to a saline lock and is functioning properly.
- Client's gown is changed while maintaining IV placement.
- IV is discontinued intact; site remains free of infection or bleeding.

Unexpected Outcomes/Alternative Actions

Pearson Nursing Student Resources

Find additional review materials at
nursing.pearsonhighered.com.
Prepare for success with NCLEX®-style practice questions and Skill Checklists.

Skill 28.2.1 | Regulating Infusion Flow Rate

Procedure

1. Perform hand hygiene. Check manufacturer's drip-rate calibration on administration set package. Macrodrip sets vary from 10 to 15 gtt per 1 mL. Microdrip factor is 60 drops/mL.
2. Check physician's order for amount of fluid to be delivered per unit of time (e.g., 1 L every 8 hr, or hourly flow rate such as 100 mL/hr).
3. Calculate flow rate.

   a. To find the number of milliliters to be given per hour:

   $$\frac{\text{Total solution}}{\text{No. of hours to run}} = \text{mL/hour}$$

   b. To find drops per minute:

   $$\frac{\text{mL/hr} \times \text{drop factor}}{60 \text{ min}} = \text{gtts/min}$$

4. Note drip chamber; count the drops in 1 min (or in 15 seconds and multiply by 4). See Box 28-3 ■ for IV calorie calculation.
5. Adjust tubing clamp until the chamber drips the desired number of drops per minute (or 15-second increment).
6. Monitor flow rate frequently. Adjustments to maintain desired delivery are often necessary (Box 28-4 ■).

Box 28-3 IV CALORIE CALCULATION

- 1,000 mL of D_5W provides 50 g of dextrose.
- 50 g of dextrose provides 4 cal/g; therefore, multiply 50 g × 4 cal.
- 1,000 mL of D_5W provides 200 cal.
- Usual IV fluid maintenance is 2,000–3,000 mL/day (400–600 cal/day).
- 4 cal/g is used in calculation; however, it is actually 3.4 cal/g.

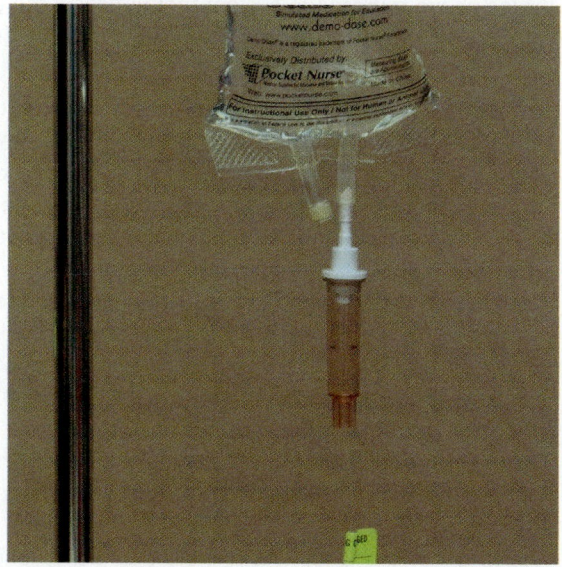

Count drops per minute to check accuracy of drip rate.

Box 28-4 FACTORS THAT INFLUENCE IV FLOW RATES WHEN USING GRAVITY FOR INFUSION

- Warm fluids drip faster than cold fluids.
- The higher the bag is above insertion site, the faster the content infuses.
- The more the IV administration set is tilted, the larger each drop from drip chamber will be.
- The larger the catheter diameter, the faster the flow rate.
- The longer the catheter, the slower the flow rate because of resistance.
- Increased blood pressure or coughing will slow the flow rate (usually just temporarily).

Note: Because of these variables, manual control of IVs is not recommended. IV pumps are the most predictable method of infusing fluids.

Skill 28.2.2 | Using an Electronic Flow-Control Device

Equipment

Electronic infusion device (pump; Box 28-5 ■)
Device-compatible IV administration set
Needleless access device
Gloves

Preparation

1. Introduce self and verify client using two identifiers.
2. Attach controller to IV pole.
   a. Attach controller to the IV pole so it is below and in-line with IV container.
   b. Plug machine into electric outlet (unless using battery-operated).

Note: Batteries last up to 6 hr. Keep device plugged into electric outlet unless it is necessary to move device.

Box 28-5 INFUSION PUMP

In contrast to gravity flow devices, positive-pressure infusion pumps are more accurate in the preselected volume delivery by adding pressure to overcome resistance to fluid flow produced by tubing diameter, filter, viscosity of infusing fluid, cannula, and so on. Pumps usually require use of specially designed administration sets. When the system is working with normal resistance, delivery pressure is minimal. When resistance (5 psi over baseline) develops in the catheter or tubing, the pump adds pressure (within limits) to maintain the infusion. Changes in resistance at an insertion site due to infiltration or thrombosis may not set off the system's alarm, and site problems could become serious. When the pump's maximum pressure limit is reached, an occlusion pressure alarm sounds. The nurse must become familiar with infusion devices by reading the manufacturer's literature and adhering to all instructions to ensure safe, efficient operation.

Procedure

1. Explain procedure to client and discuss the various sounds that can be heard during the use of the equipment (Box 28-6 ■).
2. Perform hand hygiene.
3. Close the regulating clamp on the set tubing before hanging the bag.
4. Spike IV solution bag.
5. Fill the drip chamber to minimum one-third full.
   ➤ *Rationale:* This amount allows sufficient air space in the drip chamber.
6. Prime tubing by opening the regulating clamp slowly and allowing tubing to fill with IV solution. If using a cassette-type tubing, follow package instructions to correctly prime the cassette portion of the tubing that engages into the control device.

Note: Check if tubing has an anti–free-flow device that must be opened before the primary tubing.

7. Follow manufacturer's instructions to load the administration set into the device, taking care to fit tubing and cassette into appropriate receptor sites.
8. Close device door and latch it.
9. Perform hand hygiene and don gloves.
10. Check that client's venipuncture site is free from signs of vein irritation or infiltration.

Box 28-6 IF ALARM SOUNDS, CHECK THE FOLLOWING

Most devices have a message system that specifies the exact problem. You should be prepared to troubleshoot various components of the system.

- *Infusion Complete*: When the exact volume to be delivered is set and the volume limit has been reached, an alarm sounds and the machine goes to a KVO "keep-open" mode. Establish if the total volume of the container has been delivered; change the solution container if needed, and reset the volume to be infused.
- *Occlusion*: All devices sound an alarm when they cannot maintain delivery in the face of increasing resistance. In this instance, check the insertion site for infiltration and look for position problems, pinched tubing, closed clamp, turned stopcock, or clogged filter.
- *Other Problems*: Other messages may indicate "air in the line," "low battery," "cassette" (improperly loaded), or "free flow."
- *Nursing Action*: Check trouble spot carefully, readjust, and restart the infusion.

CLINICAL ALERT

Observe IV site frequently when pumps are used. IV pumps do not normally detect infiltration at the IV site. Infiltration does not produce enough pressure to trigger an alarm. Check for **edema**, cool skin, discomfort, and tenderness at the IV site.

11. Connect the administration set tubing to the established infusion site.
12. Open the regulating clamp on the administration set.
13. Turn the device ON.

14. Set device parameters for operation, again following manufacturer's instructions or machine's setup prompts. Parameters may include:

    a. Infusion (e.g., primary)
    b. Volume to be infused
    c. Rate (mL/hr)
    d. Pressure (measure can vary; e.g., mm Hg, cm H_2O, or psi)

15. START device when parameters are set.
16. Observe that infusion is running properly.
17. Remove gloves and perform hand hygiene.
18. Check client's infusion site frequently (Box 28-7 ■).

Box 28-7 INFUSION SITE EVALUATION CRITERIA

Catheter sites are evaluated at least each shift for both phlebitis and infiltration using evaluation criteria established by the Intravenous Nurses' Society (2011).

Phlebitis

0 = no clinical symptoms
1+ = erythema at access site with or without pain
2+ = pain at access site with erythema or edema
3+ = pain at access site with erythema or edema, streak formation
4+ = pain at access site with erythema or edema, streak formation, palpable venous cord longer than 2.5 cm (1 in.), **purulent** discharge

Note: No catheter should remain in place with signs of phlebitis, even with good blood flow and IV infusion rate.

Infiltrations

0 = no symptoms
1 = skin blanched, edema

2 = skin blanched, edema 2.5–15 cm (1–6 in.) in any direction, cool to touch, with or without pain
3 = skin blanched, translucent, gross edema more than 15 cm (6 in.) in any direction, cool to touch, mild to moderate pain, possible numbness
4 = skin blanched, translucent; skin tight, leaking; gross edema more than 15 cm (6 in.) in any direction or deep pitting tissue edema; skin discolored, bruised, or swollen; circulatory impairment; moderate to severe pain; infiltration of any amount of blood product, irritant, or vesicant.

Note: Infiltrations should be diagnosed well before obvious swelling occurs. Most infiltrations should be warm packed to promote reabsorption of fluid into vascular bed and out of tissues, except in case of infiltration by a vesicant drug, then follow facility policy or drug manufacturer's directions.

Skill 28.2.3 | Using a "Smart" Pump

Equipment
Point-of-care computer specific to nursing unit
IV tubing
IV fluids and/or IV medications

Procedure
1. Introduce self, identify client using two identifiers, and explain the pump's function (Box 28-8 ■).
2. Assemble equipment and bring to client's bedside.
3. Perform hand hygiene.

4. Verify IV site is patent and without signs of infiltration.
5. Plug pump into electrical outlet.
6. Insert the pump module into the point-of-care computer ("brain").
7. Spike IV fluid bag.
8. Prime IV tubing with appropriate solution.
9. Insert the IV tubing into the pump module and close the door to the pump. (Follow photos for inserting tubing into cassette.) ❶ ❷ ❸ ❹

(continued)

Skill 28.2.3 | Using a "Smart" Pump *(continued)*

❶ Hang IV on pole. Prime tubing and insert into pump module cassette.

❸ Insert white slide clamp into cassette and listen for click.

❷ Place top of IV tubing into top of cassette and listen for click indicating it is seated.

❹ Close pump module door and lower locking lever.

10. View screen will ask which client care area is being used.
    ➤ *Rationale:* The pump automatically configures itself to provide the infusion parameters for that area (e.g., pediatrics, ICU).
11. Choose the intended drug and concentration from the list outlined on the screen. ❺

12. Enter the ordered dose and infusion rate; the pump checks this information against the drug library. ❻ If what was programmed matches the pump's drug library, the pump allows the infusion to begin (Box 28-9 ■). Follow manufacturer's directions on how to program the pump. Each manufacturer's equipment is somewhat different.

❺ Select medication to be infused.

❻ Check screen for drug name and infusion rate.

Box 28-8 SMART IV PUMPS

- Smart pumps have a "brain" (computer).
- Nurses are alerted when a pump setting does not match the facility's drug administration guidelines.
- Data is logged from pump to pharmacy computer: time, date, drug that was infused, concentration, programmed rate, and volume infused are recorded. Data about all alerts is also collected to help shape practice guidelines.
- Individual facility pharmacists create the database of information for their own facility, and then the information is programmed into the pump.
- Facilities program pumps with specific data sets or "profiles." Each area of the facility (such as OB, pediatrics, ICU) develops its own drug library. When the specific client care area is designated (e.g, pediatrics), the pump automatically configures itself to give the infusion parameters for that area.
- Manufacturers of smart pumps offer different features:
  - Add-on syringe pumps for small-volume IV push or **bolus** infusions.
  - Multiple infusions through one pump.
  - Administration of patient-controlled analgesia (PCA).

(continued)

Skill 28.2.3 | Using a "Smart" Pump *(continued)*

13. If an audible and visual alert occurs, the programmed data are outside the specified limits. The alert informs you about which parameter is out of the recommended range.

14. Depending on the medication or client care area, the pump will sound a "soft" alarm or a "hard" alarm. ➐ Some facilities allow a "soft" alarm to be overridden. If you override the alarm, the infusion will begin. This alarm is considered a minor error.

15. When "hard" alarm occurs, the pump shuts down. It cannot be overridden. Reprogram the pump with settings that are within your facility's specified limits to begin infusing when a "hard" alarm sounds.

Note: The smart pump's software logs and tracks all alerts, recording the time, date, drug, concentration, and infusion rate, as well as any action taken and whether the pump is overridden or not.

> **CLINICAL ALERT**
>
> Check the facility's policies and procedures to determine whether the pump can be run with the override.

16. Observe the screen to ensure medication is infusing at the prescribed rate.

➐ Check the screen when "soft alert" sounds to determine the problem.

Box 28-9 USING A BAR CODE MEDICATION ADMINISTRATION SYSTEM

- Most facilities use a bar code medication administration (BCMA) system, a computerized prescriber order entry (CPOE), automatic medication dispensing, and electronic medication records. Smart pumps can provide a very high level of client safety, providing information on which IV medications were ordered via a CPOE and when each medication is due.

- When the nurse enters the client's room with the scanning device, he or she scans the bar-code labels on the medication, the client's identification band, and the nurse's ID badge. The information from the bar-code label attached to the medication IV bag is transmitted wirelessly and is programmed into the infusion pump.

- The pump will begin infusing only when scanning of all information is complete.

- The pump automatically communicates with a computer in the pharmacy, providing the status of the infusion.

EVIDENCE-BASED PRACTICE
Smart Infusion Pumps are Selectively Intelligent

In earlier studies it was found that after the implementation of Smart Pump Technology and the electronic drug library, there was a 50% reduction in the number of drug administration errors involving syringe pumps. However, in an article first published in 2011, research indicated there are still potential errors associated with this technology.

1. Drug libraries require knowledge and understanding of pump technology for safe use.

2. Updating of pump libraries needs close coordination between pharmacy and nursing staff to ensure that the product is prepared the way the drug is presented in the drug library.

3. Setting appropriate "hard" and "soft" limits on drugs requires close communication between pharmacy and nursing.

4. Smart pumps do not replace hospital procedures and clinical client monitoring.

Source: DiTrapano (2013)

Skill 28.2.4 | Using a Syringe Pump

Equipment
Battery or electronic operated syringe infusion pump ➊
Pharmacy-prepared and labeled syringe with prescribed medication
Microbore tubing with needleless access device
Chlorhexidine gluconate

Procedure
1. Check the syringe label against the physician's order for drug, dosage, and amount of drug to be delivered over a specified time.

2. Ensure that medication is compatible with the primary infusing solution.

❶ Smart pumps have syringe modules available to be attached to the point-of-care computers. To attach a module, follow the manufacturer's directions.

3. Calculate the amount of medication to be delivered per minute.
4. Attach microbore tubing to the syringe. Holding the syringe upright, expel air from the medication syringe before priming tubing.
5. Holding the syringe downward, carefully prime microbore tubing with medication (about 0.5 mL).
6. Insert the syringe into the cradle of the pump, squeezing the clamp around designated parts of the syringe; attach pusher to plunger.
7. Verify that the IV site is free from infiltration or vein irritation.
8. Swab primary IV tubing port closest to the client.
9. Insert the microbore cannula into the port.
10. Set rate for drug delivery according to pharmacy specifications on the syringe label, or as prescribed. Drug will be infused *independent* of the primary infusion rate.
11. Start the syringe pump.
12. Check the infusion indicator to verify pump is infusing.
13. Monitor the site and pump function frequently.
14. For subsequent doses, pharmacy dispenses a new syringe, but microbore tubing may be reused for 48 to 72 hr (according to agency policy). A sterile cap is used each time the client's primary tubing is accessed.

Note: For other brands of syringe pumps, follow directions for setup and delivery of meds with their product.

Skill 28.2.5 | Managing the IV Site

Equipment
Appropriate tubing for IV site
IV cap (according to hospital policy)
Clean gloves
Transparent dressing
Sterile tape
Stabilizing device

> **CLINICAL ALERT**
> Clients receiving hypertonic, acidic, or irritating agents; older adult clients with fragile veins; and pediatric clients who are active are at particular risk for IV site problems.

Procedure
1. Evaluate every 2 hr for site-related complications (Table 28-3 ■).

> **CLINICAL ALERT**
> To check for extravasation, place a constrictive band proximal to the infusion site tight enough to restrict blood flow through the vein. Set tubing roller clamp to a "keep open" (or slow) rate, and remove tubing from the infusion pump. If the infusion continues to drip, fluid is extravasating into the surrounding tissue.

2. Identify the client using two forms of identification and perform hand hygiene.

3. Include gentle palpation through an intact transparent dressing.
4. Remove the IV cannula in the periphery, and change to a new, more proximal site every 72 to 96 hr. (CDC recommends 72–96 hr; INS Standards of Practice recommend 72 hr.)
5. Assess the IV site every 4 hr if client's status prohibits changing IV site.

IV Administration Sets
1. Change administration sets, including all stopcocks, access devices, and extension tubings, every 96 hr (according to agency policy). This can be done routinely at the same time a new container of IV solution is started.
2. Change IV tubing according to use.
   a. Primary intermittent tubing, every 24 hr
   b. Hyperalimentation, every 24 hr
   c. Secondary infusion tubing, every 24 hr ➤ **Rationale:** Once a secondary tubing is disconnected, it must be treated as a primary tubing according to INS Standard 54.
   d. Blood and blood component tubing, every 4 hr or after 2 units of blood
   e. Hemodynamic and arterial pressure monitoring tubing, every 96 hr
3. Use separate secondary tubing for each "piggy-backed" agent if agents are incompatible.

(continued)

Skill 28.2.5 | Managing the IV Site *(continued)*

Table 28-3 Complications of IV Therapy

Assessment: Signs and Symptoms	Implementation: Nursing Action
Phlebitis	
Pain along the vein, tenderness	Discontinue infusion, and remove needle.
Erythema—red streak at vein site	Apply warm compresses.
Edema at insertion site	Start IV at another site. Select a large vein when administering irritating agents. Anchor cannula to prevent movement in vein.
Sluggish flow rate	Do not use positive irrigation with sluggish flow rate—there may be a clot at the end of the needle and it could be flushed into bloodstream. Reposition extremity. Note where the IV catheter is in relationship to joint, such as wrist, antecubital.
Area warm to touch	Document description and location of site.
Infiltration of fluid	
Edema around insertion site—swelling of cannulated extremity	Discontinue infusion and remove needle.
Blanching of infusion site	Apply warm compresses to encourage absorption.
Coolness of skin around site	Notify physician if solution contains potassium or other irritating component (e.g., 10% dextrose). Do not rely on backflash of blood to determine location of catheter or needle in vein.
No backflow of blood when tubing is pinched or fluid container lowered below IV site (Tubing must be removed from infusion device.)	Lower container below IV site—if blood returns, needle is in vein, *but* fluid may be leaking into tissue if bevel has pierced posterior wall of vein. Restart IV at another site.
Extravasation of medication	
Pain, stinging, or burning at site	Discontinue infusion; attempt to **aspirate** the drug.
Redness and swelling	Apply ice compress to area Research the medication—some agents have specific antidotes for extravasation injury. Notify physician. Administer irritating or vesicant medications through a central venous device.

① Flush the site, then attach needleless cannula into needleless cap.

② Using the needleless cannula reduces risk of needle sticks during IV procedures.

Converting From Continuous IV to a "Lock"

1. Ensure site is patent and functional.
2. Perform hand hygiene and don clean gloves.
3. Clamp infusion tubing.
4. Disconnect IV tubing from catheter.
5. Attach needleless injection cap or primed T connector extension tubing with needleless injection cap to catheter hub (Box 28-10 ■). **① ②**

Box 28-10 NEEDLELESS IV ACCESS DEVICES

Split Septum Technology–Needleless Access System

The system consists of a pre-split injection cap that requires a blunt cannula to access the fluid path. One new version of the split septum is accessed with a standard male Luer syringe or administration set.

Luer Access Mechanical Valve

This is a needleless access device that consists of a valve that is opened by the insertion of a standard male Luer syringe or administration set to access the fluid path. There are two types:

1. Compression seal is depressed by male Luer, opening the fluid path.
2. Open Luer that houses a valve is activated by the male Luer; it requires a new cap on the Luer after each use.

Luer Access Mechanical Valve With Positive Displacement-Needleless Access Device

The system consists of a valve and a fluid reservoir. The valve is opened by the insertion of a standard male Luer syringe tip or administration set, accessing the fluid path. When the male Luer is disconnected, the compression seal reseats, causing the reservoir to empty and creating positive displacement of fluid into the catheter lumen.

Source: Hadaway (2006)

---

6. Prep, then inject port with 1 mL of sterile normal saline to maintain patency.

CLINICAL ALERT

Some facilities use a single secondary tubing for all agents. The tubing is back-flushed with the primary solution before administering a new agent, providing the agents are compatible.

Applying a Securement Device

1. Prepare skin area according to facility policy—chlorhexidine recommended.
2. Apply skin prep provided with device. ➤ *Rationale:* This increases adhesion of device and protects skin.
3. Place IV catheter into the device before adhering anchor pad to skin.

---

4. Assess the site daily. ➤ *Rationale:* This is to ensure placement of the device on the skin.
5. Assess skin under the device for skin tears.
6. Change device every 7 days by gently stroking under device surface with alcohol swab while continuing to lift pad off skin.

EVIDENCE-BASED PRACTICE

Comparison of Two Stabilization Systems

An open-label, prospective, randomized, noninferiority study was conducted at a large academic, magnet-designated, Level I trauma center to compare the peripheral intravenous catheter securement-related complication rates of two different stabilization systems. The control stabilization system included the StatLock device with a nonwinged catheter, and the investigational stabilization system included a closed catheter system with a specially designed Tegaderm dressing. Data from 302 subjects indicated that the investigational stabilization system was noninferior or similar to the control stabilization system with respect to the overall securement-related complications. The cost of the investigational stabilization system was approximately 75% of the cost of the control stabilization system.

Source: Bausone-Gazda, Lefaiver, & Walters (2010)

Applying a Transparent Dressing

1. Cover IV insertion site with transparent dressing.
   a. Line up slit in the frame with the catheter hub.
   b. Apply the dressing over the insertion site just to the top edge of the hub.
   c. Do not stretch the dressing during application.
   d. Firmly smooth down the dressing edges as the frame is slowly removed.
   e. Gently pinch and seal the dressing around the catheter hub.
   f. Smooth down the entire dressing from the center out to the edges, using firm pressure to enhance adhesion.
   g. Label dressing with date of insertion, date of change, gauge used, and initials of nurse.
2. Document catheter insertion and dressing information.

CLINICAL ALERT

Regard IV systems as closed sterile systems and maintain as such. All entries into the tubing should be made through injection ports that are disinfected just before entry.

Skill 28.2.6 | Converting IV to Saline Lock

Equipment

Extension tubing with needleless connector
Needleless syringe
Clean gloves
Saline flush syringes with 0.9% preservative-free normal saline
2×2 sterile gauze

Procedure

1. Gather equipment and perform hand hygiene. Introduce self and identify client using two identifiers.
2. Assess that IV is infusing and there are no signs of phlebitis or infiltration.
3. Don gloves.

(continued)

Skill 28.2.6 | Converting IV to Saline Lock *(continued)*

4. Prime extension tubing. ❶
5. Turn off IV and disconnect from pump if necessary.
6. Disconnect IV tubing and attach extension tubing. Check drip chamber. ❷ ❸ ❹ A 2×2 gauze can be placed under IV site to catch drops from IV tubing disconnect.

7. Redress the IV site.
8. Discard equipment.
9. Remove gloves and perform hand hygiene.

❶ Prime the extension tubing.

❸ Attach IV tubing to threaded lock cannula.

❷ Attach extension tubing to IV catheter. Back priming.

❹ Check drip chamber.

Skill 28.2.7 | Changing Gown for Client With IV

Equipment
Clean gown
Bathing supplies, if needed

Procedure
1. Check client care plan for infusion drip rate, type of solution, and any special considerations.
2. Perform hand hygiene. Take equipment to client's room.
3. Introduce self and identify client using two descriptors.
4. Explain procedure to client. Provide privacy.
5. Untie back of gown and remove gown from unaffected arm.

6. Support arm with IV and slip gown down arm to IV tubing.
7. Place clean gown over client's chest and abdomen.
8. Use tubing clamp to slow infusion to "keep open" rate and remove tubing from infusion pump if in use.
9. Remove IV bag from hook and slip sleeve over bag, keeping bag above client's arm. Do not jar or pull tubing.
   ➤ *Rationale:* Maintaining the bag's height prevents backflow of blood into tubing. If the IV tubing is pulled or jarred, it may become dislodged and infiltrate into surrounding tissue.

10. Place your hand up through distal end of clean gown sleeve and grasp IV bag. Pull bag and tubing out through clean gown sleeve.
11. Rehang bag on hook and check to see that infusion is running according to ordered drip rate.
12. Replace tubing into infusion pump, unclamp, and reestablish prescribed infusion flow rate.
13. Guide sleeve of gown up client's arm to the shoulder.
14. Assist client to put the other arm through the remaining sleeve.
15. Tie gown at the back.

16. Check IV infusion rate and IV tubing to determine that solution is flowing unimpeded into client's vein. ➤ *Rationale:* Kinks in tubing impede flow.
17. Return bed to a comfortable position for the client.
18. Remove dirty linen from the room.
19. Perform hand hygiene.

Note: Most facilities provide "IV gowns" that snap from the shoulder down the sleeve of the gown for ease in removal without disturbing the IV.

Skill 28.2.8 | Discontinuing an IV

Equipment
Sterile 2×2 gauze pads (3–4)
Sterile tape
Clean gloves

Procedure
1. Gather equipment.
2. Perform hand hygiene and don gloves.
3. Introduce self, identify client using two descriptors, and explain the procedure to the client.
4. Turn off the infusion.
5. Loosen transparent dressing and securement device. ❶ ❷ Use alcohol swabs or hold the center while stretching the dressing to release the dressing and prevent skin tears.
6. Stabilize catheter while removing dressing and securement device. ❸ ❹ ➤ *Rationale:* Stabilizing the site prevents unnecessary movement that could injure the vein.
7. Hold sterile gauze, pressing the skin 3 cm (1⅛ in.) above the insertion site. Remove catheter carefully and smoothly, keeping it almost flush with skin. ❺ Observe catheter for breakage and ensure it is intact.
8. Quickly press a sterile pad over the venipuncture site and hold firmly until bleeding stops. ❻

> **CLINICAL ALERT**
> Assess whether the client has been receiving antithrombotic (aspirin) or anticoagulant (Coumadin, heparin) therapy. Hold pressure for several minutes if the client has prolonged bleeding caused by drug therapy.

9. Hold pressure for several minutes if client's drug therapy prolongs bleeding.
10. Apply sterile pad and tape in place. ❼
11. Elevate arm to reduce venous pressure and help collapse vein to facilitate clot formation. Do not bend arm at elbow. ➤ *Rationale:* Bending elbow causes **hematoma** formation.
12. Observe venipuncture site for redness, swelling, or hematoma.
13. Dispose of equipment and gloves.
14. Perform hand hygiene.
15. Check site again in 15 min.
16. Record volume infused on I&O sheet or in the electronic health record. ❽

Note: If there are signs of infection or inflammation at catheter site or client complains of symptoms related to infection, cut tip of catheter with sterile scissors, place in sterile container, and send to lab for culture.

❶ Remove tape carefully from the tubing site.

(continued)

Skill 28.2.8 | Discontinuing an IV *(continued)*

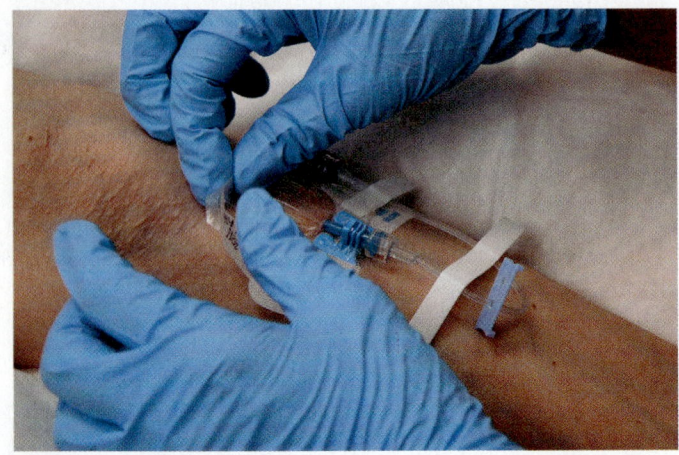

2 Remove occlusive dressing, starting at top and pulling down toward the IV site.

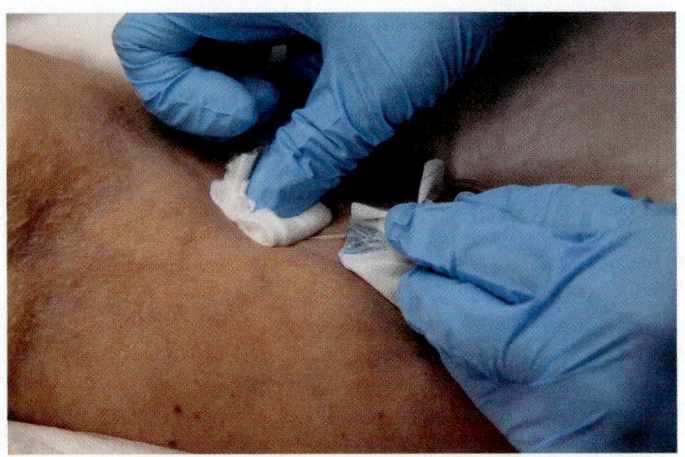

5 Remove IV cannula carefully by pressing the skin 3 cm (1⅛ in.) above the insertion site.

3 Holding cannula in place, continue to pull the dressing toward the IV site.

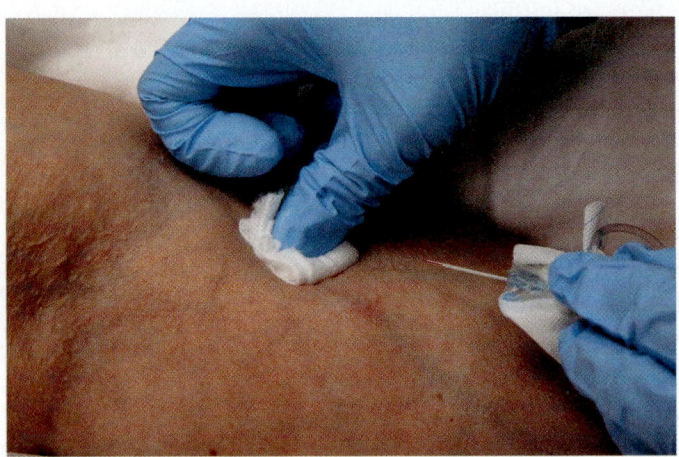

6 Place sterile gauze directly over IV site and press firmly until bleeding stops.

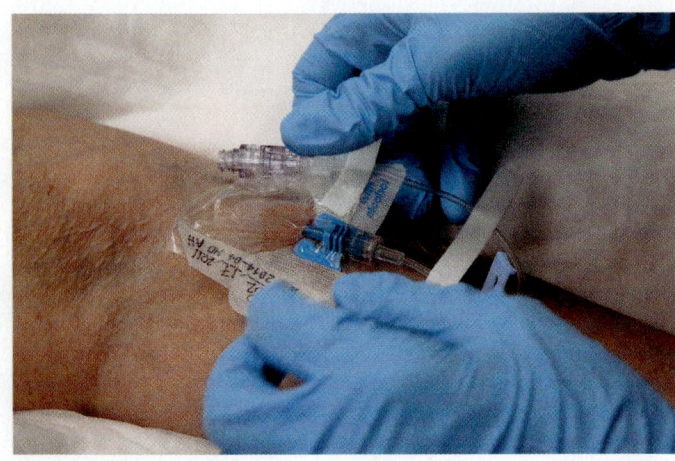

4 Lift dressing off the skin.

7 Tape gauze dressing in place.

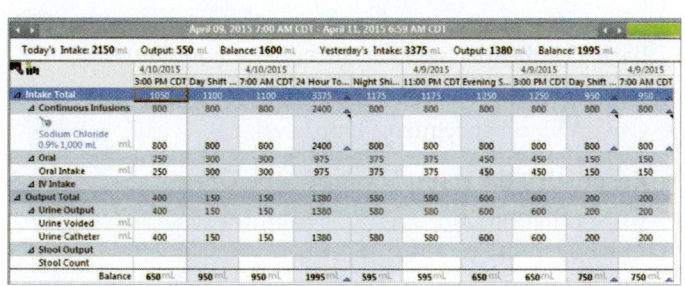

8 Portions of intake and output record.

Source: From Cerner Electronic Health Record. © Cerner Corporation. Pearson has restricted permission to reproduce and distribute this copyrighted work. Further reproduction or distribution is strictly prohibited without written consent of Cerner Corporation.

Unit 28.2 Documentation and Evaluation

DOCUMENTATION for Intravenous Management

IV Insertion

- Date and time
- Location of insertion site
- Gauge and length of catheter inserted
- IV solution and flow rate
- Site care given
- Condition of site
- Client response to procedure

IV Discontinued

- Date and time
- Note condition of the catheter—"intact"
- Assess catheter length
- Condition of site
- Client response to procedure
- Catheter tip to lab if appropriate

EVALUATION/Critical Thinking

Excepted Outcomes

- Fluids are administered without adverse effects.
- IV site remains clean, without signs of infection or infiltration.
- IV is converted to a saline lock and is functioning properly.
- Client's gown is changed while maintaining IV placement.
- IV is discontinued intact and site remains free of infection or bleeding.

(continued)

Unexpected Outcomes	**Alternative Actions**
• Client develops unexplained fever with chills and rising pulse rate.	• Unexplained fever may be associated with catheter-related sepsis. Report to physician.
	• Assess IV site for signs of infection.
	• Ensure that IV solutions hang for no more than 24 hr.
	• Check client's vital signs: temperature usually above 37.8°C (100°F) when caused by IV-related sepsis.
	• Check for other symptoms of pyrogenic reactions (e.g., backache, headache, malaise, nausea, and vomiting).
	• Stop the infusion.
	• Obtain blood specimens, if ordered.
• IV solution does not flow properly.	• Ensure that the control clamp is open.
	• Check that blood pressure readings are not taken on arm in which IV is running, as flow is impeded and a clot can form on the end of the catheter.
	• Ensure that IV administration set is properly loaded. Check pump for flow problem indicator (e.g., cassette seating, air in line).
	• Check IV tubing from insertion site to IV solution for kinks and obstructions.
	• Check for extremity causing positional obstruction to flow (e.g., elbow bent, arm rotated).
• IV solution appears to be infiltrating, resulting in tissue swelling.	• Decrease the flow rate. (Remove from pump for "keep open" rate.)
	• Lower bag of IV solution; if blood returns, cannula may be in the vein but fluid may be leaking into surrounding tissue via existing puncture in vein wall.
	• Discontinue infusion and establish a new site.
• Phlebitis is suspected at infusion site (tenderness, warmth, erythema, and pain).	• Check infusion solution and medications being administered. (Potassium chloride and hypertonic solutions are particularly irritating to veins.)
	• Discontinue IV.
	• Apply warm compress per hospital policy.
• Postinfusion phlebitis may also occur after the IV has been discontinued in response to either chemical or mechanical factors of the preexisting IV.	• Check IV solution; hypertonic solution causes irritation necessitating use of large veins and changing IV sites more frequently.
	• Follow hospital policy for treatment. Warm compresses to the site are generally recommended.
	• Elevate extremity.

Monitoring Fluid Balance

Nursing Process Data

ASSESSMENT Database

- Assess client's need for intake and output recording.
- Assess client's ability to keep intake and output fluid records.
- Evaluate client for any factors that might affect his or her intake and output (e.g., preexisting disease states, concurrent disease, drug therapies, and current physical status).
- Determine all measurable sources of fluid intake: fluids with and between meals, tube feeding, liquid medications, IV fluids, and IV medications.
- Determine all measurable sources of fluid output: urine, emesis, **diarrhea**, and drainage sites.
- Determine alterations in nonmeasurable sources of fluid intake and loss: food, increased metabolism (e.g., fever), rapid respirations, and perspiration.
- Determine balance of daily intake and output.

PLANNING Objectives

- To establish a written record of the client's total fluid intake (oral, parenteral, and feeding tubes) and fluid output (urine, wound/tube drainage, diarrhea, and vomiting)
- To plan fluid replacement or appropriate therapy by assessing deficits or excesses of fluid and electrolytes
- To ensure a fluid intake of at least 2,000 to 2,600 mL unless contraindicated by diagnosis
- To monitor the client's fluid status, vital signs, and mental state to determine homeostasis

IMPLEMENTATION Procedures

DOCUMENTATION AND EVALUATION

Expected Outcomes

- Client's intake and output are maintained within expected parameters of 200–300 mL of each other.
- Fluid intake is at least 2,600 mL unless contraindicated by diagnosis.
- Client's fluid status, vital signs, and mental status are within normal range.
- Output is maintained at more than 30 mL/hr.
- IV flow rate is maintained at prescribed rate.

Unexpected Outcomes/Alternative Actions

Pearson Nursing Student Resources

Find additional review materials at
nursing.pearsonhighered.com.
Prepare for success with NCLEX®-style practice questions and Skill Checklists.

Skill 28.3.1 | Monitoring Intake and Output

Equipment

Graduated container in client's bathroom

I&O bedside record sheet and computer to record intake and output

Urinal or bedpan; bedside commode or underseat basin for toilet

Hourly in-line urine measurement device for clients requiring frequent monitoring

Posted measurement standards for commonly used drinking and eating utensils (e.g., glasses, mugs, bowls)

Posted signs, dietary slips, and other communication devices to notify hospital personnel about how client's I&O is to be measured

Procedure

1. Determine whether client needs I&O measurements by checking client's chart or care plan. All clients with an IV need I&O measurement (Table 28-4 ■). ❶
2. Introduce self, identify client using two identifiers, and wash hands.
3. Instruct client and/or family about the need to measure all intake and output. Keep I&O sheet at the bedside for the family to record I&O.
4. Measure intake from all sources.

   a. Oral fluids
   b. IV fluids (see Box 28-11 ■ for types of IV solutions)
   c. Fluid medications (oral, enteral, or IV)
   d. Tube feedings and water used to clear tubing

> **CLINICAL ALERT**
> Measurement of all fluids is done in milliliters (mL).

❶ The majority of facilities use an electronic health record. Follow hospital protocol for documentation.

5. Measure output from all sources to establish a record and plan fluid therapy (Table 28-5 ■).

   a. Urinary catheters
   b. Bedpans and urinals
   c. Nasogastric drainage
   d. Drainage tubing (e.g., T-tubes, wound, or chest tube)
   e. Diarrheal stools
   f. Draining wounds
   g. Emesis

Table 28-4 Body Sites for Assessment of Fluid Status

Site	Fluid Excess	Fluid Deficit
Head and Neck		
Face	Eyeballs firm or protruding	Eyeballs soft or sunken
	Edema, especially around eyes	Decreased **skin turgor** over forehead
Mucous membranes	Excessive salivation	Dry or sticky mucosa with thick mucous secretions
	Swollen tongue	Shrunken tongue with multiple longitudinal furrows
Neck	Jugular vein distention	Crusted lips
Trunk		
Chest	Crackles in lung bases	Decreased skin turgor over sternum
Abdomen	**Ascites** (measure **girth** at umbilicus)	Dry, flaking skin
Sacrum	Edema	
Extremities		
Arms	Distended veins	Flattened veins
	Edema, particularly of the hands	Delayed capillary refill
	Delayed capillary refill	Dry, flaking skin
	Pulse bounding	Pulse weak and thready
Legs	Edema	Poor skin turgor, especially across shins
	Taut shiny skin	Dry, flaky skin, especially on feet
	Peripheral **cyanosis**	Weak pedal pulse or decreased capillary refill

6. Record I&O on record each time you check on client's intake or measure output.

CLINICAL ALERT

Check all drainage receptacles such as Foley bag and NG canister at the beginning of each shift to ensure they were emptied from the previous shift and that there has not been excessive drainage. NG canisters may not be emptied, but mark at the beginning and end of the shift to indicate how much output has occurred through the NG tube.

7. Correlate intake and output with daily weight. Weight is measured in kilograms (1 kg = 2.2 lb).
8. Record 24-hr totals of I&O on bedside record and place in client's chart, or enter data into computer.
9. Notify physician of any significant imbalance; more intensive monitoring may be indicated. ➤ **Rationale:** Hourly urine output less than 25–30 mL/hr for 2 consecutive hr or 24-hr urine output less than 500 mL can indicate dehydration or internal bleeding and can result in acute renal failure.

Box 28-11 **FLUID REPLACEMENT SOLUTIONS**

Hypertonic Solution—a solution with higher osmolality than blood serum

- Causes cells to shrink
- Used in severe salt depletion (very rare)
- Used as nutrient source (10% dextrose)
- Examples of solutions: 5% dextrose in 0.45% normal saline; 10% dextrose in water; 3% normal saline

Hypotonic Solution—a solution with lower osmolality than blood serum

- Hydrates cells, causes them to expand
- Used to correct dehydration
- Examples of solutions: 0.45% normal saline; 0.2% normal saline; 2.5% dextrose

Isotonic Solution—a solution with the same osmolality as blood serum

- Cells remain unchanged.
- Used for replacement or maintenance (expands extracellular volume), and especially for expanding circulating (intravascular) volume
- Examples of solutions: 5% dextrose in water; 0.9% normal saline (NS); Lactated Ringer's

Note: One liter of normal saline (0.9% NaCl) meets the usual daily requirement of these **electrolytes** in an adult.

Table 28-5 Objective Data Associated With Fluid Status

Data	Fluid Excess	Fluid Deficit
Vital Signs		
Blood pressure	Increased*	Decreased (especially on standing)
Pulse	Increased rate	Increased rate
Temperature	Unchanged	Elevated
Respirations	Increased rate	Unchanged or increased
Laboratory Findings		
Urine-**specific gravity**	Decreased, approaching 1.003	Increased, approaching 1.025 or greater
Blood hematocrit	Less than 3 times the hemoglobin	Greater than 3 times the hemoglobin
Serum sodium (Na)	Less than 135 mEq/L or normal	Greater than 145 mEq/L or normal
Blood urea nitrogen (BUN)	Decreased (except in heart or renal failure)	Proportionately greater than the serum creatinine
Hourly Urine Output	More than 60 mL/hr	Less than 30–60 mL/hr
Weight	A 5% or greater gain	Mild: 2% loss Moderate: 3–5% loss Severe: 6% or greater loss

*If the heart is unable to pump the increased blood volume, the blood pressure (reflecting cardiac output) may decrease. Polyuria can also be seen with fluid volume deficit (FVD) as in diabetic states.

Skill 28.3.2 | Monitoring IV Intake

Equipment

Electronic infusion device
I&O record
IV container marked with timed intervals
IV flow sheet or computer recording

Procedure

1. Introduce self, identify client using two client identifiers, and perform hand hygiene.
2. Place I&O worksheet at bedside unless using computer to record I&O (Table 28-6 ■).

(continued)

Skill 28.3.2 | Monitoring IV Intake *(continued)*

3. Determine time interval required for monitoring IV intake.
4. Mark time intervals on IV container according to facility policy (use tape to mark, or use preprinted time strips). The IV pump can be used to determine how much fluid was given to the client during the time period.
5. Set IV drip rate according to physician's orders.
6. Observe IV container and read IV solution level.
7. Record amount of IV solution infused at prescribed time (e.g., every hour, every shift).

8. If using electronic infusion device, push "total volume infused" for shift amount, then "clear."
9. Record total IV intake on I&O record at end of each shift or record in computer.
10. Record 24-hr IV total according to facility policy. Take into account all sources of IV fluid (all IV sites, IV medications).

Table 28-6 Intake and Output Flow Sheet (Sample)

Date	Time	IV No.	IV Started	Description	IV Intake	Oral Intake	Urine Output	Other	NG
1/9/16	9 A			Full liquid breakfast		620			
	9:45 A			Vomitus				400	
	10:30 A	#1	1,000						
	12 N						500		
	2:30 P						400		
				7–3 Total	600	620	900	400	100
	6:30 P	#2	1,000						
	9 P						500		
				3–11 Total	1,000	NPO	500		350
1/10/16	2:30 A	#3	1,000		450				
	5 A				550		350		
				11–7 Total	1,000	NPO	350		375
				24-hr Total	2,600	620	1,750	400	825

Unit 28.3 Documentation and Evaluation

DOCUMENTATION for Monitoring Fluid Balance

- Amount and description of all measurable I&O
- Approximate volume of loss when unable to measure contents (e.g., incontinent of urine in bed)
- Dietary intake (food that liquefies at room temperature, as well as liquids)
- 8-hr (or 12-hr) and 24-hr totals

- Signs and symptoms of client's fluid status, including vital signs, mucous membranes, daily weight, etc.

Note: I&O records are frequently inaccurate due to numerous possibilities for error, estimation being a common source of inaccuracy. It is important to maintain these records accurately.

EVALUATION/Critical Thinking

Expected Outcomes

- Client's intake and output are maintained within expected parameters of 200–300 mL of each other.
- Fluid intake is at least 2,600 mL unless contraindicated by diagnosis.

- Client's fluid status, vital signs, and mental status are within normal range.
- Output is maintained at more than 30 mL/hr.
- IV flow rate is maintained at prescribed rate.

Unexpected Outcomes	Alternative Actions
• Recorded I&O do not balance.	• Correlate I&O imbalance with weight changes.
	• Emphasize importance of accurate measures to client and family.
	• Check that entries into computer are accurate (i.e., entering 100 mL instead of 1,000 mL).
	• Identify possible nonmeasurable sources of I or O.
	• Report to charge nurse so she can ensure that all nurses are keeping accurate records.
	• Check if client or family can help with keeping the I&O record.
	• Check the addition on the I&O record to see if an error was made.
• Client unable to maintain an intake of at least 1,500 mL/day.	• Ensure that fluid restriction is not ordered.
	• Offer fluids in small amounts more frequently.
	• Determine client's fluid preferences.
	• Determine client preference for fluid to be hot, cold, or room temperature.
	• Consider "other" fluids such as Jell-O, Popsicles.
	• Assess client's ability to use a straw (hemiplegic client is often unable to suck through a straw).
	• Check if client is able to drink fluids independently or if assistance is needed.
	• Ensure that adequate fluids are accessible at the bedside for the client.
	• Do not administer fluids with a bulb syringe.
	• Address client's toileting needs every 2 hr—some clients restrict their fluid intake for fear of incontinence.
	• Use a thickening additive to liquids to facilitate swallowing for the client with aspiration precautions.
• IV flow not maintained at appropriate rate.	• Monitor IV fluid intake hourly.
	• Observe IV site for complications.
	• Restart IV immediately when infiltrated to ensure continuous IV fluid intake.
	• Document IV fluid intake every shift.
	• Account for interruption of primary infusion and the delivery of intermittent infusions of medications.
	• Check accuracy of IV administration equipment: electronic device, dial-a-flow, and others.
	• Inform physician of alterations in fluid received from what was ordered.

Nursing Process Data

ASSESSMENT Database

- Note client's allergies.
- Note any drug or solution incompatibilities.
- Assess amount and type of diluent needed to prepare medications.
- Assess client's general status to establish a baseline.
- Assess patency of infusion set and condition of IV insertion site.
- Assess physical parameters as indicated such as blood pressure, heart rate.

PLANNING Objectives

- To maintain a therapeutic level of medication in the client's bloodstream
- To administer medication safely over a specific period of time
- To prevent complications associated with medication administration

IMPLEMENTATION Procedures

DOCUMENTATION AND EVALUATION

Expected Outcomes

- Solutions from secondary IV bags infuse without difficulty.
- Therapeutic blood levels of medication are maintained.
- Complications of medication administration are prevented.
- Medication is infused over appropriate time span using volume control set.
- Saline lock inserted for medication administration without complications.

Unexpected Outcomes/Alternative Actions

Pearson Nursing Student Resources

Find additional review materials at
nursing.pearsonhighered.com.
Prepare for success with NCLEX®-style practice questions and Skill Checklists.

Skill 28.4.1 | Adding Medication to IV Solution

Equipment
IV solution bag
Syringe with medication
Antimicrobial swab
Label with medication dosage, date, time, and initials

> **CLINICAL ALERT**
> Only under unusual circumstances will the nurse be asked to add medications to parenteral solution. Refer to the facility's policy and procedure manual to determine which medications can be added by the nurse or if this is allowed. Medications may be added by the nurse only in an emergency.

Preparation
1. Introduce yourself. Identify client using two forms of identification.
2. Perform hand hygiene.
3. Gather equipment

Procedure
1. Check physician's orders, MAR, and agency policy.

Note: The addition (admixture) of medication to an IV solution for continuous administration is usually performed by the pharmacist, according to standards established by the American Society of Health System Pharmacists (ASHP) and Occupational Safety and Health Administration (OSHA). Special precautions for this procedure include preparation in a laminar airflow environment, strict adherence to requirements of asepsis, safety regarding components' stability and compatibility, proper dilution of agents, and control of extraneous particle addition to the admixture.

2. Check to ensure that prescribed drug is compatible with IV solution.
3. Draw up medication into syringe according to directions on medication insert (or *Physicians' Desk Reference*, the *PDR*).
4. Check all medications to be added to IV solutions with a second RN before injecting into the IV solution.
5. Wipe injection port on IV bag with antimicrobial swab.
6. Inject medication into the bag while maintaining aseptic technique.
7. Mix IV solution and medication by gently agitating the bag to mix thoroughly.
8. Affix medication label to the IV bag.
9. Hold the bag against both dark and light backgrounds to inspect for any precipitate.
10. Insert IV tubing into the bag, and proceed with the appropriate method of administration as ordered.

> **CLINICAL ALERT**
> Some drugs are incompatible with saline solution; these include diazepam (Valium), chlordiazepoxide hydrochloride (Librium), and amphotericin B. These drugs should be flushed with D_5W. Check compatibility of all IV drugs with solutions infusing.

Skill 28.4.2 | Using a Secondary ("Piggyback") Bag

Equipment
Primary IV set, consisting of compatible IV solution bag and IV administration set with injection port
Short secondary administration set with needleless cannula and extension hook or lowering hanger for primary bag (if indicated; Box 28-12 ▪)
Pharmacy-prepared medication bag with label, including name of medication, date, time, rate for infusion, and client's name
2% Chlorhexidine gluconate swab

Preparation
1. Check medication with physician's orders and MAR.
2. Perform hand hygiene.
3. Gather equipment.
4. Introduce self and identify client using two forms of identification.

Procedure
1. Ensure medication compatibility with primary infusing solution.

Note: If medication is incompatible with primary IV solution, temporarily discontinue primary infusion. Flush client's injection port, initiate a normal saline (or other compatible) solution as the primary, then proceed with "piggyback" into the "new" compatible primary. When complete, restart the original primary solution (use new needleless cannula to access the client's injection sites).

2. Spike the bag with secondary administration set.
3. Cleanse the injection port of primary tubing with chlorhexidine gluconate or alcohol swab.
4. Insert needleless connector of secondary "piggyback" tubing into primary tubing port (port above pump). ❶

Note: If using the same tubing from a previous administration, change the needleless connector before inserting into primary tubing.

5. Hang the secondary bag on the IV pole. ❷
6. Use an extension hook to lower primary bag below secondary bag if indicated (some infusion devices do not require this). ➤ *Rationale:* Primary solution ceases

(continued)

Skill 28.4.2 | Using a Secondary ("Piggyback") Bag (continued)

flow because of increased hydrostatic pressure in higher secondary bag.

7. Clear tubing of the medication bag by opening clamp, temporarily placing secondary bag lower than the primary solution bag, and allowing primary solution to flow retrograde into secondary bag tubing (back-priming). ❸

8. Backfill until the secondary tubing chamber is one-third full. Clamp secondary tubing. ➤ *Rationale:* This ensures that no medication is lost during priming.

9. Program secondary settings into infusion device if used.

10. Open clamp on secondary bag tubing. The secondary solution should begin to flow. ❹

11. Check that the primary infusion resumes at its "set" rate when secondary volume has been infused.

Note: Some infusion devices control secondary infusions without necessitating bag height differentials.

❶ Insert needleless cannula of secondary tubing into distal primary tubing port.

❸ Lower medication bag to clear tubing and back-prime tubing.

❷ Hang secondary bag on IV pole; lower primary bag.

❹ Unclamp secondary tubing.

12. When the secondary bag is empty, readjust rate of administration in the primary solution to desired flow (unless infusion device controls this).
13. To add a new secondary bag, ensure that medication is the same as previously administered since some drug remains in the secondary tubing. A *different* medication requires its own secondary tubing. ➤ *Rationale:* This prevents admixture of potentially incompatible drugs.
14. Remove old secondary bag, and spike new "piggyback" medication bag.
15. Lower partial-fill bag below the injection port of the primary IV.
16. Open clamp on the secondary tubing and allow solution from the primary IV set to enter tubing, backfilling the tubing to the drip chamber. ➤ *Rationale:* This procedure displaces air in the secondary tubing.
17. Replace new secondary bag on the IV pole and proceed with administration.
18. Change the secondary tubing every 24 hr if disconnected from the primary IV bag.

CLINICAL ALERT

Always document all fluids as intake that are used for administering medications in piggyback or volume control sets.

Box 28-12 **USING A MINI-INFUSER PUMP**

A mini-infuser pump is a tandem device that allows a small amount of medication to be given (5–60 mL) as a controlled infusion.

- The prefilled syringe is added to the battery-operated mini-infuser and connected to the main IV line.
- A needleless system is connected to the primary IV line.
- The infusion pump is hung with the primary IV bag and activated by an ON button.
- After infusion of medication, the primary infusion automatically begins to flow as the pump stops.
- The primary infusion should be checked and the flow regulated when the mini-infusion pump stops.

Skill 28.4.3 | Using a Volume Control Set

Equipment
Primary IV set (IV solution bag and IV administration set)
Calibrated volume control set
Medication prepared in syringe
2% Chlorhexidine gluconate swab or alcohol swab
Label with medication, date, time, and nurse's initials

Preparation
1. Check physician's orders and MAR.
2. Introduce self. Identify client using two descriptors.
3. Determine compatibility of medication with primary infusion.
4. Perform hand hygiene.

Procedure
1. Add extension tubing to the volume control set if needed and close clamps on the volume control set, both above and below the volume chamber. ❶
2. Open air vent by turning the clamp located on top of the volume chamber.
3. Spike the IV bag with the volume control set and then hang the bag. Attach IV tubing to the volume control set.
4. Open the upper clamp (between the bag and volume chamber) and fill the chamber with IV solution so that chamber is one-third full.
5. Close upper clamp.
6. Open lower clamp and squeeze the drip chamber (located underneath the volume chamber) until it is one-half full.
7. Allow solution to flow down tubing.
8. Prime tubing and cannula affixed to end of tubing. If volume control set has membrane filter instead of floating valve filter, follow manufacturer's instructions for priming so that you do not damage the filter.

❶ Add extension tubing, if necessary.

(continued)

Skill 28.4.3 | Using a Volume Control Set *(continued)*

9. Close clamp.
10. Swab off injection port (located on top of the volume chamber) with antimicrobial swab. ❷
11. Inject prepared medication into the chamber and agitate gently to mix medication with solution in the chamber. ❸
12. Dilute medication, if necessary, by opening the upper clamp and adding additional fluid from the IV bag.
13. Open the clamp on the volume control set and adjust the drip rate to desired rate of administration.
14. Place a medication label on the volume control set. Include client's name, medication, dose, and time medication infusion began.

❷ Swab injection port before infusing medication.

❸ After instilling medication, gently mix with solution in volume control chamber.

Skill 28.4.4 | Using a Peripheral Saline Lock

Equipment

Needleless injection cap with primed extension tubing and port (if one is not in place)
Needleless access device
Syringe for medication and diluent (if indicated)
Two 0.9% preservative-free normal saline prefilled syringes (3–5 mL each; preferred method)
2% Chlorhexidine gluconate swab or alcohol swab
Clean gloves
Stethoscope and sphygmomanometer (if indicated)

Preparation

1. Check physician's orders and MAR.
2. Gather equipment.
3. Perform hand hygiene and don gloves.
4. Introduce self. Identify client using two descriptors.

5. If client does not have peripheral lock in place, proceed with venipuncture, selecting veins that are both large enough to receive the medication and away from areas of movement (e.g., the elbows and wrists).

Procedure

1. Prepare medication with appropriate diluent according to manufacturer's instruction for IV injection and draw it up into a syringe. (See drug insert or *PDR*.)
2. Fill two syringes, each with 1 mL of 0.9% preservative-free normal saline or have prepackaged saline flush available.
3. Explain procedure to client.
4. Check client's vital signs if agent to be given has hemodynamic effects.
5. Prep needleless injection port with antimicrobial swab.
6. Insert *first* saline syringe into port, briefly aspirate to check patency, then flush system and observe for site swelling.

➤ *Rationale:* Presence of blood and absence of swelling at site indicate that needle is probably in vein, not in surrounding tissue.

7. Insert medication syringe into port and inject medication into vein, timing injection administration rate according to drug manufacturer's instruction (see insert or *PDR*).
8. Observe client for any adverse reactions.
9. Remove medication syringe.
10. Flush with *second* saline syringe to clear line and maintain patency of lock. Administration of saline should take same time period as the medication administration. ➤ *Rationale:* This prevents a bolus of medication or "speed shock" when fluid is administered.
11. Dispose of equipment and gloves and perform hand hygiene.
12. Recheck client's vital signs if indicated.

> **CLINICAL ALERT**
> Studies indicate that there is no significant difference in the use of saline or heparin to maintain catheter patency, maintain dwell time, and avoid phlebitis. Some hospitals still use a small amount of dilute heparin for flushing peripheral locks; it is usually prepared with 1 mL of heparin (1,000 units/mL) added to 9 mL of normal saline to produce 100 units/mL solution. Prefilled syringes of heparin and saline for infusion come in 10 units of heparin/mL. Caution should be exercised because heparin-induced thrombocytopenia can occur with as little as 500 units of heparin per day.

Skill 28.4.5 | Flushing a Peripheral Saline Lock

Equipment
Two prefilled syringes with 0.9% preservative-free normal saline
2% Chlorhexidine gluconate swab or alcohol swab
Clean gloves

Preparation
1. Check physician's order and MAR including allergies.
2. Gather equipment.
3. Perform hand hygiene.
4. Introduce self. Identify client using two descriptors.

Procedure
1. Explain procedure to the client.
2. Don clean gloves.
3. Prep injection port with chlorhexidine gluconate or alcohol swab according to facility policies. ❶ ➤ *Rationale:* When prepping with an antimicrobial swab, it is the pressure and friction applied that produce the antimicrobial effect. Scrub the hub for a minimum of 15 seconds.
4. Insert or connect the first saline syringe into the injection port and gently aspirate for blood. ❶
5. Observe for blood in the syringe. ❷ ➤ *Rationale:* Blood will indicate catheter is not occluded.

> **CLINICAL ALERT**
> If the gauge of the catheter is small, that is, 22 gauge or smaller, it is possible that you may not get a blood return. This can be due to the collapse of the tip of the catheter as negative pressure is applied when attempting to aspirate blood. This does not always mean that the catheter is occluded. You may attempt to inject the saline gently while feeling for resistance. If resistance is felt, the catheter may be occluded; it needs to be removed and a new catheter inserted.

6. Remove and discard the used syringe in an appropriate sharps container. ❸ Be careful not to contaminate the injection port. If the port is contaminated, prep again with an antimicrobial swab.
7. Insert or connect the second syringe into the injection port and gently flush with saline. Assess IV insertion site for tissue swelling or pain when injecting saline. ➤ *Rationale:* These could be a sign of infiltration.
8. Disconnect the syringe and discard in appropriate sharps container.
9. Remove and discard gloves.
10. Perform hand hygiene.
11. Document flush on the MAR.

❶ After swabbing injection port, attach syringe with normal saline.

(continued)

Skill 28.4.5 | Flushing a Peripheral Saline Lock (continued)

❷ After checking for blood return, discard the syringe and attach a second syringe with saline into the port and gently irrigate the lock.

❸ Remove the syringe and discard in sharps container.

Skill 28.4.6 | Administering Medications by Peripheral IV Line Injection "Push"

Equipment

Medication prepared in syringe with needleless access device, according to pharmaceutical instruction for IV administration

2% Chlorhexidine gluconate swab or alcohol swab

Clean gloves

Stethoscope and sphygmomanometer (if indicated by drug action)

Two prefilled 0.9% normal saline solution syringes

Preparation

1. Check physician's orders and MAR.
2. Gather equipment.
3. Perform hand hygiene.
4. Prepare medication according to pharmaceutical company's instructions for IV administration according to drug insert or *PDR*.
5. Check package insert or other references for drug's compatibility with the primary infusing solution.
   ➤ *Rationale:* Flushing the primary infusion tubing will be necessary both before and after administering the drug if incompatibility exists. Alternatively, a secondary "piggyback" bag of normal saline can be hung and used for flushing the primary line during the drug injection.
6. Check medication according to the *Six Rights*.
7. Take medication to client's bedside.
8. Check that client is not allergic to the drug.

Procedure

1. Introduce self. Identify client using two identifiers.
2. Obtain vital signs if agent to be given has hemodynamic effects.
3. Don gloves.
4. Validate placement using the first prefilled syringe.

> **CLINICAL ALERT**
>
> Before any IV push, or if drug is irritating, validate the intravenous line placement. Place a tourniquet proximal to the primary infusion; slow the drip rate and remove tubing from the pump. Ensure that infusion slows or stops before injecting the IV medication. This action validates the intravenous status of infusion. Blood flashback is not a reliable indicator.

5. Prep the primary tubing injection port closest to client.
6. Insert the medication syringe cannula into the line port.
7. Pinch primary tubing between the port and the infusion bag while injecting medication slowly in calculated increments (e.g., inject one-fourth of medication over a 20-second period). Always check the literature to determine injection times for specific medication.
8. After injecting small increments, unpinch the primary tubing to allow flushing of medication.
9. Observe the client for any adverse effects.
10. Deliver the next increment, using your watch and timing drug injection according to the drug insert instructions.
11. Withdraw the syringe when medication injection is complete.

12. Prep the primary tubing injection port again.
13. Insert the second saline syringe to flush all medication from IV tubing. Use the same time rate as medication administration.
    ➤ *Rationale:* This is to prevent adverse reactions.
14. Discard equipment.
15. Remove gloves and perform hand hygiene.
16. Recheck client's vital signs and document if indicated.

> **CLINICAL ALERT**
>
> In contrast to IV "push," an IV bolus of a drug is injected rapidly in order to achieve an immediate desired drug level—usually for emergency situations. Always refer to pharmaceutical company's instructions for *IV drug injection* before administering.

> **LEGAL ALERT**
>
> Up to 90% of all clients receiving healthcare services require some form of IV therapy. As a nurse, you will most likely be involved in starting, monitoring, and discontinuing IV therapy.
>
> Administering drugs is a major problem related to IV therapy. Medication errors account for 2 in 1,000 hospital deaths and are frequent causes of malpractice actions. The most frequent errors are incorrect dose, wrong drug, and improper technique (such as infusing the medication too quickly).
>
> Ensure that you administer IV therapy according to the acceptable nursing standards established by your facility, as well as state and federal guidelines. Keeping up with new standards and reading journal articles will assist you in keeping current. In order to accomplish this, you will need to update your skills yearly.
>
> Documentation must be appropriate, accurate, and concise in case of lawsuits regarding client injuries.
>
> **Documentation: "Do and Don't"**
> - Document only what you observed firsthand, what the client stated, and what was done. Do not offer opinions.
> - Use the word "observed," not "noted," because "noted" could mean something was written in the medical record.
> - Do write "no IV-related complications observed." If you document only parts of the assessment, such as "no redness noted," it could be interpreted that you did not observe for any other signs of infection.
> - Document details about complications: nursing interventions, physician orders, client's comments about complications or responses to treatments.
> - Document catheter length when removing a peripheral venous access device or PICC line.
> - Do not write "client tolerated procedure well." Provide statement from clients as to how they felt.
> - DO NOT rely solely on charting by exception or check-off flow sheets to document. They do not provide proper client assessment and may or may not be considered valid in court.

Unit 28.4 Documentation and Evaluation

DOCUMENTATION for IV Medications

- Amount of medication administered
- Method of drug administration
- Flush (e.g., NS) if indicated for compatibility
- Flush solutions documented on I&O flow sheet
- IV site status
- Client's response to medication
- Parameters such as vital signs, as indicated

EVALUATION/Critical Thinking

Expected Outcomes

- IV solutions from secondary IV bags infused without difficulty.
- Therapeutic blood levels of medication are maintained.
- Complications of medication administration are prevented.
- Medication is infused over appropriate time span using volume control set.
- Saline lock inserted for medication administration without complications.

(continued)

Unexpected Outcomes	Alternative Actions
• Secondary bag solution does not infuse adequately.	• Check that primary IV bag is lower than secondary bag (if infusion device requires). • Ensure that secondary needleless connector is properly attached in the primary injection port and secondary bag is sufficiently spiked. • Check that the roller clamp of the secondary tubing is open fully.
• Solution in primary IV tubing is incompatible with medication to be administered via secondary "piggyback."	• Turn primary infusion off. • Before administering medication, flush primary tubing with solution compatible with medication (e.g., normal saline, 5% D/W). • Hang a separate solution compatible with medication and run through line to flush during drug administration.
• Solution does not infuse through peripheral lock.	• Gently turn lock to establish flow. • Reposition client's extremity. • Initiate a new IV site.

Blood Transfusions

Nursing Process Data

ASSESSMENT Database

- Assess that client has signed informed consent for transfusion.
- Assess if client has an established IV site.
- Assess client's vital signs, especially temperature, for baseline data.
- Ensure that client's number and blood type on unit match client's blood ID bracelet name and number before administration to ensure compatibility. (Validate consistency with another nurse.)

PLANNING Objectives

- To provide blood or blood components (e.g., platelets, fresh-frozen plasma) for clients with a demonstrated deficiency
- To ensure compatibility between client's blood and the blood or blood component to be transfused
- To prevent the infusion of microaggregates or leukocytes
- To prevent febrile reaction to the transfusion
- To monitor and ensure a timely transfusion
- To monitor for potential complications during and after the blood transfusion

IMPLEMENTATION Procedures

DOCUMENTATION AND EVALUATION

Expected Outcomes

- Transfusion of blood is performed in a timely manner.
- Client's blood deficiency is corrected.
- Transfusion reaction does not occur.

Unexpected Outcomes/Alternative Actions

Pearson Nursing Student Resources

Find additional review materials at
nursing.pearsonhighered.com.
Prepare for success with NCLEX®-style practice questions and Skill Checklists.

Skill 28.5.1 | Administering Blood Through a Y-Set

Equipment
Blood unit (packed RBCs)

Note: Few conditions require the transfusion of whole blood. Most whole blood is used to prepare separate components to meet specific client needs (e.g., RBCs, plasma, platelets).

250-mL bag of normal saline
Y-set blood tubing with filter
Venipuncture supplies if client does not have established site, at least an 18- or 20-gauge needle or catheter
Needleless injection cap (if not in place)
2% Chlorhexidine gluconate swabs or alcohol swabs
Tape
Clean gloves

Preparation
1. Check physician's order for number and type of transfusion units (order must dictate "transfusion"). The order will include warming if the blood is to be warmed (Box 28-13 ■).
2. Introduce self. Identify client using two descriptors.
3. Explain procedure to client and confirm that client has signed consent form for transfusion. ❶
4. Check that type and crossmatch have been completed and that blood is ready in the blood bank.

> **CLINICAL ALERT**
> In emergency situations, when time does not allow ABO determination, group O negative red blood cells may be given. Whole blood, however, *must* be administered ABO identical.

Box 28-13 **WARMING BLOOD FOR TRANSFUSION**

Routine transfusions are not usually warmed. Warming is required in massive transfusions or, more commonly, may be ordered in maternity or the post-anesthesia care unit. A blood warming device is used. Never warm a blood bag in hot water or a microwave. Once blood is warmed, it must be used or disposed of, as it cannot be returned to the blood bank. Hemolysis of the blood occurs at temperatures above 40°C (104°F).

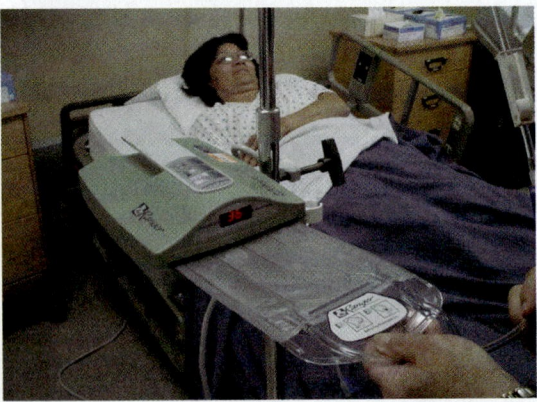

5. Determine patency of client's IV and needle or catheter gauge. Begin infusion of NS with appropriate blood tubing.

> **CLINICAL ALERT**
> Always determine patency of the IV line before obtaining blood from the blood bank.

6. Obtain client's pretransfusion vital signs. ► *Rationale:* If client has temperature above 37.8°C (100°F), physician must be notified before proceeding.
7. Obtain ordered typed and matched blood component bag from blood bank, or notify blood bank to deliver unit (according to agency policy). Both nurse and lab tech check transfusion number and sign transfusion form. ❷
8. With another nurse, validate that client's ID bracelet number matches the blood bank number on the unit of blood to be transfused.
9. Validate client's name, ID number, blood group/Rh, blood product, unit number, and expiration date. ❸

Transfusion of Blood or Blood Product (s)

Transfusion of Blood or Blood Product (s)

I understand that the risks of transfusion are low, and include but are not limited to: infection (HIV, hepatitis, other uses), antibody development and immune reactions, contamination by bacteria, difficulty breathing related to antibodies in the donor blood, temporary reduction In my natural immunity*.

I understand that there are alternatives to transfusion that include administration of hormones that stimulate the bone marrow (takes weeks to be effective), mineral supplementation (takes weeks to months to be effective), collection of my own blood during surgery (for certain surgical patients only).

I understand that the benefits of blood transfusion include improved oxygen delivery to vital organs (red blood cell transfusions) , improved blood clotting (plasma, platelets, cryoprecipitate).

The procedure(s) , risks and alternatives listed above were explained to me. I had the opportunity to ask questions and all of my questions about the procedure (s), risks and alternatives were answered to my satisfaction. I understand I have the right to accept or refuse transfusion of blood or blood products.

I consent to the Transfusion of Blood or Blood Products:

_____   _____   _____
(Patient's Signature**)   (Printed Name)   (Date and Time)

**Patient is unable to consent because: _____

I therefore consent for patient: _____   _____
                                               (Authorized Consenter's Signature)   (Printed Name)

_____   _____
(Witness' Signature**)   (Printed Name)

I Have Explained the Above Procedure(s) to the Patient or Authorized Consenter:

_____   _____   _____
(Physician's/Credentialed Provider's Signature)   (Printed Name)   (Date and Time)

Blood Transfusion Consent Form	PATIENT IMPRINT (Name and ID)

❶ Consent for blood transfusion.

Source: From Cerner Electronic Health Record. © Cerner Corporation. Pearson has restricted permission to reproduce and distribute this copyrighted work. Further reproduction or distribution is strictly prohibited without written consent of Cerner Corporation.

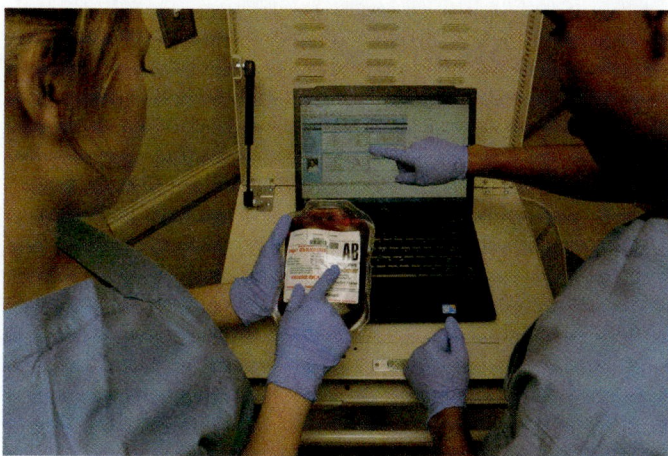

2 Obtain ordered typed and matched blood/component bag from blood bank.

3 Ascertain that client's name, ID number, blood group, number/Rh, unit expiration date, and hospital number match the number on the record on the blood bag.

CLINICAL ALERT

If transfusion requires electronic monitoring device to control blood flow, only pumps designed for the infusion of whole blood and RBCs may be used. These pumps require the use of special tubing and filter. Other types of pumps may cause hemolysis of RBCs.

---

10. Take and record client's vital signs on transfusion record 5 min before starting, 5 min and 15 min after starting infusion, and then every 30 min until transfusion is completed (1–1.5 hr), and immediately after the transfusion.
11. Remember that blood cannot be returned to the blood bank after it has been checked out for 20 min.
12. Check the blood bag for bubbles, cloudiness, dark color, or sediment. ➤ *Rationale:* These signs indicate bacterial contamination.
13. Perform hand hygiene and don clean gloves.

CLINICAL ALERT

Most clients can tolerate a flow rate of one unit of packed cells in 1.5–2 hr. For older adult clients or those with respiratory or cardiac conditions, the nurse may need to adjust the flow rate according to the client's status.

Procedure

1. Close all clamps on the Y-set tubing.
2. Spike a bag of normal saline with one arm of the Y-tubing. **4**
3. Open clamps on both arms of the Y-tubing to flush.
4. Close clamp on the free arm of the Y-set (blood side) and open clamp below the tubing filter to prime the main tubing.
5. Close the main clamp when tubing is primed.
6. Close clamps.
7. Gently agitate blood unit bag. ➤ *Rationale:* Agitation suspends the red cells in the anticoagulant.
8. Pull back tabs on the blood unit bag, and expose the port.
9. Spike blood bag port with the free arm of Y-tubing, then hang the unit.
10. Prep the client's injection port.
11. Connect blood tubing via needleless connection.
12. Open the clamp to the blood bag.
13. Start the blood infusion, administering slowly for the first 15 min. ➤ *Rationale:* Slow administration allows time to

4 Prime blood administration Y-set tubing with sterile normal saline before starting infusion.

(continued)

Skill 28.5.1 | Administering Blood Through a Y-Set *(continued)*

observe for adverse reactions. Most reactions occur in the first 15 min. The total transfusion should not take more than 4 hr.

> **CLINICAL ALERT**
> Blood must be hung within 30 min after taking it from the blood bank. Usually only 1 unit of blood is dispensed at a time.

14. Take vital signs 5 min *before*, and 5 min, 15 min, and every 30 min *after* starting transfusion and record on the Transfusion Record portion of the electronic health record. Check hospital policy and procedures (may vary).

15. Observe the client closely for adverse signs: chilling, backache, headache, nausea or vomiting, tachycardia, tachypnea, respiratory distress, skin rash, itching, or hypotension.

16. Agitate blood bag each time the client is checked.

17. If venous spasm occurs with cold blood infusion, apply a warm pack to the site to improve flow rate.

18. Complete the blood transfusion in less than 4 hr.
    ➤ *Rationale:* Blood deteriorates rapidly after a 2-hr exposure to room temperature and increases risk of bacterial infection.

19. Check that transfusion is completed, then flush the line with normal saline.

20. Obtain post-transfusion vital signs.

21. Report a 1°C (2°F) rise in temperature to the physician.
    ➤ *Rationale:* This could be indicative of a transfusion reaction.

22. Complete documentation on the electronic health record. If using paper charting, complete the Transfusion Record: Place one copy on client's chart, and send the remaining copy of the Transfusion Record to the Blood Bank as soon as the transfusion is complete.

23. Discard the administration set within 4 hr of use.

24. Place all transfusion-related equipment in a biohazard waste receptacle.

25. Remove gloves and perform hand hygiene.

26. Continue to observe the client. **❺**

❺ Observe the client carefully for first 15 min and frequently throughout the blood transfusion. It is recommended to stay at the client's side during the first 15 min of the transfusion.

Skill 28.5.2 | Administering Blood Through a Straight Line

Equipment
Blood unit
Blood administration straight-line set with 170-micron filter microaggregate or leukocyte-depleting filter
Needleless cannula
Electronic infusion device (optional)
Clean gloves

Procedure

1. Obtain and check blood as stated in the Preparation for Skill 28.5.1, Administering Blood through a Y-Set.

2. Introduce self and identify the client using two forms of identifier. Explain the procedure.

3. Perform hand hygiene and don gloves.

4. Spike blood bag port carefully and hang unit.

5. Gently agitate the unit, and suspend on the IV pole.

6. Open the clamp and fill the drip chamber, making sure filter is totally submerged in the blood.

7. Open clamp on the tubing and run blood through the tubing, then clamp.

8. Load tubing into the infusion pump, if used.

9. Carefully connect blood tubing to client's IV site catheter or lock.

10. Begin blood transfusion.

11. Observe the client closely and obtain vital signs 5 min before, 5 min after start, then after 15 min, then every 30 min or per hospital policy and procedures (Box 28-14 ■).

12. When blood bag is empty, close all clamps and remove blood tubing cannula from IV site.
13. Dispose of equipment in biohazard waste receptacle.

14. Remove gloves and perform hand hygiene.
15. Continue to observe the client.

Box 28-14 BLOOD TRANSFUSION PROTOCOL

The nurse is responsible for early assessment of possible transfusion reactions by completing the following interventions.

- Identify client and blood bag.
  - Ident-A-Band number matches transfusion record number.
  - Name is spelled correctly on the transfusion record.
  - Blood bag number and pilot tube number are the same.
  - Blood type matches on transfusion record and blood bag.
- Double-check blood with another RN before infusing; record on transfusion record.

- Determine client allergy history and previous blood reactions.
- Establish baseline vital sign data.
- Start transfusion slowly to observe for severe reactions. Stay with client for first 15 min of the transfusion. Monitor vital signs frequently per facility policy.
- Maintain aseptic technique during procedure.
- Observe time rules for administering blood. (Hang no longer than 4 hr.)
- Observe blood bag for bubbles, cloudiness, dark color, or black sediment, which indicates bacterial invasion.

Skill 28.5.3 | Administering Blood Components

Equipment
Blood component (Box 28-15 ■ and Table 28-7 ■)
Appropriate IV administration set
Filter, if indicated
Clean gloves

Procedure
1. Check physician's orders and client's signed consent for transfusion.
2. Obtain blood component from the blood bank.
3. Obtain an appropriate administration set.
4. Introduce self and identify client using two client identifiers. Explain the procedure.
5. Perform hand hygiene and don gloves.
6. Read directions for proper administration of the solution.
7. Identify the rate at which blood component should infuse.
8. Check for appropriate rate, risk factors, and possible complications.

Box 28-15 MODIFIED BLOOD PRODUCTS

In addition to the usual blood components such as platelets and cryoprecipitate, modified blood products are becoming more popular. Washed, irradiated, or leukocyte-removed blood is being used for clients at risk because of multiple transfusions or a weakened immune system. Testing for cytomegalovirus and matching RBC or human leukocyte antigens is also done to ensure safe transfusions.

CLINICAL ALERT
When infusing a blood product that has undergone leukocyte reduction, the product must be filtered again through a standard blood administration set in order to trap cellular debris that may have accumulated since the original filtration.

Table 28-7 Blood Component Therapy

Type	Use	Alerts	Administration Equipment
Fresh plasma	To replace deficient coagulation factors To increase intravascular compartment	Hepatitis is a risk. Administer as rapidly as possible. Use within 6 hr.	Any straight-line administration set
Platelets	To prevent or treat bleeding problems, especially in surgical clients To replace platelets in clients with acquired or inherited deficiencies (thrombocytopenia, aplastic anemia) To replace when platelets drop below 20,000 mL/mm (normal 150,000–350,000 mL/mm)	Administer at rate of 10 min a unit (usually comes in multiple platelet packs).	Platelet transfusion set with special filter to allow platelets to infuse through filter

(continued)

Skill 28.5.3 | Administering Blood Components *(continued)*

Table 28-7 Blood Component Therapy *(continued)*

Type	Use	Alerts	Administration Equipment
Granulocytes	To treat oncology clients with severe bone marrow depression and progressive infections To treat granulocytopenic clients with infections that are unresponsive to antibiotics To treat clients with gram-negative bacteremia or infections where marrow recovery does not develop	Administer slowly, over 2–4 hr. Give one transfusion daily until granulocytes increase or infection clears. Use within 48 hr after drawn. Observe for shaking, fever, or chills. Observe for hives and laryngeal edema (treat with antihistamines).	Use Y-type blood filters and prime with physiologic saline. A microaggregate filter is not used as it filters out platelets
Serum albumin	To treat shock To treat hypoproteinemia	Available as 5% or 25% solution Infuse 25% solution slowly 1 mL/min to prevent circulatory overload. Administer 100–200 mL (25% solution) for shock clients and 200–300 mL for hypoproteinemia.	Special tubing accompanies albumin solution in individual boxes
Gamma globulin	To treat agammaglobulinemia To act as a prophylaxis for hepatitis exposure	Pooled plasma contains antibodies to infectious agents. Administer 0.25–0.50 mL of immune serum globulin/kg of body weight every 2–4 weeks.	Given IM
Coagulation factors	To treat clients with von Willebrand's disease	Made from fresh-frozen plasma	Standard syringe or component drip set only
Factor VIII (cryoprecipitate)	To treat clients with factor VIII, hemophilia A	Administer one unit cryoprecipitate for each 6 kg of body weight initially, followed by 1 unit/3 kg of body weight at 6–12-hr intervals until treatment is discontinued. Administer 1 unit/5 min. Observe for febrile reactions.	
Factor IX	To treat clients with factor IX, hemophilia B	Administer in 12–24-hr cycle. Preparation for administration is 400–500 units/vial. Must reconstitute in 10–20 mL diluent One unit/pound of body weight increases the circulating factor activity by 5%. Serum hepatitis can be transmitted.	Any straight-line set—drip or by IV push—not to exceed 10 mL/min

Skill 28.5.4 | Monitoring for Potential Complications

Equipment
Sphygmomanometer
Stethoscope
Thermometer

Procedure

1. Check temperature, blood pressure, pulse, and respiration before transfusion is started.
2. Check vital signs 5 min before, then 5 and 15 min and every 30 min for the first 100 mL after transfusion has started.
   ➤ *Rationale:* Most blood transfusion reactions occur during this time. (Facility monitoring policies may vary.)
3. Maintain vital sign assessment throughout blood infusion according to hospital policy.
4. Monitor client for possible transfusion reactions (see Table 28-8 ■).
   a. **Hemolytic** or incompatibility reaction—most severe reaction
   b. Bacterial contamination
   c. Allergic reaction
5. If any severe untoward sign occurs (increase in temperature, pain in kidney region), STOP transfusion immediately.
6. Remove blood and any blood-filled tubing and replace with saline bag and new tubing to keep line open. Return blood bag and administration set to blood bank or laboratory.
7. Notify physician immediately after stopping IV for signs of transfusion reaction. Also notify physician if any unusual sign (itching or hives) occurs.

Table 28-8 Transfusion Reactions

Type	Clinical Manifestations	Nursing Interventions
Bacterial	Sudden increase in temperature Hypotension Dry, flushed skin Abdominal pain Headache Lumbar pain Sudden chill	Stop transfusion immediately and remove blood tubing. Maintain IV site; change tubing and start infusion of normal saline. Observe for shock. Monitor vital signs every 5 min. Insert Foley catheter and monitor urine output hourly. Notify physician and obtain order for antibiotic and steroids/shock management. Draw blood cultures before antibiotic administration. Send remaining blood and tubing to laboratory for culture and sensitivity.
Allergic	Mild: **urticaria** and hives, **pruritus** Severe: respiratory distress, wheezing Anaphylactic reaction: shock, loss of consciousness	Stop transfusion immediately if symptoms are severe—immediate resuscitation may be necessary. Monitor vital signs for possible anaphylactic shock. If symptoms are mild, stop transfusion or follow hospital policy and obtain physician's orders. Monitor for signs of progressive allergic reaction as transfusion continues.
Hemolytic	Severe pain in kidney region and chest Pain at needle insertion site Fever (may reach 40.5°C [105°F]), chills, flushing **Dyspnea** and cyanosis Oozing of blood at IV site Headache Hypotension **Hematuria** Nausea	Stop transfusion immediately and remove blood tubing. Start normal saline infusion at "keep open" rate with a new IV tubing. Obtain vital signs. Notify blood bank STAT. Administer oxygen. Notify physician. Obtain orders for IV volume expansion and **diuretic** or vasopressor to dilate renal blood vessels to prevent acute renal tubular necrosis. Complete transfusion reaction form. Send two blood samples (from different sites), urine specimen, remaining blood and tubing, and transfusion record to laboratory. Monitor vital signs every 15 min for shock. Monitor urine output hourly for possible acute renal failure.

Unit 28.5 Documentation and Evaluation

DOCUMENTATION for Blood Transfusions

- Type, unit number, and amount of blood product administered
- Name of healthcare provider who verified information with nurse
- Amount of normal saline used
- Type and gauge of catheter or needleless access device
- Time transfusion began and ended
- Vital signs 5 min before transfusion begins; 5, 15, 30, and 60 min after infusion begins (or per facility policy); and then hourly until infusion completed (check hospital blood administration policy and procedure for vital sign frequency)
- I&O record documentation
- Vital sign information on transfusion tag if there is space
- Client's response to procedure
- Any unusual clinical manifestations; any nursing interventions
- Warning device if used
- Infusion device used and flow rate setting
- Filter if used

EVALUATION/Critical Thinking

Expected Outcomes
- Transfusion of blood is performed in a timely manner.
- Client's blood deficiency is corrected.
- Transfusion reaction does not occur.

(continued)

Unexpected Outcomes	Alternative Actions
• Transfusion reaction occurs.	• Stop blood administration and begin infusion of normal saline or ordered solution to keep IV open. • Check transfusion reaction form for appropriate nursing intervention. • Complete all relevant nursing actions.
• Blood does not flow through tubing.	• Check client's IV site and gauge of needle or catheter (at least 18 or 20 gauge). • Gently agitate blood bag to mix blood cells with the anticoagulant. • Raise blood bag higher on IV pole. Squeeze flexible tubing to promote blood flow. • Adjust clamp on tubing. As the blood passes over the filter, more blood microaggregates clog the filter and slow drip rate. • Replace tubing. • Utilize an infusion pump, especially if administering blood through a small catheter or lock. • Consider using blood warmer.
• Blood has been hanging for more than 4 hr.	• Take down blood bag and send to laboratory. • Document amount of blood administered. • Maintain IV with normal saline or ordered IV solution. • Monitor vital signs for complications. • Notify physician.
• Potential circulatory overload occurs.	• Monitor symptoms: sudden dyspnea, tachypnea, tachycardia, chest discomfort, distended neck veins, moist crackles and rales, restlessness, sudden increase in blood pressure. • Stop transfusion and place client in Fowler's position. • Start oxygen at 2 L/min per nasal cannula. • Be prepared for ECG and chest x-ray. • Be prepared to administer Lasix and morphine sulfate.

Chapter Wrap-Up

GERONTOLOGIC Considerations

Older Adult Clients' Veins Are Fragile and Roll Easily, and Frequently the Needle Punctures the Wall of the Vessel

• Insert small-gauge winged catheter in distal vein first to preserve proximal vessel.
• Tourniquet (constricting band) may not be necessary for venipuncture. If used, it should be applied loosely.
• If used, release tourniquet as soon as venipuncture yields blood return to prevent excessive pressure in vein.
• Maintain close assessment of IV sites to promote long-term use of vessel.

Older Adult Clients Are Prone to Fluid and Electrolyte Disorders as a Result of the Normal Aging Process

• Thirst mechanism is decreased.
• Renal threshold is altered.
• Total body fluid is less due to decreased lean muscle mass.
• Fluid replacement therapy requires close monitoring to prevent fluid overload, leading to pulmonary edema and electrolyte imbalance.

- Dehydration is a common reason for IV therapy.
- When infusing IV fluids, monitor closely for signs of fluid volume overload.
- Monitor BUN and electrolytes regularly for signs of overload.
- Use IV pump whenever infusing fluids into older adult clients. If dextrose solution is being infused, IV pumps *must* be used. Dextrose overload can lead to cerebral edema if infused too rapidly.

Stabilizing IV Catheter and Dressing Is Problematic Due to Client's Fragile Skin

- Avoid excessive use of tape.
- Apply skin protector solution before dressing site.
- Use stretch mesh gauze to cover site and tubing to prevent catching on bed (avoid roll-type gauze).

Protect Fragile Skin That Is More Susceptible to Injury, Infiltration, and Discomfort From Irritating Drugs

- Observe IV site carefully for signs of infiltration. Because of skin's loose folds and decreased tactile sensation, a large amount of fluid can sequester in subcutaneous tissue and go unnoticed before client complains of pain.
- Check IV site frequently when client is receiving drugs that can cause irritation and even necrosis if they infiltrate.
- At first sign of phlebitis or infiltration, remove IV and restart in a new site.
- If client complains of discomfort during IV therapy, apply a moist and warm pack to site, decrease rate of fluid infusion.

MANAGEMENT Guidelines

Each state legislates a Nurse Practice Act for RNs and LVN/LPNs. Healthcare facilities are responsible for establishing and implementing policies and procedures that conform to their state's regulations. Verify the regulations and role parameters for each healthcare worker in your facility.

Delegation

- Each state identifies the scope of practice for RNs and LPN/LVNs. Several states have identified that the LPN/LVN has a specific role in IV therapy, but the scope of practice is always dictated by each agency (e.g., initiating, regulating, discontinuing IVs).
- Daily weighing of clients is usually assigned to the CNA or UAP. The RN should verify that weights are taken in the morning before breakfast, using the same scale each time. The client should urinate before weighing for accuracy. Since a client's weight changes are frequently taken into consideration for prescribing fluid allowances or medication adjustments, accuracy in measurement and documentation is imperative.
- All care providers must be aware of clients whose intake and output are monitored and must conscientiously participate in accurate measurement.
- All care providers must be aware of clients for whom fluid restriction is ordered and carefully adhere to designated allowances.
- CNAs and UAP report vital data to the professional nurse by monitoring vital signs. This skill can be delegated for the pre-, intra-, and post-blood transfusion, and results should be given immediately to the nurse. The professional nurse then validates and acts upon any abnormal findings accordingly. This can vary by state; in some states only the RN can take vital signs.
- The CNA/UAP providing personal hygiene must understand that the IV system is a closed one and must be able to give care without disrupting this system. The components of the system must never be disconnected for the convenience of care (e.g., changing gown). The CNA/UAP should receive training in changing the client's gown without disrupting the IV system.
- It is the nurse's responsibility to monitor and document intravenous fluid volume administered.
- It is the nurse's responsibility to evaluate the client's total balance of intake and output and to investigate significant imbalances for further decision making.
- While the professional nurse monitors the IV infusion site regularly, the CNA/UAP must communicate observations of swelling, client reports of concern (e.g., pain), and infusion device signals that prompt the professional to further assess the client.

Interprofessional Communication

- All care providers participate in accurate recording of the client's intake and output. Records are usually kept at the bedside. All must be familiar with the standard capacities for frequently used vessels (bowls, cups) to facilitate accurate recording of intake.
- Likewise, careful recording of measurable output and best estimation of unmeasurable losses (e.g., incontinence) will facilitate care decisions.
- The nurse must ensure that CNA/UAP know to report any unusual fluid loss the client is experiencing (e.g., vomiting). It is the nurse's responsibility to evaluate alterations in fluid loss (e.g., vomiting, scant urine output) and act upon these findings accordingly. Knowledge and judgment cannot be delegated.
- It is the nurse's responsibility to document vital client information on the Transfusion Record, which is placed into the client's hospital chart.

CASE STUDY Applications

Scenario 1

Mrs. Beatty is a 40-year-old client, 5-ft-1-inch tall and weighing 300 lb. She had emergency abdominal surgery for lysis of adhesions. You are assigned to care for her on her first postoperative day. As you begin your assessment, you note she has an NG tube that is draining bile-colored return. Her IV is D5% in 0.45NS infusing at 125 mL/hr. The IV is on a pump. As you observe the IV site, you find it difficult to determine whether the site is edematous or it is just her normal appearance. It seems like the area surrounding the site is cooler to the touch than the remaining part of the arm. Mrs. Beatty states the IV area is sore. A gauze dressing is placed directly over the IV site, making it difficult to visualize it. The IV fluid seems to be infusing at the prescribed amount and the IV pump alarm is not ringing.

1. What is your priority action in this situation?
2. After completing the first priority, what is your second priority?
3. While assessing the IV site, what would you look for if you suspect phlebitis or infiltration? With the initial information provided in the scenario, which of these potential complications do you suspect? Provide rationale for your answer.
4. How will you check the IV to determine whether the client does have an infiltration?
5. Indicate your priority intervention if you determine the client has an IV that has infiltrated.
6. Indicate your priority intervention if you determine the client has beginning signs of phlebitis.

Scenario 2

The head nurse comes to you, a new RN, and tells you that Mr. Jones' physician has ordered whole blood for his client, to be given immediately, and hands you a unit of blood.

1. What is your first action after this interaction with the head nurse?
2. What additional data should be collected before implementing this order?
3. After starting the transfusion, the client develops urticaria, hives, and slight respiratory distress. From these symptoms, what would you conclude about the client's status and what intervention would you make?

NCLEX® Review Questions

Unless otherwise specified, choose only one (1) answer.

1. For which one of the following IV infusions are in-line filters *not* recommended?
   A. Ringer's lactate
   B. TPN
   C. PCA
   D. Blood platelets

2. The nurse begins to assess the client's arms to determine the most appropriate site for the venipuncture. Which of the following principles should be kept in mind when determining this site?
   A. The veins that are deeper in the forearm should be assessed first.
   B. The antecubital fossa is a primary site.
   C. The most appropriate site is below an infiltrated area to save the vein.
   D. The distal end of the vein should be selected first.

3. When preparing for a venipuncture, what nursing actions are completed?
   Select all that apply.
   A. Lightly tap the vein to distend it.
   B. Instruct the client to relax the arm and keep the hand loose and open.
   C. Apply a cool cloth to the arm for 10 min before attempting venipuncture.
   D. Position the arm on a pillow to increase blood flow to the area.

   E. Instruct the client to open and close the fist to distend the vein.

4. What skin prep is recommended before attempting venipuncture?
   A. Alcohol swab
   B. Betadine swab
   C. Iodine swab
   D. Chlorhexidine gluconate swab

5. When preparing to change IV tubing as required during your shift, which of the following should you recall?
   A. Primary and secondary tubing is changed every 24 hr.
   B. Primary intermittent tubing is changed every 96 hr.
   C. TPN and lipids are changed with each bottle.
   D. Blood or blood-product tubing is changed every 4 hr or 2 units.

6. Which of the following is a step in inserting an over-the-needle catheter?
   A. Check catheter with the bevel in a "downward" position to examine the integrity of the end of the catheter.
   B. Place the bevel of the needle in the "up" position and insert the catheter at a 45-degree angle into the skin.
   C. Insert the needle into the anterior surface of the vein.
   D. After hearing the "pop" sound in the vein, remove the plastic catheter hub.

7. The client's IV order is: Administer 2,500 mL of normal saline in 24 hr. The administration set delivers 10 gtt/mL. The IV will deliver _____ mL/hr.

   A. 10

   B. 15

   C. 60

   D. 104

8. You walk into the room of a client whose Smart Pump is sounding a "hard" alarm. What is your initial action?

   A. Reset the pump after checking for possible air in tubing.

   B. Reset the rate of the medication infusion on the pump.

   C. Notify the client's nurse.

   D. Reprogram the pump after scanning your badge into the system.

9. The client has an isotonic IV solution ordered for the next 24 hr. If the faculty asks you to explain the rationale for this solution, what would your answer be?

   A. Isotonic solution hydrates the cells, causing them to expand.

   B. It corrects dehydration.

   C. Isotonic solution is used as a nutrient source.

   D. It is used to expand intravascular volume.

10. One of your clients has a medication ordered to be infused through the primary tubing injection port. Which of the following safety steps must be taken when administering IV drugs through this method?

    A. Administer the medication over 20 seconds.

    B. Flush the primary infusion tubing before and after administering any drug.

    C. After injecting a small amount of drug, unpinch the primary tubing and flush the medication.

    D. Administer IV drugs using only a dextrose solution to ensure drug compatibility.

QSEN Activity

Domain: Knowledge

Activity:

Review the Joint Commission National Patient Safety Goal

NPSG.01.03.01—Eliminate transfusion errors related to patient misidentification.

Elements of Performance for NPSG.01.03.01

1. Before initiating a blood or blood component transfusion:

   a. Match the blood or blood component to the order.

   b. Match the patient to the blood or blood component

   c. Use a two-person identification process or a one-person verification process accompanied by automated technology, such as bar coding.

2. Using a two-person verification process, one individual conducting the identification verification is the qualified transfusionist who will administer the blood or blood component to the client.

3. When using a two-person verification process, the second individual conducting the identification is qualified to participate in the process, as determined by the hospital.

By using the following KSA, discuss the impact of this NPSG when applying the QSEN competency of Safety:

Knowledge

1. Discuss potential and actual impact of national safety resources, initiatives, and regulations.

Skills

2. Use national patient safety resources for own professional development and to focus attention on safety in the care setting.

Attitude

3. Value relationship between national safety campaigns and implementation in local practices and practice settings.

Bibliography

Anderson, B., Mitchell, M. D., Williams, K., & Umscheid, D. (2010, Feb. 12). A comparison of heparin and saline flush to maintain patency in central venous catheters. *Nursing Times*. Retrieved from http://www.nursingtimes.net/nursing-practice/specialisms/haematology/a-comparison-of-heparin-and-saline-flush-to-maintain-patency-in-central-venous-catheters-/5011482.article

Bausone-Gazda D., Lefaiver, C. A., & Walters, S. A. (2010, Nov./Dec.). A randomized controlled trial to compare the complications of 2 peripheral intravenous catheter-stabilization systems. *Journal of Infusion Nursing*, 33(6), 371–384.

Bertolino, G., Pitassi, A., Tinelli, C., Staniscia, A., Guglielmana, B., Scudeller, L., & Balduini, C. L. (2012, Nov.). Intermittent flushing with heparin versus saline for maintenance of peripheral intravenous catheters in a medical department: A pragmatic cluster-randomized controlled study. *Worldviews on Evidence-Based Nursing*, 9(4), 221–226.

Billingsley, L., & Kinchen, L. (2014). Peripheral intravenous catheter protection: Are we using best practice? *Journal of Continuing Education in Nursing*, 45(8), 338–339.

Carson, J. L., Grossman, B. J., Kleinman, S., Tinmouth, A. T., Marques, M. B., Fung, M. K., ... & Djulbegovic, B. (2012). Red blood cell transfusion: A clinical practice guideline. *Annals of Internal Medicine* 157(1), 49–58.

Centers for Disease Control and Prevention. (2011). 2011 Guidelines for the prevention of intravascular catheter-related infections. Retrieved from http://www.cdc.gov/hicpac/bsi/bsi-guidelines-2011.html

Dal Molin, A., Allara, E., Montani, D., Milani, S., Frassati, C., Cossu, S., ... Rasero, L. (2014, Aug.). Flushing the central venous catheter: Is heparin necessary? *Journal Vascular Access*, 15(4), 241–248.

DiTrapano, C. (2013). Smart infusion pumps are selectively intelligent. Retrieved from http://www.medsafetyonline.org/smart-infusion-pumps-are-selectively-intelligent/

Fung, M. K., Grossman, B. J., Hillyer, C. D., & Westhoff, C. M. (2015). *Technical manual*, 18th ed. American Association of Blood Banking (AABB). Retrieved from http://www.aabb.org/programs/publications/Documents/pubscatalog.pdf

Hadaway, L. (2006). Principles of flushing vascular access devices. *Becton Dickinson (BD) Medical Clinical Resource* [CD-ROM]. Franklin Lakes, NJ: BD Service Department.

Hendler, C. (2008, Jun.). A perfect match: Preventing blood incompatibility errors. *NurseWeek California*, Sunnyvale, CA, 24–28.

Hepzibha, A. (2010) Heparin versus normal saline as flush solutions. *Journal for the Advancement of Science and Arts*, 1(1), 63–75.

Infusion Nursing Society. (2011). Infusion nursing standards of practice. *Journal of Infusion Nursing*, 34(1S), 1533–1548.

Lopez-Briz, E., Ruiz Garcia, V., Cabello, J. B., Bort-Marti, S., Carbonell Sanchis, R., & Burls, A. (2014, Oct. 8). Heparin versus saline solution flushing for prevention of occlusion in central venous catheters in adults. Cochrane. Retrieved from http://www.cochrane.org/CD0084662/PVD_heparin-versus-saline-solution-flushing-for-prevention-of-occlusion-in-central-venous-catheters-in-adults

Mathers, D. (2011). Evidence-based practice: Improving outcomes for patients with a central venous access device. *Journal of the Association for Vascular Access*, 16(2), 64, 67, 70–72. Accessed through ProQuest. Web. Oct. 3, 2014.

McCartney, P. (2014). Evidence for practice with smart infusion pumps. American Journal of Maternal/Child Nursing, 39(4), 270.

NovaCath Integrated IV Catheter System. Tangent Medical. http://tangentmedical.com/novacath/

Reed, S., Brock, A. J., & Tyler, A. (2014, Sep.). Champions for central line care. *American Journal of Nursing*, 114(9), 40–48.

Rosenthal, K. (2007). Reducing the risks of infiltration and extravasation. *Nursing*, 37(Fall), 4–6. Retrieved from http://journals.lww.com/nursing/Fulltext/2007/11001/Reducing_the_risks_of_infiltration_and.1.aspx

Scales, K. (2014). IV fluid therapy. *Nursing Standard*, 28(23), 19. Retrieved from http://dx.doi.org/10.7748/ns2014.02.28.23.19.s25

Self, W., White, S. J., McNaughton, C. D., Storrow, A. B., Slovis, C. M., & Collins, S. P. (2013). Warming intravenous fluids for improved patient comfort in the emergency department. *Western Journal of Emergency Medicine*, 14(5), 542–546.

Trimble, T. (2003). Peripheral I.V. starts: Securing and removing the catheter. *Nursing*, 33(9), 26.

U.S. Food and Drug Administration. (2011, Aug.). Guidance for industry: Bar code label requirements: Questions and answers. Retrieved from http://www.fda.gov/downloads/biologicsbloodvaccines/guidancecomplianceregulatoryinformation/guidances/ucm267392.pdf

Wicker, S., Stirn, A. V., Rabenau, H. F., von Gierke, L., Wutzler, S., & Stephan, C. (2014). Needlestick injuries: Causes, preventability and psychological impact. *Infection*, 42(3), 549–552. Retrieved from http://dx.doi.org/10.1007/s15010-014-0598-0

Chapter 29
Central Vascular Access Devices

Learning Objectives

29.1 Identify the common types of central vascular access devices (CVADs).

29.2 Discuss the rationale for using central vascular catheters for long-term IV therapy.

29.3 Discuss the special needs of clients with central vascular catheters (prevention of infection, air embolism).

29.4 Describe the role of the nurse in the insertion of CVADs.

29.5 Explain the nurse's responsibility for assisting the physician with a percutaneous central vascular catheter insertion.

29.6 Compare and contrast features of various central vascular access devices.

29.7 Describe initiation and discontinuation of infusions via CVADs.

29.8 Differentiate protocols for maintaining patency of intermittently used CVADs.

29.9 Outline steps for dressing and protecting the CVAD insertion site.

29.10 Discuss the advantage of using a BIOPATCH at the catheter insertion site.

29.11 Outline the steps in changing an access cap.

29.12 Discuss the data included in client education for the care and maintenance of vascular access devices.

Chapter Outline

Terminology

Antimicrobial preventing the development of pathogenic action of microbes.

Aspiration application of negative pressure (as when checking for blood return).

Calorie the amount of heat necessary to raise the temperature of 1 kilogram of water 1°C (1.8°F). One thousand (1 kcal) of these calories equals 1 dietary calorie (or calorie).

Carbohydrates a group of chemical substances, including sugars, glycogen, starches, dextrins, and cellulose, that contain only carbon, oxygen, and hydrogen.

Central vascular access device (CVAD) catheter, centrally placed in the superior vena cava, to provide medication, fluid, and nutrition.

Central venous pressure (CVP) measurement monitoring central venous return (volume) and right ventricular function.

Catheter-related bloodstream infection (CRBSI) fourth most common hospital-acquired infection with central line catheter placement.

Cyanosis slightly bluish, grayish, slate-like, or dark purple discoloration due to desaturation of hemoglobin.

Dyspnea a subjective feeling of difficulty breathing.

Electrolytes substances that develop an electrical charge when dissolved in water.

Erythema redness of the skin produced by capillary congestion, as in a sunburn.

Extravasation leakage of fluid out of a vessel.

Fat substance made up of carbon, hydrogen, and oxygen, occurring naturally in foods (especially meats, dairy).

Gastrointestinal pertaining to the stomach and intestines.

Huber needle a right-angled (90-degree) or straight, noncoring needle.

Hyperalimentation the process of nourishing the body through parenteral means.

Hyperglycemia condition characterized by an increase in blood glucose levels.

Hypertonic having a higher osmotic pressure or tonicity than a solution with which it is compared.

Hypovolemia diminished circulating fluid volume.

Implanted (as in medication ports) inserted under the skin.

Implanted infusion port device placed in subcutaneous tissue with a tunneled catheter that goes into the central venous system.

Infusion (in nursing) a liquid substance introduced into the body via a vein for therapeutic purposes.

Intravascular related to within blood vessels.

Irrigate to rinse or wash out with a fluid.

Isotonic having the same concentration of salts, or tonicity, as another solution with which it is compared.

Lipids fats; emulsion containing fats, used to correct fatty acid deficiencies via parenteral nutrition.

Lumen the inner open space of a tube or blood vessel.

Minerals inorganic elements or compounds.

Nutrients nourishing food items that supply the body with necessary elements.

Palpate to examine by touch; to feel.

Peripherally inserted central catheter (PICC) long, soft, flexible catheter placed through an arm vein to the superior vena cava.

Phlebitis inflammation of a vein.

Port subcutaneously implanted plastic or metal case that provides access to the venous system.

Protein substance that contains amino acids essential for growth and repair of tissues.

Sepsis pathologic state, usually febrile, resulting from the presence of microorganisms or their poisonous products in the bloodstream.

Thrombophlebitis an inflammation of a vein due to the presence of a thrombus.

Transfusion injection of blood or blood component from client (autologous) or from another individual into the blood vessels of a client.

Tunneled catheter a long single- or multilumen catheter inserted into a central vein, with the remainder tunneled subcutaneously to a distant exit site on the chest or abdomen.

Valsalva maneuver attempt to forcibly exhale with the glottis closed.

Venipuncture insertion of a needle into a vein.

Viscosity resistance offered by a fluid; property of a substance that is dependent on the friction of its component molecules as they slide by each other.

Vitamins a group of organic substances essential for life.

Venous Access Devices

Peripheral Catheters

Intravenous therapy is administered through a variety of catheters and devices. Several factors are considered when selecting the proper catheter: duration of therapy, pH, and osmolarity of solution to be infused. Solutions that are not appropriate for short catheters include continuous solutions with pH less than 5 or greater than 9, and osmolarity greater than 600 mOsm/L. Medications that cannot be infused in short catheters include vancomycin, penicillin, ganciclovir, dilantin, and promethazine (Phenergan) because of their pH. In addition, vasoactive drug infusions such as norepinephrine cannot be infused in short catheters. Nitroprusside and dopamine should not be infused because of the possibility of extravasation.

The most common type of venous access device is the peripheral catheter, inserted into veins of the hands, arms, or antecubital area. These are short catheters, less than 7.5 cm (3 in.) in length. They are intended for short-term IV therapy, usually lasting no more than 7 days. It is usually hospital policy to change peripheral catheters every 72 to 96 hr, although the Centers for Disease Control and Prevention (CDC) does not specify when the catheters should be replaced. The recommendation is that they be replaced only for clinically unresolved issues. For children, replacement is only for clinically indicated issues (Brown & Rowland, 2013).

In children, indications for obtaining vascular access are divided into broad categories, peripheral and central venous. Peripheral, short-term catheters are safe for giving many IV medications, such as antibiotics; for providing IV fluids; or for blood sampling for lab tests. (Fluids and medications that cannot be given were described previously.) Central venous access sites are indicated for children requiring long-term treatment with antibiotics, emergency medications such as inotropes, medications to manage cardiopulmonary arrest, chemotherapy, or TPN.

Site selection is based on four factors: condition of the selected vein, type of infusate, rate of infusion, and duration of infusion. When considering the vein, keep in mind that if it has been used previously, you must select a site more proximal than the previous site, especially if there was an infection. It is best to place the first catheter at the lowest point on the upper extremity; this allows for further catheter placement, if needed. In addition, the American Nephrology Nurses Association recommends that all clients with chronic kidney disease should have the hands used first for cannulation and that the client should have one designated arm that will have peripheral IVs in case there is a need to place an AV fistula or graft in the other at a later time. Some clients may have a wrist band that reads "Save the Vein" to indicate there is the possibility of creating an AV fistula or graft at a later date.

Areas above the flexion of a joint, such as wrist and elbow, should be avoided. Use of these sites can result in mobility problems and catheter dislodgement due to movement of the extremity. Because of the risk of deep vein thrombosis and pulmonary embolism, lower extremities are used only if necessary and require a physician's order in most facilities.

Midline Catheters

Midline catheters are 7.5 to 20 cm (3–8 in.) in length. They are inserted 2.5 to 3.8 cm (1–1.5 in.) above or below the antecubital fossa and terminate in one of the client's arms in a proximal vein. The basilic, cephalic, or median antecubital sites are also used. They are similar to the **peripherally inserted central catheter (PICC)** but are shorter in length. Both catheters are used for long-term IV therapy. Midline catheters are used only for administering nonirritating, normal pH solutions or medications, whereas the PICC can be used to infuse vesicants, hyperosmolar solutions, and total parenteral nutrition (TPN). Clients with midline catheters should not receive any medications or IV fluids with pH below 5 or above 10, or with osmolarity greater than 600 mOsm/L, since these could damage the vessel walls and lead to **phlebitis** or thrombosis.

Because they are placed in larger veins, midline catheters usually can be left in longer than peripheral catheters. The recommendation is that they be replaced only when there is a specific indication. However, because of the longer dwell time as compared with the peripheral catheter, complications such as thrombosis at the catheter site can occur. Phlebitis, infection, occlusion, clotting, breakage, and leakage at the insertion site of the catheter are associated with use of the midline catheter. Unfortunately, complications are more difficult to assess in clients with midline catheters than in clients with peripheral lines. For example, it takes longer for symptoms of phlebitis to appear in the client with a midline catheter. The short peripheral or midline catheters are not checked by x-ray for placement because they do not enter the superior vena cava as do the central vascular catheters.

Central Vascular Access Devices

Long-term **intravascular** therapy is best accomplished through use of medically placed **central vascular access devices** (CVADs). The specific type of device used depends on the type and duration of treatment, as well as client variables (Box 29-1 ■). CVADs are placed both in clients who are actively involved and at home and in critically ill hospitalized clients. Clients requiring chemotherapy, nutritional supplements, blood products, medications, frequent blood draws, and fluids can benefit from CVADs. These devices allow repeated access to the vascular system without **venipuncture**.

Central vascular catheters are categorized into three types: central catheters, subcutaneously **implanted** ports, and PICC lines. The specific type of device used depends on the type and duration of treatment, as well as client

---

Box 29-1 CLIENT SELECTION FOR CVADs

- Long-term intravenous therapy
- Need for frequent venous access
- Central venous pressure (CVP) monitoring
- Administration of total parenteral nutrition (TPN)
- Self-administration of intravenous therapies
- Sclerosed peripheral veins
- Limited peripheral venous access
- Irritating IV solutions

---

variables. Central catheters are further classified as tunneled or nontunneled catheters.

Central Venous Catheters

NONTUNNELED CENTRAL VENOUS CATHETERS Nontunneled catheters are large-bore catheters that vary in length from 15 to 20 cm (6–8 in.) and have one to four **lumens**. The catheters are made of soft silicone or polyurethane. Some of the newer catheters are impregnated with heparin, chlorhexidine, or an antibiotic. In most cases, physicians, physician assistants, or advanced practice nurses insert these catheters. Inaccurate placement of any central vascular catheter that is threaded to the superior vena cava can cause a potentially life-threatening arrhythmia if the catheter lodges against the myocardium.

Nontunneled central venous catheters are placed percutaneously into the subclavian, jugular, or femoral vein as a last resort. The preferred site is the subclavian area. They are used for fluid or blood administration, obtaining blood specimens, and administering medications and parenteral nutrition. Catheter extension into the superior vena cava minimizes vessel irritation and sclerosis of the vessel due to infusion. Because of the high volume of blood that normally flows through this portion of the superior vena cava (2,000 mL/min) the risk of complications is lessened. Central catheters can be single or multilumen catheters typically used for days to weeks.

TUNNELED CATHETERS Hickman, Broviac, and Groshong catheters are **tunneled catheters.** The closed-ended or Groshong-type catheter is designed to prevent backflow into the catheter when it is not in use. The Groshong catheter is used when low flow rates will be infused. In the Groshong, fluids infuse through a slit valve on the side of the tip. When there is no infusion of fluids into the catheter, the slit valve remains closed.

CLINICAL ALERT
Groshong catheters are never clamped, because of the design feature that prevents backflow. Pressure from clamping the catheter or extension tubing can force the slit valve to open, allowing a blood leak back into the lumen. Heparin flushing is not routinely done because of the design of the catheter tip.

The Hickman catheter is open-ended with a silver ion–impregnated cuff in the subcutaneous tract. This promotes growth of a connective tissue seal, reducing the risk of microbial immigration from the exit site along the catheter tract. The catheter has a reinforced sleeve of silicone on which the catheter clamp is used.

Hickman catheters are flushed with heparin. The client may shower and swim once the exit site has healed, but the hub of the catheter must be covered.

Tunneled catheters are used for long-term replacement therapy, medication administration, nutritional supplementation, and blood specimen withdrawal. These catheters can remain in place for months or even years. The catheter's tip is inserted into a central vein (e.g., subclavian or internal jugular vein) and advanced to the distal area of the superior vena cava. The remaining portion of the catheter is threaded subcutaneously to exit at a convenient distal site (chest, abdomen). A Dacron cuff on the catheter promotes scar formation to seal the tract to prevent ascending tract infection. Only physicians may discontinue a tunneled catheter.

Subcutaneously Implanted Ports

These implanted **ports** are surgically placed under the skin in a subcutaneous pocket in the chest, arm, abdomen, or, occasionally, the back. The newer ports are MRI compatible and available as a titanium port or titanium dome. Implanted ports are used for long-term and complex IV therapy such as chemotherapy. The septum of the port is made of silicon or polyurethane rubber latex, allowing more than 2,000 punctures with a 19-gauge noncoring needle. The attached catheter enters the superior vena cava. Single and dual septal ports are available with open-end or closed catheter endings.

Access to the port is by placement of a noncoring needle through the skin, into the self-sealing injection port housed in a plastic or metal case. This needle can remain in place for 7 days, then be replaced. Since the entire unit is implanted subcutaneously, risk for infection and maintenance requirements are greatly reduced.

A regular port cannot be used for high-pressure IV contrast in the radiology area, because the material of the catheter is too soft. A Power Port can be used in these situations for IV contrast radiological procedures. The pressure that is exerted during the injection of the contrast, for example in a CAT scan with contrast, is at 300 psi. A regular port is unable to handle that level of pressure during the injection process.

Peripherally Inserted Central Catheters (PICC)

Peripheral (antecubital) insertion of a central vascular catheter (PICC) to the superior vena cava is easier and less risky than entering a central vein through the chest wall, neck, or groin. The basilic vein is the usual choice for catheter insertion because it provides the straightest pathway to the superior vena cava and has a blood flow rate of 95 mL/min. The tip of the catheter resides in the lower third of the superior vena cava, not in the right atrium. The usual length of the catheter is 40 to 60 cm (16–24 in.).

PICC lines result in fewer problems than other types of access devices; however, common problems associated with PICC lines include phlebitis and infection. PICC lines have a tendency to occlude frequently due to their small diameter. They need to be assessed thoroughly for breakage and phlebitis.

A PICC line is the most appropriate method for infusing vesicants such as dopamine HCl hyperosmolar solutions such as TPN or blood products, and antibiotics that are potentially irritating drugs. These drugs and solutions can be infused through the PICC line because the superior vena cava is large and the volume of blood dilutes these medications before they enter the systemic circulation. Studies have indicated that PICC lines have been in place for up to 1 year. The average time is 6 months.

These access devices may be inserted by specially trained nurses who complete a certification process. The PICC line is inserted at the bedside using a bedside ultrasound, which makes it possible to visualize and access the veins in the upper arm accurately. The PICC line is inserted in the upper arm 95% of the time. Upper arm insertion has a lower rate of thrombosis, phlebitis, and catheter migration. A small-gauge (21–22 gauge) needle can be used that reduces the incidence of hematomas and damage to the vein. Most facilities use PICC-certified nurses to insert the line.

As with all centrally placed catheters, a chest x-ray is taken to verify placement of the radiopaque catheter to validate that the tip is in the superior vena cava. The catheter must not be used until IV placement is verified. Trained healthcare workers may discontinue the line when it is no longer needed.

A regular PICC line cannot be used for high pressured IV contrast in the radiology area because the catheter material is too soft. A Power PICC line has addressed this issue and it can be used for IV contrast radiological procedures. There is a dedicated lumen for the IV contrast and it is marked so. Other infusions still may be infused in the designated lumen when not used for IV contrast.

Securement devices such as the StatLock are routinely used to prevent complications and restarts in hospitalized clients. The manufacturer (Bard) indicates there is a 45% decrease in these problems since the securement device has been instituted. When compared with suture securement, these devices have eliminated sharps injuries when securing the central catheter lines. Arterial catheter restarts have been decreased by 49%. Using the StatLock device has lowered the rate of total IV complications by approximately 67%, decreased IV total complications from 48% to 16%, decreased phlebitis rate by approximately 80%, and decreased the rate of tape-related skin damage, which is documented to be as high as 54%.

Maintaining CVADs

Sterile technique must be maintained throughout all procedures associated with CVADs and PICC lines. Infection may occur if contamination results from poor technique in maintaining insertion sites, flushing catheters, or inserting the noncoring needle. Transparent dressings are placed over the insertion site for better stabilization and easy assessment and monitoring. Table 29-1 ■ provides guidelines for maintaining CVADs.

Catheter-Related Bloodstream Infections

Catheter-related bloodstream infections (CRBSIs) are the fourth most common hospital-acquired infections with central line catheter placement, and as such, reimbursement to hospitals is decreased or eliminated for these clients. Until recently, over 250,000 CRBSIs occurred every year in the United

Table 29-1 Maintaining CVADs: General Guidelines

CVAD	Frequency of Irrigation	Flush Solution
Single- or multilumen percutaneous catheter Short-term Long-term	q 12 hr to daily, after each use Daily to weekly and after each use	10–20 mL of normal saline 2–5 mL of dilute heparin (10 units) per lumen
Implanted port	Weekly and after each use	10 mL of normal saline after each infusion 3–5 mL of dilute heparin in 10-mL syringe monthly (100 units/mL)
Groshong valve device	Weekly and after each use	10–20 mL of normal saline ONLY in 10-mL syringe
PICC	q 4–12 hr and after each use	Normal saline (twice the normal volume of the catheter and access device) followed by 5 mL of dilute heparin (10 units/mL)

Note: Check frequency and flush solutions according to agency protocols.

States, and more than 80,000 of these were in the ICU. These infections increased the average length of hospital stay from 10 to 12 days and average cost of care from $4,000 to $56,000. Whether and how these infections are associated with an increased risk of death remains unknown. As of January 2011, the CMS has required acute care hospitals that wish to receive compensation under its conditions of participation program to report their ICU CRBSI incidence densities to National Healthcare Safety Network (NHSN). They are displayed by standardized infection ratios (SIRs) on the Centers for Medicare and Medicare Services (CMS) Hospital Compare website. Over 1,000 hospitals report the number of CLABSIs and the number of line days attributed to specific locations within the facility to NHSN (Shah, Bosch, Thompson, Hellinger, 2013).

Hospitals have developed central line bundle procedures to reduce the rates of infection, usually following the Institute for Healthcare Improvement (IHI) or Centers for Disease Control guidelines. Actions to prevent CRBSIs are provided in Box 29-2 ■.

Box 29-2 CENTRAL LINE BUNDLE

"Bundles" are groupings of best practices that individually improve care, but when used together, greatly increase the outcome or prevention of CRBSIs. The central line bundle has five key components:

- Hand hygiene
- Maximal barrier precautions
- Chlorhexidine gluconate or alcohol swab skin antisepsis
- Optimal catheter site selection, with avoidance of the femoral vein for central venous access in adult clients
- Daily review of necessity with prompt removal of unnecessary lines

Use of Antimicrobial Central Venous Catheters

Antimicrobial central venous catheters (CVCs) have been recommended for clients at risk for CRBSIs and clients for whom the expected duration of use is between 1 and 3 weeks. There are several types of antimicrobial CVCs. There is concern that the use of these catheters may encourage the emergence of resistant microorganisms; however, there is no evidence to support this at this time.

The most common type of antimicrobial CVC is coated with chlorhexidine and silver sulfadiazine. The newest available catheter has a strong concentration of chlorhexidine, with silver sulfadiazine on the external CVC surface. It has a coating of chlorhexidine on the internal surface of the CVC lumen. The results of a meta-analysis have demonstrated that the earlier type of CVC shows a significant reduction in CVC colonization and a trend toward reduction in CRBSIs (Casey, Mermel, Nightingale, & Elliott, 2008). There have been insufficient numbers of studies to form a conclusion on their effectiveness.

Total Parenteral Nutrition

Parenteral nutrition is a method whereby **nutrients** are introduced intravenously. Bypassing the normal **gastrointestinal** system, this route provides a nitrogen source for those with a nonfunctional gastrointestinal tract (enteral starvation) or those with high caloric requirements (burn client), or acute hypoalbuminemia.

Balanced blends of nutrients, including **vitamins** and **minerals**, can be administered both by central line and peripherally using **isotonic** concentrations of glucose (no greater than 10% dextrose). In contrast, **hypertonic** solutions that are irritating to veins are administered through a central, high-flow vein. Rapid dilution of the solution decreases risk of phlebitis, clot formation, and hemolysis. This technique requires special handling and management, presents greater risk for complications, and is the most expensive method of feeding.

Nursing Diagnoses

The following nursing diagnoses may be appropriate to include in a client care plan when the components are related to intravascular therapy.

NURSING DIAGNOSIS	RELATED TO . . .
Activity Intolerance	Change in setting—intensive care, catabolic state Compromised cardiac reserve
Anxiety	Lifestyle modification, pain, chronic condition Uncertainty related to illness and diagnosis, placement of a CVAD
Decreased Cardiac Output	Impaired myocardial function, hypovolemia
Excess Fluid Volume	Excess fluid replacement, medications, renal and cardiac dysfunction
Infection, Risk for	Invasive procedures, inadequate site care, use of hypertonic glucose solutions
Deficient Knowledge	Ability to care for intravenous catheter or administer TPN
Imbalanced Nutrition: Less Than Body Requirements	Chronic fatigue states, nausea and vomiting, inadequate absorption, faulty metabolism, eating disorders, side effects of chemotherapy
Ineffective Peripheral Tissue Perfusion	Altered blood supply, arterial or venous, impaired myocardial contractility, hypovolemia

Source: Herdman, T. H. & Kamitsuru, S. (Eds.) *Nursing Diagnoses – Definitions and Classification 2015-2017.* Copyright © 2014, 1994–2014 by NANDA International. Used by arrangement with John Wiley & Sons Limited. Companion website: www.wiley.com/go/nursingdiagnoses. In order to make safe and effective judgments using NANDA-I nursing diagnosis it is essential that nurses refer to the definitions and defining characteristics of the diagnoses listed in this work.

Unit 29.1
Percutaneous Central Vascular Catheters

Nursing Process Data

ASSESSMENT Database

- Determine client's level of consciousness so explanation of procedure can be done to allay anxiety.
- Assess level of anxiety to determine need for possible premedication.
- Assess skin and surrounding tissue for erythema, edema, and warmth.
- Assess circulating volume status and right heart function.
- Assess StatLock site for potential complications.

PLANNING Objectives

- To assist the licensed practitioner with percutaneous central vascular catheter insertion
- To maintain patency of central vascular catheter
- To change central venous catheter dressing without complications
- To maintain the insertion site free of infection
- To prevent air embolism
- To monitor central venous pressure

IMPLEMENTATION Procedures

DOCUMENTATION AND EVALUATION

Expected Outcomes

- Central vascular line is properly placed without complication.
- Central vascular line remains patent and free of infection.
- CVP monitoring guides fluid management.
- Central vascular catheter dressing is changed without complications.
- BIOPATCH is applied and potential infection prevented.
- Access cap replaced, maintaining sterile technique.
- StatLock prevents catheter displacement.

Unexpected Outcomes/Alternative Actions

Pearson Nursing Student Resources

Find additional review materials at
nursing.pearsonhighered.com.
Prepare for success with NCLEX®-style practice questions and Skill Checklists.

Skill 29.1.1 | Assisting With Percutaneous Central Vascular Catheterization

Equipment

Specific nontunneled catheter

Routine IV setup (tubing and solution)

Through-the-needle radiopaque central catheter

Local anesthetic, syringes, and needles

Sterile gloves, sterile gown, masks, full body drapes, and sutures or securement device.

Note: A securement device is preferred because sutures are another break in the skin that can cause infection.

Antimicrobial 2% chlorhexidine gluconate swabs

Intermittent infusion caps or positive pressure device

Prefilled syringes with preservative-free normal saline

Transparent semipermeable dressing

Securement device

Ultrasound device per provider request

Note: National Guidelines encourage the use of an ultrasound device to easily locate the vein. AccuVein is the most common device.

Procedure

1. Identify client using two descriptors and validate signed consent for catheter insertion. Introduce self.
2. Perform hand hygiene and explain procedure to client, including rationale for mask, positioning, and **Valsalva maneuver**.
3. Place client in Trendelenburg position. ➤ **Rationale:** This position prevents air embolism and helps distend subclavian and jugular veins.
4. According to licensed practitioner's preference, extend client's neck and upper chest by placing a rolled pillow or blanket between shoulder blades. ➤ **Rationale:** Usual insertion sites are either subclavian or right jugular vein.
5. Place mask on client and turn client's head away from side of venipuncture. ➤ **Rationale:** This facilitates filling the vessel with blood and prevents contamination.

❶ Central line "Blue Guard." Triple lumen catheter—subclavian vein.

6. Maintain sterility while opening glove packet and sterile drape pack.
7. Open antimicrobial prep pads.

Note: Guidelines to prevent catheter-related bloodstream infection recommend that licensed providers don cap and sterile gown in addition to mask and sterile gloves.

CLINICAL ALERT

Required drying time needed in order to prevent skin breakdown as a result of chemical reaction between solutions and dressings is as follows:

Solutions	Required Drying Time
Chlorhexidine gluconate 2% with alcohol	30 seconds
Chlorhexidine gluconate without alcohol	2 min
Povidone–iodine	2 min
70% isopropyl alcohol	Dries quickly, kills bacteria only when first applied. No lasting bactericidal effect; can excessively dry the skin.

Source: Dychter, Gold, Carson, & Haller (2012)

8. Don mask and gloves and assist with central catheter insertion.
   a. Licensed provider dons mask, gown, and sterile gloves for this procedure.
   b. Licensed provider prepares the client's skin, drapes area, and, using a sterile syringe and needle, draws up anesthetic to infiltrate the site.
   c. As a licensed provider inserts the catheter, the client is instructed to perform Valsalva maneuver to prevent air embolism (Box 29-3 ■).
      1. Instruct client to exhale against a closed glottis or to hum.
      2. If client is unable to do this, compress client's abdomen. ➤ **Rationale:** Both of these actions help to decrease the chance of air embolism.

Note: A 14-gauge needle is inserted into the subclavian vein, using the clavicle as a guide. When blood returns in syringe, the syringe is removed from the needle and a wire is threaded through the needle into the subclavian vein. The needle is removed and the catheter is fed over the wire into the subclavian and brachiocephalic vein. The wire is removed when the tip of the catheter rests in the superior vena cava. Current guidelines recommend using an ultrasound device to locate the vein being accessed. The device identifies vein placement and indicates veins that have occlusions that need to be avoided.

(continued)

Skill 29.1.1 | Assisting With Percutaneous Central Vascular Catheterization *(continued)*

9. When catheterization is complete, insert injection cap, flush with 5 mL of normal saline (according to agency policy).
10. Apply securement device to skin and place catheter in clamp.
11. Cover securement device and catheter with sterile transparent dressing (according to hospital policy) to prevent infection (Box 29-4 ■).
12. Label insertion site dressing with date, nurse's initials, and time of insertion.
13. Obtain x-ray for validation of placement into superior vena cava before initiating infusion (unless emergency placement performed).
14. Monitor client's vital signs. ➤ *Rationale:* Bleeding or pneumothorax may occur.

Box 29-3 PREVENTION OF AIR EMBOLISM IN CLIENTS WITH CENTRAL LINES

- Clear central line of air before insertion.
- Use IV pumps with in-line air detectors.
- Use the head-down position and Valsalva maneuver during both insertion and removal.
- Use screw-on connections and secure with tape.
  ➤ *Rationale:* Hemostats or other clamps can crack the hub and open the system.
- Use transparent dressing during the time the catheter is in place and after removal of a central catheter. Leave in place for at least 24 hr.

Box 29-4 GUIDELINES TO PREVENT CATHETER-RELATED BLOOD STREAM INFECTIONS (CRBSIS)

Hand Hygiene

- Decontaminate hands with alcohol-based hand cleaner; if hands are visibly contaminated with blood or body fluids, use antimicrobial soap and water.
- Use hospital-provided hand lotions compatible with antiseptic agents to maintain integrity of skin. Home lotions may neutralize antibacterial agents in antiseptic agents used in hospitals.
- Decontaminate hands before and after putting on or removing gloves, providing direct client care, assisting with insertion of central venous catheter, inserting peripheral catheter, changing central venous dressing, or accessing catheter to administer medication or flush.
- Do not use artificial nails when working in the healthcare facility.

Barrier Precautions

- Use maximum barrier precautions when inserting or assisting with insertion of central venous catheters, including PICC lines. Include cap that covers all hair, mask covering mouth and nose, sterile gown, and sterile gloves.
- Cover client from head to toe with large sterile drape, leaving a small opening for insertion of catheter.
- Place mask on client when PICC insertion is done, and cover face if subclavian or jugular vein is placement site for central venous catheters.
- Keep all supplies together on nursing unit to prevent need to look for additional supplies after CVC insertion is begun.

Site Preparation Using Chlorhexidine Gluconate

- Prepare site using 2% chlorhexidine gluconate.
- Pinch wings on chlorhexidine applicator to break open the ampule. Hold applicator down to allow solution to saturate pad.

- Press sponge against the skin.
- Swab with applicator using a gentle back-and-forth motion. This motion creates friction and lets the solution more effectively penetrate epidermal layers.
- Swab site for 30 seconds and then allow it to dry thoroughly, approximately 2 min. Do not wipe or blot area.

Catheter Site Selection

- Use central venous catheters (CVCs) impregnated with antimicrobial agents, if available.
- Nontunneled percutaneously inserted CVCs are available with three different agents: chlorhexidine/silver sulfadiazine; rifampin/minocycline; and silver/platinum ionic metals. PICC brand uses rifampin/minocycline agents.
- Catheter should be inserted in the subclavian vein for nontunneled catheter.
- These catheters should be used for clients with dwell time of more than 5 days and in healthcare facilities where catheter-related bloodstream infection rates are high.
- There is inconclusive evidence that multiple-lumen catheters should not be used; even though they have higher infection rates, they also have fewer mechanical complications than single-lumen catheters.

Daily Assessment

- Evaluate need to determine when lines are no longer necessary and should be removed.
- Provide site care when needed.

EVIDENCE-BASED PRACTICE
Antimicrobial Swabs

Studies have shown that 2% chlorhexidine gluconate solution significantly lowers catheter-related bloodstream infection rates when compared with 70% povidone–iodine and 70% isopropyl alcohol.

Source: Data from American Society of Anaesthesiologists (2012) and Labeau, Vereecke, Vandijck, Claes, & Blot (2008)

CLINICAL ALERT

To decrease pressure in the catheter, use a 10-mL syringe. Some facilities use a 5-mL syringe that is the same diameter as the 10-mL syringe. The rationale is to decrease the amount of saline that is used.

All continuous IV infusions administered via a central line must have an electric infusion controller device in place. In addition, the drug library must be used for all infusions so that the type of infusion is displayed at all times on the controller device.

EVIDENCE-BASED PRACTICE
Chlorhexidine Gluconate-Impregnated Sponges Reduced Rate of Catheter-Related Infections in ICU

Using chlorhexidine-impregnated sponge dressings with intravascular catheters reduced the risk for major catheter-related infections by 60% among clients treated in the ICU. Changing unsoiled, adherent dressings weekly was not inferior to a 3-day changing schedule, according to data from a randomized controlled trial.

A randomly assigned study consisted of 1,636 clients over the age of 18 in an ICU setting. The clients were expected to need an arterial catheter, central vein catheter, or both for 48 hr or longer. Some of the clients received chlorhexidine-impregnated sponges and some the standard dressings,

scheduled for change either once every 7 days or once every 3 days. The rate for major catheter-related infection decreased from 1.40 per 1,000 catheter days to 0.60 per 1,000 catheter days with the use of the chlorhexidine-impregnated sponge. The 3-day group had a 7.8% rate of catheter colonization versus 8.6% for the 7-day group, which proves the 7-day dressing schedule is not inferior compared with the 3-day dressing schedule. Use of chlorhexidine gluconate-impregnated dressings decreases the rate of major catheter-related infection when the baseline rate is lower than two per 1,000 catheter days.

Source: Timsit (2009)

Skill 29.1.2 | Changing a Central Line Catheter Dressing

Equipment

2% Chlorhexidine gluconate or according to facility policy
Antimicrobial hand soap
Tape or transparent dressing
Needleless access caps
Receptacle for soiled dressing
Clean gloves
Sterile gloves
Mask
Sterile long-sleeved gown, according to facility policy

Preparation

1. Review facility policy and procedure manual to determine protocol for skin prep.
2. Review the client's chart for last dressing change (recommended every 7 days for clear dressings and 2 days for gauze, unless the dressing becomes soiled or loose).
3. Gather equipment.
4. Introduce self and identify client using two descriptors and explain procedure to client.
5. Perform hand hygiene.
6. Position client flat on back. ❶ ➤ *Rationale:* This position reduces risk of air embolism.

7. Turn client's head away from the insertion site and mask the client's nose and mouth. ➤ *Rationale:* This decreases exposure to microorganisms at site.
8. Make sure that all personnel don masks and/or gloves according to hospital policy.

❶ Positioning client flat on back for dressing change. Nurse will apply mask to client and have client turn away from site. Gauze dressings are used only if the site is oozing. Gauze dressing must be changed every 48 hr or if soiled.

(continued)

Skill 29.1.2 | Changing a Central Line Catheter Dressing *(continued)*

Procedure

1. Don clean gloves and gown, according to facility policy.
2. Carefully remove old dressing or tape without pulling on catheter. Remove edges toward insertion site. ➤ *Rationale:* This prevents stress on insertion site.
3. Discard old dressing and gloves in proper receptacle.
4. Inspect site for loose sutures, signs of infection (Table 29-2 ■), inflammation, or infiltration, and check length of exposed catheter.
5. Remove clean gloves, perform hand hygiene, and don sterile gloves.
6. Cleanse insertion site, sutures, and catheter with 2% chlorhexidine in 70% alcohol or according to facility policy.
7. Cleanse site using back-and-forth scrubbing motion for 30 sec.
8. Cover site with a sterile transparent dressing.
9. Change IV tubing according to hospital policy.

   a. Clamp central catheter using on-line slide or squeeze clamp.
   b. Use aseptic technique to change needleless access cap.
   c. Prepare cap with antimicrobial swab.
   d. Insert new tubing with needleless connector.
   e. Place protective connector cap per agency policy (usually impregnated with alcohol).

10. Label dressing and tubing with date and your initials.

11. Change dressing if it becomes loose, wet, or soiled or according to facility policy. ➤ *Rationale:* If it is wet, soiled, or loose, it is considered contaminated.
12. Discard equipment, gown, and gloves, and perform hand hygiene.

CLINICAL ALERT

All primary and secondary continuous IV administration sets should be replaced at least every 96 hr (according to facility policy) or immediately if signs or symptoms of infection are present. Intermittent sets should be changed every 24 hr.

Table 29-2 Infusion Site Complications

Signs and Symptoms	Possible Indications
• Redness, swelling at CVAD infusion site	• Infiltration, hematoma, or sepsis
• Crepitus on chest	• Subcutaneous emphysema that can lead to respiratory distress
• Respiratory distress with recent placement of a central line	• Pneumothorax
• Arm, shoulder, or neck pain	• Infiltration or thrombosis
• Temperature elevation	• Catheter-related infection
• Fluid leaks from IV site	• Hole or break in catheter

Skill 29.1.3 | Infusing IV Fluids Through a Central Line

Equipment

Primed IV fluid administration set with needleless Luer Lok connector
Infusion delivery pump
Antimicrobial swabs
10-mL needleless syringe with 5 mL of preservative-free 0.9% normal saline solution
CLC2000 Positive Pressure Cap (or another brand)
Clean gloves
Protective connector cap

Preparation

1. Check physician's order sheet and client's Medication Record for IV order (Table 29-3 ■).
2. Check IV order against IV solution bag.
3. Take equipment to client's room.
4. Introduce self and identify client using two descriptors.
5. Explain procedure to client and provide privacy.

Procedure

1. Perform hand hygiene and don gloves.
2. Hang IV solution on IV stand and attach point-of-care module. ❶ ❷
3. Wipe access port with antimicrobial swab for 30 sec; allow to air dry. ❸ Ensure clamp is open. Then attach syringe.

Table 29-3 Administration Set Change According to Solution Type

Solution Type	Set Change Frequency
• Not receiving blood or blood products, or **fat** emulsions	• No more frequently than 96-hr intervals
• Parenteral nutrition (amino acids)	• q 72 hr or when integrity compromised
• **Lipids**, parenteral nutrition solutions containing lipids	• q 24 hr or when integrity compromised
• Whole blood and components (platelets, red blood cell concentrate, plasma, cryoprecipitate)	• 4 hr or 2 units or immediately upon suspected contamination
• Fractionated products (IVIG, clotting factors, albumin)	• Upon completion of infusion

Source: Centers for Disease Control and Prevention (2011)

4. When all fluid is flushed from syringe, the tip on the plunger is compressed. Detach syringe from catheter hub. The force on the plunger is released and the tip rebounds, pulling blood into the catheter lumen. (Clamp is not found on PICC lines or Groshong valve catheter.) ❹ ❺
5. Aspirate for blood return, using very little force, to check for lumen patency and placement. ❻

❶ Hang IV solution on IV stand.

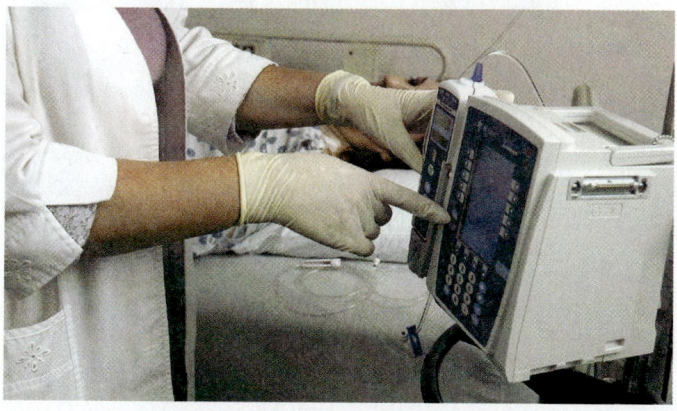

❷ Attach point-of-care module and program.

❸ Wipe access cap or positive pressure clamp with antimicrobial swab and allow to dry.

❹ Ensure clamp is open before attaching syringe.

❺ Attach 10-mL needleless syringe with saline to pressure valve.

❻ Aspirate and check for blood return before infusing saline solution.

6. Instill saline solution slowly. The CVD and tubing has a volume of 1–3 mL; therefore, about 5 mL of solution in a 10-mL syringe should be used to flush the catheter thoroughly. ➤ *Rationale:* This is to clear the lumen of in-line dilute heparin if used.
7. Maintain positive pressure when withdrawing syringe by clamping catheter before removing syringe, by maintaining pressure on syringe plunger before you clamp, or by using the CLC2000 Positive Pressure Cap. ❼ ➤ *Rationale:* This prevents **aspiration** of blood into lumen and decreases risk of catheter occlusion.
8. Swab the access port again with antimicrobial swabs.
9. Insert IV tubing with Luer Lok connector into the access port. Unclamp lumen.

(continued)

Skill 29.1.3 | Infusing IV Fluids Through a Central Line *(continued)*

❼ Positive fluid displacement and positive end-pressure prevent blood reflux into catheter lumen. The device provides the saline flush to prevent clotting of catheter. (See also Skill 29.4.2, Using a Positive Pressure Device.)

10. Set electronic device to prescribed rate and begin infusing IV fluids. ❽
11. Ensure central line dressing is clean and intact.
12. Remove gloves and perform hand hygiene.

> **CLINICAL ALERT**
> To minimize pressure on the catheter during injection, NEVER use less than a 10-mL syringe for central lines *unless* the 5-mL syringe has the same diameter as a 10-mL syringe. Smaller syringes increase pressure within the catheter, which can damage the catheter.
>
> ───────────────────────────
>
> Nontunneled central vascular access devices have the highest infection rate of all types of CVADs; therefore, it is crucial that aseptic technique be used in all aspects of catheter care.

❽ After connecting IV to catheter, set electronic device to prescribed rate.

Skill 29.1.4 | Drawing Blood From a Central Venous Access Device

Equipment
Two 10-mL Luer Lok syringes filled with sterile preservative-free
  normal saline
3-mL Luer Lok syringe with 3 mL of heparinized saline
  (10 units/mL heparin) **ONLY** if policy of facility
  Note: Many facilities have stopped using heparin for routine
  flush of central access devices except for ports.
Two 10-mL syringes (or larger if needed)
Antimicrobial swabs
Blood tubes appropriate for tests ordered
Sterile injection cap
Protective connector caps
Clean gloves

Preparation
1. Check physician's orders and MAR.
2. Introduce self. Identify client using two descriptors.

Procedure
1. Explain procedure to the client.
2. Perform hand hygiene and don gloves and mask.
3. If fluids are infusing through the catheter, turn off infusion for at least 1 min before drawing blood specimen.
4. Swab cap and hub with antimicrobial swabs for 30 seconds and allow to air dry. ❶ Use most distal lumen of catheter for blood draw. ▶ *Rationale:* Proximal port specimen will not be contaminated if fluids are infusing distally.
5. Remove cap from syringe, insert 10-mL saline-filled syringe, and unclamp catheter. ❷

❶ Unclamp catheter; clean cap and hub with antimicrobial swab, and allow to dry.

❷ Insert 10-mL needleless syringe into cap and unclamp catheter.

6. Flush catheter with 3–5 mL of normal saline. ➤ *Rationale:* This is to determine patency of catheter.

Using the Vacutainer Method

> **CLINICAL ALERT**
> Some facilities do not allow Vacutainers to be used for blood draws from central lines because of increased pressure buildup in the catheter.

a. Clamp catheter.
b. Attach needleless connector to Vacutainer barrel holder.
c. Place blood tube into Vacutainer holder.
d. Disinfect injection or access cap with antimicrobial swab for 30 sec.
e. Remove needle cover and insert Vacutainer needleless connector into injection or access cap.
f. Unclamp the catheter.
g. Advance blood tube inside Vacutainer holder to activate retrograde blood flow.
h. Hold tube in place until blood flow ceases; this is considered the "discard." The volume should be 1.5–2 times the fill volume of the CVAD.
i. Clamp catheter and remove blood tube from Vacutainer holder, leaving needles and holder connected to injection or access cap.
j. Discard blood tube immediately into appropriate container.
k. Insert another blood tube, unclamp catheter, and obtain blood specimens as ordered.
l. After all specimens are collected, clamp catheter.
m. Remove Vacutainer holder and needleless connector from injection or access cap.
n. Disinfect injection or access cap with antimicrobial swab.
o. Flush catheter using 5 to 10 mL of preservative-free 0.9% sodium chloride.
p. Change injection or access cap and extension set, if needed (Alexander, Corrigan, Gorski, Hankins, & Perucca, 2010).

Using the Syringe Method

a. Clamp catheter.
b. Remove injection or access cap and discard.
c. Disinfect catheter hub with alcohol.
d. Attach empty 10-mL syringe to catheter hub.
e. Unclamp catheter.
f. Withdraw 1.5–2 times the fill volume of the CVAD of blood and discard. ❸ ❹

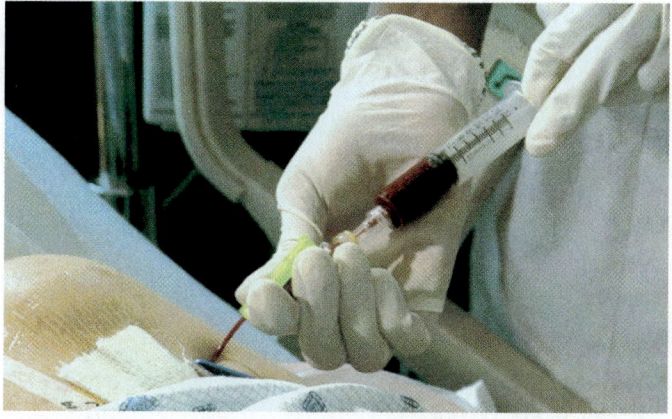

❸ Withdraw 1.5–2 times the fill volume of the CVAD of blood for discard before drawing blood sample, unless specimen is for culture.

❹ Dispose of blood waste in biohazard container.

(continued)

Skill 29.1.4 | Drawing Blood From a Central Venous Access Device (continued)

g. Reclamp catheter.

h. Remove and discard syringe into biohazard container.

i. Attach second syringe to catheter hub and unclamp catheter. Withdraw blood into syringe.

j. Reclamp catheter. Remove syringe.

k. Replace caps of the central line of the lumen in which the blood was drawn per facility policy.

l. Cleanse catheter hub with alcohol.

m. Attach prefilled injection or access cap attached to 10-mL syringe with 5–10 mL of preservative-free 0.9% sodium chloride.

n. Unclamp catheter and flush with sodium chloride solution.

o. Transfer blood from syringe into collection tube using needleless transfer device (Alexander et al., 2010).

7. Clamp catheter, remove syringe, and attach new 10-mL empty syringe. Unclamp catheter.

8. Withdraw 1.5–2 times the fill volume of the CVAD; discard volume of blood from catheter slowly and then clamp the catheter. Discard syringe. ➤ **Rationale:** It's important to clear the catheter of fluids or medications, particularly heparin, before blood samples are obtained.

CLINICAL ALERT
Do not discard any blood if drawing blood for cultures. Blood from the first draw is always used for blood cultures.

Specimens obtained from central catheter lines have been reported as inaccurate in some studies, especially coagulation studies. Heparin molecules can bind within the catheter to cause abnormal results. If lab values are significantly different from earlier values or from the normal range, assess client to determine whether additional lab tests need to be drawn. In this case, draw specimens from a direct vein, if possible.

9. Discard syringe in biohazard box.

10. Remove gloves and discard.

11. Perform hand hygiene.

Note: Withdraw 8–10 mL of blood if coagulation studies have been ordered.

Skill 29.1.5 | Applying a BIOPATCH

Equipment
BIOPATCH Antimicrobial Dressing with Chlorhexidine Gluconate
BIOCLUSIVE Transparent Dressing or other similar dressings
Sterile gloves
Clean gloves
Mask

Procedure
1. Check the client chart to determine last dressing change.
2. Gather equipment.
3. Identify client using two descriptors. Introduce self and explain procedure to client.
4. Remove dressing using clean gloves.
5. Perform hand hygiene and don sterile gloves.
6. Prepare skin surrounding percutaneous device according to hospital protocol. Ensure sufficient space is left between hub of catheter and insertion site for placement of dressing.
7. Remove dressing from sterile package using aseptic technique.
8. Place the BIOPATCH dressing around catheter so catheter rests on slit portion of patch. Ensure GRID side of patch is facing upward. The smooth foam side of patch is next to the skin.

CLINICAL ALERT
The patch is made of a hydrophilic polyurethane absorptive foam with chlorhexidine gluconate (CHG). The patch absorbs up to 8 times its own weight in fluid and the CHG inhibits bacterial growth under dressing.

9. Ensure edges of slit approximate each other to ensure efficacy of patch.

10. Apply transparent dressing over patch and catheter insertion site. Ensure complete contact between skin and transparent dressing. ❶

11. Discard equipment packages.

12. Remove gloves and place in receptacle.

13. Perform hand hygiene.

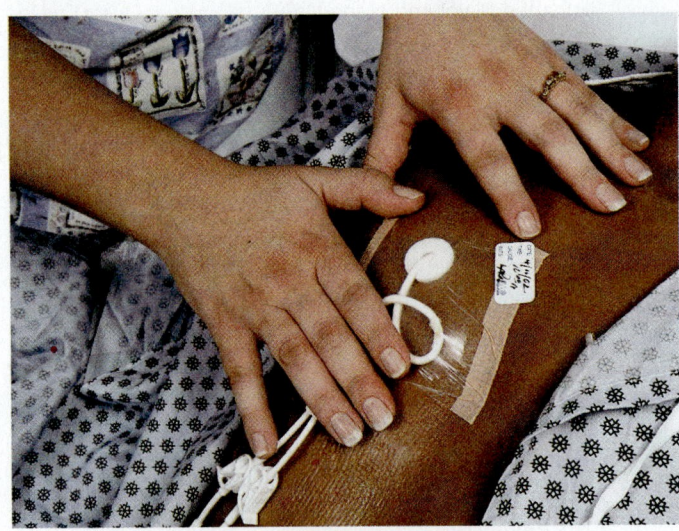

❶ BIOPATCH with transparent dressing over insertion site.

14. Change BIOPATCH as necessary. Follow facility policy; however, dressing change should be at a minimum of every 7 days.

   a. Don clean gloves.
   b. Remove patch by picking up corner of dressing and stretching dressing away from catheter while holding catheter in place. Dressing should partially lift off skin when stretching dressing.

   c. Peel back dressing until resistance is felt.
   d. Repeat stretch and peel action until dressing is removed. Both the dressing and the patch will be removed together with this action.
   e. Discard old dressing in biohazard container.
   f. Discard gloves in appropriate receptacle and perform hand hygiene

EVIDENCE-BASED PRACTICE

Skin Reactions with Chlorhexidine Gluconate-Impregnated Central-Line Dressings

The use of chlorhexidine gluconate (CHG) in clients requiring central line insertion does reduce the incidence of central line–associated bloodstream infections. However, a potential negative outcome in using CHG is skin necrosis or contact dermatitis at central venous line sites. In a small study of six adult clients with complicated skin disorders, erosions were observed 4 to 14 days after disk placement (Wall, 2014); reepithelialization took 2 to 10 weeks to

occur. A review of use of CHG-impregnated dressings in neonates reported a distinct increase in contact dermatitis among infants with gestation less than 27 weeks and very low birth weight versus infants of normal weight born after 27 weeks (Safdar et al., 2014). Another report (Ruiz et al., 2011) stated that CHG-impregnated central line dressings are effective in the prevention of CRI, but suggested cautious use in children because of their immature skin.

| **Skill 29.1.6** | Applying a Securement Device (StatLock) |

Equipment
Securement devices (Box 29-5 ■)
Sterile gloves
Antimicrobial skin prep, according to facility policy
Transparent dressing

Procedure
1. Identify client using two identifiers.
2. Introduce yourself to client and explain procedure.
3. Open device package, sterile skin prep, and gloves.
4. Perform hand hygiene and don gloves.
5. Cleanse insertion and securement site with antimicrobial skin prep for 30 sec. Allow to completely dry.
6. Apply protectant (in package) to securement site. Allow to dry completely, about 10 to 15 sec.
7. Align anchor pad so directional arrow points toward insertion site.

   a. **Using Post Version:** Place suture hole in catheter wing over first post, then slide catheter to capture second post.
   b. **Using Fixed Version:** Place suture holes in catheter wings over fixed posts.

8. Support under surface of anchor pad and catheter while closing retainer doors.
9. Peel away paper backing from anchor pad, one side at a time, then place on skin.
10. Apply transparent dressing per facility policy.
11. Apply both provided dressing change labels.
12. Discard equipment in appropriate receptacle.
13. Perform hand hygiene.

Note: Monitor the device daily, and replace when clinically indicated, at least every 7 days. Treat insertion site according to facility policy. This device is sterile and latex-free; however, clients with known adhesive allergies should not use the device.

Box 29-5 RECOMMENDATIONS FOR USE OF CATHETER SECUREMENT DEVICES

Infusion Nurses Society
The Infusion Nurses Society has published major guidelines that state a preference for using a securement device such as the StatLock for stabilizing catheters.

Centers for Disease Control and Prevention (CDC)
The CDC states that sutureless securement devices are an advantage over sutures in preventing bloodstream infections and complications.

The Joint Commission and National Patient Safety Foundation
The Joint Commission and the National Patient Safety Foundation identify securement devices as a major contributor to client safety because they reduce catheter-related infections and overall complications. This is in addition to improving safety for healthcare providers.

Occupational Safety and Health Administration
The Occupational Safety and Health Administration (OSHA) has issued directives that instruct healthcare employers to consider using securement devices to reduce needle-stick injuries in healthcare providers.

Skill 29.1.7 | Removing a Securement Device

Equipment
Sterile gloves
New securement device (StatLock)
3–4 alcohol pads

Preparation
1. Introduce self and identify client using two client identifiers.
2. Perform hand hygiene, and explain the procedure to the client.

Procedure
1. Open new device package.
2. Don gloves.

3. Remove transparent dressing using the "stretch technique." Lift edge of anchor pad using three to four alcohol pads. Fold alcohol pad to squeeze out alcohol. ➤ *Rationale:* This will dissolve the undersurface of the pad away from skin. Do not pull or force pad to remove.
4. Fold adhesive anchor pad underneath.
5. Stabilize catheter while holding the StatLock device.
6. Use thumb of opposite hand to lift retainer door gently from behind, while pressing down with index finger.
7. Reposition hands and repeat process to open second door.
8. Remove PICC from retainer and carefully reapply new device or discontinue the line.

Skill 29.1.8 | Changing an Access Cap

Equipment
Antimicrobial swabs
Sterile resealable injection cap
10-mL syringe with 5–10 mL of preservative-free 0.9% normal saline for flush, or
10-mL syringe with 2–3 mL of heparin solution for maintenance according to agency policy (Many facilities have discontinued the use of heparin for routine flushing of central venous access devices.)
Clean gloves

Procedure
1. Check client's chart to determine time of last access cap change.

> **CLINICAL ALERT**
> The ideal time interval is not scientifically known at this time, but it is suggested that the access cap be changed at least every 7 days, when the cap has been accessed more than the manufacturer's recommendations, if the integrity of the port is compromised, if residual blood remains within the port, or after blood draw or blood administration. Positive pressure caps (such as the CLC2000) are changed after blood draws.

2. Identify client using two descriptors. Introduce self.
3. Explain procedure to client, and provide privacy.
4. Gather equipment.
5. Perform hand hygiene and don gloves.
6. Open access cap package, maintaining sterility, and place it near the working area.
7. Assess access cap to determine whether cap should be changed even if time frame is not met.
8. Place client in supine position. Clamp catheter using on-line slide or squeeze clamp. ➤ *Rationale:* This is to prevent air embolism during cap change. Client can be instructed to perform Valsalva maneuver during cap change as an alternative to lying supine.
9. Stop any IV infusion and disconnect IV tubing from access cap.
10. Remove existing cap using aseptic technique.
11. Take new access cap out of package, flush access cap with saline to prime, maintaining sterility, and place on catheter hub.
12. Cleanse injection cap with antimicrobial swab for 30 sec.
13. Flush catheter using 10-mL syringe with normal saline or insert new IV fluid tubing and begin infusion at prescribed rate.
14. Infuse heparin solution if central line is used for intermittent infusions ONLY if agency policy.
15. Remove gloves and perform hand hygiene.

Skill 29.1.9 | Measuring and Monitoring Central Venous Pressure (CVP)

Equipment
Disposable CVP manometer with stopcock
IV solution according to facility policy.
Extension tubing with needleless Luer connector
IV pole
Carpenter's level, laser
Antimicrobial swabs
Prefilled 10-mL syringe with 5 mL of preservative-free
    0.9% normal saline
Marker

Preparation
1. Check physician's order.
2. Identify client using two descriptors. Introduce self.
3. Explain procedure to the client and provide privacy.
4. Determine client's previous CVP parameters.
    ➤ *Rationale:* Trends are more relevant than isolated pressure readings.

Central venous pressure (CVP) is a measure of venous return or the pressure of blood in the right atrium. Used to guide fluid administration, it is measured in centimeters of water pressure (normal is 5–10 cm H_2O).

Procedure

1. Perform hand hygiene.
2. Spike IV solution bag with IV administration set using sterile technique.
3. Prime tubing with solution.
4. Close clamp on tubing.
5. If you are using a one-piece disposable manometer and stopcock, affix unit to IV pole.
6. Push male end of IV administration set into female end of stopcock, connecting the IV set to stopcock.
7. Turning stopcock so that manometer and IV solution are open to each other, open clamp on IV tubing and fill manometer with IV solution to between 18 and 20 cm (7–8 in.). ➤ *Rationale:* Overfilling the manometer may expose the client to contamination resulting from overflow.
8. Close clamp and rotate stopcock so that IV solution is open to client.
9. Prime the rest of IV tubing that extends from stopcock to client's central line.
10. Place client flat in bed, without a pillow, if client can tolerate this position. If not, place client in position of comfort (e.g., head of bed at 15–30 degrees).

11. Record position so that same position can be used each time a CVP reading is made. ➤ *Rationale:* This allows accurate CVP trending.
12. Locate client's right atrium (midaxillary at fourth intercostal space). Mark this location on client's skin using marking pen.
13. Adjust level of CVP manometer (using carpenter's level) so that zero on manometer is at the same level as client's right atrium, 5 cm on manometer level to sternal notch. ❶ ➤ *Rationale:* Using level at right atrium reflects blood volume and cardiac function of client.
14. Turn stopcock to open position for manometer, filling manometer with additional solution if needed. ❷
15. Turn stopcock to the manometer→client position and watch level of the solution in the manometer fall to the pressure level existing in the right atrium. ➤ *Rationale:* Normally this pressure should be between 5 and 10 cm. Remember, however, there are no absolute values and trends—the rise and fall of CVP readings are more important than one isolated pressure reading.
16. Observe meniscus at eye level and watch rise (with exhalation) and fall (with inhalation) of fluid column in response to client's breathing. ❸ ➤ *Rationale:* Fluctuations reflect changes in intrathoracic pressures during respiratory cycle and indicate that manometer is functioning properly.
17. Take reading at end of exhalation (rise of fluid in manometer).
18. Turn off stopcock to manometer, and adjust rate of infusion to reestablish IV solution flow to client.
19. Return client to desired position and record CVP reading.

❶ When a CVP reading is taken, the zero of the manometer must be level with client's right atrium, regardless of client's position.
Source: © / Alamy

❸ Take CVP reading.

❷ *Left stopcock*: Fill the manometer by turning stopcock OFF to the client. This allows solution to flow from the container to the manometer. *Middle stopcock*: Measure CVP by turning stopcock OFF to the IV solution, allowing fluid to flow from manometer to client. *Right stopcock*: Reinstitute flow from IV container to the client by turning stopcock OFF to the manometer.

Unit 29.1 Documentation and Evaluation

DOCUMENTATION for Central Vascular Catheterization

- Location of insertion site
- Type and size of cannula used for insertion
- Time of insertion
- Assessment of site and dressing every 8 hr
- Name of physician performing catheterization
- Types of solutions infused
- Amount of solution infused

- Time x-ray was performed to check position of catheter
- Time, initials, and the date the dressing and tubing changed
- Date and time of CVP reading (record subsequent CVP readings on appropriate flow sheets)
- Client's response to treatment
- Any unusual conditions or reactions

EVALUATION/Critical Thinking

Expected Outcomes

- Central vascular line is properly placed without complication.
- Central vascular line remains patent and free of infection.
- CVP monitoring guides fluid management.
- Central vascular catheter dressing is changed without complications.
- BIOPATCH is applied and potential infection prevented.
- Access cap replaced, maintaining sterile technique.
- StatLock prevents catheter displacement.

Unexpected Outcomes

- Air enters central vein, producing air embolism from system being open to atmosphere.

Alternative Actions

- Immediately clamp catheter and place client in Trendelenburg's position (turned to the left so right ventricle is uppermost).
- Immediately inform physician and monitor until physician arrives. Assess vital signs and breath sounds.
- Administer high-flow O_2 as necessary.
- Prevent air embolism by having client perform Valsalva maneuver any time catheter is open to air, or use in-line catheter clamp.
- Ensure client has a patent peripheral IV line.

- Infection at insertion site.

- Prepare for catheter removal and possible reinsertion at another site.
- If catheter is removed, cut off catheter tip with sterile scissors and place in sterile container; send tip to laboratory for culture.
- Administer antibiotics as ordered.
- Observe client carefully for signs of systemic infection.

Unexpected Outcomes	**Alternative Actions**
• Dysrhythmia detected.	• Change client's position. • Notify physician. • Verify catheter position on chest x-ray (right atrium placement causes dysrhythmias). • Prepare for catheter repositioning or removal of catheter by physician.
• Catheter becomes dislodged.	• Check the exact length of catheter to determine extent of problem. • Secure catheter and extension tubing with securement device to prevent further migration of tube. • Notify physician immediately.
• Catheter appears to be or becomes occluded.	• Reposition client. • Ask client to raise arms overhead. • Follow facility policy and procedure. • Assess mechanical problem: tubing, pumps, catheter, clamps, insertion site, or securement device. • Assess nonthrombotic problem: medications infused, fluids, or withdrawal of blood. Use of precipitate clearance agent is established by individual facility policies and procedures. • Assess thrombotic problem. Use of thrombolytic clearance agents is established by individual facility policy and procedures. • Perform Valsalva maneuver. Turn head to one side. • Attempt to flush catheter with normal saline, using gentle pressure. • Notify physician for order to administer fibrinolytic agent or other agents.
• CVP system does not infuse.	• Check line for kinks. Change client's position. Check to make sure the manometer stopcock is in the IV → client position. • Obtain order for placing heparin in IV bag to maintain patency. • Notify physician and prepare for possible reinsertion.
• CVP readings vary greatly.	• Assess patency of setup. • Assess client's level of pain; pain increases the CVP reading. • Assess if position of client has been changed; raising the head of the bed alters the reading unless setup is adjusted. • Check that the marked area at midaxillary level is at the level of the client's right atrium (4th ICS). • If client has COPD, heart failure, or **hypovolemia**, expect readings to differ from normal range. However, once baseline is established for individual client, trends should be watched and evaluated against goals of therapy.

Total Parenteral Nutrition/Total Nutrient Admixture

Nursing Process Data

ASSESSMENT Database

- Complete a physical assessment and client history.
- Assess client's nutrition status.
- Identify any condition that would affect TPN (renal or cardiac disease).
- Assess nutritional needs of clients who are unable to process nutrients normally (gastrointestinally).
- Observe for correct additives in each hyperalimentation bag or container.
- Check rate of infusion on physician's orders.
- Monitor catheter insertion site for signs of infection or possible infiltration.
- Monitor regularly client's blood sugar response to hyperalimentation.

PLANNING Objectives

- To provide a nutrition source for clients unable to process nutrients normally
- To provide nutrients for clients requiring bypass of the gastrointestinal tract (bowel rest)
- To provide increased calories for clients in a catabolic state
- To prevent or correct a deficiency of essential fatty acids
- To provide a contamination-free mode of delivering parenteral nutrition
- To regularly administer sliding scale insulin according to client's glucose level

IMPLEMENTATION Procedures

DOCUMENTATION AND EVALUATION

Expected Outcomes

- Catheter is placed correctly.
- Dressing remains dry and intact.
- Catheter insertion site remains free of infection and inflammation; sepsis does not occur.
- TPN infuses at prescribed rate and client receives nutrients necessary for tissue repair.
- Client's blood glucose is maintained within normal parameters.
- Client's electrolytes, protein, renal, and liver function maintained within normal parameters.

Note: Total Nutrient Admixture (TNA) is being used more frequently in healthcare facilities. Skills are the same as for TPN; only the solution composition is different.

Unexpected Outcomes/Alternative Actions

Pearson Nursing Student Resources

Find additional review materials at
nursing.pearsonhighered.com.
Prepare for success with NCLEX®-style practice questions and Skill Checklists.

Skill 29.2.1 | Assisting With Catheter Insertion

Equipment

Multi-lumen catheter
Antimicrobial swabs, 2% chlorhexidine gluconate
Transparent dressing
Sterile 4×4 gauze pads
Sterile gloves
Sterile drapes
Sterile gown
Two masks
3-mL syringe with 25-gauge needle
Lidocaine (Xylocaine—local anesthetic agent)
Suture material, only if securement device not used
Syringe with 5 mL of normal saline
Syringe with 2 mL of dilute heparin
IV administration set with appropriate filter
Hyperalimentation solution (Box 29-6 ■)
Blanket or pillow to provide roll under shoulders

Preparation

1. Identify client using two descriptors. Introduce self and validate signed consent for catheter insertion.
2. Reinforce procedure explanation to client to allay anxiety.
3. Teach Valsalva maneuver for use during catheter-insertion procedure. ➤ *Rationale:* This maneuver prevents air from entering the catheter during catheter-insertion or tubing changes.
   a. Ask client to take a deep breath and bear down without exhaling.
   b. This action produces increased intrathoracic pressure.

Box 29-6 COMPOSITION OF TPN SOLUTIONS

- Amino acids
- **Carbohydrates**—10%–35% glucose
- Vitamins (become inactive when exposed to light)
- Minerals and trace elements
- **Electrolytes** (individualized)
- Water
- Hyperalimentation solution is prepared aseptically in the pharmacy under a laminar flow hood

4. Review physician's orders for correct hyperalimentation solution.
5. Inspect TPN container for layering, turbidity, or precipitates. If there are layers, return to pharmacy.
6. Assemble IV system with in-line filter. Tubing with a 1.2 micron filter is used for TPN with lipids; a 0.2 micron filter is used for TPN without lipids.

Note: Many facilities use interventional radiology to insert central venous catheters. See also illustrations ❶ ❷

7. Perform hand hygiene.
8. Prime IV tubing and filter with solution.
9. Insert IV tubing into infusion pump.

Procedure

1. Position client in head-down position with head turned to opposite direction of catheter insertion site. Place a small roll between client's shoulders to expose insertion site.

❶ Right subclavian vein is preferred access to right atrium.

❷ Central venous catheter inserted via right jugular vein.

(continued)

Skill 29.2.1 | Assisting With Catheter Insertion (continued)

➤ *Rationale:* This position increases intrathoracic venous pressure and reduces risk of air embolism.

2. Assist physician to put on gown, mask, and gloves before beginning procedure.
3. Don mask and sterile gloves.
4. Cleanse insertion area with antimicrobial swab.

   a. Cleanse a large area around insertion site, using a scrubbing back-and-forth motion for 30 seconds.

5. Assist physician as needed during catheter insertion.
6. Instruct client in Valsalva maneuver when stylet is removed from catheter and injection cap is connected to catheter.

   a. Instruct client to exhale against a closed glottis.
   b. If client is unable to do this, compress client's abdomen.

      ➤ *Rationale:* Both these actions help decrease possibility of air embolism.

7. After cap is connected, instruct client to breathe normally.
8. Flush catheter with saline, and heparinize with dilute heparin according to agency policy.
9. Apply transparent dressing over insertion site.
10. Obtain portable chest x-ray to verify correct catheter placement.
11. After confirmation of catheter placement, initiate hyperalimentation solution and adjust flow rate as ordered.
12. Observe for signs of complications (Box 29-7 ■ and Table 29-4 ■).

Box 29-7 MONITORING GUIDELINES FOR TPN

- Monitor for signs of infection or **sepsis** at the insertion site—the most common complication of TPN.
- Weigh client daily—observe for fluid gain or loss (0.5–1.5 kilograms or 1–3 pounds per week). Weight gain may indicate fluid overload rather than nutritional gain.
- Monitor electrolyte and **protein** levels. Electrolyte imbalances may occur.
- Regularly monitor blood glucose levels observing for **hyperglycemia** (thirst, polyuria).
- Assess blood urea nitrogen and creatinine levels—increases may indicate excess amino acid intake.
- Check liver function test results—abnormal values may indicate an excess of lipids or problems in protein or glucose metabolism.

13. Take vital signs every 4 hr. ➤ *Rationale:* If signs change or temperature rises significantly, the client may be developing complications.

CLINICAL ALERT
TPN and lipids are frequently infused together in the same bottle to prevent microorganism growth from lipid emulsion.

Table 29-4 Complications With Total Parenteral Nutrition

Complication	Symptoms	Prevention	Nursing Action
			Implementation
Air embolism Air enters catheter during catheter insertion or tubing changes.	Potentially fatal Respiratory distress, apprehension Chest pain, **dyspnea** Hypotension Pulse weak and rapid Churning heart murmur (classic sign)	Instruct client in Valsalva maneuver for tubing and cap changes. Check all catheter connections. Place client in head-down position with head turned opposite direction of insertion site (increases intrathoracic venous pressure).	Clamp catheter. Place client in left Trendelenburg position (to trap air in right side of heart). Notify physician. Administer oxygen as ordered.
Catheter-related infection (sepsis) Because the TPN solution is high-concentrate glucose, it is a medium for bacterial growth.	Fever (early sign), chills Insertion site—**erythema** or drainage Elevated white blood cell count Septic shock	Use strict aseptic technique. Change solution every 24 hr. Change tubing as ordered (every 24 hr using aseptic technique). Change dressing every 7 days or when soiled or loose.	Remove tip of catheter, send to laboratory for culture. Administer antibiotics as ordered.
Hyperglycemia: Increased blood glucose level due to infusion, stress, medications, diabetes	Elevated glucose levels (more than 200 mg/dL) Excessive thirst, fatigue, restlessness, confusion, weakness, diuresis When severe—coma	Check history for glucose intolerance; frequent glucose monitoring—check medications (e.g., steroids). Begin infusion at slow rate (usually 40 mL/hr). Increase proportion of **calories** as lipids. Do not "catch up" if infusion rate falls behind.	Start sliding-scale insulin therapy as ordered. Monitor blood glucose levels every 4–6 hr. Maintain blood glucose < 200 mg/dL.
Hypoglycemia TPN is discontinued abruptly or client is receiving too much insulin.	Client is shaky, weak, anxious, diaphoretic. May be hungry Decreased blood glucose (less than 70 mg/dL)	Continue blood glucose monitoring. Gradually decrease infusion when discontinuing TPN. Use infusion pump.	Infuse 10% dextrose in water (50% may be needed; restart IV if necessary). Assess blood glucose 1 hr after discontinuing TPN.

Skill 29.2.2 | Maintaining Total Parenteral Nutrition (TPN) Infusions

Equipment

Parenteral nutrition solution (TPN) (refrigerated) **❶**
IV tubing, filter, and infusion pump
Extension tubing with filter per agency protocol
Glucometer
I&O record
Securement device

Procedure

1. Introduce self, identify client using two client identifiers, and wash hands.
2. Store TPN solution in refrigerator until 30 min before use. (Some pharmacies deliver the solution before each infusion.) ➤ *Rationale:* Solution is refrigerated to prevent growth of organisms, but should be left at room temperature 1 hr before use.
3. Ensure central line is patent when infusing TPN. Check for patency according to facility policy.
4. Change IV tubing and filter every 24 hr. This is completed when entire system is changed. **❷ ❸** ➤ *Rationale:* This is recommended for TPN infusions to prevent infection.
5. Maintain IV flow rate as prescribed. Use infusion pump for infusion.

❷ Nontunneled catheter used to deliver parenteral nutrition.

❸ In-line filter used when administering TPN solution.

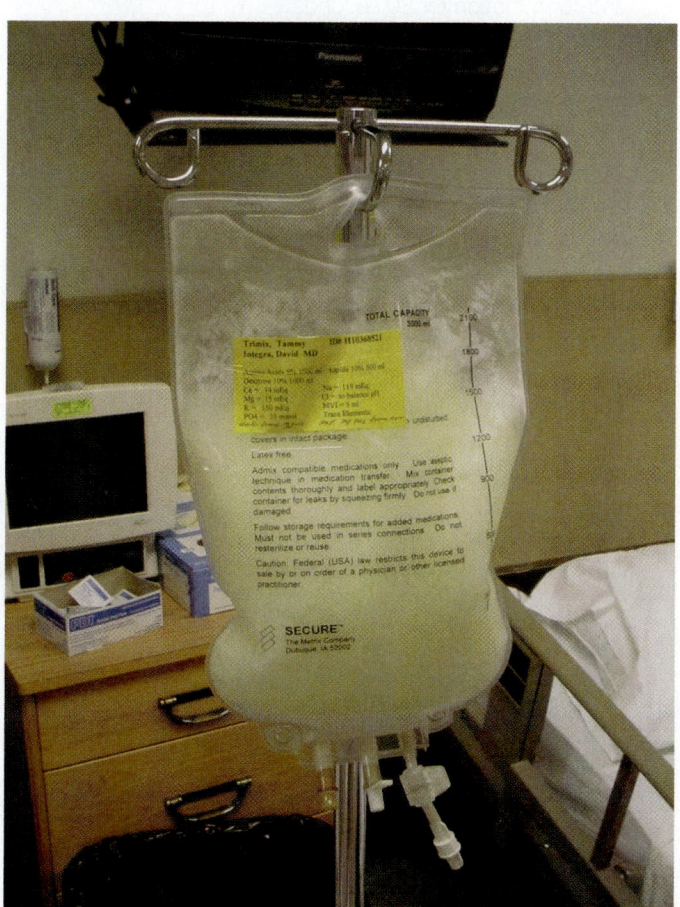

❶ Total parenteral nutrition.

> **CLINICAL ALERT**
> Do not "catch up" on a deficit in infused volume, as doing so could result in complications for the client. To ensure constant flow rate, check rate every 2 hr.

   a. If rate is too rapid, hyperosmolar diuresis occurs (excess glucose and water is excreted); if severe enough, intractable seizures, coma, and death can occur.
   b. If rate is too slow, little benefit is derived from the calories and nitrogen.
6. Change solution every 24 hr. ➤ *Rationale:* Changing the solution prevents growth of bacterial organisms that proliferate in glucose solution.

(continued)

Skill 29.2.2 | Maintaining Total Parenteral Nutrition (TPN) Infusions *(continued)*

7. Monitor client's blood glucose regularly (e.g., every 6 hr).
8. If necessary, administer Regular insulin according to prescribed "sliding scale."
9. Maintain accurate I&O.
10. Observe for complications, such as air embolus, hyperglycemia, osmotic diuresis, infiltration, or sepsis.

> **CLINICAL ALERT**
>
> No medication or blood products are to be added or piggybacked into TPN line. Use portless tubing for administration.
>
> No blood specimen should be withdrawn from an IV line infusing TPN.
>
> TPN is never stopped abruptly. It should be tapered off.

Skill 29.2.3 | Changing Total Parenteral Nutrition (TPN) Dressing and Tubing

Equipment
Clean and sterile gloves
Mask
IV tubing and filter (0.22 micron)
TPN solution
2×2 sterile gauze pads and tape
Antimicrobial swabs, 2% chlorhexidine gluconate
Transparent semipermeable dressing
Securement device

Preparation
1. Check to determine when tubing was last changed.
2. Gather equipment and perform hand hygiene.
3. Verify client ID using two descriptors. Introduce self and explain procedure to client.
4. Connect IV tubing and filter to parenteral hyperalimentation (TPN) solution container.
5. Flush tubing to clear air.
6. Place IV tubing through infusion pump.
7. Prepare dressing: antimicrobial swabs, sterile 2×2 gauze pads and tape, or sterile transparent dressing.
8. Place client supine with head turned in opposite direction of insertion site. Instruct client not to talk or cough. (Place mask on client if client cannot cooperate.) ➤ *Rationale:* These steps reduce risk of contamination.

Procedure
1. Don mask (according to institutional policy) and clean gloves.
2. Remove old dressing and discard both dressing and gloves in appropriate receptacle.

3. Don sterile gloves.
4. Observe insertion site for signs of erythema, drainage, or swelling.

> **CLINICAL ALERT**
>
> When central-line dressings are loose, wet, or soiled, they are considered contaminated and must be changed. Dressings are routinely changed every 7 days.

5. Cleanse insertion site with antimicrobial swabs, using back-and-forth motion for 30 seconds.
6. Allow 30 seconds for drying.
7. Apply securement device following package instructions and according to agency policy.
8. Place sterile transparent dressing over insertion site.
9. Change IV tubing.
   a. Clamp catheter using slide clamp.
   b. Loosen tubing in catheter hub.
   c. Insert new primed tubing, *or*
   d. Cap catheter and insert new IV tubing using needleless connector or use positive pressure device.
10. Remove gloves and perform hand hygiene.
11. Label dressing with date and your initials.

> **CLINICAL ALERT**
>
> Transparent dressings are changed every 7 days. Transparent dressings are preferred unless the site is draining.

Skill 29.2.4 | Maintaining Total Parenteral Nutrition (TPN) for Children

Equipment
Same as for adult parenteral nutrition with these additions:
Intracath, 22-gauge needle
Microdrip IV tubing administration set
0.22-micron in-line filter
Restraints, only if necessary and ordered

Preparation
1. Identify client using two descriptors. Introduce self.
2. Gather equipment for blood glucose monitoring and dressing change.
3. Perform hand hygiene.

Procedure

1. Verify solution with physician's orders.
2. Examine solution. Generally, there is a higher concentration of calcium, phosphorus, magnesium, and vitamins. Either a 10% dextrose/2% amino acids or 5% dextrose/4% amino acids solution can be infused peripherally. Higher concentrations are infused centrally, as is long-term therapy.
3. Monitor patency of catheter. Stopcocks are never used. Monitor infusion pump and filter.
4. Obtain finger stick or urine glucose samples every 8 hr. Glucose level rises, but usually exogenous insulin is not required as the pancreas adapts to high glucose loads.
5. Monitor intake and output and daily weight.
6. Change the dressing every 7 days and the tubing every 24 hr using aseptic technique. Stockinette can be used to keep scalp dressing secure. Tight-fitting T-shirt can keep chest site secure.

7. Monitor for accurate rate of infusion. Do not "catch up" if infusion is behind. Pumps can be used to maintain infusion rates, particularly when small amounts of solution are being infused.
8. Observe the child when ambulating for twisting or kinking of tubing, getting the tubing caught in the crib, or stepping on it.
9. Instruct parents on rationale for treatment and methods to prevent accidental dislodging of the tubing.
10. Provide play therapy and sources of stimulation to distract the child from the catheter.
11. If discontinuing TPN, taper infusion for 1 hr (decrease rate every 30 min). ➤ **Rationale:** Abrupt discontinuation may cause a hypoglycemic reaction since insulin production is increased.

Unit 29.2 Documentation and Evaluation

DOCUMENTATION for Total Parenteral Nutrition

- Charting in the computer per protocol
- Catheter type, insertion site, physician's name
- X-ray, following insertion
- Type of parenteral nutrition solution and flow rate
- Results of blood glucose monitoring
- If insulin administered, type, amount, and site

- Date and time of dressing and tubing change with name or initials of individual who did the change
- Condition of insertion site
- Client's tolerance of procedure
- Daily weights
- Intake and output

EVALUATION/Critical Thinking

Expected Outcomes

- Catheter is placed correctly.
- TPN infuses at prescribed rate and client receives necessary nutrients for tissue repair.
- Dressing remains clean, dry, and intact.
- Catheter insertion site remains free of infection and inflammation; sepsis does not occur.
- Client's blood glucose remains within normal parameters.
- Client's electrolytes, protein, renal, and liver function maintained within normal parameters.

(continued)

Unexpected Outcomes	Alternative Actions
• Parenteral nutrition solution is not infused at the prescribed rate.	• Observe filter to ensure patency. A plugged filter is the most common cause of infusion failure. Change the filter and tubing. • Ensure that the next parenteral nutrition bag is ready to be superimposed. • Observe for signs of hypoglycemia caused by sudden change in dextrose concentration—weakness, trembling, sweating, hunger. Check blood glucose. • Adjust flow rate to that which was ordered. Do not attempt to "catch up" on the amount not infused as this action could lead to osmotic diuresis from hyperglycemia.
• Catheter insertion site becomes inflamed.	• Notify physician immediately so catheter can be discontinued if catheter-related sepsis is suspected. • Cut tip of catheter off with sterile scissors and place in sterile container. Send to laboratory for culture and sensitivity for specific causative organism. • Cleanse site of catheter insertion with antimicrobial swab and place sterile dressing over site. • Obtain order for and administer antibiotics as needed.
• The dressing becomes wet or loose.	• Change the dressing as soon as moisture is observed, using aseptic technique. • If the dressing will be exposed to moisture (e.g., showering) or secretions, cover with transparent dressing.
• TPN solution temporarily unavailable.	• Infuse D10W IV solution at prescribed rate until TPN solution is available.

Lipid Emulsion Therapy

Nursing Process Data

ASSESSMENT Database

- Observe for signs of essential fatty acid deficits: rash; eczema; dry, scaly skin; poor wound healing; sparse hair.
- Assess pancreatic function.
- Assess client for predisposing factors that could promote fat emboli, such as anemia, coagulation disorders, abnormal liver, or pulmonary function.
- Check IV site for patency, erythema, and edema before infusing solution.
- Assess vital signs to establish baseline.

PLANNING Objectives

- To spare protein in clients who are critically ill
- To provide a source of energy for clients with deficient protein intake
- To provide essential fatty acids

IMPLEMENTATION Procedures

DOCUMENTATION AND EVALUATION

Expected Outcomes

- Lipids infused within time frame.
- Adequate calories and essential fatty acids are provided to clients unable to ingest orally.
- Parenteral nutrients are provided without complications or adverse effects.
- Normal pancreatic function is maintained.

Unexpected Outcomes/Alternative Actions

Pearson Nursing Student Resources

Find additional review materials at
nursing.pearsonhighered.com.
Prepare for success with NCLEX®-style practice questions and Skill Checklists.

Skill 29.3.1 | Infusing IV Lipids

Equipment

IV lipid solution in container

Nonphthalate vented IV tubing infusion set (to prevent pooling of fat in IV tubing)

Needleless cannula

2% chlorhexidine gluconate swabs

Volume control device

IV filter

Note: Many facilities do not infuse lipids alone but combine with TPN.

> **CLINICAL ALERT**
>
> Administration sets that contain di-(2-ethylhexyl) phthalate (DEHP) plasticizers extract lipids from infusion set. It is recommended to use a separate administration set, glass infusate containers, or special non–polyvinyl chloride (non-PVC) IV bags.
>
> ---
>
> Lipid emulsions alone promote growth of specific bacteria and yeasts as soon as 6 hr after the infusion. Combination of lipids with TPN (solution of amino acids, lipid emulsion, and glucose) in the same bag does not appear to support any greater microbial growth than non–lipid-containing TPN fluids. Thus, TPN solution can hang safely for 24 hr.

Preparation

1. Review physician's orders and MAR. For guidelines for IV lipid infusion, see Box 29-8 ▪.
2. Obtain lipid emulsion (refrigerated) from the pharmacy and allow to warm to room temperature (may take 1 to 2 hr).
3. Examine solution for separation of emulsion into layers or fat globules or for accumulation of froth. Do not use if any of these appear.

Box 29-8 **GUIDELINES FOR IV LIPID INFUSION**

- IV lipid solutions are isotonic and provide 1.1 kcal/mL of solution in a 10% solution or 2.0 kcal/mL in a 20% solution.
- Do not put additives into IV lipid bottle.
- A filter is not required because the particles are large and cannot pass through.

For Adults

- Lipid 10%: Up to 500 mL 4–6 hr on first day to maximum of 2.5 g/kg body weight per day. Do not exceed 60% of client's total caloric intake per day.
- Liposyn 10%: Do not exceed 500 mL/day in 4–6 hr.

For Children

- Lipid 10%: Up to 1 g/kg in 4 hr. Do not exceed 60% of total caloric intake.

4. Label bottle/bag with client name, medical record number, room number, date, time, flow rate, bottle number, and start and stop times.
5. Introduce self and identify client using two forms of identification.
6. Explain procedure to client.

Procedure

1. Take vital signs for baseline assessment. ➤ *Rationale:* Baseline information is needed because an immediate reaction can occur.
2. Perform hand hygiene and then swab stopper on IV bottle with antimicrobial swab and allow it to dry.
3. Attach vented non-PVC infusion set to bottle, twisting the spike to prevent particles from stopper falling into the emulsion, or spike bag with regular IV tubing. ❶ ❷
4. Hang IV bottle at least 76 cm (30 in.) above IV site. ➤ *Rationale:* Due to solution **viscosity**, lipid emulsion needs to be at this height to prevent backing up into infusion tubing.
5. Fill drip chamber two-thirds full, slightly open clamp on the tubing, and prime the tubing slowly. ➤ *Rationale:* Priming more slowly reduces chance of air bubbles with this solution.
6. Attach the tubing to the IV site.

❶ Lipids are administered from glass container or non-PVC infusion sets.

7. If piggybacking lipids into hyperalimentation, use port closest to client, below tubing filter.

8. Infuse lipid solutions initially at 1 mL/min for adults and 0.1 mL/min for children for first 15–30 min. Then increase rate to 2 mL/min for adults and 0.2 mL/min for children.
9. Monitor vital signs according to facility policy and observe for side effects during first 30 min of the infusion. If side effects occur, stop the infusion and notify the physician.
10. Adjust flow to prescribed IV rate if no adverse reactions occur.

❷ Vented tubing is required for lipid infusion.

11. Monitor and maintain the infusion at the ordered rate.
12. Monitor serum lipids 4 hr after discontinuing infusion. ➤ *Rationale:* If you draw blood too soon after infusion is completed, incorrect blood values result.
13. Monitor liver function tests for evidence of impaired liver function. ➤ *Rationale:* These tests indicate the liver's ability to metabolize the lipids.
14. Discard partially used bottles/bags. ➤ *Rationale:* This action prevents contamination.
15. Discard administration set after each unit unless additional units are administered consecutively.
16. Continue to monitor vital signs and observe client for adverse reactions during the entire process of infusion.
17. Answer any questions the client may have about the procedure and make client comfortable before leaving room.

❸ Check facility policy regarding use of in-line filters for lipid administration. Filters are not recommended by CDC, but Infusion Nurses Society uses them.

Unit 29.3 Documentation and Evaluation

DOCUMENTATION for Lipid Emulsion Therapy

- Type of solution infused
- Rate of infusion
- Site of infusion

- Vital signs monitored
- Adverse clinical manifestations and appropriate nursing intervention

EVALUATION/Critical Thinking

Expected Outcomes

- Lipids infuse within time frame.
- Adequate calories and essential fatty acids are provided to clients unable to ingest orally.
- Parenteral nutrients provided without complications or adverse effects.
- Normal pancreatic function is maintained.

Unexpected Outcomes	Alternative Actions
• Client experiences side effects and cannot continue with lipid infusion.	• Reassess client's ability to tolerate fat solution. • Notify physician for order to discontinue fat solution, and administer hyperalimentation solution. • Monitor liver function test results.
• Client develops dyspnea, cyanosis, or allergic reaction, such as nausea, vomiting, increased temperature, or headache.	• Stop infusion immediately and notify physician.
• Client's serum triglyceride and liver function test results remain elevated.	• Continue IV lipid infusion. • Begin the feeding with a weaker concentration of formula and increase the concentration slowly as ordered. • Repeat lab values.
• Client develops hyperlipemia or hypercoagulability.	• Monitor laboratory results, particularly liver function tests, and notify physician when any abnormality occurs.

Tunneled Central Vascular Access Devices (CVADs)

Nursing Process Data

ASSESSMENT Database
- Assess patency of catheter.
- Assess insertion site for signs of infection.
- Assess the tubing for accidental breaks.
- Assess injection cap at the end of catheter to ensure tightness.

PLANNING Objectives
- To provide a patent catheter
- To clear a nonpatent catheter
- To provide an access for blood drawing
- To provide an access for infusions

IMPLEMENTATION Procedures

DOCUMENTATION AND EVALUATION

Expected Outcomes
- IV catheter remains patent using CLC2000 device.
- The catheter site remains infection-free.
- Blood samples are obtained without difficulty.
- Infusions of medications or fluids are accomplished without difficulty.

Unexpected Outcomes/Alternative Actions

Pearson Nursing Student Resources

Find additional review materials at
nursing.pearsonhighered.com.
Prepare for success with NCLEX®-style practice
questions and Skill Checklists.

Skill 29.4.1 | Maintaining the Hickman or Broviac CV Catheter

Equipment

10-mL Luer-Lok syringe with 3 mL of dilute heparin (100 units/
   mL solution or 10 units/mL) or tissue plasminogen activator
   (t-PA) 2 mg/2 mL (Anteplase)
2% chlorhexidine gluconate swab
Clean gloves
Syringes (size per facility policy)
10-mL syringe prefilled with preservative-free 0.9% sodium
   chloride
CLC2000 (or other brand) positive pressure device

Preparation

1. Check client care plan and type of tunnelled central vascular
   access device (Box 29-9 ■). **1**
2. Identify client using two forms of identification. Introduce self
   and explain procedure to client.
3. Provide privacy for client.
4. Perform hand hygiene and don gloves.

Procedure

Flushing Intermittently Used Line

1. Wipe catheter cap with antimicrobial swab for 30 sec.
2. Insert syringe cannula into needleless access cap or
   CLC2000 device and unsnap catheter squeeze clamp.
3. Inject heparin solution slowly through catheter until almost
   empty.

Box 29-9 TUNNELED CENTRAL VASCULAR ACCESS DEVICES (CVADs)

- Tunneled central vascular access devices (CVADs) provide
  long-term access to a central vein for the purpose of drawing blood, administering drugs (chemotherapy, antibiotics),
  administering total parenteral nutrition (TPN), or administering blood and blood products.
- Catheters are soft, silicone elastomers, thermoplastic polyurethane, or PVC. Used because of tensile strength and
  biocompatibility.
- Long-term catheters have one, two, or three lumens.
- The tip is inserted into a central vein and advanced to the
  superior vena cava. The remainder of the catheter passes
  through a subcutaneous track and exits on the chest wall
  or abdomen for easy access. A Dacron cuff on the catheter elicits scar formation that prevents ascending tract
  infection.
- Three common tunneled CVADs are the Hickman, Broviac,
  and Groshong.
- Clients with tunneled CVADs are advised to display
  medical-alert information.

---

1 The tunneled Broviac catheter (single, double, or triple lumen) is commonly used for children.

4. Remove syringe while still moving plunger forward, or
   clamp catheter before removing syringe if not using positive
   pressure device (see Skill 29.4.2, Using a Positive Pressure
   Device). ➤ *Rationale:* This maintains positive pressure in
   the catheter and prevents clotting by preventing backflow of
   blood into catheter.
5. Withdraw syringe.
6. Flush nonused capped lines daily.

Irrigating a Nonpatent Catheter

1. Follow facility policy for irrigating catheter.
2. Obtain 10-mL syringes with dilute heparin (usually prepared
   by pharmacy). ➤ *Rationale:* The size of this syringe
   decreases pressure exerted in the system.
3. Swab catheter cap with antimicrobial swab for 30 sec unless
   protective cap is in place; then remove protective cap.
4. Insert syringe with Luer-Lok and unclamp catheter.
5. Inject heparin from syringes, 1 mL at a time or per facility
   policy.
6. Leave heparin in catheter tubing for prescribed time.
7. Check that dwell time is completed, then use a 10-mL
   syringe to aspirate solution from catheter by gently pulling
   back on plunger.
8. Follow with an irrigation of 5–10 mL of heparinized solution
   if aspiration is successful. Use same solution for irrigation as
   with maintenance solution.
9. Repeat procedure once. If unsuccessful, notify physician
   and be prepared to instill thrombolytic agent, t-PA (t-PA
   is infused at 2 mg/2 mL). Alteplase is the only approved
   thrombolytic agent for treatment of catheter occlusion.
10. Discard equipment and gloves and perform hand hygiene.

Skill 29.4.2 | Using a Positive Pressure Device

Equipment

Positive Pressure Device; CLC2000 (Box 29-10 ■) or FloStar, or
 SmartSite
Antimicrobial swab
Gloves
10-mL prefilled saline syringe

Preparation

1. Check physician's orders.
2. Identify client using two forms of identification.
3. Introduce yourself and explain the procedure.
4. Perform hand hygiene and gather equipment.

Procedure

1. Assess peripheral or central venous access site for signs of infection.
2. Perform hand hygiene and don gloves.
3. Use aseptic technique to open package, remove device, and remove cap without contaminating.
4. Prepare positive pressure device by attaching prefilled saline syringe and priming through device with saline. Leave syringe attached.
5. Attach the syringe to the female Luer and prime the CLC2000 device according to facility policies and procedures. Invert the device to expel air.
6. Attach the male spin lock to the venous access device. Push and twist the male spin lock of the CLC2000 into the VAD until it is tight. ❶
7. Cleanse the female Luer vigorously with an antimicrobial swab for 30 seconds or per facility protocol. ❷
8. Attach the prefilled saline syringe; push and twist the Luer into the CLC2000 until there is a tight fit; unclamp catheter.
9. **Irrigate** with saline as ordered (Boxes 29-11 and 29-12 ■).
10. Remove the syringe and dispose of it in the sharps container.
11. Remove gloves and discard.

Box 29-10 POSITIVE PRESSURE DEVICE

The positive pressure device (CLC2000) creates positive pressure within the central venous access device, preventing blood from being drawn back into the catheter when the flush syringe is removed. The CLC2000 is a Luer-Lok that replaces the other needleless caps and should be used when a CVAD cannot be flushed with heparin. The device is only flushed with saline, and the line must not be clamped, nor should extension sets be added as these actions negate the anti-reflux action of the device.

Positive pressure devices are applied to PICC line.

12. Perform hand hygiene.

Note: If using device for IV fluid infusion, cleanse female Luer and attach IV tubing. Open clamp on catheter and begin IV flow.

Attach Positive Pressure Device

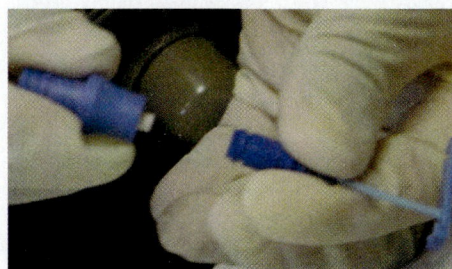

A. Clamp catheter and remove cap from line, maintaining sterility of device.

❶ Attach positive pressure device.

B. Cleanse proximal adapter tip with chlorhexidine for 30 sec; air dry; attach device.

C. Attach male spin lock to venous access device by screwing device into catheter

(continued)

Skill 29.4.2 | Using a Positive Pressure Device (continued)

Flushing Catheter Using Positive Pressure Device

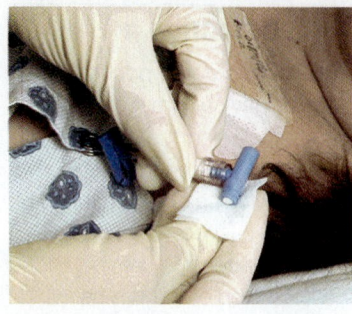

A. Cleanse female Luer vigorously for 30 sec.

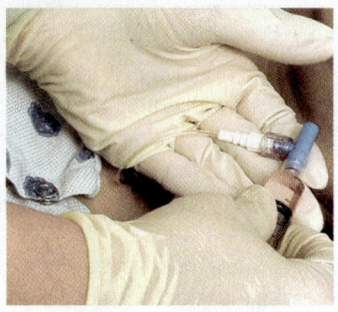

B. Attach 10-mL prefilled saline syringe, infuse saline, and aspirate for blood return.

C. Remove syringe from device and cleanse Luer.

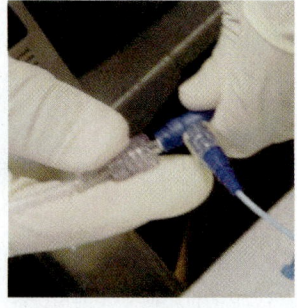

D. Attach IV tubing to device.

❷ Flushing catheter using positive pressure device.

Box 29-11 FLUSHING PROTOCOLS

Using 10 mL of Saline

- Flush catheter weekly when not in use.
- Flush catheter after every use.

Using 20 mL of Saline

- Flush catheter before and after any aspiration of blood, after **transfusion** of blood, or when blood is seen in the catheter (client straining or lifting may cause blood to back up into catheter).

- Flush catheter after infusion of lipids or hyperalimentation solutions.

Note: Regardless of the volume of saline used, ALWAYS flush in a stop–start action, pushing about 2 mL of solution at a time. ➤ **Rationale:** This creates a swirling effect at the distal end of the catheter.

Box 29-12 FLUSHING TUNNELED CATHETERS

Flush catheter with 3–5 mL of heparin (10 units/mL) daily when catheter is not used and before and after each use. The SASH protocol is used (saline, administer drug or withdraw blood, saline, and heparin).

This type of flushing is *not* done with a closed-ended (Groshong) catheter. Its internal valve is designed to prevent blood reflux into the catheter.

Skill 29.4.3 | Changing the Hickman or Broviac CV Catheter Dressing

Equipment
Antimicrobial swabs, 2% chlorhexidine gluconate
Transparent, semipermeable dressing
Clean gloves
Sterile gloves
Mask (if client is neutropenic and per agency policy)

Procedure

1. Identify client using two descriptors. Introduce self and explain procedure.
2. Apply mask as needed.
3. Perform hand hygiene and don gloves.
4. Remove old dressing and place in appropriate receptacle.

5. Observe for signs and symptoms of infection and crepitus at insertion site. ➤ **Rationale:** Signs most frequently observed are erythema, edema, and drainage for infection. Crackling under the skin denotes crepitus due to air in the subcutaneous tissue; this finding should be reported to the physician.
6. Remove and discard gloves.
7. Set up supplies on a sterile field and don sterile gloves. ❶
8. Clean exit site using antimicrobial swabs. Swab with back-and-forth movement for 30 seconds.
9. Clean catheter tubing at exit site. Allow to air dry.
10. Apply sterile transparent dressing; change weekly or if soiled. When cuff heals into place, dressings are not necessary.
11. Remove gloves and discard.

1 Hickman catheter.

12. Sign and date dressing.
13. Secure catheter to prevent dislodging; tape to chest.
14. Perform hand hygiene.

Note: Nonhospitalized clients who are not immunosuppressed may protect the exit site with a Band-Aid or leave the site undressed. They should cleanse daily with antibacterial soap and water, palpate site daily to check for signs of infection, and tape catheter to the chest to prevent accidental dislodgement.

> **CLINICAL ALERT**
> To prevent a potentially life-threatening mistake, never use scissors near central venous catheters.

Skill 29.4.4 | Maintaining the CV Catheter With Groshong Valve

Note: The Groshong valve (Box 29-13 ■) is available in a variety of CVADs, including ports and PICCs. The Groshong allows infusion but prevents backflow of blood unless negative pressure is applied. There is no need for heparin flush, and external clamps are not used. Clamping could force the slit valve open, allowing blood to leak into the lumen.

Equipment
Normal saline, preservative-free
Antimicrobial swab, 2% chlorhexidine gluconate
Sterile injection cap
Appropriate syringe: 10 mL or 20 mL
Clean gloves
Sterile gloves
Positive pressure device

Preparation
1. Check physician's orders.
2. Gather equipment.
3. Identify the client using two descriptors. Introduce self.
4. Perform hand hygiene and don gloves.

Procedure
1. For non–positive pressure device, wipe injection cap and catheter connection with antimicrobial swab for 30 sec.
2. While holding catheter, remove catheter cap and attach hub of syringe directly to catheter hub.
3. Inject normal saline rapidly into lumen.
4. Maintain positive pressure on syringe plunger as last 0.5 mL is injected and syringe is withdrawn. ➤ **Rationale:** Keeping pressure on the plunger prevents backup of blood into catheter.

Box 29-13 **THE GROSHONG CATHETER**

The Groshong catheter offers an alternative to the Hickman and Broviac catheters. It is distinguished by a rounded, blunt catheter tip with a three-way pressure-sensitive valve that remains closed at normal vena caval pressure. When closed, it restricts air from entering the venous system or a backflow of blood from the catheter. When a syringe is inserted to create a vacuum, it allows the valve to open inward for blood aspiration. Positive pressure into the catheter by infusion forces the valve to open outward. The primary advantages of this type of catheter are:

- Decreased risk of air emboli or bleeding
- Elimination of heparin to flush the catheter
- Elimination of catheter clamping
- Reduced flushing protocols between use

Note: It is recommended that a positive pressure device be used for irrigating CVADs. See Skill 29.4.2, Using a Positive Pressure Device.

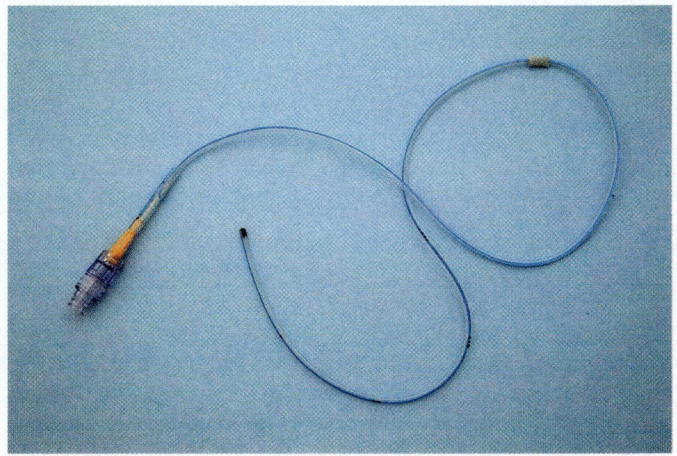

The tunneled CV catheter with Groshong valve is ideal for long-term therapy.

(continued)

Skill 29.4.4 | Maintaining the CV Catheter With Groshong Valve *(continued)*

5. Remove cap by holding catheter connector between thumb and forefinger of one hand and grasping barrel of cap with other hand.
6. Twist and pull counterclockwise to separate cap from connector.
7. Continue to hold connector with one hand. ➤ *Rationale:* Holding connector prevents inadvertent contamination by placing connector on dirty surface.
8. Discard old cap.
9. Clean liberally around connector using antimicrobial swab.
10. Holding new sterile injection cap, twist clockwise and insert into connector.

10- or 20-mL Flushing

1. Remove syringe from package.
2. Remove injection cap carefully from connector and discard.
3. Clean connector with chlorhexidine gluconate wipe for 30 sec. DO NOT let go of connector. ➤ *Rationale:* Holding connector prevents inadvertent contamination.
4. Insert syringe barrel directly into catheter connector, twisting slightly to ensure good connection.

5. Flush lumen with preservative-free normal saline using stop–start action. ➤ *Rationale:* Heparin is not used because clotting is not a factor with catheter tip design of the Groshong.

CLINICAL ALERT

Nursing attention to the catheter during dressing change is important to ensure the catheter is not pinched, kinked, occluded, cut, or dislodged. It is recommended that the external portion of the catheter be coiled and taped to avoid a straight pull on the catheter insertion site.

6. Maintain positive pressure on syringe barrel as syringe is removed from connector. DO NOT clamp the catheter after flushing. ➤ *Rationale:* The Groshong CV catheter does not require clamping to keep blood from entering the lumen. Clamping the catheter damages it.
7. Change injection cap.
8. Remove gloves and perform hand hygiene.

Skill 29.4.5 | Drawing Blood From the CV Catheter With Groshong Valve

Equipment

Sterile injection cap
Three 10-mL Luer-Lok syringes for drawing blood
One 20-mL Luer-Lok syringe filled with preservative-free normal saline
Blood tubes appropriate for tests ordered
Antimicrobial swabs, 2% chlorhexidine gluconate
Clean gloves

Note: Vacuum tubes should not be used with the Groshong valve because they can cause it to malfunction.

Preparation

1. Introduce self and identify client using two client identifiers.
2. Explain procedure to the client.

Procedure

1. Perform hand hygiene and don gloves.
2. Clean cap and outside of connector with swabs for 30 sec and allow to air dry.
3. Remove and discard injection cap while holding connector so that it does not make contact with any surface.

4. Insert first 10-mL syringe with saline directly into catheter, twisting slightly to ensure connection.
5. Flush with stop–start action. Groshong catheter must be flushed with stop–start action with at least 10 mL of normal saline before blood sample removal.
6. Pull back plunger 0.5 mL, pause 2 seconds, and then continue aspirating until 5 mL of blood is in syringe.
7. Remove syringe, set aside; continue to hold connector.
8. Connect second 10-mL syringe directly to catheter connector, twisting slightly to ensure connection.
9. Proceed to aspirate blood volume needed for sample after same aspiration procedure of pulling 0.5 mL and waiting for 2 seconds.
10. Remove syringe and continue to hold connector.
11. Flush catheter briskly with 20 mL of preservative-free normal saline and attach new sterile injection cap.
12. Transfer blood sample from second syringe into appropriate tube(s), and label. Do not hold receiving tube during transfer.
13. Discard syringe containing first aspirated blood into biohazard container.
14. Remove gloves and perform hand hygiene.

Unit 29.4 Documentation and Evaluation

DOCUMENTATION for CVADs

- Flush frequency and solution used
- Dressing changes and type applied
- Site condition
- Condition and patency of catheter
- Medications or solutions administered through catheter

- Amount of blood withdrawn for testing and the amount discarded.
- Infusion cap change
- Positive pressure device in place

EVALUATION/Critical Thinking

Expected Outcomes

- IV catheter maintains patency with use of CLC2000 device.
- Catheter site remains free of infection.
- Blood samples are obtained without difficulty.
- Infusions of medications or fluids are accomplished without difficulty.

Unexpected Outcomes	Alternative Actions
CV Catheter:	
• Nurse is unable to aspirate blood even though solution flows through the catheter.	• Use less negative pressure on syringe when aspirating blood. Tip of catheter may be sucking against wall of vessel. • Have client raise arms above head. This can alter position of catheter. • Have client perform Valsalva maneuver. • Change client's position.
• Clotting of catheter occurs (client develops arm or neck swelling on catheter side of body).	• Do not force plunger with Groshong; this may rupture catheter. • Make sure clamps are open and tubing is not kinked. • Use flushing procedure for catheter with a recently developed clot. Instill 1 mL of normal saline. • Allow 15 min before aspirating to see if declotting occurs. Repeat if necessary. • Prevent occlusion due to drug sludge by flushing carefully after administration. • Thrombolytic agent is required for fibrinous clot. • FDA approved use of t-PA (tissue plasminogen activator) for thrombolytic protocol. Follow facility policy regarding instillation of drug. • Instill 2 mg of t-PA in a 10-mL syringe. Wait 60 min. Aspirate; if unable to obtain blood flow, instill a second dose of t-PA. If this does not produce blood flow, notify physician.

(continued)

Unexpected Outcomes	Alternative Actions
• Catheter breaks or is pierced by clamp.	• Immediately clamp catheter proximal to break site, if necessary (Groshong may be clamped using rubber band). • Obtain repair kit for catheter.
• Air enters catheter when open to atmosphere; client experiences chest pain, shortness of breath, or coughing.	• Clamp catheter (use rubber band if Groshong device). • Turn client on left side with head lower than rest of body to trap air in right heart. • Notify physician immediately. • Administer oxygen.
• Signs of infection develop at exit site (redness, pain, fever, chills).	• Notify physician immediately. • Catheter will have to be removed and cultures taken.

Implanted Subcutaneous Port

Nursing Process Data

ASSESSMENT Database

- Assess site.
- Assess patency of port.

PLANNING Objectives

- To provide an access for blood withdrawal
- To provide an access for drug or blood/fluid administration

IMPLEMENTATION Procedures

DOCUMENTATION AND EVALUATION

Expected Outcomes

- Subcutaneous implanted port remains patent to facilitate medication administration.
- Implantation site remains infection-free.
- Blood samples are obtained without difficulty.

Unexpected Outcomes/Alternative Actions

Pearson Nursing Student Resources

Find additional review materials at **nursing.pearsonhighered.com.**
Prepare for success with NCLEX®-style practice questions and Skill Checklists.

Skill 29.5.1 | Accessing and Flushing an Implanted Port Using a Huber Needle

Note: Implanted venous access ports, such as Port-a-Cath, are usually placed in a subcutaneous pocket on the chest wall, require minimal maintenance, and may be used for months to years before the maximum 2,000 punctures are achieved. Ports are best utilized for cyclic therapies like chemotherapy or antibiotic therapy. They are well suited for care of clients with cancer or others with long-term illnesses requiring IV medications. Ports can be used for either bolus or continuous infusions.

Equipment

Noncoring needle (Huber) with attached extension tubing and
  clamp (Box 29-14 ■)
Intermittent infusion cap or CLC2000
Two 10-mL Luer-Lok syringes
Preservative-free normal saline or prefilled syringes
Heparin (100 or 10 units/mL) according to facility policy
Antimicrobial swabs, 2% chlorhexidine gluconate
Sterile gloves
Clean gloves
Mask

Preparation

1. Check physician's orders and client care plan. Review specific hospital policy and procedure for care of implanted port. ❶ ❷
2. Gather equipment.
3. Perform hand hygiene.
4. Draw up 10 mL of normal saline into 10-mL syringe, or use prefilled syringes.
5. Draw up 5 mL of dilute heparin (10 mL or 100 units/mL according to facility policy) into 10-mL syringe.
6. Identify client using two forms of identification. Introduce self.
7. Explain procedure to client.
8. Don clean gloves.

❶ Implanted subcutaneous port.

A   **B**

❷ **A.** Huber needle. **B.** Placement of Huber needle.

Box 29-14 NONCORING NEEDLES (HUBER)

- Noncoring needles, such as the **Huber needle,** are the only ones used to access the port.
- Huber needle and tubing are usually changed every 7 days or per agency policy.
- This specially designed needle (bent at 90-degree angle to its hub or wings) has a sharp-angled bevel and attached extension tubing with clamp and needleless cap. Huber needles can also be straight.
- It is inserted through the skin and into the rubber septum for central venous access.
- It prevents coring of the port.
- It produces an insertion tract that seals itself when it is removed.

Procedure

1. **Palpate** skin over **implanted infusion port.** ➤ *Rationale:* This identifies location and contours of the device.
2. Place thumb and forefinger of left hand on port (right hand if left-handed) and feel for septum with right hand. ➤ *Rationale:* This position stabilizes the port.
3. Numb the area with a topical anesthetic cream or ice, according to facility policy. Depending on the product used, the time for effective anesthesia may vary from a few minutes to 1 hr.
4. Clean skin with antimicrobial swab using a back-and-forth movement. Scrub for 30 sec.
5. Allow site to air dry for 30 sec. ➤ *Rationale:* Drying permits solution to work best against bacteria, fungi, and spores.
6. Affix syringe with 10 mL of normal saline into Huber needle extension tubing cap and prime tubing; leave syringe attached.

7. Remove clean gloves and dispose in appropriate container.
8. Apply mask according to facility policy, perform hand hygiene, and don sterile gloves.
9. Stabilize port using thumb and index finger or index finger and middle finger.
10. Insert needle into port at a 90-degree angle until it meets resistance from the stainless steel back of the port.
11. Check for correct placement by aspirating for blood return.
    a. Withdraw flash of blood to check needle position. If no blood is obtained, try repositioning client (sit up, raise arms, cough.)
    b. If still unable to obtain blood, try flushing port with small amount (2–3 mL) of normal saline.
    c. If no blood return, remove noncoring needle and reaccess port.
    d. If still unable to obtain blood, call the physician. (X-ray for placement may be required.)
12. If placement is correct, stabilize needle and inject remaining normal saline. There should be no sign of infiltration into surrounding tissue.

13. Close clamp of needle extension tubing.
14. Exchange syringe of normal saline for syringe filled with dilute heparin flush, then open clamp.
15. Instill 5 mL (in 10-mL syringe) of heparin flush (100 units/mL).
16. Clamp extension tubing before removing syringe.
17. Remove needle by pulling straight out from port while stabilizing port with free hand.
18. If needle is to be left in place for intermittent use, secure wings with tape for hub (chevron style) and apply sterile transparent dressing over all.
19. Dispose of equipment.
20. Remove gloves and perform hand hygiene.

Note: If CLC2000 device is used, follow directions for use in Skill 29.4.2, Using a Positive Pressure Device.

> **CLINICAL ALERT**
> Implanted ports have the lowest risk of infection of all chest-accessed central lines.

Skill 29.5.2 | Administering Drugs via a Subcutaneous Implanted Port

Equipment
Syringe filled with medication
Equipment as listed in previous skill
Syringe filled with 10 mL of saline
Syringe with 10 mL of dilute heparin solution

Procedure
1. Follow procedure listed in previous skill. (Using sterile gloves, verify correct placement of access port, i.e., blood return on aspiration, ability to infuse normal saline flush, and no infiltration.) ❶
2. Clamp short needle extension tubing. ❷
3. Exchange saline syringe for syringe filled with ordered medication.
4. Unclamp tubing.
5. Administer medication at prescribed rate.

6. Flush port between drugs with 5 mL of saline if giving more than one drug. ➤ *Rationale:* This prevents the possibility of drug–drug interactions.
7. Flush system with saline, then with dilute heparin.
8. Inject last 0.5 mL of heparin flush while simultaneously withdrawing needle and stabilizing port.
9. Wipe skin gently with dry swab to remove any solution.
10. If client is to receive intermittent IV drugs or solution, the Huber needle may remain in place for 1 week. After intermittent administration, clamp tubing, insert new sterile protective cap into extension tubing, open clamp to flush and heparinize, then reclamp tubing.
11. Flush used port with 5 mL heparin (100 units/mL) daily; if unused, flush monthly.
12. Dispose of equipment (including gloves) and perform hand hygiene.

Note: Change port dressing weekly or when wet or soiled.

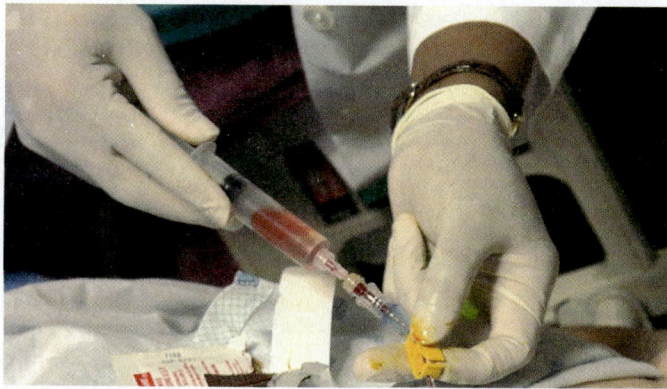

❶ Check for blood flashback when flushing CVAD (unless Groshong valve present).

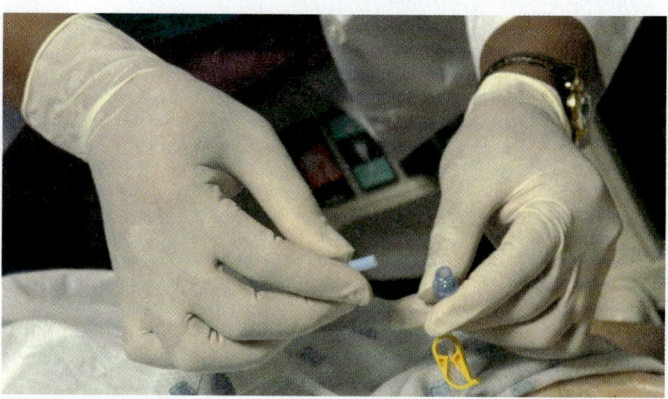

❷ Always have CVAD clamped when changing infusion cap (Groshong valve does not require clamp).

Skill 29.5.3 | Administering Infusions via a Subcutaneous Port

Equipment

Huber needle with attached extension tubing and in-line clamp
Intermittent infusion cap
5-mL syringe with needleless cannula
Two 10-mL syringes with needleless connector
Normal saline
Heparin (10 units/mL or 100 units/mL, according to facility policy) or normal saline
Antimicrobial swabs, 2% chlorhexidine gluconate
Sterile and clean gloves
Mask
Sterile gauze squares
Transparent dressing
Sterile tape
Prescribed IV solutions, drugs, or blood products

Preparation

1. Check physician's orders.
2. Gather equipment.
3. Identify client using two descriptors. Introduce self and explain procedure to client.
4. Provide privacy and raise bed to comfortable working position.
5. Perform hand hygiene.
6. Don clean gloves.

Procedure

1. Remove dressing, prepare site, and access port using sterile technique (sterile gloves and mask) as previously described.
2. Secure needle hub with sterile tape, or wings with tape or Steri-strips.
3. Place transparent dressing over insertion site, needle, and proximal IV tubing; date and initial.
4. Flush port with 10 mL of saline solution.
5. Proceed with administration of ordered solution, drug, or blood.

> **CLINICAL ALERT**
> Electrical controller device (pump) should be used for continuous IV infusion via CVAD.

6. Upon completion, flush with 10 mL of normal saline, followed by 5 mL of dilute heparin flush.
7. Clamp tubing before removing syringe to maintain positive pressure; cap tubing.
8. For continuous infusion, change tubing daily and dressing every 96 hr.
9. Dispose of equipment (including gloves) and perform hand hygiene.

Note: If using CLC2000 device, refer to Skill 29.4.2, Using a Positive Pressure Device.

Skill 29.5.4 | Drawing Blood From an Implanted Subcutaneous Port

Equipment

Huber 19-gauge needle with short extension tubing
Needleless injection cap or CLC2000 device
Two 10-mL syringes
Blood collection tubes
Heparin 3-mL and normal saline 10-mL flush solutions
Antimicrobial swabs, chlorhexidine gluconate
Sterile tape
Sterile gloves

Procedure

1. Gather equipment.
2. Check physician's orders for type of blood test.
3. Identify client using two descriptors and explain procedure to client. Introduce self.
4. Perform hand hygiene and don sterile gloves.
5. Access implanted port using Huber needle with capped extension tubing as discussed previously.
   a. Prep tubing cap or CLC2000 device with antimicrobial swab.
   b. Clean around junction of cap and hub with antimicrobial swab for 30 sec before removing cap or before inserting syringe into CLC2000 device.
6. Insert syringe into hub of extension tubing.

7. Unclamp tubing.
8. Withdraw 5–10 mL blood, remove syringe, and discard.
   > *Rationale:* This discards the filling volume of the catheter.
9. Maintain aseptic technique—attach new syringe to hub of extension tubing or insert into CLC2000 device. Withdraw appropriate amount of blood for tests and remove syringe.

> **CLINICAL ALERT**
> When drawing blood, attach syringe directly to hub of extension tubing. Never draw through an older type cap, as hemolysis can occur. Always place a new cap on extension tubing after withdrawing blood samples. Check the newer caps to determine if blood can be drawn through the cap.

10. Fill appropriate type of blood tubes with specified amount of blood according to tests ordered.
11. Flush catheter with 10 mL of saline solution after obtaining blood specimens.
12. Place new cap on extension tubing. CLC2000 device is changed every 24 hr.
13. Discard equipment.
14. Remove gloves and perform hand hygiene.

Unit 29.5 Documentation and Evaluation

DOCUMENTATION for Implanted Subcutaneous Port

- Condition of port implantation site
- Frequency and type of flushes
- Name and dosage of drugs or solutions administered
- Presence of Huber needle, if left in place
- Document gauge and length of Huber needle
- Dressing type
- Amount of blood withdrawn
- CLC2000 device if used

EVALUATION/Critical Thinking

Expected Outcomes

- Subcutaneous implanted port remains patent to facilitate medication administration.
- Client's subcutaneous port implantation site remains infection-free.
- Blood samples are obtained without difficulty.

Unexpected Outcomes	Alternative Actions
• Needle entry is painful.	• Use topical anesthetic or apply ice before accessing. • Use local anesthetic injected intradermally before inserting needle (check client sensitivity and agency policy).
• Occluded catheter.	• Change needle. If no improvement, suspect occluded catheter. • Try gentle aspiration to dislodge clot. • Never try to forcefully flush system—clot may mobilize; catheter may rupture. • Thrombolytic agent may be required to lyse fibrin clot (specialty nurse skill). • Transfuse packed red blood cells along with continuous infusion of normal saline; use an infusion pump; flush catheter well with 20 mL of normal saline after infusion to prevent occluded catheter.
• Inability to aspirate blood when checking placement.	• Needle may not be in port reservoir. • Tip of catheter may be against vessel wall. Try changing client's position from sitting up to lying or ask client to raise one or both arms. If appropriate, have client bear down or cough using Valsalva maneuver while irrigating with normal saline. • Heparinize catheter and return in 40 min to aspirate. • Removal of a fibrin clot, thrombolysis, is done by a certified IV nurse (according to agency policy).

(continued)

Unexpected Outcomes	Alternative Actions
• Pain, swelling at site.	• Suspect catheter rupture. Report to physician. • Suspect port migration and infusion infiltrating subcutaneously.
• Port becomes movable.	• Port may not be anchored securely. Port could be flipped under skin. • Silicone tubing has separated from port. • Always check for blood return to ensure accurate needle placement, before injecting medications. • Notify physician and prepare for removing port.

Peripherally Inserted Central Catheter (PICC)

Nursing Process Data

ASSESSMENT Database

- Assess length of exposed catheter.
- Assess that catheter is secure.
- Assess insertion site.
- Assess catheter patency.

PLANNING Objectives

- To provide access for infusion, parenteral nutrition, or drugs
- To provide access for blood sampling
- To provide patent access

IMPLEMENTATION Procedures

DOCUMENTATION AND EVALUATION

Expected Outcomes

- PICC remains patent without sign of infection.
- Catheter is irrigated at designated time frames.
- Transparent dressing remains intact for 7 days.

Unexpected Outcomes / Alternative Actions

Pearson Nursing Student Resources

Find additional review materials at
nursing.pearsonhighered.com.
Prepare for success with NCLEX®-style practice questions and Skill Checklists.

Skill 29.6.1 | Maintaining the PICC

Equipment

Pre-filled syringe with 10 mL of preservative-free normal saline (0.9%)

Pre-filled syringe with 20 mL of preservative-free normal saline

Pre-filled syringe with 3–5 mL of dilute heparin (10 units/mL) solution (per hospital policy)

Optional CLC2000

Sterile gloves

Antimicrobial swabs, 2% chlorhexidine gluconate

Transparent dressing

StatLock securement device

For Medication Administration

Medication IV bag

Two 10-mL syringes pre-filled with preservative-free 0.9% normal saline

Heparin flush according to facility policy

2% Chlorhexidine gluconate swabs

Note: Midline catheters are very similar to PICC lines, except they are shorter. The same policy and procedures apply to the care and maintenance of these lines (Box 29-15 ■).

Preparation

1. Check client care plan and MAR.
2. Introduce self and identify client using two descriptors.
3. Explain procedure to client and provide privacy.

Procedure

1. Perform hand hygiene and don gloves.
2. Assess IV site and surrounding area for signs of infection (i.e., erythema, tenderness, edema, and drainage).
3. Assess securement device site for stability, cleanliness, and intact dressing.

Box 29-15 PERIPHERALLY INSERTED CENTRAL CATHETER

PICCs are long, soft, flexible, single or multilumen catheters placed in basilic, cephalic, or brachial vein and advanced into the superior vena cava (SVC) for central venous access. The length of catheter is documented. Placement is less invasive and less expensive than other CVADs since they can be inserted by specially educated certified IV nurses. As with tunneled catheters, exit site below heart level decreases risk of air embolism when system is open to the atmosphere. PICC lines need to be checked by x-ray to verify tip placement if inserted into a proximal arm. Clients receiving TPN or vesicants should have tip inserted into SVC, and x-ray should be done to confirm position. Research has shown that PICC lines inserted into SVC have fewer complications such as inflammation or thrombosis.

Securement devices are now recommended to prevent catheter migration. These catheters may be used for long-term therapy. PICC lines can be left in place for at least 1 year.

Preservative-free 0.9% saline is recommended for flushing. Heparin is usually not recommended. Check facility policy regarding heparin usage and dose.

CLINICAL ALERT

If catheter tip is resting in the right atrium or pericardium instead of the superior vena cava, the tip can move across the muscle to the sinoatrial node (SA node) and can cause cardiac arrhythmias, cardiac rupture, or other associated conditions. The PICC catheter must be withdrawn 2.5 cm (1 in.) and a repeat x-ray taken to check for catheter placement.

All continuous infusions using a PICC line should be connected to an electric infusion device to maintain infusion and patency of line.

4. Swab catheter port with chlorhexidine swab for 30 sec. Allow to air dry for 30 seconds.
5. Inject pre-filled syringe with preservative-free 0.9% normal saline into catheter hub and aspirate. ➤ *Rationale:* This checks for patency.
6. Inject solution of 0.9% preservative-free sodium chloride (twice the internal volume of the CVD and injection cap) slowly; flush with minimal force using a pulsatile motion until syringe is almost empty. ➤ *Rationale:* This action creates turbulence for catheter cleansing. ❶ ❷

❶ Maintain PICC line with cleaning and irrigation.

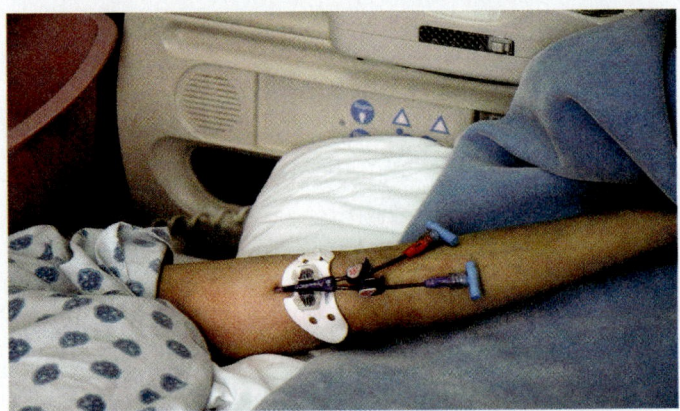

❷ Double-lumen PICC with positive pressure device.

7. Continue to inject flush while removing syringe from catheter port.
8. For medication administration:
   a. Perform hand hygiene.
   b. Check client using two identifiers.
   c. Don gloves, if facility policy.
   d. Remove protective tab from both the PICC tubing and the IV bag. (The tabs are usually brightly colored so you can easily identify them.)
   e. Push the pointed end of the tubing into the opening on the IV bag. Hold the bag up high and squeeze the drip chamber until it is half full.
   f. Open roller clamp and observe fluid run through tubing until all air is removed from tubing. Close roller clamp.
   g. Flush PICC line using saline solution and a push–pause technique.
   h. Attach needleless connector on PICC tubing to rubber cap of IV catheter. Unclamp catheter and adjust the roller clamp to prescribed rate.
   i. When IV bag is empty, clamp PICC tubing and remove tubing from rubber cap.
   j. Clean lumen with 2% chlorhexidine gluconate swab by vigorously rubbing port.
   k. Flush PICC line with saline using push–pause technique.
      ➤ **Rationale:** This avoids buildup of precipitates, which can occur in catheter occlusions.
   l. Flush PICC line with heparin according to facility policy.
   m. Clamp IV catheter.
9. Flush nonused catheter at least every 12 hr using push–pause technique. Times when flushing should be performed are listed in Box 29-16 ■.

10. Place discarded equipment in appropriate receptacle. Place syringe in sharps container.
11. Remove gloves and perform hand hygiene.

Note: The use of positive pressure devices is now suggested for catheter care.

EVIDENCE-BASED PRACTICE
Peripheral Intravenous Catheter Dwell Times
In 2010, the CDC indicated that peripheral IVs could remain in place for 96 hr or more as long as they were functioning properly and there were no signs of infection. The review described current research on the effectiveness of IV securement devices. Overwhelmingly, results demonstrated use of IV securement devices decreased complications associated with peripheral IV catheters, and prolonged their longevity and patency.

Source: Alekseyev et al. (2012)

Comparison of Three Types of Valved and Nonvalved Peripherally Inserted Central Catheters
Randomized studies investigated the impact of valved and nonvalved power-injectable, peripherally inserted central catheters (PICCs) in terms of three types of third-generation polyurethane PICCs that were compared. One hundred and eighty adult clients undergoing chemotherapy were randomly placed into three groups: power-injectable PICCs with a proximal valve, power-injectable PICCs with a pressure-activated safety valve, and nonvalved power-injectable PICCs. All PICCs were single lumen 4 Fr. and inserted according to a defined protocol. They were placed using maximal barrier protection and ultrasound guidance, and, according to recent guidelines for antisepsis, with 2% chlorhexidine. All catheters were flushed with 10-mL saline before and after each infusion or with 20 mL following blood sampling. No heparin was used.

No clinical advantage between the valved or nonvalved PICCs was found. There were no complications at insertion, PICC-related blood-stream infections, nor dislocations. There were five cases of transient occlusion and two cases of persistent withdrawal occlusion evenly distributed among the three groups. There were several other complications among the groups.

Source: Pittiruti et al. (2014)

CLINICAL ALERT
Pulsatile (Push–Pause) Flushing
Use a rapid succession of push–pause–push–pause movements exerted on the plunger of the syringe barrel. This motion creates a turbulence within the catheter lumen, which causes a swirling effect that moves fibrin, lipids, medications, or other adherents attached to the catheter lumen and prevents occlusions to the catheter.

Box 29-16 **TIMES FOR FLUSHING PROCEDURE**

Frequency
1. Check facility policy and follow protocol.
2. Suggested recommendations:
   a. Every 4–6 hr for no. 2 French or smaller catheters and after each use
   b. Every 8–12 hr for larger size catheters and after each use

Other Times
1. When LOCK is applied
2. After blood draws
3. After intermittent medication administration
4. After blood or blood component administration
5. After administration of TPN

Skill 29.6.2 | Changing the PICC Dressing

Equipment

Antimicrobial swabs, 2% chlorhexidine gluconate or alcohol swab

Securement device

Transparent semipermeable dressing

BIOPATCH disc (optional)

Clean gloves

Sterile gloves

Mask

Procedure

1. Identify client using two descriptors and check electronic medical record and client care plan for last dressing change (review facility policy and procedure).
2. Introduce self and explain procedure to client.
3. Perform hand hygiene and don mask and clean gloves.
4. Remove old transparent dressing by gently pulling in an upward direction. ❶ ➤ *Rationale:* This prevents dislodgement of the catheter.
5. Check site for bleeding, infection, or signs of phlebitis. ➤ *Rationale:* Bleeding may occur with arm use. Phlebitis is the most common complication.
6. Discard old dressing and gloves. Perform hand hygiene.

CLINICAL ALERT

Unless absolutely necessary, avoid blood pressure measurement in the arm with a PICC and avoid venipunctures on the extremity with a PICC line.

---

7. Prepare sterile supplies.
8. Don sterile gloves.
9. Clean exit site and catheter with antimicrobial swabs for 30 sec using back-and-forth movement. ❷

Note: The catheter is anchored by a securement device, which does not require suturing of the PICC line. Approximately 2.5 cm (1 in.) of catheter extends from the insertion site.

10. Allow time for antimicrobial solution to air dry. ❸ Do not blow on arm or wave your hand to hasten drying.
    ➤ *Rationale:* Waving a hand or blowing may contaminate the site; antibacterial action does not take effect until solution is dry.
11. Place securement device over catheter. ❹ ➤ *Rationale:* Catheter is not sutured in place, so securement device is used to prevent catheter migration. (Refer to Skill 29.1.6, Applying a Securement Device.)
12. Cover exit site with transparent semipermeable dressing. Avoid stretching the dressing. Press down on dressing to seal catheter site. No part of actual catheter should be outside transparent dressing.

Note: Transparent dressings are not occlusive; they allow air to circulate through the semipermeable dressing and thus prevent perspiration from collecting under the dressing.

13. Remove gloves, mask, and perform hand hygiene.
14. Initial and date dressing.
15. Change initial transparent dressing in 24 hr and then every 7 days or whenever it is soiled or loose. ➤ *Rationale:* First dressing change is done to check insertion site.

❶ Remove dressing by gently pulling in an upward direction.

❷ Cleanse site with chlorhexidine gluconate swab or alcohol swab using back-and-forth motion.

❸ Allow site to dry before applying dressing. Place transparent dressing over the site.

❹ StatLock device, the only evidence-based catheter stabilization device that meets national standards.

Skill 29.6.3 | Drawing Blood From the PICC

Equipment
Antimicrobial swabs—2% chlorhexidine gluconate
Two 10-mL syringes with needleless connector
20-mL syringe with needleless connector filled with saline
Two 10-mL syringes with preservative-free normal saline, 10–mL syringe with 3–5 mL of dilute heparin (check hospital policy as heparin is not usually used), and needleless connector
Clean gloves

Preparation
1. Check physician orders.
2. Identify client using two descriptors. Introduce self and explain procedure to client.
3. Perform hand hygiene and don gloves.

Procedure
1. Stop all infusing fluids for at least 1 min before drawing a specimen.

2. Swab catheter cap with antimicrobial swab for 30 sec and allow to air dry.
3. Use 10-mL syringe and withdraw 5 mL of blood and discard appropriately in biohazard container. Check facility policy and procedure for amount to discard.
4. Use 10-mL syringe with needleless connector and withdraw required amount of blood for laboratory tests. Do not use Vacutainer. ➤ **Rationale:** Catheter will collapse with intense vacuum.
5. Change cap after all blood draws and transfusions. Flush with 20 mL of saline solution to clear catheter.
6. Complete procedure with dilute heparin flush (unless Groshong valve present).
7. Discard equipment and gloves; perform hand hygiene.
8. Handle blood sample appropriately. Transfer to collection tube.

Skill 29.6.4 | Removing the PICC

Equipment
Gloves
10-mL syringe pre-filled with 0.9% preservative-free sodium chloride
Sterile 2×2 gauze
Tape

Procedure
1. Check healthcare provider's order.
2. Introduce self and identify client using two descriptors.

3. Explain the procedure to the client. Client may be in bed or sitting in a chair, however, the preferred position is lying flat in bed to prevent air embolism.
4. Perform hand hygiene and don gloves.
5. Clean exit site and catheter with antimicrobial swab for 30 sec and allow to air dry.
6. Flush catheter with 0.9% sodium chloride.
7. Carefully remove dressing, loosening edges toward insertion site. Remove Steri-strip on securement device.
8. Grasp catheter at insertion site.
9. Gradually pull catheter parallel to skin 2.5 cm (1 in.) at a time.

(continued)

Skill 29.6.4 | Removing the PICC (continued)

10. Continue inching catheter out. If resistance is felt, stop and reposition arm, wait 15 seconds.
11. After removal, measure length of catheter and compare to documented length on chart.
12. Culture tip according to facility policy. Cut tip with sterile scissors and place in sterile container. Be careful not to contaminate tip when withdrawing blood from vein.
13. Hold gauze at exit site for hemostasis.
14. Apply tape to gauze securely, making an occlusive dressing. Leave in place for 24 hr.
15. Dispose of catheter in biohazard container.
16. Document length of catheter removed.
17. Monitor site and notify physician or IV therapist if needed (Box 29-17 ■)

CLINICAL ALERT
NEVER FORCE catheter removal (apply warm, moist pack to upper arm to relax vein for approximately 15 min).

Box 29-17 **WHEN TO NOTIFY PHYSICIAN OR IV THERAPIST**

- Infusion leaking from insertion site
- Inconsistent flow rates
- Inability to infuse fluids
- Excessive bleeding or drainage at insertion site
- Chest, neck, or ear pain; numbness or tingling of affected arm
- Swelling, pain, redness, palpable cord at or above insertion site

Unit 29.6 Documentation and Evaluation

DOCUMENTATION for the Peripherally Inserted Central Catheter

- Site labeled "PICC" to ensure proper use of line.
- Frequency of flush and type of solution
- Type of dressing applied and labeled date, time, initials, and "PICC"
- Site assessment
- Length of exposed catheter
- Amount of blood withdrawn for specimen

- Solutions or drugs administered, including flow rate
- Electronic infusion device utilized

For Discontinuing PICC
- Condition and length of catheter
- Site assessment
- Client's response to treatment and procedure
- Catheter tip sent to lab for culture, if appropriate

EVALUATION/Critical Thinking

Expected Outcomes
- PICC remains patent without signs of infection or migration.
- Catheter is irrigated at designated time.
- StatLock remains in place.
- Transparent dressing remains intact for 7 days.

Unexpected Outcomes	**Alternative Actions**
Mechanical phlebitis (pain, redness spreading to surrounding tissue) occurs.	Apply warm, moist compresses for 20 min 4 times a day. Elevate the arm and encourage mild exercise. Report problem—anti-inflammatory drugs may correct problem and prevent PICC removal.
Bleeding occurs at insertion site.	Apply direct pressure on insertion site. Check client's coagulation profile (bleeding time, platelet count, PT, PTT) for coagulation problem. Consider removal if excessive bleeding persists after using pressure.

Unexpected Outcomes	Alternative Actions
• Exudate occurs at insertion site.	• Notify physician or IV therapist. • Send specimen to lab for culture. • Maintain aseptic technique during site care.
• Solution does not infuse.	• Increase volume of flush solution. • Utilize infusion pump or elevate infusion bag for gravity pressure. • Flush with a push–pull motion and clamp catheter before removing syringe. • Report problem—thrombolytic declotting may be necessary.
• Pain in shoulder or neck occurs during infusion—or client hears gurgling sound with flush.	• Report so x-ray can validate catheter placement (catheter may have migrated with client maneuvers).
• Sepsis occurs (rare).	• Monitor client for fever and assess insertion site for drainage, tenderness, and redness. • PICC may be removed—send tip to lab for culture.

Chapter Wrap-Up

GERONTOLOGIC Considerations

Older Adult Clients Requiring Chemotherapy or Parenteral Nutrition Are Good Candidates for Implanted Vascular Access Devices

With an implanted vascular access device:

• Decreased amounts of fluids can be administered to prevent fluid overload.
• Risk of infection is decreased, which is a concern in older adults. Frequency and severity of infection tend to increase with age due to a decline in the immune response.

• Repeated IV punctures are not necessary, so veins are preserved and discomfort minimized.
• Greater client mobility is achieved.

With Aging, Epidermal Turnover Decreases and Skin Fragility Increases; Even Minimal Trauma May Result in Serious Erosion
Healthcare Providers or Family Members Can Be Instructed to Provide Medication Administration, Fluid Therapy, or Parenteral Nutrition at Home

MANAGEMENT Guidelines

Each state legislates a Nurse Practice Act for RNs and LVN/LPNs. Healthcare facilities are responsible for establishing and implementing policies and procedures that conform to their state's regulations. Verify the regulations and role parameters for each healthcare worker in your facility.

Delegation

• Each state identifies the scope of practice for RNs and LVN/LPNs. Several states have identified that the LVN/LPN has a specific role in IV therapy, but the scope of practice is always dictated by each agency (e.g., initiating,

regulating, discontinuing IVs). The LPN/LVN educated in IV therapy is the minimum level practitioner to assist in tasks delegated by the RN for the delivery of IV therapy. The RN may be assisted by an LVN/LPN educated in IV therapy, but the RN remains responsible for the care given.

• Policies outlining the responsibility of the IV nurse vary significantly among agencies. A written policy should clearly outline all aspects of this role, and all staff should be familiar with its scope. Policies and procedures should follow national guidelines and standards of practice established by the Centers for Disease Control and

Prevention, the American Association of Blood Banks, and the IV Nurses Society. All nurses must be aware of the many physical hazards associated with IV therapy and related OSHA rules to be observed.

- Central line catheter management must be done by an RN.
- The nurse who delivers IV therapy must be qualified by specific knowledge and experience to perform such highly specialized skills.
- TPN and lipids may be administered only by an RN according to specific physician's orders.
- The CNA/UAP providing personal hygiene must understand that the IV system is a closed one and must be able to give care without disrupting the system. The components of the CVAD system must never be disconnected. Doing so places the client at risk for infection and air embolism. The CNA/UAP should receive training in changing the client's gown without disrupting the CVAD system.
- For the client with a CVAD allowed to shower, the RN should disconnect infusion lines, place a dry sterile gauze (4×4) over the dressed site and exposed tubing(s), then cover all with a large transparent dressing for waterproofing. Post-shower removal of the covering and inspection of the dressing should also be performed by the RN.

Interprofessional Communication

While the professional monitors the IV infusion site regularly, the CNA/UAP provides vital data to the professional nurse by immediately reporting:

- Observations of redness or swelling around the CVAD insertion site (signs of possible infiltration, hematoma, sepsis)
- Presence of crepitus (bubble-wrap feeling) on the client's chest (sign of possible subcutaneous emphysema that can lead to respiratory distress)
- Observations of respiratory distress in any client with recent (24 hr) placement of a central line (symptoms of possible pneumothorax)
- Any client complaint of arm, shoulder, or neck pain (symptom of possible thrombosis or infiltration)
- Temperature elevation (fever—a sign of possible catheter-related infection if otherwise unexplainable)
- Infusion device alarms to prompt the professional to further assess the client
- Presence of blood backup in the catheter
- A loose or soiled/wet dressing

CASE STUDY Applications

Scenario 1

Mr. John Baker is a 68-year-old retired pharmacist who has just returned from surgery after placement of a tunneled CVAD with a Groshong valve. He will be started on a long-term intermittent chemotherapy regimen for acute lymphocytic leukemia. His wife is a retired RN who worked in the operating room for many years.

1. Identify at least three advantages for inserting the tunneled catheter for his treatment.
2. His wife is very concerned about the initial care of the catheter. What explanation will you give her?
3. After the explanation regarding the care of the catheter, Mrs. Baker asks you how they can prevent an infection of the catheter.
4. The client needs to be instructed on how to flush the catheter. What are the most important directions you should provide to him?

5. Mrs. Baker asks you to describe what symptoms require reporting to the physician. What is your best response to this question?

Scenario 2

Seth Eley, age 24, has been admitted to your unit with the diagnosis of inflammatory bowel disease with exacerbation of fever, severe diarrhea, right lower quadrant pain, weight loss, and anemia. Short-term total parenteral nutrition and bowel rest are planned. A triple-lumen central venous catheter has been placed for these purposes.

1. Based on these data, what generalizations can you make about the purpose of hyperalimentation for this client?
2. Why is central venous access necessary?
3. Develop several scenarios about the most common complications of central catheter placement.
4. How does TPN affect fluid and electrolyte balance?

NCLEX® Review Questions

Unless otherwise specified, choose only one (1) answer.

1. What is the best device for long-term IV therapy?
   A. Peripherally inserted central vascular catheter
   B. Midline catheter placed in the basilic vein
   C. Peripheral catheter placed in the antecubital vein
   D. Long-line catheter threaded into the right atrium

2. Which of the following is included in guidelines to prevent catheter-related bloodstream infections?
   A. Using good hygiene principles
   B. Using a catheter impregnated with an antibiotic agent
   C. Preparing the IV site with Betadine or alcohol swabs
   D. Placing a mask on the client when inserting a PICC line

3. You are preparing the site for an IV insertion of a PICC line. Which one of the following drying times is required when using chlorhexidine gluconate 2% with alcohol?

A. 30 seconds
B. 1 min
C. 2 min
D. 3 min

4. How often should primary and secondary continuous IV administration sets be replaced if there are no signs and symptoms of infection?

A. 24 hr
B. 48 hr
C. 72 hr
D. 96 hr

5. When assessing the client's IV that is infusing a parenteral nutrition solution, you find it is not infusing at the prescribed rate. What is your priority intervention?

A. Recalculate the amount of solution and time remaining for the infusion and set the flow rate at that newly calculated rate.
B. Notify the physician immediately and have a new IV catheter available for insertion by the physician.
C. Change the dressing to ensure it was not too tight, causing the change in IV flow rate.
D. Observe the filter, because a plugged filter is the most common cause of infusion failure.

6. Place in sequence the steps for obtaining a central venous pressure reading.

A. Turn stopcock so manometer and IV solution are open to each other.
B. Close clamp and rotate stopcock so IV solution is open to client.
C. Open clamp on IV tubing and fill manometer to 18–20 cm (8 in.).
D. Turn stopcock to the manometer → client position and obtain reading.

7. A client is admitted to the healthcare facility and has an implanted port in place for chemotherapy. How often do instructions for care of the port say to flush the port?

A. Weekly with heparin
B. Daily with normal saline
C. Monthly and after each use
D. Every 12 hr

8. The physician has ordered a blood sample using a central line catheter. Which one of the following steps will be implemented after turning off the IV flush infusion for 1 min?

A. Flush the catheter with normal saline.
B. Swab the cap and hub with antimicrobial swabs.
C. Remove the cap from the syringe.
D. Flush the catheter with 10 mL of normal saline.

9. The client has a medication order to be administered through a subcutaneous implanted port. Which one of the following steps is appropriate for this procedure?

A. Scrub the site over the port using a Betadine solution for 1 min.
B. Insert a 10-mL syringe with a large-bore needle and withdraw 10 mL of blood and discard the sample.
C. Insert a Huber needle into the port at a 90-degree angle until it meets resistance.
D. After infusion is complete, flush the port with normal saline and remove the needle by pulling it out at a 60-degree angle.

10. What is the major advantage of using a positive pressure device, such as a CLC2000?

A. The positive pressure device ensures ease of obtaining blood samples from the IV site.
B. The device maintains an accurate IV solution at the prescribed rate.
C. It maintains sterility at the junction of the IV tubing and the cap.
D. It prevents blood from being drawn back into the catheter when the flush syringe is removed.

QSEN Activity

Domain: Evidence-Based Practice

KSA: Attitudes

Activity:

Select one of the following topics and review an evidence-based research project: flushing a Hickman or Broviac catheter or drawing blood from an implanted subcutaneous port. After reading the article, be prepared to discuss the changes in nursing care that have occurred within the last 5 years related to the skill. Discuss changes in equipment, in irrigation of the port or catheter, and in methods to prevent infection that have occurred as examples.

Be prepared to demonstrate the findings of your research, such as cleansing the port or irrigating the port.

Bring the research article to class and obtain the equipment to demonstrate the skill.

Bibliography

Alekseyev, S., Byrne, M., Carpenter, A., Franker, C., Kidd, C., & Hulton, L. (2012). Prolonging the life of a patient's IV: An integrative review of intravenous securement devices. *Medsurg Nursing, 21*(5), 285–92.

Alexander, M., Corrigan, A., Gorski, L., Hankins, J., & Perucca, R. (2010). *Infusion nursing: An evidenced-based approach* (3rd ed.). St. Louis, MO: Saunders/Elsevier, Ch. 25, p. 503.

Alexandrou, E., Ramjan, L. M., Spencer, T., Frost, S. A., Salamonson, Y., Davidson, P. M., & Hillman, K. M. (2011). The use of midline catheters in the adult acute care setting—Clinical implications and recommendations for practice. *Journal of the Association for Vascular Access, 16*(1), 35–38, 40–41.

American Society of Anaesthesiologists. (2012, Mar.). Practice guidelines for central venous access. *A Report by the American Society of Anesthesiologists Task Force on Central Venous Access, 116*(3), 539–573.

Association of Professionals for Infection Control and Epidemiology (APIC). (2009). *Guide to the elimination of catheter-related bloodstream infections. An APIC guide.* http://www.apic.org/Resource_/EliminationGuideForm/259c0594-17b0-459d-b395-fb143321414a/File/APIC-CRBSI-Elimination-Guide.pdf

Bard Access Systems (n.d.). StatLock IV stabilization device for BD INTIMA™ catheters: Clinical outcomes. Retrieved from http://www.bardaccess.com/statlock-piv-bd-intima-cath.php?section=Clinical Outcomes

Bartock, L. (2010). An evidence-based systematic review of literature for the reduction of PICC line occlusions. *Journal of the Association for Vascular Access, 15*(2), 58–63.

Biggs, T. C., Mohammed, A., & Mulvihill, D. (2012). Importance of securing central venous catheters. *Anaesthesia and Intensive Care, 40*(2), 366–367.

Brown, D., & Rowland, K. (2013). Optimal timing for peripheral IV replacement. *The Journal of Family Practice, 62*(4), 200–202.

Camp-Sorrell, M., & Camp-Sorrell, D. (2010). *Access device guidelines: Recommendations for nursing practice and education* (3rd ed.). Pittsburgh, PA: Oncology Nursing Society.

Casey, A. L, Mermel, L. A, Nightingale, P., Elliott, T. S. (2008, Dec.). Antimicrobial central venous catheters in adults: A systematic review and meta-analysis. *The Lancet Infectious Diseases, 8*(12), 763–776. doi:10.1016/S1473-3099(08)70280-9

Centers for Disease Control and Prevention. (2011). Checklist for prevention of central line associated blood stream infections. Retrieved from http://www.cdc.gov/HAI/pdfs/bsi/checklist-for-CLABSI.pdf

Daniels, K. R., & Frei, C. R. (2012). Antimicrobial-impregnated discs for prevention of intravenous catheter-related infections. *American Journal of Infectious Diseases, 8*(1), 50–59.

Dychter, S. S., Gold, D. A., Carson, D., & Haller, M. (2012). Intravenous therapy: A review of complications and economic considerations of peripheral access. *Journal of Infusion Nursing, 35*(2), 84–91.

Gabriel, J. (2013, Oct.). Preventing and managing complications of CVADs. *Nursing Times, 109*, 20–23.

Genentech. (n.d.) About central venous access devices. Retrieved from http://www.gene.com/patients/disease-education/central-venous-access-devices-cvads

Institute for Healthcare Improvement. (2012). How-to guide: Prevent central line infections. Retrieved from http://www.ihi.org/resources/Pages/Tools/howtoGuidePreventCentralLineAssociatedBloodstreamInfection.aspx

Kayyali, A., & Joy, S. D. S. (2014). Preventing central line infections with 'Quality Nurse.' *The American Journal of Nursing, 114*(7), 55.

Labeau, S., Vereecke, A., Vandijck, D. M., Claes, B., & Blot, S. I. (2008). Critical care nurses' knowledge of evidence-based guidelines for preventing infections associated with central venous catheters: An evaluation questionnaire. *American Journal of Critical Care, 17*(1), 65–71.

Miller, D. L., & O'Grady, N. P. (2012, Aug.). Guidelines for the prevention of intravascular catheter-related infections: Recommendations relevant to interventional radiology for venous catheter placement and maintenance. *Journal of Vascular and Interventional Radiology, 23*(8), 997–1007.

Mutters, N. T., Günther, F., Heininger, A., & Frank, U. (2014). Device-related infections in long-term healthcare facilities: The challenge of prevention. *Future Microbiology, 9*(4), 487–495. http://dx.doi.org/10.2217/fmb.14.12

New, K. A., Webster, J., Marsh, N., & Hewer, B. (2014). Intravascular device use, management, documentation and complications: A point prevalence survey. *Australian Health Review, 38*(3), 345–349.

O'Grady, N. P., Alexander, M., Burns, L. A., Dellinger, E. P., Garland J., Heard, S. O., . . . & the Healthcare Infection Control Practices Advisory Committee (HICPAC). (2011). Guidelines for the prevention of intravascular catheter-related infections. HICPAC Publications. Centers for Disease Control and Prevention. http://www.cdc.gov/hicpac/pdf/guidelines/bsi-guidelines-2011.pdf

Paolucci, H., Nutter, B., & Albert, N. (2011). RN knowledge of vascular access devices management. *Journal of the Association for Vascular Access, 16*(4), 221–225.

Pittiruti, M., Emoli, A., Porta, P., Marche, B., DeAngelis, R., & Scoppettuolo, G. (2014). A prospective, randomized comparison of three different types of valved and non-valved peripherally inserted central-catheters. *The Journal of Vascular Access, 15*(6), 519–523.

Ruiz, R. R., Keever, M. A. V., Novales, M. G. M., Martinez, D. C., Muñoz, G. C. B., & Clark, P. (2011, Sep.–Oct.). Efficacy of a chlorhexidine-gluconate impregnated patch for prevention of catheter-related infections in pediatric patients: Systematic review and meta-analysis. *Boletin Medico del Hospital Infantil Mexico, 68*(5), 349–355.

Sacks, G. D., Diggs, B. S., Hadjizacharia, P., Green, D., Salim, A., & Malinoski, D. J. (2014). Reducing the rate of catheter-associated bloodstream infections in a surgical intensive care unit using the Institute for Healthcare Improvement central line bundle. *The American Journal of Surgery, 207*(6), 817–823. http://dx.doi.org/10.1016/j.amjsurg.2013.08.041

Safdar, N., O'Horo, J. C., Ghufran, A., Bearden, A., Didier, M.E., Chateau, D., Maki, D. G. (2014, Jul.). Chlorhexidine-impregnated dressing for prevention of catheter-related bloodstream infection: A meta-analysis. *Critical Care Medicine, 42*(7), 1703–13. Retrieved from doi:10.1097/CCM.0000000000000319.

Save the Vein Campaign. (n.d.) http://www.annanurse.org/resources/save-the-vein-campaign

Shah, H., Bosch, W., Thompson, K. M., & Hellinger, W. C. (2013, Jul.). Elucidation of the pathogenesis of catheter-related bloodstream infections. *Neurohospitalist. 3*(3), 144–151.

Spratt, D., Dutton, R. P., Dellinger, E. P., Bird, B., Guglielmi, C. L., Farber, M., & Groah, L. (2012). The role of the healthcare professions in preventing surgical site infection. *AORN Journal, 95*(4), 430–440.

Timsit, J. F. (2009, Apr. 14). Chlorhexidine gluconate-impregnated sponges reduced rate of catheter-related infections in ICU. *JAMA, 301*, 1231–1241.

Toomey, M. (2013). Preoperative chlorhexidine anaphylaxis in a patient scheduled for coronary artery bypass graft: A case report. *AANA Journal, 81*(3), 209–214.

Wall, J. (2014, Jun. 7). Chlorhexidine gluconate-impregnated central-line dressings and necrosis in complicated skin disorder patients. *Journal of Critical Care, 29*(6), 1130.e1–4. http://www.ncbi.nlm.nih.gov/pubmed/25035049

Zhani, E. A. (2014). Joint Commission alerts organizations to tubing misconnection risks. Retrieved Sep. 10, 2014, from http://www.jointcommission.org/joint_commission_alerts_organizations_to_tubing_misconnection_risks/

Chapter 30
Respiratory Care

 Learning Objectives

30.1 Outline the three processes of respiration.

30.2 Identify three nursing diagnoses for clients with ventilatory dysfunction.

30.3 Describe the steps for teaching a client deep breathing and coughing exercises.

30.4 Discuss the purpose of using an incentive spirometer.

30.5 Describe the steps for peak flow measurement.

30.6 Describe positions for postural drainage and chest percussion and vibration.

30.7 Differentiate modes of oxygen delivery and describe nursing care relevant to each mode.

30.8 Differentiate various modes of airway maintenance.

30.9 Outline the care needs of the intubated client.

30.10 Describe the nursing actions included in tracheostomy care.

30.11 Explain the procedure for inflating a tracheal tube cuff.

30.12 Describe safety measures used when suctioning clients.

30.13 List measures to promote safe, effective care for clients with chest tubes.

Chapter Outline

Terminology

Acidosis accumulation of acids (metabolic or respiratory), potentially disturbing acid–base balance and causing acidemia (low pH).

Adventitious abnormal extra sounds (crackles, wheezes) superimposed on breath sounds.

Alkalosis condition in which the alkalinity of the body tends to increase beyond normal, potentially resulting in alkalemia (high blood pH).

Apnea cessation of breathing, usually of a temporary nature.

Atelectasis collapse of alveoli, which may lead to hypoxemia, increased PCO_2, and pneumonia.

Crackles discontinuous popping (opening) sounds indicative of hypoventilation of alveoli, usually auscultated at end of inspiration in dependent lung areas.

Cyanosis bluish or grayish discoloration of the skin resulting from significant reduction of oxygen saturation of hemoglobin.

Dyspnea a subjective feeling of having difficulty breathing.

Expectorant an agent that facilitates the removal of airway secretions.

Hyperventilation abnormally deep breathing that results in a decrease in PCO_2 (respiratory alkalosis).

Hypoventilation reduced rate and depth of breathing resulting in retention of carbon dioxide (respiratory acidosis).

Hypoxemia insufficient oxygenation of the blood (decreased PO_2).

Hypoxia lack of adequate amount of oxygen transported to the tissues.

Intubation insertion of a tube into a body opening, as into the trachea.

Narcosis unconscious state due to narcotics or other depressing agent (e.g., elevated PCO_2).

Peak flow meter device measuring maximum rate of air flow out of lungs during forced expiration; used to monitor lung capacity in asthma—called also *peak expiratory flow meter.*

PEP an abbreviation that means positive expiratory pressure.

Percussion rhythmic striking of the thorax to loosen pulmonary secretions.

Pneumothorax presence of air in the intrapleural space resulting in lung collapse.

Postural drainage the use of gravity to drain secretions from the airways.

Spirometer a device used for measuring inhalation and exhalation volumes.

Sputum substance expelled by coughing.

Tension pneumothorax lung collapse with potential contralateral shift of mediastinal structures resulting from accumulation of air or fluid in the intrapleural space.

Tracheostomy surgical opening into the trachea, usually for insertion of a tube to provide airway patency.

Ventilation the acts of inspiration and exhalation for the exchange of oxygen and carbon dioxide between the lungs and the atmosphere.

Vibration therapeutic high-frequency shaking of a body part.

Vital capacity breathing capacity of lungs expressed as inches^3 or centimeters^3 of air that can be forcibly exhaled after a full inspiration.

Wheezes musical adventitious sounds heard on inspiration or expiration due to airway spasm, retained secretions, or other obstruction.

The Respiratory System

The respiratory system provides for the exchange of gases between the blood and the external environment so that cellular respiration can occur. The respiratory structures involved include the nose, pharynx, larynx, trachea, bronchi, lungs, diaphragm, intercostal muscles, and ribs (Figure 30-1 ■).

The upper respiratory tract includes the nose, pharynx, and larynx. These structures filter, warm, and humidify the air before it passes into the lower airways. When the upper respiratory tract is bypassed by **intubation** or **tracheostomy**, these protective processes are lost.

The lower respiratory tract is considered a sterile environment. It begins below the larynx. The trachea is composed of smooth muscle reinforced by C-shaped rings of cartilage lined with a membranous sheath. It branches into the right and left mainstream bronchi. The right bronchus extends vertically from the trachea, whereas the left bronchus branches from the trachea at an angle. The right and left bronchi divide further and further into terminal bronchioles and finally into respiratory bronchioles, alveolar ducts, and alveoli.

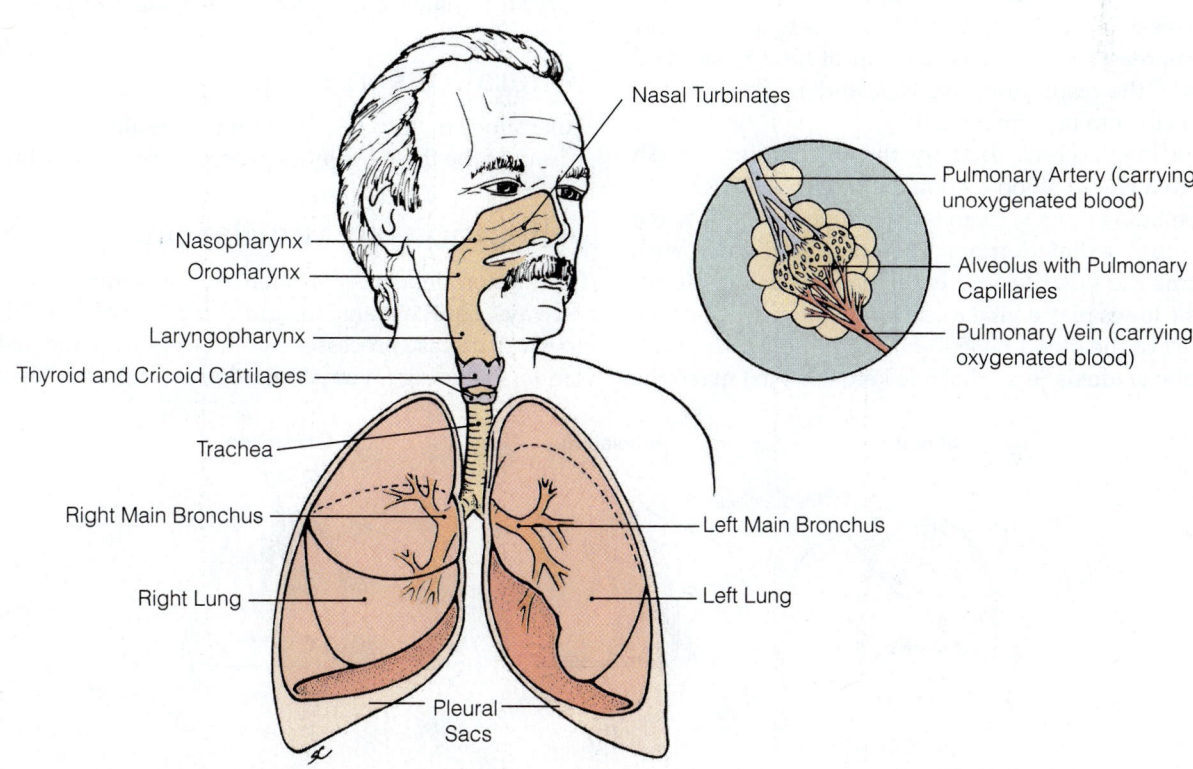

Nasal Turbinates

Pulmonary Artery (carrying unoxygenated blood)

Alveolus with Pulmonary Capillaries

Pulmonary Vein (carrying oxygenated blood)

Nasopharynx

Oropharynx

Laryngopharynx

Thyroid and Cricoid Cartilages

Trachea

Right Main Bronchus

Right Lung

Left Main Bronchus

Left Lung

Pleural Sacs

FIGURE 30-1 Anatomy of the respiratory system.

Because of the anatomical difference of the bronchi, migration of an endotracheal tube (ET) into the right bronchus occurs more frequently. Such a migration would result in ventilation of only the right lung. Chest x-rays are taken to ensure proper placement of ET tubes in the trachea. Auscultation of *bilateral* breath sounds also helps to verify optimal ventilation of intubated clients.

Protective processes of the lower airway include mucus secretion and the presence of special hairlike cells (cilia). This "mucociliary escalator" continuously traps and moves inhaled irritants up toward the pharynx to be removed by swallowing or coughing. Drying pharmacologic agents and pathophysiologic states (e.g., immobility) interfere with these protective processes and place the client at risk for pulmonary complications.

Processes of Respiration

Cellular respiration occurs when oxygen is transported from the atmosphere to tissue cells, and carbon dioxide is removed and carried from the cells to the atmosphere. RBC hemoglobin is the carrier for these gases. Three processes—ventilation, diffusion, and perfusion—are essential for this to occur.

Ventilation is the mechanical exchange of air between the lungs and the atmosphere. *Inspiration* is the *active* phase of ventilation. It requires contraction of the diaphragm and external intercostal muscles to expand the thorax (Figure 30-2 ■). When thoracic expansion occurs, intrapulmonic pressure becomes negative compared with atmospheric pressure, and air flows into the lungs. *Exhalation* is the *passive* phase of ventilation. It occurs when alveolar pressure increases due to elastic recoil of lung tissue and relaxation of the respiratory muscles, and air flows out of the lungs back into the atmosphere.

Ventilation is controlled by the brainstem, which responds to a rise in blood carbon dioxide level (PCO_2). As breathing eliminates CO_2, there is a negative feedback to the brain. Through exhalation of carbon dioxide (which with water forms the volatile acid carbonic acid in the bloodstream), the lungs play a vital role in maintaining the normal alkaline pH of the blood (7.35–7.45). Conditions that result in metabolic **acidosis** (e.g., diabetic ketoacidosis) make the

blood more acidic, also stimulating the brainstem to increase the rate and depth of breathing. The resultant lowering of PCO_2 (exhalation of volatile acid or respiratory **alkalosis**) helps return the blood pH to an alkaline state. This process is called respiratory compensation for metabolic acidosis.

Although CO_2 is the major stimulus for breathing, high sustained levels of carbonic acid depress the respiratory center, and respiratory arrest can occur. Individuals who have chronically elevated PCO_2 levels due to chronic obstructive pulmonary disease (COPD) may become insensitive to PCO_2 as a stimulus for breathing. Instead, their brain responds to a lower than normal PO_2 (less than 60 mm Hg) to stimulate breathing. The administration of high flows of oxygen to such "hypoxic-dependent breathers" can eliminate their stimulus to breathe. Such individuals are at high risk for CO_2 **narcosis**.

Diffusion is the process of gas exchange between the alveolar air and the blood. The respiratory unit (respiratory bronchiole, alveolar ducts, and alveoli) is surrounded by capillaries, which allow for this exchange of oxygen and carbon dioxide. Alveoli must be ventilated and must remain diffusible for gas exchange to prevent respiratory failure. Oxygen tension in blood flowing through alveolar capillaries is *lower* than the oxygen tension in the alveoli. This pressure gradient causes oxygen to pass from the alveoli to the blood, thus increasing the PO_2 and "arterializing" the blood. Conversely, carbon dioxide tension is *higher* in the capillary blood than it is in the alveoli, thus promoting its diffusion into alveoli and the elimination of carbon dioxide on exhalation.

Perfusion is the process of circulating oxygen and carbon dioxide between the lungs and tissue cells. Without this blood transport and exchange of gases at both the pulmonary and tissue capillary levels, survival is impossible.

Alterations in Respiration

Alterations in tissue respiration can result from dysfunction of any of the three essential processes previously outlined.

Alterations in Ventilation

Ventilation depends on patent airways, the ability to clear airways, chest expansion, and compliant alveoli. Many factors and disease processes can interfere with adequate ventilation, including (1) any limitation in ability to clear airways

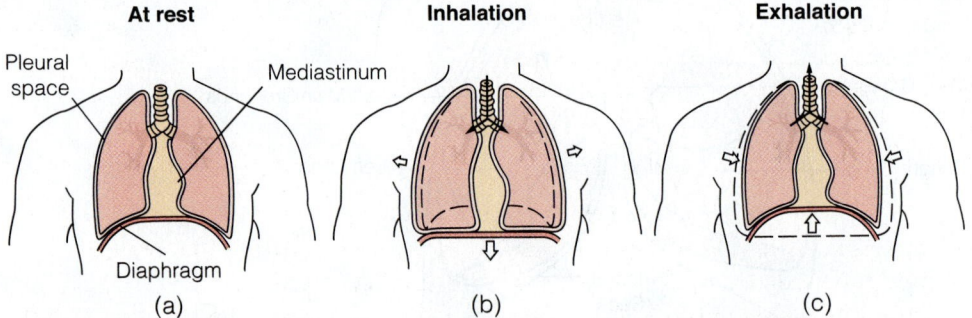

FIGURE 30-2 Diaphragm contracts and descends on inspiration. Diaphragm relaxes and ascends on expiration.

(ineffective cough, intubation, decreased level of consciousness); (2) any limitation of alveolar expansion (pneumonia, congestive heart failure, fractured ribs, pain, thoracic deformity, neurologic disease, respiratory depressants, immobility); and (3) factors that interfere with surfactant activity, which is essential for alveolar inflation (narcotics, anesthetics, **hypoventilation**, high oxygen flow rates). Inadequate ventilation results in abnormal arterial blood gases (ABGs) (low PO_2 and low SaO_2, and eventually, an increase in PCO_2).

Pathologic processes that cause ineffective exhalation due to loss of elasticity (overcompliance) of small airways and alveoli also result in an increased PCO_2 (respiratory acidosis). COPD is an example.

Alterations in Diffusion

Diffusion is dependent on a partial pressure difference in gases and an adequate amount of permeable alveolar surface area. Any disease that thickens the alveolar membrane (fibrosis, congestive heart failure) reduces alveolar permeability and leads to a reduced PO_2 (**hypoxemia**). Alveolar surface area can be reduced by lobectomy or pneumonectomy.

Alterations in Perfusion

For cells to receive oxygen and give off their wastes, blood must flow at both the pulmonary and tissue capillary levels. Adequate perfusion depends on a normal blood volume, an adequate amount of hemoglobin capable of combining with oxygen and carbon dioxide, effective cardiac function, and competent vasculature. Any pathology that interferes with blood cell production, maintenance of blood volume, cardiac function, or vascular patency can result in inadequate tissue perfusion. Likewise, any factor that prevents blood from flowing through pulmonary capillaries (pulmonary embolism) disrupts the process of gas exchange for replenishment of oxygen and the elimination of carbon dioxide.

Assessment of Respiratory Function

ABGs and pulmonary function tests reflect pulmonary capacity. The pH of the blood is affected by pulmonary function. If carbon dioxide is not eliminated by the lungs due to hypoventilation for any reason, the PCO_2 rises. Since CO_2 creates an acid in the bloodstream, its accumulation (respiratory acidosis) causes the blood pH to decrease (acidemia). See Box 30-1 ■ for manifestations of hypoventilation. *Hypoventilation* is the only mechanism for PCO_2 accumulation and is encountered when factors depress the respiratory center, inhibit breathing, or a client has a disease, such as COPD, that prevents efficient exhalation. The peak flow meter measures maximum expiratory flow rates. These units are used by asthma clients to regularly self-assess. A declining flow rate (by 20%) may indicate a worsening condition. Serial measurements help the healthcare provider to adjust the client's medical regimen. **Hyperventilation** (due to anxiety, neurologic dysfunction, or iatrogenic over ventilation) causes the PCO_2 to fall below normal (respiratory alkalosis) and the blood pH to rise above normal (alkalemia).

ABG studies also evaluate diffusion and perfusion as reflected by the PO_2 and SaO_2. Pulse oximetry is often preferred over ABGs as a cost-effective laboratory test of SaO_2.

It is essential that ventilation of alveoli is matched with blood flowing through alveolar capillaries. If alveolar ventilation occurs without matched perfusion (e.g., pulmonary embolism), the PO_2 falls, but the PCO_2 remains normal because of the greater solubility of CO_2; the PCO_2 may even decrease due to hyperventilation (respiratory alkalosis). Conversely, if the alveoli are perfused but not ventilated (as in **atelectasis**), the blood is not adequately oxygenated. This condition results in a low PO_2 and a normal PCO_2, because carbon dioxide is highly diffusible. Continued hypoventilation, however, eventually results in an increased PCO_2 (respiratory acidosis).

Normal pulmonary ventilation and perfusion are reflected by *normal blood gas values*. Note: Pulse oximetry (SpO_2) allows noninvasive estimation of SaO_2.

pH	7.35–7.45
$PaCO_2$	35–45 mm Hg
HCO_3^-	24–28 mEq/L
PaO_2	75–100 mm Hg (breathing room air)
SaO_2	> 95%

Pulmonary function (spirometry) tests measure lung volumes and capacity and help differentiate restrictive and obstructive defects of ventilation.

VC (vital capacity)	75–80% of that predicted by age, gender, and height (decreased in restrictive disease)
FEV (forced expiratory volume)	65–85% of VC in 1 sec and 95% in 3 sec (decreased in obstructive disease)
FEV_1 (forced expiratory volume in 1 sec)	Normal = 75% VC (decreased in obstructive disease)
FEV 25–75	Measures expiratory flow capacity of small airways; most sensitive measure of small airway disease

Nursing Interventions

The goal of respiratory nursing interventions is to maintain, restore, or to artificially provide the vital functions of the respiratory system.

Nursing interventions are used routinely to help prevent pulmonary complications for clients with known pulmonary problems, for clients at risk for pulmonary complications

MANIFESTATIONS OF INADEQUATE VENTILATION

The most common clinical manifestations of inadequate ventilation are:

- Tachycardia (heart rate over 100/min)
- Tachypnea (breathing rate over 24/min)
- Anxiety reflected in facial expression
- Restlessness or confusion
- Use of accessory muscles for breathing
- Change in cognition or level of response
- Increased blood pressure
- Change in oxygen saturation
- Change in end tidal CO_2

Early recognition of these indicators of possible hypoxemia should prompt further investigation and appropriate intervention.

(e.g., immobility), or for surgical clients who have undergone general anesthesia and who experience pain.

These interventions include pain management; maintaining adequate hydration (2–3 L of water/day unless contraindicated); turning to help ventilate dependent lung areas; deep breathing to stimulate surfactant and inflate hypoventilated alveoli; coughing to remove retained secretions; airway suctioning to assist ineffective airway clearance; and early ambulation. Protective splinting of operative sites promotes client comfort, adherence, and prevents wound strain.

Continuous positive airway pressure (CPAP)/bilevel positive airway pressure (BiPAP) is the noninvasive application of positive pressure to upper airways to prevent their obstruction by the soft tissues that surround them. This mode improves alveolar ventilation and decreases PCO_2,

respiratory rate, and the work of breathing. Clients with obstructive sleep **apnea**, central sleep apnea, or respiratory insufficiency may benefit from this therapy. It can also provide life support for clients who have decided to forego endotracheal intubation.

Similarly, oscillating positive expiratory pressure (**PEP**) devices function as a cough support to assist COPD clients to clear their airways.

Techniques such as **postural drainage**, chest **percussion**, and **vibration** (CPT) utilize gravity and mechanical energy to help mobilize secretions. These measures are reserved for the client who produces excessive amounts (>25 mL/day) of thick secretions that are difficult to mobilize.

A variety of devices are used to deliver supplemental oxygen to the hypoxic client (SaO_2 under 90%). These devices differ in the degree that they control the client's inspired air.

Artificial means to establish and maintain patent airways include oral/pharyngeal and endotracheal devices. Bypassing the body's natural protective airway and communication processes, these devices render the client dependent and at risk for serious respiratory complications. Clients with artificial airways require additional nursing measures to ensure ventilation and to protect the respiratory system. Such skills include suctioning, tracheostomy care, providing a means for communication, and regular oral hygiene.

If air or fluid accumulates in the intrapleural or mediastinal space due to trauma, disease, or surgery, the lung cannot expand. Cardiac tamponade with decreased cardiac output can occur due to decreased venous return secondary to compression of mediastinal structures. Chest tubes are placed to evacuate air and fluid from the pleural or mediastinal space to facilitate lung re-expansion and prevent increased mediastinal pressure. In certain postoperative settings, chest drainage may be reinfused to replace blood lost.

Nursing Diagnoses

The following nursing diagnoses may be appropriate to use on client care plans when the components are related to respiratory conditions.

NURSING DIAGNOSIS	RELATED TO . . .
Activity Intolerance	Imbalance between oxygen supply and demand
Ineffective Airway Clearance	Fatigue; excessive secretions; pain; immobility; neuromuscular disease; chronic obstructive pulmonary disease
Aspiration, Risk for	Depressed airway protective mechanisms; presence of artificial airway; enteral feeding, neuromuscular disease
Ineffective Breathing Pattern	Immobility; fatigue, pain; neuromuscular impairment; chronic respiratory disease; pharmacologic agents
Impaired Gas Exchange	Ventilation–perfusion imbalance; hypoventilation, chronic obstructive pulmonary disease, airway obstruction, heart failure, pulmonary edema
Disturbed Sleep Pattern	Obstructive airway (sleep apnea)

Nursing Process Data

ASSESSMENT Database

- Observe client's physical ability to perform exercise (e.g., to assume Fowler's position, energy level, degree of pain experienced, and need for pain medication).
- Observe rhythm, rate, and depth of breathing.
- Auscultate breath sounds.
- Note client's report of dyspnea or signs of increased work of breathing.
- Note presence of adventitious sounds.
- Note proximity of incision to muscles necessary for breathing and coughing.
- Assess need for supported ventilation or resuscitation.

PLANNING Objectives

- To improve pulmonary ventilation
- To conserve energy and decrease the work of breathing
- To loosen secretions and promote clear airways
- To prevent hypoventilation and hypoxemia

IMPLEMENTATION Procedures

DOCUMENTATION AND EVALUATION

Expected Outcomes

- Breath sounds are normal; adventitious sounds are cleared.
- Vital capacity, pulmonary ventilation, and gas exchange are improved or supported.
- Client reaches predetermined tidal volume level when using incentive spirometer.
- Client's energy is conserved and work of breathing is eased.
- Secretions are loosened and airways are clear.
- Client monitors peak flow appropriately.
- Client experiences an improved sleep pattern.

Unexpected Outcomes/Alternative Actions

Pearson Nursing Student Resource

Find additional review materials at **nursing.pearsonhighered.com.**
Prepare for success with NCLEX®-style practice questions and Skill Checklists.

Skill 30.1.1 | Instructing Client to Deep Breathe

Equipment
Straight chair or hospital bed at 90-degree elevation

Preparation
1. Introduce self and identify client with two identifiers.
2. Perform hand hygiene.
3. Provide privacy.
4. Explain the rationale for the procedure.
5. Help client to sit straight up in bed with knees slightly flexed or on side of bed. ➤ *Rationale:* This position promotes maximum lung expansion.

Procedure
1. Demonstrate the deep breathing steps, allowing time for client to practice each step.
2. Place your hands on your ribs or have client place hands palm down around the sides of client's lower ribs ❶.
   ➤ *Rationale:* This action supports deep breathing and assists you to evaluate depth of inspiration.
3. Tell client to breathe in slowly through nose until chest expands and abdomen rises visibly.
4. Have client hold a sustained maximal inspiration 3–5 sec, and then exhale slowly through the mouth.
5. Evaluate client's response to determine how often exercise should be performed—diminished breath sounds or presence of **crackles** indicates need for frequent deep breathing, turning, and early ambulation.

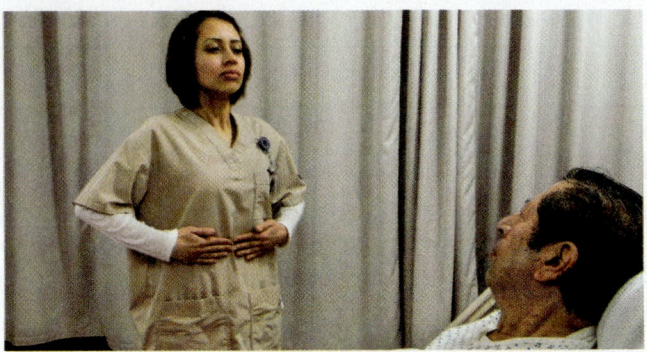

❶ Nurse demonstrates deep breathing.

EVIDENCE-BASED PRACTICE
Reducing Respiratory Complications in Medical Clients With a Respiratory Care Bundle
Nurses on a general medicine unit implemented a respiratory care bundle that included incentive **spirometer** use by clients 10 times every 2 hr and brushing teeth twice daily. For those clients who were dependent, the head of the bed was elevated 30–45 degrees; they were repositioned every 2 hr and were given mouth care every shift. The results showed fewer transfers to the intensive care unit due to respiratory complications after the bundle was implemented.

Source: Lamar (2011)

Skill 30.1.2 | Instructing Client to Cough

Equipment
Straight chair or hospital bed at 90-degree elevation
Pillows for positioning and incisional support
Tissues for secretions
Protective gear (gloves, gown, goggles, mask) as indicated

Preparation
1. Introduce self and identify client with two identifiers.
2. Premedicate client if indicated for pain relief.
3. Perform hand hygiene.
4. Provide privacy.
5. Explain procedure to client.
6. Don protective gear if indicated.
7. Provide client with tissues.

Procedure
1. Place client in upright position, upper body positioned slightly forward. ➤ *Rationale:* This position assists client to cough more effectively.
2. Ask client to slowly take two or three deep breaths through the nose and exhale through the mouth.
3. Instruct client to inhale deeply, hold breath for several seconds, lean forward, and cough, using abdominal, thigh, and buttock muscles. ➤ *Rationale:* This promotes a more effective cough.
4. Instruct client with pulmonary condition to exhale through pursed lips and to "huff" while coughing in mid-exhalation (not at end of deep inspiration). ➤ *Rationale:* The "huff cough" maintains an open glottis; it helps prevent high expiratory pressures that collapse diseased airways, thus facilitating movement of secretions along the tracheobronchial tree; it reduces fatigue.

CLINICAL ALERT
Deep breathing is indicated, but coughing may be *contraindicated* for the client after eye, ear, brain, or neck surgery, or if efforts are nonproductive. Check with the healthcare provider for specific orders.

❶ Holding pillow against incision when coughing prevents incision strain.

5. Support any incision with the palms of your or client's hands, or place a rolled pillow firmly against the incision (called splinting the incision). **❶ ➤ Rationale:** This prevents incisional strain and encourages client to cough more effectively.
6. Encourage client to deep breathe and cough more frequently if cough is productive. Explain why coughing is beneficial and keep tissues and disposal receptacle handy. **➤ Rationale:** Accumulated secretions in airways promote bacterial growth and interfere with ventilation.

Skill 30.1.3 | Teaching Diaphragmatic Breathing

Equipment
Hospital bed in flat position

Preparation
1. Introduce self and identify client with two identifiers.
2. Check healthcare provider's orders and client care plan.
3. Perform hand hygiene.
4. Provide privacy.
5. Inform client that the purpose of this exercise is to learn how to breathe by using abdominal muscles.

Note: Clients with COPD tend to overwork the upper chest muscles and suck in the abdomen on inspiration, making it difficult for the diaphragm to descend. This exercise improves breathing efficiency.

Procedure
1. Place your hands on client's abdomen, below ribs.
2. Have client breathe in through the nose and try to push stomach outward against your hands.
3. Instruct client to hold breath for 3–5 sec to keep alveoli open.
4. Have client breathe out slowly through the mouth as you apply slight pressure at the base of the ribs.
5. Encourage client to practice diaphragmatic breathing frequently, using own hands to feel the abdomen rise.

Skill 30.1.4 | Teaching Use of Incentive Spirometer (IS)

Equipment
Hospital bed or straight chair
Incentive spirometer with flow rate indicator (save bag for storage of device)
Tissues for secretions

Preparation
1. Introduce self and identify client with two identifiers.
2. Check healthcare provider's orders and client care plan.
3. Gather equipment.
4. Perform hand hygiene.
5. Explain purpose and procedure to client.
6. If preoperative measurement was not done, use guide in spirometer package to determine client's volume goal, and set marker at this goal.
7. Attach open end of tubing to stem on front of exerciser.
8. Auscultate lungs before and after using IS. **➤ Rationale:** This evaluates effectiveness of spirometry.

Procedure
1. Instruct client to hold exerciser, place mouth tightly around mouthpiece, and breathe in a trial breath through the mouth. **❶ ➤ Rationale:** Client can see the flow rate indicator on side of unit to visualize appropriate *rate* for inhalation.
2. Explain that a slow deep breath is better than a fast breath.
3. Instruct client to exhale completely, and then place mouth tightly around mouthpiece.
4. Instruct client to inhale slowly to raise and maintain yellow flow rate indicator at the "best" flow rate range, and continue inhaling to try to raise piston to prescribed (or preoperative measured) volume level.
5. Instruct client to remove mouthpiece but hold breath at maximum inspiration for 3–5 sec, and then exhale through pursed lips. Repeat a few times, and then cough.

(continued)

Skill 30.1.4 | Teaching Use of Incentive Spirometer (IS) *(continued)*

1 Client places mouth tightly around mouthpiece and inhales slowly, while watching yellow flow rate indicator, to promote lung expansion.

6. Encourage client to use spirometer hourly, coordinating use with TV program breaks, for instance, as a reminder.
7. Provide positive feedback as client uses IS to reattain predetermined inspiratory capacity, using marked goal as an incentive.
8. Replace unit in bag when not in use and keep in accessible place for client.

EVIDENCE-BASED PRACTICE
Incentive Spirometry and Pulmonary Complications
Incentive spirometry alone has not been found to be sufficient in the preoperative and postoperative setting to prevent pulmonary complications. The Agency for Healthcare Research on Quality National Guideline Incentive Spirometry recommends that incentive spirometry be used with deep breathing techniques, directed coughing, early mobilization, and optimal analgesia to prevent postoperative pulmonary complications.

Source: Restrepo, Wettstein, Wittnebel, & Tracy (2011)

Skill 30.1.5 | Teaching Peak Flow Measurement

Equipment
Peak flow meter with instructions for client

Preparation
1. Introduce self and identify client with two identifiers.
2. Check healthcare provider's orders or client care plan.
3. Gather equipment.
4. Perform hand hygiene.
5. Explain purpose of procedure and provide instruction sheet to client.

Procedure
1. Assist client to follow product instructions to assemble meter.
2. Instruct client to attach mouthpiece to peak flow meter, if desired. ➤ *Rationale:* Most meters can be used with or without mouthpiece.
3. Slide indicator to zero position. 1
4. Instruct client to inhale as deeply as possible, and then place mouth around mouthpiece, forming a tight seal. If possible, client should be standing.

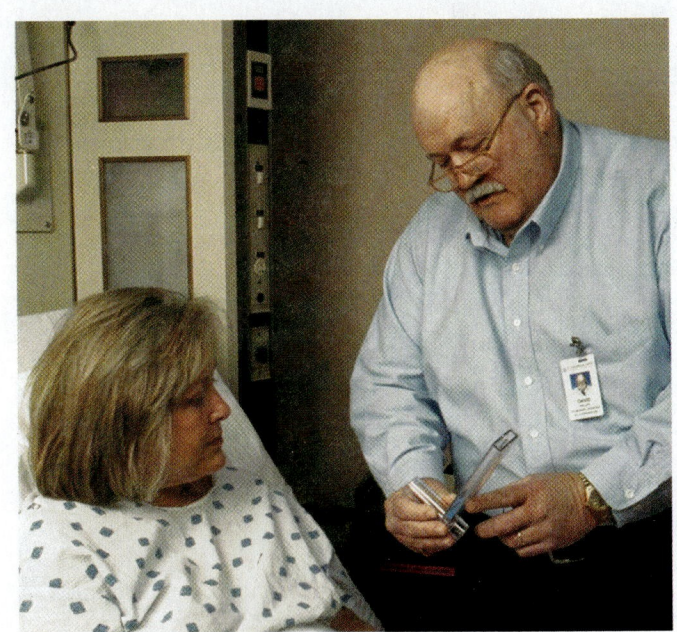

1 Slide indicator to bottom of meter scale to bring indicator to zero point.

5. Have client blow out through mouth as hard and fast as possible. ❷ ➤ *Rationale:* As client forcefully exhales, indicator moves up scale to record client's peak expiratory flow (L/min).

6. Repeat peak flow measurement three times and record highest value. ➤ *Rationale:* Client may keep daily record of peak flow values and report significant changes.

7. Instruct client to clean unit weekly, following manufacturer's instructions.

EVIDENCE-BASED PRACTICE

Peak Flow Monitoring

Color-coded zones indicate forced expiratory volume. The green zone indicates 80–100% of the individual's best, yellow zone indicates 60–80%, and red zone is less than 60%. Clients with asthma should develop an asthma action plan with their healthcare provider, which specifies actions to take when they are in the yellow and red zones. Blank plans can be downloaded from the CDC or American Lung Association websites and taken to the clinic visit to be filled out with the healthcare provider.

Source: National Heart, Lung, and Blood Institute (2014)

❷ Have client blow out through mouth as hard and fast as possible—indicator moves up scale to record peak expiratory flow (L/min).

Skill 30.1.6 | Teaching Use of Oscillating Positive Expiratory Pressure (PEP) Cough Support Device

Equipment

"Flutter valve system" with adjustment dial, one-way inspiratory valve, and detachable mouthpiece

Preparation

1. Introduce self and identify client with two identifiers.
2. Explain use and purpose of device. ➤ *Rationale:* The device functions to maintain positive pressure throughout exhalation to facilitate pulmonary secretion removal—cough support device.
3. Open packet and save for device storage.
4. Secure all device connections.
5. Adjust vibration frequency dial clockwise to low resistance setting when initiating therapy. ➤ *Rationale:* Higher frequency of vibrating pressure waves and higher resistance of opening changes produce higher resistance to exhalation.
6. Position client sitting with elbows resting on table.

Procedure

1. Instruct client to place mouthpiece in mouth with tight seal during exhalation.
2. Have client take a deep breath in and hold it for 2–3 sec.

3. Instruct client to exhale through the device, prolonging exhalation actively (not forcefully, but three to four times longer than inhalation) as the device vibrates.
4. If client cannot maintain exhalation for 3–4 sec, adjust dial clockwise to increase resistance and allow client to exhale at a lower flow rate. ➤ *Rationale:* Proper resistance range produces an inspiratory to expiratory (I:E) ratio of 1:3 or 1:4.
5. Once a proper range is determined, the client may change adjustments for harder or softer exhalation to meet a subjective comfort with the device. ➤ *Rationale:* Adjustments may be necessary to meet client needs.
6. Clean mouthpiece and return device to storage bag.
7. Encourage client to use the "PEP" device for 10–20 min, four times a day.

Note: This device directs exhaled air through an opening that alternately closes and opens the path of air flow. This maintains a vibratory positive pressure through exhalation (common lay term is *flutter valve*).

Equipment

Nasal mask, full face mask, or nasal pillows of proper
    size (S, M, L)
Indelible marker
Airflow generator
Delivery tubing
If ordered:
    Oxygen source
    Oxygen tubing
    Pulse oximetry

Preparation

1. Introduce self and identify client with two identifiers.
2. Check healthcare provider's orders or client's care plan.
3. Gather equipment.
4. Perform hand hygiene.

> **CLINICAL ALERT**
> Clients with obstructive sleep apnea are at risk for
> cardiovascular complications including hypertension, stroke,
> arrhythmias, heart failure, and myocardial infarction.

5. Explain purpose of procedure to client and provide written
   instructions for home use (Box 30-2 ■).
6. Assess the client's ability to communicate a need for help or
   to remove the mask themselves. ➤ *Rationale:* If a client is
   unable to remove a mask or communicate a need for help,
   the client should be placed in the intensive care unit.
7. Determine the reason for CPAP/BiPAP.

   a. Clients with obstructive sleep apnea should wear their
      device at night and are usually cared for on acute care units.
   b. Clients who are receiving noninvasive positive pressure
      breathing support in which cessation of support would

Box 30-2 CPAP AND BIPAP

- CPAP provides single positive pressure to establish minimal airway value (e.g., 5 mm Hg) at end of exhalation.
- BiPAP provides two positive airway pressures, one to
  assist peak pressure on inhalation (e.g., 10 cm H_2O) and
  a lower one (e.g., 5 cm H_2O) to establish minimal airway
  value at end of exhalation.
- Monitoring for clients on CPAP and BiPAP needs to include
  both continuous pulse oximetry and end tidal CO_2 monitoring, especially for those clients who are postoperative.
  End tidal CO_2 is a more sensitive indicator of hypoventilation and hypoxemia than pulse oximetry and can provide
  the nurse with an early indication that the client is having
  respiratory distress.
- Postoperative clients are often sent to a monitored unit
  where staffing ratios are 2:1 or 3:1 for the first 24 hr
  (Gammon and Ricker, 2012).

---

lead to respiratory decompensation should be cared
for in an intensive care environment where they can be
monitored closely.

8. Have client wash face or assist client to wash face.

Procedure

1. Connect CPAP/BiPAP device delivery tubing to pressure
   generator.
2. Plug pressure generator into grounded outlet.
3. Connect oxygen delivery tubing into device tubing adapter
   port (if ordered).
4. Turn on pressure generator.

> **CLINICAL ALERT**
> Respiratory therapy and biomedical engineering departments
> must check to ensure proper functioning and electrical safety
> of outside equipment (e.g., CPAP) that is brought from home
> to be used in an agency.

5. Establish CPAP/BiPAP parameters based on
   healthcare provider orders. In many institutions, a respiratory
   therapist is responsible for setting up the CPAP/BiPAP
   devices initially.
6. Apply device over the client's nose or face, avoiding a tight
   fit, and mark straps for future proper fit. ❶ ❷ ➤ *Rationale:*
   Tight fit is uncomfortable for the client and unnecessary for
   proper functioning.
7. Establish continuous pulse oximetry if ordered.

   a. ABGs may be obtained before and within the first hour of
      BiPAP initiation.
   b. Per agency protocol, monitor vital signs, level of
      consciousness, sedation score, and work of breathing.
   c. Monitor pulse oximetry and end tidal CO_2 (eTCO_2).

8. Tell client to detach tubing from face device if getting up
   during the night.

❶ Client receiving CPAP via face mask. Machine is capable of
CPAP and BiPAP.

9. Monitor client periodically.
10. Teach client to clean device according to manufacturer's instructions.

❷ The BiPAP Vision noninvasive ventilator support system has most features of any standard mechanical ventilator.

Skill 30.1.8 | Providing Bag–Valve–Mask Ventilation

Equipment
Manual resuscitator bag with nonrebreathing valve
Oxygen source and tubing
Airway adapter or face mask

Preparation
1. Determine that client's breathing is absent or inadequate.
2. Summon an assistant if client is not intubated. ➤ *Rationale:* If no artificial airway is present, two responders are preferred. Assistant holds mask while nurse compresses resuscitator bag.
3. Gather equipment (Box 30-3 ■).
4. Place client in supine position.
5. Connect mask or airway adapter to bag.
6. Connect oxygen tubing and oxygen flow meter to bag inlet.

Procedure
1. Turn oxygen flow meter wide open to 15 L/min ("flush").
2. Stand at client's head and hyperextend client's neck.
3. Place apex of mask over client's nose and place base of mask between client's lower lip and chin. ❶ ➤ *Rationale:* This ensures a tight seal.
4. Use dominant hand to compress central portion of resuscitator bag until client's chest rises (1–2 sec), and then allow exhalation. ➤ *Rationale:* Overinflation may result in gastric distention.
5. Provide ventilations every 5 sec for an apneic adult, noting rise and fall of client's chest with each compression.

CLINICAL ALERT

If client's chest does not rise with ventilations, suspect foreign body airway obstruction. See Chapter 31 for abdominal thrust maneuvers.

Box 30-3 **BAG–VALVE–MASK WITH RESCUE POD**

The bag–valve–mask with rescue pod (circulatory enhancer) is used only for clients who are *unable to breathe spontaneously* (e.g., during CPR). This device with a one-way valve is attached between the resuscitator bag and mask or airway tube. It allows the rescuer to deliver air to the client.

The system accepts attachment of an expiratory filter for epidemiologic considerations and an external PEEP device for maintaining PEP to enhance diffusion (PO_2) during its use. A pressure manometer indicates pressure from resuscitator bag compression. Desired pressure is sufficient to achieve adequate chest wall movement (normally 15–25 cm H_2O). Maintaining minimal necessary ventilation pressure helps prevent barotraumas to lung tissue and gastric air insufflation. The rescue pod device must be removed *immediately* if the client is able to resume spontaneous breathing.

❶ Compress central portion of resuscitator bag until client's chest rises, then allow exhalation.

(continued)

Skill 30.1.8 | Providing Bag–Valve–Mask Ventilation (continued)

6. Check to see if client breathes spontaneously; if so, give compressions in synchrony to support ventilation.
7. Observe for possible gastric distention. ➤ *Rationale:* Gastric insufflation may result in regurgitation and aspiration.

8. Reposition client's head if gastric distention is present and reduce compression volume, noting whether client's chest rises.
9. Notify healthcare provider or respiratory care practitioner for further client evaluation.

Unit 30.1 Documentation and Evaluation

DOCUMENTATION for Respiratory Preventive and Maintenance Measures

- Pre- and postintervention breath sounds and adventitious sounds
- Frequency of deep breathing exercises or use of IS
- Whether cough is productive or not
- Amount and character of secretions expectorated
- Changes in vital signs, SpO_2, or other client responses
- Inspiratory capacity attained with IS
- Circumstances necessitating use of mask and bag resuscitator
- Client outcome after manual breathing

- Peak flow measurement: highest of three therapy sequential measures
- Client teaching and return demonstration

For CPAP/BiPAP
- Type of CPAP/BiPAP device used
- Established parameters
- Respiratory rate if programmed
- FiO_2 if ordered
- SpO_2 findings pre- and posttherapy
- Client's tolerance of therapy

EVALUATION/Critical Thinking

Expected Outcomes
- Client coughs effectively, supporting incision to prevent strain.
- Client is able to breathe through nose without distress.
- Client demonstrates appropriate use of incentive spirometer.
- Client experiences benefits of CPAP/BiPAP with undisturbed sleep.

Unexpected Outcomes
- Client is unwilling to complete exercise because of misunderstanding or fear of pain or wound dehiscence.

Alternative Actions
- Inform client that fresh incision is secure.
- Instruct again on rationale and necessity for procedure.
- Support incision area more fully, using the palms of your hands or a firmly rolled pillow to allay fears of dehiscence.
- Medicate 30–60 min before using spirometer and coughing.

- Nasal congestion inhibits client's breathing capability.

- Ask client to blow nose before the breathing exercise.
- Check with healthcare provider to prescribe medications, such as saline spray to open nasal passages.

Unexpected Outcomes	Alternative Actions
• Client is unable to master use of incentive spirometer device.	• Instruct client to start slowly and increase volume over several exercise sessions. • Supervise practice with encouragement. • Provide positive reinforcement with increments in volume. • Ensure that client does regular deep breathing if device interferes with client adherence. • Turn client every 2 hr and encourage ROM and early ambulation to help stimulate deep breathing and secretion mobilization. • Instruct client to deep breathe effectively without using the spirometer: to inhale slowly and deeply through the nose, hold the breath several seconds, and then exhale.
• Client does not tolerate BiPAP therapy.	• Loosen the appliance since some leakage is acceptable and does not compromise function of the device. • Consult respiratory therapy to adjust settings. • Use nasal spray (saline solution) to reduce nasal congestion. • Find a more individually suited device. • Reassess true need for BiPAP.

Chest Physiotherapy (CPT)

Nursing Process Data

ASSESSMENT Database

- Note any contraindicating conditions for CPT: acute exacerbation of COPD, pneumonia *without* evidence of significant **sputum** production, osteoporosis, lung cancer, and cerebral edema.
- Determine rate and depth of breathing and heart rate and rhythm.
- Auscultate breath sounds and check for adventitious sounds or excessive sputum production (over 25 mL/day).
- Note time elapsed since eating (perform CPT between meals to prevent regurgitation).
- Observe quality of secretions. Thick, tenacious secretions may require aerosol therapy before treatment.
- Note client's ABGs/SpO$_2$ and changes on chest x-ray report.

PLANNING Objectives

- To decrease respiratory rate and improve ventilation and gas exchange
- To reduce client's feeling of shortness of breath
- To facilitate clearance of retained secretions
- To assist client to cough more productively and effectively
- To decrease adventitious lung sounds
- To decrease risk of infection due to stasis of secretions

IMPLEMENTATION Procedures

DOCUMENTATION AND EVALUATION

Expected Outcomes

- Chest x-ray shows improvement.
- Breath sounds and adventitious sounds improve on auscultation.
- Shortness of breath is reduced.
- Sputum production is over 25 mL/day (to justify continuation of CPT).
- ABGs/SpO$_2$ values are improved.

Unexpected Outcomes/Alternative Actions

Pearson Nursing Student Resources

Find additional review materials at
nursing.pearsonhighered.com.
Prepare for success with NCLEX®-style practice questions and Skill Checklists.

Skill 30.2.1 | Preparing Client for CPT

Equipment

Hospital bed or other surface to place client in head-down
  position
Gown or towel (optional)
Tissues
Container for sputum
Clean gloves
Stethoscope
Pulse oximeter (if indicated)
Mouthwash/oral hygiene product

Procedure

1. Validate healthcare provider's order for CPT. ➤ *Rationale:*
   These procedures are tiring to clients, time-consuming,
   and contraindicated in cases of osteoporosis, pulmonary
   embolism, cardiac conditions, lung cancer, or other
   conditions not associated with excessive sputum
   production.
2. Perform hand hygiene.
3. Introduce self and identify client using two identifiers.
4. Administer CPT before or at least 2 hr after meals to prevent
   vomiting.
5. Establish the location of lung segments if the entire lung field
   is to undergo CPT; the affected segment should be drained

first. ❶ ➤ *Rationale:* Usually, the lower areas are the most
affected.
6. Provide privacy.
7. Prepare client by explaining CPT and purpose.
8. Auscultate chest for breath sounds and **adventitious**
   sounds before therapy.
9. Obtain pulse oximetry (SpO_2) if indicated before therapy.
10. Place towel over skin when performing CPT (optional).

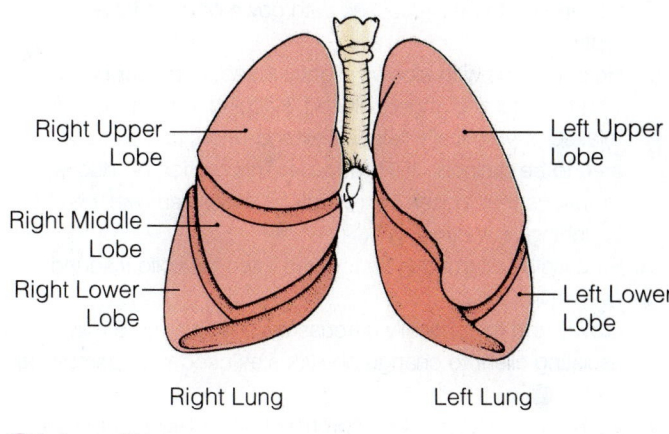

❶ Lobes of lungs.

Skill 30.2.2 | Performing Postural Drainage

Equipment

See Skill 30.2.1, Preparing Client for CPT.

Preparation

1. See Skill 30.2.1, Preparing Client for CPT.
2. Introduce self and identify client with two client identifiers.
3. Perform hand hygiene.

Procedure

1. Loosen any tight clothing.
2. Lower head of bed slowly so that client's head is positioned
   at no greater than a 25-degree downward angle.
   ➤ *Rationale:* Gravity helps mobilize secretions.
3. Place sputum container and tissues in client's reach.
4. Tell client to remain in position for 3–15 min. ➤ *Rationale:*
   Percussion and vibration may be added to help mobilize
   secretions (*skills to follow*).
5. Instruct client to expectorate secretions.
6. Instruct client to turn to other side, then to supine position,
   and then repeat procedure.

Note: Clients should take a deep breath between position
changes.

7. Assist client to slowly return to normal sitting position after
   coughing in dependent positions.
8. Determine pulse oximetry if ordered.
9. Auscultate chest areas for improved breath sounds.
10. Note characteristics, measure sputum, and then discard.
11. Remove gloves and perform hand hygiene.
12. Offer oral hygiene after secretion expectoration.

EVIDENCE-BASED PRACTICE

Manual Chest Physiotherapy

Manual chest physiotherapy (MCP) involving chest percussion
and vibration was evaluated in clients hospitalized with acute
exacerbation of COPD. The study evaluated MCP techniques
on quality of life at six months postexacerbation. Results of this
study did not support the use of MCP in the routine management
of acute exacerbation of COPD.

Source: Cross et al. (2012)

| **Skill 30.2.3** | Performing Chest Percussion |

Equipment
See Skill 30.2.1, Preparing Client for CPT.

Preparation
1. See Skill 30.2.1, Preparing Client for CPT.
2. Introduce self and identify client using two identifiers.
3. Perform hand hygiene.

Procedure
1. Cover area to be percussed with gown or cloth towel (optional).
2. Holding arms with elbows slightly flexed, cup your hands with thumbs and fingers closed. Keeping wrists loose and relaxed, rhythmically flex and extend wrists to clap over area to be drained. ➤ *Rationale:* This motion produces vibrations that loosen secretions for easier removal with coughing or suctioning.
3. Percuss by alternating hands and listen for hollow sound with strikes.
4. Slowly and rhythmically percuss each area for 3–5 min assisting client to change positions as needed to percuss all areas. ❶
5. Do not percuss over bony prominences, breasts, or tender areas. ➤ *Rationale:* Vibrations are not transmitted to the chest wall through bone or breast tissue and percussion in these areas can cause discomfort.
6. Encourage client to "huff" cough after percussion of lung areas.
7. Auscultate all lung areas for changes in breath sounds.
8. Don gloves, assist client to cough or suction as needed, note character and measure quantity of sputum, and discard.
9. Remove gloves and perform hand hygiene.

❶ Perform percussion and vibration with each position change.

10. Offer oral hygiene.
11. Document procedure and client's response.

> **CLINICAL ALERT**
> Since chest percussion is taxing and time-consuming for both client and nurse, it is indicated only in clients with serious secretion retention (e.g., client with cystic fibrosis).

| **Skill 30.2.4** | Performing Chest Vibration |

Equipment
See Skill 30.2.1, Preparing Client for CPT.

Preparation
1. See Skill 30.2.1, Preparing Client for CPT.
2. Introduce self and identify client using two identifiers.
3. Perform hand hygiene.

Procedure
1. Perform vibration after postural drainage and percussion in each position.
2. Cover area to be vibrated with gown or towel (optional).
3. Instruct client to breathe in through nose and exhale slowly through pursed lips.
4. Place your hands flat over area to be vibrated, or place one hand on top of the other. ❶ Keep your arms and shoulders straight and wrists stiff.
5. Have client inhale deeply.

❶ Place hands flat over area to be vibrated, keeping wrists stiff.

6. As client exhales through pursed lips, use moderate pressure to vibrate chest by quickly contracting and relaxing your arms and shoulders. ➤ *Rationale:* This increases the turbulence and velocity of exhaled air and loosens and mobilizes secretions from peripheral airways.

7. Vibrate for three or four exhalations over the area.

8. Encourage clients to "huff" cough before changing positions.

9. Assess vital signs, pulse oximetry, and auscultate breath sounds.

10. Don gloves.

11. Measure and note character of expectorated secretions, and then discard.

12. Remove gloves and perform hand hygiene.

13. Provide oral hygiene.

14. Document procedure and client's response.

Skill 30.2.5 | Using an Airway Clearance System (Wrap)

Equipment

See Skill 30.2.1, Preparing Client for CPT

Disposable inflatable chest wrap of appropriate size (small, medium, large, or extra large)

Air pulse generator with connecting tubes

Preparation

1. Validate healthcare provider's order for high-frequency chest wall oscillation therapy (HFCWO), frequency, and duration of therapy. ❶ ➤ *Rationale:* Vest or wrap HFCWO increases mobilization of secretions while requiring no caregiver skill and no special positioning, and many clients require no assistance.

2. Notify nurse before initiating therapy to determine that it is safe to have monitoring compromised for the time period of therapy. ➤ *Rationale:* The ECG and hemodynamic monitoring are distorted with artifact during airway clearance with vest or wrap therapy.

3. Perform hand hygiene.

4. Introduce self and identify client using two identifiers.

5. Provide privacy.

6. Explain function and purpose of vest/wrap.

7. Assess lung sounds before therapy.

Procedure

1. Elevate head of bed or have client sit in chair. Alternately, place wrap on bed and roll client onto wrap.

2. Apply wrap over single layer of clothing, wrapping deflated vest around client's chest, just beneath axillae; have client inhale deeply; and secure with Velcro fasteners. ➤ *Rationale:* Wrap should fit snugly, but not be uncomfortable.

3. Adjust generator to a comfortable working height.

4. Lock generator castors. ➤ *Rationale:* This is to prevent movement.

5. Slide air hose into connector port on front of generator using a twist and push motion.

6. Slide other end of hose into disposable vest slits.

7. Fasten Velcro loops to secure air hoses in position.

8. Plug the power cord into the power inlet on back of air pulse generator.

9. Plug power cord into grounded outlet.

10. Adjust arrows up or down to set frequency, pressure, and treatment time, confirming that setting on screen matches those prescribed.

11. Press "ON" button to inflate disposable vest. ➤ *Rationale:* Air pulsation provides vibration to client's chest. Treatment will last 10 min, but then must be restarted if indicated. Usual treatments are 10–20 min qid.

12. Press "OFF" button to end treatment before set time and wrap will deflate.

13. "Session complete" message will show on screen when treatment set time is complete and wrap will deflate.

14. Unplug system and remove disposable air hoses and vest from client.

15. Store vest and air hoses in client's area and return generator to storage for future use.

16. Reassess client's breath sounds; note character and amount of coughed/suctioned secretions.

17. Assist client to a comfortable position.

18. Perform hand hygiene.

EVIDENCE-BASED PRACTICE

High-Frequency Chest Wall Oscillation Therapy Preferred Over Chest PT

Clients undergoing lung transplant surgery had less pain when using HFCWO for secretion mobilization as compared to chest physiotherapy. This has important implications because when secretions are not effectively mobilized, it can lead to respiratory complications and poor client outcomes.

Source: Esguerra-Gonzalez et al. (2013)

---

❶ Vest or wrap high-frequency chest wall oscillation therapy increases mobilization and clearance of airway secretions.

CLINICAL ALERT

Strenuous coughing should be avoided with head-down position since it raises the client's intracranial pressure.

Unit 30.2 Documentation and Evaluation

DOCUMENTATION for Chest Physiotherapy (CPT)

- Time, specific treatment, and duration of therapy
- Pre- and posttherapy vital signs, breath sounds, and pulse oximetry
- Quantity and character of sputum produced
- Client's physical tolerance of procedures

EVALUATION/Critical Thinking

Expected Outcomes

- Client tolerates postural drainage.
- CPT facilitates expectoration of secretions.

Unexpected Outcomes	Alternative Actions
Client experiences dyspnea during postural drainage.	Change client's position, so head is no lower than 25 degrees below horizontal.
Client vomits with CPT treatment and coughing.	Perform treatments between or before meals.
Client tires with manual chest vibration.	Notify healthcare provider to alter therapy with a mechanical device for chest vibration.
	Limit total CPT time.
Slapping sounds produced with percussion.	Cup hands more and ensure that clapping is with wrist flexion and extension only.

Oxygen Administration

Nursing Process Data

ASSESSMENT Database

- Review client's ABG or pulse oximetry values.
- Assess client's vital signs.
- Observe client for signs of increased work of breathing.
- Assess skin under oxygen mask for irritation.
- Assess for signs of carbon dioxide narcosis.

PLANNING Objectives

- To return arterial PaO_2 or SpO_2 values to normal or acceptable range
- To correct hypoxic condition
- To assist breathing to return to normal rate and effort
- To increase client's comfort, breathing efficiency, and activity tolerance

IMPLEMENTATION Procedures

DOCUMENTATION AND EVALUATION

Expected Outcomes

- Arterial PO_2 and SpO_2 values return to normal or acceptable range.
- Signs and symptoms of hypoxia are relieved.
- Comfort, breathing efficiency, and activity tolerance increased.
- Complications of oxygen use do not occur.

Unexpected Outcomes / Alternative Actions

Pearson Nursing Student Resources

Find additional review materials at
nursing.pearsonhighered.com.
Prepare for success with NCLEX®-style practice questions and Skill Checklists.

Skill 30.3.1 | Monitoring Clients Receiving Oxygen

Equipment

Oxygen supply source
Oxygen delivery device

Procedure

1. Check healthcare provider's orders for mode of oxygen delivery and prescribed oxygen liter flow. **❶**
2. Introduce self and identify client using two client identifiers.
3. Perform hand hygiene.
4. Employ safety precautions for oxygen administration (Box 30-4 ■).
5. Place client in semi- or high-Fowler's position to facilitate lung expansion.

❶ Oxygen flow meter indicates liters per minute delivered to administration setup.

Box 30-4 SAFETY PRECAUTIONS FOR OXYGEN ADMINISTRATION

- Set up "No Smoking" and "Oxygen in Use" signs at the site of administration and at the door, according to agency policy.
- Provide cotton gown—synthetics and wool may generate sparks of static electricity.
- Remove matches, lighters, and ashtrays from bedside (these items should NOT be present as hospitals are smoke-free facilities).
- Remove any friction-type or battery-operated toys or devices.
- Disconnect ungrounded electric equipment.
- Remove all volatile or flammable materials (alcohol, oils, petroleum products).
- Make sure that all electrical monitoring equipment are properly grounded.
- Locate fire extinguishers and unit or area oxygen meter turn-off lever.

6. Turn and reposition client frequently to promote ventilation.
7. Encourage deep breathing and coughing exercises unless directed otherwise.
8. Ensure adequate fluid intake, especially if secretions are thick.
9. If ordered, humidify oxygen.
10. Assess client's progress by frequently checking vital signs, color, level of consciousness, and presence of **hypoxia**—the best indicator of oxygen delivery problems. Monitor for manifestations of hypoxia (Box 30-5 ■).
11. Assess clients with COPD frequently for signs of carbon dioxide narcosis:
    a. Bounding peripheral pulses
    b. High blood pressure
    c. Altered sensorium
    d. Increased pulse pressure
    e. Warm, clammy skin
12. Evaluate SpO_2 30 min after any change in oxygen flow rate.

CLINICAL ALERT

Oxygen is indicated for clients with COPD, but is used conservatively. High levels of oxygen may suppress breathing stimulus, cause hypoventilation and CO_2 retention, and lead to respiratory arrest due to CO_2 narcosis.

Box 30-5 SIGNS AND SYMPTOMS OF HYPOXIA (SAO_2 <90% OR BELOW DESIRED RANGE FOR CLIENT'S SITUATION)

Early Symptoms

- Restlessness
- Headache
- Visual disturbances
- Confusion or change in behavior
- Tachypnea
- Tachycardia
- Hypertension
- **Dyspnea**
- Anxious face

Advanced Symptoms

- Hypotension
- Bradycardia
- Metabolic acidosis (production of lactic acid)
- **Cyanosis**

Chronic Hypoxia

- Polycythemia
- Clubbing of fingers and toes
- Peripheral edema
- Right-sided heart failure
- Chronic PaO_2 less than 55 mm Hg; O_2 saturation less than 87%
- Elevated $PaCO_2$ (respiratory acidosis)

Skill 30.3.2 | Using Pulse Oximetry

Equipment
Oximeter (battery or line power operated)
Sensor (clip-on or disposable adhesive sensor)

Preparation
1. Evaluate client's health status before using oximetry.
   ➤ *Rationale:* Inaccurate oximetry readings can be found in clients with:
   a. Alkalosis, acidosis
   b. Fever, hypothermia
   c. Poor peripheral blood flow
   d. Carbon monoxide poisoning
   e. Recent dye injection studies
   f. Shivering or excessive movement
2. Remove dark nail polish or artificial nails, if using finger for sensor placement. ➤ *Rationale:* These substances can distort readings.
3. Obtain appropriate sensor. ➤ *Rationale:* Sensor probes are designated for specific sites (clips for finger or earlobe, wraps for toes or across the nose).

Procedure
1. Identify client and explain purpose of procedure for pulse oximetry (Box 30-6 ■).
2. Plug unit into electric outlet.
3. Turn on power.
4. Apply sensor probe to selected site flush with skin and secure. ❶ Make sure both sensor probes are aligned directly opposite each other. ➤ *Rationale:* Oximeter sensors contain both red and infrared light-emitting diodes (LEDs) and a photo detector. The photo detector registers light passing through vascular bed, the basis for microprocessor determination of oxygen saturation.

CLINICAL ALERT
- Avoid placing SpO_2 clip sensor on the thumb or edematous site. Wrap sensors can be used on the thumb or great toe.
- Avoid extremity with an intra-arterial catheter or noninvasive automatic BP cuff.

---

5. Set alarms to predetermined saturation levels or pulse rate.

Note: New motion-tolerant pulse oximeters are associated with fewer false alarms.

6. Read oxygen saturation level on digital readout monitor.
7. Evaluate findings with previous saturation levels and changes in oxygen therapy.
8. Rotate site of clip-on probes every 4 hr. Replace disposable probes every 24 hr. ➤ *Rationale:* Skin irritation can occur with continuous usage.

9. Validate that oximeter pulse rate is consistent with manually assessed pulse rate.
10. Document findings on appropriate hospital record.

Box 30-6 PULSE OXIMETRY SPO_2

ABG analysis has been used for decades to determine a client's gas exchange and oxygenation transport ability. Pulse oximetry technology allows for more cost- and time-efficient prn or continuous monitoring of arterial oxygen saturation (SaO_2). The primary advantages of this method are:

- It is cost-effective.
- It is a noninvasive evaluation tool.
- Minute-to-minute changes in saturation can be assessed and timely intervention made to meet client needs.
- The client's response to treatment can be evaluated immediately and continuously.

---

❶ Sensor probe placed on finger provides continuous oximeter unit display of hemoglobin oxygen saturation (SpO_2) and pulse rate. Alarms are set at predetermined limits.

EVIDENCE-BASED PRACTICE
Effectively Monitoring Postoperative Clients
The alarm feature on the pulse oximetry system is often used postoperatively to monitor clients on general care units who are receiving opioids. When this alarm sounds, the nurse should be able to respond in a timely manner to ensure that client safety is not compromised. A study conducted on an acute care unit in a large tertiary care setting found that one-third of the alarms were for clinically relevant concerns and that the nurses were able to respond within 1 min on average. However, they cautioned that there is a need to further refine the systems to reduce the number of false positive alarms to avoid nurses becoming desensitized to the alarms.

Source: Voepel-Lewis et al. (2013)

Skill 30.3.3 | Using an Oxygen Cylinder

Equipment
Steel cylinder portable oxygen tank
Regulator/flow meter
Oxygen delivery tubing

Procedure
1. Place oxygen cylinder in carrier in secure upright position. ➤ *Rationale:* If cylinder of compressed air falls accidentally, unit becomes a projectile with uncontrollable force and direction.
2. Using hexagon key, slowly turn cylinder release valve clockwise (left is loose) to crack tank open for a brief period, and then close (right to tighten). ➤ *Rationale:* This action removes lint from system.
3. Check pressure gauge on front of tank to determine amount of oxygen pressure in tank. ➤ *Rationale:* Full status is 2,200 psi.
4. Attach flow meter regulator unit over neck of cylinder, ❶ aligning pins with green "O" ring openings.
5. Use turn key to tighten regulator to cylinder neck.
6. Connect delivery tubing to "Christmas tree" adapter on regulator unit.
7. Open cylinder release valve using hexagon key on top of cylinder. ➤ *Rationale:* This allows oxygen flow.
8. Slowly open regulator/flow meter and adjust to prescribed rate of oxygen delivery in liters per minute.

> **CLINICAL ALERT**
> Oxygen cylinders are mandated by the Compressed Gas Association to be green or incorporate a green collar at the gauge and flowmeter mechanism. Wall outlets are also green for oxygen, yellow for air, and white for suction.

❶ Attach regulator to cylinder neck, attach tubing, open cylinder release valve, and adjust oxygen flow rate (L/min) as prescribed.

Skill 30.3.4 | Using a Nasal Cannula

Equipment
Oxygen source
Oxygen flow meter
Disposable humidifier if ordered (flow rate over 4 L/min or per agency policy)
Nasal cannula and tubing

> **CLINICAL ALERT**
> Humidification of low-flow oxygen through nasal cannulae is not considered essential and is contraindicated because it supports bacterial growth.

Preparation
1. Check healthcare provider's order for oxygen prescription (flow rate).
2. Gather equipment.
3. Insert oxygen flow meter into wall outlet.
4. Connect cannula tubing to flow meter.
5. Place disposable humidifier unit between flow meter and cannula tubing if humidification is ordered.
6. Perform hand hygiene.

Procedure
1. Introduce self and identify client with two forms of identification.
2. Explain purpose and procedure of oxygen use to client.
3. Place nasal prongs of cannula into client's nares. ❶
4. Fit cannula tubing around client's ears and adjust tubing slide under client's chin.

5. Adjust flow of oxygen. Should be limited to 6 L/min or less, FiO_2: 24–44%, flow: 1–6 L. ➤ *Rationale:* Since atmospheric air mixes with prescribed oxygen concentration as client inhales, the FiO_2 varies depending on the flow and nature of client's breathing. Deep breathing dilutes rather than enhances the FiO_2 because more room air is inhaled.

Note: Oxygen therapy is not corrective for hypoxia caused by anemia, abnormal hemoglobin, or vascular insufficiency.

6. Monitor vital signs and check client's condition regularly.
7. Provide nares care every 4 hr—use ONLY water-soluble products and avoid petroleum products. ➤ *Rationale:* Petroleum products are combustible, not absorbed by the body, and difficult to clear from the mucosa.
8. Monitor for pressure around ears and pad cannula tubing for comfort if indicated.

❶ Oxygen administration by nasal cannula.

Skill 30.3.5 | Using an Oxygen Face Mask

Equipment
Oxygen mask
Four types of masks:
   Simple face mask
   Partial rebreather mask with reservoir bag
   Nonrebreather mask with reservoir bag
   Venturi mask used to specifically control oxygen
   concentration

Oxygen source
Oxygen flowmeter
Disposable humidifier (if indicated)

Preparation
1. Check healthcare provider's orders for oxygen.
2. Gather equipment (Table 30-1 ■).
3. Perform hand hygiene.

Table 30-1 Oxygen Delivery Devices (FiO_2 Numbers Are Approximate)

Nasal Cannula

This equipment is easily tolerated by most clients. It is also simpler than a mask. The fraction of inspired oxygen (FiO_2) varies depending on the oxygen liter flow and the rate and depth of client breathing.

FiO_2:	24–38%	Flow:	1–2 L
FiO_2:	30–35%	Flow:	3–4 L
FiO_2:	38–44%	Flow:	5–6 L

Simple Face Mask

This equipment ❶ requires fairly high oxygen flow to prevent rebreathing of carbon dioxide. About 75% of the inspired volume is room air drawn in through side holes in the mask. Accurate FiO_2 is difficult to estimate.

FiO_2	35–65%	Flow:	8–12 L

Mask With Reservoir Bag

The reservoir allows higher FIO_2 to be delivered. At flows of less than 6 L/min, the risk of rebreathing carbon dioxide increases. Two types are available:

Partial rebreather mask: ❷ No inspiratory valve so that the beginning portion of exhaled air returns to the bag and mixes with the inspired air. Ports are present so that the most expired air escapes. The reservoir bag remains one-third to one-half inflated.

FiO_2	40–60%	Flow:	6–10 L

Nonrebreather: Valve closes during expiration so that exhaled air does not enter reservoir and is not rebreathed. Valves on mask side ports allow exhalation but close on inspiration to prevent inhalation of room air.

FiO_2	60–100%	Flow:	6–15 L

(continued)

Skill 30.3.5 | Using an Oxygen Face Mask *(continued)*

Table 30-1 Oxygen Delivery Devices (FiO$_2$ Numbers Are Approximate) *(continued)*

Venturi Mask
This system ❸ utilizes different-sized adapters to deliver a fixed or predicted FiO$_2$. The FiO$_2$ is dependent on liter flow and/or entrainment port size. It is used effectively on clients with COPD when accurate FiO$_2$ is necessary. Carbon dioxide buildup is kept at a minimum. Humidifiers usually are not used. FiO$_2$ is dependent on liter flow and/or entrainment port size.
FiO$_2$ 24–50%

Face Tent
This soft aerosol mask fits loosely around the face and neck. ❹ It is an alternative to an aerosol mask for clients who feel claustrophobic, but it is sometimes difficult to keep in place. It is convenient for providing humidification and oxygenation; however, oxygen concentration cannot be controlled.
FiO$_2$:   28–100%   Flow: 8–12 L

Oxygen Hood
This disposable vinyl box fits over a child's head to provide warm humidified oxygen at a controlled temperature.
FiO$_2$:   28–40%   Flow: 5–8 L FiO$_2$:   40–85%   Flow: 8–12 L
Less than 5 L flow may lead to carbon dioxide narcosis.

Oxygen Tent
This canopy encloses the child and is used to provide oxygen, humidification, and/or a cool environment to control temperature.
FiO$_2$:   Up to 50%   Flow: 10–15 L

Hyperbaric Chamber
See Box 30-7 ∎.

❶ Simple face mask delivers moderately high flow of oxygen.

❷ *Left:* Partial rebreather mask provides higher FiO$_2$ than a simple mask, but is seldom used. *Right:* Nonrebreather mask provides highest FiO$_2$.

Procedure

1. Introduce self and identify client using two identifiers.
2. Explain procedure and rationale for administration of oxygen to client.
3. Check size of face mask to make sure it fits client.
4. Turn on oxygen flow to liters prescribed. If reservoir bag is attached, partially inflate it with oxygen.
5. Place client in semi- or high-Fowler's position.
6. Fit mask to client's face from nose downward during expiration. If reservoir bag is attached, oxygen flow must be at a level to prevent bag from collapsing. ➤ **Rationale:**

A tight fit prevents oxygen from escaping around eyes or nose.

7. Place elastic band around client's head.
8. Stay with client until client feels at ease with mask.
   ➤ **Rationale:** Clients may be afraid of suffocating.
9. Assess client's condition by checking vital signs and oxygenation status.
10. Change mask and tubing according to agency policy and provide skin care to face.
11. Check equipment frequently. If humidifier is attached, check water level, dispose, and change prn.

❸ Venturi mask with oxygen percent control pieces.

❹ Oxygen face tent delivers unpredictable oxygen flow with high humidity.

Box 30-7 NEW TRENDS: HYPERBARIC OXYGEN THERAPY (HBOT)

Intermittent HBOT supports healing and alleviates symptoms in a number of acute and chronic health problems where blood flow and tissue oxygenation are reduced. This modality:

- Increases oxygen concentration in body tissues, even those with inadequate blood flow
- Reduces local tissue edema
- Stimulates growth of new blood vessels
- Causes rebound vasodilation after therapy
- Stimulates the body's immune response, production of antioxidants, and free radical scavengers
- Enhances WBC activity and potentiates effects of antibiotics

HBOT is used intermittently to deliver 100% oxygen at greater than normal atmospheric pressure (1 atmosphere absolute). The client reclines on a cot in a transparent cylinder ("chamber") with room air and breathes 100% O_2 through a hood or mask while pressure in the chamber is increased 1.5–2 times atmospheric pressure. Treatments usually last 1 hr, during which the client can watch TV, read, sleep, or converse with others outside of the chamber. At completion of treatment, the client is gradually decompressed to normal atmospheric pressure. Studies regarding the usefulness of HBOT are ongoing.

Delivery of 100% oxygen at greater than atmospheric pressure is used for a number of acute and chronic health problems where blood flow and tissue oxygenation are reduced.

Source: ERproductions Ltd

Skill 30.3.6 | Using an Oxygen Hood

Equipment
Disposable oxygen hood
Oxygen source
Oxygen analyzer
Flexible oxygen tubing

Procedure
1. Check healthcare provider orders for oxygen level.
2. Perform hand hygiene.
3. Introduce self and identify client using two identifiers.
4. Explain procedure as appropriate.

(continued)

Skill 30.3.6 | Using an Oxygen Hood *(continued)*

5. Place hood around child's head and/or upper body and attach tubing to oxygen supply.
6. Close ports and lid, but do not obstruct neck opening. ➤ *Rationale:* Obstructing neck opening can lead to carbon dioxide accumulation.
7. Infants are cared for through portholes or lid. ➤ *Rationale:* This prevents excessive oxygen leakage.
8. Maintain oxygen levels at 40–50%, and check for moisture that accumulates inside hood.
9. Observe usual oxygen administration precautions.

LEGAL CONSIDERATIONS

Gordon v. Presbyterian Hospital: In this case, a client was being received for emergency surgery. Available oxygen tanks were empty in the holding area, so the nurse obtained a tank from one of the surgical suites. The room was dark, color of the tank was not appreciated, and the client received CO_2 (gray tank) rather than O_2 (green tank). When discovered, a CODE BLUE was called. The client remained comatose for several weeks before her death.

Manning v. Twin Falls Clinic & Hospital, Inc.: There was substantial evidence in medical malpractice action against a nurse to support award of punitive damages where the plaintiff's expert witness concluded that the nurse's conduct in disconnecting supplemental oxygen to the client during the client's transfer to another room was extreme deviation from the standard of care. Evidence was also present that the nurse disconnected oxygen despite pleadings from family members present who claimed that the client could not survive without his oxygen and who requested that he be provided with a portable oxygen unit preparatory to the move. From this evidence, the jury could have found that the nurse's conduct was grossly negligent and that she acted with disregard for consequences that were likely to follow.

Unit 30.3 Documentation and Evaluation

DOCUMENTATION for Oxygen Administration

- Type of equipment used for oxygen administration, liter flow, FiO_2
- Arterial PaO_2 and SaO_2 or pulse oximetry results
- Vital signs
- Client's tolerance of device
- Client and family teaching and indication of understanding

EVALUATION/Critical Thinking

Expected Outcomes

- Client breathes without distress.
- Oxygen administration does not have adverse effects.
- Breath sounds are normal in all lung fields.
- Client's respiratory rate remains within normal limits.
- SpO_2 values do not vary significantly.
- SpO_2 false alarms do not occur.
- Client remains comfortable with oxygen therapy delivery.

Unexpected Outcomes

- Client reports having difficulty breathing (dyspnea).

Alternative Actions

- Check SpO_2 and compare with previous findings.
- Encourage client to describe what he or she is experiencing.
- Place client in Fowler's position.
- Assist with all activities of daily living (ADLs) to conserve client's energy.
- Employ measures to alleviate pain or anxiety.

Unexpected Outcomes	Alternative Actions

• Client shows these abnormal signs and symptoms: changes in blood pressure, tachycardia, tachypnea, abnormal color, restlessness, or altered sensorium.	• Check ABGs for drop in blood pH (acidemia) or rise in $PaCO_2$ (respiratory acidosis) and report if found. These conditions can occur if hypoxic drive is blunted by the administration of high oxygen concentration.
	  • Check oxygen delivery setting.
	  • Reduce oxygen concentration as ordered.
	• Clients who chronically retain carbon dioxide may require controlled oxygen concentration delivery device (e.g., Venturi mask).

• Client develops atelectasis.	• Encourage deep breathing, range of motion, frequent position changes, and early ambulation if possible. • Use sedatives or other respiratory depressants carefully. • CPT may be ordered. • Check breath sounds. (They are usually decreased with this condition and crackles are frequently heard at the end of inspiration in dependent lung areas and may clear after client coughs.)
• Client develops tachypnea.	• Report change and check SpO_2 immediately, since inadequate flow rates may be causing the problem. • Increase flow rate as ordered and monitor. • Monitor vital signs and correlate with client findings as pulmonary embolus may be the cause. • Check client's breathing pattern and breath sounds and report significant change.
• Oxygen toxicity occurs.	• Toxicity occurs soon after initiation of oxygen use and is directly related to the FiO_2. • Monitor closely for nausea, restlessness, pallor, lethargy, weakness, and dyspnea. • Validate that sensor and oximeter are from the same manufacturer. • Do not exceed 40% oxygen concentration (FiO_2) unless using continuous monitoring of SpO_2.
• Oxygen saturation (SpO_2) findings are erratic.	• Check that sensor probes are aligned to prevent photodetector picking up light from sources other than sensor. • Check that appropriate sensor site was selected for specific probes (e.g., finger site for finger sensor).
• Pulse oximeter alarm sounds frequently.	• Do not disarm the system. • Encourage client to immobilize sensor site. Movement scrambles signals from photodetector, interfering with readings. • Obtain wrap sensor if thumb or toe is used. • Place sensor on different site. • Avoid placing sensor on hand of arm used for continuous blood pressure monitoring.
• Client experiences discomfort with nasal prongs.	• Obtain smaller-gauge pediatric cannula. • Obtain mustache pad or foam wrap for easing tube pressure behind ears.

Intubated Airways

Nursing Process Data

ASSESSMENT Database

- Assess client's level of consciousness.
- Determine whether gag–swallow reflex is present.
- Assess breath sounds in all lung fields, SpO$_2$, ABGs.
- Observe for shortness of breath, labored breathing, tachypnea, or tachycardia.
- Note presence of adventitious sounds.
- Note character of secretions.

PLANNING Objectives

- Oropharyngeal or nasopharyngeal intubation:
  - To provide patent airway
- Endotracheal intubation:
  - To provide patent airway
  - To provide route for mechanical ventilation
  - To facilitate removal of airway secretions
  - To improve gas exchange

IMPLEMENTATION Procedures

DOCUMENTATION AND EVALUATION

Expected Outcomes

- Patent airway is established.
- Intubation assessment parameters indicate correct placement.
- Accidental extubation does not occur.

Unexpected Outcomes/Alternative Actions

Pearson Nursing Student Resources

Find additional review materials at
nursing.pearsonhighered.com.
Prepare for success with NCLEX®-style practice
questions and Skill Checklists.

Skill 30.4.1 | Inserting an Oropharyngeal Airway

Equipment
Oropharyngeal tube
Tongue depressor
Clean gloves
Suction catheter
Suction source

Procedure
1. Ensure that client is unresponsive and has NO gag reflex.
   ➤ *Rationale:* Conscious client may vomit and aspirate or develop laryngospasm during tube insertion.
2. Select appropriate size airway—length should be from corner of mouth to corner of ear tragus.
3. Perform hand hygiene; don gloves.
4. Gently open client's mouth with crossed finger technique, placing your thumb on client's lower teeth and index finger on the upper teeth and gently pushing them apart. You may need to use modified jaw thrust to insert tube.
5. Perform oral suctioning.
6. Hold tongue down with tongue depressor and advance airway to back of tongue OR advance airway upside down (curved upward) ❶ and, as airway passes uvula, rotate the airway 180 degrees.
7. Check that concave curve fits over tongue. It should extend from the lips to the pharynx, displacing the tongue anteriorly.
   ➤ *Rationale:* Proper positioning helps prevent injury to lips, teeth, tongue, and posterior pharynx.
8. Tape top and bottom of airway in position. ➤ *Rationale:* Stabilization of the tube prevents injuries.
9. Position client on side to facilitate drainage.

❶ Oropharyngeal airway is initially inserted upside down (curved upward), then rotated 180 degrees.

10. Remove gloves, discard, and perform hand hygiene.
11. Observe position of airway and evaluate quality of client's spontaneous breathing.

Skill 30.4.2 | Inserting a Nasopharyngeal Airway (Nasal Trumpet)

Equipment
Flexible nasopharyngeal airway
Water-soluble lubricant
Clean gloves

Procedure
1. Select appropriate size tube (length from tip of nose to earlobe and lumen slightly narrower than client's naris).
2. Perform hand hygiene; don gloves.
3. Introduce self and identify client using two identifiers.
4. Lubricate entire length of tube.
5. Explain procedure to client. ❶
6. Insert entire tube gently through naris, following anatomic line of nasal passage. If obstructed, try other naris.
7. Validate position by:
   a. Feeling exhaled air through tube opening
   b. Inspecting for tube tip behind uvula.
8. Position client on side to facilitate drainage of secretions.
9. Remove gloves, discard, and perform hand hygiene.

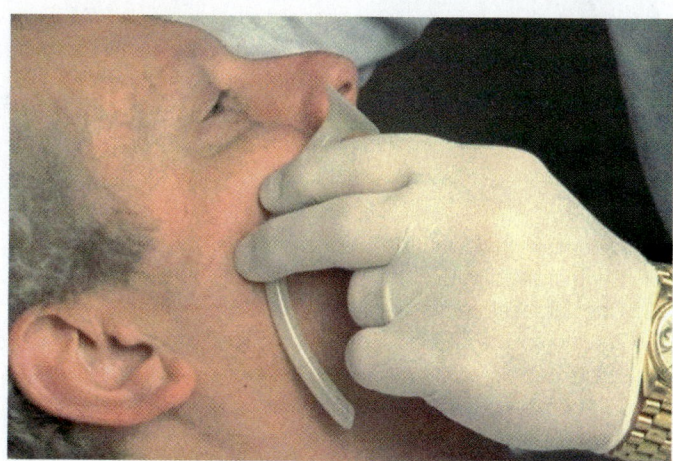

❶ Nasal trumpet protects airway from repeated trauma with upper airway (nasopharyngeal) suctioning.

10. Continue to monitor position of airway and client's response.
11. Suction upper airway prn using clean technique.

Skill 30.4.3 | Assisting With Endotracheal Intubation

Equipment

"Crash cart" (contains most needed supplies)

Laryngoscope with several blade sizes

Stylet to guide endotracheal tube (*ONLY for oral intubation*)

Endotracheal tubes

Water-soluble lubricant

McGill forceps

Suction source

Oxygen source

Bag–valve–mask

Twill, adhesive tape, or Velcro holder

10-mL syringe for cuff inflation

Stethoscope

CO_2 detector (for airway placement validation)

Oral airway or bite block

Clean gloves and personal protective equipment (PPE), including face shield

Established pulse oximetry and cardiac monitoring if available

Wrist restraints (if ordered by healthcare provider)

Prepared sedative as ordered

Labeled container for client's dentures if needed

Note: Noninvasive positive pressure ventilation methods (CPAP, BiPAP) provide an appropriate alternative to intubation for many clients with ventilatory insufficiency. Intubated clients require a higher level of care than clients receiving CPAP or BiPAP for obstructive sleep apnea.

> **CLINICAL ALERT**
>
> The presence of an endotracheal tube bypasses defenses that normally protect the lower airways (filtration, humidification, and hydration of inspired air and epiglottal closure). In addition, mucociliary transport of secretions and trapped pathogens is impaired. These alterations place intubated clients at risk for aspiration pneumonia. Use of care bundles such as the ventilator-associated pneumonia (VAP) bundle—a set of best practices that includes frequent mouth care and keeping the head of bed at 30–45 degrees—will help prevent this complication.

Preparation

1. Determine that client has *no protective airway reflexes*.
2. Bring crash cart to client's doorway.
3. Check that all necessary equipment is functioning (oxygen or suction source and delivery systems, laryngoscope batteries).
4. Inflate and deflate airway cuff to determine whether it is intact.
5. Perform hand hygiene and don gloves. Don PPE.
6. Insert stylet into tube (only for oral intubation); ensure that stylus does not extend beyond tube tip.
7. Lubricate tube.
8. Administer medication as ordered.
9. Remove client's dentures or bridgework if present and place in labeled container.

10. Prepare tape to secure endotracheal tube or obtain endotracheal tube holder.
11. Review, See Skill 30.1.8, Providing Bag–Valve–Mask Ventilation.

Procedure

1. Don clean gloves and PPE.
2. Place client in flat supine position with pillow under shoulders to hyperextend neck and help open airway. Position so that mouth, pharynx, and trachea are aligned. ➤ *Rationale:* Proper positioning facilitates intubation.
3. Restrain client's wrists only if necessary.
4. Premedicate client as ordered.
5. Preoxygenate client for several minutes, using bag–valve–mask. ➤ *Rationale:* This is to create an "oxygen reserve."

> **CLINICAL ALERT**
>
> While cuff pressures are typically maintained at 20–25 mm Hg, an individual client's tracheal capillary pressure cannot be determined; excessive cuff pressure is the best predictor of tracheolaryngeal injury.

> **CLINICAL ALERT**
>
> Even if spontaneously breathing, the client should be preoxygenated with 100% O_2 for endotracheal tube placement. Ventilation must not be interrupted for over 30 sec.

6. Using thumb and index finger, apply cricoid pressure during tube insertion if requested to do so by healthcare provider. ➤ *Rationale:* This facilitates tracheal placement and protects against aspiration of gastric contents.
7. Maintain cricoid pressure while inflating cuff to "minimal leak" inflation by placing stethoscope at client's suprasternal notch and noting a slight hissing sound at peak of inspiration. ❶
8. Attach bag–valve–mask, provide ventilation, and look for chest to rise. ➤ *Rationale:* If chest does not rise, esophageal intubation is likely.
9. Check tube placement using CO_2 detector. ➤ *Rationale:* Presence of CO_2 indicates tracheal intubation.
10. Place stethoscope over epigastrium. ➤ *Rationale:* If gurgling is heard and abdominal distention is noted, esophageal placement is likely.
11. Auscultate lung fields for bilateral breath sounds. ➤ *Rationale:* This ensures that accidental right main stem intubation has not occurred.

> **CLINICAL ALERT**
>
> Cricoid pressure may be used only if the client:
> - Is nonresponsive
> - Is not vomiting
>
> It may only be done by someone skilled in the procedure.

❶ CASS-ETT has a lumen that opens above the tube cuff. Lumen (white tip) is connected to continuous suction to remove subglottic secretions that accumulate above the cuff in order to prevent pneumonia due to aspiration of these secretions.

❷ Endotube stabilizer distributes equipment weight and pressure evenly on the client's face and facilitates easy periodic relocation of tube from side-to-side to prevent oral tissue trauma.

> **CLINICAL ALERT**
> CDC guidelines recommend orotracheal over nasotracheal intubation to reduce the incidence of sinus infection.

12. Mark tube at level of client's front teeth and tape securely with twill or adhesive tape or endotube stabilizer. ❷
    ➤ **Rationale:** Securement prevents tube displacement.
13. Recheck tube placement with the previous measures (steps 9–11).
14. Place bite block or oral airway if ET tube has been positioned orally.
15. Attach O_2 source to ET tube.
16. Discard disposable equipment, remove protective gear and gloves, and perform hand hygiene.

17. Position client in position as ordered.
18. Obtain chest x-ray to confirm tracheal placement of ET tube.
19. Place call bell and writing material within client's reach (as indicated).
20. Reposition ET tube (using Velcro or endotube stabilizer) right, center, and left, and then repeat as needed to prevent pressure ulcers. Refer to agency protocol for frequency.

> **CLINICAL ALERT**
> Low-pressure tracheal tube cuffs provide adequate blood flow to trachea, thus decreasing potential of tracheal tissue necrosis. These cuffs do not need periodic deflation.

Skill 30.4.4 | Inflating a Tracheal Tube Cuff

Equipment
10-mL syringe
Suction equipment
Stethoscope
Clean gloves

Note: The tracheostomy tube with foam cuff (Binova) does not require injected air. Air enters the balloon when port is open.

Procedure
1. Introduce self and identify client with two identifiers.
2. Don clean gloves.
3. Attach 10-mL syringe to distal end of inflatable cuff port, ❶ making sure seal is tight.

4. Inflate cuff for a minimal leak or minimal occlusive volume detected by auscultating over the suprasternal notch for a hissing sound at peak of inspiration. ❷ ➤ **Rationale:** This provides an adequate seal without risking tracheal pressure necrosis.
5. Ask client to speak—if voice is heard, inflation is inadequate for mechanical ventilation.
6. Connect ventilator or T-piece to tracheal tube opening if indicated.
7. Assess breath sounds every 2 hr. ➤ **Rationale:** Presence of bilateral breath sounds indicates proper tube position in trachea.

(continued)

Skill 30.4.4 | Inflating a Tracheal Tube Cuff *(continued)*

1 Attach 10-mL syringe to inflate tube cuff.

2 Inflate endotracheal or tracheostomy tube cuff to minimal occlusive volume.

8. Monitor cuff pressure regularly. ➤ *Rationale:* This may detect inadvertent cuff overinflation and prevent potential necrosis of tracheal tissue. Pressure is usually maintained at 20–25 mm Hg to prevent tracheal necrosis. However, an individual client's tracheal capillary pressure cannot be determined.

CLINICAL ALERT
Tracheal tube cuff inflation is essential for mechanically ventilated clients. Without cuff inflation, delivered air diverts out through the nose and mouth, and lungs are not ventilated.

Skill 30.4.5 | Providing Care for Client With Endotracheal Tube

Procedure

1. Monitor breath sounds every 4 hr. Breath sounds should be heard equally throughout lung fields bilaterally.
2. Check marked points on tube at insertion level. ➤ *Rationale:* This determines whether tube has moved.
3. Inspect positioning and stabilization of tube. ➤ *Rationale:* A change of position can obstruct airway or cause erosion and necrosis of tissues.
4. Inspect and clean mouth and nose. Observe for pressure areas or ulceration.
5. Reposition ET tube every 4 hr (right, center, left), noting tube depth each time.
6. Support client's head and tube when turning. ➤ *Rationale:* This prevents tube from becoming dislodged or airway from becoming obstructed.
7. Place call bell within reach and provide alternative means of communication when cuffed tube is in place. ➤ *Rationale:* No air passes over larynx, so client is not able to summon help or communicate.
8. Support client by spending extra time, using touch, and anticipating client's needs.
9. Ensure adequate hydration. ➤ *Rationale:* Artificial airways bypass the humidifying process of normal breathing.
10. Provide suction tooth brushing every 12 hr, oral swabbing every 2 hr, and oropharyngeal subglottal suctioning every 6 hr. ➤ *Rationale:* This reduces oropharyngeal bacteria and helps prevent pulmonary infection.

CLINICAL ALERT
Even with appropriate cuff inflation, intubated clients receiving gastric or enteral tube feedings are at high risk for aspiration.

Skill 30.4.6 | Extubating an Endotracheal Tube

Equipment
Suction source
Oral suction catheter (or Yankauer)
Sterile suction catheter set
Clean gloves

Sterile gloves
PPE
Oxygen source
Postextubation oxygen delivery device
Syringe for cuff deflation

Preparation

1. Introduce self and identify client with two identifiers.
2. Assess client's readiness for extubation per agency protocol.
3. Determine who needs to be present during extubation and who can perform extubation per agency protocol. ➤ *Rationale:* This skill is generally performed by an advanced practitioner.
4. Obtain vital signs.
5. Explain procedure to client.
6. Prepare postextubation oxygen administration device.
7. Place client in Fowler's position.

Procedure

1. Perform hand hygiene and don clean gloves and PPE.
2. Perform oral or nasopharyngeal suctioning.
3. Have client take several slow deep breaths. ➤ *Rationale:* This hyperoxygenates client in preparation for extubation.
4. *Deflate* tube cuff using syringe.
5. *Untie* the endotracheal tube.
6. Remove gloves, perform hand hygiene, and don sterile gloves.

7. Connect sterile catheter to suction source.
8. Insert sterile suction catheter into airway until resistance is met, and then retract slightly.
9. Leave suction catheter in place.
10. Have client take a deep breath. ➤ *Rationale:* This dilates the vocal cords and makes removal easier and less traumatic.
11. Apply suction while removing catheter and airway at the same time.
12. Immediately apply supplementary oxygen device.
13. Monitor client frequently at first, then regularly.
14. Dispose of equipment, remove gloves, protective gear, and perform hand hygiene.

> **CLINICAL ALERT**
>
> Do not feed client by mouth immediately after extubation. Check swallow reflex and seek consult for a feeding trial for clients at risk for aspiration.

Unit 30.4 Documentation and Evaluation

DOCUMENTATION for Intubation

- Clinical manifestations indicating need for intubation
- Specific reason for intubation
- Premedication administered
- Size and type of inserted endotracheal, nasopharyngeal, or oropharyngeal tube
- Where the tube was taped (e.g., 22 cm at the lips)
- Minimal occlusive pressure for cuff inflation or measured mm Hg pressure
- Preoxygenation and postoxygenation when suctioning
- Quantity and character of secretions
- Pre- and post-procedure vital signs
- Client's tolerance of procedure
- Settings of ventilator or other oxygen mode

EVALUATION/Critical Thinking

Expected Outcomes

- Patent airway is established.
- Intubation assessment parameters indicate correct placement.
- Accidental extubation does not occur.

(continued)

Unexpected Outcomes	Alternative Actions
• Naso/oropharyngeal airway cannot be placed.	• Change size of tube; change naris; do not force insertion. • Hyperextend client's neck. • Direct insertion of nasopharyngeal tube more medially. • Insert oropharyngeal rather than nasopharyngeal airway. • Use tongue depressor to facilitate insertion of oropharyngeal tube. • Relubricate airway and attempt to reinsert. • Call Rapid Response Team if indicated.
• Laryngospasm occurs when endotracheal tube is inserted.	• Remove tube and wait a few minutes. • If severe, administer sedation per healthcare provider order. • Possibly prepare for immediate cricothyroidotomy or tracheotomy.
• Tube placement is incorrect: Air movement heard over epigastrium; bilateral breath sounds not heard; CO_2 indicator does not register.	• Withdraw tube and assist with reintubation. • Verify tube placement with x-ray (tube tip should be between larynx and carina). • Recheck CO_2 indicator for correct placement. • Recheck for bilateral breath sounds and SpO_2 status. • Ensure that mark is visible at insertion level for monitoring ETT placement.
• Accidental extubation occurs.	• Immediately call a CODE or Rapid Response Team for airway replacement. • Call for crash cart and emergency supplies. • Immediately seek assist to provide bag–valve–mask ventilations. • Assess marker on tube frequently to ensure proper placement.

Nursing Process Data

ASSESSMENT Database

- Assess client's need for suctioning.
- Observe vital signs for increases in pulse and respiration.
- Auscultate breath sounds and for presence of adventitious sounds.
- Observe respiratory status for tachypnea, shortness of breath, and restlessness.
- Observe for signs of hypoxia.

PLANNING Objectives

- To provide patent airway
- To remove secretions
- To improve ventilation
- To decrease breathing rate
- To increase tissue oxygenation

IMPLEMENTATION Procedures

DOCUMENTATION AND EVALUATION

Expected Outcomes

- Secretions removed without complication.
- Tube-fed client does not aspirate feeding.

Unexpected Outcomes/Alternative Actions

Pearson Nursing Student Resources

Find additional review materials at **nursing. pearsonhighered.com.**

Prepare for success with NCLEX®-style practice questions and Skill Checklists.

Skill 30.5.1 | Suctioning With Catheter in Sleeve

Note: For Suctioning Using Single-Use Catheter for Tracheostomy, see Skill 30.6.1.

Equipment

Portable suction machine or wall suction unit with receptacle and tubing

Appropriate length suction catheter in protective sleeve packet (with pop-up cup)

Clean gloves

Sterile saline/water

Receptacle for used equipment

Oxygen source and administration device (e.g., bag–valve device with tube adapter)

PPE—gown, goggles, mask if splash anticipated

Stethoscope

Preparation

1. Check healthcare provider's orders. Gather equipment.
2. Introduce self and identify client with two identifiers.
3. Recruit an assistant for manual ventilation, if indicated.
4. Attach resuscitator bag to oxygen tubing, if indicated. ❶
5. Perform hand hygiene.
6. Assess lung sounds and heart rate and rhythm.
7. Open saline flush solution bottle.
8. Set suction control regulator at 100–120 mm Hg vacuum.
9. Don protective gown, mask, and goggles. ➤ *Rationale:* This is for self-protection if splash is anticipated.

Procedure

1. Explain procedure and rationale to client regardless of client's level of consciousness.
2. Place client in semi-Fowler's or Fowler's position.
3. Turn on suction.
4. Remove cap from saline bottle.

5. Open catheter kit. Pour sterile saline/water flush solution into pop-up cup.
6. Don gloves.
7. Administer 100% oxygen (oxygen flowmeter to maximum "flush") for 1–2 min. Use resuscitator bag with tracheal tube adapter to hyperoxygenate client. ➤ *Rationale:* Suction removes residual lung volume, resulting in hypoxemia and potential cardiac arrest. Hyperoxygenation prevents these complications.
8. Hold catheter in protective covering and attach end to suction tubing. ❷
9. Retract sleeve enough to lubricate sterile catheter tip by dipping it into cup with sterile saline/water.
10. Advance catheter into client's artificial airway approximately 28 cm (11 in.), or 1 cm beyond tip of ET tube or trach tube, while retracting protective sleeve before applying suction. ➤ *Rationale:* Suctioning during insertion deprives client of oxygen and inhibits catheter advancement. Deep suctioning traumatizes tissue.
11. Apply suction and withdraw catheter using a rotating motion as the catheter is retracted back into protective sleeve.
12. Suction intermittently by placing and releasing thumb over catheter suction port. ➤ *Rationale:* Intermittent versus continuous application of suction may help to reduce airway injury.
13. Limit suction to no more than 10 sec. ➤ *Rationale:* This prevents hypoxemic complications induced by suctioning.
14. Reattach oxygen delivery device to artificial airway and have client take several deep breaths, or hyperoxygenate client's lungs with resuscitator bag for 30 sec.
15. Flush suction catheter and tubing with sterile saline/water and retract back into protective sleeve.
16. Catheter remains in sleeve and attached to suction tubing. ➤ *Rationale:* This is to allow prn use. Reuse same catheter (according to agency policy).
17. Replace catheter in sleeve packet at time interval according to agency policy (e.g., 24 hr).

Note: A separate catheter must be used for pharyngeal suctioning.

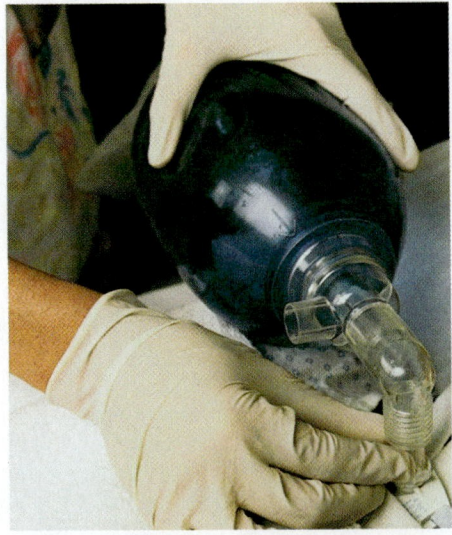

❶ Connect resuscitator bag to hyperoxygenate before and after suctioning.

❷ Hold catheter in protective covering and attach to suction tubing.

18. Perform hand hygiene.
19. Assess lung sounds and heart rate and rhythm for changes.
    ➤ *Rationale:* Suctioning usually causes tachycardia, but hypoxemia and vagal response may cause serious bradycardia or cardiac arrest.
20. Don clean gloves to empty suction receptacle prn or at end of every shift, noting character of secretions.
21. Ensure call bell is within client's reach.

CLINICAL ALERT

Instillation of normal saline should not be performed with endotracheal suctioning. No studies have found this practice to be beneficial; it places clients at risk for healthcare-associated pneumonia. Saline does not liquefy or mobilize secretions; it acts as a vehicle to wash bacteria that normally cling to the inner aspects of the artificial airway into the lung. Instillation of saline also adversely affects arterial oxygenation.

EVIDENCE-BASED PRACTICE
Importance of Oral Suctioning

Clients who are on ventilators have an increased risk for VAP. One of the key risk factors is the aspiration of oral secretions that accumulated in the oral cavity. Good oral hygiene has been shown to decrease that risk but another practice is also important: oral suctioning. Clients who are intubated build up oral secretions that need to be regularly suctioned so they do not aspirate those secretions into their lungs. A study found the minimum frequency needed was every 4 hr and some clients needed oral suctioning as often as every 2 hr.

Source: Sole et al. (2011)

Skill 30.5.2 | Suctioning With Closed Suction System

Equipment

In-line closed system (ET or tracheostomy connected) suction unit with catheter enclosed by plastic sleeve
10 mL of normal saline in unit dose vial
Suction source
Connecting tubing
Oxygen source and side-arm connector (e.g., bag–valve device or ventilator)
Clean gloves

Note: In-line closed system suctioning allows rapid suctioning for intubated clients and does not interrupt ventilator–client interface.

Procedure

1. Introduce self and identify client with two identifiers.
2. Explain procedure and rationale to client regardless of client's level of consciousness. ❶
3. Perform hand hygiene and don gloves. See Box 30-8 ■ for information on safe practice when suctioning.
4. Place client in semi-Fowler's or Fowler's position.
5. Turn on suction source.
6. Connect oxygen source to side arm of tube connector.
7. Hyperoxygenate client with 100% oxygen, using manual bag or mechanical ventilator (100% oxygen source with several manual sighs, if indicated.)
8. Open access valve and advance catheter ❷ within plastic sleeve into client's artificial airway using your dominant hand.
    ➤ *Rationale:* Sterility is maintained because catheter is enclosed by plastic cover and slides within it.
9. With nondominant hand, activate suction valve. Intermittently apply suction (for no more than 5–10 sec) while rotating and withdrawing catheter *completely* back into plastic sheath.
    ❸ ➤ *Rationale:* If not totally out of the airway, the catheter impairs client ventilation.

❶ Mechanical ventilator provides 100% oxygen for hyperoxygenation.

Box 30-8 PREVENTING INFECTION DURING RESPIRATORY CARE

- Maintain sterile technique during suctioning.
- Maintain good hand hygiene.
- Change gloves when providing respiratory care to prevent cross-contamination from another part of the client's body.
- Administer oral care routinely per protocol.
- Avoid instillation of saline into airways.
- Change ventilatory equipment only when visibly soiled or malfunctioning.
- Do not allow condensation in circuit to drain toward client.

(continued)

Skill 30.5.2 | Suctioning With Closed Suction System *(continued)*

2 Intubated client with in-line closed suction catheter being advanced.

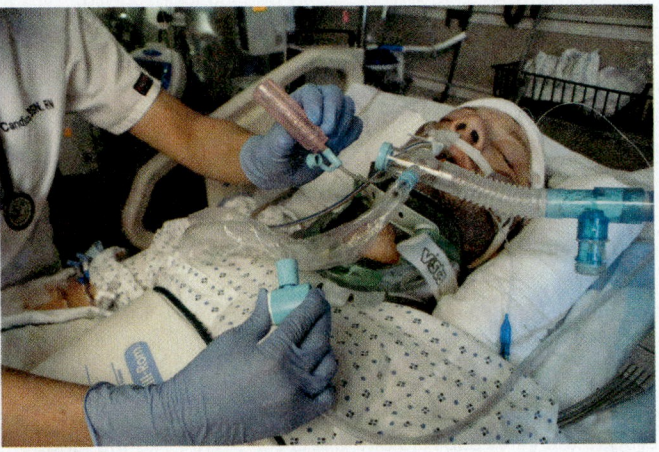

4 Apply suction while instilling saline to flush catheter and tubing.

3 Note black indicator to ensure that catheter is completely withdrawn.

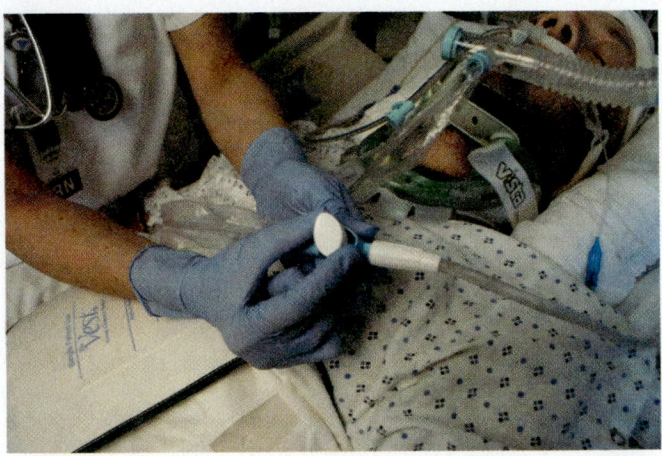

5 Lock access valve when suctioning is complete.

10. Repeat steps 7–9 as necessary to clear secretions; allow time between suctioning for hyperoxygenation. ➤ *Rationale:* Repeated suctioning without hyperoxygenation causes complications such as hypoxemia and cardiac dysrhythmias.
11. Attach saline vial to catheter irrigation port; inject saline while applying suction to rinse catheter and tubing, and then close irrigation port and suction valve. **4** ➤ *Rationale:* Rinsing prevents catheter occlusion by dried secretions.
12. Remove syringe, release suction, and lock mechanism. **5** ➤ *Rationale:* Locking catheter prevents inadvertent catheter advancement and occlusion of client's airway.

13. Remove gloves and perform hand hygiene.
14. Ensure that call bell is within client's reach.
15. Ensure the head of the bed is at 30 degrees. ➤ *Rationale:* This prevents VAP.

CLINICAL ALERT
Monitor client closely and suction prn, as coughed secretions may accumulate at the suction catheter–client's airway interface and obstruct airflow to client's lungs.

Unit 30.5 Documentation and Evaluation

DOCUMENTATION for Suctioning

- Frequency of suctioning
- Amount and character of secretions
- Pre- and postsuctioning hyperoxygenation
- Breath sounds, respiratory rate, heart rate and rhythm, and SpO_2
- Client's tolerance of procedure
- Reestablishment of oxygen therapy and L/min

EVALUATION/Critical Thinking

Expected Outcomes

- Secretions are removed without complication.
- Tube-fed client does not aspirate feeding.

Unexpected Outcomes	Alternative Actions
Hypoxemia and tachycardia or bradycardia occur with suctioning.	• Suction only as needed. • Preoxygenate before and postoxygenate after suctioning, seeking assistance if necessary. • Limit suctioning time to no more than 10 sec. • Ensure that catheter diameter is no larger than half the inner diameter of the airway it enters.
Excessive secretions necessitate frequent suctioning.	• Suction more frequently but administer 100% oxygen before and after suctioning. • Establish in-line catheter in sleeve, check frequently and suction secretions prn. • Allow rest period before suctioning again. • Turn client regularly to mobilize secretions. • Notify healthcare provider for CPT or other therapy. • Maintain adequate hydration.
Aspiration is suspected in enterally tube-fed intubated client.	• Check suctioned secretions for presence of glucose. (Secretions should not contain blood for accurate determination.) • Recommend use of continuous aspiration of subglottic secretions ET tube. • Maintain 30- to 45-degree elevation of head of bed (HOB) at all times if feeding is continuous. • Monitor gastric residuals regularly. • Advocate small-bore enteral versus gastric tube feeding.

Tracheostomy Care

Nursing Process Data

ASSESSMENT Database

- Note presence of dried or moist secretions surrounding cannula or on tracheal dressing.
- Note excessive coughing or expectoration of secretions.
- Assess whether routine tracheal care is adequate for this client.
- Assess respiratory status: breath sounds, respiratory rate, and use of accessory muscles for breathing.
- Observe for signs of respiratory distress while tracheal tube is capped: labored breathing, anxious face, flaring of nares, tachypnea, and tachycardia.
- Monitor pulse oximetry (SpO_2).
- Auscultate for minimal occlusive cuff inflation pressure.

PLANNING Objective

- To ensure a patent airway
- To suction secretions more easily
- To improve ventilation
- To prevent infection
- To prevent aspiration while feeding

IMPLEMENTATION Procedures

DOCUMENTATION AND EVALUATION

Expected Outcomes

- Tracheostomy tube remains stable.
- Tracheostomy tube provides a patent airway.
- Client is able to communicate with speaking valve placement.

Unexpected Outcomes/Alternative Actions

Pearson Nursing Student Resources

Find additional review materials at
nursing.pearsonhighered.com.
Prepare for success with NCLEX®-style practice
questions and Skill Checklists.

Skill 30.6.1 | Suctioning Using Single-Use Catheter for Tracheostomy

Equipment

Portable suction machine or wall suction unit with receptacle and tubing

Oral suction catheter (e.g., Yankauer)

Suction catheter set with suction catheter, sterile gloves, and container (or pop-open cup) for sterile saline

Select catheter of appropriate length—15–20 cm (6–8 in.)

Sterile saline or sterile water (mark time and date bottle is opened and discard in 24 hr)

Receptacle for used equipment

Oxygen source and administration device (e.g., bag–valve device with tracheal tube adapter)

PPE—gown, goggles, mask if splash anticipated

Stethoscope

Preparation

1. Check healthcare provider's orders and client care plan. Box 30-9 ■ provides indications for suctioning.
2. Gather equipment.
3. Recruit an assistant for manual ventilation if indicated.
4. Attach resuscitator bag to oxygen tubing, if indicated.
5. Perform hand hygiene.
6. Assess lung sounds and heart rate and rhythm.
7. Set suction control regulator at 100–120 mm Hg vacuum.
8. Don protective gown, mask, and goggles. ➤ *Rationale:* This is for self-protection if splash anticipated.

Note: This skill is more safely performed with an assistant who manages the resuscitator bag for hyperoxygenation while the nurse performs suctioning.

> **CLINICAL ALERT**
>
> Suction catheter diameter should be no larger than one-half the inner diameter of the artificial airway. To determine catheter diameter size, multiply the artificial airway's diameter times 2 (e.g., for 8-mm tube, use a 16-French suction catheter).

Procedure

1. Explain procedure and rationale to client regardless of client's level of consciousness.
2. Place client in semi-Fowler's or Fowler's position.
3. Turn on suction (100–120 mm Hg vacuum). ❶
4. Remove cap from saline bottle.
5. Open catheter kit using wrapper as sterile field.

Box 30-9 INDICATIONS FOR SUCTIONING

- Ineffective cough
- Client with depressed level of consciousness
- Thick, tenacious mucus
- Impaired pulmonary function

❶ Turn wall suction or other source to 100–120 mm Hg vacuum.

6. Carefully open container (pop open cup) and fill with sterile saline/water.
7. Administer 100% oxygen (oxygen flowmeter to maximum "flush") for 1 min, or have assistant use resuscitator bag with adapter to hyperoxygenate client. ➤ *Rationale:* Suction removes oxygen, resulting in hypoxemia and potential cardiac arrest. Hyperoxygenation prevents these complications. ❷
8. Don sterile gloves. *Dominant* hand will remain sterile, and *nondominant* hand becomes "clean."
9. Holding catheter connecting end with *dominant* (sterile) hand, attach to suction tubing held with nondominant hand (*nondominant* hand is no longer sterile at this point). ❸

> **CLINICAL ALERT**
>
> Hyperoxygenate the client before and after each time the airway is entered for suctioning, and wait 1 min before suctioning again to prevent severe hypoxemia.

10. Lubricate sterile catheter tip by dipping it into cup with sterile normal saline/water.
11. Using *dominant* (sterile gloved) hand, insert catheter into tracheostomy without applying suction. ❹ ➤ *Rationale:* Suctioning during insertion deprives client of oxygen and inhibits catheter advancement.

(continued)

Skill 30.6.1 | Suctioning Using Single-Use Catheter for Tracheostomy *(continued)*

12. Advance catheter quickly 1–2 cm (½–1 inch) beyond end of trach tube until resistance is felt, even if client coughs. ➤ *Rationale:* Deep suctioning traumatizes tracheal mucosa.
13. Suction intermittently by placing and releasing *nondominant* thumb over catheter suction port while withdrawing catheter using a rotating motion. ➤ *Rationale:* Intermittent versus continuous application of suction may help to reduce airway injury.
14. Limit suction to no more than 10 sec. ➤ *Rationale:* This prevents hypoxemic complications induced by suctioning.
15. Reattach oxygen delivery device and have client take several deep breaths, or hyperoxygenate client's lungs with resuscitator bag.
16. Flush suction catheter and tubing with sterile saline/water. ❺
17. Use same catheter (according to agency policy) and repeat suctioning procedure one time, if necessary.

Allow 1 min between suctioning attempts for hyperoxygenation.
18. After lower airway suctioning, use the same catheter to suction client's oropharyngeal secretions. ➤ *Rationale:* Lower airway is sterile; upper airway is not.
19. Coil suction catheter around hand and deglove over it to discard. ❻
20. Discard gloves and catheter and remove PPE.
21. Turn off suction source.
22. Assess lung sounds and heart rate and rhythm for changes. ➤ *Rationale:* Suctioning usually causes tachycardia, but hypoxemia and vagal response may cause serious bradycardia or cardiac arrest.
23. Perform hand hygiene.
24. Empty suction receptacle prnor at end of every shift, noting character of secretions.
25. Ensure call bell is within client's reach.

❷ Connect resuscitator bag to hyperoxygenate before and after suctioning.

❸ Hold sterile catheter with dominant (sterile) hand and connect suction tubing to catheter.

❹ Guide catheter into tracheostomy tube using sterile hand.

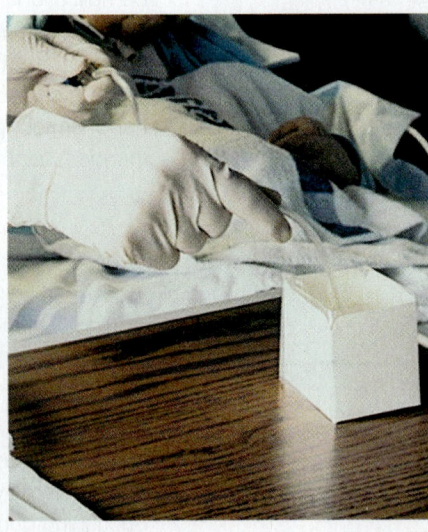

❺ Rinse catheter and connecting tubing to clear.

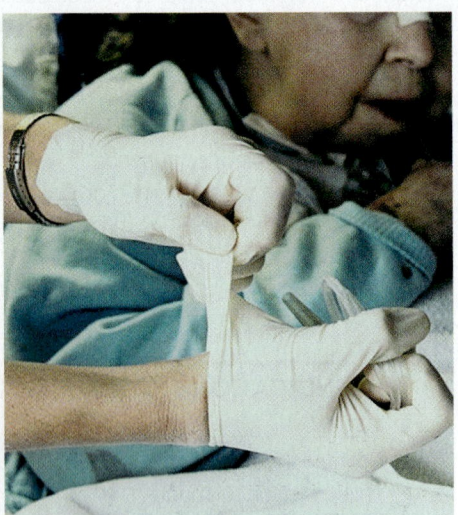

❻ Coil catheter around fingers and pull glove over it for disposal.

Skill 30.6.2 | Cleaning the Inner Cannula and Ostomy

Equipment

Note: Most agencies use disposable inner cannulas that eliminate the need for cleaning.

Tracheal cleaning tray (includes two sterile basins, pipe cleaners, 4×4 gauze pad)
Sterile gloves
Suction equipment
Complete tracheal tube set for emergency use
Disposable inner cannula of same size ❶
Sterile normal saline
Sterile nonraveling presplit dressings
Clean tracheal ties or commercial tube holder

Preparation

1. Check healthcare provider's orders.
2. Assemble equipment.
3. Make sure suction equipment and additional tracheal tubes are available. Suction trach tube before cleaning if indicated.
4. Perform hand hygiene.

Procedure

1. Explain procedure and rationale to client.
2. Open trach tray and put on one sterile glove.
3. With gloved hand, separate basins; with ungloved hand, pour saline into basin.
4. Don second sterile glove. Secure outer cannula neck plate with index finger and thumb. Unlock inner cannula by turning left about 90 degrees.
5. Gently pull the inner cannula slightly upward and out toward you. ❷
6. Soak nondisposable cannula in sterile basin with saline to remove dried secretions. ❸
7. Cleanse the lumen and outer surface of the cannula with pipe cleaners moistened with saline. ➤ *Rationale:* This is to remove dried secretions.

❷ Gently pull inner cannula upward and outward to remove.

8. Rinse cannula thoroughly with saline.
9. Place clean tube on sterile 4×4 gauze pad and dry tube thoroughly.
10. Replace inner cannula carefully, stabilizing outer flange of the cannula with your other hand.
11. Lock the inner cannula by turning the lock to the right so that it is in an upright position.

CLINICAL ALERT

An obturator is kept at the bedside for emergency use. If the tracheostomy tube is inadvertently dislodged, it can be reinserted immediately using the obturator.

❶ Disposable inner cannula eliminates need for cannula cleaning.

Step 1

Step 2

Step 3

❸ Inner nondisposable cannula is removed for cleaning. Outer cannula is not.

(continued)

Skill 30.6.2 | Cleaning the Inner Cannula and Ostomy (continued)

12. Clean around tracheostomy site with applicator soaked in normal saline. ④
13. Cleanse outer cannula with separate applicator.
14. Apply precut, nonraveling trach dressing around insertion site (flaps pointing up), and change tracheal ties if needed.

⑤–⑦ ➤ *Rationale:* Nonraveling dressing prevents fibers from entering trach tube.

15. Discard soiled dressings, tapes, cleaning equipment, and gloves.
16. Perform hand hygiene.
17. Ensure call bell is within client's reach.

④ Clean around tracheostomy site and outer cannula.

⑥ A precut, nonraveling sponge is used for the trach dressing to prevent fibers from entering trach site.

⑤ Apply precut, nonraveling dressing around tracheostomy.

⑦ Folded 4×4 trach dressing for use if presplit dressing is not available.

Skill 30.6.3 | Changing Tracheostomy Tube Ties

Equipment

Scissors
Forceps
Twill tape or commercial tracheostomy tube holder.

Preparation

1. Seek assistance from another individual. ➤ *Rationale:* It is safer to have someone hold the trach tube in place when changing ties.

2. Explain procedure to client.
3. Perform hand hygiene.
4. Gather equipment.
5. Place client in semi- to high-Fowler's position.

Procedure
Twill Tape Ties

1. Cut trach ties length you desire, if not precut.
2. Fold ends of the trach ties over 3–4 cm (1.5 in.) and cut a slit in the piece starting at the folded edge.
3. Have assistant hold the trach tube in place. Cut the old trach ties, remove, and discard. ➤ *Rationale:* Securing tube helps prevent accidental extubation if client coughs.

CLINICAL ALERT

Some agencies recommend that tracheostomy tube and ties not be changed for the first 72 hr because of risk for stoma closure.

---

4. Pass the slit end of the ties through the flange loop of the trach tube about 5–7.5 cm (2–3 in.) (you may use Kelly

forceps to grab tie). ❶ ➤ *Rationale:* Leave the old trach tie in place if you are changing the ties without assistance. This prevents accidental dislodging of the trach tube.
5. Thread the other end of the tie all the way through the slit. Pull it firmly in place. ❷ ➤ *Rationale:* This action anchors the tie around the flange loop.
6. Repeat steps 4 and 5 on other flange loop.
7. Bring ties around client's neck and tie in a square knot to one side of neck, leaving one finger-breadth slack under tie. ❸ ➤ *Rationale:* Slack prevents pressure on the neck and jugular vein.
8. Cut off soiled trach ties if not already done and discard.
9. Position client for comfort.
10. Perform hand hygiene.

Alternate Method

1. Using a long piece of twill, pull end of tape through flange slit. ❹
2. Double tape around back of neck.
3. Thread one end through other flange slit and tie to other end.
4. Apply new tape before old one is cut off and removed (doesn't require an assistant).

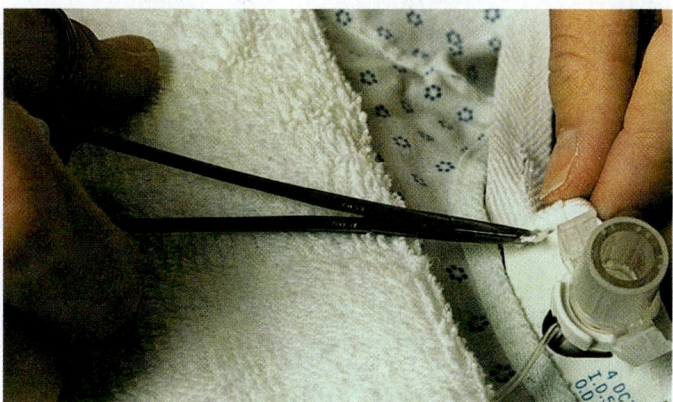

❶ Use forceps to thread tape through tracheostomy neck plate flanges.

❸ Allow one finger-breadth slack under trach ties to prevent pressure on neck and jugular vein. ***Note:*** Velcro is frequently used for track ties in place of twill tape.

❷ Thread other end of tie through slit and pull into place.

❹ (*left*) Use a long piece of twill. Pull end through flange slit and double tape around back of neck. (*right*) Thread one end through other flange slit and tie to other end of twill in square knot.

Skill 30.6.4 | Capping With a Passey–Muir Speaking Valve

Equipment

Passey–Muir speaking valve and storage container
Fenestrated uncuffed tracheostomy tube (preferred)
Suction source
Two suction catheters
Clean gloves
10-mL syringe

Note: A fenestrated uncuffed tracheostomy tube has openings that allow the client's exhaled air to flow through the upper airway as well as the tracheostomy opening. When the outer cannula is capped with a one-way valve, exhaled air flows over the vocal cords for speech production.

Preparation

1. Check healthcare provider's orders and client care plan.
2. Determine that client has been screened with trial for candidacy by a speech pathologist and respiratory care practitioner. See Box 30-10 ■.
3. Determine type of tracheostomy tube present. ➤ ***Rationale:*** A fenestrated, uncuffed tube is preferred. The valve is *not* used with endotracheal tube.
4. Review client's vital signs, SpO$_2$, breath sounds, and work of breathing.
5. Perform hand hygiene.
6. Gather equipment.
7. Explain procedure to client.
8. Place client in Fowler's position. ➤ ***Rationale:*** This assists with lung expansion and helps to maintain a patent airway.
9. Don clean gloves.

> **CLINICAL ALERT**
> The speaking valve should be removed during sleep.

Box 30-10 PASSEY–MUIR SPEAKING VALVE

The Passey–Muir Speaking Valve can be used on or off a ventilator and is safe for infants and adults in acute or home care. The valve expedites mechanical ventilation weaning and reduces decannulation time.

The speaking valve opens only during inspiration and closes automatically before the beginning of the expiratory cycle, restoring exhaled airflow through the oronasopharynx. The valve restores a more normal "closed respiratory system," resulting in many benefits including hands-free, clear, uninterrupted speech production; improved swallowing; reduced aspiration; and stronger, more effective cough. Additionally, use of the valve restores the sense of smell and taste, thus improving appetite and promoting nutritional intake.

EVIDENCE-BASED PRACTICE
Use of Talking Tracheostomy Tubes

Clients who are unable to tolerate having their cuffs deflated on their tracheostomy tubes should be considered candidates to have a special tracheostomy placed to assist them in communicating with the cuff inflated. This allows the client to feel more independent and in control of their care. These "talking tracheostomy tubes" are often not considered, but they are critically important to allow a higher quality of life for clients who are in critical care units or are at risk for aspiration if their cuffs are deflated.

Source: Pandian et al. (2014)

Procedure

1. Using clean technique, suction nasopharynx *if cuffed tube in place.* ➤ ***Rationale:*** This removes secretions that have pooled above cuff and prevents their mobilization into lower airways upon cuff deflation.
2. Attach syringe and deflate tracheal cuff, if present.
   ➤ ***Rationale:*** If tracheostomy tube is capped, ❶ a deflated cuff allows an airway.

> **CLINICAL ALERT**
> If a cuffed tracheostomy tube is capped and cuff is *not* deflated, client has no airway. Place notice: *Do not inflate cuff with cap in place* on pilot balloon, over bed, and on client's chart. An uncuffed fenestrated tube is preferred when speaking valve is used.

❶ Tracheostomy tube is capped with a one-way valve to allow client to speak.

3. Allow the client to adjust to cuff deflation. ➤ *Rationale:* Initiation of upper airway breathing increases resistance to airflow.
4. Place speaking valve over opening of tracheostomy tube.
5. Place notice: "Do not inflate cuff with speaking valve in place" on pilot balloon, over bed, and on client's chart.

6. Gently stabilize the tracheostomy tube to remove the valve and place in container.
7. When the valve is removed, reinflate tube cuff (if indicated).
8. Discard gloves and perform hand hygiene.

Unit 30.6 Documentation and Evaluation

DOCUMENTATION for Tracheostomy Care

Tracheostomy Tube Suctioning
- Frequency of client suctioning
- Before and after suctioning hyperoxygenation
- Amount, color, and consistency of secretions
- Client's tolerance to procedure
- Unanticipated problems and client's response

Cleaning the Inner Cannula and Ostomy
- Time and date of care
- Ostomy site status
- Cannula cleaning or disposable cannula replacement
- Tracheostomy ties or holder replacement

Capping Tracheostomy Tube
- Type of tracheostomy tube in place
- Type of speaking valve utilized
- Tracheal tube DEFLATION status
- Baseline data before procedure
- Client's tolerance of valve placement
- Respiratory and O_2 status during valve use
- Client's ability to speak and swallow

Tracheal Tube Cuff Inflation
- Cuff inflation auscultated for minimal occlusive pressure.
- Bilateral breath sounds present on auscultation.

EVALUATION/Critical Thinking

Expected Outcomes
- Tracheostomy tube remains stable.
- Tracheostomy tube provides a patent airway.
- Client is able to communicate with speaking valve placement.

Unexpected Outcomes
- Client experiences tracheostomy tube decannulation.

Alternative Actions
- Call a "CODE" immediately.
- For new stoma:
- If present, pull tracheal retention sutures apart to lift the trachea and hold the stoma open.
- *Or*: Cover stoma and have assistant provide bag–mask ventilations.
- *Or*: Obtain new tracheostomy tube, place obturator and insert tube into client's stoma, and then remove obturator.

(continued)

Unexpected Outcomes

- Client experiences distress—tracheostomy tube is obstructed; breath sounds not heard.

Alternative Actions

- Call Rapid Response Team or "CODE" immediately.
- Deflate cuff.
- Cut tracheostomy ties.
- Remove tube.
- See above options.

- Client experiences distress with speaking valve placement.

- Request repeat assessment by speech pathologist and respiratory care practitioner.
- Monitor client's SpO_2.
- Downsize tracheostomy tube.
- Reduce time of valve use.
- Remove speaking valve if respiratory distress occurs.
- Administer O_2 per nasal cannula if desaturation occurs.
- Obtain Passey–Muir valve with oxygen adapter to administer O_2 if indicated.
- Remind client that use of the speaking valve is a step toward trach tube removal.

Chest Drainage Systems

Nursing Process Data

ASSESSMENT Database

- Assess client's respiratory status, vital signs.
- Note placement site of chest tube (intrapleural or mediastinal).
- Assess that all drainage system connections are securely taped.
- Note prescribed amount of negative pressure to be established.
- Check patency of chest drainage system.
- Assess for signs of mediastinal shift.
- Note character and amount of chest drainage.

PLANNING Objectives

- To evacuate air and/or fluid from intrapleural space to promote lung re-expansion
- To reestablish negative intrapleural pressure
- To facilitate drainage of fluid from the mediastinum after cardiac surgery
- To administer autotransfusion after cardiac surgery

IMPLEMENTATION Procedures

DOCUMENTATION AND EVALUATION

Expected Outcomes

- Chest drainage system is patent.
- Mediastinal shift does not occur.
- Chest tube remains securely placed.

Unexpected Outcomes/Alternative Actions

Pearson Nursing Student Resources

Find additional review materials at
nursing.pearsonhighered.com.
Prepare for success with NCLEX®-style practice questions and Skill Checklists.

| **Skill 30.7.1** | Setting Up and Maintaining a Disposable Water Seal Chest Drainage System |

Equipment

Disposable water seal chest drainage system and stand
Suction source
Connecting tubing and adapter
60-mL sterile syringe with catheter tip
Sterile water in pouring bottle
Tape
Gloves
PPE

Note: Placement of chest tubes in the mediastinum for drainage after cardiac surgery is common. Intrapleural pressure is not affected.

Procedure

1. Introduce self and identify client with two identifiers.
2. Gather equipment.
3. Perform hand hygiene; don gloves and PPE.
4. Unwrap water seal chest drainage system.
5. Place unit in stand on floor at bedside or hang from foot of bed frame.
6. Remove plastic connector on short tube attached to water-seal chamber.
7. Remove plunger from 60-mL syringe and attach barrel of syringe to short tube.
8. Pour specified amount of sterile water into barrel of syringe, filling water seal chamber to 2-cm (0.8-in.) level (according to package directions). ➤ ***Rationale:*** This level provides sufficient fluid to create a one-way valve to prevent atmospheric air from entering client's intrapleural space.

❶ Disposable water-seal chest drainage system. The suction control chamber regulates the amount of negative pressure applied to the chest. The water seal chamber allows air to escape from the intrapleural space and prevents air from reentering. Box 30-11 ■ provides information on checking for chest tube air leaks.

9. For gravity drainage: Leave suction control source tubing open to air.

Box 30-11 CHECK POINTS FOR CHEST TUBE AIR LEAKS

Check Insertion Site

- Pinch or briefly clamp with padded hemostat tube at chest insertion site. Bubbling stops in the water seal chamber if there is an air leak at insertion site.

Check Tubing

- Pinch rubber connecting tubing. Bubbling stops if there is a leak at chest tube connector site.

Check Water Seal Drainage System

- Pinch rubber connecting tubing. Bubbling continues if there is a leak in water seal connection.

Observe water seal chamber. There should not be excessive continuous bubbling. A small amount of bubbling is seen in the water seal:

- When suction is first initiated
- As air is displaced by drainage in the collection chambers
- As client exhales and coughs and air is forced out of intrapleural space
  When lung has re-expanded, the bubbles cease.

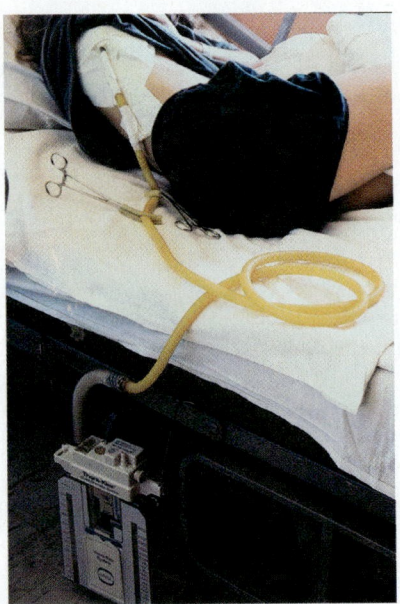

Padded hemostat or plastic tube clamp is used for clamping chest tube. Tube clamped only if ordered.

10. For suction drainage: Remove plastic plug from atmosphere vent to suction control chamber.
11. Attach 60-mL syringe barrel to atmosphere vent and pour sterile water into suction control chamber.
12. Fill suction control chamber to 20-cm (8-in.) level.
    ➤ *Rationale:* Fluid level controls amount of negative pressure created throughout system.

Note: Some chest drainage systems do not require water in either chamber, or only in the suction control chamber. ❷ See manufacturer's instruction for waterless system use. Dry suction is quieter and capable of achieving greater degrees of negative pressure (up to 40 cm H_2O). These units may have a "dry suction control" dial, usually set at 20 cm H_2O. Turn on suction source until orange bellows appears in indicator window to establish suction (Kane, York, & Minton, 2013).

CLINICAL ALERT

Subcutaneous emphysema (air in tissue) may be felt around the chest tube insertion site but should be reported if it extends beyond this.

---

13. Remove long tube adapter from collection chamber and connect it to client's chest tubing.
14. Tape connection.
15. Coil tubing loosely on the bed, but provide a straight line of tubing from bed to collection system. ➤ *Rationale:*

❷ This dry suction system requires that water be added to the water seal, but does not require water in the suction chamber. The suction is wall regulated. These systems are quieter and easier to use.

Straight-line tubing prevents pooling of fluid pressure alterations and system obstruction.

16. Make sure tubing is free and not kinked. Do not use pins or restrain tubing. ➤ *Rationale:* Pins could puncture tubing, causing an air leak.
17. Attach short rubber tube on water-seal chamber to wall suction tubing using an adapter.
18. Turn suction device on slowly until bubbling occurs in suction control chamber.
19. Monitor water levels daily in both water seal chamber and suction control chamber.
20. Maintain pressure.

    a. Keep drainage system at least 30–61 cm (12–24 inches) below client's chest level. ➤ *Rationale:* Raising the unit can cause backflow of drainage into client's intrapleural space. Keeping it low maintains an adequate water seal.
    b. Maintain wall suction to create gentle bubbling in suction control chamber.
    c. Maintain water seal level (2 cm [0.8 in.]). ➤ *Rationale:* Water seal prevents room air from entering pleural space.
    d. Maintain suction control chamber water level at 20 cm (8 in.) or as ordered.

CLINICAL ALERT

Stripping and milking chest tubes are controversial practices used by healthcare providers to clear obstructions in the drainage tubes. Milking involves massaging or twisting the tube to loosen the clots. Milking is still performed by nurses; in some agencies, it requires a healthcare provider's order. Stripping—compressing lubricated finger and thumb on the tube near the body and sliding them down toward the drainage chamber—is no longer considered an acceptable practice.

Source: Kane et al. (2013)

---

21. Maintain chest tube patency. Milk chest tubes to maintain drainage and tube patency *only if healthcare provider orders.*

    a. If ordered, milk tube by alternately folding or squeezing and then releasing drainage tubing. ➤ *Rationale:* This provides intermittent suction to the chest tube but generates extreme negative pressure in intrapleural space.
    b. Milk tube away from client toward the drainage receptacle (disposable system or bottles).

22. Keep rubber-tipped hemostat at the client's bedside.
    ➤ *Rationale:* In an emergency, tube can be clamped nearest to chest insertion site.
23. Keep collection system at least 30–61 cm (12–24 inches) below client's chest level. ➤ *Rationale:* This enables fluid to flow by gravity.
24. Mark drainage on disposable system collection chamber hourly, or every shift. Drainage should be measured at eye level. Report drainage exceeding 50 mL/hr after the first 2 hr. Drainage may be up to 100–300 mL/hr for the first few hours after insertion.

(continued)

Skill 30.7.1 | Setting Up and Maintaining a Disposable Water Seal Chest Drainage System *(continued)*

25. Assess client's status.

   a. Instruct client to deep breathe and cough at frequent intervals. ➤ *Rationale:* Frequent deep breathing helps to expand the lungs. Coughing helps evacuate air from intrapleural space.

   b. Encourage client to change positions frequently (Box 30-12 ■). Chest tube drainage does not limit client activity.

   c. Observe and report any adverse change in SpO$_2$, vital signs, or client's tolerance.

Box 30-12 SMALL MOBILE CHEST DRAINS

Small mobile chest drains allow mobility and early discharge from the hospital. Examples include:

Heimlich one-way valve, which, attached to the client's chest tube, allows *air* to escape but not enter; the distal end of the valve remains open. It, and the chest tube, should be taped to the client's chest. The Heimlich valve is not used for chest tube drainage.

Pneumostat is a plastic device that has a one-way valve and a gravity drainage collection chamber. The unit can be clipped to the client's clothing.

Skill 30.7.2 | Administering Autotransfusion Using Pleur-Evac ATS

Equipment

Sterile disposable Pleur-Evac ATS, ❶ including blood collection bag
Replacement bag
Microaggregate filter
Clean gloves
Sterile saline or water in parking bottle

Note: A variety of sterile chest drainage systems provide evacuation of air and/or fluid from the chest or mediastinum. Evacuated blood may be simultaneously reinfused or collected and reinfused in postoperative or trauma cases.

❶ Pleur-Evac autotransfusion system (ATS) is frequently placed in cardiac surgery.

Procedure

1. Perform hand hygiene and don gloves.

2. Connect client's pleural or mediastinal chest tube by following steps 1–3 printed on Pleur-evac unit. ➤ *Rationale:* Tight connection establishes water-seal drainage system.

3. Check that ALL clamps are open on blood collection bag and drainage tubing and that connections are airtight.

4. Check that blood begins collecting in bag.

5. Mark time and amount of drainage on bag.

6. Close clamp on chest drainage tubing and collection bag and connect new bag to drainage system. Make sure all connections are tight.

7. Depress button on high-negativity relief valve and release it when negativity drops to desired level. ➤ *Rationale:* This reduces excess negativity before removing first collection bag.

8. Close white clamp on client tubing, and then close two white clamps on top of collection bag, and disconnect all connectors on first bag.

9. Remove protective cap from collection tubing on replacement bag. Maintain aseptic technique when changing tubing.

10. Use red connectors to connect unit's collection tubing to client's chest drainage tube.

11. Remove protective cap from replacement bag's suction tube.

12. Use blue connectors to attach replacement bag's suction tube to Pleur-Evac unit.

13. Open all clamps, and check that system is airtight.

14. Attach red (female) and blue (male) connector sections on top of autotransfusion bag.

15. Move out and disconnect metal support arms, and disconnect foot hook. ➤ *Rationale:* Releasing these connections allows you to remove bag from drainage unit.

16. Attach replacement bag by using foot hook and support arm.

17. Slide bag off support frame and invert bag with spike port pointing up. ➤ *Rationale:* This position allows blood to be reinfused from original collection bag.

18. Remove protective cap from spike port, and insert a microaggregate filter. Twist filter into position. ➤ *Rationale:* Filter is essential for reinfusion.
19. Prime filter by gently squeezing inverted bag until drip chamber is half full.
20. Close clamp on reinfusion line, and remove residual air from bag.
21. Invert bag on IV pole.
22. Flush IV tubing to remove air, and then reinfuse blood by gravity or pump according to hospital policy. Blood should be totally reinfused within 6 hr from *start of collection*.
23. Remove gloves and perform hand hygiene.
24. Assess neurologic signs and pulmonary status every 4 hr. ➤ *Rationale:* Microemboli can occur with autotransfusion.

> **CLINICAL ALERT**
>
> Reinfusion is not indicated unless system is primed with drainage and an additional 50 mL of drainage has been collected for reinfusion.
>
> No more than 6 hr should elapse from time of *beginning* collection to *completion* of reinfusion.
>
> Refer to evacuation/reinfusion system manufacturer's package insert for indications, contraindications, and instructions for use.

Skill 30.7.3 | Assisting With Removal of Chest Tube

Equipment

Suture removal set
Rubber-tipped hemostat
Disposable underpad
Sterile 4×4 gauze for mediastinal tube
 Or
Sterile petrolatum gauze dressings for intrapleural tube
Tape (elasticized foam tape for intrapleural tube)
Sterile gloves
PPE (face mask or shield)
Prescribed premedication

Preparation

1. Identify client using two forms of identification and introduce self.
2. Gather equipment and prepare client for procedure, including instruction to take a deep breath and hold it or to hum during tube removal.
3. Premedicate client (as ordered), allowing time for peak effect upon tube removal.

> **CLINICAL ALERT**
>
> The chest tube can be removed when drainage is less than 50–100 mL in 24 hr, or, if inserted for blood removal, drainage has become serous or serosanguineous and less than 100 mL in the past 8 hr.

Procedure

1. Perform hand hygiene and don PPE.
2. Place client in semi-Fowler's position.
3. Don sterile gloves.
4. Assist healthcare provider to remove dressing, clip suture securing chest tube, ❶ and clamp chest tube.

❶ Sutures anchoring chest tube are cut.

5. Instruct client to take a deep breath and hold their breath or hum as the tube is removed.
6. Cover the site with sterile petroleum gauze and tape securely.
7. Dispose of chest tube and drainage equipment.
8. Remove personal protective gear, gloves, and discard.
9. Perform hand hygiene.
10. Reevaluate client's status regularly. ➤ *Rationale:* Client should be assessed for unstable vital signs, diminished or absent breath sounds, or respiratory distress (**pneumothorax**, mediastinal shift) after removal of chest tube.

Unit 30.7 Documentation and Evaluation

DOCUMENTATION for Chest Drainage Systems

Chest Drainage System

- Site and size of chest tubes inserted and drainage system established
- Negative pressure established
- Client's tolerance of procedure
- Vital signs
- Breath sounds
- Drainage—amount, color
- Any problem with the system and its management
- Client activity (turning, ambulation)
- Chest-tube milking or stripping, if performed

Autotransfusion

- Amount of blood reinfused
- Time collection started to completion of reinfusion
- Signs and symptoms of any complications encountered
- Changes in coagulation times or hemoglobin, hematocrit
- Client's response to treatment

Chest Tube Removal

- Breath sounds
- Premedication administered
- Name of physician removing tube
- Status of insertion site and dressing applied
- Client's tolerance of procedure

EVALUATION/Critical Thinking

Expected Outcomes

- Chest drainage system is patent.
- Mediastinal shift does not occur.
- Chest tube remains securely placed.

Unexpected Outcomes	Alternative Actions

• Air leak is present.	• Check for specific leak area by briefly clamping chest drainage tube between client and bottle closest to client.
	  a. If water-seal chamber continues to bubble, the leak is in the tubing.
	  b. If water-seal chamber stops bubbling, the leak is in the client's chest tube at insertion site.
	• Secure all connections with tape.
	• Change tubing if necessary (obtain healthcare provider's order).
	• Apply sterile petrolatum gauze around chest tube insertion site if leak is at that site.

• Drainage system is obstructed.	• Assess tubing for kinks or clots. • Loop tubing on bed to allow straight drainage to collection system. • Obtain healthcare provider's order to milk tubing.
• Client develops signs of mediastinal shift (trachea deviated to unaffected side, paradoxical pulse develops, jugular veins distend, cardiac output decreases).	• Note signs of respiratory distress and call Rapid Response Team or "CODE" immediately. Check drainage tube for patency. Prepare to assist with thoracentesis.

Unexpected Outcomes	Alternative Actions

• Chest tube becomes disconnected from drainage system.	• Clamp chest tube near chest insertion site.
	   a. Replace extension tubing leading from chest tube and submerge into open bottle of sterile water to create underwater seal.
	   b. Unclamp chest tube as soon as extension tubing is placed underwater or connected to new system.
	• Secure connecting sites with tape to prevent disconnection.
	• Assess client for signs of respiratory distress due to pneumothorax and report.

• Chest tube becomes dislodged.	• Notify healthcare provider. • Instruct client with external chest disruption to exhale and apply sterile nonporous 4×4 gauze dressing with tape on three sides to allow air to escape on exhalation but inhibit air intake on inspiration.

Chapter Wrap-Up

GERONTOLOGIC Considerations

Physiologic Changes That Occur in Older Adults Affect Respiratory System

- The respiratory muscles lose their strength and the rib cage becomes more rigid.
- The alveoli increase in size and decrease in number as well as become less elastic and more dilated.
- Gas exchange is reduced; the PaO_2 decreases 1 mm/year after age 60, so a reading of 77 mm Hg is not unusual in an older adult client.
- Skeletal alterations affect posture and may restrict lung expansion.

Pulmonary Disorders More Common in Older Adults; COPD the Fourth Leading Cause of Death

- Respiratory reserves are reduced with aging; older adults are at greater risk for respiratory failure.
- Pneumonia may develop primarily or secondary to other conditions. Because it is a major cause of death in older adults, pneumonia vaccine, influenza vaccine, and other preventive measures should be employed.

- Asthma may occur as a problem in older adults who have never had the disease.
- Cancer of the lung is the leading cause of cancer death in older adults.

Important Nursing Actions That Support the Respiratory System in Older Adults

- Deep breathing and exercise help promote ventilation.
- Hydration helps to liquefy secretions and reduce risk for infection.
- Monitor oxygen therapy closely with older adults—note signs of hypoxia and decreased responsiveness due to possible carbon dioxide narcosis.
- Older adults are at risk for hypoxemia with bed rest (PO_2 may drop to 40 mm Hg even with a night's sleep). Position change, range of motion, and early mobilization all stimulate ventilation and must be encouraged in all clients.

MANAGEMENT Guidelines

Each state legislates a Nurse Practice Act for RNs and LVN/LPNs. Healthcare facilities are responsible for establishing and implementing policies and procedures that conform to their state's regulations. Verify the regulations and role parameters for each healthcare worker in your facility.

Delegation

- Each state identifies the scope of practice for RNs, LVN/LPNs, and respiratory care practitioners. States may differ in defining responsibilities of respiratory care by these practitioners. Usually, the respiratory care practitioner is licensed to perform invasive procedures such as suctioning, changing tracheostomy inner cannulas, and administering medication by aerosol. The initiation of oxygen administration by various modes and utilization of biophysical parameters (ABGs and such) and standard protocols in decision making and management of the mechanically ventilated client are also within the scope of respiratory care practice.

- All professionals collaborate in the care planning and evaluation of client responses to respiratory care interventions. The nurse must be aware of the unique role competencies, responsibilities, and accountabilities of specialty personnel when a variety of care providers are involved.

- The nurse should ensure that regular turning and deep breathing are encouraged by the CNA/UAP to promote ventilation and prevent complications of immobility in bedfast clients.

- The CNA/UAP should be familiar with appropriate client positioning to promote airway patency and reduce risk for aspiration of oral intake.

- Even though hospitals are "smoke free" today, all personnel must take precautions when oxygen is in use: No petrolatum products are used around nose or mouth; no battery-operated equipment or friction-type toys can be used. The area surrounding the client is oxygen-rich and can support combustion.

- All personnel should be able to locate the main oxygen supply valve to the area for discontinuation of oxygen flow in case of fire.

- The nurse must verify that the CNA/UAP understands the importance of oxygen administration so that it is appropriately maintained. The nurse ensures that the CNA/UAP seeks assistance so portable oxygen can be provided if it is required during client ambulation.

- Unlicensed personnel should be informed that aspiration is an ever-present danger for the client with a tracheostomy tube.

- Clients who require oxygen administration may be unable to perform ADLs independently. The CNA/UAP providing basic care should be *instructed to assist* the client with these activities (e.g., set up food tray, provide bed or partial bath).

- All care providers must be familiar with the location of emergency supplies and should be prepared to retrieve equipment and assist with manual respiratory resuscitation if necessary.

Interprofessional Communication

- The CNA/UAP usually performs routine vital signs assessment and documentation (including respiratory rate). The nurse should request that respiratory rates less than 12 or greater than 20 be reported immediately, as more specific assessment may be indicated.

- The CNA/UAP should know to *report* any change in the client's breathing status or tolerance of activity. The character and amount of sputum production should also be reported and saved for the nurse's inspection and documentation.

- While the nurse or respiratory care practitioner is responsible for suctioning clients, the CNA/UAP must recognize the client's need for such and *report* it immediately.

- The PO status of intubated clients must be clearly communicated to all personnel. NPO status should be clearly posted at the bedside.

- All care providers must ensure that the intubated client has nonvocal means for summoning help (call bell) and communicating (paper and pencil).

- There should be clear postings at the bedside of the client for swallowing precautions, oxygen precautions, communication through nonvocal means, and intubation precautions.

CASE STUDY Applications

Scenario 1

Mrs. Harvey, age 72, has a history of COPD with components of emphysema and chronic bronchitis. She has frequent recurrence of respiratory infection requiring hospitalization. With her most recent hospitalization, she has developed pulmonary hypertension and right-sided heart failure with weight gain and systemic edema. After treatment with IV antibiotics, she is ready for discharge, but will be sent home with continuous low-flow (1.5 L) oxygen therapy. Her ABGs at the time of discharge show elevated PCO_2 (respiratory acidosis), elevated bicarbonate level (metabolic alkalosis), PO_2 of 60 mm Hg, and O_2 saturation of 90% on oxygen. Her blood pH is low normal due to the *compensated* respiratory acidosis.

1. What is the rationale for home oxygen therapy for Mrs. Harvey?

2. What are the hazards that accompany home oxygen therapy?

3. What should the client know about home oxygen therapy?

4. What are the expected outcomes of home oxygen therapy (ABGs)?

Scenario 2

Joe Snodgrass has been referred to the sleep laboratory for an overnight polysomnogram (sleep study) due to his complaints of excessive fatigue, daytime sleepiness, awakening with a headache, and his heart racing. In addition, his wife reports that he snores a lot and has breathing pauses when he is sleeping that frighten her.

Outcomes of his study reveal that Mr. Snodgrass has obstructive sleep apnea (OSA). His healthcare provider has prescribed nasal continuous positive airway pressure (nCPAP) for nighttime use. As his nurse, you are to obtain follow-up assessment data regarding your client's tolerance, adherence, and response to this therapy.

1. What is OSA?

2. What are the risk factors for developing OSA?

3. What are potential complications of untreated OSA?

4. How does CPAP benefit the client with OSA?

5. Why do many clients fail to adhere to CPAP therapy?

6. Are there other treatment options available for the client who cannot tolerate CPAP?

NCLEX® Review Questions

Unless otherwise specified, choose only one (1) answer.

1. Which instructions about inhaling through the mouthpiece should be given for use of an incentive spirometer device?

    A. Inhale quickly to maximum level, and then exhale slowly through the nose.

    B. Inhale slowly to maximum level, hold several seconds, and then exhale forcefully.

    C. Inhale quickly to maximum level, hold for several seconds, and then exhale slowly with mouth open.

    D. Inhale slowly to maximum level, hold for several seconds, and then exhale through pursed lips.

2. Which clients benefit from chest physiotherapy (CPT)?

    A. Clients with pneumonia

    B. Clients with retained secretions

    C. COPD clients with acute exacerbation

    D. Mechanically ventilated clients

3. Which clients should not be selected for CPAP/BiPAP mask application?

    A. Clients allergic to latex

    B. Sedated clients

    C. Clients who are asleep

    D. Claustrophobic clients

4. Which system provides the greatest oxygen delivery (FiO$_2$)?

    A. Nasal cannula

    B. Face mask

    C. Venturi mask

    D. Nonrebreathing mask with reservoir bag

5. In which clients is hemoglobin saturation by pulse oximetry (SpO$_2$) a less reliable measurement?

    Select all that apply.

    A. Anemic clients

    B. Clients with low blood glucose

    C. Hypovolemic clients

    D. Hypertensive clients

    E. Clients post dye injection

6. What is the purpose of tracheal intubation or tracheostomy tube placement?

    A. To provide mechanical ventilation

    B. To establish a patent airway

    C. To prevent aspiration

    D. To provide oxygenation

7. The proper inflation of an endotracheal or tracheostomy tube cuff is necessary to prevent what complications?

    Select all that apply.

    A. It prevents aspiration of food.

    B. It prevents aspiration of pharyngeal secretions.

    C. It prevents tube migration.

    D. It prevents mechanical ventilation.

    E. It prevents talking.

8. The nurse knows which of the following are early signs and symptoms of hypoxia?

    Select all that apply.

    A. Headache

    B. Tachycardia

    C. Visual disturbances

    D. Auditory hallucinations

    E. Confusion

9. What is needed for the client with a tracheostomy tube that is capped with a speaking valve?

    A. Mechanical ventilation

    B. Tube cuff deflated

    C. Tube cuff inflated

    D. A Bivona Fome Cuf tube

10. Place the following steps in correct sequence for suctioning a client's airway with a single-use catheter:

    A. Hyperoxygenate client.

    B. Suction client's oropharynx.

C. Pour catheter flush solution into container.

D. Attach catheter to end of suction tubing.

E. Set suction source to 100 mm Hg.

F. Don sterile gloves.

G. Apply suction.

H. Advance catheter into client's airway.

QSEN Activity

Encouraging Evidence-Based Practice

Domain: Evidence-Based Practice

KSA: Describe how the strength and relevance of available evidence influences the choice of interventions in provision of client-centered care.

Activity:

You are working on an intensive care unit and you notice several nurses instilling normal saline while suctioning their clients who are intubated. When you question the practice, you are told that it helps loosen up the secretions, so they can be suctioned out more effectively. You remember reading that best practice is not to instil normal saline. You decide to gather some evidence so that you can help the nurses understand why this is not the best way to suction clients.

Project:

1. Gather evidence from guidelines and research articles.
2. Put together a short PowerPoint presentation highlighting suctioning best practices.
3. Cite the evidence used in supporting your best practice.

Bibliography

American Sleep Apnea Association. (2015). Health care professional. Retrieved from http://www.sleepapnea.org/i-am-a-health-care-professional.html

Cross, J. L., Evender, F., Barton, G., Clark, A., Shepstone, L., Blyth, A., Bachman, M. O., & Harvey, I. (2012). Evaluation of the effectiveness of manual chest physiotherapy techniques on quality of life at six months post exacerbation of COPD (MATREX): A randomised controlled equivalence trial. *BMC Pulmonary Medicine, 12*(33), 1–9.

Esguerra-Gonzalez, A., Ilagan-Honorio, M., Fraschilla, S., Kehoe, P., Lee, A. J., Marcarian, T., . . . & Gawlinski, A. (2013). CNE article: Pain after lung transplant: High-frequency chest wall oscillation vs chest physiotherapy. *American Journal of Critical Care, 22*(2), 115–124.

Gammon, B. T., & Ricker, K. F. (2012). An evidence-based checklist for the postoperative management of obstructive sleep apnea. *Journal of PeriAnesthesia Nursing, 27*(5), 316–322.

Kane, C. J., York, N. L., & Minton, L. A. (2013). Chest tubes in the critically ill patient. *Dimensions of Critical Care Nursing, 32*(3), 111–117.

Lamar, J. (2011). Relationship of respiratory care bundle with incentive spirometry to reduced pulmonary complications in a medical general practice unit. *Medsurg Nursing: Official Journal of the Academy of Medical-Surgical Nurses, 21*(1), 33–36.

McIlwaine, M. P., Alarie, N., Davidson, G. F., Lands, L. C., Ratjen, F., Milner, R., . . . & Agnew, J. L. (2013). Long-term multicentre randomised controlled study of high frequency chest wall

oscillation versus positive expiratory pressure mask in cystic fibrosis. *Thorax, 68*(8), 746–751.

National Heart, Lung, and Blood Institute. (2014). Expert panel report 3: Guidelines for diagnosis and management of asthma. Retrieved from http://www.nhlbi.nih.gov/health/health-topics/topics/asthma

Pandian, V., Smith, C. P., Cole, T. K., Bhatti, N. I., Mirski, M. A., Yarmus, L. B., & Feller-Kopman, D. J. (2014). Optimizing communication in mechanically ventilated patients. *Journal of Medical Speech-Language Pathology, 21*(4), 309.

Regan, E. & Dalachiesa, L. (2009). How to care for a patient with a tracheostomy. *Nursing, 39*(8), 34–39.

Restrepo R. D., Wettstein R., Wittnebel L., & Tracy, M. (2011, Oct.). AARC clinical practice guideline: Incentive spirometry: 2011. *Respiratory Care, 56*(10), 1600–1604.

Sole, M. L., Penoyer, D. A., Bennett, M., Bertrand, J., & Talbert, S. (2011). Oropharyngeal secretion volume in intubated patients: The importance of oral suctioning. *American Journal of Critical Care, 20*(6), e141–e145.

Voepel-Lewis, T., Parker, M. L., Burke, C. N., Hemberg, J., Perlin, L., Kai, S., & Ramachandran, S. K. (2013). Pulse oximetry desaturation alarms on a general postoperative adult unit: A prospective observational study of nurse response time. *International Journal of Nursing Studies, 50*(10), 1351–1358.

Chapter 31
Circulatory Maintenance

Learning Objectives

31.1 Identify four properties of the cardiac muscle and define cardiac output.

31.2 Define the words *inotropic* and *chronotropic*.

31.3 Locate the following sites to palpate the pulse: temporal, carotid, brachial, radial, femoral, popliteal, posterior tibial, and dorsalis pedis.

31.4 Outline the assessment actions for a client who is hemorrhaging.

31.5 Identify two interventions for treating heart failure.

31.6 Define the term *ischemia*.

31.7 List the nine pressure points in the body that can be used to control bleeding if hemorrhage occurs.

31.8 Identify two potential problems that could occur in clients who are bleeding, and state one suggested intervention for each problem.

31.9 Describe how to measure for appropriate-size graduated compression stockings.

31.10 List at least four potential problems for clients requiring CPR and two suggested interventions for each problem.

31.11 Outline the steps in administering CPR with one rescuer and with two rescuers.

31.12 Demonstrate performing the abdominal thrust.

31.13 Describe four steps in using the automatic external defibrillator (AED).

31.14 State two nursing diagnoses relevant to clients with alterations in circulation.

31.15 Differentiate between a normal and abnormal ECG pattern.

31.16 Describe lead placement for a 12-lead ECG.

31.17 Describe the rationale for use of a permanent pacemaker versus a temporary pacemaker.

31.18 Compare and contrast the various types of pacemakers.

31.19 Identify three benefits of internal cardiac defibrillator (ICD).

31.20 Discuss teaching for home care clients with cardiac pacemakers.

31.21 Determine symptoms requiring healthcare provider notification when reviewing the diary of a client using a Holter monitor.

Chapter Outline

Terminology

Aberrancy abnormally conducted beat or cardiac rhythm.

Afterload resistance or impedance to blood flow during ventricular systole.

Antiembolic related to a preventive measure used to help prevent the formation of an embolism, such as elastic hosiery.

Arrhythmia an abnormality in cardiac rhythm.

Atherosclerosis accumulations of lipid-containing material within inner and middle layers of the arterial wall forming a fixed atheromatous plaque.

Cardiovascular pertaining to the heart and blood vessels.

Chronotropic pertaining to factors known to alter the heart rate through external causes (e.g., medication).

Conductivity the electrical conducting capability of a substance.

Congestion excessive accumulation of blood or fluid within a blood vessel, tissue, or organ.

Contractility the ability to contract or shorten.

Cyanosis bluish, purplish discoloration of the skin resulting from reduced hemoglobin or oxygen in the blood.

Diastole relaxation filling phase of the cardiac cycle.

Dilatation expansion of an organ or vessel.

Dorsiflexion flexion of the foot in an upward direction so as to bend the joint toward the dorsum.

Ecchymosis escape of blood into the tissues from a ruptured blood vessel causing a discoloration of the skin; color is blue-black, changing to greenish brown or yellow.

Ectopy beat originating in the heart other than from the sinoatrial node.

Edema an excessive accumulation of fluid within tissue or bodily cavity.

Embolism sudden obstruction of a blood vessel by debris (e.g., a blood clot, plaque).

Endocardial arising from the endocardium.

Endocardium serous lining membrane of the inner surface and cavities of the heart.

Endotracheal within the trachea.

Epistaxis hemorrhage from the nose.

Heart failure a condition whereby the heart is unable to pump sufficient blood at either an adequate rate or volume to meet the metabolic demands of the body.

Hematemesis vomiting of blood.

Hematoma a swelling or mass of blood, usually clotted, confined to a specific space and caused by a break in a blood vessel.

Hemodynamic the study of blood flow within the systemic circulation.

Hemoptysis expectoration of blood from the larynx, trachea, bronchi, or lungs.

Hemorrhage abnormal internal or external bleeding.

Hypotension a low systolic blood pressure that is insufficient to maintain adequate tissues and organ perfusion.

Immobilize to fix part or all of the body to reduce or eliminate motion.

Inotropic influencing the contractibility of muscle tissue.

Ischemia a decrease in circulation to tissue, organ, or limb due to obstruction of the inflow of arterial blood, which is reversible if blood flow is reestablished promptly.

Manubrium the sternum articulating with the clavicle and first pair of costal cartilages.

Pacemaker a device that provides electrical stimulation to the heart muscle.

Perfusion passing of fluid through spaces; the circulation of blood through tissues.

Petechiae small, purplish, hemorrhagic spots on the skin.

Phlebitis inflammation of a vein.

Precordial pertaining to the precordium or occurring in front of the heart.

Preload length or stretch of the cardiac muscle fiber imposed by the volume of blood in the ventricles at the end of diastole.

Purpura hemorrhage into the skin, mucous membranes, internal organs, and other tissues, which causes a deep purple color.

Resuscitation act of bringing someone back to consciousness.

Shock term used to designate a clinical syndrome with varying degrees of disturbances of reduced blood flow and oxygen supply to the tissues.

Stasis standing still; stagnation of normal flow of fluids.

Syncope fainting, transient loss of consciousness due to inadequate blood flow to the brain.

Thrombosis formation of a blood clot.

Vertigo sensation of moving or having objects moving around when they are actually still.

The Circulatory System

The heart is a three-layered organ, approximately the size of an adult fist, weighing approximately 250–350 g. The pericardium is a double-walled, strong nondistensible sac that encloses the heart, the aorta, and the other great vessels attached to the heart. The pericardium contains a fibrous and a serous layer, the function of which is to restrict excessive movement of the heart and act as a lubricated container during cardiac contraction. The pericardium protects the heart from positional changes and infection and prevents friction between the heart and other organs. There are two layers of the serous pericardium, the parietal and visceral layers. These two layers are separated by a thin, fluid-containing cavity, the pericardial sac, which contains about 50 mL of pericardial fluid that lubricates and facilitates the movement of the heart. The fibrous pericardium and parietal layer of the serous pericardium are supplied by the phrenic nerve, whereas the visceral layer of the serous pericardium is innervated by the sympathetic nervous system and the vagus nerve. Both influence reflex changes in the heart rate and blood pressure. The myocardium is the thickest layer of the heart and is composed of cardiac muscle cells. Cardiac muscle cells are unique and possess four properties: (1) automaticity—ability of some cardiac cells to initiate an impulse spontaneously and repetitively;

(2) **conductivity**—ability to transmit electrical impulses; (3) **contractility**—trait characterizing all muscle; however, a cardiac contraction is an all-or-nothing response to an impulse as opposed to partial contractions in skeletal muscles; and (4) **excitability**—the ability to respond to an external stimuli, resulting in a contraction. The **endocardium** is the innermost lining of the heart and is continuous with the endothelium that lines arteries, veins, and capillaries.

The heart serves as a pump and is made up of four chambers: the right atrium, right ventricle, left atrium, and left ventricle. Unidirectional blood flow is regulated through the heart by four valves: the tricuspid, pulmonary, mitral, and aortic valves (Figures 31-1 ■ and 31-2 ■). Venous blood enters into the right atrium of the heart from the superior and inferior vena cava. Blood flows from the right atrium into the right ventricle through the tricuspid valve, and then into the lungs for oxygenation through the pulmonary artery. After gases exchange in the pulmonary system, the blood enters the left atrium, the left side of the heart, by way of four pulmonary veins. These are the only veins within the body that carry oxygenated blood. From the left atrium, blood flows into the left ventricle via the mitral valve, and then out into the aorta via the aortic valve. Blood flows to all parts of the body through the systemic circulation system. The heart pumps the entire circulating volume each minute (4–7 L of blood).

FIGURE 31-1 Blood flow pattern through the right and left sides of the heart.

FIGURE 31-2 Blood flow in coronary arteries.

```
Superior
        Vena Cava → Right Atrium → Tricuspid Valve →
Inferior
                    Right Ventricle → Pulmonary Valve →
                Pulmonary Artery → LUNGS (oxygenation)

LUNGS → Pulmonary veins → Left Atrium → Mitral Valve →
                Left Ventricle → Aortic Valve → Aorta – BODY
```

Arteries carry oxygenated blood from the heart throughout the body from the largest vessel, the aorta, to the smallest, arterioles and capillaries. Arteries have three layers: endothelium, smooth muscle, and connective tissue. Capillaries join the arterial system to the venous system and are a single cell layer that allows for the exchange of gases, nutrients, and waste material.

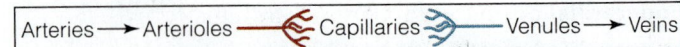

Capillaries are also known as capacitance vessels, which serve to regulate blood flow within the venous system by returning it to the right side of the heart.

Cardiac Output

Cardiac output (CO) is the amount of blood flow ejected by the heart, and it is measured in liters per minute. Heart rate (HR) and stroke volume (SV) determine cardiac output. Cardiac output is determined by multiplying the amount of volume ejected from the heart with each contraction by the heart rate.

$$CO = SV \times HR$$

Cardiac Output = Stroke Volume × Heart Rate

In order to maintain its continuous pumping activity, the heart muscle itself must receive oxygen and nutrients. Approximately 5% of blood leaving the heart and pumped into the aorta enters the coronary circulation for oxygenation and waste removal from cardiac tissue. The coronary arteries branch from the aorta, extend over the surface of the heart, supply blood to all areas of the heart muscle, and fill during **diastole**. The major coronary arteries are the right coronary artery and the left coronary artery, which divides into two branches, the anterior descending artery and the circumflex artery.

If the blood flow in the coronary arteries to the heart muscle is severely reduced, **ischemia** or injury can occur, but it is reversible. If the flow is blocked completely for a prolonged period, necrosis will occur; necrosis is irreversible. This is referred to as a myocardial infarction (MI) or "heart attack."

After supplying the heart muscle, 15% of the cardiac output (600–500 mL) travels to the brain, 25% (1000–1750 mL) goes to the kidneys, and another 25% to the other viscera. The extremities and skin normally receive approximately 30% of the cardiac output.

Electrical Conduction

Specialized cardiac electrical tissues have the ability to spontaneously generate an electrical impulse, previously mentioned as automaticity. The rate and rhythm of cardiac impulses are primarily determined by this specialized tissue (pacemakers). The intrinsic rate is influenced by the autonomic nervous system. Sympathetic stimulation increases heart rate, speeds the conduction through the atrioventricular (AV) node, and increases force of myocardial contraction (Figure 31-3 ■). Parasympathetic stimulation slows the heart rate by decreasing firing rate of the sinoatrial (SA) node and decreasing the speed of conduction through the AV node.

Normally, the electrical impulse originates within specialized cells within the SA node located on the posterior wall of the right atrium, just right of the opening of the superior vena cava. It functions as the **pacemaker** for the heart. The SA node initiates approximately 60–100 impulses each

Bundle of His

SA Node

Left Bundle Branch

AV Node

Right Bundle Branch

Purkinje Fibers

FIGURE 31-3 Intrinsic conduction system of the heart.

minute. The impulse travels to the AV node, located in the right atrial wall near the tricuspid valve. If there is a problem with the impulse being generated in the SA node, the AV node can actually take over as the pacemaker. The intrinsic rate of the AV node is only 40–60 impulses per minute, and the heart's mechanical response (contraction) fails to receive the additional volume of atrial contraction. The AV node relays the electrical impulse to the ventricles through the bundle of His's specialized conduction fibers, which divide into the right and left bundle branches. Then, the impulse continues to the Purkinje fibers. Depolarization of the ventricular myocardium takes place by impulse conduction through the muscle fibers themselves. If both the SA and AV node are dysfunctional, or there is blockage in the bundle of His, the Purkinje fibers are capable of maintaining their own intrinsic rate, but the rate is less than 20 beats/min.

Electrocardiogram

The electrocardiogram (ECG) is used to detect abnormalities associated with the electrical system of the heart. The waveforms, which indicate depolarization and repolarization of the myocardium, are analyzed using the ECG tracing.

P wave—represents atrial depolarization. The P wave is usually smooth and upright, or "positive."

PR interval—is measured from the beginning of the P wave (onset of atrial depolarization) to the R wave. It represents the time required for atrial depolarization and for the impulse to travel through the entire conduction system, including the Purkinje fiber network. Normal PR interval is 0.12–0.20 sec.

QRS complex—represents depolarization of the ventricles. It is measured from the beginning of the Q wave (or

the R) to the end of the S wave. Not all leads have a Q wave but if present, it is very narrow and not deep. The normal QRS duration is 0.06–0.12 sec and represents the time required for depolarization of both ventricles.

ST segment—represents the period of early ventricular repolarization. The ST segment is normally isoelectric (the line is flat). The segment normally is not elevated >1 mm or depressed >0.5 mm from the isoelectric line.

QT interval—represents the total time required for ventricular depolarization and repolarization. It is measured from the beginning of the QRS complex to the end of the T wave and corresponds with ventricular systole (contraction). The normal QT interval is 0.34–0.43 sec.

T wave—represents rapid ventricular repolarization or the return of the ventricles to a resting state. The wave is normally asymmetrically rounded and upright, or "positive." The end of the T wave corresponds with the end of systole.

Segments and waves are measured for duration (time) and configuration. Abnormalities in duration or configuration may indicate that a problem is occurring in that specific area of the heart.

Any disturbance in the rate or rhythm of the heartbeat is termed **arrhythmia**. The term *dysrhythmia* is also used in the literature. Arrhythmias are classified according to their site of origin. The sites include sinus, atrial, junctional, and ventricular. A sinus arrhythmia reflects a change in rate or rhythm. An atrial arrhythmia results from a disturbance with atria, indicated by an abnormality in the P wave configuration. A junctional dysrhythmia occurs when there is a problem associated with the AV node, as indicated by a change in the PR interval. A ventricular arrhythmia results from a problem within the ventricle and is indicated by an abnormality in the configuration of the QRS complex. Although many arrhythmias have no clinical manifestations, many others have serious consequences. A ventricular arrhythmia is the most life-threatening.

Cardiac Monitoring

The selection of a particular monitoring lead (view) is guided by the client's clinical condition determined by the arrhythmias most likely to occur and the potential severity of the arrhythmia. Any lead that displays a clear P wave and QRS complex can identify premature atrial complexes, abnormal sinus rhythms, and most heart blocks. Most leads recognize atrial fibrillation by the irregular R-R intervals and chaotic atrial activity. When the QRS complex becomes wide, as it does when the client is in bundle branch block or has ventricular rhythms, the lead that best differentiates these findings is selected. The V1 and V6 leads are the best leads to differentiate wide QRS rhythms. Multiple lead monitoring is best for observing and detecting these arrhythmias. Bedside monitors allow monitoring of two leads simultaneously, but only allow monitoring of one **precordial** (V) lead at a time; some systems still may use a three-lead system.

ST-segment monitoring is now being used in clients with a potential for ischemia (clients admitted with chest discomfort, or possible acute coronary syndrome, or clients having a surgical procedure who have a history of cardiac disease). If the 12-lead ECG is not available, the American Association of Critical-Care Nurses recommends leads III and V3 for monitoring clients for changes in the ST segment.

Refer to Chapter 33, Advanced Nursing Skills, for discussion of life-threatening dysrhythmias.

Pacemakers

Pacemakers are devices that stimulate the heart with electrical impulses to produce a heartbeat or to override an abnormally fast rhythm. Most commonly, pacemakers are used for a slow heart rate (bradycardia) or when the conduction system is diseased and unable to conduct electrical impulses to the atria or ventricles (heart block). The use of a temporary or permanent pacemaker may be necessary to provide an electrical impulse to pace the heart when the inherent electrical system fails.

Temporary pacemaker A temporary pacemaker is inserted invasively to stimulate cardiac contraction until the underlying pathology is treated or a permanent pacemaker can be placed. Clients with temporary pacemakers require hospitalization with continuous monitoring. The pulse generator of the temporary pacemaker is located outside the body, and the leads are positioned to provide low-voltage electrical stimuli to the myocardium. The leads are positioned in one of several ways:

- The pacemaker wires are threaded percutaneously through the subclavian, external jugular, or femoral vein or through a cutdown in the brachial vein. The lead is advanced through the vena cava, to the right atrium, or advanced through the tricuspid valve and positioned in the right ventricle on the **endocardial** surface. The lead is then attached to the external pulse generator.
- During cardiac surgery, the pacing leads are attached to the outer surface of the heart (epicardially). This type has wires (electrodes) located in the lower chest and can be attached to an external pulse generator if pacing the heart postoperatively is necessary.

In emergency situations, such as in cases of symptomatic bradycardia, external pacing pads are applied to the chest wall (transcutaneously).

Permanent pacemaker The decision to place a permanent pacemaker and the type of pacemaker selected depends on multiple factors, including:

- The exact nature and underlying cause of the conduction disturbance
- The presence or absence of symptoms and the impact on activities of daily living
- The potential risk for life-threatening dysrhythmias

Permanent pacemakers are intended for long-term use. The pulse generator is implanted into the subcutaneous tissue of the upper chest. The pacemaker leads are typically inserted through the subclavian vein (transvenously),

advanced into the right side of the heart, and secured in the right ventricle. The other ends of the leads are attached to the implanted pulse generator that continuously monitors the heart's electrical activity. The type of pacemaker selected is designed to meet different needs. The three basic types of permanent pacemakers include:

- *Demand Pacemaker*—monitors the heart's natural rate and discharges an electrical impulse only when the rate falls below a programmed minimum rate.
- *Fixed-rate Pacemaker*—discharges a steady electrical impulse at a programmed rate, regardless of the underlying heart rate. These devices are rarely used today.
- *Rate-responsive Pacemaker*—increases or decreases the discharge electrical impulse rate (pacing rate) to meet the body's demands. The pacemaker monitors various physical changes in the body and alters the rate of discharge according to changes in the client's activity and rest. These also work on demand.

Pacemakers can send electrical impulses to the right atrium or right ventricle to stimulate the heart chambers to depolarize in a regular rhythm.

Types of Pacemakers

Types of pacemakers include atrial, ventricular, or dual-chamber pacemakers.

Single-chamber In a single-chamber pacemaker (Figure 31-4 ■), one lead is located in either the right atrium or right ventricle. Atrial pacemakers are indicated when the SA node is diseased or damaged but the remaining conduction system through the heart is normal. A pacemaker spike precedes the P wave because the pacing electrode is placed within the atria. Ventricular pacemakers are indicated when conduction abnormalities occur above the ventricles. The pacing lead is located in the ventricle and when discharged

FIGURE 31-4 Permanent pacemaker: single chamber.

FIGURE 31-5 Permanent pacemaker: double chamber.

results in a pacemaker spike before the QRS complex, producing a wide QRS complex because of the abnormal conduction pathway.

Dual-chamber In a dual-chamber pacemaker (Figure 31-5 ■), two leads, one in the right atrium and one in the right ventricle, can monitor and initiate impulses to one or both chambers. The dual-chambered pacemaker can produce an atrial contraction followed closely by a ventricular contraction, thereby mimicking the normal cardiac cycle while preserving atrial contraction and thus ventricular filling.

Triple-chamber or biventricular pacing With this type of pacemaker, one lead in the right atrium, one in the right ventricle, and one in the coronary sinus stimulate the lateral wall of the left ventricle. These pacemakers are inserted in clients who have a weakened myocardium (heart muscle) or a severely depressed myocardial function, causing problems with shortness of breath and inability to tolerate physical activity. With left ventricle enlargement, the wave of depolarization and repolarization is prolonged. Placing a third lead in the coronary sinus facilitates a coordinated wave of depolarization and repolarization simultaneously within the myocardium, allowing for the heart to contract in a more unified manner, thus improving the cardiac output.

Alterations in Circulation

The closed circulatory system is made up of the heart, arteries, veins, and capillaries. Alteration in the structure or function of any part of the system will result in impaired circulation. There are many ways to categorize circulatory disorders. For the purposes of this chapter, alterations in circulation will include hemorrhage, **shock**, pump failure, ischemia, **thrombosis**, and **embolism**.

Hemorrhage

Hemorrhage may occur when trauma or disease disrupts the closed circulatory system. Normally, when a blood vessel ruptures or is severed, compensatory mechanisms protect the body from significant blood loss. The wall of the injured vessel contracts immediately. A platelet plug forms at the site, blood clots, and new connective tissue penetrates the clot for permanent closure of the injured site.

For the client with hemorrhage, the nurse assesses the nature of the bleeding as external, internal, or both. An assessment is made to determine the body's response and establish baseline data, including vital signs and urinary output (Table 31-1 ■). A priority of care is to monitor the client frequently and regularly and minimize the client's stress, thus decreasing the sympathetic response. Sympathetic nervous system stimulation will increase heart rate (**chronotropic** effect) and force of contraction (**inotropic** effect), thereby increasing bleeding.

Interventions for clients who are hemorrhaging include restricting activity, elevating involved body areas above the heart if possible, applying direct pressure, and replacing lost fluid volume. A tourniquet is generally not used unless there has been a traumatic amputation, because a tourniquet crushes the underlying tissues and results in ischemia to the affected limb. But, if used, it is placed proximal to the site of the traumatic limb amputation.

Shock

Hemorrhage is the most common cause of hypovolemic shock, a potentially life-threatening condition, which is the most common cause of preventable postinjury deaths.

Table 31-1 Assessment Guide for Hemorrhaging

1. Observable bleeding from skin and mucous membranes. Check under the individual's clothing, dressing, and casts.

2. Observable bleeding into the skin and mucous membranes. Check for **petechiae**, **ecchymosis**, **hematomas**, and **purpura**.

3. Observable bleeding from body orifice. Check for **epistaxis**, **hematemesis**, and **hemoptysis**.

4. Observable bleeding from tubes. Check drainage tubes, **endotracheal** tubes, suction drainage, and urinary catheters.

5. Generalized signs and symptoms of bleeding.

   a. Thirst
   b. Narrow pulse pressure
   c. Positional vital sign changes
   d. Low blood pressure (systolic below 90 mm Hg and diastolic below 50 mm Hg)
   e. Tachycardia
   f. Weak pulses or absence of pulses
   g. Clammy skin and central **cyanosis**
   h. Deep, rapid respirations (above 24/min)
   i. Low body temperature (one or more degrees below 98.6°F [37°C], oral temperature)
   j. Reduced urine output (less than 30 mL/hr)
   k. Behavioral changes
   l. **Syncope** and visual disturbance
   m. Loss of consciousness

Hypovolemic (hemorrhagic) shock means there is insufficient intravascular volume (insufficient venous return) to maintain adequate tissue **perfusion**. Rapid assessment of the client's **hemodynamic** status is mandatory. Level of consciousness (LOC), skin color, pulse, and urinary output are four elements that can be determined rapidly during clinical observation. LOC is impaired when blood flow to the brain is reduced because of lack of circulating blood volume. The earliest signs include anxiety, agitation, and dizziness coupled with orthostatic **hypotension**. Skin color is important to immediately assess because clients with pink skin are rarely critical, whereas clients with ashen gray facial color or a white, exsanguinate extremity are ominous hypovolemic signs of shock. Pulse is determined by accessing central pulse, either the carotid or femoral artery, and assessing the quality, rate, and rhythm. If the client's pulse is slow, regular, and full, these are indications that the client is normovolemic, whereas if the pulse is rapid (tachycardic) and thready, then the client is hypovolemic, although other factors may also contribute to this sign. If the pulse is rapid and irregular, then cardiac dysfunction is occurring. This sign is a signal for rapid assessment, immediate **resuscitation** measures, and rapid replacement of volume. Urinary output is a good indicator for kidney perfusion. If blood flow is normal to the kidneys, then hourly urine output is maintained greater than 30 mL/hr. However, if blood flow to the kidneys is compromised, the first indication is decreased urinary output less than 30 mL/hr.

Children, because of their remarkable physiologic reserve, display very minimal early signs of hypovolemic shock even after severe volume depletion. However, when symptoms are manifested in a child, these symptoms are precipitous and may be catastrophic.

Hemorrhagic shock occurs on a continuum. In the initial phases, there are subtle changes in the hemodynamic status of the client. However, as blood loss continues and the intravascular blood volume continues to decrease, organ involvement worsens because of lack of perfusion. For example, in the kidneys, the client initially becomes oliguric, but as the blood flow continues to be reduced to the kidneys, the client becomes anuric. The pulse gradually increases, whereas the blood pressure continues to drop precipitously. If rapid interventions are not implemented immediately to stop this downward spiral of events, then death will be the eventual outcome. Interventions for hypovolemic shock are provided in Box 31-1 ■.

CLINICAL ALERT

Do Not Use Trendelenburg Position

Placing shock clients in Trendelenburg position or a modified Trendelenburg position (client lying flat with the lower extremities raised) has not been proven to significantly raise the systolic pressure in prehospital hypotensive clients. Of the 30 articles written on Trendelenburg positioning, only nine articles were peer reviewed. Trendelenburg or modified Trendelenburg did increase the risk of aspiration, and in cardiogenic shock clients, pulmonary **edema** worsened.

Additionally, although CVP and PAP pressures increase with Trendelenburg position, intrathoracic blood volume and cardiac function do not increase.

Heart Failure

Heart failure results from any condition that reduces the ability of the heart to effectively pump blood. When this occurs, the cardiac output is decreased, which impedes adequate blood flow to all tissues. Causes of heart failure are numerous, with coronary artery disease being the most common cause. Other causes of heart failure include valvular heart disease, myocardial infarctions, myocardial infections, and toxins.

Heart failure may involve either right, left ventricle, or both ventricles. Although most heart failure begins on the left side, as the disease process progresses, the right ventricle may become involved; this is known as *bi-ventricular failure*.

Cardinal manifestations of heart failure are dyspnea and fatigue, with limited activity tolerance. When the heart is unable to adequately pump, the blood begins to back up. In left-sided failure, the left ventricle is unable to pump effectively, which leads to the buildup of fluid in pulmonary capillaries, termed *pulmonary edema*. Pulmonary edema is the most common result of left ventricle pump failure and is a life-threatening condition. As fluids accumulate in alveoli of the lungs, gas exchange is impaired. Clinical manifestations of left-sided failure include dyspnea; moist, hacking cough; bibasilar crackles; distended neck veins; and orthopnea. Increased pulmonary vascular pressure may cause right-sided heart failure with resultant reduction of circulation into the pulmonary artery, causing a backup of fluid in the systemic venous circulation. Clinical manifestations

---

Box 31-1 **INTERVENTIONS FOR HYPOVOLEMIC SHOCK**

- Maintain airway.
- Place client in supine position.
- Administer supplemental oxygen.
- Keep client warm.
- Immediately establish two large-bore intravenous catheters—the loss of significant blood volume requires rapid infusion of at least 2–3 L of warmed intravenous solution.
- Fluid and blood replacement: isotonic crystalloids, such as Ringer's solution, are preferred over 0.9% normal saline

to replace extracellular volume. Colloid solutions, such as blood transfusions or serum albumin, may also be given to expand intravascular space. Packed RBCs are used for acute blood loss.

- Drug administration: only occurs after adequate fluid replacement. Vasopressor agents, such as vasopressin, norepinephrine, or dopamine, may be given, if volume replacement is unsuccessful.

Source: Halm (2012)

of right-sided heart failure include weight gain, peripheral edema, oliguria, hepatomegaly, ascites, and fatigue.

The goal of treatment for heart failure is to reduce workload on the heart, increase efficiency of contractions, and reduce fluid retention. Both physiological and pharmacological interventions are necessary to meet this goal. Bed rest during the most critical time may be ordered to reduce the workload on the heart. Oxygen therapy is essential to maximize the oxygen available to the tissues, as well as both reduced sodium intake and restricted fluid intake to decrease fluid volume and edema. Pharmacological interventions include:

- Diuretics—furosemide, spironolactone
- Nitrates—nitroglycerine because of vasodilating properties
- Antihypertensive agents
- Angiotensin-converting enzyme (ACE) inhibitors
- Antidysrhythmics, if needed
- Inotropic medications—digitalis
- Beta-blockers
- Potassium chloride (KCl)—client cannot be on potassium-sparing diuretics, such as spironolactone

Ischemia

Tissue ischemia results when blood flow is reduced to a critical level. Hypotension can cause relative ischemia because blood flow is insufficient to meet the metabolic demands. Absolute ischemia is usually due to a sudden, complete occlusion of a blood vessel, resulting in tissue necrosis. Leaving a tourniquet on an extremity for more than 15 min may cause tissue necrosis. Other causes of ischemia due to decreased blood flow include Raynaud disease, Buerger disease, thromboembolism, mechanical obstruction, arteriosclerosis, and **atherosclerosis**.

Deep Vein Thrombosis (DVT)

Venous thromboembolism and the resulting complication of pulmonary embolus (PE) is a frequent cause of preventable illness and death in hospitalized clients. Deep vein thrombosis (DVT) can result in complications such as PE. The incidence of DVT in clients without DVT prophylaxis is unacceptably high in both surgical and medical hospitalized clients. As a result, this is considered a high client safety indicator by The Joint Commission, the Agency for Healthcare Research and Quality (AHRQ), and the Center for Medicare and Medicaid Services because of the underutilization of simple, cost-effective prophylactic measures.

Most hospitalized clients, whether medical or surgical, have multiple risk factors for developing DVT. Risk factors include thrombophilia; hypercoagulability states regarding clotting factors; cancer; obesity; pregnancy; smoking; surgery; trauma; head injury; medications (birth control pills, hormone replacement therapy, tamoxifen); surgical conditions involving the hip, pelvis, or knee; prolonged sitting for more than 6 hr in aircraft; or when on bed rest.

According to the Centers for Disease Control, approximately 300,000–600,000 people each year will be affected by DVT or PE, and approximately 60,000–100,000 will die. Among those people who have a DVT, half will have long-term complications such as swelling, pain, discoloration, and scaling in the affecting limb (Centers for Disease Control, 2014). The classic symptoms of a DVT, if present, include swelling, pain, warmth, and redness in the involved extremity. Some may experience a dull ache or tightness in the calf upon walking and may show slight edema, a palpable cord, venous collateral distention, low-grade fever, cyanosis, and a positive Homans sign. Homans sign, which was previously a mainstay for the diagnosis of DVT, is no longer considered accurate. It is present in less than one-third of clients with confirmed DVTs and is found in more than half of clients without DVTs.

Hypercoagulable state, thrombophilia, venous **stasis**, and vascular (endothelial) injury are factors that may lead to platelet aggregation, fibrin, WBC and RBC deposition, and eventual formation of a free-floating clot. In 80% of cases, clots begin in deep veins of the calf. Within 7–10 days, the clot adheres to the vein wall, **phlebitis** develops, the clot is invaded by fibroblasts, scar is formed, and blood flow is restored, but the vein valves are usually permanently damaged. The clot propagates proximally; pieces can break off and embolize to the heart and obstruct the pulmonary circulation, with resultant right heart failure, atelectasis, hypoxemia, decreased cardiac output, or cardiac arrest.

DVT prophylaxis is indicated for all moderate- to high-risk medical and surgical clients. Low-molecular-weight heparin and unfractionated heparin decrease incidence of asymptomatic or symptomatic DVT and pulmonary emboli by 50–65%.

Compression stockings, also known as TED hose, reduce venous stasis and reduce the incidence of postoperative venous thrombosis in low-risk surgical clients and moderate-risk neurosurgical clients. Mechanical devices (sequential compression devices [SCDs]) prevent venous thrombosis by improving blood flow through the deep leg veins, which prevents venous stasis. Additionally, SCDs reduce plasminogen activator inhibitor, which increases fibrinolytic activity, although the exact mechanism is not known. SCDs are effective in reducing the incidence of DVT in moderate-risk surgical clients, including neurosurgical and coronary artery bypass clients. They are not as effective in calf vein thrombosis in orthopedic surgical clients. SCDs are beneficial when used in conjunction with anticoagulant therapy. Other interventions to prevent development of DVT in clients on bed rest include:

- Assessment of risk factors
- Early ambulation
- Adequate hydration
- Foot and leg exercises while in bed
- Minimal interruptions during application
- Accurate assessment, measurement, and application of devices

Note: These measures help venous flow, but do not decrease the incidence of pulmonary embolism.

The goal of treatment for *existing* thrombophlebitis is to prevent clot propagation, pulmonary emboli, and thrombus recurrence. Care interventions include early ambulation, avoidance of rubbing or massaging the affected extremity, and adequate hydration. Pharmacological (systemic) intervention includes anticoagulation with heparin drip to a goal of 1.5–2 times normal PTT, or use of low-molecular-weight heparin to stop propagation of the clot. This is followed by oral warfarin therapy for 3 or 6 months or longer, with a therapeutic international normalized ratio goal of 2.0–3.0.

Altered Circulation

Assessment

Alterations in circulation are indicated by a variety of signs and symptoms. If bleeding exists, external and/or internal sites must be identified. Attention is given to disease conditions of major organs or coagulation and the family history. Although a variety of sophisticated devices are available to monitor the client's circulatory status, direct observation is also reliable. Baseline data are obtained for vital signs and arterial blood pressure. Note the color, temperature, and condition of the skin. Abnormalities of superficial veins often indicate obstruction or pooling. Additional assessment data include:

- Vein distention
- Edema (fluid retention)
- Petechiae (platelet abnormalities)
- Homans sign (calf tenderness with **dorsiflexion**); positive in less than 50% of cases; therefore, not frequently used

Information obtained from the client's medical history, medications, and lifestyle influences selection of nursing interventions. Trauma victims require especially close inspection since more overt signs and symptoms may not appear until days later. Table 31-1 illustrates an assessment of a hemorrhaging client.

Emergency Life Support Measures

The 2010 American Heart Association Guidelines for Cardiopulmonary Resuscitation (CPR) and emergency **cardiovascular** care (ECC) are recommendations designed to improve survival from sudden cardiac arrest (SCA) and acute life-threatening cardiopulmonary incidents (Table 31-2 ■). According to the AHA, *basic life support* includes recognition

Table 31-2 Summary of Basic Life Support ABCD Maneuvers for Infants, Children, and Adults (Newborn Information Not Included)

Maneuver	Adult 8 Years and Older	Child 1–8 Years	Infant Under 1 Year of Age
Compression Compression landmarks	Lower half of sternum (center between the nipples to prevent compression over the xiphoid)		Just below nipple line (lower half of sternum)
Compression method (Push hard and fast; allow complete recoil.)	Heel of one hand, other hand on top	Heel of one hand or as for adults (depending on size of the child)	One rescuer: 2 or 3 fingers 2 rescuers: 2 thumb-encircling hands
Compression depth	5–6 cm (2–2.4 in.)	5 cm (2 in.)	3.8 cm (1.5 in.)
Compression rate	Approximately 100–120/min		
Compression–ventilation ratio	30:2	30:2 15:2 (2 rescuers)	30:2 15:2 (2 rescuers)
Airway	Jaw thrust		
Breathing Initial	2 breaths at 1 sec/ breath; after 30 compressions, use airway device	One rescuer: 2 effective breaths at 1 sec/breath after 30 compressions Two rescuers: 2 effective breaths after 15 compressions	
HCP: Rescue breathing without chest compressions	10–12 breaths/min (approximate)	One rescuer: 2 effective breaths at 1 sec/breath after 30 compressions Two rescuers: 2 effective breaths after 15 compressions	
HCP: Rescue breaths and CPR with advanced airway	30 compressions, 2 breaths	1 breath every 3–5 sec	
Foreign body airway obstruction (conscious) (unconscious)	Abdominal thrusts CPR with compressions first	Child abdominal thrusts Infant: 5 back blows, 5 chest thrusts Infant and child: CPR with chest compressions first	
Defibrillation AED	Shock as soon as AED available. You cannot use pediatric pads.	Use AED as soon as available. Use child pads for child 1–8 years if available. Otherwise you can use adult pads.	Use as soon as available. Use child pads for child 1–8 years if available. Otherwise you can use adult pads.

Note: Maneuvers used by only healthcare providers are indicated by "HCP."

Sources: Travers, et al. (2010), Berg, R. A., et al. (2010), & Berg, M. D., et al. (2010)

of signs of SCA, MI (heart attack), cerebral vascular accident (stroke), and foreign-body airway obstruction (FBAO); CPR; and defibrillation with an automated external defibrillator (AED).

The 2010 Guidelines focus on giving chest compressions first, but added an upper limit on rate and depth to ensure adequate time for recoil between compressions. Chest compressions act like an artificial heart by pumping blood to the heart and brain.

There is a significant amount of oxygen in the bloodstream capable of sustaining brain tissue for several minutes even without breathing. Many who believe doing only chest compressions as a sufficient solution for adequate blood flow feel that interrupting compressions with rescue breathing does not allow oxygen to reach vital organs.

Studies published in the *American Journal of Medicine* and *The Lancet* have shown that there was a better outcome of victims who had only chest compressions. Not all cardiac arrests are from heart disease. Victims of drowning, drug overdose, or respiratory problems that lead to cardiac arrest will need rescue breathing.

To provide the victim with the best chance of survival, these actions must occur within the first moments of a cardiac arrest.

1. Activate the EMS System (Emergency Medical Services) by calling 911 and send for the AED.
2. Begin chest compressions at 100–120 compressions/min with a depth of at least 5–6 cm (2–2.4 in.) in adult clients.

The CPR Guidelines are termed CAB: compression, airway, breathing.

Use of airway devices by trained medical personnel will deliver air to the lungs rather than the stomach, greatly reducing complications such as aspiration and pneumonia. Lay rescuers are taught the skills of hands-only CPR unless they have access to airway devices and are trained in their use.

After 30 compressions, the trained CPR individual will open the victim's airway using the jaw-thrust method and using an airway device. Infants and children may still require mouth-to-mouth resuscitation by a trained CPR individual as breathing issues are more common in this age group, but a barrier device (Box 31-2 ■) is still recommended. The American Heart Association guidelines place priority on caring for victims of stroke as well as those with an acute MI. Early fibrinolytic treatment for the MI client is necessary; also, clients with a stroke require treatment within 4.5 hr of onset of symptoms for a quality outcome.

Box 31-2 BARRIER DEVICES

Face Shield: Clear plastic or silicon sheet placed over victim's face to prevent direct contact with victim during rescue breathing. Face shields are small, flexible, and portable.

Face Mask: Hard plastic device that fits over mouth and nose. They cost more than face shields and are bulkier, preventing people from carrying them on their person.

EMS personnel are trained to provide stroke screening tools and then rapidly transport stroke clients to the nearest hospital where fibrinolytic therapy can be administered quickly upon arrival at the facility.

The *AED* is a battery-operated computerized defibrillator that analyzes the heart rhythm, recognizes a shockable rhythm, and advises the operator when the victim should be shocked. Outside the hospital facility, AEDs should be accessible in areas where there is a high probability of cardiac arrest situations and when EMS is 5 min or more away from the location. Lay individuals, properly trained, can recognize signs of cardiac arrest and apply and operate the AED.

Early Defibrillation Programs in Hospitals

The American Heart Association standard-of-care recommendation is that the collapse-to-shock interval be less than 3 min in all areas of the hospital and ambulatory care facilities. Even though emergency (crash) carts with defibrillators are available in hospitals, AEDs should be available on the nursing units if the cart is more than 3 min away. It is estimated that time from collapse to first defibrillation in hospitals can be 5–10 min.

The major benefit for AED usage throughout noncritical care units within the hospital is that other healthcare providers and noncritical care nurses can easily provide defibrillation within the AHA standard of 3 min. Every minute is crucial if the individual is in ventricular fibrillation, the most common cause of sudden death in adults. Survival decreases 7–10% for each minute that normal heart beat is not restored.

Planning and Intervention

Once an initial assessment of a client for alterations in circulation has been made, the nurse develops a plan of care and prioritizes interventions. Interventions for circulatory problems usually fall into three broad categories: inputs, outputs, and pressure supports. Inputs include arterial lines, venous lines, fluids, drug regimens, transfusions, and blood component therapies. Outputs include suctioning with specialized equipment such as Hemovacs and chest tubes and procedures such as thoracentesis. Pressure supports include dressings, direct compression, tourniquets, and CPR. An evaluation of the planned actions, based on the client's response, should be continuous and modified as the client's condition dictates.

In coping with alterations in circulation, care should be directed toward promoting, maintaining, or regaining the best possible cardiopulmonary function. The design for nursing action is to assess the situation and client for stressors. The client should be interviewed if possible, observed, and examined to identify actual and/or potential circulatory problems. The client's responses are appropriate, deficient, or excessive, and interventions should be planned accordingly. The nurse attempts to reduce client stress, supports adaptive behaviors, replaces deficiencies, modifies or removes excessive responses, and prevents injury and complications. The nurse should always assist in the evaluation of planned actions, report client responses, and assist in modifying the interventions as indicated.

Adaptations to Home Care

Circulatory skills performed in the home setting are similar to those in the hospital. Vital signs are taken using the same equipment and procedures. CPR and abdominal thrusts are performed exactly the same way. Care of the pacemaker client, however, is somewhat different.

Clients with permanent pacemakers are expected to monitor pacemaker function on a daily basis. While in the hospital, the client is taught how to monitor pulse, vital signs, symptoms of pacemaker failure, and indications of infection at the pacemaker insertion site. When the client returns home, the home health nurse needs to reinforce the teaching that was initiated in the hospital. Pacemaker batteries generally last up to 12 years depending on the type and the demand placed on the pacemaker. During discharge, the client will be taught how to use the telephone monitoring system that will be used to monitor the pacemaker after discharge.

Clients will also need to be educated about the use of cell phones and other electric devices that might affect their pacemaker. Cell phones can be used but should be used on the opposite side of where the pacemaker is implanted. With modern pacemaker technology, microwaves, modern electronic home appliances and airport metal detectors will not affect pacemaker function.

A Holter monitor, also called an ambulatory electrocardiology (ECG) monitor, is a small battery-operated device that the client wears. The monitor shows the heart's electrical activity while the client performs usual activities. The monitor will show how fast a heart beats, and if it beats in a regular pattern. If the client has a heart problem, the signals in the heart may not function properly, resulting in **vertigo**, chest pain, or death. As with the pacemaker, the Holter monitor is now being replaced by Event Monitoring and Signal-Averaged ECG monitoring. These monitors can measure the heart function periodically and do not necessarily measure only for 24–36 hr.

Nursing Diagnoses

The following nursing diagnoses may be appropriate to use on a client care plan when the components are related to circulation.

NURSING DIAGNOSIS	RELATED TO . . .
Decreased Cardiac Output	Cardiac disease states, altered electrical conduction, altered contractility, altered preload and afterload drug side effects, hypovolemia
Deficient Fluid Volume	Blood loss from hemorrhage, dehydration
Ineffective Peripheral Tissue Perfusion	Altered blood supply, arterial or venous, hypovolemia, shock
Impaired Gas Exchange	Ventilation–perfusion imbalance, abnormal blood gases, tachycardia
Excess Fluid Volume	Compromised regulatory mechanism, heart failure
Deficient Knowledge	Understanding pacemaker function, corrective lifestyle habits for heart failure

Unit 31.1
Control of Bleeding

Nursing Process Data

ASSESSMENT Database

- Observe the amount of bleeding.
- Check for the source of bleeding.
- Observe the extent of the wound.
- Identify familial history of bleeding disorders.
- Assess baseline vital signs and blood pressure readings.
- Observe color, temperature, and condition of the skin.
- Obtain list of current medications taken by client.

PLANNING Objectives

- To detect source of bleeding
- To stop or control bleeding or hemorrhage before large blood loss occurs
- To provide pressure as an assist (adjunct) to stop bleeding
- To minimize capillary seepage, hematoma, and serum accumulation

IMPLEMENTATION Procedures

DOCUMENTATION AND EVALUATION
Expected Outcomes

- Early detection of bleeding occurs and loss of blood is minimized.
- Pressure dressing is applied and bleeding is controlled.
- Peripheral circulation is preserved.
- Vital signs are within normal limits.

Unexpected Outcomes / Alternative Actions

Pearson Nursing Student Resources

Find additional review materials at
nursing.pearsonhighered.com.
Prepare for success with NCLEX®-style practice
questions and Skill Checklists.

Skill 31.1.1 | Using Digital Pressure

Equipment
Towels or gauze dressing if available
Gloves

Procedure
1. Perform hand hygiene and don gloves (sterile preferred).
2. Identify the closest artery proximal to the bleeding site. ❶ ➤ *Rationale:* The rapid loss of more than 40% of the total blood volume will lead to death if rapid aggressive intervention is not implemented.
3. Apply direct pressure to artery using your gloved finger.
4. If towels or 4×4 gauze pads are available, apply direct pressure to site if wound does not contain glass particles. ➤ *Rationale:* If pressure is placed on wound when glass is present, additional tissue damage can occur.
5. Raise the affected limb above the level of the heart about 30 degrees. ➤ *Rationale:* This decreases arterial blood flow to area and promotes venous return.
6. Maintain direct pressure on site for 5 min. ➤ *Rationale:* This action promotes clot formation.

> **CLINICAL ALERT**
> Determine whether individual is receiving medications or herbal therapies that affect blood coagulation (e.g., Coumadin). If so, increase time of applying pressure.

7. When bleeding has subsided, proceed to gently clean and dress the wound.
8. To control nose bleeds (epistaxis), place client in sitting position, with head tilted forward. Pinch nose for 5 min. Apply ice pack to back of neck. ➤ *Rationale:* This assists in vasoconstriction.

❶ Pulse sites that may be used to control bleeding.

9. Remove gloves when bleeding subsides.
10. Perform hand hygiene immediately. ➤ *Rationale:* This is to protect yourself from possible contamination should any leakage have occurred through the gloves.

Skill 31.1.2 | Using Pressure Dressing

Equipment
4×4 gauze pad
Sterile dressings—number and size depend on wound
Sterile gloves
Cleansing solution
Tape

Preparation
1. Check healthcare provider's orders.
2. Assemble necessary supplies according to extent of wound.
3. If time permits, explain procedure to client and provide light and privacy.
4. Perform hand hygiene thoroughly if time permits.
5. Set up sterile field and prepare cleansing solution if time permits.

Procedure

1. Put on sterile gloves.
2. Cleanse wound and apply dressing. Use several layers of 4×4 gauze pads.
3. Place tape tightly over entire dressing to provide an occlusive dressing. Do not completely circle an extremity or the body. ➤ *Rationale:* Encircling an extremity with a bandage acts like a tourniquet and may prevent blood flow.
4. Check for pulses distal to pressure site. ➤ *Rationale:* This is to ensure that collateral blood flow is maintained.
5. Place all soiled materials in biohazard bag. ➤ *Rationale:* This is to prevent cross-contamination and ensure proper disposal.
6. Remove gloves and perform hand hygiene.
7. Monitor vital signs and observe for signs of shock.
8. Continue to monitor extremity distal to pressure dressing. ➤ *Rationale:* This ensures adequate circulation.
9. Position client for comfort.
10. Elevate extremity. ➤ *Rationale:* This is to minimize bleeding.
11. Monitor frequently for signs of bleeding and hematoma.

Note: Hematomas feel spongy even under bandages.

Unit 31.1 Documentation and Evaluation

DOCUMENTATION for Control of Bleeding

- Size (in centimeters), location based on anatomical landmark, condition of wound
- Color, odor, amount of drainage
- Type and number of dressings used
- Approximate amount of blood loss
- Condition of dressing when removed (e.g., saturated with drainage)

EVALUATION/Critical Thinking

Expected Outcomes

- Early detection of bleeding occurs and loss of blood is minimized.
- Pressure dressing is applied and bleeding is controlled.
- Peripheral circulation is preserved.
- Vital signs are within normal limits.

Unexpected Outcomes

- Even with direct pressure and application of pressure dressing, bleeding continues.

Alternative Actions

- Reinforce pressure dressing.
- Maintain IV infusion.
- Notify healthcare provider and be prepared to send client to surgery for wound closure.
- Monitor closely for signs of shock (LOC, vital signs, oliguria or anuria, tachycardia, narrow pulse pressure, hypotension).
- Apply pressure directly or proximal to wound.
- Place tourniquets proximal to site of hemorrhage to control bleeding if all other actions are unsuccessful, notify healthcare provider immediately, and prepare for surgery.

(continued)

Unexpected Outcomes	**Alternative Actions**
• Wound edges do not approximate.	• Notify healthcare provider. • Be prepared to assist with wound closure or to send client to surgery.
• Glass particles are evident in wound.	• Irrigate wound profusely with sterile saline solution as ordered. • If large amount of glass or if glass is difficult to extract, notify healthcare provider and be prepared to send client to surgery for wound cleansing and debridement. • Do not apply direct pressure or pressure dressing to wound containing glass.

Circulatory Maintenance

Nursing Process Data

ASSESSMENT Database

- Evaluate client's overall physical status, particularly client's risk for venous thrombus formation.
- Assess baseline vital signs before procedures are initiated.
- Determine whether client is at risk for pooling of blood in extremities or decreased venous return. Clients who require use of graduated stockings or SCDs are postoperative clients, those who are immobile, and those with a history of venous insufficiency.
- Assess peripheral pulses, observing skin color and temperature, and fluid accumulation or edema.
- Compare findings with contralateral extremity.

PLANNING Objectives

- To prevent venous stasis
- To prevent thrombus formation and subsequent emboli
- To use compression stockings or SCDs to prevent venous stasis

IMPLEMENTATION Procedures

DOCUMENTATION AND EVALUATION

Expected Outcomes

- Compression stockings remain wrinkle-free, and pressure is evenly distributed.
- Peripheral pulses are present during use of sequential stockings and elastic hosiery.
- Compression devices function properly.
- Client's skin remains intact while using compression stockings.

Unexpected Outcomes/Alternative Actions

Pearson Nursing Student Resources

Find additional review materials at
nursing.pearsonhighered.com.
Prepare for success with NCLEX®-style practice questions and Skill Checklists.

Skill 31.2.1 | Applying Graduated Compression Stockings (Elastic Hosiery)

Equipment
Tape measure
Specific type of hosiery (e.g., below-the-knee or above-the-knee) (Box 31-3 ■)

Preparation
1. Check healthcare provider's orders for type and specifications.
2. Gather supplies, and explain procedure.
3. Perform hand hygiene, and provide for client's privacy and comfort.
4. Identify client using two client identifiers.
5. Assess client for contraindications to use of compression stockings (signs and symptoms of DVT).
6. Apply drape as top linens are removed. Bathe and ensure legs are dry before applying stockings.
7. Assess lower extremities for edema, dry skin, and palpable pulses.
8. Position client in dorsal recumbent position, and elevate bed to working height.
9. Measure client for hosiery size (Table 31-3 ■). Length is determined by measuring distance from gluteal fold to bottom of the heel.
   a. For thigh-high stockings, measure midcalf and midthigh circumference to determine size.
   b. For below-the-knee stockings, measure from the Achilles tendon to the popliteal fold, and measure the midcalf circumference.
10. Compare your measurements with manufacturer's chart to obtain correct hose size.

Procedure
1. Invert foot of stocking back to heel area.
2. Holding both sides of hose at inverted foot area, pull hose over toes, and ease gently toward top of foot.
3. Gather top of hose down to heel area, and with curving motion, cover heel. ❶ ❷ Pull hose up leg, positioning support section on inner thigh. ❸
4. Reposition client, lower bed, and perform hand hygiene.

5. Observe that stockings are wrinkle-free and correctly placed on extremity. ▶ *Rationale:* Stockings tend to roll down and create a tourniquet effect that inhibits venous return.
6. Check client in 30 min for adequate circulation, assessing for warmth, color of feet, blanching of nail beds, and edema above level of stockings.
7. Remove hose two to three times daily for 30 min. Assess skin integrity and peripheral circulation and perform neurovascular checks for circulation, motion, and sensation.
8. Wash hose in mild detergent and warm water daily and hang to dry.

Note: A second pair of hose should be available to use when hose are drying.

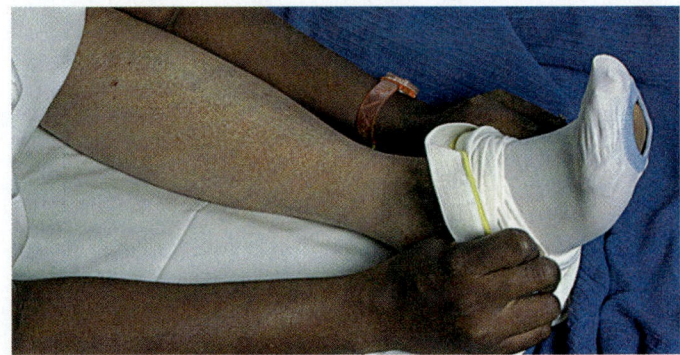

❶ Gather elastic hose and pull over toes and then to top of foot.

Box 31-3 EFFECTIVENESS OF ELASTIC COMPRESSION STOCKINGS

Hospitalized clients can develop DVT after surgery or if they are immobile due to their medical condition. The use of elastic compression stockings has been shown to be effective in reducing the incidence of DVT according a review published in the Cochrane Library. The review looked at 18 randomized control trials (one of the highest levels of evidence in research) and found that elastic compression stockings were effective at preventing DVTs in hospitalized clients.

Source: Sachdeva (2010)

Table 31-3 Measuring for Graduated Compression Stockings (Elastic Hosiery)

Thigh-High Measuring		Knee-High Measuring	
Circumference	Length	Circumference	Length
Measure mid-thigh circumference	Measure leg from bottom of heel to fold of buttocks	Measure calf at largest circumference	Measure leg from Achilles tendon to popliteal fold

2 Ensure hose fits properly without wrinkles over toe or heel.

3 Position support section on inner thigh.

EVIDENCE-BASED PRACTICE

Compliance in Using Compression Stocking and Intermittent Compression Devices

A survey of 29 nurses found several concerns that interfered with consistent use of both compression stockings and intermittent compression devices. Top among those concerns in compression stockings were concern for skin breakdown around the ankle and thigh due to rolling outside, difficulty getting them onto unconscious clients, and damage due to compression of banding in thigh. The majority of the concerns expressed with the intermittent compression devices were failure to sustain the Velcro part of the device, complaints of discomfort (by client), and getting soggy due to sweat. The authors suggest that issues related to the devices need to be addressed along with more education for nurses on how to prevent some of the problems they encountered to ensure good compliance.

Source: Kim & Lee (2015)

Skill 31.2.2 | Applying Sequential Compression Devices (SCDs)

Equipment

Disposable leg wraps (knee- or thigh-length) or foot wraps (Box 31-4 ■)
Tubing set
Pump controller

Preparation

1. Review healthcare provider's order for type/length of SCD.
2. Determine that device is not contraindicated for client.
3. Review product information for application and use.
4. Gather equipment.
5. Perform hand hygiene.

Procedure

1. Introduce yourself and identify client using two client identifiers.
2. Provide privacy.
3. Perform neurovascular assessment noting circulation, motion, and sensation in lower extremities. ➤ **Rationale:** This is to provide a baseline of ongoing assessment of neurovascular status after devices are in place.

4. Explain the purpose of the SCD:
   a. They are used to reduce risk of developing DVT by improving blood flow through the leg veins.
   b. The wraps must be used continuously (unless ambulating) in order to be effective.
5. Plug the pump into the electrical wall outlet but leave unit turned *off*.
6. Remove wraps from plastic bag (leg wraps and foot wraps can be used on either leg).

Box 31-4 **COMPRESSION PATTERN**

Each sleeve in the sequential devices is inflated in sequence. The inflation begins at the ankle and progresses to the knee or mid-thigh. Pressures range from a maximum pressure in the ankle of 45–50 mm Hg, 35 mm Hg at the calf, and 30 mm Hg at the thigh. Compression duration is 11 sec, with a 60-sec relaxation time between compressions.

For intermittent devices, sleeve inflates, then deflates, alternating from one leg to the other.

(continued)

Skill 31.2.2 | Applying Sequential Compression Devices (SCDs) *(continued)*

7. Connect tubing set to the pump, making certain a connecting click is heard.
8. Unfold wrap and place the inflatable bladder directly behind client's calf. ❶
9. Wrap the device around client's leg and secure the fastener tabs. Repeat process on other leg.
10. For foot (venous plexus) wraps (Box 31-5 ■):

    a. Place foot in center of wrap with back of wrap in line with client's heel.
    b. Bring large wrap over top of foot, holding it in place.
    c. Bring the two narrower wraps over foot and secure.
    d. Bring the heel strap around back of heel and fix in place to secure wrap.

11. Check that wrap is not too tight by slipping two fingers underneath. ❷ ➤ *Rationale:* This is to validate that wraps do not constrict circulation distally.
12. Attach the wraps to the tubing set, making certain a connecting click is heard. ❸
13. Adjust pump pressure regulator to product-recommended pressure or as the healthcare provider has ordered.

❸ Attach tubing from wrap to tubing connected to pump.

➤ *Rationale:* Intermittent compression and relaxation reduces venous stasis and thus improves the body's natural fibrinolytic activity.

14. Ensure that tubing is free of kinks. ➤ *Rationale:* Kinks can restrict airflow through the system.
15. Turn the pump on, noting that green light illuminates.
16. Place client in position of comfort; place call bell in reach.
17. Inform client to notify nurse if tingling, numbness, or discomfort develops. ➤ *Rationale:* Wraps should be removed should any of these occur.
18. Perform hand hygiene.
19. Regularly remove wraps for skin inspection and neurovascular assessment.

❶ Place inflatable bladder directly behind client's calf.

❷ Slip two fingers under wrap to ensure that it is not too tight.

CLINICAL ALERT

Contraindications to Use of Sequential Compression Devices

- Known or suspected acute DVT, phlebitis, severe atherosclerosis, or ischemic peripheral vascular disease
- DVT within last 6 months
- Pulmonary embolism
- Any condition where an increase in venous return to the heart might be detrimental
- Local conditions such as dermatitis, gangrene, recent skin graft, infected leg wound, or ulcer.

Box 31-5 **FOOT PUMPS**

Foot pumps gently squeeze the sole of the foot to mimic circulatory effects of walking. The plexus of veins in the foot act as a powerful venous pump in the weight-bearing phase of ambulation. The foot pump is designed to mimic natural effects of walking on blood circulation in feet and legs. These pumps increase circulation and decrease edema and pain to the lower extremities in clients who are not ambulatory.

Unit 31.2 Documentation and Evaluation

DOCUMENTATION for Circulatory Maintenance

Elastic Hosiery

- Size and type of elastic hose applied
- Condition of skin
- Presence of pulses
- Capillary refill time
- Edema formation below or above hose
- Time and length of time hose removed

Compression Devices

- Neurovascular assessment baseline data
- Neurovascular assessment after application
- Condition of skin
- Presence of SCDs
- Type of sleeve used; thigh high, knee high

EVALUATION/Critical Thinking

Expected Outcomes

- Compression stockings remain wrinkle-free, and pressure is evenly distributed.
- Peripheral pulses are present during use of sequential stockings and elastic hosiery.
- Compression devices function properly.
- Client's skin remains intact while using compression stockings.

Unexpected Outcomes

For Graduated Compression Stockings

- Graduated compression stockings are not available.

Alternative Actions

- If ordered, use elastic (Ace) bandages. Anchor bandages on top of the foot and proceed up the leg. Bandage should overlap one-third of bandage width; for a 10-cm (4-in.) width, each turn overlaps by 3.8 cm (1.5 in.). Ensure pressure is evenly distributed throughout bandage application.
- Assess that elastic bandages are tight enough for support but do not obstruct arterial flow. Assess neurovascular status 20 min after bandages applied and every 2–4 hr thereafter.
- While making each turn, place a finger between the bandage and skin with rotation to prevent bandage from becoming too tight.

- Graduated compression stockings are loose and do not provide support.

- Remeasure legs and compare with chart to determine correct size.
- Hosiery may be old with no elasticity and should be discarded; ensure line drying rather than with electric dryer.

(continued)

Unexpected Outcomes	**Alternative Actions**
• Graduated compression stockings do not provide support.	• Need to order different knit design and elastomeric yarn denier that will increase pressure. Pressure ranges from less than 15 mm Hg to 30–40 mm Hg at the ankle. Double check healthcare provider's order to ensure accuracy of original order.

For Compression Devices

• Client complains of numbness or tingling in leg.	• Remove devices immediately.
	• Suggest use of foot pulse device as alternate.
	• Complete neurovascular assessment.
	• Notify healthcare provider of assessment findings.
• Buildup of excess sleeve pressure (above 80 mm Hg).	• Check tubing for kinks or twists.
	• Turn power switch to OFF position and then ON to restart system.

Nursing Process Data

ASSESSMENT Database

- Determine whether there is preexisting cardiac disease or chest pain.
- Assess client's level of understanding and cooperation with procedure.
- Determine client's fear or anxiety regarding diagnosis, procedure, or outcome.
- Identify pharmacologic agents currently prescribed.
- Determine other factors that may precipitate conditions, such as fever, anxiety, alcohol, tobacco, or caffeine ingestion.
- Determine subjective complaints of diaphoresis, palpitations, dizziness, or fainting.
- Identify electrolyte abnormalities affecting the electrocardiogram, particularly potassium and calcium deficiencies or excesses.

PLANNING Objectives

- To obtain 12-lead ECG
- To continuously monitor a client on telemetry
- To identify ECG changes
- To determine cardiac dysrhythmias
- To identify and treat potentially dangerous rhythms accordingly

IMPLEMENTATION Procedures

DOCUMENTATION AND EVALUATION

Expected Outcomes

- ECG leads applied appropriately and without difficulty.
- Abnormal ECG findings interpreted accurately.
- Heart rate calculated correctly.
- Monitor wave forms are distinct and readable.

Unexpected Outcomes/Alternative Actions

Pearson Nursing Student Resources

Find additional review materials at
nursing.pearsonhighered.com.
Prepare for success with NCLEX®-style practice questions and Skill Checklists.

Skill 31.3.1 | Monitoring Clients on Telemetry

Equipment
Telemetry transmitter box battery
Electrode pouch or gown with transmitter pocket
Five-lead electrode cable and wires
Electrodes
Skin prep pad or alcohol swab

Preparation
1. Review the client's cardiac assessment (Box 31-6 ■).
   ➤ *Rationale:* The choice of monitoring lead is based on the client's assessment and potential arrhythmias that could occur.
2. Gather equipment and perform hand hygiene. ❶
3. Place a fresh 9-volt battery in the telemetry transmitter box, if needed.

Box 31-6 CARDIAC ASSESSMENT FINDINGS

- **Abnormal sinus rhythms**, premature atrial complexes, and most heart blocks can be recognized in any lead that displays a clear P wave and QRS complexes.
- **Atrial fibrillation** can be recognized in most leads by the irregular R-R intervals and chaotic atrial activity.
- **Bundle branch block** and ventricular rhythms are depicted by a widened QRS complex. Leads V_1 and V_6 (or MCL_1 and MCL_6) are the best leads for differentiating a widened QRS rhythm. These leads aide in differentiating ventricular tachycardia from supraventricular tachycardia with aberrant conduction. It is best to monitor the client with multiple leads or a 12-lead ECG.
  i. The V_1 and V_6 leads are obtained by using the five-lead bedside monitoring cable and limb electrodes. Arm electrodes are placed on the shoulders as close as possible to where the arms join the torso. Leg electrodes are placed at the level of the lowest ribs on the thorax or on the hips.
  ii. To monitor lead V_1, place the chest electrode in the fourth intercostal space (ICS) at the right sternal border and select "V" on the bedside monitor.
  iii. To monitor lead V_6, place the chest electrode in the fifth ICS at the left midaxillary line and select "V" on the bedside monitor.
- A second method used to diagnose the widened QRS complex is to use the V_1 and the bipolar lead MCL_6 together by placing the electrodes accordingly:
  i. Arm electrodes placed on shoulders.
  ii. Right leg electrode placed on right thorax or right hip.
  iii. Left leg electrode placed in the V_6 position (fifth ICS, left midaxillary line).
  iv. With the electrodes in place, select "V" on the first channel of the monitor to display "v1" and select lead III on the second channel to display MCL_6.

4. Attach lead wire securely into color-coded transmitter box, ensuring colors match. ❷
5. Introduce self and identify the client with two identifiers.
6. Explain procedure to client. Radio waves transmit the heart's electrical activity to a central monitoring station. This system allows the client to move around while his or her heart is constantly being monitored. Explain that the telemetry range is limited; therefore, client cannot wander out of the range, which is usually the nursing unit. If client goes off the unit, nurse must be notified.
7. Instruct the client to notify the nurse if the electrode falls off.

Procedure
1. Check the expiration date on the electrode packet.
   ➤ *Rationale:* This is to ensure electrode gel is moist.
2. Select electrode sites according to leads to be used for monitoring (Table 31-4 ■). Ensure they are not over bony prominence, muscular area, joints, breasts, or skin creases.
   ➤ *Rationale:* Placing electrodes on these areas can lead to artifact on the monitor screen. See diagrams for lead placements (Box 31-7 ■). ❸

Note: If client is overly obese, electrodes may have to be placed on the bones, since a large amount of adipose tissue results in poor image on the oscilloscope.

❶ Transmitter box, cable, and lead wires for telemetry.

❷ Insert electrode cable into transmitter box.

❸ Color-coded lead wires and placement of electrodes for ECG monitoring.

Box 31-7 ELECTRODE PLACEMENT

White to right shoulder

Black to left shoulder

Red to left midclavicular upper abdominal area (lead II positive electrode)

Brown to fourth ICS, right sternal border (MCL_1 or precordial lead V_1), or left sternal border, or alternatively at left fifth ICS, anterior axillary line (V_5 position)

Green to right abdomen or other convenient area (ground electrode)

Note: Limb leads and any one chest lead can be monitored using these electrode positions.

3. Assess skin site before placing electrode. Wipe skin areas using alcohol swab. Allow site to dry thoroughly before affixing electrode. ➤ *Rationale:* This removes oily substances and dead skin for better adherence of electrodes. Rub skin until slightly red. If client's chest is hairy, then clip hair. ➤ *Rationale:* This enables electrode to adhere well to skin and minimizes artifact.

4. Attach lead wires to chest electrodes.

5. Apply electrodes to client's chest: Peel off paper backing on electrode disc. Check that sponge pad in center of electrode is moist with conductive jelly. Place electrode on skin with adhesive side down. Press edges down to secure.

6. Attach wire into transmitter box, matching the color codes of the cable wires to the telemetry box. ➤ *Rationale:*

Mismatch of the colors will cause the client's rhythm pattern to appear inverted.

7. Have base station run an ECG strip to check clarity of transmission.

8. Set HIGH and LOW alarm limits on the monitor. Turn alarm buttons to ON per agency/unit protocol (e.g., 50 low, 100 high).

9. Assess skin surrounding electrode for signs of irritation regularly.

10. Check lead placement at least once a shift unless notified by client or monitoring station that electrodes are not functioning properly.

11. Change electrodes at least every 3 days or if ECG strip indicates poor conduction of wave form.

Table 31-4 Telemetry Electrode Placement

- Lead I: Records activity between a negative electrode (below right clavicle) and a positive electrode (below left clavicle). This lead looks at the heart's left lateral wall. Atrial arrhythmic activity is poorly identified.

- Lead II:* Records activity between a negative electrode (below right clavicle) and a positive electrode (midclavicular line on left flank). This lead looks at left inferior wall. It is used to diagnose supraventricular rhythms that arise from the atrial and junctional nodes. It best detects atrial activity.

(continued)

Skill 31.3.1 | Monitoring Clients on Telemetry *(continued)*

Table 31-4 Telemetry Electrode Placement *(continued)*

- **Lead III:** Records activity between a negative electrode (below left clavicle) and a positive electrode (lowest rib, left midclavicular line). It looks at left inferior wall.

- **Lead MCL₁:*** Records activity between a negative electrode (below left clavicle) and a positive electrode (fourth ICS, right of sternum). It is used to differentiate between **ectopy** versus abnormally conducted beats such as supraventricular tachycardia with **aberrancy** versus ventricular tachycardia.

- **Lead MCL₆:** Records activity between a negative electrode (below left clavicle) and a positive electrode (fifth ICS, left midaxillary line). It monitors ventricular conduction changes much like MCL₁. Not as frequently used.

*Most popular leads for telemetry.

Note: Check frequency and flush solutions according to agency protocols.

Skill 31.3.2 | Interpreting an ECG Strip

Equipment
Calipers (optional) ❶
ECG rhythm strip

Procedure

1. Assess ECG grid. ❷
   a. Each small square represents 0.04 sec (horizontal measurement).
   b. Each large block (five small squares) represents 0.20 sec.
   c. Fifteen large blocks represent 3 sec.
2. Determine heart rate by calculating ventricular rate; normal is 60–100/min (Table 31-5 ■).

   a. Count the number of R waves in a 6-sec period (30 large blocks) and multiply this by 10 to obtain the heart rate.
   b. For true accuracy, count client's apical heart rate for 1 full minute.
3. Determine the regularity of ventricular rhythm (R waves should be equally spaced).
4. Determine the P wave rate (atrial depolarizations). ❸
   a. There should be one P wave in front of each QRS complex.
   b. Note if there are more P waves or fewer P waves than QRS complexes. ❹
5. Determine the regularity of the P waves; are they all equally spaced?

Table 31-5 Normal Sinus Rhythm

Regular configuration, uniform P wave precedes each QRS

Atrial rate 60–100

PR interval 0.12–0.2 sec

QRS width <0.12 sec

Ventricular rate 60–100

❸ It is important to determine configuration and location of wave pattern to interpret an ECG accurately.

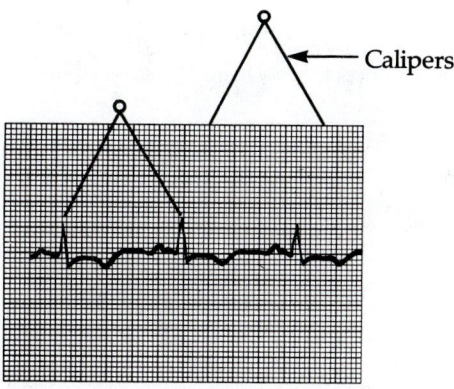

Calipers

❶ Use calipers to measure heart rate.

0.5 mV (5 mm)   0.1 mV (1 mm)

0.20 second   0.04 second

3 seconds

❷ ECG grid.

❹ ECG pattern and lead placement are depicted on oscilloscope.

6. Measure the PR interval (beginning of the P wave to the beginning of the QRS complex); represents conduction time through the electrical tissue to the ventricles (from the SA node, through the AV node, bundle of His, bundle branches, and Purkinje fibers); normal is 0.12–0.20 sec., and it generally shortens as the heart rate increases.

7. Measure the QRS duration from beginning of the Q wave, if present, to end of the S wave (normal is less than 0.12 sec).

8. Interpret the client's cardiac rhythm and place ECG rhythm sample strip in client's chart, according to hospital policy. See Table 31-6 ■ for selected cardiac rhythms and dysrhythmias.

CLINICAL ALERT

Always assess client to determine whether the abnormal rhythm is potentially life-threatening and emergency measures should be taken. Signs of hemodynamic instability include:

• Ongoing chest pain

• Shortness of breath

• Change in mental status

• Systolic blood pressure (SBP) less than 90 mm Hg

• Heart rate less than 150/min.

(continued)

Skill 31.3.2 | Interpreting an ECG Strip *(continued)*

Table 31-6 Selected Cardiac Rhythms and Arrythmias

Sinus Tachycardia	Sinus Bradycardia

Regular rhythm >100/min P waves—normal Atrial rate—>100/min PR interval—>0.12–2.0 sec QRS complex width—0.06–0.08 sec usually normal ***Note:*** A moderately faster heart rate can be a physiological normal variant.	Regular rhythm <60/min P waves—normal Atrial rate—<60/min PR interval—0.20 sec QRS complex width—0.08 sec usually normal ***Note:*** A slow heart rate can be physiologically normal for some clients.
Etiology	**Etiology**
Underlying causes such as anxiety, fever, shock, drugs, exercise, electrolyte disturbances	Drugs, hypoxia, altered metabolic states (hypothyroidism), cardiac diseases, athletes
Initial Treatment	**Initial Treatment**
Immediately initiate cardioversion if unstable. Treatment dependent on elimination of cause Decreasing anxiety Pain relief Antipyretics O_2 Medications (sedatives, tranquilizers, antianxiety, and such) Calcium channel blockers	Maintain patent airway; assist breathing as needed. Oxygen IV Atropine 0.5–1 mg bolus IV while awaiting pacemaker May repeat to a total dose of 3 mg Consider epinephrine (2–10 mg/min) or dopamine (2–10 mg/kg/min) infusion while awaiting pacer Transcutaneous pacing

Multifocal Premature Ventricular Contraction (PVCs)	Ventricular Tachycardia

Irregular rhythm P waves—none with premature beat, impulse originates in ventricle Atrial rate—undetermined PR interval—none with premature beat QRS width—>0.12 sec for premature beat Ventricular rate—varies ***Note:*** Each PVC has different configuration because foci are from different areas of heart. PVCs may be the result of an imbalance between oxygen demand versus supply, thereby making the myocardium irritable.	Regular rhythm Atrial rate—cannot differentiate PR interval—none QRS width—>0.12 sec Ventricular rate—130–250 ***Note:*** Ventricular tachycardia is a result of myocardial irritability and is life-threatening.
Etiology	**Etiology**
• Heart disease, MI • Hypoxia • Acidosis • Myocardial ischemia • Electrolyte imbalance	• Acute MI • Coronary artery disease, cardiomyopathy • Electrolyte imbalances • Drug toxicity (especially digitalis) • Drug intoxication (digitalis)

Table 31-6 Selected Cardiac Rhythms and Arrythmias *(continued)*

Initial Treatment

- Oxygen
- Potassium or magnesium if electrolytes dictate
- Lidocaine bolus—1–1.5 mg/kg; may repeat doses of 0.5–0.75 mg/kg every 5–10 min up to 3 mg/kg
- Refractory to lidocaine: amiodarone or procainamide
- Correct underlying cause

Initial Treatment

- Lidocaine 1.5 mg/kg bolus; may repeat in 3–5 minutes to maximum dose of 3 mg/kg
- Amiodarone 300 mg IV/IO can be followed by 150 mg IV/IO
- Cardioversion if cardiac output is compromised
- Pulseless ventricular tachycardia—follow treatment for ventricular fibrillation (epinephrine)

Atrial Fibrillation

Irregularly irregular rhythm
Disorganized atrial activity—>350 beats/min
P waves—none identifiable
PR interval—not measured
QRS—variable
QRS complex: irregular

Etiology

Heart failure
Rheumatoid heart disease
Coronary heart disease
Hypertension
Hyperthyroidism

Initial Treatment

Cardioversion
Diltiazem
Beta-blocker: Carvedilol or Toprol Xl
Digoxin
Quinidine
Procainamide
Amiodarone or dronedarone
Ibutilide
Anticoagulant to reduce risk of clot formation and stroke if atrial fibrillation duration new in onset but >48 hr

Atrial Flutter

Regular or irregular rhythm (depending on block)
Atrial rate >250 beats/min
P wave usually sawtooth pattern; PR interval cannot calculate
PR interval—regular
Ventricular rate can be irregular
QRS complex—0.6–0.10 sec

Etiology

Sympathetic nervous system stimulation (e.g., anxiety), caffeine, and alcohol intake
Thyrotoxins
Coronary heart disease; MI; pulmonary embolism

Initial Treatment

Cardioversion—if symptomatic
Diltiazem
Calcium channel blocker (Cardizem) or beta-blocking agents to slow ventricular response
Followed by ibutilide, quinidine, procainamide

Ventricular Fibrillation

Irregular, totally chaotic rhythm
Atrial rate—cannot differentiate
PR interval—none
QRS width—fibrillating waves only
Ventricular rate—cannot differentiate
Note: There is ineffective quivering of ventricles with no audible heartbeat, pulse, or respirations.

Third-Degree Heart Block

Regular atrial and ventricular rhythm
Atrial rate—greater than ventricular rate
PR interval—varies
QRS width—<0.12 sec if pacemaker cell in junction; >0.12 sec if cell in ventricle
Ventricular rate—40–60 beats/min if pacemaker from bundle of His; <40 if from Purkinje fibers in ventricle.
Note: Electrical impulse originates in SA node but is blocked in either the AV node, the bundle of His, or Purkinje fibers. There is no correlation between the atrial rate and the ventricular rate.

Skill 31.3.2 | Interpreting an ECG Strip *(continued)*

Table 31-6 Selected Cardiac Rhythms and Arrythmias *(continued)*

Ventricular Fibrillation	Third-Degree Heart Block
Etiology	**Etiology**
• Myocardial ischemia, acute MI • Coronary artery disease • Cardiomyopathy • Acid–base imbalance • Severe hypothermia • Electrolyte imbalance	• Digitalis toxicity • MI: inferior or anterior wall • Organic heart disease
Initial Treatment	**Initial Treatment**
• Immediately defibrillate, shock. • CPR—100 chest compressions/min • Ventricular fibrillation continues—give a vasopressor (epinephrine 1 mg IV push), repeat 3–5 min. • Defibrillate again and continue CPR. • Second-line drugs may be used, such as amiodarone (300 mg IV), lidocaine.	• Transcutaneous pacing • Dopamine, dobutamine, or epinephrine • Prepare for pacemaker insertion.

Skill 31.3.3 | Recording a 12-Lead ECG

Equipment
Electrodes
Skin prep pad or alcohol swab
ECG machine
Cable

Preparation
1. Review healthcare provider's order for ECG and perform hand hygiene.
2. Introduce self, identify client using two client identifiers, and explain the procedure. Reassure the client that the machine will not cause discomfort or electrocution.
3. Assess chest for placement of electrodes.
4. Determine whether skin site care is necessary. If so, cleanse areas with skin prep pad, alcohol swab, or clip hair if needed. Allow area to dry thoroughly before placing electrodes. ➤ *Rationale:* This will ensure a more secure fit for the electrodes and provide a better ECG tracing.
5. Attach wires to electrodes before pressing onto client's chest. ➤ *Rationale:* This prevents pressure being applied to chest area. This is particularly necessary after open heart surgery or chest trauma.
6. Check the color coding on the manufacturer's directions before placing electrodes to ensure they are correct.

Procedure
1. When placing electrodes, ensure lead wires are all going in the same direction.
2. Place electrodes on fleshy areas, avoiding bone and muscle. ➤ *Rationale:* This ensures good electrical conduction and clear ECG tracings.

3. Place the four limb leads, one on each limb, according to the color coding. Three standard leads will be recorded on the 12-lead ECG.
   a. **Lead I:** Right arm wrist (negative electrode) white; and left arm (positive electrode) black. Records activity between the two arms.
   b. **Lead II:** Right arm (negative electrode) and left leg ankle (positive electrode) red. Records activity between arm and leg.
   c. **Lead III:** Left arm (negative electrode) black and left leg (positive electrode) green. Records activity between arm and leg.
4. Three augmented limb lead tracings are obtained on the ECG as follows.
   a. **aVR:** Records activity between the center of the heart and right arm.
   b. **aVL:** Records activity between the center of the heart and left arm.
   c. **aVF:** Records activity between the center of the heart and the left leg or foot.
5. Place the chest leads as follows. ❶
   a. **V₁:** Fourth ICS, right sternal border. Records activity between the center of the heart and the fourth ICS; P wave is shown best here.
      i. Palpate the jugular notch above sternum (feels like a depression).
      ii. Move finger down and palpate the **manubrium** of sternum (feels solid).
      iii. Continue to move finger down to the angle of Louis, which is at the top of the sternal body.

iv. Move finger to the right of the angle of Louis to the second right rib.

v. Below the rib is the second ICS.

vi. Move fingers down, palpating the next two ribs. Below the fourth rib and to the right of the sternal body is the fourth ICS. Place electrode in this area.

b. **V₂:** Fourth ICS, left sternal border.

c. **V₃:** Midway between V₂ and V₄, between fourth and fifth ICS.

d. **V₄:** Fifth ICS, left midclavicular line.

e. **V₅:** Fifth ICS, anterior axillary line.

f. **V₆:** Fifth ICS, left midaxillary line.

6. Begin taking the ECG according to manufacturer's directions on machine. ❷

7. Place tracing copy on client's chart. ❸

8. Remove electrodes; perform hand hygiene.

❷ Portable ECG machine for taking 12-lead ECG tracing.

Source: Simon Fraser / Science Source

❶ Electrode placement for chest leads V₁–V₆.

❸ Normal 12-lead ECG.

| **Skill 31.3.4** | ST-Segment Monitoring |

Equipment

12-Lead ECG machine
Electrodes
Cable
Skin Prep

Procedure

1. Check healthcare provider's orders for type of ST-segment monitoring. If the 12-lead ECG is not available, then the lead selected is based on the coronary artery involved in the acute infarction or interventional procedure being performed.
   ➤ *Rationale:* The best ST-segment monitoring is done using the 12 lead, as it provides a global view of the heart.

2. Use the most appropriate leads based on client's needs and risk for ischemia or dysrhythmia if 12-lead monitoring is not available.

   a. Acute coronary syndromes (ACS) with a known "ST fingerprint," obtained during ST-Segment Elevation, myocardial infarction (STEMI), or percutaneous coronary intervention (PCI), use the lead(s) that best display the client's "ST fingerprint" when monitoring. ❶

   i. If the "ST fingerprint" is not known in ACS, use leads III and V₃.

   ii. If the client's diagnosis is not confirmed as ACS, but it is being ruled out, use leads III and V₅.

   iii. In noncardiac clients undergoing surgical procedures or admitted to the ICU, lead V₅ is the best lead to identify demand-related ischemia, which appears to be more common in these clients.

   b. Use the lead selection for ST-segment monitoring if specific coronary artery injury is known.

   i. Circumflex (lateral wall injury): Use lead I, aVL, V₅, or V₆. V₅ is preferred for noncardiac clients undergoing surgery.

   ii. Right coronary (inferior wall): Lead III is preferred, then a VF or II.

(continued)

Skill 31.3.4 | ST-Segment Monitoring *(continued)*

1 ST-segment and J point ECG waveform.

iii. Left anterior descending (anterior wall): Lead V_2 or V_3 preferred, then V_4. V_1 and V_2 are associated with the septal wall. V_3 is preferred for clients with ACS who do not have an ST fingerprint.

3. Introduce yourself and identify client using two forms of identification.
4. Explain the monitoring procedure to the client (Box 31-8 ■).
5. Perform hand hygiene.
6. Connect cable to ECG machine and turn on the machine.
7. Clean skin before applying electrodes to skin. Cleanse skin with alcohol and clip hair where electrodes are placed, if needed. ➤ **Rationale:** This is to rid skin of oil and hair to provide a secure adherence of the electrodes to the skin.
8. Attach lead wires in chest electrodes.
9. Place electrodes in appropriate area of the chest with the adhesive side down. Ensure the electrodes are placed on

Box 31-8 **ST-SEGMENT MONITORING**

This monitoring is used to detect myocardial ischemia, electrode imbalance, and coronary artery reocclusion in clients who have received thrombolytic therapy or interventional cardiology procedures such as atherectomy, stents, or rotablation. It is also used to detect silent ischemia and in evaluating chest pain in clients presenting with atypical pain and nondiagnostic ECGs.

the site for leads being used in ST-segment monitoring. ➤ **Rationale:** Appropriate placement is imperative as just a 1 cm (⅜ in.) change in the placement of the lead can interfere with the waveform patterns. This is particularly a problem when the precordial leads are not properly positioned.
10. Press edges of electrode pad down on skin. ➤ **Rationale:** This is to secure the electrode to the skin to provide a good ECG waveform.
11. Attach wire into transmitter box.
12. Check the clarity of the waveform transmission.

CLINICAL ALERT
Ischemia can be easily detected by observing the T wave. If it is inverted or the ST segment is depressed, it indicates ischemia has occurred. The ST segment depression is often seen in combination with a sharp angle at the junction of the ST segment and the T wave.

Evaluate ST segment with the client in the supine position, set the ST alarm parameter 1–2 mm above and below the client's baseline ST segment, and measure ST segment changes 60 ms beyond the J point of the ECG complex. ST depression or elevation of 1–2 mm that lasts for at least 1 min can be clinically significant, and further assessment is necessary.

Unit 31.3 Documentation and Evaluation

DOCUMENTATION for ECG Monitoring

- 12-lead ECG taken
- Telemetry initiated
  - ST-segment monitoring initiated and monitoring leads used
  - Findings based on the interpretation of the ECG strip
- Nursing interventions carried out, based on the ECG findings
- Rhythm strips entered into client's record at least once each shift

- Telemetry strip documentation:
  - Lead monitored
- Interpretation of ECG strip to include:
  - Rate
  - Rhythm
  - PR interval
  - QRS complex
  - Q-T interval

- Document a telemetry strip for:
  - Any change in client condition
  - Client symptoms during procedures as appropriate
  - Administration of medications as appropriate (i.e., lidocaine)

- Health teaching completed
- Healthcare provider notification of abnormal findings

EVALUATION/Critical Thinking

Expected Outcomes

- ECG leads applied appropriately and without difficulty.
- Abnormal ECG findings interpreted accurately.
- Heart rate calculated correctly.
- Monitor wave forms are distinct and readable.

Unexpected Outcomes	Alternative Actions
For ECG Interpretation	
• ECG is not clearly displayed on monitor.	• Ensure that electrodes are applied in correct position and are securely attached. • Observe for electrical interference resulting in a 60-cycle interference on oscilloscope. • Observe for excessive client activity resulting in artifact display on oscilloscope.
• Electrodes do not adhere to skin and interference appears on oscilloscope.	• Recleanse skin thoroughly using skin prep or alcohol and allow to dry.
• Alarms ring without change in pattern.	• Check HIGH and LOW parameters. They may need to be changed. • Check GAIN. It may be too low to sense pattern.
• ECG pattern is abnormal.	• If client is asymptomatic, recheck lead placement and ensure cables are attached properly. • Check if pattern is a life-threatening arrhythmia (for ventricular tachycardia, call rapid response team (RRT); for ventricular fibrillation, call code). • If PVCs are increasing—notify RRT. • Notify healthcare provider immediately.
• Electrical interference appears on monitor.	• Check all other electric equipment in the immediate environment. • Check for proper grounding of monitor. • Change electrodes and cable; poor conduction may cause 60-cycle interference. • Check that monitor is calibrated.
• Electrodes cause skin irritation.	• Remove electrodes, cleanse site, and reapply electrodes on new site.
• Chaotic rhythm appears on monitor.	• Assess client's vital signs and level of consciousness. • Check electrode contact on skin, and ensure that wires are in contact with cable.

(continued)

Unexpected Outcomes	Alternative Actions
• High or low alarms on monitor continue to sound.	• Check for loose electrodes or try a different lead. • Observe activity level of client. • Check that alarm parameters on monitor are not set too close to client's pulse. • Check client's position. • Reposition electrodes, avoiding large muscle masses or bone.
• Electrodes conduct poorly on diaphoretic client.	• Clean skin sites as usual; apply benzoin to the skin and let dry and apply electrodes. • Clean skin sites as usual; apply spray deodorant to the skin, allow skin to dry, and apply electrodes.
• Asystole displays on monitor.	• Check client's LOC and electrodes, wires, and cable connection. • If the client has an arterial line, check for an arterial waveform in the absence of an ECG waveform.

For Telemetry

• ECG only provides partial information on heart activity.	• Obtain 12-lead ECG. It portrays activity in all areas of heart except posterior aspect—monitor different lead (e.g., MCL).
• Client experiences life-threatening arrhythmia.	• Begin treatment for arrhythmia. Notify RRT. Obtain 12-lead ECG when client is stable.
• Telemetry signal not picked up at base station.	• Check that client has not wandered to an area where transmission is not available. • Check that transmitter battery is functioning. • Check that transmitter is ON. • Change wires. • The usual cause is a dry electrode. Replace electrodes.

For 12-Lead ECG

• Interference apparent on ECG tracing.	• Ensure that lead wires are hanging in same direction on corresponding extremities. • Assess chest to determine whether chest dressing is interfering with ECG electrode placement or signal. • Breast tissue may be interfering with ECG signal. Reapply electrodes under the breast as close to the heart as possible. • Instruct client to remain still.

Unit 31.4
Emergency Life Support Measures

Nursing Process Data

ASSESSMENT Database

- Assess client for signs of cardiac or respiratory arrest (responsiveness, breathing, circulation, and so on).
- Know emergency number to summon help and identify location of AED.
- Identify location of emergency cart.
- Identify procedure for activation of RRT.

PLANNING Objectives

- To provide adequate oxygenation of lungs through mechanical support
- To support ventilation and circulation
- To reestablish a patent airway for client with foreign body airway obstruction

IMPLEMENTATION Procedures

DOCUMENTATION AND EVALUATION

Expected Outcomes

- Basic life-support measures established within 3 min after arrest.
- Emergency measures performed according to established protocol.
- Client is stabilized or resuscitated with basic life-support measures.
- No permanent neurologic damage is sustained.
- Obstructed airway is reestablished.

Unexpected Outcomes/Alternative Actions

Pearson Nursing Student Resources

Find additional review materials at
nursing.pearsonhighered.com.
Prepare for success with NCLEX®-style practice questions and Skill Checklists.

Skill 31.4.1 | Administering Basic Life Support to an Adult or Child

Equipment
Cardiac board
AED
CPR mask or Ambu bag (Box 31-9 ■)

Procedure
Unresponsiveness
1. Quickly approach client.
2. Check responsiveness. Tap shoulders. Shout, "Are you OK?"
   ➤ *Rationale:* This is to determine responsiveness of client. ❶

> **CLINICAL ALERT**
> Institute CPR within 3 min. Cardiopulmonary resuscitation is usually not effective in preventing brain damage unless initiated within 4 min of an arrest.

3. Call out or phone for help. Get AED. ❷
4. Move victim to flat, firm surface and position yourself next to victim, left side near head of victim. ❸ ➤ *Rationale:* Left side is preferred when using AED. A firm surface enhances effective compression between chest wall and sternum.

❶ Check for response: Tap victim, and speak loudly and clearly.

❷ Call for help and retrieve AED before starting CPR.

Box 31-9 **HANDS-ONLY CPR**
The American Heart Association has a new campaign—Two Steps to Staying Alive with Hands-Only CPR.
Step 1 Call 911
Step 2 Push hard and fast at the center of the chest (100 beats/min)
AHA is no longer recommending rescue breathing for anyone performing CPR outside of the hospital until EMS first responders arrive. You can find their campaign information at the American Heart Association website.

5. Place heel of hand in middle of chest. Place other hand on top of first with fingers interlaced.
6. Start chest compressions at 100/min with a depth of 5 cm (2 in.) for adults. ❹

Airway
1. Use head tilt-chin lift (if there is no suspicion of neck injury). ❺
   ➤ *Rationale:* This will safely open the client's airway.
2. Lift chin by placing three fingers under chin. Lift chin up and forward until teeth are nearly closed.

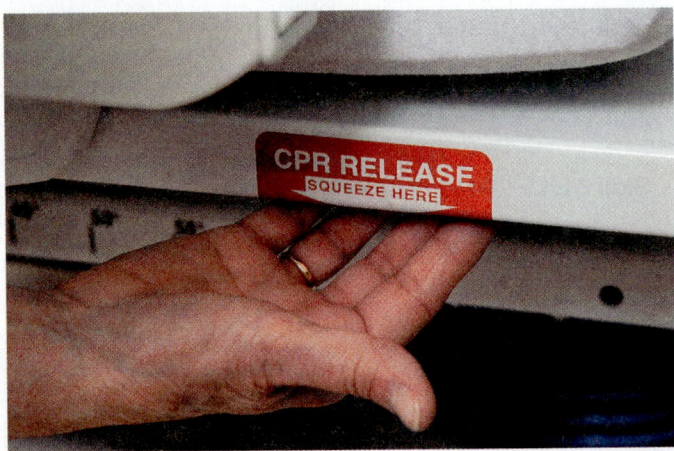

❸ Place bed in flat position for CPR.

❹ Begin compressions at 100–120/min, unless other instructions are provided.

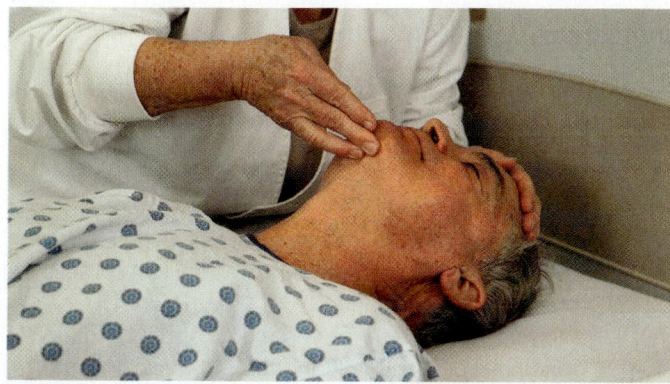

5 Open airway by using head tilt-chin lift method.

6 Reposition head and try ventilation again, if chest does not rise.

7 Ventilate with 2 rescue breaths using bag–valve–mask or CPR mask.

3. Use an airway device such as a CPR mask or Ambu bag.
4. Perform 30 compressions; open airway if trained in CPR. Otherwise, continue chest compressions.
5. Apply AED immediately upon arrival.

Rescue Breathing

1. Evaluate respiratory function:

   a. Check for rise and fall of chest. ➤ *Rationale:* If chest movement occurs but you cannot feel or hear air, then airway is obstructed. **6**

   b. Repeat rescue breath.

2. Repeat 30 compressions and 2 breaths for five cycles. **7**
3. Stop compressions after 2 min and check for breathing. If not breathing, continue compressions and breathing until help arrives or AED is activated.

EVIDENCE-BASED PRACTICE
Chest Compressions for CPR

Chest compressions are the most important aspect of CPR. The chest is able to fully recoil during each compression, thereby lowering intrathoracic pressures. This promotes improved cardiac **preload** and improved filling of the coronary arteries. Interruptions in chest compressions, even if brief, produce a dramatic decline in coronary perfusion pressures and worsen outcomes. It is critical to minimize disruptions to chest compressions and in hospital code situations to change often, so that the individual doing chest compressions does not become too fatigued, and the quality of the compressions is maintained.

Source: Field, et al. (2010)

Skill 31.4.2 | Administering Basic Life Support to an Infant (Under 12 months)

Note: Basic life support guidelines for healthcare providers defines "infant victims" as less than 12 months old, whereas "pediatric victims" are defined as victims from about 1 year of age to the onset of adolescence or puberty, as defined by the presence of secondary sex characteristics.

Procedure

1. Try to wake the infant by gently tapping infant. Small infants respond to rubbing and tapping the soles of their feet.
2. If infant does not wake up, have someone call 911. If no one is available, call 911 and then begin CPR.

3. Begin chest compressions, place two fingers on the breastbone directly between the baby's nipples. Push straight down 3 cm (1–½ in.) and one-third depth of baby's chest.
4. Allow chest to rise back to usual position. Complete 30 compressions, about 2 compressions/sec.
5. Trained CPR rescuers begin rescue breathing. If not trained, continue compressions until help arrives.
6. Airway devices are recommended; however if you chose to do mouth to mouth, then cover the baby's entire mouth and nose with your mouth and gently blow until you see

(continued)

Skill 31.4.2 | Administering Basic Life Support to an Infant (Under 12 months) *(continued)*

the chest rise. Let the air escape and the chest go back to normal. Give a second breath.

7. Continue to give 2 min of CPR; if no help has arrived, call 911 again.

8. Continue CPR until help arrives.

> **CLINICAL ALERT**
>
> AEDs can be now be used in both infants and children. Child pads are calibrated to be used in infants.

Foreign Body

1. If foreign body or aspiration is suspected:

   a. *Infant:* Clear airway by administering back and chest thrusts.

   b. *Conscious Infant*

      i. Position infant over your forearm, head lower than trunk. Support the head by holding it firmly while resting your arm on your thigh.

      ii. With free hand, deliver five sharp blows to infant's back, over spine and between shoulder blades. If object is not expelled, then:

   iii. Turn infant as a unit to supine position, maintaining head support. Deliver five chest thrusts by placing two fingers over sternum and providing thrusts.

   c. Unconscious Infant

      i. Attempt to ventilate. If unable, reposition head and try again. Lift chin. ➤ *Rationale:* Trachea can collapse if neck is hyperextended.

      ii. Form tight seal by encircling mouth of child and mouth and nose of infant. ➤ *Rationale:* Maintain tight seal.

      iii. If unable to ventilate, commence CPR.

2. Administer 2 breaths.

   a. Give breaths slowly—1 sec/breath.

   b. Fill cheeks with air and use short puffing breaths for infants. Do not use full breaths for children or infants. ➤ *Rationale:* Small breaths prevent overinflation of the lungs and abdominal distention.

3. Between breaths, release seal for exhalation, and turn your head to side.

4. Administer 1 breath every 3–5 sec.

5. Continue ventilations until infant is intubated or Ambu bag is available.

Skill 31.4.3 | Placing Victim in Recovery Position

Procedure

1. Assess for potential head or neck trauma; if you suspect injury, do not tilt or turn client's head. If no trauma and client has a pulse and is breathing adequately, place in recovery position (see following steps).

2. Straighten victim's legs.

3. Place victim's arm nearest to you at right angles to his or her body with elbow bent and palm upward.

4. Place other arm across chest and place hand near his or her cheek.

5. Grasp victim's far-side thigh above knee; pull thigh up toward his or her body.

6. Roll victim onto his or her side. ❶

7. Ensure upper leg (including knee and hip) is bent at right angles over the lower leg.

8. Use jaw thrust to maintain open airway, place hand under cheek to maintain jaw-thrust, if necessary. (This is hand that was placed near cheek.)

9. Monitor victim closely until transported to facility.

❶ Place client on side to assume recovery position.

Skill 31.4.4 | Providing Bag–Valve–Mask (BVM) Ventilation

Equipment

Manual resuscitator bag with nonrebreathing valve, clear face mask, and reservoir bag

Oxygen source and tubing
Airway adapter or face mask

Preparation

1. Determine that client's breathing is absent or inadequate.
2. Summon an assistant if client is not intubated.
   ➤ *Rationale:* If no artificial airway present, two responders are essential. Assistant holds mask while nurse compresses resuscitator bag.
3. Gather equipment.
4. Place client in supine position.
5. Connect mask, airway adapter to bag, attach reservoir bag if not attached.
6. Connect oxygen tubing and oxygen flowmeter to bag inlet.

Procedure

1. Turn oxygen flowmeter wide open to 15 L/min ("flush") and ensure reservoir bag is filled with oxygen. ➤ *Rationale:* Reservoir bag delivers 90–100% concentration of oxygen at 15 L/min.
2. Standing at client's head, hyperextend client's neck, if no suspected trauma.
3. Clear airway of any secretions or vomitus, and then place apex of mask over client's nose and place base of mask between client's lower lip and chin. ➤ *Rationale:* This reduces incidence of aspiration, improves oxygenation, and provides for tight seal.
4. Using dominant hand, compress central portion of resuscitator bag just until client's chest rises, and then allow exhalation. ❶ ➤ *Rationale:* Overinflation may result in gastric distention.
5. Provide ventilations every 5–6 sec for an apneic adult, noting that client's chest rises and falls with each compression.
6. If client breathes spontaneously, give compressions in synchrony to support ventilation.
7. Observe for possible gastric distention. ➤ *Rationale:* Gastric insufflation may result in regurgitation and aspiration.

❶ Compress central portion of resuscitation bag.

8. If gastric distention is suspected in the unresponsive client, have assistant apply pressure to the cricoid cartilage in the trachea. ➤ *Rationale:* Protect airway from aspiration of client's gastric secretions. Anticipate insertion of naso–oro gastric tube to remove gastric secretions.

CLINICAL ALERT

Cricoid pressure may be used only if the client:

- Is nonresponsive—deeply unconscious (no cough or gag reflex)
- Is not vomiting
- Does not have a cuffed tracheal tube

---

9. Notify healthcare provider or respiratory care practitioner for further client evaluation.

Skill 31.4.5 | Using an Automated External Defibrillator (AED)

Equipment

AED unit

Procedure

1. Place AED near head on left side of victim. ➤ *Rationale:* This placement facilitates easy use of machine by rescuer.
2. Open AED. This automatically turns on power in some devices.
3. Press power button on, if not automatically part of opening AED. Sound alerts, lights, and voice prompts will tell you that power is on and will direct you in use of the AED.
4. Remove victim's clothing on torso.
5. Ensure chest is dry. ➤ *Rationale:* This ensures electrode pads will stick to chest.
6. Open package of adhesive electrode pads. Most defibrillation electrode pads are preconnected to cables.
   ❶ If pads are dry, then discard and obtain new adhesive electrode pads. ➤ *Rationale:* Dry pads will prevent accurate rhythm analysis and conduction.

❶ After setting up the AED unit, remove backing and apply pads to victim's chest.

(continued)

Skill 31.4.5 | Using an Automated External Defibrillator (AED) *(continued)*

7. Peel off protective plastic backing from pads to expose adhesive surface.

8. Place two adhesive electrode pads directly on chest skin following pictures on pads. ❷

   a. First pad goes on upper right side of victim's chest, with top edge touching bottom of clavicle.

   b. Second pad (marked with a ♥) goes to outside of left nipple, with top margin of pad at anterior axillary line, or may be placed posteriorly between the two scapulas.

   c. Do not place pads directly over nitroglycerin patches.

   d. Do not place pads within 2.5 cm (1 in.) of implanted devices such as pacemakers or ICDs. If ICD is in process of delivering a shock and the rescuer is in contact with the client, he or she will feel the shock. Wait for 30–60 sec for device to complete the shock cycle.

   ➤ *Rationale:* ICDs are designed to shock the client's lethal rhythm back into their normal rhythm. If effective, then AED shock may not be required.

9. Stop CPR if CPR is being performed. Instruct everyone to not touch the victim, in order for AED to analyze rhythm. You may need to push ANALYZE button to start the analysis. Some machines begin analyzing rhythm as soon as pads are applied.

10. If analysis indicates and commands a shock, push SHOCK on AED. ❸ (It may automatically charge when the rhythm indicates the need to shock. A voice message will inform everyone to "stay clear.")

Note: A voice prompt will inform you if electrode pads are not securely attached to chest.

11. Give one shock, and then immediately begin CPR for five cycles or 2 minutes. Press ANALYZE button on AED. Repeat this procedure.

12. If victim is not in need of shock, rescuer immediately checks for pulse and begins CPR, beginning with chest compressions (30:2 ventilations).

13. When shockable rhythm is not present, AED will signal *no shock indicated* or *no shock advised*.

14. Check for presence of pulse—if none found, resume CPR.

15. Leave AED electrodes attached to victim's chest and leave AED in ON position.

16. Follow protocol for rescue breathing or CPR as victim's condition warrants.

> **CLINICAL ALERT**
>
> The AutoPulse, an automated, noninvasive cardiac support pump, delivers chest compressions using a "hands-free" approach to restore blood flow faster and at a higher rate than manual resuscitation after a cardiac arrest.
>
> The number of shocks an AED delivers and the energy level for each shock are preset by the manufacturer. Follow the AED voice and visual prompts. The shock sequence is usually completed three times if the client remains in fibrillation.

❷ Apply pads to chest, one below right clavicle, one below and lateral to heart.

❸ If AED indicates need for shock, push SHOCK on AED.

Skill 31.4.6 | Administering the Abdominal Thrust to Adult or Child

Procedure

1. Be familiar with choking signs (Box 31-10 ■):

   a. Ask client if he or she can speak.

   b. Ask client to hold hand on neck if choking. ❶

   ➤ *Rationale:* This is the universal sign for choking.

2. If unable to talk or coughing becomes ineffective, begin abdominal thrusts.

3. Stand behind client. Place your arms around the client's waist.

4. Position hands halfway between xiphoid process and umbilicus. (Identify area by placing thumb near xiphoid and index finger on umbilicus.)

Note: For pregnant or obese client, chest thrusts rather than abdominal thrusts are used.

5. Make a fist with one hand and press thumb side of fist into victim's abdomen above umbilicus. Place other hand over the fist. ❷

6. Press your fist into client's abdomen.

7. Using a rotating motion of the hands, forcefully thrust your hands in an upward direction to assist in expelling the foreign body. (Client will probably fall over your arms.)

8. Repeat measures until foreign body is expelled or the client becomes unconscious.

> **CLINICAL ALERT**
> Foreign bodies may partially block airway but still allow good air movement. When victim remains conscious and can forcefully cough and speak—do nothing!

Box 31-10 **AIRWAY OBSTRUCTION SIGNS**

- Poor air exchange
- Weak, ineffective cough
- Inability to speak
- High-pitched noise with inhalation
- Cyanosis

❷ Position hands to perform abdominal thrust making a fist and placing the other hand on top of it.

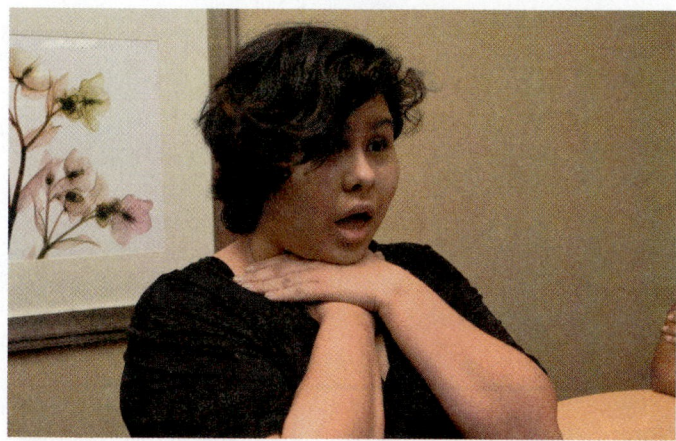

❶ Determine whether client is choking.

Skill 31.4.7 | Administering the Abdominal Thrust for Unresponsive Client

Procedure

Unresponsive Adult

1. Immediately activate EMS system.
2. Begin cardiac compressions at 100–120/min until foreign object is ejected. ❶ ➤ *Rationale:* Chest compressions have been shown to increase intrathoracic pressure higher than abdominal thrusts.
3. Attempt 2 rescue breaths. Check if chest rises.
4. Look in mouth for foreign body each time the airway is opened for rescue breath.
5. Continue compressions and rescue breaths.

Unresponsive Child

1. Activate EMS. Begin cardiac compressions at 100–120/min, continuing for five cycles (2 min) before summoning EMS (unless another rescuer is available to do so immediately).
2. Activate EMS after five cycles, and then return to child to continue CPR until EMS arrives.

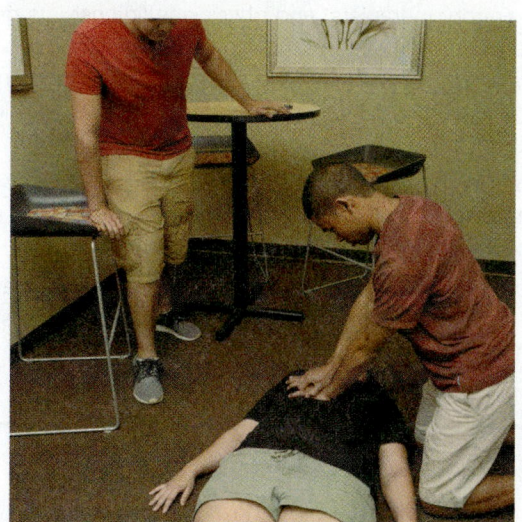

❶ If client is unresponsive, begin CPR.

Skill 31.4.8 | Calling for Rapid Response Support

Preparation

1. Be familiar with facility's RRT policy. ➤ *Rationale:* This team is summoned to assist the bedside nurse in managing a deteriorating client and prevent avoidable deaths. The facility's RRT team may consist of the bedside nurses, ICU nurses, respiratory therapists, and physicians or nurse practitioners (Box 31-11 ■).
2. Identify location of emergency equipment and medications.

Procedure

1. Identify clients at risk for prearrest at the beginning of each shift.
2. Monitor client frequently and closely for signs of a potentially serious complication. ➤ *Rationale:* Most in-hospital arrests are preceded by a change in the client's physiological or mental responses.
3. Establish a flow sheet for more intensive monitoring of client's vital signs, neurological assessment, urinary output, and so on, as indicated.
4. Anticipate need for emergency equipment (e.g., bag–valve–mask, oxygen) and crash cart and place close at hand in case crisis occurs.

5. Check that identified client has established venous access. ➤ *Rationale:* IV access is necessary for infusion of fluids and administration of emergency medications.
6. Recognize deteriorating trends or patterns of signs and symptoms that require resources to stabilize the client (physician and other specialized personnel on RRT) (Box 31-12 ■).
7. Request a more experienced colleague to assist in validation of concerns, if indicated. ➤ *Rationale:* Novice nurses may be uncertain of findings and inexperienced in recognizing a "pattern" of change in clients.
8. Act upon findings and intuition by calling RRT for early intervention to stabilize the client if indicated.
9. Set up O_2 and suction if not already at bedside.
10. RRT takes action: orders blood tests, x-ray, medications, transfers client to intensive care setting, or calls a code if indicated.

Box 31-11 RAPID RESPONSE SYSTEMS

Rapid response systems were developed to improve the recognition of and response to clients who were deteriorating on general care units. The goal was to improve the outcomes of these clients. There are three components of a rapid response system:

1. The afferent limb—the activation criteria (vital sign changes, client condition changes, and so on) and the notification system to activate the RRT.

2. The efferent limb—the team itself. This response team is often called either a RRT or a medical emergency team (MET). It is generally comprised of ICU-trained personnel (nurses and respiratory therapists) and physicians (intensivists or hospitalists are often used). They are either nurse led or physician led. Nurses on the general care units are often the ones who initiate the call to RRTs, but in some agencies families may also call the team.

3. A quality improvement component—this part of the system collects and analyses data, provides feedback, and ensures improvement in performance over time.

The actual benefits of RRTs on overall client outcomes have been mixed in the studies that have been done and further research is ongoing.

Source: Winters, et al. (2013)

EVIDENCE-BASED PRACTICE

Nurse Practitioner–Led RRTs as Effective as Intensivist Led Teams

A study done in two Canadian hospitals found that RRTs led by NPs were just as effective in managing the care of clients during an RRT intervention. The study also found the nurses were very satisfied with the care provided by RRT. Services provided by the RRT most often included monitoring and stabilization of the clients, with 18% requiring transfer to an ICU setting.

Source: Scherr, Wilson, Wagner, & Haughian (2012)

Note: See Skill 33.3.1, Maintaining the Emergency Cart; Skill 33.3.2, Checking Contents of the Emergency Cart; and Skill 33.3.3, Performing Defibrillation.

Box 31-12 WHEN TO ACTIVATE THE RAPID RESPONSE SYSTEM

The RRS, also called the RRT or MET, is initiated when the following conditions are met:

- Heart rate is >140 beats/min or <40/min.
- Systolic blood pressure is >180 mm Hg or <90 mm Hg.
- Respiratory rate is over 28/min or <8/min.
- Oxygenation saturation is <90% despite O_2 supplementation.
- There is an acute change in mental status.
- Urinary output is <50 mL over 4 hr.
- Staff has significant concern about the client's condition.

Source: Ehlenbach, et al. (2009)

Unit 31.4 Documentation and Evaluation

DOCUMENTATION for Emergency Life Support

- Time victim found in prearrest or unresponsive state
- Description of victim when found
- Time emergency measures were initiated
- Nature or description of emergency life-support measures provided (e.g., CPR, use of AED, abdominal thrusts, RRT actions, and medications administered, including name, dosage, and route)
- Names and titles of rescue participants (i.e., RRT)
- Duration of emergency measures provided
- Outcome of prearrest interventions or resuscitation efforts (client outcome)
- Recorded data from AED, monitors used, and strips placed on chart per hospital policy

EVALUATION/Critical Thinking

Expected Outcomes

- Basic life-support measures established within 3 min after arrest.
- Emergency measures performed according to established protocol.
- Client is stabilized or resuscitated with basic life-support measures.
- No permanent neurologic damage is sustained.
- Obstructed airway is reestablished.
- Unresponsive client is rescued by timely intervention (calling EMS, retrieving the AED, and initiating CPR).
- Choking victim expels foreign body in response to abdominal thrusts.
- Client has a positive outcome after emergency life support.

Unexpected Outcomes	Alternative Actions
• Client is revived but maintained on life-support system.	• Assist in transferring client to ICU. Provide support for family and explain where ICU is and visitation policy.
• Attempts at ventilation for rescue breathing are ineffective, chest does not rise, and no air is felt.	• Perform CPR.
• Rescuer cannot continue efforts at what appears to be unsuccessful CPR.	• Stop CPR if exhaustion or endangerment to rescuer.
• AED fails to analyze rhythm after 15 seconds.	• Resume CPR at 100 chest compressions/minute and attempt to analyze rhythm after five cycles or about 2 minutes.
• Pulse does not return after AED shock.	• Resume CPR at 100 chest compressions/min for five cycles or 2 minutes, reanalyze rhythm, check for pulse, and deliver shock if ventricular fibrillation continues.
• There is no response to your EMS call for help (e.g., 911).	• Suspect that your location is not programmed into EMS system. Try local area dial for highway patrol. • Be familiar with your local emergency response system's summoning directives.

(continued)

Unexpected Outcomes	Alternative Actions
• AED prompt says "no shock indicated."	• Immediately resume CPR, starting at 100 chest compressions/min; if CPR trained can start with ventilations, continue for five cycles (2 min) before reanalyzing heart rhythm per AED. • Suspect client has nonshockable rhythm such as pulseless electrical activity (PEA); hypovolemia is most common cause. • Rule out possible causes: hypovolemia, hypoxia, hypothermia, hypoglycemia.
• Choking client becomes unresponsive after several attempts at abdominal thrusts.	• Initiate CPR (30 compressions to 2 ventilations).
• Client is obese or pregnant, making abdominal thrust impossible or inappropriate to perform.	• Perform chest thrusts rather than abdominal thrusts.
• Client develops complications (signs of stroke, heart attack, hypotension, altered mental status, dyspnea, tachycardia).	• Monitor client intensely, using flow chart to trend changes in status (tachypnea, decreased urinary output). • Note client's condition and document findings. • Determine and locate equipment or anticipate procedures client might require if deterioration continues. • Initiate RRT for decision making and early intervention before crisis occurs. • Be cognizant of client's advance directives regarding resuscitation measures.

Nursing Process Data

ASSESSMENT Database

- Assess preexisting cardiovascular status.
- Assess cardiac monitor rhythm and rate.
- Assess heart sounds.
- Observe client's general appearance for pallor, dyspnea, or edema.
- Assess for hemodynamic abnormalities related to low cardiac output, including dizziness, weakness, altered level of consciousness, low blood pressure, and decreased urinary output.
- Ensure intravenous access for administration of fluids and medications.
- Identify client's or family's knowledge of procedure.

PLANNING Objectives

- To provide temporary cardiac electrical stimulation for conditions resulting in alterations of heart rate
- To prevent bradycardia
- To overdrive fast heart rates
- To improve cardiac output

IMPLEMENTATION Procedures

DOCUMENTATION AND EVALUATION

Expected Outcomes

- Client's cardiac rate is maintained through use of a pacemaker.
- Client is prepared psychologically and physically for insertion of the pacemaker.
- Pacemaker is inserted without complications.
- Heart rate and cardiac output improve.

Unexpected Outcomes/Alternative Actions

Pearson Nursing Student Resources

Find additional review materials at
nursing.pearsonhighered.com.
Prepare for success with NCLEX®-style practice questions and Skill Checklists.

Skill 31.5.1 | Monitoring Temporary Cardiac Pacing (Transcutaneous, Transvenous, Epicardial)

Equipment
Cardiac monitor

Transcutaneous: pacing generator, pacing electrodes

Appropriate temporary pulse generator (select for single- or dual-chamber pacing)

Battery for pulse generator (single- or dual-chamber)

Bridging cable for epicardial wires

Clean gloves

Established continuous cardiac monitoring—see Skill 31.3.1, Monitoring Clients on Telemetry

Preparation
1. Validate that informed consent has been obtained for temporary pacing.
2. Introduce self, and identify client by checking two forms of client ID.
3. Explain rationale for temporary pacing and necessary restrictions/precautions, and provide reassurance of close continuous monitoring.
4. Perform a baseline assessment: vital signs, urinary output, LOC, heart rate, rhythm, and skin color. If life-threatening dysrhythmia is assessed, prepare for pacemaker insertion (Box 31-13 ■). ➤ *Rationale:* Transcutaneous pacemakers are used for symptomatic bradycardia unresponsive to atropine or high-degree atrioventricular block causing hemodynamic compromise. If transcutaneous pacing is ineffective, then prepare for transvenous pacemaker insertion.
5. Assess IV site for patency; if no IV, establish line. ➤ *Rationale:* IV access is needed for drug administration.
6. Document client's cardiac rhythm according to hospital policy.
7. Perform hand hygiene.

Procedure

Transcutaneous Pacing (TCP)
1. Sedate client. ➤ *Rationale:* TCP causes discomfort.
2. Clip hair, if necessary. Do not shave under electrode placement. Do not use alcohol or tincture of benzoin because they can cause burns. ➤ *Rationale:* Improve conduction between electrode and skin. Shaving may cause nicks in skin, which may increase discomfort with pacing.

3. Ensure client is on cardiac monitoring with either lead I, II, or III. Lead II is customary as it assesses atrial activity.
4. Connect ECG cable to input connection on pacing generator. ❶
5. Turn switch selector to "Monitor On." ECG waveform will appear.
6. Set alarm, press "Alarm On." Ensure alarm parameters are set 20 beats higher and lower than client's desired rate.
7. Record waveform by pressing "Start/Stop" button.
8. Apply pacing pads as marked, first removing posterior pad covering, and then placing posterior (back) pad left of spine between the scapulas. Place anterior "front" pad to left side of lower sternum.
9. Press firmly on and around pacing electrodes. ➤ *Rationale:* This ensures good skin contact.
10. Attach pacing cable to pace connector on defibrillator/monitor.
11. Select "Pacer" button and green light will appear.
12. Set pacing rate to 60–80 beats/min.
13. Assess cardiac rhythm on oscilloscope and observe the QRS for sensing marker.

❶ Type of external pacemaker.

Box 31-13 REVISED NASPE/BPEG GENERIC CODE FOR ANTIBRADYCARDIA PACING

I	II	III	IV	V
Chamber(s) Paced	**Chamber(s) Sensed**	**Response to Sensing**	**Rate Modulation**	**Multisite Pacing**
0 = None	0 = None	0 = None	0 = None	0 = None
A = Atrium	A = Atrium	T = Triggered	R = Rate modulation	A = Atrium
V = Ventricle	V = Ventricle	I = Inhibited		V = Ventricle
D = Dual (A+V)	D = Dual (A+V)	D = Dual (T+I)		D = Dual (A+V)
S = Single (A or V)	S = Single (A or V)			

Source: Data from Hayes (2009) and Bernstein, et al. (2002)

14. Set milliamperes (mA) threshold initially at 0. ➤ *Rationale:* This prevents pacemaker discharge while setting adjustment.
15. Activate pacing by depressing "Start–Stop" button.
16. Increase mA slowly, increasing it until capture appears.
17. Assess pulse and blood pressure ➤ *Rationale:* These parameters assess for perfusion.
18. Record ECG strip and document pacing parameters.
19. Continually assess client's need for sedation. ➤ *Rationale:* Pacing causes discomfort.

CLINICAL ALERT

Transcutaneous pacing is not beneficial in asystole or PEA. If transcutaneous pacing fails to capture or increase the pulse, then transvenous pacing is required. If defibrillation is required because of ventricular defibrillation, immediately select "Charge" button, as pacing will cease and defibrillation will occur.

CLINICAL ALERT

Transvenous single-chamber (ventricular) pacing is most commonly used as an emergency measure to support ventricular contraction and cardiac output. Epicardial pacing occurs when pacing electrodes are inserted into the epicardium of the right ventricle during cardiac surgery. If the surgeon wants to initiate atrioventricular sequential pacing, then the surgeon places an additional electrode in the right atrium. The pacing wires are then pierced through the chest wall and may be attached to the external pulse generator, which is placed on standby mode should pacing become necessary. If no pacing is indicated at this time, insert the pacing wires in either a sterile rubber glove or a finger cot. Place sterile gauze and occlusive dressing over pacing wires and insertion site to prevent microshock or infection. Epicardial pacing electrodes provide either single-chamber atrial pacing, single-chamber ventricular pacing, or dual-chamber pacing, known as A-V sequential pacing, which is used to simulate normal pump function (atrial followed by ventricular stimulation–contraction).

Epicardial Pacing

1. Don clean gloves. ➤ *Rationale:* Gloves are worn to prevent microshock to client.
2. Locate epicardial pacing wires on client's chest wall.
3. Securely connect pacing wires to external generator. ➤ *Rationale:* This promotes pacemaker impulse reception from and transmission to the myocardium.
4. Connect cable to pulse generator (positive to positive, negative to negative). ➤ *Rationale:* Pacing stimulus goes from pulse generator to the negative terminal and back to pulse generator by the positive terminal.
5. Remove protective cover to dial settings.
6. Select pacing mode (e.g., atrial, ventricular, AV synchronous, or demand).

Transvenous or Epicardial Pacing

1. Set dial at prescribed pacing rate (atrial or ventricular).
2. Set energy *output* (milliamperes or mA) on pulse generator to prescribed level (set for both atrial and ventricular pacing). ➤ *Rationale:* Energy output setting ensures that pacemaker stimulates the client's myocardium.
3. Return plastic cover to protect generator dial settings and hang generator from pole at client's bedside.
4. Monitor pacemaker function for *sensing* (light indicates client's QRS complexes), *capture* (pacemaker spike is followed by QRS complex), and pacemaker *rate*.
5. Monitor client's heart rhythm, vital signs, and other responses to pacing, including femoral pulsation palpable with captured beats. ➤ *Rationale:* These demonstrate effectiveness of pacemaker support.
6. Remove gloves and perform hand hygiene.
7. Evaluate electrode insertion and exit sites and dress according to agency protocol.

Skill 31.5.2 | Assisting With Pacemaker Insertion

Equipment

Emergency cart with defibrillator
External pacemaker pulse generator
Pacing catheter electrodes
ECG monitor
Client cable
Rubber glove
Sterile antiseptic solution
Sterile gloves, gown, and mask
Sterile towels
Lidocaine, 1–2%
Alcohol wipes
Syringe
Needles
Suture with attached needle
Sterile 4×4 gauze pads
Tape
Cutdown tray
Gloves

Preparation

1. Introduce self. Identify client with two IDs. Complete hand hygiene.
2. Provide sedation as necessary. Conscious sedation may be used.
3. Connect client to a continuous ECG monitor.

(continued)

Skill 31.5.2 | Assisting With Pacemaker Insertion *(continued)*

4. Place the client in the appropriate position for central line insertion and provide appropriate sterile draping.
5. If either the subclavian or external jugular vein is to be used, place a towel roll under the client's shoulders to provide better exposure of the insertion site.

Procedure

1. Assist physician as needed.

   a. Physician dons mask, sterile gown, and gloves.
   b. Insertion site is cleansed with sterile antiseptic solution.
   c. Drape area with sterile towels.
   d. Break single-dose vial of lidocaine and hold at angle for physician withdrawal.
   e. Physician withdraws lidocaine, using filtered needle, then changes to 25-gauge needle and injects skin.
   f. Insertion is accomplished (transvenous method via cutdown or percutaneously). Catheter electrode wires are positioned, and skin sutures are applied.

2. Continuously monitor the ECG and client status during the insertion.
3. Don gloves to prevent microshock to client.
4. Connect the pacing electrode to the appropriate outlet terminal (unipolar to negative and bipolar to both the positive and negative terminals).
5. Turn on power switch on external pacemaker.
6. Set rate according to physician's orders.
7. Set mA by determining threshold. To do this, observe the ECG while slowly increasing the number of milliamperes from its lowest setting to a point where each QRS complex is captured and preceded with a pacing spike.

8. Multiply the threshold level according to hospital policy (usually two to four times) to adjust the milliampere setting.
9. Set sensitivity mode according to physician's order (usually 1.5 mV).
10. Secure all connections. Put plastic cover back over pacemaker controls if required.
11. Place external pacemaker and exposed wires in a rubber glove to ensure insulation against electric shock to client.
12. Apply sterile dressings to insertion site, and tape securely.
13. Obtain chest x-ray after insertion to validate lead placement if pacemaker not inserted using fluoroscopy.
14. Obtain 12-lead ECG.

> **SAFETY ALERT**
> **Electrical Safety**
>
> - Use only grounded equipment; use common ground.
> - Remove and tag any defective equipment.
> - Maintain environmental humidity at 50–60%.
> - Do not roll equipment over electrical cords.
> - Avoid placing wet articles on electrical equipment.
> - Insulate exposed pacing electrodes at all times.
> - Wear rubber gloves when handling pacing electrodes or terminals.
> - Do not touch any electric equipment while handling wire or terminals.
> - Discharge static electricity by touching faucets or other metal that communicates with ground.
> - When temporary transvenous pacemakers are used, the balloon air port is *not* to be used for IV access.

Skill 31.5.3 | Maintaining Temporary Pacemaker Function

Equipment ❶ ❷
Battery
Oscilloscope

❶ Temporary pacemakers have two parts, the pulse generator and the electrode. The pulse generator is external to the body. (A) Epicardial ventricular pacemaker. (B) Transvenous ventricular pacemaker.

❷ Equipment for external monitoring includes belts, gel, and transducers.

Procedure

1. Perform hand hygiene. Introduce self and identify client with two identifiers.
2. Observe for failure to sense.
   a. Observe the oscilloscope for presence of pacemaker artifact (spikes): artifact before QRS complex in ventricular paced or preceding the P waves and QRS waves in AV sequential pacing. ❸ ❹
   b. Check connections for secure, tight fit.
   c. Observe that pace–sense needle deflects to right, indicating pacing is occurring.
   d. Check sensitivity dial to determine whether sensitivity threshold is set correctly.
3. Observe for failure to pace.
   a. Check that external generator is ON.
   b. Check battery to ensure it is functioning.
   c. Check lead connector sites.
   d. Check pace–sense indicator. (Absence of or slight deflection of the pace–sense indicator reveals battery failure.)

❸ ECG tracing showing pacemaker spike triggering ventricular depolarization (QRS).

❹ ECG showing examples of pacemaker spikes.

4. Observe for failure to capture.
   a. Observe for pacing artifact not followed by QRS complex. ➤ **Rationale:** This indicates a failure of the stimulus to trigger a ventricular response.
   b. Check the setting of the mA, or output dial, to determine whether setting should be increased. ➤ **Rationale:** The myocardial threshold may be altered as a result of disease or drugs.
   c. Check all connector sites for secure, tight fit.
5. Observe that sutures are intact.
6. Assess insertion site for bleeding, hematoma formation, or infection.
7. Obtain chest x-ray post insertion.
8. Monitor client's response to therapy.
   a. Assess urine output. ➤ **Rationale:** Decreased urine output indicates poor cardiac output.
   b. Observe for dyspnea, crackles, heart rate, or decreased blood pressure.
   c. Monitor temperature.
   d. Observe client for signs of anxiety. Complete pacemaker teaching as necessary.

CLINICAL ALERT

Observe for indications of pacemaker failure:

   Decreased urine output
   ECG pattern change
   Decreased blood pressure
   Bradycardia
   Shortness of breath

---

9. Obtain and analyze a strip for functioning of pacemaker.
10. Observe for battery failure.
11. Observe for electrical interference and development of microshocks.
    a. Ground all electrical equipment in close proximity to client.
    b. Cover exposed wires with nonconductive material.
    c. Wear gloves when handling generator and lead wires.
12. Complete pacemaker teaching as necessary.

Skill 31.5.4   Providing Permanent Pacemaker Client Teaching

Equipment

Audiovisual aids
Written material

Procedure

1. Perform hand hygiene.
2. Introduce self and identify client using two forms of identification.
3. Ascertain what client already knows and understands.
4. Determine client's ability and level of interest in learning about pacemaker.
5. Recognize client's fears, and provide opportunity to talk about them.
6. Review facts: heart anatomy and physiology and pacemaker information. Use illustrations and audiovisual aids.
7. Clarify misconceptions and allay fears.
8. Provide rationale for any mobility restrictions.

(continued)

Skill 31.5.4 | Providing Permanent Pacemaker Client Teaching *(continued)*

9. Answer questions and provide additional opportunities to discuss procedure.
10. Check pacemaker function regularly per instructions. With new pacemakers, healthcare providers check them on routine visits.
11. Instruct client in clinical manifestations related to pacemaker failure and when to contact healthcare provider or pacemaker clinic (Box 31-14 ■).
12. Provide client with pacemaker information ID card (provided by manufacturer) and instruct to carry in wallet.
13. Suggest that a Medical Alert band be worn at all times.

Note: Inform client of electromagnetic interference restrictions:

a. No MRI; do not place cell phone or cardiovert over generator.
b. If dizziness is experienced, move away from area.

Box 31-14 **PACEMAKER CLINICS**

Some clients use telephone transmission of the generator's pulse rate to determine status of pacemaker function. Special equipment is used to transmit information concerning function of the pacemaker over the telephone to a receiving system in a pacemaker clinic. The equipment converts information to electronic signals that are permanently recorded on ECG strip. Physicians monitor client's records and can intervene quickly when abnormalities appear on ECG strip. This type of clinic is very common in outlying areas where clients are unable to go to a clinic easily.

Unit 31.5 Documentation and Evaluation

DOCUMENTATION for Pacemaker Management

- Date and time of temporary pacing
- Pacemaker settings (rate, outputs, sensitivity, AV interval)
- Client's response to treatment
- Vital signs, heart rhythm
- Rhythm strips of pacing obtained during insertion

EVALUATION/Critical Thinking

Expected Outcomes

- Client's cardiac rate is maintained through use of a pacemaker.
- Client is prepared psychologically and physically for insertion of the pacemaker.
- Pacemaker is inserted without complications.
- Heart rate and cardiac output improve.

Unexpected Outcomes

- Temporary pacing is ineffective.

Alternative Actions

- Check for battery depletion and change if necessary (9-V batteries).
- Record rhythm strip and correlate to client's signs and symptoms.
- Monitor vital signs, mental status.
- Check sensitivity setting. (If too high, P or T wave may be sensed; if too low, fixed-rate pacing occurs.)
- Check mA setting (may be too high).
- Check pace indicator for movement.
- Check rate setting.
- Check all connections.
- Check catheter insertion site for swelling, hematoma.

Unexpected Outcomes	Alternative Actions
• Client does not understand function of pacemaker.	• If client is frightened, reassure him or her that a pacemaker is not dangerous. • If client does not understand pacemaker or procedure, use illustrated learning aids. • Allow time for questions and further explanations. • Orient your teaching to the client's intellectual and interest level.
• Electromagnetic interference occurs.	• Check all electric equipment for proper grounding. Use common ground. • Remove unnecessary electric equipment from vicinity of client. • Insulate generator terminals and exposed electrodes in a rubber glove.
• Inflammation occurs at insertion site.	• Provide daily site care using strict aseptic technique. • Keep dressings dry at all times. • Monitor vital signs. • Instruct client to limit extremity movement.
• Diaphragmatic pacing occurs.	• Observe for hiccoughs or muscle twitching. • Change client's position. • Decrease the amperage (mA). • Notify healthcare provider that endocardial perforation may have occurred.
• Failure to capture is suspected.	• Check client's heart rate. If heart rate less than the rate set on generator, and if pace indicator shows firing, suspect failure to capture. • Check all connections. • Anticipate that pacer wires are dislodged. • Check battery. • Change position of extremity. • Turn client on left side; catheter may float back to epicardial wall. • Increase amperage (mA) after checking threshold. • Obtain chest x-ray and 12-lead ECG. • Anticipate change of batteries, electrode terminals, or generator.
• Battery depletion occurs.	• Have atropine and isoproterenol available. • Anticipate possible CPR. • Turn on power switch, and observe pace indicator. If there is little or no movement, replace battery immediately. • Record clock hours of battery usage. (Record should be taped to back of generator.) • Determine rate fluctuations. • Label each pacemaker with the date battery is inserted. • Store extra batteries in refrigerator and put new battery in pacemaker before use. • Disconnect catheter from pacemaker before replacing battery. Contact with battery terminal may be dangerous to the client.

Chapter Wrap-Up

GERONTOLOGIC Considerations

Stressful Physical and Emotional Conditions May Have an Especially Adverse Effect on the Older Adult Client

- The heart may be unable to respond to these changes with an adequate increase in rate, which could precipitate heart failure.
- Changes in the heart lead to decreased myocardial contractility, increased left ventricular ejection time, and delayed conduction, which plays a role in this phenomenon.

Cardiac Output Is Decreased as a Result of Tachycardia or Atrial Fibrillation, Which Is Evidenced on the ECG

- Tachycardia causes a shortened ventricular filling time.
- Atrial fibrillation causes the loss of the atrial kick (blood volume delivered to the ventricle as a result of a coordinated atrial contraction).

ECG May Be Abnormal Due to a Chronic Disease Such as Heart Failure

- Assess client for behavioral changes, changes in level of consciousness, palpitations, dyspnea, fatigue, and falls. These are indicators of a dysrhythmic heart.
- Dysrhythmias, such as PVCs and premature atrial contractions (PACs), may be very common and not cause for alarm unless they change in number or configuration.
- Pacemaker spikes are evident on ECGs for clients with pacemakers.

Geriatric Changes in Cardiovascular System

- Exercise— ↓ cardiac response.
- Cardiac valves—thicker and stiffer.
- Sinoatrial node— ↓ of pacemaker cells;
- Sympathetic nervous system:
  ↓ response to physical stress
  ↓ response to emotional stress
  Less sensitive to β-adrenergic agonist drugs
- Arterial blood vessels—thicker, ↓ elasticity = ↑ BP.
- Hypertension should NOT be considered a normal consequence of aging.

Client Requiring CPR Has Dentures in Place

- Keep dentures in place to provide for good seal around mouth.
- Bag-valve breathing is more effective when tight seal around mouth is maintained.

Peripheral Vascular Assessment Is Essential When an Older Client Is Using Elastic Hosiery or Sequential Stockings

- Older adult clients may very well have altered peripheral circulation before this treatment is started.
- Stockings that are too tight can interfere with the already compromised vascular blood flow, leading to ulceration of the lower extremity.
- Check color, warmth, capillary refill, and presence of pedal pulses every 4 hr when client is using these devices.

MANAGEMENT Guidelines

Each state legislates a Nurse Practice Act for RNs and LVN/LPNs. Healthcare facilities are responsible for establishing and implementing policies and procedures that conform to their state's regulations. Verify the regulations and role parameters for each healthcare worker in your facility.

Delegation

- All healthcare workers are trained in basic cardiac life support or CPR and Heimlich maneuver; therefore, anyone can initiate CPR or perform the Heimlich maneuver.
- CPR training renewal is provided frequently in the healthcare facility to ensure all employees stay current in the skill.
- RN staff assigned to the critical care units, emergency department, and operating room may also be certified in

advanced cardiac life support (ACLS). These staff members can be delegated as members of the Code Team in the facility. The operating room staff does not respond to codes outside the operating room.
- RN staff may be assigned to a RRT for the hospital.
- It is not the usual protocol that LVN/LPNs are assigned to the critical care unit. If they do have responsibility for client care in these settings, additional education regarding ECG monitoring must be provided.
- All healthcare workers assigned to the team can measure and apply elastic hosiery.
- Ancillary staff members may have additional training in monitoring ECGs (monitoring technicians) and in taking a 12-lead ECG (ECG technician). These individuals can be delegated to perform these tasks.

Interprofessional Communication

- If the RN is not directly involved in monitoring the ECG, it is imperative that the technician have specific parameters for reporting the findings. These parameters must be defined during the staff report at the beginning of each shift.
- For clients on telemetry, it is critical that the staff nurse assigned to care for the client on the nursing unit be apprised of any unusual ECG findings. The telemetry nurse must place an ECG tracing on the client's chart according to hospital policy.
- During a code, the nurse caring for the client should be relieved from performing CPR duties to answer questions, obtain information, and assist others in the code team to perform the necessary skills to promote a positive outcome of the event.
- During shift report, ensure that the oncoming shift is apprised of any client who is at risk for developing cardiac complications or is considered a potential "code."
- Orders for a code or no-code status should be addressed so that all staff are aware of the client's status. The code cart should be placed near the client's room if the code is imminent.
- Call the RRT if client is decompensating.
- Copy of advance directives should be placed in client chart.

CASE STUDY Applications

Scenario 1

You work day shift in the transitional care unit (TCU) and have been assigned two clients who require total care. Each client is on a cardiac monitor.

Client 1: A 65-year-old male in heart failure, responding well to drug therapy of furosemide (Lasix) and digoxin. His lungs are clear, and he has lost 5 lb since yesterday.
Client 2: A 70-year-old female with a MI 2 days ago. She is considered unstable and is receiving close monitoring.

1. What is your first nursing action of the morning?
2. What alterations will you expect in the assessment of Client 2? Provide rationale for your answer.
3. Which client will you attend to first? Provide rationale.
4. Complete the interpretation of the ECG for Client 1.
5. Determine the following:
   a. HR
   b. Regularity of rhythm
   c. PR interval
   d. QRS duration
6. Identify the rhythm based on the information in question 5.
7. Is this a life-threatening arrhythmia?
8. What is your priority intervention?
9. Identify the rhythm strip for Client 2.
10. What are implications for the condition of this client?
11. Identify why this client may have this type of ECG reading.

12. Identify the most effective drug treatment for this arrhythmia and provide the pharmacologic action to support your answer.
13. Identify the possible side effects of the drug and the clinical manifestations you will be monitoring in your assessment.
14. As you are preparing to provide hygienic care to Client 2, you look at the monitor and see the following ECG findings.
    a. What rhythm is depicted on the above strip?
    b. Describe what is happening to the client in this rhythm.
    c. What priority intervention should be done?
    d. What is the second intervention if the priority intervention is not effective?

Scenario 2

During nursing report the nurse indicates she is very concerned about a client who has been unstable all night. You decide to check that client first on your rounds.

1. What is the initial client assessment you will make when you enter the room?
2. Is this a client who might be a candidate for the RRT? Provide rationale for your answer.
3. Describe the function of the RRT.
4. What role does the RN taking care of the client assume on the RRT?

NCLEX® Review Questions

Unless otherwise specified, choose only one (1) answer.

1. The client you are caring for is placed on telemetry. As you assess the ECG findings, what do you remember the QRS complex represents?
   A. Atrial depolarization
   B. The time it takes for atrial depolarization
   C. Depolarization of the ventricles
   D. Ventricular repolarization

2. An atrial arrhythmia results from a disturbance where?
   A. With an SA node
   B. In the AV node
   C. In the Purkinje fibers
   D. In the bundle of His

3. For which one of the following cardiac needs is a demand pacemaker used?
    A. To alter the rate of discharge according to changes in activity and rest
    B. To discharge a steady electrical impulse at a certain rate regardless of the underlying HR
    C. To discharge an electrical impulse only when the HR falls below a programmable HR
    D. To discharge an electrical impulse only when a ventricular dysrhythmia occurs

4. The morning report indicates the client you are assigned to care for is at risk for hemorrhage. When assessing the client, which one of the following symptoms would *not* lead you to suspect a hemorrhage is occurring?
    A. Urine output of 30–40 mL/hr for the last 4 hr
    B. Diastolic pressure of 90 mm Hg for the last 2 hr
    C. Respirations of 18–20 and shallow
    D. Clammy skin and central cyanosis

5. As you go by a client's room, the client's son comes running out and says, "My dad isn't breathing!" You go quickly to the bedside and determine he needs CPR. What is your first step?
    A. Activate the emergency response or code team
    B. Administer 30 chest compressions and 2 breaths
    C. Defibrillate the client with the AED
    D. Check for breathing by opening the mouth and listening for breaths

6. The preoperative client has an order for thigh-high graduated compression stockings before surgery. Your first action is to measure the client for the correct hosiery size. How will you measure?
    A. By first checking the circumference of the largest area of the calf
    B. By measuring from the Achilles tendon to the popliteal fold

    C. By measuring from the gluteal fold to bottom of the heel
    D. By checking the distance between one handbreadth above the knee to the ankle

7. Which of the following conditions are contraindications to the use of SCDs?
    Select all that apply.
    A. Heart failure
    B. Dermatitis
    C. Conditions that increase venous return to the heart
    D. Pulmonary embolism
    E. Pressure ulcer

8. While making a home visit, you find a client who seems to be choking on food. What is your initial response in this emergency?
    A. Perform an abdominal thrust.
    B. Begin CPR at the rate of 30 compressions and 2 breaths.
    C. Ask the client if he can speak.
    D. Strike the client on the back.

9. What does the nurse know when using a bag valve mask?
    A. Rescue breathing is more effective when a tight seal around the mouth is maintained.
    B. The flowmeter is turned to 6 L/min.
    C. A backboard is placed under the client.
    D. Cricoid pressure is used as needed to obtain good chest rise.

10. In which circumstance is an RRT called?
    Select all that apply.
    A. HR great than 140 beats/min or less than 40 beats/min
    B. Urine output less than 30 mL/hr over 4 hr
    C. RR greater than 28/min or less than 8/min
    D. Oxygen saturation less than 90%
    E. Acute change in mental status

QSEN Activity

Domain: Teamwork; Respect the centrality of the client and family as core members of any healthcare team.

KSA: Attitude

Activity:

Get together in groups and discuss the pros and cons of having family be present at the bedside during code situations.

Get together in groups and discuss the pros and cons of having family members initiate a call to the RRTs.

Bibliography

American Heart Association. (2015). Advanced cardiac life support—classroom. Retrieved from http://www.heart.org/HEARTORG/CPRAndECC/HealthcareProviders/AdvancedCardiovascularLifeSupportACLS/Advanced-Cardiovascular-Life-Support—Classroom_UCM_306643_Article.jsp

American Heart Association. (2010). Basic life support. Retrieved from http://www.heart.org/HEARTORG/CPRAndECC/HealthcareProviders/BasicLifeSupportBLS/Basic-Life-Support-BLS_UCM_001281_SubHomePage.jsp

American Heart Association. (n.d.) CPR in schools. Retrieved from www.heart.org/cprinschools

Berg, R. A., Hemphill, R., Abella, B. S., Aufderheide, T. P., Cave, D. M., Hazinski, M. F., . . . & Swor, R. A. (2010). Part 5: Adult basic life support 2010: American Heart Association guidelines for cardiopulmonary resuscitation and emergency cardiovascular care. *Circulation, 122*(18 suppl 3), S685–S705.

Berg, M. D., Schexnayder, S. M., Chameides, L., Terry, M., Donoghue, A., Hickey, R. W., … & Hazinski, M. F. (2010). Pediatric basic life support: 2010 American Heart Association guidelines for cardiopulmonary resuscitation and emergency cardiovascular care. *Pediatrics, 126*(5), e1345–e1360.

Bernstein, A. D., Daubert, J. C., Fletcher, R. D., Hayes, D. L., Lüderitz, B., Reynolds, D. W., . . . & Sutton R. (2002). The revised NASPE/BPEG generic code for antibradycardia, adaptive-rate, and multisite pacing. *Pacing and Clinical Electrophysiology, 25*(2), 260–264.

Centers for Disease Control. (2014). Deep vein thrombosis (DVT)/pulmonary embolism (PE)—blood clot forming in a vein. Retrieved from http://www.cdc.gov/ncbddd/dvt/data.html

Ehlenbach, W. J., Barnato, A. E., Curtis, J. R., Kreuter, W., Koepsell, T. D., Deyo, R. A., & Stapleton, R. D. (2009). Epidemiologic study of in-hospital cardiopulmonary resuscitation in the elderly. *New England Journal of Medicine, 361*(1), 22–31.

Field, J. M., Hazinski, M. F., Sayre, M. R., Chameides, L., Schexnayder, S. M., Hemphill, R., . . . & Hoek, T. L. V. (2010). Part 1: Executive summary: 2010 American Heart Association guidelines for cardiopulmonary resuscitation and emergency cardiovascular care. *Circulation, 122*(18 suppl 3), S640–S656.

Francis, C. W. (2007). Prophylaxis for thromboembolism in hospitalized medical patients. *New England Journal of Medicine, 356*(14), 1438–1444.

Halm, M. A. (2012) Trendelenburg position: Put to bed or angled toward use in your unit. *American Journal of Critical Care, 21*, 449–452.

Hayes, D. L. (2009, Jul. 19). Modes of cardiac pacing: Nomenclature and selection. Retrieved from http://www.uptodate.com/online/content/topic.do?topicKey=carrhyth/26065&view=print.htm

Institute for Healthcare Improvement. (2009, Jul. 15). Establish a rapid response team. Retrieved from http:ihi.org/IHI/Topics/CriticalCare/IntensiveCare/Changes/EstablishaRapidResponseTeam.htm

Kim, H. & Lee, E. S. (2015). Major difficulties and information needs recognised by nurses in applying graduated compression stocking and intermittent pneumatic compression for deep vein thrombosis prophylaxis. *Journal of clinical nursing, 24*(1–2), 308–311.

National Heart, Lung, and Blood Institute, NIH. (2011). How to use an automated external defibrillator. Retrieved from http://www.nhlbi.nih.gov/health/health-topics/topics/aed/howtouse

Neumar, R. W., Shuster, M., Callaway, C. W., Gent, L. M., Atkins, D. L., Bhanji, F., . . . Hazinski, M. F. 2015 American Heart Association guidelines update for cardiopulmonary resuscitation and emergency cardiovascular care. Part 1: Executive summary. *Circulation, 132*: 132:S315-S367; doi:10.1161/CIR.0000000000000252

Pozner, C. N. (2015). Advanced cardiac life support (ACLS) in adults. Retrieved from http://www.uptodate.com/contents/advanced-cardiac-life-support-acls-in-adults

Reuter, D. A., Felbinger, T. W., Schmidt, C., Moerstedt, K., Kilger, E., Lamm, P., & Goetz, A. E. (2003). Trendelenburg positioning after cardiac surgery: Effects on intrathoracic blood volume index and cardiac performance. *European Journal of Anaesthesiology, 20*(1), 17–20.

Sachdeva, A., Dalton, M., Amaragire, S. V., & Lees, T. (2010). Elastic compression stockings for prevention of deep vein thrombosis. *Cochrane Database of Systematic Review, 7*(7), 1–55.

Scherr, K., Wilson, D. M., Wagner, J., & Haughian, M. (2012). Evaluating a new rapid response team: NP-led versus intensivist-led comparisons. *AACN Advanced Critical Care, 23*(1), 32–42.

Travers, A. H., Rea, T. D., Bobrow, B. J., Edelson, D. P., Berg, R. A., Sayre, M. R., . . . & Swor, R. A. (2010). Part 4: CPR overview 2010 American Heart Association guidelines for cardiopulmonary resuscitation and emergency cardiovascular care. *Circulation, 122*(18 suppl 3), S676–S684.

Wesley, K. (2009, Apr. 5). The myth of Trendelenburg position. *Journal of Emergency Medical Services. 6*(01), 48–49.

Winters, B. D., Weaver, S. J., Pfoh, E. R., Yang, T., Pham, J. C., & Dy, S. M. (2013). Rapid-response systems as a patient safety strategy: A systematic review. *Annals of Internal Medicine, 158*(5_Part_2), 417–425.

Chapter 32
Neurologic Management

 ## Learning Objectives

32.1 Review the structure and function of the cerebrum, cerebellum, and brainstem.

32.2 Describe the unique metabolic demands of the central nervous system.

32.3 Outline the role of structures that protect the brain.

32.4 Discuss the brain's ability to autoregulate cerebral blood flow.

32.5 Calculate cerebral perfusion pressure (CPP) based on available data: mean arterial pressure (MAP) and intracranial pressure (ICP).

32.6 Identify the three components that dictate intracranial pressure.

32.7 List physical and environmental or contextual factors that increase intracranial pressure.

32.8 Discuss physiologic compensatory mechanisms that occur with an increased intracranial pressure.

32.9 Describe the process of assessing the neurologic client experiencing increasing intracranial pressure.

32.10 Explain the rationale for monitoring intracranial pressure (ICP).

32.11 Explain rationale for therapies used to treat intracranial hypertension.

32.12 Describe the difference between ischemic and hemorrhagic stroke

32.13 Discuss limitations and alternatives to the use of the Glasgow Coma Scale in comatose clients.

32.14 Identify various assessment tools used to evaluate pain and sedation level in the nonverbal client.

32.15 State criteria used to determine brain death.

32.16 Outline nursing responsibilities in the care of a client with an ICP monitoring system or ventriculostomy for cerebrospinal fluid drainage.

32.17 Identify components of a normal intracranial pressure (ICP) waveform.

Chapter Outline

Terminology

Anisocoria pupils of unequal size.

Autoregulation ability of the brain to maintain, *within limits*, a constant blood flow despite significant changes in systemic blood pressure.

Brain death medical–clinical diagnosis based on cessation of all brain function (evidenced by unresponsiveness, absence of brainstem reflexes, apnea) when the cause is known and irreversible.

Cerebral perfusion pressure (CPP) a calculated value derived from intracranial pressure (ICP) and mean arterial pressure (MAP; MAP – ICP = CPP); an indirect method of evaluating adequacy of cerebral blood flow; normal CPP ranges from 60 to 160 mm Hg.

Cognition skill for thinking and remembering, including paying attention, being aware of surroundings, reasoning, judgment, and problem solving.

Coma clinical state of altered consciousness in which a client is nonresponsive to environmental stimuli (cannot be aroused) due to diffuse bilateral cerebral hemispheric dysfunction, involvement of the brainstem, or both; coma level based on motor response to noxious stimulus.

Concussion complex pathophysiological process affecting the brain, induced by traumatic biomechanical forces (e.g., blow to the head or elsewhere with impulsive force transmitted to the head); may or may not result in loss of consciousness. Cumulative (repeated) events affect white matter (axons).

Consciousness a state of wakefulness (arousal) *and* general awareness (cognition) of self and environment, including orientation to time, place, and person. (Terminology used to describe various levels of consciousness include full consciousness, confusion, lethargy, obtundation, stupor, and coma.)

Confused disoriented in time, place, or person; short attention span; inability to think with normal speed and clarity; impaired judgment and decision making; difficulty following commands; may have hallucinations, be agitated, restless, irritable, increasingly confused at night.

Contralateral on the opposite side.

Contusion neurologic dysfunction caused by acceleration or deceleration injury (e.g., blow to the head) often associated with *coup* (injury at site of impact) and *contrecoup* (injury at side opposite the impact) due to movement of the brain within the skull.

Craniectomy removal of a bone flap to allow decompression (expansion of edematous brain tissue) and reduce intracranial pressure.

Cushing's triad systolic hypertension, widening pulse pressure, and bradycardia indicative of medullary ischemia.

Decerebration abnormal posturing associated with mid-brain (upper brainstem) dysfunction.

Decortication abnormal posturing associated with a direct lesion of the thalamus or mass that compresses the thalamus (above the brainstem).

Diplopia seeing two separate images of the same object in visual space due to images falling on each retina at different points rather than on the same points.

Disorientation beginning stage of loss of consciousness; impaired awareness of time, then place and memory, then recognition of self.

FOUR-Score Coma Scale "Full Outline of Un-Responsiveness" grading system (0 to 4) used to assess eye response, motor response, brainstem reflexes, and respiration.

Glasgow Coma Scale assessment tool designed to standardize observations of a client's level of consciousness (comatose states).

Hydrocephalus progressive dilation of the ventricles due to overproduction of CSF or abnormalities of CSF circulation or reabsorption.

Intracranial pressure (ICP) the sum of pressures exerted by intracranial contents (cerebrospinal fluid, blood, and brain tissue); normal range is 5–15 mm Hg.

Ipsilateral on the same side.

Lethargic having limited spontaneous movement or speech but easily aroused by speech or tactile stimulation; sluggish in thought, but oriented to time, place, and person.

Level of consciousness a continuum of responsiveness ranging from arousal (wakefulness), orientation, comprehension, and expression to nonresponsiveness to bodily or environmental stimuli.

Locked-in syndrome state of normal level of consciousness but complete body paralysis except for vertical eye movements and ability to blink on command (paralysis below CN III).

MAP (mean arterial pressure) average cardiac cycle arterial pressure:

$$MAP = \frac{(SBP) + (DBP \times 2)}{3}$$

Medial longitudinal fasciculus (MLF) pathway that interconnects the vestibular nuclei (CN VIII) with motor nuclei that innervate the extraocular eye muscles (CN III, IV, VI).

Microsensor fiberoptic "transducer tipped" intraventricular or intraparenchymal bolt catheter used to monitor intracranial pressure.

Neuromuscular blockade chemical paralysis used as restraint to control increased blood pressure and ICP due to restlessness, agitation, posturing, ventilator dyssynchrony.

Nystagmus involuntary drift of the eye with rapid correction in the opposite direction; the direction of fast correction describes the nystagmus.

Obtunded being in a state of reduced awakeness or alertness and limited response to the environment; rousable but falls asleep unless stimulated orally or by touch; responds minimally to questions.

Reticular activating system center located in the brainstem that interacts with the cerebral hemispheres to maintain normal consciousness.

Rostrocaudal descending the long axis of the body (top downward).

Secondary brain injury cascade of events including brain tissue ischemia and cerebral edema that occurs, causing damage to surrounding tissue after primary traumatic brain injury.

Stuporous having minimal spontaneous movement; unresponsive except to vigorous repeated stimuli; may have unintelligible sounds or eye opening; responds appropriately to painful stimulus; may withdraw from or grab at the stimulus.

Tragus cartilaginous projection in front of the external auditory canal.

Vegetative state state in which client with bilateral hemispheric disease (metabolic encephalopathy), initially comatose, may show improvement so that the client is awake, but unaware.

Ventriculostomy a hollow ventricular catheter placed through a burr hole in the skull and advanced into the lateral ventricle of the nondominant hemisphere; used to monitor ICP, provide therapeutic CSF drainage to relieve pressure, and allow specimen sampling.

This chapter presents a nursing process approach to care, focusing on techniques of assessing the neurologic client with altered levels of **consciousness** and the management of intracranial hypertension. (See Chapter 11 for basic information and neurologic assessment.)

The Conscious State

The nervous system includes two interdependent subsystems: the central nervous system (CNS) composed of the brain and spinal cord and the peripheral nervous system (PNS) composed of nerve fibers (cranial, spinal, and autonomic) that relay information between the CNS and other parts of the body. This complex system involves automatic feedback mechanisms that allow us to respond to stimuli from the internal and external environments through cognitive, behavioral, autonomic, and motor responses in a way that enables us to maintain a steady state, or *homeostasis*.

The brain is composed of left and right cerebral hemispheres (each divided into four functional lobes), the cerebellar lobes, and brainstem (midbrain, pons, and medulla). See Figure 32-1 ■. The conscious state includes both *wakefulness* and *awareness* of one's self and the environment (*orientation* to time, place, and person) and depends on an intact interaction between the **reticular activating system** (RAS) located in the brainstem and thalamus, which controls wakefulness, and the higher cerebral cortical centers, which are responsible for orientation. Altered levels of consciousness (**coma**) can occur with intracranial (structural) or extracranial (metabolic) disorders. The vast majority (85%) of coma cases are due to metabolic disorders, such as hypoxia, respiratory failure, hypo/hyperglycemia, uremia, or drug overdose, which cause diffuse dysfunction of both cerebral hemispheres and/or involvement of the ascending RAS. Intracranial disorders such as infection (meningitis, encephalitis) or **concussion** (brain trauma) can also cause coma with diffuse dysfunction.

FIGURE 32-1 Lobes of the brain.

In contrast to diffuse dysfunction, unilateral cerebral hemispheric lesions such as infarction ("brain attack"), hematoma, hemorrhage, or tumor may cause *focal* neurologic signs of dysfunction related to the particular area or functional lobe involved. Focal lesions expand and, along with edema formation, increase **intracranial pressure (ICP)**, may decrease cerebral blood flow, displace **contralateral** structures, and exert **rostrocaudal** (downward) compression on the brainstem (RAS) such that deteriorating levels of consciousness follow.

Normal function of the cerebral lobes, diencephalon (located above the brainstem), cerebellum, and brainstem and findings associated with dysfunction of these areas are reviewed in Table 32-1 ■.

Table 32-1 Functions of the Cerebral Cortex, Cerebellum, and Brainstem

Structure	Function	Dysfunctional Behaviors
Frontal Lobe Cortex	Memory, judgment, problem solving, concentration, personality, mood Initiation of motor activity and voluntary movement Expressive (motor) speech (left hemisphere)	Difficulty with attention and problem solving; inflexible thinking; personality change; behavioral changes (emotional, social, sexual) Left CVA: contralateral hemiparesis or hemiplegia and hemisensory loss in the same distribution; expressive aphasia; contralateral homonymous hemi-anopsa; limited right conjugate gaze; shortened attention span; hesitancy Right CVA: contralateral hemiparesis or hemiplegia and hemisensory loss in the same distribution; contralateral homonymous hemianopia; left visual and sensory neglect; poor left conjugate gaze; impulsive behavior; unaware of deficits.
Temporal Lobe Cortex	Memory, hearing, understanding (receptive) language Emotional affect	Short-term memory loss; may verbalize, but unable to understand what is said by others; aggressive behavior; difficulty identifying objects; difficulty recognizing faces; disturbed selective attention; change in sexuality Auditory, visual, and sensory hallucinations
Parietal Lobe Cortex	Sense of touch, pain, position, pressure, vibration Recognition of object size, shape, texture Spatial perceptual orientation Awareness of one's body parts Visual perception Receptive speech (written, oral) function	Difficulty naming objects; problems with reading and writing; right–left **confusion**; math difficulties Inability to focus visual attention; problems with eye–hand coordination; lack of awareness or inattention to body parts Receptive language dysfunction; expressive "word salad"
Occipital Lobe Cortex	Interpretation of visual stimuli (impulses from cranial nerve [CN] II)	Visual field defects; difficulty identifying colors; hallucinations or visual distortions; word blindness; difficulty reading and writing
Diencephalon: Thalamus	Relay center for all sensory and motor pathways All sensory pathways (except olfactory, CN I) to the brain are processed here before being sent to the cerebral cortex Awareness of pain, temperature, and light touch; reticular activating system focuses attention, stimulates cortex and autonomic nervous system (ANS)	Impaired consciousness Sensory and motor dysfunction *Decorticate* (abnormal flexor) posturing associated with a direct lesion or compression from hemispheres
Diencephalon: Hypothalamus	Stimulates the autonomic nervous system: regulates temperature, water balance, thirst, appetite, visceral, and somatic activities Controls pituitary hormone release Coordinates body behavioral responses to emotion Sleep–wakefulness cycle, circadian rhythm	Impaired consciousness Alterations of body temperature Diabetes insipidus (polyuria) Syndrome of inappropriate antidiuretic hormone (water retention with hyponatremia) Cheyne-Stokes respiration (rhythmic rise and fall in rate and depth of breathing with long periods of apnea)

(continued)

Table 32-1 Functions of the Cerebral Cortex, Cerebellum, and Brainstem *(continued)*

Structure	Function	Dysfunctional Behaviors
Cerebellum	Maintains posture, balance Coordination of voluntary muscle activity and muscle tone Controls fine movement and skilled motor activity	Problems with fine movement and coordination; inability to make rapid movements Lack of coordination Inability to grasp objects, tremors, dizziness, slurred speech, inability to walk
Brainstem: Midbrain	Contains nuclei for CN III and IV Center for auditory and visual reflexes Lies directly beneath the diencephalon (thalamus and hypothalamus) Contains aqueduct of Sylvius Pathway between cerebral hemispheres and lower brain	**Ipsilateral** pupil dilation with head injury or uncal herniation Both eyes deviate medially or laterally. Neurogenic hyperventilation (sustained deep breathing with no apneic periods) *Decerebrate* (abnormal extensor) posturing
Brainstem: Pons	Contains nuclei for CN V through VIII **Medial longitudinal fasciculus** tract connects CN III, IV, and VI with vestibular portion of acoustic nerve (CN VIII), allowing coordinated eye movement in response to noise, motion, position, and arousal. Relays information to and from the brain Contains fourth ventricle Contains vital centers for breathing (length of inspiration/expiration, rate)	Alterations of extraocular movements *See* Oculocephalic and Oculovestibular Testing Apneustic breathing (prolonged inspiratory or expiratory pauses)
Brainstem: Medulla	Contains nuclei for CN IX through XII Controls vital functions: swallowing, vomiting, hiccupping, coughing, heart rate, arterial constriction, respiratory rhythm Motor tracts cross to opposite side, descend the spinal cord for contralateral voluntary movement.	Cluster breathing (irregular gasping respirations with long periods of apnea) Ataxic respiration (irregular deep and shallow breathing with periods of apnea) **"Cushing's Triad"**: bradycardia, systolic hypertension, widened pulse pressure Arrhythmias, atrioventricular block

Structures and Functions That Protect the Brain

Skull, Meninges, and Spinal Fluid

The brain is protected by an unyielding skull, the meninges that cover the brain (dura, arachnoid, and pia mater), and cerebrospinal fluid (CSF), which circulates within the subarachnoid space to provide protective shock absorption. The ventricles produce 120 mL of CSF each day, while an equal amount is reabsorbed through arachnoid projections (villi) and returned to the venous circulation such that CSF pressure remains constant. If the villi become obstructed, the ventricles may dilate, causing a "normal pressure **hydrocephalus**" with a classic triad of gait instability, urinary incontinence, and altered mental status. This problem, occurring mostly in older clients, can be relieved by placement of a VP shunt that diverts CSF from the ventricles to the peritoneal cavity.

The dura mater lies close to the skull and creates a vertical fold (falx) that separates the right and left frontal lobes and a horizontal fold (tentorium) that separates the occipital and cerebellar lobes. With increasing intracranial pressure, brain tissue may herniate around these dural folds.

Fractures of the temporal and parietal bones may be associated with epidural (between the skull and dura) meningeal artery bleed that spreads freely and causes a rapid change in **level of consciousness**. An epidural hematoma is a surgical emergency. In contrast, a subdural bleed is venous in nature, slower, and may be associated with delayed signs of altered consciousness. This type of injury is more commonly seen in older adult clients with head injury associated with a fall that may or may not have been documented or remembered.

Fractures of the basal skull bones may be missed because they are not visible on skull or sinus x-rays but are often associated with tearing of the dura, causing CSF leakage from the ear (otorrhea) or nose (rhinorrhea) or altered CN VII function. These findings may be delayed, but should be reported immediately as they increase risk for infection. Leakage is usually self-limiting, but if it persists for 4–5 days, lumbar CSF drainage may be necessary to allow the dural tear to heal.

Autoregulation

The brain requires a continuous supply of oxygen and glucose to maintain its energy requirements. While it makes up only 2% of body weight, it receives 15% of the cardiac output and uses 20% of blood oxygen. Despite fluctuations in blood pressure, the brain has **autoregulation**, meaning it is able to regulate its own blood flow by arteriolar dilation when blood pressure falls or constriction when blood pressure rises. This protective function requires a mean arterial pressure (**MAP**) of 50–150 mm Hg and is disrupted with any increase in intracranial pressure or decrease in **cerebral perfusion pressure**. Then, if blood pressure rises, cerebral blood volume increases, causing an increased intracranial pressure. While hypertension must be controlled, a MAP sufficient to provide adequate cerebral perfusion must be maintained if intracranial hypertension exists. Target cerebral perfusion pressure (CPP) is 70–80 mm Hg and is calculated by subtracting the intracranial pressure (ICP) from the MAP (MAP − ICP = CPP).

Intracranial Hypertension

Intracranial pressure, normally 3–15 mm Hg, is dictated by three components: 80% brain tissue, 10% cerebral blood volume (with 80% being venous blood), and 10% CSF. Volumes of these constituents are kept relatively constant, but pathologic conditions can cause an increase of one of these components that must be compensated for by a decrease in one or both of the other components in order to maintain a normal ICP (Monro-Kellie hypothesis).

An increase in brain tissue occurs with edema that accompanies any type of injury (trauma, CVA) or a mass such as a tumor. An increase in cerebral blood flow occurs with an intracranial bleed or subarachnoid hemorrhage, or even cerebral vasodilation due to hypoxemia, hypocarbia, or certain medications. An increase in CSF occurs with blockage of its outflow paths or obstructed reabsorption by subarachnoid villi.

The brain has limited ability to control increased ICP by: (1) shunting CSF from the intracranial to the lumbar space, where CSF reabsorption is increased; (2) by compression of the cerebral venous system to reduce cerebral blood volume; and (3) by displacement of brain tissue, but this is adaptive only with a slowly expanding mass or hematoma condition. When these compensatory mechanisms are exhausted, ICP rises exponentially, cerebral perfusion is impaired, and brain tissue displaces or herniates through available openings.

When ICP increases to a level that compresses arterial flow (ICP = MAP), the Cushing reflex (bradycardia, increased SBP with widened pulse pressure, erratic breathing pattern) is activated to protect the brain from inadequate blood flow. Unfortunately, these changes in vital signs are late indicators of rostrocaudal deterioration.

Intracranial pressure monitoring systems may be used to measure the mean pressure exerted in the skull and alert the nurse to increases in ICP before external signs such as altered level of consciousness or pupillary changes occur. Monitoring also guides early intervention before damage occurs, assists the nurse in determining effects that care measures have on the client's ICP responses, and serves as a basis for ongoing evaluation of goal achievement and maintenance of desired outcomes: for example, target ICP ≤ 20 mm Hg and CPP ≥ 70–80 mm Hg.

A number of medical and nursing measures help to control ICP by selectively manipulating the three components that dictate intracranial pressure. Brain volume can be reduced by decreasing cerebral edema with osmotic diuretics (mannitol) and hypertonic saline, which also improve cerebral blood flow by decreasing blood viscosity and reducing serum hematocrit. During the acute phase, cerebral metabolic needs, refractory elevations of ICP, and effects of **secondary brain injury** can be modulated by induced hypothermia. CSF volume is reduced by continuous or intermittent external drainage of CSF (**ventriculostomy**). Cerebral blood volume can be reduced with hyperventilation (PCO_2 25–30 mm Hg), which can cause vasoconstriction with global or localized cerebral ischemia but may be used briefly as a bridge to more appropriate therapy. Blood volume can also be reduced by supporting jugular venous return with neutral head alignment, 30-degree bed elevation, and by preventing surges in central venous pressure associated with maneuvers that increase intra-abdominal and intrathoracic pressure. Cautious use of analgesics and sedatives is an integral component of managing ICP as these modalities blunt the ANS response to noxious stimuli, decrease O_2 consumption, and enhance psychological well-being. These agents have adverse side effects that may increase ICP and necessitate continuous assessment of the client's response to their use and impact on ventilation and oxygenation.

Stroke

Stroke is the fifth leading cause of death in the United States and a leading cause of serious long-term disability (Minino, 2010; AHA, 2011). There are over 7,000,000 stroke survivors in the United States over the age of 20 years, and strokes will occur approximately every 40 seconds, affecting women more than men. The estimated total cost of stroke in the United States in 2010 was 73.7 billion dollars. There are two types of stroke: ischemic strokes and hemorrhagic strokes. Ischemic strokes occur when arteries are blocked by blood clots or by the buildup of plaque and other fatty deposits. About 87% of all strokes are ischemic. These strokes can be treated with tPA (tissue plasminogen activator) if the client can get to an emergency department that can provide treatment within 3 hours of onset of symptoms. Hemorrhagic strokes occur when a blood vessel in the brain ruptures, leaking blood into the surrounding tissues. This type of stroke is less common but accounts for 30% of all stroke deaths. Stroke is referred to as *brain attack*, and the National Stroke Association has encouraged teaching for everyone to recognize and respond to the signs of stroke using the acronym FAST (Box 32-1 ■).

Nurses should be aware of the early warning signs of stroke in their hospitalized clients, as clients can develop stroke after surgery or while they are hospitalized. The American Heart Association and The American Stroke Association provide tools for healthcare providers to assist them in caring for stroke clients.

Box 32-1 **FAST CHECK FOR STROKE**

F = Face	Ask the individual to smile. Does one side of the face droop?
A = Arms	Ask the individual to raise both arms. Does one arm drift downward?
S = Speech	Ask the individual to repeat a simple sentence. Does the speech sound strained or slurred?
T = Time	If you observe any of these signs (independently or together), call 9-1-1 immediately.

Source: www.strokeassociation.org

Nursing Care of the Neurologic Client

The **Glasgow Coma Scale** (GCS; see Glasgow Coma Scale, Chapter 11) has been used for several decades to evaluate level of consciousness (LOC) by requiring the client to hear the examiner and respond with (1) eye opening, (2) oral, and (3) motor responses. If the client is unresponsive to these, abnormal posturing response (**decortication, decerebration**) to shaking or noxious stimuli is assessed. Clients with a score of 8 or less are considered to be comatose and are typically intubated to protect the airway and facilitate mechanical ventilation if required. A "T" is added to their GCS score to indicate this functional limitation. Using this scale, a client with spinal cord injury who is paralyzed may receive a coma score of 8, be intubated, but not be comatose. It follows that the GCS cannot be used to assess neurologic signs in clients who are unable to respond orally (e.g., clients who are intubated, sedated, aphasic, have impaired hearing or altered level of consciousness).

The Full Outline of Un-Responsiveness (**FOUR-Score Coma Scale**) is an alternative tool for assessing the comatose client, especially one with an acute metabolic or other nonstructural brain injury or disorder because it detects early changes in consciousness such as inability to follow the examiner's commands, altered brainstem reflexes, and Cheyne-Stokes breathing. It is also used to differentiate **vegetative state** from minimally conscious states, **locked-in syndrome**, uncal herniation, and **brain death**.

Pain, general discomfort, fatigue, anxiety, restlessness, and agitation increase cerebral metabolism, heart rate, blood pressure, and intracranial pressure, but the neurologic client's inability to communicate confines the nurse to observing the behavioral and physiologic indicators of distress without the ability to identify or validate a potential cause. Since nonverbal responses have many possible stimuli that require different treatment, they may be misinterpreted and inadequately managed. For instance, failure to recognize that pain often leads to agitation may lead to excessive administration of sedatives, leaving pain untreated. It is essential to use reliable assessment tools to differentiate among distressful stimuli so that appropriate therapies can be provided. The Critical Care Pain Observation Tool and a number of sedation/agitation assessment scales have been determined to be valid and reliable to use with neurologic clients who are unable to communicate verbally.

Caring for neurologic clients challenges the nurse's insight and ability to appreciate the client's unique experience, to assess patiently, to identify distressful stimuli, and to respond empathically with informed actions. Comprehensive care also includes ongoing support of all body systems and prevention of a wide range of complications that can occur. Emotional support is provided by communicating with the client, whether or not he or she is responsive. This has been shown to help relieve anxiety and fear and serves as a means of preventing acute surges in ICP. Concerned others are also supported by answering questions and explaining how technical aspects of care contribute to the client's progress as they inform and help direct decision making. Once the client is stable, family members can be encouraged to participate in simple comforting care measures and engage in providing gentle sensory stimuli, which may enhance arousal and awareness as the client regains the conscious state.

Cultural Awareness

Many cultures may be wary of discussions of advance directives and organ donation, especially if the client is seriously ill. The topic of organ donation and the withdrawal of life support is a very sensitive issue for many families and is often not discussed before families are in the position where they have to deal with it. The added dimension of understanding the cultural complexities make this a very challenging situation for the nursing staff. The nurse should approach the family and ask if there are specific cultural beliefs and practices they have that will impact their decision making around these topics. This allows the family to feel more included in the discussion and decisions around the client's care. Often the nurse is able to include some of these practices in the client's care without comprising treatment.

Nursing Diagnoses

The following nursing diagnoses are appropriate to use on client care plans when the components are related to clients who require focused neurological assessment and management of increased intracranial pressure.

NURSING DIAGNOSIS	RELATED TO . . .
Aspiration, Risk for	Altered level of consciousness Airway intubation
Imbalanced Body Temperature, Risk for	Traumatic brain (hypothalamic) injury
Acute Confusion	Brain injury
Decreased Intracranial Adaptive Capacity	Increased intracranial contents (blood, tissue, spinal fluid)
Imbalanced Fluid Volume, Risk for	Traumatic brain (hypothalamic) injury
Impaired Verbal Communication	Altered level of consciousness, neuromuscular blockade, airway intubation
Ineffective Thermoregulation	Brain injury
Impaired Bed Mobility	Neuromuscular blockade; invasive monitoring
Ineffective Cerebral Tissue Perfusion, Risk for	Increased intracranial pressure
Infection, Risk for	Invasive monitoring catheters; pathologic (rhinorrhea, otorrhea) and therapeutic cerebral spinal fluid (CSF) drainage
Impaired Skin Integrity, Risk for	Sedation, neuromuscular blockade (paralysis) Restricted positioning due to monitoring devices

Source: Herdman, T. H. & Kamitsuru, S. (Eds.) *Nursing Diagnoses – Definitions and Classification 2015-2017*. Copyright © 2014, 1994–2014 by NANDA International. Used by arrangement with John Wiley & Sons Limited. Companion website: www.wiley.com/go/nursingdiagnoses. In order to make safe and effective judgments using NANDA-I nursing diagnosis it is essential that nurses refer to the definitions and defining characteristics of the diagnoses listed in this work.

Unit 32.1
Assessment of the Neurologic Client

Nursing Process Data

ASSESSMENT Database

- Determine a neurologic client's level of consciousness.
- Determine deviations and implications for care for the client with altered brainstem reflexes.
- Identify signs of basilar skull fracture.
- Recognize changes in vital signs that occur with altered level of consciousness.
- Utilize the FOUR-Score Coma Scale for nonverbal clients.
- List criteria used to determine brain death in adults.

PLANNING Objectives

- To determine a neurologic client's level of consciousness
- To assess brainstem reflexes in the neurologic client
- To employ protective measures for the client with altered brainstem reflexes
- To recognize signs of basilar skull fracture and implications for care
- To identify changes in brainstem reflexes and vital signs associated with herniation syndromes
- To compare features of the Glasgow Coma Scale with those of the FOUR-Score coma scale
- To assist the healthcare provider with determination of brain death
- To support a family/caregiver of a deceased organ donor

IMPLEMENTATION Procedures

DOCUMENTATION AND EVALUATION

Expected Outcomes

- Appropriate tools are used to evaluate a neurologic client's level of consciousness.
- Ongoing assessment of brainstem reflexes and vital signs are used to identify increasing intracranial pressure in the neurologic client.
- Signs of possible basilar skull fracture are identified.
- Established criteria are used to determine brain death.
- Supportive communication is provided for family or caregiver of a deceased organ donor.

Unexpected Outcomes/Alternative Actions

Pearson Nursing Student Resources

Find additional review materials at
nursing.pearsonhighered.com.
Prepare for success with NCLEX®-style practice questions and Skill Checklists.

Skill 32.1.1 | Assessing Levels of Consciousness (Descending Categories)

Note: There is no internationally accepted taxonomy of definition of LOC, no precise terminology, and no agreement on behaviors of various stages.

Preparation

1. Introduce self.
2. Perform hand hygiene.
3. Identify client using two client identifiers.

Procedure

1. Describe client behaviors that were assessed. ➤ *Rationale:* Behaviors are more helpful and allow others to easily note changes in client functioning.
2. Obtain information about the client's LOC (Table 32-2 ■).
3. Record client's response (e.g., responds appropriately to oral questioning).

Table 32-2 Assessing Levels of Consciousness

Category	Findings and Implications for Care
Conscious	Responds immediately to minimal external stimuli Is alert, fully awake and oriented to time, place, purpose, and person. Understands spoken and written word and expresses ideas orally or in writing Alterations in LOC reflect cerebral and metabolic disorders very quickly.
Confused	Disoriented to time, and place, but usually oriented to person. Has short attention span, impaired memory Has difficulty following instruction; may have hallucinations, be agitated, restless, irritable, and more confused at night *Frequent observation and supervision indicated*
Lethargic	Drowsy, sluggish in speech and mental and motor responses Requires increased stimulus to awaken Oriented to time, place, and person. *Frequent observation and supervision indicated*
Obtunded	Drowsy, arouses to stimulus but with minimal response Responds appropriately to painful stimulus *Needs complete care*
Stuporous	Arouses only by vigorous and continuous stimulus Has little spontaneous movement May appropriately localize or withdraw from stimulus May open eyes, make incomprehensible sounds *Needs complete care*
Comatose	Cannot be aroused Has no voluntary response to stimuli, including pain Coma level is based on motor response to painful stimulus. May or may not have protective brainstem reflexes (e.g., gag) *Needs total dependent care, with airway a priority*

Skill 32.1.2 | Assessing Cranial Nerves (Brainstem Reflexes)

Note: In most clients with increasing intracranial pressure, level of consciousness deteriorates before changes in cranial nerve reflexes, motor response, and vital signs occur. See Chapter 11, Physical Assessment, for basic assessment.

Procedure

1. Assess cranial nerves (Table 32-3 ■).
2. Record the stimulus applied and the client's response (e.g., responds appropriately to oral questioning).

> **CLINICAL ALERT**
>
> Change in pupil size, shape, or reactivity should be reported immediately. This may be an early sign of transtentorial herniation requiring immediate intervention.
>
> - Flexor (decorticate) posturing indicates loss of all function *above* the brainstem.
> - Extensor (decerebrate) posturing indicates brainstem dysfunction.
> - Loss of cough, gag, or corneal (blink) reflex indicates loss of brainstem integrity.

(continued)

Skill 32.1.2 | Assessing Cranial Nerves (Brainstem Reflexes) *(continued)*

Table 32-3 Assessing Cranial Nerves (Brainstem Reflexes)

Cranial Nerve	Significance of Alteration
CN II (sensory) and CN III (motor) **Pupil size, shape, and reactivity**	Normal pupils are round, usually 3–5 mm diameter, equal in size, and react (constrict) consensually (both pupils respond) and briskly to light. Alternately, have client look at an object 10 cm (4 in.) from the eyes and then at something on the wall behind the observer. The pupils should constrict (accommodate) when focusing on the near object. **Anisocoria** (unequal pupil size) may be found in up to 20% of healthy clients. Smaller than average pupils may occur with metabolic coma. Pinpoint pupils may indicate pontine ischemia or opiate overdose. Oval pupils are early indication of CN III compression or increased ICP (18–35 mm Hg), but pupils may be round in presence of increased ICP. Ipsilateral pupil dilation with head injury indicates uncal herniation with compression of CN III. *Bilateral* dilated (small ring of iris) and fixed pupils indicate extremely increased ICP causing pontine compression with complete CN III palsy. Absence of pupillary light reflex is consistent with comatose state. Hypothermia, barbiturate coma, and opiate overdose may mimic comatose states with unreactive pupils.
CN III, IV, and VI (all motor) **Assess extraocular movements in the conscious client**	***Note:*** See below for assessment of the conscious client (six fields of gaze, Box 32-2 ■). Inability to move the eye inward or downward may be seen with head trauma (midbrain compression of CN IV). Inability to move the eye outward (pontine compression of CN VI) may be due to intracranial hypertension. The client has **diplopia** (double vision) when turning the right eye, if affected, to the right and same for the left turning leftward. Consciousness with complete body paralysis except for vertical eye movements occurs with a lesion in the ventral pons as seen in locked-in syndrome.
CN III, IV, and VI (all motor) **Oculocephalic (doll's eyes) reflex in unconscious client**	"Doll's eye reflex" is used to test extraocular movements—integrity of the pontine-midbrain level (CN III, IV, and VI) in the *unconscious* client. Damage to the reticular activating system may damage these nerves, which pass through the midbrain to innervate extraocular movements. Reflex may be absent in severe metabolic encephalopathy. *See Skill 32.1.3, Assessing the Oculocephalic (Doll's Eye) Reflex.*
CN V (sensory) and VII (motor) **Corneal blink reflex**	Reflex is frequently absent in the comatose client. Periorbital swelling may prevent eyelid closure. Loss of ability to blink indicates need for corneal protection (instillation of eye lubricant) to prevent corneal drying and scarring. Polyethylene film may be taped over the eyes, extending beyond the eyebrows.
CN VIII (sensory) and III, IV, VI (all motor) **Oculovestibular (cold caloric) reflex in unconscious client** (test performed by healthcare provider)	These are used for final assessment of brainstem function in the unconscious client and can be used when cervical spine precautions must be maintained. Test may elicit abnormal posturing in comatose client. Reflex may be temporarily absent in client with metabolic encephalopathy. *See Skill 32.1.4, Assessing the Oculovestibular Reflex: "Cold Caloric Test" in an Unconscious Client.*
CN IX (sensory) and X (motor) **Cough and gag reflex**	Normally this medullary reflex protects the airway; its absence places the client at high risk for aspiration. Loss of this reflex is a poor prognostic sign.

Box 32-2 THE SIX CARDINAL DIRECTIONS OF GAZE

This test assesses CNs III, IV, and VI, which innervate the six extraocular muscles that move the eyes as a pair in the same direction. These eye movements interact with the internuclear pathway of the medial longitudinal fasciculus (MLF) and cerebral cortex to coordinate focus in a given direction.

Test the six extraocular muscles (conjugate eye) movement in the conscious client:

1. Ask the client to follow your finger through an "H" sequence: client looks rightward, leftward, left upward, left downward, then right upward and right downward.

2. Assess that both eyes move simultaneously, symmetrically, in the same direction, and in alignment.

3. Dysconjugate movement (one eye deviating from mid-position at rest), *diplopia* (double vision), impaired movement (gaze paresis or paralysis) or **nystagmus** (eye drift with rapid correction in the opposite direction) indicates cranial nerve injury.

Coordinated eye and *head movement* incorporates complex reflexes of the eyes plus *vestibular* systems (CN VIII) and the *cerebral cortex*. The *oculocephalic reflex* (doll's eyes response) and the *oculovestibular reflex* (caloric stimulation) are used to assess brainstem reflexes in the unconscious client.

Skill 32.1.3 | Assessing the Oculocephalic (Doll's Eyes) Reflex

Preparation

1. Identify client and perform hand hygiene.
2. The purpose of this test is to assess extraocular movements in the unconscious client by determining presence and extent of structural damage.
   a. Cranial nerves III, IV, and VI pass through the midbrain to innervate the extraocular muscles.
   b. The medial longitudinal fasciculus (MLF) also passes through the midbrain and coordinates eye movements with head and body position changes. ❶
   c. If the eyes are able to cross the midline, the medial longitudinal fasciculus and midbrain through which it passes are considered to be intact.
3. Determine that neck injury has been ruled out before this test is performed.

Procedure

1. Hold client's eyes open.
2. Briskly turn client's head to one side, then briskly turn head to the other side, noting client's eye movement.
   ➤ **Rationale:** The intact brainstem will attempt to keep the eyes looking forward even as the head is rotated laterally.
3. Assess for an intact oculocephalic reflex, when the eyes briefly remain in the direction opposite that of the head turn (positive doll's eye reflex).
4. Assess if eyes remain midline and move with the head, or if the eyes rove or move in opposite direction; this *abnormal* oculocephalic reflex indicates a lesion at the pontine-midbrain level of the brainstem.

5. *For an alternative method*: Flex the neck and note that the eyes look upward, then extend the neck and note that the eyes look downward, indicating a normal or positive "doll's eye" reflex.

Initial eye movement direction is opposite head movement

Eyes are fixed

❶ Oculocephalic reflex: Eyes briefly remain in the direction opposite to that of the head turn (positive doll's eye reflex).

Skill 32.1.4 | Assessing the Oculovestibular Reflex: "Cold Caloric Test" in an Unconscious Client

Note: This test is performed by a healthcare provider. This noxious stimulation may elicit abnormal posturing in the comatose client.

Equipment
Otoscope
Catheter tip syringe
50 mL ice water

Preparation

1. Identify client and perform hand hygiene.
2. Purpose of test is to assess brainstem integrity in the unconscious client.
3. Inspect to validate that client's tympanic membrane is intact.
4. Raise client's head to a 30-degree angle.

Procedure

1. Healthcare provider injects 20–50 mL of ice water into the external auditory canal. ➤ **Rationale:** This cools the mastoid bone and disturbs the endolymph flow in the inner ear. A signal passes from the medulla to the midbrain, triggering compensatory eye movements.
2. Check both eyes that tonically move toward the side of the cold water infusion, then rapidly correct back toward midline with bursts of nystagmus, indicating an intact brainstem.
   ❶ ➤ **Rationale:** In the unconscious client, the cold caloric test is used to test brainstem reflex presence or absence. With cold irrigation, vestibular pathway mediates a slow deviation towards the irrigated ear, indicating the brainstem is intact. This is followed by a rapid corrective movement back to baseline via the cortical pathway on the ipsilateral

(continued)

Skill 32.1.4 | Assessing the Oculovestibular Reflex: "Cold Caloric Test" in an Unconscious Client *(continued)*

cerebral hemisphere. In the presence of cerebral damage, the fast phase of nystagmus is absent, so the eye deviates towards the side being irrigated.

3. Healthcare provider test may repeat in the other ear to test integrity of the *contralateral* side of the brainstem.

❶ Oculovestibular reflex: Both eyes tonically move toward the side of cold water infusion, then rapidly back toward midline, with bursts of nystagmus (cold caloric test).

Skill 32.1.5 | Assessing Signs of Basilar Skull Fracture

Note: Fractures of basal skull bones usually are not visible on skull or sinus x-rays but are often associated with tearing of the dura. A possible basilar skull fracture is suspected if the client develops leakage of CSF from the nose (rhinorrhea) or ears (otorrhea) or exhibits altered facial nerve (CN VII) function. These findings should be reported immediately as they are associated with increased risk for infection.

Preparation

1. Introduce self and identify client using two client identifiers.
2. Wash hands.

Procedure

1. Assess for *rhinorrhea* (leakage of blood or CSF from client's nose): Look for milky CSF ring around bloody drainage on drip pad ("halo sign"). ➤ *Rationale:* Drainage may indicate a basilar skull fracture with dural tear and risk for infection (meningitis). Drainage should not be obstructed but allowed to drip freely from the nose onto a sterile "mustache" dressing. Nasal suctioning and nose blowing must be avoided.
2. Assess auditory canal for *otorrhea* (leakage of blood or CSF from the client's ear). Look for milky CSF ring around bloody drainage on drip pad ("halo sign"). ❶ ➤ *Rationale:* Drainage may indicate a basilar skull fracture with dural tear, ruptured tympanic membrane, and risk for infection (meningitis). Drainage should not be obstructed.
3. Place client on side of drainage and allow fluid to drain freely from the ear onto a sterile towel (drip pad).
4. Assess for *Battle's sign*. Look for ecchymosis or bruising behind the ear. ➤ *Rationale:* This may indicate a basilar skull fracture and associated with CN VII defect. Finding may be delayed and should be reported.

❶ "Halo" sign showing a milky CSF ring around bloody drainage.

CLINICAL ALERT

Otorrhea and rhinorrhea are suggestive of CSF leakage, but drainage is often combined with blood, so glucose determination is unreliable to detect presence of CSF. Laboratory analysis of chloride content of drainage is more reliable because CSF chloride concentration is greater than that of serum.

If basilar skull fracture is suspected, do not insert a nasogastric tube. Orogastric placement is indicated and should be performed before orotracheal intubation in order to prevent aspiration.

5. Assess for *raccoon eyes*. Look for ecchymosis or bruising around the eyes, which may be accompanied by *rhinorrhea*. ➤ *Rationale:* These signs may indicate a basilar skull fracture. Finding may be delayed and should be reported.

Skill 32.1.6 | Assessing Vital Signs

Note: Changes in vital signs are late indicators of decompensation.

Preparation
1. Gather equipment. Wash hands.
2. Introduce self and identify client using two client identifiers.

Procedure
1. Measure temperature. ➤ *Rationale:* Hyperthermia or hypothermia may indicate hypothalamic injury, infection, or noninfectious fever.
2. Assess heart rate and rhythm. ➤ *Rationale:* Various arrhythmias occur with abrupt changes in ICP. Bradycardia develops in high spinal cord injury and with medullary ischemia.
3. Assess respiratory rate, and pattern. ➤ *Rationale:* Respiratory changes occur early, even before alterations of LOC. *Note:* See Chapter 10, Vital Signs, for respiratory patterns. For example:

- Cheyne-Stokes respiration (an exaggerated pattern of normal breathing) is associated with structural disorders above the midbrain, may be present in metabolic encephalopathy, and may be observed in healthy individuals during sleep or those with heart failure.
- Hyperventilation may indicate acidemia (low blood pH) or may occur early with pontine pathology.
- Erratic breathing patterns, which may include periods of apnea, develop with midbrain and pontine (upper brainstem) injury.

Note: It is best to describe the breathing pattern as it is seen rather than to use names of breathing patterns. Description of the pattern clarifies the assessment finding and helps others to recognize changes.

4. Measure blood pressure. ➤ *Rationale:* Hypotension (SBP ≤ 90 mm Hg) relates directly to cerebral ischemia and secondary brain injury.

> ### CLINICAL ALERT
> Systolic hypertension and widening pulse pressure are responses to maintain cerebral blood flow in the presence of pressure on the brainstem (medullary ischemia).

Note: Loss of autoregulation occurs with any type of brain injury. If blood pressure increases, cerebral blood flow, blood volume, and ICP also increase. Systemic hypertension must be controlled, but the MAP must be maintained to support adequate cerebral blood flow (CPP near 80 mm Hg) when ICP is increased.

EVIDENCE-BASED PRACTICE
Caring for Client With Increased Intracranial Pressure (ICP)
Clients in the intensive care unit with high ICPs require nursing interventions to prevent complications that have often been thought to cause increases in their ICP. Oral care, suctioning, and turning are three common interventions that were associated with increases in ICPs. A recent review of the evidence recommends oral care can be safely administered without any increase in ICP. Endotracheal suctioning should be limited to two passes. Clients should be hyperoxygenated but not hyperventilated, and clients can be safely repositioned.

Source: McNett & Olson (2013)

Skill 32.1.7 | Assessing Coma in the Neurologic Client (FOUR-Score Coma Scale)

Procedure
1. Determine score for each of the four components: 0 is worst response and 4 is best response. Scores are not totaled (Box 32-3 ■).

   a. **Assess eye response:** E4 = eyelids open or opened, tracking, or blinking to command; E3 = eyelids open but not tracking; E2 = eyelids closed but open to loud voice; E1 = eyelids closed but open to pain; E0 = eyelids remain closed with pain.

   b. **Assess motor response:** M4 = thumbs-up, fist, or peace sign; M3 = localizing to pain; M2 = flexion response to pain; M1 = extension response to pain; M0 = no response to pain or generalized myoclonus status.

   c. **Assess brainstem reflexes:** B4 = pupil and corneal reflexes present; B3 = one pupil wide and fixed; B2 = pupil or corneal reflexes absent; B1 = pupil and corneal reflexes absent; B0 = absent pupil, corneal, and cough reflex.

   d. **Assess respiratory pattern:** R4 = not intubated, regular breathing pattern; R3 = not intubated, Cheyne-Stokes breathing pattern; R2 = not intubated, irregular breathing; R1 = breathes above ventilatory rate; R0 = breathes at ventilator rate or apnea.

(continued)

Skill 32.1.7 | Assessing Coma in the Neurologic Client (FOUR-Score Coma Scale) *(continued)*

Box 32-3 ASSESSING COMA IN THE NEUROLOGIC CLIENT USING THE FULL OUTLINE OF UN-RESPONSIVENESS (FOUR) SCORE COMA SCALE

This tool scores four components of impaired consciousness: eye response, motor response, brainstem reflexes, and respiration. It differs from the Glasgow Coma Scale by not requiring a verbal response. It is useful for assessing agitated and confused clients without impaired consciousness and those who are alert but unable to respond verbally, including clients who are intubated, stuporous, or comatose. It is also useful for sedated clients (since sedation affects eye opening and motor response, but not brainstem reflexes and respiration) and for clients developing early changes in consciousness who are unable to follow commands, to track examiner's finger movements, and have Cheyne-Stokes respirations.

FOUR (Full Outline of Un-Responsiveness) Score Coma Scale is used to assess coma in the neurologic client.

Skill 32.1.8 | Determining Brain Death—Assessing for Apnea (CO_2 Challenge)

Note: Institutional protocol may vary slightly.

Preparation

1. Determine that client lacks all evidence of responsiveness (Box 32-4 ■). ➤ *Rationale:* This confirms coma.
2. Determine that cause of coma has been established and is irreversible.
3. Before diagnosis of brain death is attempted, clinical conditions such as acid–base or electrolyte or endocrine disturbance, hypothermia, presence of CNS depressant drugs or alcohol, and recent administration of **neuromuscular blockade** should be normalized, if possible, since these conditions can complicate attempts to diagnose brain death.
4. Adjust therapies so that client is normotensive (SBP 100 mm Hg), normothermic, euvolemic, eucapnic (PCO_2 35–45 mm Hg), without history of COPD or severe obesity and has normal PO_2. ➤ *Rationale:* The objective of the test is to determine apnea.

Box 32-4 DETERMINING BRAIN DEATH

The diagnosis of brain death is a medical–clinical diagnosis based on "irreversible cessation of all functions of the entire brain, including the brainstem: coma (unresponsiveness) with a known cause, absence of brainstem reflexes, and apnea."

- Recovery of neurologic function has not been reported after the clinical diagnosis of brain death has been established using these criteria.
- Minimally acceptable observation period has not been determined.
- Non–brainmediated spontaneous movements (e.g., spinal and deep tendon reflexes) can falsely suggest retained brain function.
- Ventilator triggering may falsely suggest client-initiated breathing.

Source: Wijdicks, Varelas, Gronseth, Greer, & American Academy of Neurology (2010)

5. Determine that client has absence of brainstem reflexes:

   a. Pupil, oculocephalic, oculovestibular, and corneal reflexes
   b. Pharyngeal (gag) and tracheal (cough) reflexes
   c. Facial muscle movement to noxious stimulus
   d. Absence of motor response to noxious stimuli in all four limbs

Procedure

1. Preoxygenate client with 100% oxygen for 10 min. ➤ *Rationale:* This is to achieve a PO_2 200 mm Hg.
2. Reduce ventilation rate to 10 breaths per min. ➤ *Rationale:* This is to achieve eucapnia.
3. Reduce ventilator PEEP mode to 5 cm H_2O. (See Chapter 33, Advanced Nursing Skills.)
4. Obtain baseline ABGs if SPO_2 is 95%.
5. Disconnect client from ventilator. ➤ *Rationale:* This is the only way to determine apnea.
6. Immediately change to T-Tube with 100% FiO_2 or place small catheter through endotracheal tube to level of carina and deliver 100% O_2 at 6 L/min. ➤ *Rationale:* This is to maintain oxygenation.
7. Healthcare provider continuously observes for respiratory effort (chest, abdominal excursion) for 8–10 min.
   ➤ *Rationale:* If client shows *any* effort to breathe, respiratory support is reestablished according to agency protocol or consistent with measures predecided by client's family and agency's client advocate.
8. Abort test if SBP decreases to <90 mm Hg or if SpO_2 is <85% for more than 30 seconds and retry procedure with T-piece, CPAP 10 cm H_2O, and 100% O_2 at 12 L/min.

➤ *Rationale:* Deterioration of vital signs and oxygenation should not precede proof of apnea.

9. Repeat ABGs after 8 min if no respiratory drive is observed.
10. If no respiratory drive is observed and PCO_2 is 60 or 20 mm Hg over baseline, apnea test result is positive. ➤ *Rationale:* These findings support a clinical diagnosis of brain death.
11. Brain–death re-examination is not required, but may need to be repeated depending on etiology of coma. Recommended minimal time intervals between first and second clinical examinations:

    a. 6 hr after trauma or hemorrhage
    b. 24 hr after an anoxic injury
    c. Time interval may decrease to 12 hr if ancillary test is utilized.
    d. If there is obvious evidence of bilateral brain injury, potentially only one exam is needed to declare brain death.

12. An ancillary test may be performed to confirm brain death.
    ➤ *Rationale:* These may be indicated if uncertainty exists or apnea test cannot be fully performed, but these tests cannot replace a neurologic examination.

    a. Cerebral angiography: positive if there is no intracerebral filling at carotid bifurcation or circle of Willis
    b. Electroencephalography (EEG): positive if there is no electrical activity throughout 30 min of recording
    c. Transcranial doppler ultrasonography
    d. Cerebral radionuclide perfusion scan: positive if there is no isotope uptake in brain tissue
    e. CT angiogram
    f. MRI/MRA

Skill 32.1.9 | Supporting the Family or Caregiver

Procedure

1. Introduce self. Respectfully reinforce to family that brain death is determined according to established and specific medical–legal criteria. ➤ *Rationale:* Some believe that brain death is recoverable or comparable to a coma.
2. Discontinue all medical interventions after brain death is declared. ➤ *Rationale:* This is ethically and legally justified.
3. Refer to the remains as a "body" rather than a "client."
4. Avoid the words "client," "care," and "treatment" while talking to family members. ➤ *Rationale:* It should not be implied that treatment or care is being provided or continued after an individual has died.
5. Discontinue conversation with the "body." ➤ *Rationale:* Directing thoughts away from the body and toward the family helps the family to understand and accept the reality of death.
6. Encourage the family to talk, touch, and hold if they choose; allow private time.

7. Contact grief counselor or clergy as indicated.
8. Clarify concerns about the deceased donor receiving artificial support:

   a. Use the term "artificial support" in place of "life support."
   b. Clarify that the only justification for continuing artificial support is to maintain organs for transplant.
   c. Reinforce that even though artificial support continues, the equipment is not supporting life, but maintaining body organs.
   d. Reinforce that the time of death is when the client was declared dead, not when donated organs are removed.

Note: As many as 60% of deaths from stroke, heart disease, and traumatic brain injury may involve some kind of treatment withdrawal, making it one of the most common pathways to death in the United States.

(continued)

Skill 32.1.9 | Supporting the Family or Caregiver *(continued)*

LEGAL ALERT
- Brain death is a medical diagnosis made by a healthcare provider. State laws and hospital policy may vary on criteria for this diagnosis.
- According to the Uniform Anatomical Gift Act (revised in 2006 in many states), a donor's declared intent to be an organ donor (documented on driver's license) is sufficient evidence of consent for organs removal. Consent of spouse or family, regardless of their objections, is not necessary. This act also requires that hospital personnel ask clients on admission if they would consider being organ donors. If an individual dies and did not declare himself or herself to be a donor, hospital or medical personnel must ask the individual's relatives or surrogates whether they would be interested in donating the individual's organs.
- The act allows medical personnel to remove organs without receiving explicit consent from a potential donor or donor's relative as long as medical personnel have made a reasonable effort to discover any objection by the donor or donor's family.

Unit 32.1 Documentation and Evaluation

DOCUMENTATION for Assessment of the Neurologic Client

- Level of consciousness:
  Description of stimulus applied and client's response
  Healthcare provider notification of significant changes
  Care measures provided if indicated
- Brainstem reflexes:
  Healthcare provider notification of significant changes
  Protective care measures provided if indicated
- Signs of basilar skull fracture:
  Presence of otorrhea, rhinorrhea, Battle's sign, or raccoon eyes
  Altered function of CN VII
  Healthcare provider notification
  Protective care measures implemented
- Vital signs:
  Frequency according to agency protocol
  Healthcare provider notification of significant changes

- FOUR-Score Coma Scale:
  Record score for each individual component: eye response, motor response, brainstem reflexes, and respiration.
  Scores are not totaled.
- Brain-death determination: Healthcare provider completes an extensive checklist for determination of brain death, including:
  Prerequisites for brain-death determination testing
  Neurologic examination
  Apnea testing
  Ancillary testing
  Time of brain death (time PCO_2 reached target value or time ancillary test is officially interpreted)

EVALUATION/Critical Thinking

Expected Outcomes
- Appropriate tools are used to evaluate a neurologic client's level of consciousness.
- Ongoing assessment of a client's brainstem reflexes and vital signs are used to determine compensated versus decompensating neurologic status.
- Signs of possible basilar skull fracture are identified.
- Established criteria are used to determine brain death.
- Supportive communication is provided for family or caregiver of a deceased organ donor.

Unexpected Outcomes	Alternative Actions
• Neurologic client's comatose state cannot be determined using Glasgow Coma Scale due to inability to respond verbally.	• Recognize that a nonverbal client cannot respond to parameters assessed using the Glasgow Coma Scale. • Utilize the FOUR-Score Coma Scale to assess separate components of eye response, motor response, brainstem reflexes, and respiration for the nonverbal client.
• Client shows signs of decreasing level of consciousness.	• Reassess to validate findings. • Notify healthcare provider of findings immediately.
• Head injury client with NG tube is having watery drainage from the nose.	• Report finding of rhinorrhea as it may indicate spinal fluid leakage and unrecognized basilar skull fracture. • Change to orogastric tube placement to allow fluid drainage and prevent infection. • Request drainage fluid analysis for chloride level to determine presence of CSF. • Allow fluid to drain freely onto a drip "mustache" dressing.
• Family of brain-dead organ donor has difficulty understanding why cardiac monitoring and mechanical ventilation are continued.	• Reinforce that the deceased client has been declared to be brain dead but donated organs are being maintained by supportive measures until time of removal.

Nursing Process Data

ASSESSMENT Database

- Identify signs and symptoms of increasing intracranial pressure.
- Relate signs of intracranial hypertension to rostrocaudal changes in levels of consciousness.
- Identify factors that increase, prevent, or manage intracranial hypertension.
- Recognize a normal intracranial pressure waveform.
- Assess indicators of pain in the nonverbal client.
- Utilize a variety of scales to assess a client's level of sedation.
- Monitor functioning and client response to ventricular CSF drainage.

PLANNING Objectives

- To identify early signs of increasing intracranial pressure in the neurologic client
- To differentiate a normal ICP waveform from one indicating decreased cranial compliance
- To provide care that prevents or manages increased ICP
- To respond to indicators of pain in the nonverbal client
- To provide adequate but minimal depth of sedation in the client with intracranial hypertension

IMPLEMENTATION Procedures

DOCUMENTATION AND EVALUATION

Expected Outcomes

- Signs and symptoms of increasing intracranial pressure are recognized.
- Factors that increase intracranial hypertension are identified.
- Client responds favorably to measures provided to prevent or manage intracranial hypertension.
- Microsensor displays client's intracranial pressure waveform.
- Client responses to pain management and sedation are evaluated.
- Ventriculostomy drains CSF appropriately to manage client's ICP.

Unexpected Outcomes/Alternative Actions

Pearson Nursing Student Resources

Find additional review materials at
nursing.pearsonhighered.com.
Prepare for success with NCLEX®-style practice questions and Skill Checklists.

Skill 32.2.1 | Recognizing Signs and Symptoms of Increasing Intracranial Pressure

Note: Some of these changes are subtle and may be confused with contextual factors (e.g., interpreting that client is drowsy from fatigue rather than an increasing intracranial pressure).

Preparation

1. Introduce self.
2. Perform hand hygiene.
3. Identify client using two client identifiers.

Procedure

1. Assess change in level of consciousness (LOC). ❶
   ➤ **Rationale:** Change in LOC is the most sensitive indicator of increasing ICP. Change may be sudden, dramatic, or very subtle (Box 32-5 ■).

> **CLINICAL ALERT**
>
> It is always best to rule on the side of caution and notify the attending healthcare provider of changes so that appropriate care decisions can be made.

2. Assess for headache. ➤ **Rationale:** Headache can be due to pressure on surrounding tissues, including the cerebral arteries, veins, and cranial nerves. Headache due to increased ICP worsens with activities that increase intrathoracic or intracranial pressure: coughing, straining, bearing down, and such.

3. Assess for vomiting. ➤ **Rationale:** Vomiting that is due to increased ICP typically occurs *without nausea*, is unexpected, is projectile, and is due to direct pressure on vagal motor centers located in the fourth ventricle in the medulla.

4. Assess for change in visual responses. ➤ **Rationale:** Altered responses of cranial nerves (II, III, IV, and VI) that are under pressure from brain swelling cause loss of visual acuity or eye movement. Altered pupillary (CN III) response, ipsilateral (same side) pupil dilation due to head injury, early sign of uncal herniation on side of injury, and altered level of consciousness may accompany or soon follow.

5. Assess for decrease in motor function. ➤ **Rationale:** Contralateral (opposite side) hemiparesis (weakness) and hemiplegia (paralysis) due to pressure increases in right and left hemispheres.

6. Assess for abnormal posturing that occurs due to noxious stimuli or spontaneously. ➤ **Rationale:** Decorticate (abnormal flexion) response indicates lesion above the brainstem (see Chapter 11, Physical Assessment, for description). Decerebrate (abnormal extension) response indicates brainstem lesion.

7. Assess for change in vital signs. ➤ **Rationale:** Change in vital signs can be due to increased pressure on thalamus, hypothalamus, pons, and medulla. Changes in respiratory pattern occur early. Cushing's triad: increasing systolic blood pressure, widened pulse pressure, and slow heart rate indicating medullary ischemia are late signs of decompensation.

> **CLINICAL ALERT**
>
> Cushing's triad (bradycardia, systolic hypertension, and widening pulse pressure) may indicate intracranial hypertension or herniation syndrome. The presence of any component calls for further assessment and intervention.
>
> ───────────────────
>
> Hyperventilation ($PaCO_2$, 25 mm Hg) was utilized in the past to manage increased ICP. A lowered $PaCO_2$ constricts cerebral arteries, and by the rules of the Monro-Kelly Doctrine, the ICP is lowered. This is used only briefly as a bridge to more appropriate therapy because constricting the cerebral arteries leads to ischemia, further damage, and edema.

❶ Central herniation differs: Deterioration of LOC precedes contralateral hemiparesis.

Note: Sensitivity to and ongoing communication with the neurologic client and family are important aspects of care. Help the family understand that a healing brain needs little stimulation (avoid constant hand-holding and stimuli such as television, limit visitation, and so on). Family members may experience an extreme feeling of powerlessness; the client's injury may result in disabilities that have far-reaching implications on family dynamics.

(continued)

Skill 32.2.1 | Recognizing Signs and Symptoms of Increasing Intracranial Pressure *(continued)*

Box 32-5 FACTORS THAT AFFECT INTRACRANIAL PRESSURE

Factors That Increase ICP (Goal Is 20 mm Hg)	Measures to Prevent or Manage Increased ICP
Nursing care activities	Note client's ICP response to various activities and organize activities and procedures to allow ICP to return to baseline. This could include clustering activities to allow for longer rest periods or spacing out activities.
Hypotension SBP ≤ 120 mm Hg *(Goal is 140–160 mm Hg.)* MAP < 85 mm Hg *(Goal is to support CPP > 60–70 mm Hg.)* CPP < 60 mm Hg *(Goal is >60–70 mm Hg.)*	Administer IV fluids, pressor agents (norepinephrine), osmotic diuretic, hypertonic saline, and CFS drainage if ICP is >20 mm Hg.
Hypoxemia *(Goal is SpO_2 > 90 mm Hg.)* Increased or decreased PCO_2 *(Goal is 35 mm Hg.)* Acidemia (low arterial blood pH) Ventilator dyssynchrony Noxious stimuli, emotional upset	Promote oxygenation: Monitor and maintain SpO_2, 90% with supplemental oxygen; determine whether desaturation occurs with a particular client position; maintain patent airway; suction prn. Monitor breath sounds for atelectasis or infiltration. Provide chest percussion therapy; obtain chest x-ray; consult respiratory care practitioner regarding client–ventilator harmony.
REM sleep	Manage pain: Assess for signs of pain in nonverbal client, provide analgesia, and provide sedation at lowest doses with daily interruption.
Factors that increase intrathoracic pressure and impede venous return from the brain: isometric muscle movement, Valsalva's maneuver coughing, vomiting, straining, neck or hip flexion, abnormal posturing, suctioning	Control environment: maintain calm, quiet room; minimize stimulation; limit visitation; avoid prolonged hand-holding; no television. Maintain positioning: head in neutral alignment without flexion or rotation. Head of bed (HOB) elevation 30 degrees if hemodynamically stable and CPP maintained; avoid hip flexion. Promote elimination: Administer stool softeners; initiate a bowel program.
Fever	Administer antiemetics, antipyretics; initiate early enteral nutrition. Provide prophylactic induced hypothermia for 48+ hr for traumatic brain injury; cooling blanket for increased temperature (avoid shivering).

EVIDENCE-BASED PRACTICE
ICP Monitoring
The high-tech world of the ICU has historically introduced technology before its effects on outcome could be studied. Intracranial pressure (ICP) monitoring has not been proven to clearly improve outcomes in all client populations in which it is utilized. Further testing of ICP versus CPP as treatment goals is another area for future research.

Source: Littlejohns & Bader (2009)

Skill 32.2.2 | Assisting Surgeon to Insert ICP Microsensor (Fiberoptic Transducer-Tipped Catheter)

Equipment
PPE: Sterile surgical gown, mask with face shield or eye protection, cap
Sterile gloves for surgeon and nurse
Sterile tray
Prepared medication for sedation, if ordered
Hair clippers
Cranial access kit with hand drill

1% or 2% lidocaine without epinephrine
3-mL syringe with 18-gauge needle for withdrawal
25-gauge needle for topical anesthetic injection
Chlorhexidine-based antimicrobial scrub or wipes
Scalpel with #11 blade
Sterile drape/towels
Clean gloves
Microsensor (fiberoptic transducer-tipped bolt catheter)

❶ ICP microsensor (fiberoptic catheter) senses changes in ICP. This system may be used to measure intraventricular parenchymal, subdural, or epidural pressure.

❷ Monitor displays digital readouts and pressure waveforms of the ECG, arterial BP, SPO₂ and calculated CPP (MAP – ICP = CCP).

External ICP microsensor monitor and monitoring cable to
   connect microprocessor to primary bedside monitor system ❷
Needle drivers
2.0 silk suture
Sterile 2×2 gauze
Sterile clear occlusive dressing
Permanent marker

Preparation

1. Validate that client's informed consent has been obtained.
2. Perform hand hygiene.
3. Check client's identification band and have client state name and birth date, if possible.
4. Explain rationale for procedure to client.
5. Validate that client has an established peripheral IV site.
   ➤ **Rationale:** This is for administration of emergency fluids or medication if needed.
6. Validate that client has established arterial blood pressure monitoring. ➤ **Rationale:** This is to determine the MAP, which is used along with the ICP to calculate cerebral perfusion pressure (CPP).
7. Prepare and assemble external monitoring system following manufacturer's instructions.
8. Raise the bed height to comfortable working position.
9. Don clean gloves.
10. Clip and save client's hair and scrub selected site with antimicrobial solution. ➤ **Rationale:** Client's hair should not be discarded, but should be returned to client or family.
11. Administer additional medication for sedation if ordered.

Procedure

1. Open sterile gloves and gown for surgeon.
2. Open sterile drape for surgeon.
3. Place cranial access kit, microsensor, and suturing materials on sterile tray within surgeon's reach.
4. Assist the surgeon to numb client's scalp.
5. Maintain cervical alignment while surgeon dissects the skin, drills the skull, and places microsensor. ❸

❸ Sites for ICP monitoring.

a. Before the microsensor is placed in the parenchyma, it must be zeroed. This can only be done once before the microsensor is placed and secured. ➤ **Rationale:** After insertion, there is no need for zero-referencing while the catheter is in use.
b. Surgeon submerges the end of the sensor in an aqueous solution that is inside the sterile field.
c. Zero the sensor by surgeon's request. The microsensor will give a reference number.
d. Document reference number on the transducer using a permanent marker. ➤ **Rationale:** This is used as reference if cables are disconnected for transport.
6. Don sterile gloves to assist surgeon as necessary.

(continued)

Skill 32.2.2 | Assisting Surgeon to Insert ICP Microsensor (Fiberoptic Transducer-Tipped Catheter)
(continued)

7. After insertion, surgeon sutures microsensor in place. (Microsensor can be inserted into the lateral ventricle, subarachnoid space, subdural space, brain parenchyma, or under a bone flap.)

> **CLINICAL ALERT**
> Increased intracranial pressure can decrease blood flow to the brain. Pressures within various locations in the cranium vary. The closer the ventricular catheter to the pathology, the higher the ICP and more accurate and reliable the reading.

8. Site is covered with clear occlusive dressing (2×2 gauze optional).
9. Hand external monitor cable to surgeon.

10. Connect the external monitor to a central monitoring system to verify that a waveform is present.
11. Record ICP and calculated CPP (MAP – ICP = CPP; Box 32-6 ■).
12. Discard disposable equipment.
13. Dispose of gloves and perform hand hygiene.

EVIDENCE-BASED PRACTICE
ICP and Chest Percussion
A study sample of 28 clients undergoing ICP monitoring demonstrated that mechanical chest percussion used to treat and prevent pneumonia does not increase intracranial pressure and can be performed safely on neurologically injured clients at risk for intracranial hypertension.

Source: Olson, Thoyre, Bennett, Stoner, & Graffagnino (2009)

Box 32-6 INTRACRANIAL PRESSURE WAVEFORMS

Intracranial pressure waveforms reflect transmission of arterial and venous pressure through cerebrospinal fluid and brain tissue. A normal ICP waveform has three pressure peaks:

P1 reflects myocardial systole (arterial blood flow).

P2 reflects myocardial diastole (drop in systolic blood flow) and coincides with the arterial dicrotic notch.

P3 follows the dicrotic notch (closure of the aortic valve) and correlates with venous pressure.

Intracranial pressure waveforms.

Increased P2 wave.

Note: P2 elevation greater than P1 (P2:P1 0.8) demonstrates an increase in intracranial pressure and loss of intracerebral compliance, especially when ICP is greater than 10 mm Hg. Frequent neurologic assessments are indicated. Changes in client status should be reported to the healthcare provider immediately.

Skill 32.2.3 | Monitoring Client Response to Sedation

Equipment
Sedation scales

Preparation
1. Introduce self and identify client using two forms of client identifier.
2. Perform hand hygiene.

Procedure
1. Consider nonpharmacologic interventions: (gentle touch, reassuring voice; frequent repositioning; use of distraction, music therapy, environmental control; use of complementary therapies such as massage) before sedation is initiated. ➤ *Rationale:* This may reduce or eliminate the need for sedation and muscle relaxation.
2. Select sedation scale to use for ongoing assessment and documentation of client response to pharmacologic intervention. ➤ *Rationale:* The selected scale should be used consistently and routinely by all caregivers.

   a. *Ramsay Sedation Scale* (goal 2–3) assesses rousability and is useful whenever sedative drugs or narcotics are administered, but cannot be used for the client receiving neuromuscular blocking drugs.

   b. *Riker Sedation–Agitation Scale* (goal 3–4) differs from the Ramsay Sedation Scale by defining degrees of agitation.

   c. *Richmond Agitation–Sedation Scale* (goal –2 to –3) distinguishes between responses to verbal and physical stimuli. This 10-level scale has confirmed validity and reliability for use in sedated and nonsedated clients.

   d. *AACN Sedation Assessment Scale* is most comprehensive, evaluating five domains: consciousness, agitation, anxiety, sleep, and client-ventilator synchrony.

CLINICAL ALERT
Most neurologic clients have normal lungs, but may require mechanical ventilation due to lack of airway protection (swallow, cough) secondary to neuronal injury, the secondary effects of increased ICP due to the primary injury or pathology, neurogenic pulmonary edema, a concomitant pulmonary process, or management with sedative medication. ICP and CPP can be adversely affected by positive pressure ventilation and must be monitored closely. Extubation should not be delayed solely on the basis of depressed neurologic function.

---

3. The Institute for Healthcare Improvement recommends "the use of dosing protocols and automatic dose reductions for benzodiazepines and other sedatives and hypnotics in target (e.g., ICU) populations." Daily sedation interruption is conducted to allow assessment of neurologic status.

EVIDENCE-BASED PRACTICE
Sedation Holiday
Intermittent lightening of sedation and daily interruption of sedation (withholding all sedative and analgesic medications until clients are awake) limits excessive sedation, reduces duration of mechanical ventilation and length of ICU stay, reduces the number of neurodiagnostic tests, and reduces frequency of complications associated with critical illness. This practice has benefits, but is underutilized due to a number of barriers that prevent its incorporation into clinical practice.

Source: Dotson (2010)

Skill 32.2.4 | Assisting Surgeon to Insert a Ventriculostomy Catheter

Note: ICP-lowering therapy is initiated with pressures above 20 mm Hg.

Equipment
PPE: sterile surgical gown, mask with face shield or eye protection, cap
Sterile gloves for surgeon and nurse
Clean gloves
Sterile tray
Hair clippers
Cranial access kit with hand drill
2% lidocaine with epinephrine (local anesthetic)
3-mL syringe with 18-gauge needle for withdrawal
25-gauge needle for topical anesthetic injection
Sedative to be administered if indicated
Chlorhexidine-based antimicrobial scrub or wipes
Sterile drape or towels
Twist drill and bits
Scalpel with #11 blade
Needle drivers
2.0 silk suture
Intraventricular catheter
Sterile 2×2 gauze (optional)
Sterile clear occlusive dressing
20-mL syringe filled with preservative-free sterile saline for flushing system
IV pole
CFS drainage system (collection tubing, chamber, and bag)
Transducer

(continued)

Skill 32.2.4 | Assisting Surgeon to Insert a Ventriculostomy Catheter *(continued)*

Preparation

1. Validate that client's informed consent has been obtained.
2. Perform hand hygiene.
3. Introduce self. Check client's identification band and have client state name and birth date, if possible.
4. Explain rationale for procedure to client (Box 32-7 ■).
5. Validate that client has an established peripheral IV site. ➤ *Rationale:* This is for administration of emergency fluids or medication if needed.
6. Prepare and assemble monitoring system (transducer and stopcocks) following manufacturer's instructions.
7. Level and zero monitoring system with air–fluid interface of zeroing stopcock level with client's foramen of Monro (level of client's **tragus**) or higher as determined by surgeon. ➤ *Rationale:* For accuracy, the same point should be used consistently for all ICP readings.

Note: The transducer must be releveled with any change in client's head position if continuous drainage is performed.

8. Remove tubing attached to an IV bag that establishes a pressurized flush system and discard.
9. Replace flush system with a 20-mL syringe filled with preservative-free sterile saline. ➤ *Rationale:* Preservatives added to medication vials are neurotoxic.
10. Flush all lumens and transducer with flush solution and leave syringe attached.
11. Raise bed to a comfortable working position.
12. Don clean gloves.
13. Clip and save client's hair. ➤ *Rationale:* Client's hair should be returned to client or family.
14. Scrub selected site with antimicrobial solution.
15. If applicable, administer additional medications for sedation.

Procedure

1. Open sterile gloves and gown for surgeon.
2. Open sterile drape for surgeon.
3. Place cranial access kit, ventriculostomy, and suturing materials on sterile tray within surgeon's reach.
4. Don sterile gloves to assist surgeon as necessary.
5. Assist surgeon to numb client's scalp.
6. Maintain cervical alignment while surgeon dissects the skin, drills the skull, and places ventriculostomy drain.
7. Surgeon caps the drain once it is in place.
8. Surgeon sutures drain in place and applies clear occlusive dressing (2×2 gauze optional).
9. Hand surgeon the primed line to the drainage system to attach it to the client.
10. Position drain as directed by the surgeon.
11. Calculate and record ICP/CPP readings hourly. ➤ *Rationale:* This is to determine adequate cerebral blood flow.
12. Return drain to open position for continuous drainage of excess CSF or open closed system intermittently to drain CSF when ICP exceeds set limits. ➤ *Rationale:* Reducing CSF volume improves cerebral perfusion.

> ### CLINICAL ALERT
> Never flush a ventriculostomy or lumbar drain toward the client. This would increase risk for infection. Additionally, instilling medications (including saline) is not within the scope of nursing practice.

13. Discard disposable equipment.
14. Dispose of gloves and perform hand hygiene.

Note: If leakage persists for 4–5 days, lumbar CSF drainage may be necessary to allow resolution of dural tear. (See Box 32-8 ■.)

Box 32-7 VENTRICULOSTOMY DRAINAGE SYSTEM

This external drainage system is used to intermittently or continuously drain CSF from the ventricles of the brain or the lumbar subarachnoid space to a drainage bag. System components facilitate CSF drainage, CSF sampling, and ICP monitoring.

Components of the system include:
- Closed sterile fluid path
- Height-adjustable, calibrated burette with stopcock that provides view of flow and clarity of the CSF, and allows reading volume of CSF before fluid enters the drainage bag
- Drainage bag with needleless sampling site
- Fluid-filled ICP monitoring transducer can be attached to the *red* capped port of the client stopcock at the zero reference position to show drainage pressure.

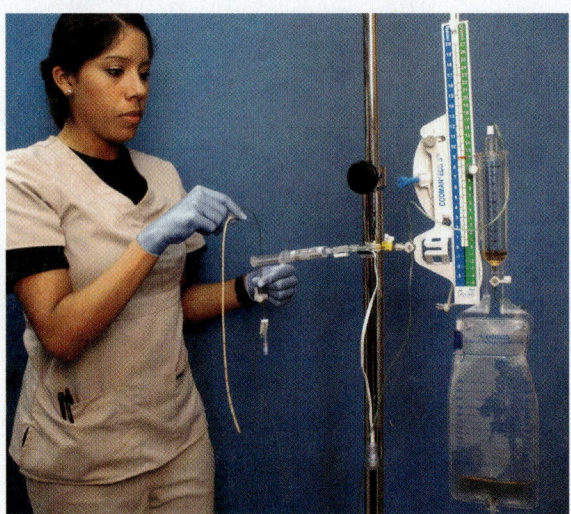

Ventriculostomy catheter: nurse with drainage system.

Box 32-8 **LUMBAR SUBARACHNOID CSF DRAINAGE**

Based on the same principles and setup as ventriculostomy drainage, lumbar puncture placement (L4–L5) of a catheter into the subarachnoid space may be performed to lower CSF pressure to allow a dural tear to heal (e.g., basilar fracture with otorrhea that persists 4–5 days).

1. The catheter is connected to a closed system to allow intermittent or continuous CSF drainage to divert CSF away from the site of the leak, lower CSF pressure, and allow the site to heal.

2. The zero reference point is the insertion site with the bed flat and client supine.

3. Drainage bag height is manipulated to drain the prescribed volume each hour (e.g., 10–20 mL/hr) based on CSF production of 20–30 mL/hr.

4. If the drainage bag is lowered, more CSF is drained.

5. The drain must be clamped if the client sits up.

Unit 32.2 Documentation and Evaluation

DOCUMENTATION for Intracranial Pressure Monitoring and Management

- Surgeon placing the microsensor or CSF drain (ventriculostomy)
- Location of microsensor or CSF drain placement
- Medications administered
- Client's tolerance of procedure
- Appearance of insertion site
- Dressing applied

- Client position during obtained measurements
- Obtained measurements: ICP and calculated CPP
- Amount and color of CSF drainage from ventriculostomy
- Appearance of the site, dressing, and length of monitoring and appearance of the drainage catheter insertion site
- Interventions used to manipulate ICP/CPP if indicated

EVALUATION/Critical Thinking

Expected Outcomes
- Signs and symptoms of increased intracranial pressure are recognized.
- Factors that increase intracranial hypertension are identified.
- Measures to prevent or manage intracranial hypertension are initiated.
- Microsensor displays intracranial pressure waveform.
- Client responses to pain management and sedation are evaluated.
- Ventriculostomy drains appropriately to manage client's ICP.

Unexpected Outcomes
- Client is very agitated with frequent nonpurposeful movements, despite increased frequency of sedative administration.

- Microsensor fails to display a waveform.

Alternative Actions
- Try to find a cause for the client's change in behavior.
- Attempt an analgesic trial to determine whether the client's pain is managed. This trial may be therapeutic as well as diagnostic.

- Verify that cable to the monitor and monitor cable are functioning appropriately and all connections are secure.
- Reassess length of microsensor exiting insertion site. If microsensor has migrated from the parenchyma, it will no longer give an appropriate waveform.

(continued)

Unexpected Outcomes	Alternative Actions
• Ventriculostomy drain shows a waveform but does not drain.	• Client may not have excess CSF that needs to be drained. Lower drain below the tragus until two to three drops of CSF are drained to ensure patency still remains. If patent, return drain to the ordered position. If no drops of CSF are released, notify the healthcare provider. • Do not strip tubing even if clots are visible. Stripping causes increased negative pressure and microbleeds and tears can occur.
• The ventriculostomy drain fails to display a waveform.	• The drain might be clotted; lower drain as directed above to verify patency. • Verify all clamps and stopcocks are positioned in an open to the monitor position. • Verify that the cable to the monitor and monitor cable are functioning appropriately and all connections are secure. • Reassess length of drain exiting the insertion site. If the drain has become dislodged from the ventricle, it will no longer give an appropriate waveform. In this instance, it is rare that there will still be drainage of excess CSF.
• Ventriculostomy drain insertion site dressing is damp.	• Inspect system for leaks. • Suspect CSF leak (test for glucose in fluid or chloride concentration if draining includes blood). • Apply new sterile occlusive dressing over insertion site. • Notify healthcare provider.
• Ventriculostomy drainage bag has sudden increase in CSF.	• Immediately check for inadvertent placement of bag below prescribed level; rapid drainage can cause ventricular collapse and intracerebral hemorrhage. • Immediately reposition drainage bag to appropriate level. • Discuss benefits of intermittent rather than continuous drainage.

Chapter Wrap-Up

GERONTOLOGIC Considerations

Neurologic Disorders Are the Most Common Cause of Disability in Older Adults

• While age-related changes do not follow a predictable course, normal neurologic system changes due to aging include:

Decreased brain size but no decline of intelligence with age

Alterations of thermoregulation (reduced heat production, increased heat loss)

Slower fine-motor movement

Diminished deep tendon and gag reflexes and vibratory sense

Reduced ability to respond to multiple stimuli

Slowed righting reflexes

Smaller pupil size

Reduced stage 3 and 4 sleep

Modest reduction in ability to learn new things

- The brain atrophies with age, leading to an increase in space between the skull and the brain and an increase in size of ventricles. This increased space can result in greater risk for cerebral contusions and cerebral vessel damage with acceleration–deceleration injuries. Damage can also be compounded if the client is taking an anticoagulant.

- Older clients are less likely to experience common symptoms of increased intracranial pressure (e.g., headache) and more likely to demonstrate mental status changes.
- Pathology of any organ system can precipitate neurologic dysfunction in an older client.
- As many as 60% of older hospitalized clients may experience delirium.
- Lethargy and confusion may be indications of infection in the older adult.

MANAGEMENT Guidelines

Each state legislates a Nurse Practice Act for RNs and LVN/LPNs. Healthcare facilities are responsible for establishing and implementing policies and procedures that conform to their state's regulations. Verify the regulations and role parameters for each healthcare worker in your facility.

Delegation

- All personnel in the critical care setting must know how to quickly summon assistance and locate and use emergency and resuscitation equipment.
- In advanced care settings, the RN simultaneously assesses, analyzes, makes decisions, intervenes, and evaluates clients on a continual basis. Complexities of care and unpredictability of outcomes necessitate *intense* ongoing client monitoring and evaluation and personal continuing education. Detection and interpretation of subtle areas of change in the client's status require the knowledge and skill of the professional nurse.
- Collaboration with the healthcare provider and respiratory care practitioner helps to support client's weaning from mechanical ventilation.
- The nurse should not assume care for any client who requires care beyond the caregiver's expertise.
- Many agencies provide emergency care protocols or standing orders of action responses to specified changes in client status. The professional nurse must be familiar with conditions for which the nurse is delegated medical care decisions guided by such protocols.
- It is the responsibility of nursing faculty to ensure that students participating in client care (in any setting) are prepared to do so. Likewise, it is the duty of the student to refuse to perform a function he or she is not qualified or competent to perform.
- The unlicensed assistive personnel (UAP) providing personal care for the neurologic client must space activities and maintain a controlled environment to prevent overstimulation and fatigue.

- The UAP must understand that continuous HOB elevation with the neck in neutral position is to be maintained for the neurologic client with external ventricular drainage, while the client with a lumbar drain remains supine with the bed flat.
- The UAP must know to leave an arterial catheter site uncovered for easy observation.
- The UAP must not move tubing drainage receptacles (e.g., ventriculostomy drip chamber).
- The UAP must understand that IVs, drainage systems, and ventilator circuits and systems are closed, and must be able to give care without disrupting system integrity or disconnecting components for the convenience of care (e.g., as in changing the client's gown or position).
- The UAP has a limited role in the care of clients who require invasive monitoring. The UAP can offer valued assistance in moving or positioning clients and providing personal hygiene and comfort measures under the direction of the professional nurse.
- The UAP assists the client, preserving an interface between technology and reality, by providing a human dimension of tactile presence while providing basic physical care for clients requiring sophisticated technological monitoring. This link assists all caregivers in their attempts to minimize client's feelings of alienation.

Interprofessional Communication

Although certain tasks may be delegated, the UAP also can provide vital data to the professional nurse by immediately *reporting*:

- Disconnected systems, loose electrodes, tubing leaks, wet or soiled dressings
- Subjective or objective change in the client's status (e.g., pain, restlessness, respiratory distress, acute change in **cognition**)
- Equipment alarms (e.g., ventilator alarms)
- Near-empty infusion bags
- Near-full collection devices

CASE STUDY Applications

Scenario 1

A 27-year-old male has been admitted to the neurotrauma ICU after surgical evacuation of a right parietal epidural hematoma that occurred secondary to a linear skull fracture sustained in a motorcycle injury.

1. Where does an epidural bleed occur and what is the typical source of bleeding?
2. How does an epidural hematoma differ from a subdural hematoma?
3. What behaviors or deficits might occur with injury to the right parietal lobe?
4. What signs would indicate uncal herniation due to increasing intracranial pressure?
5. List five nursing interventions that can help prevent increased intracranial pressure.

Scenario 2

A young man has been admitted to the trauma unit after evaluation in the emergency department (ED) and repair of a scalp laceration sustained when he was struck in the back of the head with a baseball. No cervical spine injury, internal injury, or skull fracture was identified. He had no motor or sensory deficits. Ongoing observation and neurologic assessments were indicated since the client had experienced a brief loss of consciousness and continued to have vertigo, irritability, and nausea. His Glasgow Coma Score was 13.

At 0400 the nurse awakened him for vital signs and neuro assessment and noticed a bloody stain circled by yellow discoloration on his pillowcase. It had apparently come from his ear. Drainage from the ear (otorrhea) typically results from head injury involving basal skull fracture.

1. Why was the diagnosis of basilar skull fracture missed on initial evaluation in the ED?
2. How can it be determined that the drainage includes CSF?
3. What is the major potential complication of CSF leakage?
4. How should the client be positioned?
5. How should the drainage be managed?
6. What is the typical medical management if CSF leakage persists?
7. Compare the principles of lumbar drainage and external ventricular drainage.
8. Contrast the care of a client with a lumbar drain versus one with a ventriculostomy.

NCLEX® Review Questions

Unless otherwise specified, choose only one (1) answer.

1. What cerebral perfusion pressure would a client with a blood pressure of 130/80 and an intracranial pressure of 12 mm Hg have?
   A. 65
   B. 80
   C. 85
   D. 97

2. The nurse caring for a neurologic client obtains an ICP reading of 12 mm Hg. What does this reading reflect?
   A. A severe decrease in cerebral perfusion pressure
   B. A marked decrease in the CSF production
   C. Normal balance of brain, blood, and CSF
   D. A malfunction of autoregulation

3. A client has been admitted to the hospital with a suspected brain tumor. The family members report him being hateful, having outbursts of cursing, and right-sided hemiparesis. What area of the brain do these behaviors indicate the tumor is affecting?
   A. Frontal lobe
   B. Parietal lobe
   C. Occipital lobe
   D. Temporal lobe

4. Metabolic causes of coma can be differentiated from structural causes. What characterizes metabolic causes of coma?
   A. Rostrocaudal deterioration
   B. Asymmetric motor deficits
   C. Motor deficits preceding coma
   D. Preserved pupil reflexes

5. What factor leads to cerebral vasodilation and increased intracranial pressure?
   A. Hypocapnea (low PCO_2)
   B. Alkalemia (low blood pH)
   C. Hypoxemia (low blood O_2)
   D. Hypothermia

6. What is expected to accompany pressure on the midbrain?
   A. Loss of gag reflex
   B. Loss of pupil response
   C. Widening pulse pressure
   D. Loss of blink reflex

7. What is the most sensitive indicator of increasing intracranial pressure?
   A. Altered level of consciousness
   B. Change in respiratory pattern
   C. Lack of pupil response to light stimulus
   D. Increase in blood pressure with slowed heart rate

8. A ventriculostomy is the most reliable system used to monitor intracranial pressure. What does this method include?

   A. A subarachnoid bolt or screw

   B. An intraventricular catheter with external drainage system and transducer

   C. An intraparenchymal fiberoptic transducer-tipped catheter

   D. A subdural or epidural catheter

9. ICP monitoring provides guidance in managing ICP elevations and hemodynamic status. What characterizes normal intracranial pulse waveforms?

   A. P-2 waveform greater than P-1 and P-3

   B. All waveforms of equal elevation

   C. P-3 waveform greater than P-1 and P-2

   D. P-1 waveform greater than P-2 and P-3

10. The following ancillary tests are used to confirm brain death.

    Select all that apply.

    A. Spinal fluid analysis

    B. Cold caloric test

    C. EEG

    D. Cerebral angiography

    E. MRI/MRA

    F. Brainstem reflexes

    G. Deep tendon reflexes

QSEN Activity

Domain: Patient-Centered Care

KSA: Acknowledge the tension that may exist between client rights and the organizational responsibility for professional, ethical care. Participate in building consensus or resolving conflict in the context of client care.

Activity:

You are the nurse caring for a client who was in an motor vehicle crash and sustained a significant head injury. You have just completed the brain death protocol and the client is declared legally brain dead. The client had indicated on his driver's license that he wished to be an organ donor. You are making preparations for this finding as his family arrives. They are very upset. They were unaware of his request to be an organ donor. They are opposed to his wishes and demand the process be stopped.

How should you handle this situation?

What are your legal and ethical responsibilities?

Bibliography

American Association of Critical-Care Nurses. (2008). *American Journal of Critical Care.*

American Heart Association. *Heart Disease and Stroke Statistics.* (2013 Update). Dallas, Texas: American Heart Association.

American Heart Association/American Stroke Association. (2015). Spot a stroke. Retrieved from http://www.strokeassociation. org/STROKEORG/WarningSigns/Stroke-Warning-Signs-and-Symptoms_UCM_308528_SubHomePage.jsp

Caloric stimulation. (2013). Retrieved from http://www.nlm.nih.gov/medlineplus/ency/article/003429.htm

Centers for Disease Control and Prevention. (2015). Leading causes of death. Retrieved from http://www.cdc.gov/nchs/fastats/leading-causes-of-death.htm

Dotson, B. (2010). Daily interruption of sedation in patients treated with mechanical ventilation. *American Journal of Health-System Pharmacy, 67*(12), 102–1006.

Eelco F. M., Wijdicks, E. F. M., Varelas, P. N., Gronseth, G. S., & Greer, D. M. (2010, Jun.). Evidence-based guideline update: Determining brain death in adults. Report of the Quality Standards Subcommittee of the American Academy of Neurology. *Neurology, 74:* 1911–1918.

Elevated intracranial pressure. (2013). Retrieved from http://www.uptodate.com/contents/evaluation-and-management-of-elevated-intracranial-pressure-in-adults#H30

Eliopoulos, C. (2009). *Gerontological nursing* (7th ed.). Philadelphia: Lippincott Williams & Wilkins.

Fields, L. B. (2008). Oral care intervention to reduce incidence of ventilator-associated pneumonia in the neurologic intensive care unit. *Journal of Neuroscience Nursing, 40*(5), 291–298.

Gusa, D., Miers, A., & Wkjdicks, E. (2007). More than meets the eye: The FOUR score is a new tool for assessing coma that won't miss locked-in syndrome. *RNWEB.com*, 43–47.

Littlejohns, L. R. & Bader, M. K. (2009). AACN/AANN protocols for practice: Monitoring technologies in critically ill neuroscience patients. Sudbury, MA: Jones and Bartlett.

McNett, M. M. & Olson, D. M. (2013). Evidence to guide nursing interventions for critically ill neurologically impaired patients with ICP monitoring. *Journal of Neuroscience Nursing, 45*(3), 120–123.

Miniño, A. M., Xu, J., & Kochanek, K. (2010) Deaths: Preliminary data for 2008. *National Vital Statistics Reports 59*, 2.

Olson, D. M., Thoyre, S. M., Bennett, S. N., Stoner, J. B., & Graffagnino, C. (2009). Effect of mechanical chest percussion on intracranial pressure: A pilot study. *American Journal of Critical Care, 18*(4), 330–335.

Prendergast, V., Hallberg, I., Jahnke, H., Kleiman, C., & Hagell, P. (2009). Oral health, ventilator-associated pneumonia, and intracranial pressure in intubated patients in a neuroscience intensive care unit. *American Journal of Critical Care, 18*(4), 368–376.

Wijdicks, E. F., Varelas, P. N., Gronseth, G. S., Greer, D. M., & American Academy of Neurology. (2010). Evidence-based guideline update: Determining brain death in adults: Report of the Quality Standards Subcommittee of the American Academy of Neurology. *Neurology, 74*(23), 1911–1918.

Ziegler, T. (2009). Parenteral nutrition in the critically ill patient. *New England Journal of Medicine, 361*, 11.

Chapter 33
Advanced Nursing Skills

 Learning Objectives

33.1 List hemodynamic information obtained by means of a pulmonary artery (balloon-tipped flow-directed) catheter.

33.2 Discuss the purpose and method for leveling and zeroing the monitor.

33.3 Differentiate waveforms for pulmonary artery and pulmonary capillary wedge pressures.

33.4 State three ways to troubleshoot pulmonary artery catheter problems.

33.5 Describe the rationale for arterial blood pressure monitoring.

33.6 Outline the steps in performing the Modified Allen test.

33.7 Identify a normal arterial blood pressure waveform.

33.8 Explain the procedure for obtaining a blood sample from an arterial line.

33.9 Outline safety precautions for the client with an arterial line.

33.10 Explain how the intra-aortic balloon pump assists cardiac function.

33.11 Describe nursing responsibilities in anticipating and responding to cardiac emergencies.

33.12 Ensure client and staff safety during electrical counter-shock procedures.

33.13 Differentiate various ventilator support "modes."

33.14 Discuss nursing care needs of the mechanically ventilated client.

33.15 Describe the process of weaning a client from mechanical ventilation to independent breathing.

Chapter Outline

Terminology

Afterload resistance against which the heart must pump to eject blood during systole. Pulmonary vascular resistance (PVR) presents afterload to the right heart; systemic vascular resistance (SVR) presents afterload to the left heart.

Barotrauma alveolar injury and air leak due to positive pressure mechanical ventilation.

Blood conservatory process blood sampling process that requires no blood wasting.

Bolus rapid administration of a volume of fluid or a drug intravenously.

Calibrate to check or adjust equipment, such as a transducer, to its standard measurement.

Cannulation insertion of a tube into a blood vessel for purposes of invasive pressure monitoring. The cannula is attached to a transducer, which in turn converts the pressure to a monitored waveform display.

Cardiac index (CI) the cardiac output in relation to a client's body surface area.

Cardiac output (CO) amount of blood ejected by the heart per minute. Determined by multiplying heart rate by stroke volume ($HR \times SV = CO$).

Central venous pressure (CVP) reflects filling pressure of the right heart; measures central preload.

Defibrillation process used for two lethal arrhythmias to restore heart rhythm: pulseless ventricular tachycardia, and ventricular fibrillation.

Diastole period when ventricles are relaxed; a period of ventricular filling and coronary artery perfusion.

Dicrotic notch component of the arterial waveform that represents closure of aortic valve at the end of ventricular contraction (systole).

Diffusion movement of a gas from an area of high pressure to an area of lower pressure.

Distal area farthest away from point of reference (fingers are most distal part of upper extremity; cannulated catheter tip is most distal).

Dysrhythmia abnormality of heart rate or rhythm.

ECC emergency cardiovascular care.

Electrocardiogram (ECG) graphic representation of the variations in electrical potential caused by depolarization of the heart muscles.

Electrode (in electrocardiography) a wire with an adhesive patch applied to the skin to transmit cardiac electrical activity to a machine for display.

Hemodynamic movement of blood.

Hypercarbia increased pCO_2 on ABGs.

Invasive (in medicine) involving puncturing or incising the skin for insertion of a tube or instrument into the body.

Left ventricular end-diastolic pressure (LVEDP) pressure of blood in the left ventricle at the end of diastole; a measure of left ventricular preload.

Lumen (in nursing) the inside, channel, or opening of a blood vessel or tube.

Mean arterial (blood) pressure (MAP) average pressure within the cardiovascular system throughout one cardiac cycle. Determined by adding systolic pressure to two times the diastolic pressure and dividing the sum by three.

Mixed venous oxygen saturation (SvO$_2$) hemoglobin saturation of RBCs measured in the pulmonary artery.

Modified Allen test manual test to determine patency of the ulnar or radial artery. Digital pressure is applied directly over the radial and ulnar arteries. When pressure on one vessel is released, blood flow to palm and fingers indicates obstruction is not present in that vessel.

Oscilloscope instrument that displays a visual representation of electrical activity on a monitor screen.

Perfusion blood flow to tissues.

Phlebostatic axis the crossing of two reference lines to determine the point at which the zero mark on manometer is level with this axis.

Preload (in medicine) a measure of venous return; end-diastolic filling pressure (stretch) in the ventricles.

Proximal refers to an area closest to the point of reference; humerus of upper extremity is more *proximal* to the body than the fingers.

Pulmonary artery pressure (PAP) waveform representing systolic and diastolic pressures in the pulmonary artery, usually displayed by hemodynamic monitoring. Pulmonary artery diastolic pressure is often used as equivalent to pulmonary artery wedge pressure.

Pulmonary artery wedge pressure (PAWP) also referred to as pulmonary artery occlusive pressure, or PAOP, an indirect indicator of left ventricular pressure—normal PAWP is 8 to 13 mm Hg. Elevations are seen in left ventricular failure.

Surfactant a phospholipid synthesized by the lungs that lowers alveolar tension and increases lung compliance.

Synchronized cardioversion process used to convert supraventricular tachyarrhythmias and ventricular tachycardia (with pulses) if the client shows serious signs of hemodynamic instability (e.g., ventricular rate ≥150, SBP <90 mm Hg).

Thermodilution method of calculating cardiac output by injection of solution into the proximal lumen of a pulmonary artery catheter and determining the solution's temperature change at the thermistor (distal) lumen of the catheter.

Transducer device that converts one form of energy into another (e.g., biophysical event is converted into electrical waveform, which is displayed on the oscilloscope).

Vasculature vascular system of the body.

Vasodilator causes dilation of the blood vessels. A venodilator reduces preload; an arterial vasodilator reduces afterload.

Vasopressor an agent used to increase blood pressure by constricting blood vessels.

Ventricular systole contraction phase of the cardiac cycle during which the ventricles eject blood into receiving arteries.

Volutrauma iatrogenic alveolar injury due to large tidal volumes delivered by mechanical ventilation.

Waveform pictorial representation of a pressure or electrical activity of the heart, depicted on an oscilloscope.

Weaning gradual withdrawal of mechanical ventilation and the reestablishment of spontaneous breathing.

Advanced Skills in Nursing Practice

This chapter presents a nursing process framework for nursing actions used in the maintenance of homeostasis during life-threatening conditions. Provision of competent care during critical periods requires a knowledge of physiologic monitoring techniques, skill in the analysis of data, diagnostic reasoning, and decision making. Working with monitors and providing client care at the same time can be a challenging experience for the nurse.

Monitoring techniques are useful adjunctive tools that provide the practitioner with critical information for management of select clients in intensive care settings. Interpretation and integration of this information assists in the assessment of major body systems and recognition of altered **hemodynamic** states (e.g., fluid deficit or fluid overload). Continuous surveillance of cardiovascular pressure readings and other dynamic measures serves as a guide for identifying appropriate nursing diagnoses, developing a plan of care, and evaluating the client's response to therapy.

In the clinical setting, nurses are constantly faced with new equipment, new techniques, and better and more sophisticated evaluative methods (Figure 33-1 ■). To keep pace in the area of technologic advancement can be a monumental task, one that challenges the nurse's energy, patience, and abilities. The nurse's role in assessment, planning, intervention, and evaluation is based, in part, on the nurse's familiarity with monitoring data.

FIGURE 33-1 Sophisticated technology facilitates the intensive care of clients.

Hemodynamic monitoring has evolved over the years from continuous ECG monitoring, to measuring CVP (right heart pressure), to direct determination of **cardiac output**, and indirect measurements of left heart filling pressures.

Hemodynamic monitoring techniques require that equipment be properly positioned and function correctly and that the monitor **waveforms** be representative of the client's physiologic variables and be interpreted correctly.

A multi**lumen**, balloon-tipped, flow-directed catheter (e.g., Swan-Ganz VIP) is used to measure intracardiac pressures. Individual lumens reflect measures of right atrial pressure (RAP or CVP), **pulmonary artery pressure** (PAP), and, when advanced briefly to an occlusive position, **pulmonary artery wedge pressure** (PAWP). Cardiac output (CO), systemic and pulmonary vascular resistance (SVR, PVR), and **mixed venous oxygen saturation** (SvO_2) are other valuable measures obtained with this catheter. It is simultaneously used for the infusion of fluids and medications. Placement of the catheter is verified by chest x-ray. These technologies are still considered the gold standard of monitoring. However, less **invasive** monitoring techniques, such as esophageal Doppler systems and bioimpedance systems, are currently being introduced (Vincent et al., 2011).

Waveforms (pressure signals) are transmitted from the catheter to a **transducer** by means of fluid-filled tubing (Figure 33-1). The signal is then amplified and displayed on an **oscilloscope** both as a visual (analog) waveform and a digital display. The client's physiologic pressure signals provide continuous data to help specialized nurses make critical assessments necessary for safe and effective care decisions, such as the titration of drugs and IV fluids.

Similarly, a catheter can be placed in a peripheral artery and direct blood pressure can be monitored continuously using these same principles. Therapeutically, arterial blood pressure signals can be used to trigger timing of counter-pulsation circulatory assistance (intra-aortic balloon pump) in clients with compromised cardiac output, while the client's pulmonary artery catheter hemodynamic information is used to evaluate the effectiveness of intra-aortic balloon pump (IABP) therapy. This is an example of the complementary power of technology and its value as an integrated aspect of care for clients receiving intensive care (Box 33-1 ■).

The ability to integrate all available data is essential to providing excellent nursing care. While advanced technology provides essential measures that augment more overt client data, it is important that this technology not become more important than the client. The first goal is to care for the client, not to tend the equipment. One way to achieve a balance of mastery over complex skills and the

---

Box 33-1 **INTRA-AORTIC BALLOON PUMP (IABP) CIRCULATORY ASSIST DEVICE**

An example of integrative technology is the intra-aortic balloon pump (IABP), which incorporates both hemodynamic and arterial blood pressure monitoring information. The IABP provides indirect short-term circulatory assistance for clients with compromised cardiac function due to myocardial infarction with complications, temporary left ventricular failure, cardiac injury, septic shock, or those awaiting cardiac transplantation. The goals are to decrease heart work, reduce **afterload**, improve cardiac output, enhance coronary and peripheral **perfusion**, and ultimately reduce **preload**.

The balloon catheter is inserted percutaneously into the descending aorta via the femoral artery and advanced proximally so that the balloon is positioned just below the left subclavian artery, yet above the renal artery.

The vacuum pump cyclically drives helium to inflate and deflate the balloon. Performing on the principle of counterpulsation, the catheter balloon inflates at the onset of **diastole**, enhancing perfusion and oxygen delivery to tissues antegrade and to the coronary arteries retrograde. The balloon deflates just before systole, creating a relatively negative suction effect, thereby reducing afterload and supporting ventricular ejection and antegrade blood flow.

---

attainment of high-quality client care is to become familiar with technical equipment so that it no longer causes anxiety and uncertainty. Once this level of confidence is realized, the focus is on the client, rather than the monitoring equipment.

Cultural Awareness

Some cultures view critical illness as a curse, an imbalance of heat and cold, or disharmony with the universe rather than pathology or injury to an organ system. Western medicine's healthcare system utilizes much technology and sophisticated equipment. This approach may clash with another culture's beliefs in folk medicine, rituals, and religious healing.

Individuals of the same culture will vary in response to critical illness; therefore, the nurse must explore the meaning of the experience with each individual client in order to provide sensitive care.

Nursing Diagnoses

The following nursing diagnoses may be appropriate to include in a client care plan when the components are related to advanced nursing skills.

NURSING DIAGNOSIS	RELATED TO . . .
Aspiration, Risk for	Presence of tracheostomy or endotracheal tube Incompetent lower esophageal sphincter Gastrointestinal tube Tube feedings Increased gastric residual
Ineffective Breathing Pattern	Decreased minute volume Decreased vital capacity Bradypnea (respiratory rate <11) Tachypnea (respiratory rate >24)
Decreased Cardiac Output	Altered heart rate or rhythm Altered preload (increased or decreased intracardiac pressures) Altered afterload (increased or decreased systemic or pulmonary vascular resistance) Altered contractility (low stroke volume cardiac output/cardiac index)
Impaired Verbal Communication	Physical barrier (tracheostomy, intubation) Medications Lack of information
Impaired Gas Exchange	Alveolar-capillary membrane changes (barotrauma, volutrauma) Ventilation-perfusion mismatch
Infection, Risk for	Inadequate primary defenses (broken skin, decreased ciliary action, altered pH secretions, altered peristalsis) Invasive procedures Pharmaceutical agents Trauma
Imbalanced Nutrition: Less Than Body Requirements	Inability to ingest food (e.g., presence of endotracheal tube, NPO status) Difficulty chewing or swallowing Hypermetabolic state
Powerlessness	Healthcare environment Illness-related regimen Chronic or terminal illness Impaired ability to communicate
Impaired Spontaneous Ventilation	Metabolic factors Respiratory muscle fatigue
Ineffective Peripheral Tissue Perfusion	Hypovolemia Shock (hypovolemic, cardiogenic, distributive) Decreased cardiac output Peripheral vascular disease
Dysfunctional Ventilatory Weaning Response	Inadequate nutrition Sleep pattern disturbance Ventilatory muscle atrophy/neuromuscular decline Inadequate pain management Oversedation without periodic interruption Anxiety or fear Inadequate preparation for weaning process

Source: Herdman, T. H. & Kamitsuru, S. (Eds.) *Nursing Diagnoses – Definitions and Classification 2015-2017*. Copyright © 2014, 1994–2014 by NANDA International. Used by arrangement with John Wiley & Sons Limited. Companion website: www.wiley.com/go/nursingdiagnoses. In order to make safe and effective judgments using NANDA-I nursing diagnosis it is essential that nurses refer to the definitions and defining characteristics of the diagnoses listed in this work.

Nursing Process Data

ASSESSMENT Database

- Determine purpose of hemodynamic monitoring and significance of data obtained.
- Evaluate client's understanding of the procedure.
- Assess for preexisting cardiovascular disease.
- Obtain baseline pulmonary, cardiovascular, hemodynamic, peripheral vascular, neurologic findings.
- Assess insertion site for inflammation or infection.
- Assess patency of all lines.
- Determine pressure on saline flush bag.
- Level and zero the monitoring system.
- Monitor PA systolic, PA diastolic, PA mean, and PAWP.
- Note any laboratory data abnormalities.
- Assess cardiac output using thermodilution technique.

PLANNING Objectives

- To maintain a patent pulmonary artery monitoring system
- To administer intravenous solutions and determine response to fluid therapy
- To obtain specific hemodynamic measurements for decision making
- To measure cardiac output

IMPLEMENTATION Procedures

DOCUMENTATION AND EVALUATION

Expected Outcomes

- Pulmonary artery catheter remains patent.
- Pulmonary artery, systolic, diastolic, and pulmonary artery wedge pressure measurements are measured accurately.
- Cardiac output measurements are obtained.
- Intra-aortic balloon pump circulatory assist improves cardiac output: afterload and preload are reduced.

Unexpected Outcomes/Alternative Actions

Pearson Nursing Student Resources

Find additional review materials at
nursing.pearsonhighered.com.
Prepare for success with NCLEX®-style practice questions and Skill Checklists.

Tissue oxygen consumption depends on cardiac pump performance, adequate blood volume, arterial oxygen content, and vascular distribution (perfusion). Hypovolemia, heart failure, or other conditions (e.g., sepsis) alter intracardiac pressures, tissue perfusion, and tissue oxygen consumption. Since direct measurement of left heart chamber pressures is not possible in the clinical setting, an indication of these measures is obtained by *indirect* means via the right side of the heart (Table 33-1 ■).

A balloon-tipped, flow-directed catheter (Figure 33-2 ■) is inserted into a central vein percutaneously or through a cut-down and advanced *transvenously* to the right atrium. Partial inflation of the balloon at the tip of the catheter allows the catheter to float through the tricuspid valve, the

right ventricle, and the pulmonary valve into the pulmonary artery (Figure 33-3 ■). Here the balloon is *deflated* and PAP is monitored, permitting continuous *indirect* measurement of left ventricular function for monitoring and assisting care of hemodynamically unstable clients (Figure 33-4 ■). Abnormal pressures can indicate changes in a client's fluid balance, heart pumping action, or vascular tone.

The pulmonary artery catheter typically has four or five lumens. Two lumens are used for pressure measurements. The **proximal** lumen is used to measure **central venous pressure** (CVP), assist in measuring cardiac output, and to inject selected solutions. The **distal** lumen is used to measure PAP and pulmonary artery wedge pressure (PAWP/PAOP). The third lumen is used for balloon inflation. The fourth lumen is attached to a thermistor tip that assists in the measurement of cardiac output and blood (core) temperature.

At the end of diastole (ventricular filling), the mitral valve is open, and the left ventricle, left atrium, and pulmonary **vasculature** momentarily act as a single chamber in which the pressure is equal throughout. Since the normal pressures of these chambers and vessels are known, pressure changes in the pulmonary artery can be used to reflect changes in **left ventricular end-diastolic pressure** (LVEDP). Reduced cardiac function is manifested primarily by two hemodynamic abnormalities: decreased cardiac output (or **cardiac index**) and increased LVEDP. The pulmonary artery catheter indirectly measures the LVEDP by directly measuring pulmonary artery and pulmonary artery wedge pressures.

If pulmonary artery wedge pressure measurement is required, the balloon is *briefly* inflated and the catheter is carried by blood flow through the pulmonary circulation until it "wedges." During this brief occlusion (wedge) time, pressure reflected back on the tip of the catheter allows indirect measurement of LVEDP. The balloon is then deflated passively and floats back to the pulmonary artery.

Table 33-1 Normal Pressures

Right atrial (RAP): 2–8 mm Hg

Right ventricle (RV): $\dfrac{25}{5}$ mm Hg

Pulmonary artery pressure (PAP): $\dfrac{25}{5}$ mm Hg

PA mean : $\overline{(\text{PA})}$ less than 15 mm Hg

PAWP/PAOP: 10

Left atrial (LA): 5–10 mm Hg

Left ventricle (LV): $\dfrac{130}{5\text{--}10}$ mm Hg

Aorta: $\dfrac{130}{80}$

Mean arterial pressure (MAP):

77–90 (Diastolic × 2) + (Systolic × 1), ÷ 3

or $\dfrac{(\text{SBP}) + 2(\text{DBP})}{3}$

FIGURE 33-2 Balloon-tipped, flow-directed catheter with balloon inflated briefly for pulmonary artery wedge (occlusion) pressure determination.

FIGURE 33-3 Balloon-tipped catheter has multiple lumens (internal tubes) with openings used to measure intracardiac pressures.

FIGURE 33-4 Pulmonary artery catheter provides intracardiac pressure measurements—used to derive multiple cardiac function indices.

To calculate cardiac output, a **bolus** of cold or room temperature fluid is injected into the right atrial lumen. The fluid's temperature change is then detected in the pulmonary artery by the catheter-tip thermistor. The temperature change over time is computed and represents the cardiac output. Finally, mixed venous blood oxygen saturation monitoring using a fiberoptic pulmonary artery catheter provides information about the balance between tissue oxygen delivery and tissue oxygen consumption (SvO_2), which is particularly valuable for monitoring clients with sepsis (Boxes 33-2 and 33-3 ■).

Data derived from physiologic monitoring have diagnostic and therapeutic value in the care of select critically ill (hemodynamically unstable) clients.

Box 33-2 HEMODYNAMIC MONITORING SYSTEM COMPONENTS

- **Invasive catheter** with high-pressure tubing connected to transducer
- **Flush/infusion system,** with pressure bag at 300 mm Hg, maintains patency of system.
- **Transducer**—converts physiologic wave to electrical energy.
- **Monitor**—converts electrical energy, displays pressure waveform and digital reading in mm Hg.

Box 33-3 MIXED CENTRAL VENOUS OXYGEN SATURATION (SvO_2) MONITORING

The SvO_2 reflects a dynamic relationship between tissue oxygen delivery and tissue oxygen consumption, providing an indication of overall oxygen balance. This value has diagnostic, prognostic, and therapeutic value in the care of critically ill clients, particularly those with acute MI, heart failure, and cardiogenic, hypovolemic, or septic shock.

A fiberoptic pulmonary artery catheter analyzes light absorption reflecting RBC hemoglobin saturation (similar to a pulse oximeter). An oximeter computer with microprocessor converts this information into an electrical display (graphic trend, numeric display, or both) for continuous monitoring. Since analysis occurs in the pulmonary artery, the value reflects a measurement of overall venous oxygen saturation, reflecting oxygen consumption at the tissue level. Whereas arterial oxygen content (SaO_2) is 100%, a normal

SvO_2 value is 70–80%. Clinically significant changes in SvO_2 (±5–10%) can be an early indicator of physiologic instability.

Low SvO_2 may be due to inadequate oxygen delivery caused by decreased cardiac output (increased heart rate or decreased stroke volume), reduced hemoglobin, low oxygen saturation, or excess tissue extraction of oxygen (e.g., due to pain or nursing procedures). Management will focus on optimizing preload, afterload, cardiac contractility, oxygen delivery, and increasing blood hemoglobin with transfusion. Adaptations in nursing care can reduce the client's oxygen requirement and utilization.

High SvO_2 occurs with low tissue extraction of oxygen, as seen in clients who are sedated, or may indicate hyperdynamic blood flow or tissue inability to utilize oxygen delivered, as occurs in sepsis.

Skill 33.1.1 | Leveling and Zeroing the Monitor System

Preparation

1. Introduce self.
2. Gather equipment.
3. Identify client using two client identifiers.

Procedure

1. Perform hand hygiene.
2. Reassure client and explain what you are doing.
3. **Calibrate** system.

   a. Using carpenter's level, adjust height of transducer to level of client's atrium or **phlebostatic axis.** ❶
      ➤ *Rationale:* Transducer must remain level with client's right atrium for accurate monitoring. Higher transducer position yields low readings and vice versa.

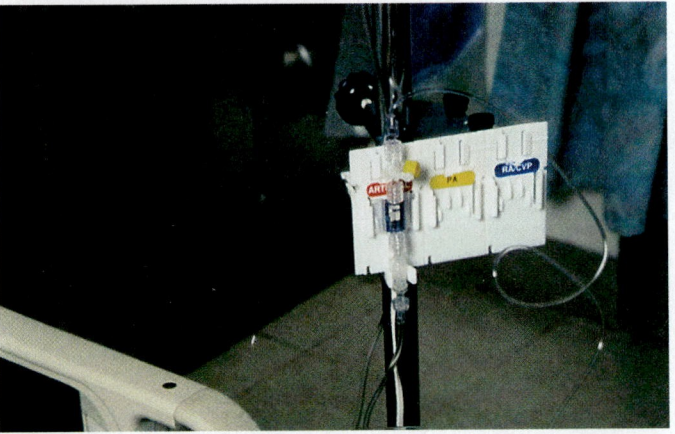

❶ Adjust height of transducer to level of client's phlebostatic axis.

> **CLINICAL ALERT**
> Level the air–fluid interface stopcock (on top of the transducer) to client's phlebostatic axis (intersection of lines at mid-anterior–posterior chest and fourth ICS) any time the bed or client's position is changed and per unit protocol.

   b. To zero monitor, remove port cap (maintain sterility), open stopcock above transducer to air, closing it to the client and the flush system. ➤ *Rationale:* This action opens transducer to atmospheric pressure.

   c. Push the "zero" monitor button, and check if monitor reading is zero. ➤ *Rationale:* When reading is zero, transducer is balanced to atmospheric pressure (actually 760 mm Hg).
4. Check that monitor shows a flat wave at zero line.
   ➤ *Rationale:* This ensures accurate reading as it changes from zero point.
5. Recap port and close stopcock to reestablish flush system.

Skill 33.1.2 | Assisting Physician With Catheter Insertion

Equipment

Sterile gloves
Percutaneous introducer kit
IV pole
Premix flush solution (usually 500 mL of normal saline) IV tubing
Pressure transducer system with pressure bag, tubing, flush device, and transducer
Pressure monitor
Clean gloves
Sterile towels
Antiseptic solution (2% chlorhexidine)
Sterile 4×4 sponges
Stethoscope
Lidocaine 1–2%
3-mL syringe with 18- and 25-gauge needle for topical anesthetic
Antimicrobial wipes
Occlusive dressing or tape
Suture with attached needle
Sterile needle holder or clamp
Cutdown tray, sterile gown, mask, and cap
Emergency cart
Sterile syringes filled with 5 or 10 mL of normal saline (cardiac output)

Preparation

1. Validate that client's informed consent has been obtained.
2. Introduce self and identify client using two client identifiers.
3. Explain rationale for procedure to client.
4. Validate that client has an established peripheral IV site.
   ➤ *Rationale:* This is for administration of emergency fluids or medication if needed.
5. Perform hand hygiene.
6. Connect IV tubing to flush fluid bag.
7. Place prepared flush solution bag in pressure bag and inflate to 300 mm Hg pressure. ➤ *Rationale:* This maintains a rate of flow through the flush device (3 mL/hr).
8. Prepare and assemble pressurized monitoring system (transducer, system flush device, and stopcocks) following manufacturer's instructions. Attach stopcocks to proximal and distal ports. Flush all lumens with flush solution.

> **CLINICAL ALERT**
> By zeroing to atmospheric pressure, the system negates the effect of atmospheric pressure on the pressure being measured.

9. Attach distal port stopcock to connecting tubing and saline flush solution, then attach to pressure monitoring unit, making sure all connections are tight.

10. Place client in Trendelenburg's position and turn client's head to opposite side. ➤ **Rationale:** This position distends central veins and prevents air embolism during the procedure.

11. Level and zero system according to manufacturer's instructions. The stopcock on top of the transducer must be at the level of client's atrium or phlebostatic axis (fourth intercostal space at the midchest line).

12. Drape entire client and prep the insertion site with chlorhexidine. ➤ **Rationale:** Full body draping during insertion and chlorhexidine skin prep have been shown to decrease bloodstream infections.

13. Cleanse lidocaine vial with antimicrobial wipe.

14. Continuously monitor client's ECG throughout insertion of catheter. ➤ **Rationale:** Rhythm changes may occur.

Procedure

1. Don sterile gloves to assist healthcare provider as necessary.

   a. Healthcare provider dons sterile mask, cap, gown, and gloves. Catheter is tested for leaks by inflating balloon with 0.5–1.5 mL (amount determined by catheter size) of *air* while balloon is submerged in a sterile basin filled with sterile irrigating solution.

   b. Healthcare provider aspirates lidocaine with 18-gauge needle, changes to 25-gauge needle, and injects lidocaine under the skin.

   c. Healthcare provider performs cutdown or percutaneous insertion.

   d. Healthcare provider aspirates and flushes the sheath with sterile normal saline before inserting the catheter. ➤ **Rationale:** This clears air and prevents air embolism.

   e. While the client performs a Valsalva's maneuver or hums, the catheter is attached to a fluid-filled transducer system. ➤ **Rationale:** This prevents inhalation and possible air embolism. Continuous pressure monitoring is observed during advancement of the catheter.

   f. Catheter is advanced with a balloon partially inflated until the correct right atrial waveform appears on monitor (❶, strip A).

   g. Healthcare provider inflates the balloon (1–1.5 mL air) to assist in the catheter's flow through the tricuspid valve into the right ventricle.

2. Observe for higher and more pronounced pressure waveform, indicating catheter's presence in the right ventricle (strip B).

3. Record right ventricular pressure (systolic and diastoles reading) and observe for **dysrhythmias**: premature ventricular contractions (PVCs) or ventricular tachycardia.

4. Observe the monitor for *higher* diastolic pressure and appearance of **dicrotic notch** on pulmonary arterial waveform (strip C). ➤ **Rationale:** Pressures of right **ventricular systole** and pulmonary artery systole are similar, but pulmonary artery *diastolic* measure "steps up."

5. Remove syringe to allow balloon to deflate passively. (A special syringe is used that prevents overinflation of the balloon.)

Right Atrial (RA) Pressure

A

Right Ventricular (RV) Pressure

B

Pulmonary Artery Pressure (PAP)

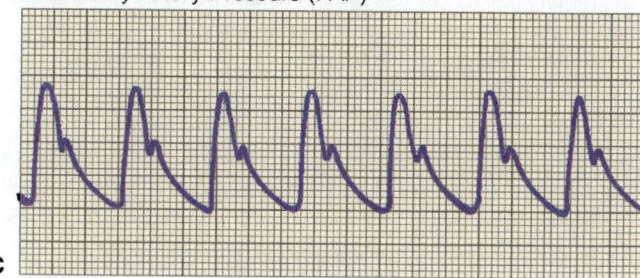

C

Pulmonary Artery Wedge Pressure (PAWP)

D

❶ Waveforms depicted on the monitor correspond with right heart chambers and pulmonary artery pressures.

EVIDENCE-BASED PRACTICE

Confirming Digital Measurements

Comparing digital readouts from the cardiac monitor of central venous pressures and pulmonary artery pressures to the values obtained from a digitized analog strip has long been considered the gold standard. A recent study with 30 adult ICU clients found measurements using the stop-cursor method from a bedside monitor can be accurately obtained, eliminating the need to print out a strip for comparison.

Source: Tyler et al. (2013)

(continued)

Skill 33.1.2 | Assisting Physician With Catheter Insertion *(continued)*

6. Record pulmonary artery systolic (PAS), diastolic (PAD), and mean pressures.

Note: Measure all pulmonary artery pressures at end of expiration.

7. Inflate balloon fully (1.5 mL maximum) or until a change is seen in waveform (pulmonary artery to artery wedge pressure; strip D). ➤ *Rationale:* Inflated balloon assists passage of catheter into distal pulmonary artery.

CLINICAL ALERT
For pulmonary artery wedge pressure (PAWP), inflate balloon *briefly* (8 to 15 sec), just until PAP changes to PAWP waveform, then allow balloon to deflate by releasing pressure on syringe plunger or removing syringe.

8. Record pulmonary artery wedge pressure (PAWP).
9. Deflate balloon by releasing pressure on syringe plunger or remove syringe to allow passive deflation. ➤ *Rationale:* Active aspiration of air from balloon with a syringe plunger can cause balloon damage.
10. Determine balloon deflation by observing return of the pulmonary artery waveform. ➤ *Rationale:* This ensures balloon deflation. Continued occlusion of vessel can cause pulmonary infarction.
11. Repeat steps and measurements to verify function.
12. Leave balloon lumen port open at all times except during advancement for wedge pressure (PAWP) measurement.
13. Clear the catheter using a fast flush device.

14. Apply an occlusive dressing to the site after the healthcare provider secures the catheter with sutures.
15. Reposition the client for comfort.
16. Auscultate the chest for presence of breath sounds.
17. Validate catheter placement by chest x-ray. ➤ *Rationale:* Pneumothorax can occur with jugular or subclavian vein **cannulation**.
18. Dispose of equipment, remove gloves, and perform hand hygiene.

EVIDENCE-BASED PRACTICE
Preventing Central Line Associated Bloodstream Infections (CLABSI)
The Institute for Healthcare Improvement recommends a set of best practices or bundles of care to prevent CLABSI. These include: hand washing, full barrier precautions when inserting a central line, chlorhexidine for skin antisepsis, avoidance of femoral catheters, and the removal of unnecessary catheters. A recent unit-based quality improvement project was done, which focused on improving CLABSI rates in clients with long-term catheters. The unit did this through several Plan-Do-Check-Act cycles and focused on each aspect of the CLABSI bundles of best practices that the nurses could directly affect. In one cycle, they focused specifically on dressing changes and blood draws to ensure the nurses performed the process according to the best practice technique. In another cycle, they included the clients in their care. After 5 cycles, they showed sustained improvement in their CLABSI rates.

Source: Jones, Stewart, & Roszell (2015)

Skill 33.1.3 | Obtaining Pressure Readings

Preparation
1. Introduce self and identify the client with two client identifiers.
2. Level transducer, and "zero" (calibrate) monitor at the beginning of every shift. ➤ *Rationale:* This ensures accurate and consistent readings.
3. Check catheter, tubing, and connection points to ensure patency and security.

CLINICAL ALERT
Do not use the PA catheter for infusion of blood or other viscous fluids, as they may occlude the catheter or alter pressure measurements.

4. Mark client's midchest level at fourth ICS for consistent readings.
5. Place client flat supine or up to 60-degree elevation.

Note: Consistent position is preferred for all readings.

6. Perform hand hygiene.

Procedure
1. Check that air reference port (stopcock) of pressure transducer is at level of client's atrium (phlebostatic axis). ➤ *Rationale:* This ensures accurate pressure reading. Level must be adjusted if client's position is changed.
2. Expose distal port to the transducer. ➤ *Rationale:* All pulmonary artery pressure readings are taken from the distal lumen of catheter, and right atrial pressures are taken from RA or proximal lumen.
3. Open balloon inflation port-locking device.

CLINICAL ALERT
Pulmonary artery diastolic pressure is an acceptable equivalent of PAWP (if correlation is determined) and it eliminates the need for occlusion (wedge) readings. Many healthcare providers prefer to use this instead and no longer use wedge readings.

4. Attach a syringe filled with the proper amount of air and align the stopcock to open position.

5. Slowly inject 0.8 or 1.5 mL of air into the balloon. Inflate sufficient volume only to support float and change in waveform.
6. Observe waveform change from pulmonary artery to pulmonary artery wedge pressure on the monitor. ❶
7. Balloon should be inflated only long enough to observe PAWP waveform (8–15 sec). ➤ *Rationale:* Longer inflation can cause overwedging (falsely high pressure readings) and damage to pulmonary tissue.
8. Allow the balloon to deflate passively. ➤ *Rationale:* Aspirating air with the syringe may damage the balloon.

❶ Monitor display of ECG, pressure waveforms, and digital readouts for continuous client assessment.

> **CLINICAL ALERT**
> Suspect balloon rupture if no resistance is encountered on inflation, syringe plunger fails to retract spontaneously, or blood returns from the balloon lumen. Mark stopcock: "DO NOT INFLATE."

9. Ensure readings are always taken at the end of expiration whether or not client is on a ventilator (document if client is on ventilator). ➤ *Rationale:* Slightly higher readings are obtained if a client is on a ventilator.
10. Use the analog strip chart recording to obtain the most valid pressure measurements.
11. Maintain empty syringe on the balloon port.
12. Flush line with fast flush device system.
13. Record readings; verify and report unusual findings to the healthcare provider if they persist.

> **CLINICAL ALERT**
> Changes in intracardiac pressures and volumes may be altered by changes in myocardial compliance. Any pressure should be interpreted in relation to the client's clinical assessment.

14. Place the client in a comfortable position.
15. Change dressings per agency policy, and observe for complications at the site of catheter insertion.

Skill 33.1.4 | Measuring Cardiac Output

Equipment
Established pressure monitoring system
Closed system cardiac output set (COSET)
Includes: 500-mL bag of NS (injectate), tubing with 3-way stopcock, syringe
Cardiac output cable

Preparation
1. Check healthcare provider's orders.
2. Introduce self and identify client using two client identifiers.
3. Perform hand hygiene.
4. Spike injectate solution bag with tubing/stopcock.
5. Unclamp injectate tubing, prime tubing and stopcock, and then reclamp tubing.
6. Connect primed system to the client's PA catheter proximal port.
7. Stop any medication being infused through the proximal port. ➤ *Rationale:* This is to prevent a medication bolus during cardiac output measurement.
8. Note the pulmonary artery waveform on the monitor. ➤ *Rationale:* This is to verify catheter position.

9. Connect computer cable to thermistor port of the pulmonary artery catheter (according to manufacturer's instructions). ➤ *Rationale:* Change in injectate temperature from proximal injectate port to thermistor port at the distal lumen is computer calculated and displayed as cardiac output in L/min.
10. Obtain the client's height and weight measures.

Procedure
1. Place the client in the same position used with previous hemodynamic readings; client should be supine, but may be elevated up to 60 degrees. ➤ *Rationale:* Consistency of position decreases measurement variability.
2. Slowly flush the proximal injectate lumen if any medications were being infused. ➤ *Rationale:* This is to prevent bolus medication delivery during cardiac output measurement.

> **CLINICAL ALERT**
> Vasoactive medications should not be infused through the proximal port; the Swan Ganz VIP catheter provides a separate proximal port for infusion.

(continued)

Skill 33.1.4 | Measuring Cardiac Output *(continued)*

3. Select *cardiac output* on the bedside monitor menu.
4. Check and set the computation constant to reflect size of the catheter, volume (5 or 10 mL) of injectate, cold versus room temperature injectate, and injectate volume (see PA catheter manufacturer's instructions). ➤ *Rationale:* These are factored into computer-derived hemodynamic measures. A 5-mL bolus may be indicated for a fluid-restricted client.
5. Unclamp the injectate solution tubing.
6. Attach syringe to the stopcock and open stopcock to withdraw 10 mL of injectate into the syringe.
7. Ensure that the client is quiet. ➤ *Rationale:* Movement may cause inaccurate readings.
8. Open the stopcock to the client and inject rapidly (2–4 seconds). ➤ *Rationale:* Slower injectate results in inaccurate readings.
9. Note and record the monitor display of the client's cardiac output measure.
10. Repeat the procedure two more times for cold injectate; repeat four more times for room temperature injectate, waiting 1–2 min between injections.

11. Obtain curves and discard abnormal curves or those with wandering baselines.
12. Record the average of the remaining cardiac output measures.
13. Clamp the injectate tubing.
14. Open the stopcock to continue previous infusion to the client.
15. Preserve closed cardiac output system by leaving tubing, stopcock, and syringe connections intact. ➤ *Rationale:* This eliminates the need to open the system each time measurements are made.
16. Determine the derived values using client's cardiac output measure: stroke volume, systemic vascular resistance, pulmonary vascular resistance, cardiac index (client's height and weight factored into the cardiac output).

Note: Routine use of pulmonary artery catheters is declining. Issues around accuracy of the data, lack of evidence to support its continued use, and the availability of less invasive and equally accurate methods of obtaining data have led to its decline.

Skill 33.1.5 | Monitoring Intra-Aortic Balloon Pump Circulatory Assistance

Preparation
1. Introduce self and identify client using two client identifiers.
2. Perform hand hygiene.

Procedure
Monitoring Balloon Pump Function
1. Validate that balloon catheter tip is at second to third ICS per daily chest x-ray.
2. Assess that balloon is precisely synchronized with the client's ECG cardiac cycle or arterial wave form:
   a. Inflation starts at the dicrotic notch of the arterial wave form (closure of the aortic valve).
   b. Deflation occurs before the QRS complex (systole).
3. Maintain frequency of assist at 1:1 or other ratio as ordered.
4. Assess IABP device timing and document by recording a strip of arterial pressure in 1:2 assist. ❶ ➤ *Rationale:* Cardiac output may decrease if timing is not precise.

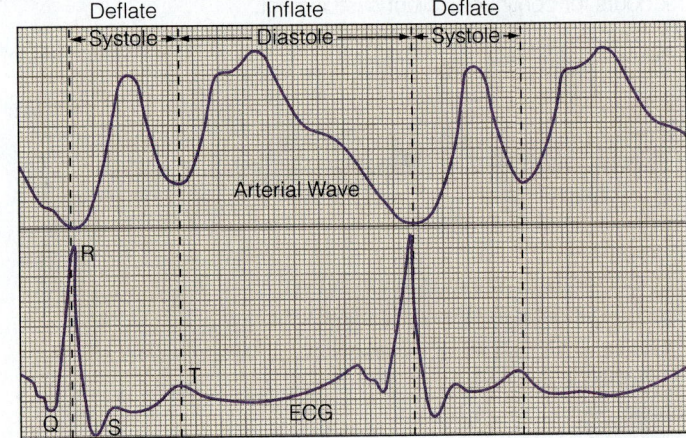

❶ Assess IABP device timing by recording strip of arterial pressure in 1:2 assist. Timing must be precise.

Monitoring Client Response
1. Check balloon insertion site hourly for bleeding, hematoma, or signs of infection.
2. Assess circulation hourly: color, temperature, capillary refill; bilateral radial, and pedal pulses. ➤ *Rationale:* This is to validate balloon position does not occlude major run-off from aorta.
3. Monitor urine output hourly; report drop in UO or UO less than 30 mL/hr × 2 hr. ➤ *Rationale:* This is to validate adequate renal perfusion.
4. Assess neurologic status per agency protocol. ➤ *Rationale:* This is to assess effect on cerebral perfusion.

5. Note CO and CI, and record per agency protocol.
   ➤ *Rationale:* This is to determine improved cardiac function.
6. Monitor bowel sounds and assess abdomen for pain.
   ➤ *Rationale:* Abnormal findings may indicate inappropriate balloon placement and should be reported.
7. Report client experience of chest discomfort or any pain, numbness, or tingling in arms or legs.
8. Report decrease in platelet count per daily CBC.
   ➤ *Rationale:* Catheter function damages platelets.
9. Monitor coagulation profile results. ➤ *Rationale:* Neither clot formation nor bleeding should occur.

Unit 33.1 Documentation and Evaluation

DOCUMENTATION for Pulmonary Artery Pressure Monitoring

- Healthcare provider who placed catheter
- Size of pulmonary artery catheter inserted
- Measurement of where catheter is (e.g., 55 cm at insertion site)
- Vessel placement and technique used to insert catheter (cutdown or percutaneous)
- Site care and dressing applied
- Client position during measurements
- Pressure readings obtained (specify digital or analog measures)
- Strip recordings attached
- Client's response to procedure
- Cardiac output results

- Problems arising and interventions performed
- IABP Circulatory Assist
- IABP assist timing ratio (e.g., 1:1)
- Femoral artery insertion site status every hour
- Peripheral circulation status every hour (pulses, color, temperature, capillary refill)
- Urine output every hour
- Abdominal and neurologic assessment per agency protocol
- Hemodynamic parameters every per agency protocol (CO, CI, SVR)
- Client reports of chest or abdominal discomfort, any pain, numbness in extremities, including problem-solving interventions

EVALUATION/Critical Thinking

Expected Outcomes

- Pulmonary artery catheter remains patent.
- Pulmonary artery systolic, diastolic, and pulmonary artery wedge pressures are measured accurately.
- Cardiac output measurements are obtained.
- Intra-aortic balloon pump circulatory assist improves cardiac output: Afterload and preload are reduced.

Unexpected Outcomes

- Pulmonary artery catheter is not patent.

Alternative Actions

- Check that tubing is not kinked.
- Ensure continuous normal saline infusion. (Check hospital policy.) Check stopcock connections. (Do not use dextrose solution.)
- Attempt to aspirate clotted blood through line by pulling back on plunger of a small syringe placed at the proximal port. Remove clot, then flush line.
- Notify healthcare provider if unable to clear the line.
- Fast flush system and flick tubing to eliminate tiny bubbles.

(continued)

Unexpected Outcomes	Alternative Actions
• Pressure waveforms are significantly abnormal.	• Check that tubing is not kinked. • Check stopcock level. • Correlate with client for possible change in clinical condition. • Tighten all connections. • Look for air in any system port. • Eliminate added stopcocks and tubing extensions. • Ask client to cough or change position to help free catheter. • If condition persists, notify healthcare provider to reposition the line and assess client.
• Analog waveform is inconsistent with digital display.	• Validate leveling at client's phlebostatic axis. • Validate zeroing of system to atmospheric pressure ("0" baseline).
• There is no pressure tracing.	• Determine that power is ON. • Check for loose connections. • Check for clotted blood in line (damping is an early sign). Try to aspirate; never flush. • Check stopcocks to make sure they are turned appropriately.
• There is no pulmonary wedge pressure tracing.	• Check and deflate balloon. • Suspect that catheter is not adequately advanced. Chest x-ray may be ordered to check placement of pulmonary artery catheter. • Reposition the client. • Suspect possible balloon rupture if no resistance is felt on inflation.
• Intra-aortic balloon ruptures.	• Turn console off and notify healthcare provider. Balloon must be removed within 30 min.
• Console fails.	• If problem not resolved in 30 min, use a syringe filled with 40 mL of room air to manually inflate and deflate balloon to move balloon folds in order to prevent clot formation.

Arterial Blood Pressure Monitoring

Nursing Process Data

ASSESSMENT Database

- Determine need for direct arterial blood pressure monitoring.
- Assess collateral perfusion of the hand using the Modified Allen Test.
- Measure arterial (direct) systolic and diastolic blood pressure readings.
- Observe the mean arterial pressure on the monitor and validate using analog strip measurement.
- Observe for trends in arterial pressure readings.
- Validate 300 mm Hg pressure on infusion system.
- Assess catheter insertion site for signs of infection or bleeding.
- Assess circulation, temperature, motion, and sensation of extremity distal to catheter insertion site.
- Monitor systemic response to circulatory assistance (IABP).

PLANNING Objectives

- To maintain a patent arterial catheter
- To directly measure systolic, diastolic, and mean arterial blood pressures
- To provide essential information regarding fluid volume, cardiac function, and perfusion to vital organs
- To provide immediate access for arterial blood gas samples
- To provide circulatory assistance (IABP) for selected clients

IMPLEMENTATION PROCEDURES

DOCUMENTATION AND EVALUATION

Expected Outcomes

- Blood supply to hand is adequate before and after arterial catheter placement.
- Arterial cannulation is accomplished without complication.
- Arterial blood pressure monitoring system functions reliably and accurately.
- Arterial blood samples are obtained.

Unexpected Outcomes/Alternative Actions

Pearson Nursing Student Resources

Find additional review materials at
nursing.pearsonhighered.com.
Prepare for success with NCLEX®-style practice questions and Skill Checklists.

Direct blood pressure monitoring allows continuous measurement of the client's systolic, diastolic, and mean arterial pressures (MAP) to facilitate evaluation of perfusion to vital organs. A short single-lumen catheter is placed in the client's radial artery, then attached to a pressure transducer and high-pressure infusion system and a display monitor (Figure 33-5 ■).

To maintain patency of the intra-arterial catheter, a continuous flush of 1–3 mL/hr of normal saline solution is administered under 300 mm Hg pressure.

Invasive monitoring is appropriate for critically ill clients requiring **vasodilator** or **vasopressor** drugs or frequent arterial blood gas studies.

Continuous arterial waveforms and values are observed on the cardiac monitor and can be downloaded into electronic health records where such technology is utilized (Box 33-4 ■). Blood pressure deviations can immediately be detected and appropriate therapy instituted without delay. It is important for alarms to be set that are specific to the client's situation and healthcare provider's orders. The arterial line also provides easy access to blood sampling for ABGs and other lab values. Arterial blood gas values assist in determining respiratory and metabolic acid–base status (Tables 33-2 and 33-3 ■) as well as lung capacity to provide oxygen. The measurements serve as a guide for implementing and evaluating treatment.

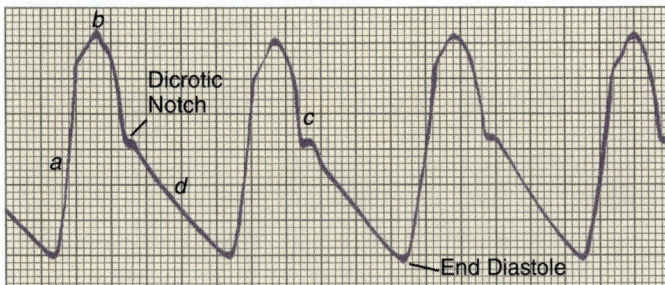

FIGURE 33-5 Arterial pressure waveform. The dicrotic notch indicates aortic valve closure (and end of systole).

Table 33-2 Arterial Blood Gas Values in Acid–Base Imbalances

Normal ABG Values		
pH	7.35–7.45	
pCO_2	35–45 mm Hg	
HCO_3^-	22–26 mEq	
Respiratory Acidosis		**Compensation**
pH: decreased	<7.35	7.35
pCO_2: increased	>45 mm Hg	
HCO_3^-: normal	24	>26 mEq
Respiratory Alkalosis		**Compensation**
pH: increased	>7.45	7.45
pCO_2: decreased	<35 mm Hg	
HCO_3^-: normal	24	<22 mEq
Metabolic Acidosis		**Compensation**
pH: decreased	<7.35	7.35
HCO_3^-: decreased	<22 mEq	
pCO_2: normal	40	<35 mm Hg
Metabolic Alkalosis		**Compensation**
pH: increased	>7.45	7.45
HCO_3^-: increased	>26 mEq	
pCO_2: normal	40	>45 mm Hg

Table 33-3 Causes of Acid–Base Imbalance

Acidemia	Alkalemia
Hypovolemia	
Hypoventilation	Hyperventilation
COPD	Hypokalemia
Cardiac arrest	Pulmonary embolus
Diabetic ketoacidosis	Diuretics/steroids
Severe diarrhea	Prolonged vomiting
Renal failure	NG suction

Box 33-4 DIRECT BLOOD PRESSURE WAVEFORM

Direct blood pressure waveform correlation to the cardiac cycle is represented by the symbols shown in Figure 33-5.

- *a* represents a sharp upstroke, correlating with ventricular systole and the QRS complex of the **electrocardiogram**.
- *b* represents peak systole; its numerical value is the systolic pressure recorded.
- *c* A label identifies the notch on the downstroke of the waveform. This notch is called the *dicrotic notch* and represents closure of the aortic valve.
- *d* represents diastole and is represented by a continuous decline in pressure. The numerical value at the lowest point is the diastolic pressure.

Skill 33.2.1 | Performing the Modified Allen Test

Preparation

1. Introduce self.
2. Perform hand hygiene.
3. Identify client using two client identifiers.

Procedure

1. Perform the **Modified Allen Test** to determine distal peripheral perfusion. ➤ *Rationale:* This procedure assesses blood supply to client's hand to determine that radial and ulnar artery are functioning before an arterial line is inserted.
2. Compress both arteries at client's wrist for about 1 min.

3. Instruct the client to clench and unclench the fist several times. ➤ *Rationale:* This causes blanching in the hand and palm.
4. With client's hand in open, relaxed position, release pressure on the ulnar artery.
5. Observe how quickly (≤10 seconds) the palm color flushes. ➤ *Rationale:* If color returns quickly, good collateral blood supply to the hand exists. If normal color does not return, there is insufficient collateral circulation to the hand should radial artery occlusion occur.
6. Report to healthcare provider if collateral blood flow is insufficient. ➤ *Rationale:* A Doppler flow study may be used to help determine collateral blood flow.

Skill 33.2.2 | Assisting With Arterial Line Insertion

Equipment

14- to 20-gauge catheter with introducer and guidewire
Single-pressure transducer system
Monitoring equipment and cables
One mL-unit dose syringe
Clean gloves, sterile gloves
Personal protective equipment (PPE)
Sterile towels and drape
Skin prep solution (2% chlorhexidine)
Sterile 4×4 gauze sponges
Lidocaine 1% (without epinephrine)
3-mL syringe with 18- and 25-gauge needles for *topical* anesthetic
Antiseptic solution
Securement device or suture material
Dressing supplies
Ultrasound device if requested

Preparation

1. Validate that informed consent has been obtained.
2. Determine whether the client has received anticoagulant therapy. ➤ *Rationale:* Coagulation studies may be indicated.
3. Introduce self and identify the client using two client identifiers.
4. Explain the rationale for the procedure.
5. Gather equipment.
6. Perform hand hygiene.
7. Connect IV tubing to the solution bag.
8. Remove *all air* from flush solution bag. ➤ *Rationale:* This will ensure accuracy in blood pressure readings.
9. Insert flush infusion bag into pressure bag and hang the bag on the IV pole.
10. Prepare and assemble the pressurized monitoring system (transducer, continuous flush device, and stopcocks) following manufacturer's instructions.
11. Level the stopcock above the transducer to client's phlebostatic axis (see Skill 33.2.1).
12. Inflate the pressure bag to 300 mm Hg using hand pump on the bag.

Procedure

1. Don gloves and PPE and prepare to assist the healthcare provider as needed.

   a. Skin is prepped briskly with 2% chlorhexidine for 3 seconds.
   b. Lidocaine vial is cleansed with alcohol wipe.
   c. Healthcare provider dons sterile gloves.
   d. Sterile drape is placed over the arterial insertion site.
   e. Healthcare provider aspirates lidocaine with 18-gauge needle, changes needle, and injects client's skin with 25-gauge needle. ➤ *Rationale:* This is for local anesthesia.
   f. Percutaneous insertion is made at the arterial insertion site, and the arterial catheter is inserted.
   g. Healthcare provider advances the catheter in the artery.
   h. Arterial catheter is sutured in place and secured with a transparent dressing. ❶

2. Observe for pulsating bright-red blood spurting retrograde into the catheter. ➤ *Rationale:* This evidence ensures arterial catheter position.
3. Attach catheter to primed pressure-monitoring system tubing—make certain all connections are secure.
4. Press the fast flush valve to clear the system.
5. Observe the monitor for arterial waveform. ❷
6. Apply a sterile transparent dressing (with date and initials) to site after the catheter is sutured into place.
7. Remove gloves and perform hand hygiene.
8. Set monitor alarms for both HIGH and LOW parameters.

> **CLINICAL ALERT**
> Arterial catheter alarms should always be enabled to detect disconnection, alterations in blood pressure, or pulseless electrical activity.

(continued)

Skill 33.2.2 | Assisting With Arterial Line Insertion (continued)

❶ Apply sterile transparent dressing (with date and initials) to the site after the catheter is sutured into place.

❷ Arterial line allows direct measurement of blood pressure—monitor displays digital and waveform.

Skill 33.2.3 | Monitoring Arterial Blood Pressure

Equipment
Disposable single-pressure transducer system
Flush valve with flush system
Display monitor (oscilloscope)
Sterile stopcock cap
Sterile transparent dressing
Gloves
Leveling device
Marker

Preparation
1. Introduce self and identify client using two client identifiers.
2. Perform hand hygiene.

Procedure
1. Leveling and "zeroing" (calibrating) the system.
   a. Calibrate system at beginning of each shift. ➤ *Rationale:* Monitor readings are altered by changes in atmospheric pressure.
   b. Position client with head of bed HOB flat or up to 45-degree elevation.
   c. Using a level, align stopcock above the transducer level with client's left atrium (phlebostatic axis). ➤ *Rationale:* Readings will be inaccurately high or low if stopcock above the transducer is not level with client's phlebostatic axis.
   d. To "zero" (calibrate) the system, turn stopcock near the transducer off to the client. Remove cap from stopcock, opening it to air, and zero the monitoring system. ➤ *Rationale:* Zero reading indicates monitor is calibrated to atmospheric pressure.

   e. Replace cap or place a new sterile cap on the stopcock.
   f. Turn stopcock so the transducer is open to the client.
2. Observe waveform at eye level for the sharp systolic upstroke, peak, dicrotic notch, and end diastole. **❶**
3. Fast flush the continuous flush system and quickly release. **❷** A sharp upstroke followed by a horizontal line, then a brisk downstroke descending below, then returning to

❶ (A) Arterial line—normal waveform. (B) Arterial line—flattened waveform. Flattened arterial waveform indicates damping. Damping results from obstruction in arterial line or imbalance of transducer.

Square wave test configuration

Observed
waveform

❷ Fast flush the continuous flush system and quickly release. A sharp upstroke, followed by a horizontal line, then a brisk down-stroke descending below and then returning to baseline indicates the system requires no adjustment (square wave test).

baseline indicates that the system requires no adjustment.

4. Ensure pressure bag is maintained at 300 mm Hg.
5. Leave cannulated extremity uncovered for easy observation. Assess the site for signs of infection every shift.
6. Assess circulation, motion, and sensation of extremity distal to cannulation site per agency protocol.
7. Immobilize extremity if necessary.

EVIDENCE-BASED PRACTICE
Monitoring Arterial Blood Pressure
The use of an indirect brachial blood pressure measurement to determine whether an arterial pressure monitoring system is accurate is not evidence based. It is more important to determine that technical aspects of the method are optimized and the blood pressure is adequate. In addition to obtaining an absolute measure, monitoring for trends or changes in blood pressure over time is equally important for guiding clinical decisions.

Source: Rauen, Chulay, Bridges, Vollman, & Arbour (2008)

8. Change flush solution and tubing every 96 hr (according to agency policy).
9. Change dressing according to agency policy if it becomes loose or soiled. ➤ *Rationale:* Loose or soiled dressings increase risk of infection at the site.

   a. Put on gloves.
   b. Remove dressing and discard in biohazard container.
   c. Apply a sterile dressing using a transparent or semitransparent. Mark the dressing with date and initials.

10. Remove gloves and PPE and perform hand hygiene.
11. Monitor the site to ensure hemostasis occurs.
12. Monitor extremity distally for adequacy of perfusion.

Skill 33.2.4 | Withdrawing Arterial Blood Samples

Equipment
One 6-mL sterile syringe
ABG kit with one 3-mL syringe with dry lithium heparin; air filter device
Or: Needleless blood sampling access device
Gloves
Face shield
Container with ice (paper cup, emesis basin)
Two specimen labels
Bubble packaging
Biohazard specimen bag
Gauze sponges or pads

Preparation
1. Introduce self and identify client using two client identifiers.
2. Gather equipment and explain procedure to client.

> ### CLINICAL ALERT
> "In-line" blood sampling systems eliminate the need for dis-carding blood, thus reducing blood loss and associated risks.

3. Attach label to specimen syringe with client's identification information. Also add client's current temperature and FiO_2.
4. For blood gas (ABG) specimen, maintain the client's current oxygen delivery setting for 20 min before obtaining the specimen.

5. Fill a paper cup with ice.
6. Perform hand hygiene and don gloves.

EVIDENCE-BASED PRACTICE
Alarm Fatigue
Alarm fatigue occurs when nurses become overwhelmed by the sheer number of alarms they are responsible for and they disable, silence, or ignore those alarms. This desensitization can lead to client safety being placed at risk. Efforts to improve alarm fatigue have found that careful assessment and customization of alarm parameters—minimizing "false" or nuisance alarms—can reduce alarm fatigue, but staff buy-in and accountability are also key factors.

Source: Graham & Cvach (2010)

Procedure
1. Momentarily disengage arterial alarms.
2. Turn stopcock off to the client.
3. Remove protective cap from open blood sampling port on the three-way stopcock closest to the arterial line insertion site.
4. Attach syringe or needleless blood sampling access device to open port of the three-way stopcock.
5. Turn the stopcock off to flush solution.

(continued)

Skill 33.2.4 | Withdrawing Arterial Blood Samples *(continued)*

6. Attach syringe or blood specimen tube into needleless blood sampling access device to establish blood draw. ❶
7. Discard obtained sample. ➤ *Rationale:* This discard ensures a specimen that is free of flush solution.

Note: For an ABG blood sample, the discard volume should be twice the dead space volume of the catheter and tubing up to the sampling site. For coagulation studies, the discard volume should be 6 times the dead space volume.

8. Obtain an arterial blood gas specimen.
9. Turn stopcock off to open port. ❷ ➤ *Rationale:* This reestablishes flow between flush solution and client.

Blood Conservatory Process or Closed Arterial Blood Sampling System

a. Don clean gloves.
b. Aspirate blood into reservoir tubing.
c. Close stopcock to reservoir tubing.
d. Access sampling port (closest to client) using blunt cannula with tube holder (Vacutainer).

e. Engage blood collection tubes into tube holder and allow them to fill. ➤ *Rationale:* Obtaining specimens using a **blood conservatory process** helps to prevent nosocomial anemia.
f. When sampling is complete, remove blunt cannula and tube holder.
g. Open stopcock to reservoir tubing and return contents to client.

10. Place arterial blood gas specimen tubes in container filled with ice.
11. Fast flush remaining blood onto gauze pad.
12. Reattach protective cap on open port.
13. Validate good arterial waveform on the monitor.
14. Reactivate monitor alarms.
15. Wrap syringe/specimen in bubble packaging and place in biohazard bag with ice.
16. Remove gloves and perform hand hygiene.
17. Send specimens to the laboratory immediately and notify the lab that tubes are being sent.

❶ Engage syringe or needleless blood sampling access device to the sample port to obtain arterial blood.

❷ When sampling is complete, open stopcock to reservoir tubing and return contents of blood conservatory system to client.

Skill 33.2.5 | Removing Arterial Catheter

Equipment
Gloves
Personal protective equipment
Two 4×4 gauze pads
Suture removal set
Tape

Preparation
1. Check healthcare provider's orders.
2. Check client's coagulation lab results (values).
3. Gather equipment.

4. Perform hand hygiene.
5. Introduce self and identify the client using two client identifiers.
6. Disarm the monitor alarms.

Procedure
1. Don gloves and PPE.
2. Remove dressing, and discard in the appropriate container.
3. Clip retaining sutures if present.
4. Apply finger pressure approximately 2 cm *above* skin puncture site. ➤ *Rationale:* The artery puncture site is proximal to the skin puncture site.

5. Place folded 4×4 gauze pad over cannula site with nondominant hand, and apply gentle pressure.
6. Pull the arterial cannula straight out of the artery with quick, even pressure.
7. Apply firm pressure over and just above the cannula site for at least 5–10 min or until hemostasis is achieved. ➤ *Rationale:* This action achieves hemostasis and prevents formation of a hematoma.

> **CLINICAL ALERT**
> Apply pressure to puncture site for at least 10 min if client is on anticoagulation or antithrombotic therapy.

8. Place folded 4×4 gauze pad over the puncture site, and tape tightly. ➤ *Rationale:* This provides additional pressure to the site to prevent bleeding.
9. Discard supplies, remove gloves, PPE, and perform hand hygiene.
10. Check the cannulation site frequently. ➤ *Rationale:* This is to observe for bleeding or thrombosis.
11. Check the distal extremity for temperature, circulation, motion, and sensation intermittently for several hours, then routinely after catheter removal. ➤ *Rationale:* Delayed complications (thrombosis) may occur.

Unit 33.2 Documentation and Evaluation

DOCUMENTATION for Arterial Blood Pressure Monitoring

- Size of arterial catheter inserted
- Name of healthcare provider inserting catheter
- Pressure readings (systolic, diastolic, and MAP)
- Direct and indirect pressure measurements
- Distal neurovascular status of cannulated extremity (temperature, color, motion, sensation)
- Position of client during readings
- Unexpected outcomes and appropriate interventions
- Client response and tolerance of procedure
- Appearance of catheter insertion site
- Monitor strip recordings

Arterial Blood Sampling
- Time specimen obtained
- Client's temperature and FiO_2 at the time blood was drawn

Arterial Site Dressing Change
- Condition of insertion site
- Type of dressing applied

Removing Arterial Catheter
- Time of removal
- Manual pressure and dressing applied
- Condition of insertion site
- Presence and quality of distal pulses
- Motion and sensation of involved extremity

EVALUATION/Critical Thinking

Expected Outcomes
- Blood supply to hand is adequate before and after arterial catheter placement.
- Arterial cannulation is accomplished without complication.
- Arterial blood pressure monitoring system functions reliably and accurately.
- Arterial blood samples are obtained.

Unexpected Outcomes
- Absence of collateral circulation noted when performing the Modified Allen Test (negative Modified Allen Test).

Alternative Actions
- Assess contralateral extremity.
- Avoid radial artery.
- Notify healthcare provider. (An alternate artery may be selected—femoral.)

(continued)

Unexpected Outcomes	**Alternative Actions**
• Cannulated extremity develops diminished distal perfusion.	• Check periphery for changes in color, temperature, motion, and sensation resulting from possible thrombus occlusion or circulatory "steal." • Notify healthcare provider immediately. • Prepare for catheter removal.
• Hematoma or bleeding occurs at arterial insertion site.	• Apply direct pressure over artery while you check for leaks in the system. • Check all stopcocks. Check if catheter is inserted in artery as it should be. • Keep cannulated extremity exposed for observation. • Remove catheter if oozing continues.
• Signs of infection or inflammation appear at insertion site.	• Use sterile transparent dressings exclusively. • Always use aseptic technique with dressing changes; change dressing per agency policy. • Cap open port on stopcock to maintain asepsis. • Change tubing, flush solution and transducer every 96 hr or with catheter change using sterile technique. • Flush open port after obtaining blood specimens. • Prepare for catheter removal if infection suspected.
• Arterial waveform loses definition and digital pressures drop.	• Perform a dynamic test if over-dampened arterial waveform is suspected. • Use low compliance (rigid), short (1–1.2 m [<3–4 ft]) monitor tubing. • Check for thrombus formation by aspirating blood through stopcock and then flushing system. • Be sure to fast-flush arterial line thoroughly after arterial blood samples are obtained or system is zeroed. • Make sure all stopcocks are closed to air. • Maintain 300-mm Hg pressure in pressure bag. • Ensure secure fit of all stopcocks and connections. Avoid adding stopcocks and line extensions. • Change position of extremity in which catheter is placed.
• Direct blood pressure readings vary significantly.	• Flick tubing system to remove tiny air bubbles escaping the flush solution. • Recheck transducer and client position to ensure accurate data. • Recalibrate transducer. • Flush system after sampling and zeroing. • Keep flush bag adequately filled and cleared of air. • Maintain bag external pressure at 300 mm Hg. • Check that connections are tightly secured.
• Arterial blood sample is unobtainable.	• Suspect arterial spasm; allow spasm of artery to stop, then attempt to aspirate blood with gentle pressure using a 6-mL syringe rather than a Vacutainer. • Reposition client's arm, making sure there is no pressure at catheter insertion site. • Check that catheter is in artery (note waveform on monitor), flush catheter, then attempt to obtain sample.

Nursing Process Data

ASSESSMENT Database

- Assess client's responsiveness, breathing, and circulation.
- Identify lethal heart rhythms on the ECG recording.
- Assess availability of emergency support response and emergency supplies.
- Identify appropriate drugs needed for an emergency situation.

PLANNING Objectives

- To be prepared to respond to the needs of unstable clients
- To locate necessary supplies and appropriate medications used in emergency situations
- To provide emergency defibrillation to convert lethal arrhythmias (dysrhythmias) to normal sinus rhythm
- To assist with cardioversion to convert rapid supraventricular rhythms or unstable ventricular tachycardia to normal sinus rhythm

IMPLEMENTATION Procedures

DOCUMENTATION AND EVALUATION

Expected Outcomes

- Supplies and medications are readily available in an emergency situation.
- Client's heart rhythm is restored to normal after defibrillation or synchronized cardioversion.

Unexpected Outcomes/Alternative Actions

Pearson Nursing Student Resources

Find additional review materials at
nursing.pearsonhighered.com.
Prepare for success with NCLEX®-style practice questions and Skill Checklists.

Early recognition is essential for prompt and effective treatment of cardiac emergencies. Interventions for treating emergencies such as hemodynamic instability and flash pulmonary edema include measures to decrease heart work, correct lethal dysrhythmias, and remove excess body fluid.

If left untreated, symptomatic bradycardias and supraventricular or ventricular tachyarrhythmias can cause reduced cardiac output and inadequate tissue perfusion. Life-threatening tachyarrhythmias are terminated by delivering an externally applied electrical countershock to the heart. This countershock depolarizes the myocardium, interrupts the dysrhythmia, and allows the normal pacemaker (sinoatrial node) of the heart to resume control of the heart rhythm. Two types of electrical counter-shock applications are used: cardioversion and defibrillation.

Defibrillation is an emergency procedure in which fairly large amounts of electric current are delivered without concern for synchronization with ventricular depolarization (QRS wave) on the ECG. Defibrillation is used to terminate ventricular fibrillation or *pulseless* ventricular tachycardia.

Cardioversion is a procedure used to convert supraventricular tachyarrhythmias and ventricular tachycardia in unstable clients. The electrical countershock is synchronized (**synchronized cardioversion**) with ventricular depolarization (QRS wave on ECG) to avoid discharge during the T wave (vulnerable period). This procedure may be elective (planned) or emergent.

The "crash cart" contains essential life support medications and supplies used in emergency situations in the hospital setting. Familiarity with its location and contents, including typical emergency drugs, will assist hospital staff to provide quick, competent care to clients during cardiac emergencies. The crash cart should be kept fully stocked and be located in an area that is accessible and obvious to all. Nurses must have a working knowledge of the contents of each drawer of the cart to find necessary supplies quickly.

Skill 33.3.1 | Maintaining the Emergency Cart

Equipment
Emergency cart with locking drawers
Emergency cart checklist
Airway equipment
Oxygen equipment
Suction equipment
Monitor leads and electrodes
Automated external defibrillator (AED)
IV equipment
Emergency drugs

Procedure
1. Identify supplies and medications commonly used in emergency situations.
2. Perform hand hygiene and gather equipment.
3. Maintain supplies in drawers according to priority use in the most commonly occurring emergency situations. Leave defibrillator plugged into electrical outlet at all times.
4. Lock drawers when cart is not in use. ➤ *Rationale:* This prevents personnel from using supplies for situations other than emergencies and not replacing them.
5. Place emergency cart checklist on outside of cart in visible area. ➤ *Rationale:* Cart contents are checked on a regular basis and often use a numbered lock system ensuring the contents are available and not outdated.
6. Place cart in designated, easily accessible, and visible area of the nursing unit. ❶ ➤ *Rationale:* This provides for less confusion if the cart is needed.
7. Familiarize all personnel with location and contents of cart, function of equipment, and emergency procedures.
8. Practice retrieving and setting up equipment in mock situations. ➤ *Rationale:* This ensures that all personnel are able to use the cart during an emergency situation.
9. Check cart daily and document; restock immediately after use. ➤ *Rationale:* If cart is not restocked, delays can occur during an emergency situation, jeopardizing client care.

❶ Fully equipped emergency cart is placed in a readily accessible area, visible to staff. Defibrillation and respiratory supplies are kept on the top of the cart.

Source: Chris Bjornberg/Science Source

Skill 33.3.2 | Checking Contents of the Emergency Cart

Equipment
Note: Emergency cart contents vary among agencies.

Top of Cart
Automated external defibrillator (AED)
Respiratory supplies
Gloves, face shield

Front or Back of Cart
Cardiac arrest board

First Drawer
Emergency medications

Second Drawer
IV access supplies
IV solutions and tubing
Syringes, special needles

Third Drawer
NG tubes
Blood pressure cuff, stethoscope
Flashlight
Suction catheter kit and supplies
Central line catheter and supplies

Side of Cart
Emergency cart checklist
Cardiac resuscitation recording sheet and clipboard
Suction unit

> **CLINICAL ALERT**
> Summon the Rapid Response Team if noting certain signs: tachypnea, hypotension, signs of shock, active bleeding, chest pain, and altered level of consciousness. For any client who becomes unresponsive, is not breathing, and has no pulse, call a "code" and get the AED.

Note: Tachypnea and hypotension frequently precede cardiac arrest. *See* procedure in Skill 31.4.5, Using an Automated External Defibrillator (AED).

> **CLINICAL ALERT**
> Sudden cardiac death is the most common cause of death, outnumbering the total number of deaths from AIDS, lung cancer, breast cancer, and stroke each year. The Joint Commission requires hospitals to track and evaluate resuscitation attempts in order to improve process and client outcomes. Development of Rapid Response Teams and in-hospital use of AEDs as well as changes in CPR/**ECC** guidelines are based on this tracking data.

EVIDENCE-BASED PRACTICE
Rapid Response Teams have been adopted by many hospitals, yet their effectiveness remains uncertain. A systematic review and meta-analysis found that the implementation of Rapid Response Teams in adults was associated with a 33.8% reduction in cardiopulmonary arrest outside of the intensive care units but was not associated with a lower hospital mortality rate.

Source: Chan, Jain, Nallmothu, Berg, & Sasson (2010)

Skill 33.3.3 | Performing Defibrillation

Equipment
Automated external defibrillator

Preparation
1. Validate that client is unresponsive.
   a. Not breathing, or not breathing normally (e.g., only gasping), and
   b. No pulse is palpable within 10 seconds (no longer).
2. Call a code and get the AED ❶ and crash cart.
3. Place back board under client, deflate air-filled mattress if present, avoiding delay to initiating CPR with chest compressions within 10 seconds.
4. Immediately begin CPR (chest compressions).

❶ Automatic external defibrillator.

(continued)

Skill 33.3.3 | Performing Defibrillation *(continued)*

Procedure

1. Plug defibrillator into electric outlet.
2. Turn defibrillator ON.

> **CLINICAL ALERT**
>
> Early defibrillation (within 3 min) is the key to successful resuscitation.
>
> ---
>
> The most common cause of PEA (pulseless electrical activity) is hypovolemia. Other contributing factors include: hypoxia, hydrogen ion imbalance (acidemia), hypo- or hyperkalemia, hypoglycemia, hypothermia, toxins, tamponade (cardiac), tension pneumothorax, thrombosis (MI, PE), and trauma.

3. Attach the defibrillator pads in the correct position to a dry chest.

> **CLINICAL ALERT**
>
> Before beginning defibrillation or cardioversion procedure, remove any transdermal medication patch on chest. Avoid placing pads or paddles over **electrodes** or leads; avoid pacemaker or ICD generator by at least 8 cm (3 in.).

4. One pad is placed on upper right sternal border directly below the clavicle and the other pad is placed lateral to the left nipple a few inches below the axilla (see pictures and directions on the AED).
5. Stop chest compressions and push analyze button on AED. ❷

❷ DEFIBRILLATION ARRHYTHMIAS

Pulseless ventricular tachycardia.

Ventricular fibrillation.

CARDIOVERSION ARRHYTHMIAS

Atrial fibrillation with rapid ventricular response.

Supraventricular tachycardia.

Ventricular tachycardia with pulses.

6. If shock is advised by the AED, clearly and loudly announce to everyone in the area to stand clear of the client and then visually inspect that everyone is clear of the client.
   > ➤ *Rationale:* This avoids someone getting a secondary shock.
7. Press the shock button.
8. Immediately begin chest compressions.
9. The AED will request another rhythm analysis in 2 min.
10. Continue to follow the directions on the AED with alternate shocks if advised and CPR until the code team arrives or the client regains a rhythm. ❸

❸ Hands-free pads provide defibrillation and protect the provider.

Skill 33.3.4 | Assisting With Synchronized Cardioversion

Equipment
Defibrillator monitor with ECG recorder set to SYNCHRONIZATION mode
Paddles—anteroposterior or anterolateral or hands-free pads
Conductive gel or conductive pads
Emergency cart with medications and supplies

Preparation for Elective Cardioversion
1. Review cardioversion orders and make sure consent form is signed. Check that equipment is functioning properly (Box 33-5 ■).
2. Review precardioversion laboratory values (electrolytes, digoxin level, ABGs). ➤ *Rationale:* Electrolyte imbalance, particularly hypokalemia, or digitalis toxicity may increase risk of dysrhythmias after cardioversion.
3. Check that client has been receiving anticoagulation therapy (Coumadin) for chronic atrial fibrillation.
4. Withhold food, medications, and fluids for 6–12 hr before elective cardioversion.
5. Obtain baseline 12-lead ECG, and label it "precardioversion."
6. Obtain baseline vital signs and ECG rhythms.
7. Assess peripheral pulses and neurologic status.
8. Notify anesthesiologist and healthcare provider of readiness.
9. Place emergency cart in the room.
10. Perform hand hygiene.

Box 33-5 SYNCHRONIZED CARDIOVERSION

Synchronized cardioversion is used for elective conversion of hemodynamically stable atrial fibrillation or atrial flutter. It is usually done under conscious/moderate sedation in cardiac catheter labs or specialized telemetry units. It is also used as emergency management for hemodynamically unstable tachyarrhythmias (narrow and wide QRS complex tachycardias with pulses).

Rhythms which may require emergency synchronized cardioversion are:

- Atrial fibrillation with rapid ventricular response
- Atrial flutter 2:1
- Paroxysmal supraventricular tachycardia with signs of instability (HR > 150, SBP ≤ 90 mm Hg)
- Ventricular tachycardia with pulses

Procedure
1. Introduce self and identify client using two client identifiers.
2. Remove any jewelry from the client. ➤ *Rationale:* Metal conducts electricity, so burns could occur.
3. Remove transdermal medication patches.
4. Establish an IV line, and administer fluids at "keep open" rate.
5. Administer oxygen if ordered.
6. Plug in the defibrillator and turn power switch ON.
7. Turn **synchronizer** switch ON. ➤ *Rationale:* Shock delivery synchronized with QRS of ECG reduces the possibility of inducing ventricular arrhythmias by the electrical shock being delivered on the T wave.
8. Test synchronization by pushing the manual synchronization button.
9. Disconnect all electric equipment from the client except ECG monitor and cardioverter.

(continued)

Skill 33.3.4 | Assisting With Synchronized Cardioversion (continued)

10. Administer conscious sedation as ordered by the healthcare provider.
11. Charge defibrillator to the level specified by healthcare provider. Note that the designated charge is reached (Table 33-4 ■).
12. Place the client in a supine position.
13. Make sure the client's chest is dry.
14. Use "hands-free" defibrillator pads and place on client's chest, or apply conductive gel to the surface of paddles.
    a. Apex-posterior self-adhesive defibrillation pads are placed over the left precordium and posteriorly below the right or left scapula.
    b. Anterolateral handheld paddles are placed as in defibrillation, one below the right clavicle and the other to the left of the cardiac apex (below and to the left of the nipple or at the 5th or 6th intercostal space at the midaxillary line).
15. Observe ECG rhythm on the monitor and start recording continuous printout using lead II to display a large R wave.
16. Discontinue oxygen. ➤ **Rationale:** This prevents combustion.
17. Ensure that synchronization indicator is superimposed on the R wave of ECG.
18. Give command to "stand clear," and stand clear yourself.
19. The healthcare provider depresses discharge buttons on paddles and keeps them depressed until cardioversion countershock is delivered. The shock may not occur instantly, since the machine waits until the next R wave in the ECG to discharge.

Table 33-4 Stepwise Energy Levels for Cardioversion

Cardioversion	Energy Level (J)*
Paroxysmal supraventricular tachycardia	50–100–200–300, then 360/J
Atrial flutter	50–100–200–300, then 360/J
Atrial fibrillation	200–300, then 360/J
Unstable ventricular tachycardia (VT with pulses)	100–200–300, then 360/J

*1 joule (J) = 1 watt second

20. Observe postcardioversion rhythm.

> **CLINICAL ALERT**
> If repeat cardioversion is necessary, reset the defibrillator to *synchronize* mode. Most defibrillators default back to unsynchronized mode (immediate shock).

21. Provide postcardioversion care.
    a. Support airway and ventilation, and oxygenate as needed.
    b. Obtain 12-lead ECG, and label it "postcardioversion."
    c. Monitor heart rhythm continuously.
    d. Evaluate vital signs, ECG, level of consciousness, peripheral pulses, and neurologic status until stable, and then routinely. ➤ **Rationale:** Thromboemboli to the brain, lungs, or systemic circulation may occur after cardioversion for atrial fibrillation. Coumadin therapy is continued indefinitely postcardioversion.
    e. Keep client under observation for 12 to 24 hr or per agency protocol. ➤ **Rationale:** Transient hypotension and minor dysrhythmias may occur.
22. Clean reusable equipment and discard used supplies.
23. Perform hand hygiene.

> **LEGAL ALERT**
> In *Odem v. State ex rel Dept of Health and Hospitals* (1999), evidence supported holding nurses negligent for improperly inactivating the client's cardiac and apnea monitors. Doctors issued orders to leave monitor alarms on at all times; no nurse heard a monitor alarm, and postdeath investigation indicated that the monitor alarm was not engaged. The electronic engineer from the monitor's manufacturer testified that the monitor was functional when he tested it after the incident. Had the monitor alarm sounded, the client might have lived.

Unit 33.3 Documentation and Evaluation

DOCUMENTATION for Cardiac Emergencies

Defibrillation
- Time of event and call for code
- Time chest compressions were started
- Client assessment before and after defibrillation
- Pre- and postdefibrillation ECG rhythm printout
- Number of defibrillation attempts and watt seconds (J) used
- Other resuscitative measures
- Time resuscitation discontinued
- Outcome of resuscitation
- Medications administered
- Record of responses and interventions (time and personnel) on Code Record
- Family support provided

Cardioversion

- Elective cardioversion client preparation completed
- Precardioversion rhythm and vital signs
- Name of healthcare provider performing elective cardioversion
- Number of cardioversion attempts
- Watt seconds (J) for each attempt
- Postcardioversion rhythm with each attempt
- Postcardioversion problems, if any
- Medications administered
- Postcardioversion monitoring

EVALUATION/Critical Thinking

Expected Outcomes

- Supplies and medications are readily available in an emergency situation.
- Client's heart rhythm is restored to normal after defibrillation or synchronized cardioversion.

Unexpected Outcomes	Alternative Actions
For Emergency Cart	
• Equipment cannot be located promptly on cart.	• After resuscitation, suggest more logical placement of item (e.g., alphabetize or place with similar equipment). • After resuscitation, practice mock codes to retrieve items and become more familiar with cart.
• Equipment malfunctions.	• Replace malfunctioning equipment immediately. • Obtain cart from the nearest unit.
For Cardioversion	
• Precardioversion laboratory findings reveal electrolyte imbalance, drug toxicity, or abnormal ABGs.	• Notify healthcare provider of findings. • Reassure client that there is not a life-threatening problem. Procedure may be delayed or postponed.
• Monitor shows asystole.	• Assess client for breathing and pulse. • View a different ECG lead; increase amplitude of lead. • Immediately institute CPR if indicated. • Assist healthcare provider in advanced cardiac life-support measures.
• Ventricular fibrillation develops after cardioversion.	• Call a code and proceed with defibrillation CPR process.

Nursing Process Data

ASSESSMENT Database

- Assess client for presence of risk factors for acute respiratory distress syndrome: sepsis, massive trauma, massive fat embolism, aspiration pneumonia, and other disorders characterized by abnormal ventilation and interstitial pulmonary edema.
- Auscultate heart and lung sounds for baseline data.
- Assess vital signs and measure arterial blood gases and hemodynamic pressures if Swan–Ganz catheter is in place.
- Identify whether need for mechanical ventilation is present. Criteria for non-COPD clients:

  Vital capacity is less than 15 mL/kg of body weight.

  Negative inspiratory pressure is less than –25 cm H_2O.

  pCO_2 is below 30 mm Hg or above 50 mm Hg.

  Alveolar–arterial oxygen difference (A–a Δ pO_2) is greater than 350 mm Hg on 100% oxygen.

  Pulmonary shunt is greater than 30%.

  Dead space-tidal volume (V_D–V_T) ratio is greater than 60%.

  pO_2 is less than 60 mm Hg on an FiO_2 of 1 (100%).

- Observe for trend of respiratory values (trend is more important than isolated measurements).
- Assess client for indications for PEEP:

  Inability to maintain arterial pO_2 of at least 70 mm Hg on 50% oxygen during continuous mechanical ventilation.

  Failure of other methods to reduce pulmonary shunt (e.g., treatment of cardiac failure or pneumonia).

  Normovolemia (normal blood volume).

- Check healthcare provider's orders for ventilator mode and other specified settings.
- Assess client's readiness for ventilator weaning.
- Assess client's response to ventilator weaning.

PLANNING Objectives

- To provide or augment pulmonary function
- To promote gas exchange and maintain acid/base balance
- To prevent ventilator-associated pneumonia
- To wean the client from mechanical support to independent breathing as safely and quickly as possible

IMPLEMENTATION Procedures

DOCUMENTATION AND EVALUATION

Expected Outcomes

- Mechanical ventilation maintains client's respiratory function.
- ABGs remain within an acceptable range during mechanical ventilation.
- Client does not develop ventilator-associated pneumonia (VAP).
- Weaning to independent breathing is accomplished safely and as quickly as possible.

Unexpected Outcomes/Alternative Actions

Pearson Nursing Student Resources

Find additional review materials at
nursing.pearsonhighered.com.
Prepare for success with NCLEX®-style practice questions and Skill Checklists.

Alterations of Ventilation and Gas Exchange

Adequate gas exchange in the lungs depends on the effective ventilation of air matched with the perfusion of blood to ventilated alveoli. The thickness and permeability of the alveolar membrane, the amount of surface area available for **diffusion**, and the pressure gradients are also factors that affect gas exchange. The pressure gradient is the difference between the partial pressures of pO_2 and pCO_2 in the alveolar air and the pulmonary capillary blood. The pressure gradients drive the inward diffusion of oxygen from alveolar air to the blood and the outward diffusion of carbon dioxide from the blood to the alveolar air for exhalation. These pressures are obtained by arterial blood gas testing.

Ventilation replenishes the supply of oxygen in the alveoli and removes the carbon dioxide released by the capillaries. If ventilation and perfusion are not matched, blood oxygenation is reduced, resulting in a right (heart) to left (heart) "shunt." Right to left shunting is characterized by a low pO_2 (hypoxemia).

Ventilation–perfusion mismatch problems are usually the result of chronic conditions such as chronic obstructive pulmonary disease (COPD). They may also occur acutely due to perfusion failure (e.g., pulmonary embolism), ventilatory failure (e.g., drug overdose, pulmonary disease, sepsis), or pulmonary edema affecting diffusion.

Mechanical ventilation provides support for the work of breathing and ensures alveolar ventilation. This intervention, however, may require intubation of the client, interferes with normal airway defenses, and increases the risk of pulmonary injury and healthcare-associated infection. It is desirable to decrease the level of controlled ventilatory support as soon as possible to assist the client to extubation and the return to independent breathing. Newer techniques of ventilation allow **weaning** by titrating from high support to minimal support modes to facilitate the transition.

Clients (especially those with underlying disease) who require mechanical ventilation for even a day may develop "ventilator dependence." All efforts focus on identifying and addressing the physiologic and psychological factors that delay successful weaning. This complex process requires the collaborative efforts of a skilled multidisciplinary team including healthcare provider, nurse, respiratory care practitioner, dietitian, and speech pathologist. Final clinical outcomes range from successful weaning to incomplete weaning (client remains on ventilatory support at home or in a subacute setting) or terminal weaning at the client's or family's request. Terminal weaning may be facilitated with a continuous infusion of morphine or a sedative to ease the client's death.

Skill 33.4.1 | Caring for the Mechanically Ventilated Client

In many agencies, respiratory therapists set up the ventilator and manage the settings and other equipment-related needs of the ventilator. The nurse should be familiar with the ventilator and how it functions. In some agencies, nursing staff may have more responsibilities in this area. It is also important to implement evidence-based practices to reduce the incidence of ventilator-associated events such as unplanned extubations and ventilator-associated pneumonia.

Equipment
Ventilator ❶
Handheld resuscitator bag connected to oxygen flowmeter
Airway connector
Sterile suction supplies
Ventilator flow sheet
Means for client communication

Preparation
1. Double-check the ventilator settings against those ordered by the healthcare provider (Box 33-6 ■). Familiarize yourself with location of alarm systems on the ventilator and make sure all alarms are activated.
2. Introduce self, identify the client, and perform hand hygiene.

❶ Computerized mechanical ventilator.

(continued)

Skill 33.4.1 | Caring for the Mechanically Ventilated Client *(continued)*

Procedure

1. Validate that tube cuff inflation is appropriate with minimal occlusive volume or minimal leak (squeak heard at end inspiration) while auscultating over the suprasternal notch.
2. Make sure the ventilator tubing is connected to client's endotracheal tube or tracheostomy tube.

Box 33-6 **INITIAL VENTILATOR SETTINGS**

- Tidal volume of 8–12 mL/kg (based on ideal body weight)

Note: Reduced volume (6 mL/kg) is indicated for clients with reduced lung compliance (e.g., ARDS) to prevent volutrauma.

- Respiratory rate of 10–15 per min
- Inspiratory–expiratory (I:E) ratio 1:2 (I:E ratio should be less than 1:1 to prevent air trapping in the lungs.)
- Pressure limit 20% above peak airway pressures delivered
- FiO_2 of 40–100%

EVIDENCE-BASED PRACTICE

Improving Nutrition in Critically Ill Clients

A recent study published in *The Lancet* found supplementing enteral feeding with parenteral nutrition in ICU clients can be beneficial if the timing is right. A randomized control trial found that when clients who were not receiving enough nutrients through enteral feedings were given supplemental parenteral nutrition starting on day 4, they had improved outcomes without the complications often seen with parenteral nutrition (bloodstream infections, nosocomial infections, and sepsis). They indicate that the timing is the important factor and that before parenteral feedings are added, clients are started on the enteral nutrition first, and support for that is maximized.

Source: Heidegger et al. (2013)

Reducing Unplanned Extubations

Clients in the intensive care unit who are intubated and on ventilators are at risk for self-extubation before it is time for the endotracheal tube to be removed. These unplanned extubations can put the client in potentially life-threatening situations. Risk factors associated with unplanned extubations are client level of consciousness, agitation, use of restraints, methods of securing endotracheal tube, and inadequate sedation. A recent study found that when nurses complied with pain and sedation protocols in addition to ventilator weaning protocols, the rates of unplanned extubations decreased. This is an important step in reducing a problem that can put clients at risk for respiratory compromise and in reducing use of restraints in intensive care units to prevent extubations.

Source: Jarachovic, Mason, Kerber, & McNett (2011)

---

3. Monitor client's vital signs as indicated by client's condition.
4. Obtain arterial blood gases as indicated by client's condition.
5. Check ventilator settings ❷ and the delivered values: tidal volume, inspiratory pressure, peak pressure, rate, FiO_2, inspiratory–expiratory (I:E) ratio, ventilatory modes. Modern ventilators monitor these parameters continuously (Box 33-7 ■). ➤ *Rationale:* As a nurse, you are responsible for knowing what the settings are for your client.

Box 33-7 **AIRWAY PRESSURE MODES**

IPPB—Intermittent positive pressure breathing—inspiration by positive airway pressure; expiration is passive.

CVM/ACV—Invasive or noninvasive continuous mandatory ventilation—total support ventilation with set ventilation rate (e.g., 12) and set tidal volume (e.g., 750 mL). Client-initiated breaths receive set volume and if client does not initiate the breath, a set rate and volume are guaranteed (sometimes referred to as ACV, meaning assist control ventilation).

SIMV—Synchronous intermittent mandatory ventilation—spontaneous ventilation is intermittently augmented by positive pressure ventilation.

PEEP—Positive end-expiratory pressure—an expiratory airway pressure modality in which the airway pressure is maintained above atmospheric at the end of expiration. Some machines may have capability to vary the PEEP level according to a preset pattern. This stimulates **surfactant** production and increases FRC (functional residual capacity).

CPAP—Invasive or noninvasive continuous positive airway pressure—spontaneous ventilation with maintenance of airway pressures above atmospheric throughout the respiratory cycle.

BiPAP—Spontaneous breathing with maintenance of bi-positive airway pressure—one set for positive inspiratory pressure and a lesser one set for positive expiratory pressure.

APRV—Airway pressure release ventilation—ventilator maintains an inspiratory pressure throughout the inspiration time. A short pressure release at the end of the respiratory cycle allows airway pressure to return to zero for a short time.

PSV—Pressure support ventilation—in addition to other ventilator settings, 6–10 cm H_2O pressure support provided to compensate for the added resistance imposed by artificial airways, making breathing easier; it also supports a larger tidal volume with less work of breathing. This is used as a major mode with pressure support level set to achieve optimal minute ventilation.

PCV—Pressure control ventilation—ventilator minimizes the pressure used to deliver an acceptable tidal volume. Some machines measure the compliance of the client–ventilator interface and calculate the ideal acceptable minimum tidal volume using the least pressure necessary. The pressure control level is adjusted to some maximum number, then the machine electronically selects the appropriate tidal volume based on PCV value set and previously calculated compliance. This is also used as a major mode.

❷ Double-check all ventilator settings with healthcare provider's orders.

6. Record intake, output, and daily weights.
7. Auscultate lungs hourly or as appropriate, and suction clients regularly to clear secretions.

Note: Continuous pulse oximetry and end tidal CO_2 facilitate constant assessment of clients receiving ventilatory assistance.

8. Observe and listen for possible cuff leaks around tracheostomy or endotracheal tubes.
9. Provide oral hygiene to clients every 4 hr (Box 33-8 ■).
   ➤ **Rationale:** This prevents ventilator-associated pneumonia.
10. Maintain HOB at 30 degrees or higher. ➤ **Rationale:** This reduces risk of ventilator-associated pneumonia (see Box 33-9 ■).

Box 33-8 ORAL AND DENTAL CARE STRATEGIES TO REDUCE RISK OF VAP

Assess client's teeth, lips, tongue, and check oral mucosa for ulcerations. Look for signs of gingival disease daily (red, spongy smooth, and shiny gingiva may be diseased).

To remove dental plaque, use a soft bristle toothbrush with antibacterial toothpaste to brush all surfaces of the teeth, gums, and tongue twice daily. Rinse with alcohol-free mouth rinse.

Note: Sponge toothettes do not remove plaque, a mass that grows by layering of bacteria on the surface of teeth and surrounding soft tissues and increases over time in the ICU setting. There is a link between increases in dental plaque and the development of VAP.

Use an oral swab with 1.5% hydrogen peroxide to cleanse the oral cavity and surrounding tissues and gums every 4 hr.

Provide suctioning of subglottic secretions continuously, or intermittently every 2 hr.

Apply moisturizer to oral mucosa and lips every 2–4 hr.

Source: Garcia et al. (2009)

Box 33-9 REDUCING RISK OF VENTILATOR-ASSOCIATED PNEUMONIA (VAP)

Note: Half of critically ill clients require mechanical ventilation. VAP occurs in 25% of clients who receive mechanical ventilation and is the leading cause of death from healthcare-associated infections.

Perform orotracheal rather than nasotracheal intubation.

Use dual lumen ET tubes (with dorsal lumen above the cuff) to allow continuous or intermittent suctioning of subglottic secretions. This decreases VAP by as much as 20–40%.

Ensure secretions are cleared from above the tube cuff before deflating the cuff.

Maintain cuff pressure at 20 cm H_2O.

Use only sterile fluid to flush the reusable suction catheter of secretions.

Prevent gastric reflux and oropharyngeal secretions aspiration by keeping the head of bed elevated 30–45 degrees.

Routinely verify placement of feeding tubes.

Change ventilator circuit only when visibly soiled or malfunctioning.

Drain tubing condensation away from the client.

Prevent or modulate oropharyngeal colonization with implementation of a comprehensive oral/dental hygiene program (see Box 33-8, Oral and Dental Care Strategies).

Don gloves upon entering the client's room.

Perform hand hygiene before and after putting on gloves, before and after contact with mucous membranes and respiratory secretions, or before and after contact with any respiratory device.

Use personal protective equipment as indicated.

Optimize sedation, interrupt it daily, and promote early mobilization (e.g., sitting on side of bed).

Perform daily assessment to wean client.

Sources: CDC (2009) and Grap (2009)

(continued)

Skill 33.4.1 | Caring for the Mechanically Ventilated Client *(continued)*

11. If necessary, discard accumulated water in the ventilator tubing via inline closed circuit drain. ➤ *Rationale:* Opening the circuit exposes client to environmental pathogens. Frequency of circuit opening should be minimized.

12. Provide client with a call bell and method of communication, such as a "magic slate" or picture board (Box 33-10 ■).

13. Administer medication (H₂ antagonists) as ordered. ➤ *Rationale:* Upper GI bleed is frequently associated with mechanical ventilation.

14. Test the nasogastric fluid and stool for occult blood if ordered.

15. Assess lung compliance frequently. ➤ *Rationale:* Lung compliance falls before changes are evident in blood gas analysis or clinical manifestations. Compliance is determined by

$$\frac{VT}{PIP - PEEP}$$

where VT = tidal volume; PIP = peak inspiratory pressure; and PEEP = positive end-expiratory pressure.

CLINICAL ALERT

In clients with reduced lung compliance (e.g., ARDS), tidal volume may be reduced to 6 mL/kg to prevent **volutrauma**. This will result in **hypercarbia** (increased pCO_2) and reduced blood pH (7.2 lowest acceptable). Sedation and paralytic agents may be necessary to control ventilation in these clients.

Box 33-10 CULTURAL AWARENESS

Touch-button voice systems are available that allow ventilated English or non–English-speaking clients to tap a touch screen that delivers preprogrammed audible words, phrases, or symbols to enable two-way communication with staff.

16. Implement methods for stress reduction, such as careful explanation of procedures, pain management, administration of sedatives or neuromuscular blocking agents as indicated.

CLINICAL ALERT

The use of sedatives in mechanically ventilated clients prolongs its duration as well as the length of hospitalization and ICU stay.

Paralytic agents have no effect on wakefulness or sensory perception, including perception of pain. With complete paralysis, pain might be manifested as increased heart rate, increased blood pressure, or sweating. Never assume that a client receiving a paralytic agent is asleep. Continually inform the client about care, offer reassurance, and provide pain relief while the paralyzing effect of the drug persists.

---

17. Monitor the client frequently to detect changes in status.

EVIDENCE-BASED NURSING PRACTICE
Delirium in Mechanically Ventilated Clients

In 2013, the American College of Critical Care Medicine updated the guidelines for the management of pain, agitation, and delirium for intensive care unit clients. An article published in the *American Journal of Critical Care* highlighted some of those recommendations. In particular, they recommended the routine monitoring of delirium in adult ICU clients using the Confusion Assessment Method for the ICU (CAM-ICU) and the Intensive Care Delirium Screening Checklist (ICDSC), both of which are valid and reliable instruments. Delirium is associated with excess morbidity, mortality, and long-term cognitive impairment.

Source: Riker & Fraser (2013)

Skill 33.4.2 | Weaning the Mechanically Ventilated Client

Equipment
Oxygen source
T-piece adaptor or tracheostomy mask, if ordered
Suctioning equipment
Arterial blood gas-sampling supplies
Continuous pulse oximetry unit
Stethoscope

Preparation

1. Validate order for weaning trial and assess client's readiness:
   Spontaneous tidal volume ≥7 mL/kg/ideal body weight (IBW)

   Respiratory rate between 12 and 20 breaths/min
   Minute ventilation (respiratory rate × VT) ≥10 L/min
   Vital signs stable (SBP ≥ 90) normal heart rate and rhythm
   Vital capacity ≥ 10 mL/kg IBW
   Negative inspiratory force is −20 cm H_2O or higher
   ABGs: pH 7.35 − 7.5, pO_2 ≥ 60 mm Hg on FiO_2 ≤ 40% or SpO_2 90%
   Able to protect airway and responsive on minimal sedation

2. Introduce self and identify the client using two client identifiers. Perform hand hygiene.

3. Note client's work of breathing and use of accessory muscles.

4. Note current ECG pattern for baseline.
5. Explain the weaning process to the client. Reassure the client that transition will be based on the client's responses. ➤ *Rationale:* When the client is included in weaning process and rationale for change, anxiety is lessened.

> **CLINICAL ALERT**
>
> Some "smart care" machines allow CPAP and PS plus an individualized weaning process based on preset client parameters, including disease process. The machine gradually decreases the degree of support as long as the client remains in a breathing comfort zone. The machine then displays a message indicating it is appropriate to extubate the client.

6. Suction the client. Hyperoxygenate client's lungs with 100% oxygen before and after suctioning.
7. Maintain endotracheal or tracheostomy cuff at minimal occlusive pressure (minimal leak) while mechanically ventilated.
8. Establish continuous oximetry. ➤ *Rationale:* Client's oxygen status should be continually assessed.

Procedure

1. Elevate head of the bed to facilitate client's diaphragmatic excursion.
2. If healthcare provider orders endotracheal tube cuff deflated during weaning, suction secretions that have accumulated above the cuff as follows:
   a. Provide positive pressure to end of tube with a handheld-resuscitation bag and 100% oxygen.
   b. Place tip of suction catheter in the posterior pharynx.
   c. Deflate cuff and apply suction to the catheter.
      ➤ *Rationale:* Positive pressure blows the secretions into the pharynx, where they can be suctioned out.

Note: Steps a–c are not necessary if a CASS-ETT tube is in place.

   d. Hyperoxygenate lungs with 100% oxygen for three to five breaths.
3. If ordered, connect T-piece to wide-bore oxygen tubing leading to the gas source.
4. Set oxygen concentration as ordered by healthcare provider, usually 10% *higher* than the ventilator FiO_2 the client has been receiving.
5. If appropriate, remove ventilator tubing from airway and connect T-piece to client's airway.
6. Cover the end of ventilator tubing with sterile gauze.
7. Observe for vital sign changes, apprehension, diaphoresis, and dysrhythmias. ➤ *Rationale:* Only a mild increase in blood pressure, pulse, and respiratory rate is normal. Mild to moderate anxiety is also normal.

> **CLINICAL ALERT**
>
> Clustering nighttime care activities to allow clients undisrupted sleep periods may facilitate the weaning process.

8. Measure arterial blood gases 1 hr after initiating weaning if client tolerates.
9. Proceed with the weaning procedure as ordered.
   ➤ *Rationale:* Gradual weaning may be necessary.
10. If the client tolerates no ventilator support (other than PSV), extubate the client. (See Skill 30.4.6, Extubating an Endotracheal Tube.)
11. After weaning, continue to monitor vital signs, vital capacity, SpO_2, end tidal CO_2, inspiratory pressure, blood gases, and subjective response.

Unit 33.4 Documentation and Evaluation

DOCUMENTATION for Mechanical Ventilation

- Type of ventilator or other device used
- Ventilator or device settings; modes used in weaning process
- Time initiated
- Any problems and actions taken
- Suctioning (i.e., frequency, amount, and character of secretions)
- Indication whether client is making spontaneous breathing efforts or is not triggering the machine

- Endotracheal tube location and minimal leak established
- Arterial blood gas and other lab values
- Vital signs and hemodynamic values
- Findings on pulmonary and cardiac assessment
- Ventilator modes utilized in weaning transition process
- Dental and oral care (type, frequency)
- HOB degree elevation
- Medications administered

EVALUATION/Critical Thinking

Expected Outcomes

- Mechanical ventilation maintains client's respiratory function.
- ABGs remain within an acceptable range during mechanical ventilation.
- Client does not develop ventilator-associated pneumonia.
- Weaning to independent breathing is accomplished safely and as quickly as possible.

Unexpected Outcomes	Alternative Actions
• Client develops signs of decreased pulmonary compliance (e.g., ARDS).	• Check for signs of fluid in lungs (x-ray, increase in PAWP, crackles on auscultation, hypoxemia). • Decrease the tidal volume being delivered. • Suction client to maintain a patent airway. • Increase the level of PEEP to prevent alveolar closure. • Consider prone positioning.
• Client needs to be transported for diagnostic testing.	• Start oxygen flow through handheld ventilating device. • Attach expiratory resistance, such as PEEP. • Disconnect ventilator tubing from airway at end of inspiration. • Attach handheld ventilator to airway during expiration. • Watch chest, and provide breaths with client's inspirations or at rate of 10–12/min. • Turn and deep breathe or sigh client several times an hour to reopen atelectatic alveoli.
• High pressure alarm is activated.	• Check for obstructions in tubing and take corrective measures. • Suction client for possible mucus obstruction of airway.
• Low pressure alarm is activated.	• Check for disconnected tubing or loose connections, and tighten them if present. • Check client for artificial airway displacement and provide emergency measures if indicated. • Deflate and reinflate the airway cuff to minimal occlusive pressure to adjust a possible cuff leak. • If unable to identify and relieve cause immediately, disconnect ventilator tubing, hand ventilate client, and summon help.
• Arterial blood gases (ABGs) are not maintained within normal range.	• Notify healthcare provider of grossly abnormal ABGs, and obtain order for alteration in ventilator settings (i.e., increased percentage of oxygen, decreased tidal volume, addition of "dead space"). • Maintain mechanical ventilation. Do not attempt to wean or extubate client. • Suction client as needed to maintain airway patency.
• pO_2 is not maintained at 80–100 mm Hg.	• Continue delivery of PEEP as ordered. If not effective, notify healthcare provider. • Do not attempt to wean client off PEEP until desired parameters are obtained.

Unexpected Outcomes	**Alternative Actions**
• Cardiac output decreases significantly.	• Anticipate that client may have difficulty adjusting to increased intrathoracic pressure during weaning process. • Decrease PEEP and notify healthcare provider for weaning adjustment.
• Weaning attempt is unsuccessful.	• Continue use of ventilator. • Cluster nighttime care activities to allow undisrupted sleep. • If client is extubated, consider noninvasive ventilation (CPAP). • Recruit skilled multidisciplinary team to identify and address physiologic and psychological factors that interfere with weaning success.
• Decreased level of consciousness, dyspnea, severe anxiety, or fatigue occurs during weaning process.	• Note client's SpO_2 (anxiety may be due to hypoxemia). • Place client on supportive ventilation. • Provide thorough explanation, and increase reassurance. • Evaluate present use of sedatives or narcotic agents administered.
• Client develops unstable vital signs.	• Place client back on more supportive ventilator mode. • Monitor vital signs more frequently, and obtain blood gases to determine oxygen concentration. • Increase FiO_2.
• Client develops ventilator-associated pneumonia.	• Use a continuous aspiration subglottic secretion ET tube. • Use closed in-line system for suctioning. • Maintain HOB elevation 30–45 degrees to prevent gastric reflux aspiration. • Discontinue mechanical ventilation as soon as possible. • Change the ventilator circuit only if soiled or malfunctioning. • Perform hand hygiene before and after contact with mucous membranes, secretions, contaminated objects. • Drain circuitry condensate away from the client. • Implement meticulous oral and oropharyngeal hygiene strategies.

Chapter Wrap-Up

GERONTOLOGIC Considerations

Older Adult Clients in the Critical Care Unit Require More Intensive Observation and Consideration

• Aging is normally accompanied by a silent physiologic decline and diminished reserve in all body systems. These changes are not pathologic, but do make older adults less adaptable to stress and illness. Older adults have a greater prevalence of chronic conditions that make them vulnerable to acute exacerbations. Over half of critical care clients are over age 65. Hospitalization is almost twice as long as that for clients under age 65 and survival is 81% compared with 98% in younger clients. However, quality of life after discharge from a critical care unit is not age-related.

• Refer to Gerontologic Considerations throughout this book for organ-system changes and other functional alterations, as well as socioeconomic and lifestyle changes, that affect care of the older client.

MANAGEMENT Guidelines

Each state legislates a Nurse Practice Act for RNs and LVN/LPNs. Healthcare facilities are responsible for establishing and implementing policies and procedures that conform to their state's regulations. Verify the regulations and role parameters for each healthcare worker in your facility.

Delegation

- All personnel in the critical care setting must know how to quickly summon assistance and locate and use emergency and resuscitation equipment.
- In advanced care settings, the RN simultaneously assesses, analyzes, makes decisions, intervenes, and evaluates clients on a continual basis. Complexities of care and unpredictability of outcomes necessitate *intense* ongoing client monitoring and evaluation and personal continuing education. Detection and interpretation of subtle areas of change in the client's status require the knowledge and skill of the professional nurse.
- The RN collaborates with the healthcare provider and respiratory care practitioner for ventilator settings.
- It is the responsibility of nursing faculty to ensure that students participating in client care (in any setting) are prepared to do so. Likewise, it is the duty of the student to refuse to perform a function he or she is not qualified or competent to perform.
- The nurse should not assume care for any client who requires care beyond the caregiver's expertise.
- Many agencies provide emergency care protocols or standing orders of action responses to specified changes in client status. The professional nurse must be familiar with conditions for which the nurse is delegated medical care decisions guided by such protocols.
- The CNA/UAP must know to leave the arterial catheter site uncovered for easy observation.

- The CNA/UAP must not move tubing drainage receptacles (e.g., Pleurevac) without supervision.
- The CNA/UAP must understand that IVs, drainage systems, and ventilator circuits and systems, are closed and must be able to give care without disrupting system integrity or disconnecting components for the convenience of care (e.g., as in changing the client's gown or position).
- The UAP has a limited role in the care of clients who require invasive monitoring. They can offer valued assistance in moving or positioning clients and providing personal hygiene and comfort measures under the direction of the professional nurse.
- The UAP assists the client, preserving an interface between technology and reality, by providing a human dimension of tactile presence while providing basic physical care for clients requiring sophisticated technological monitoring. UAP links to the client assist all caregivers in their attempts to minimize client's feelings of alienation.

Interprofessional Communication

Although certain tasks may be delegated, the CNA/UAP also can provide vital data to the professional nurse by immediately *reporting*:

- Disconnected systems, loose electrodes, tubing leaks, wet or soiled dressings
- Subjective or objective change in the client's status (e.g., pain, respiratory distress, acute change in cognition)
- Equipment alarms (e.g., ventilator alarms)
- Near-empty infusion bags
- Near-full collection devices
- Collaboration with an interdisciplinary team helps to support client's weaning from mechanical ventilation

CASE STUDY Applications

Scenario 1

Mr. Jones has a history of COPD and heart failure and has been admitted to your unit with a diagnosis of acute respiratory failure. He has the following arterial blood gas values: pH 7.2, pCO_2, 66 mm Hg, HCO_3^- 25 mEq, and pO_2 49 mm Hg. He is intubated and receiving mechanical ventilation to support his breathing and improve gas exchange and is being sedated with Versed.

On the third day of hospitalization, he is being weaned from mechanical ventilation, but attempts are unsuccessful due to difficulty breathing and development of pulmonary edema.

1. How does mechanical ventilation differ from the normal physiologic process of breathing?
2. How will resultant changes in intrathoracic pressure affect venous return and cardiac work?

3. What measures should be employed to help achieve successful weaning and extubation in this client?

Scenario 2

Mr. Hooper has been admitted to the coronary care unit with the diagnosis of anterior septal myocardial infarction with lateral ischemia and potential for infarct extension. He is being monitored by a balloon-tipped, flow-directed catheter for hemodynamic response to therapy. Myocardial infarction (tissue necrosis) results from an imbalance between heart work (demand for oxygen) and coronary supply of oxygen.

Mr. Hooper's hemodynamic measures include: cardiac index 1.8 (low), blood pressure 94/74, mean arterial pressure (MAP) 80 (normal), stroke volume 21 mL (low), pulmonary artery wedge pressure (PAWP) 24 (elevated), heart rate 110, systemic vascular resistance increased.

1. Explain the relationship between "heart work" and need for oxygen.
2. Discuss the parameters that can be monitored with the balloon-tipped catheter.
3. Identify two drugs that could be used to decrease "heart work" and nursing measures that would enhance their effectiveness.

NCLEX® Review Questions

Unless otherwise specified, choose only one (1) answer.

1. In the multilumen balloon-tipped flow-directed catheter, what is the distal lumen used to do?
   A. Measure cardiac output
   B. Measure pulmonary artery pressure
   C. Inject solutions
   D. Measure central venous pressure

2. The clients' phlebostatic axis is used for the transducer level in order to obtain accurate monitoring. The phlebostatic axis is determined by joining lines at which locations?
   Select all that apply.
   A. Midaxilla horizontally
   B. Fourth intercostal space horizontally
   C. Mid-anterior–posterior chest horizontally
   D. Manubrium horizontally
   E. Anterior axillary fold vertically
   F. Mid-anterior–posterior chest vertically
   G. Fourth intercostal space vertically

3. Which of the following statements is true regarding arterial blood pressure monitoring?
   A. Measures are less accurate, but continuous, therefore more convenient.
   B. It allows intermittent sampling of venous blood.
   C. It may interfere with distal perfusion of the extremity.
   D. It can be used for calculating the heart rate.

4. What is the rationale for use of the blood conservatory system for arterial blood sampling?
   A. It eliminates the need for blood wasting.
   B. It eliminates the need to open the tubing system.
   C. It eliminates the need to disengage alarms.
   D. It is less time-consuming than standard sampling.

5. After successful cardioversion for atrial fibrillation, what must the client continue?
   A. Antiarrhythmic therapy
   B. Anticoagulant therapy
   C. Pacemaker interrogation (monitoring)
   D. Monthly cardioversion

6. Which of the following do lethal cardiac rhythms requiring defibrillation include?
   Select all that apply.
   A. Pulseless ventricular tachycardia
   B. Unstable ventricular tachycardia
   C. Ventricular fibrillation
   D. Atrial fibrillation with ventricular response (rate over 150)
   E. Asystole
   F. Pulseless electrical activity

7. What is the most common cause of pulseless electrical activity?
   A. Peripheral vascular disease
   B. Hyperkalemia
   C. Hypovolemia
   D. Heart failure

8. Which of the following is the most supportive of all the airway pressure modes used in mechanical ventilation?
   A. PEEP (positive end expiratory pressure)
   B. SIMV (synchronous intermittent mandatory ventilation)
   C. PS (pressure support)
   D. CMV (continuous mandatory ventilation)

9. Of the following statements, what is the best rationale for the use of paralytic agents in the mechanically ventilated client?
   A. They allow the client to sleep.
   B. They eliminate the need for restraints.
   C. They allow ventilator-client synchrony.
   D. They reduce pain perception.

10. What factors contribute to ventilator-associated pneumonia?
    Select all that apply.
    A. Aspiration of subglottic secretions
    B. Accumulation of condensation in the tubing circuit
    C. Saline injection into the airway before suctioning
    D. Immobilization and inability to turn the client
    E. Maintaining the head of the bed at 30 degrees or higher

QSEN Activity

Domain: Teamwork and Collaboration

KSA: Describe examples of the impact of team functioning on safety and quality of care.

Activity:

You are caring for your client in the intensive care unit. Your client experiences a cardiac arrest. The arrest team is called and arrives to provide care for the client. Describe the various roles of a cardiac arrest team in the hospital setting. What is your role as the primary nurse? How does this team affect the safety and quality of care for the client? What training should a cardiac arrest team have?

Bibliography

2010 American Heart Association Guidelines for Cardiopulmonary Resuscitation and Emergency Cardiovascular Care Science. (2010) *Circulation, 122,* S640–S656.

Centers for Disease Control. (2009). Health-care associated infections: Ventilator-associated pneumonia. Retrieved from http://www.cdc.gov/HAI/vap/vap.html

Chan, P. S., Jain, R., Nallmothu, B. K., Berg, R. A., & Sasson, C. (2010). Rapid response teams: A systematic review and meta-analysis. *Archives of Internal Medicine, 170*(1), 18–26.

Dotson, B. (2010). Daily interruption of sedation in patients treated with mechanical ventilation. *American Journal of Health-System Pharmacy, 67*(12), 102–1006.

Garcia, R., Jendresky, L, Colbert, L., Bailey, A., Zaman, M., & Majumder, J. (2009). Reducing ventilator-associated pneumonia through advanced oral-dental care: A 48 month study. *American Journal of Critical Care, 18*(6), 523–531.

Graham, K. C., & Cvach, M. (2010). Monitor alarm fatigue: Standardizing use of physiological monitors and decreasing nuisance alarms. *American Journal of Critical Care, 19*(1), 28–34.

Grap, M. (2009). Not-so-trivial pursuit: Mechanical ventilation risk reduction. *American Journal of Critical Care, 18*(4), 299–309.

Heidegger, C. P., Berger, M. M., Graf, S., Zingg, W., Darmon, P., Costanza, M. C., . . . Pichard, C. (2013). Optimisation of energy provision with supplemental parenteral nutrition in critically ill patients: A randomised controlled clinical trial. *The Lancet, 381*(9864), 385–393.

Jabre, P., Belpomme, V., Azoulay, E., Jacob, L., Bertrand, L., Lapostolle, F., . . . & Adnet, F. (2013). Family presence during cardiopulmonary resuscitation. *New England Journal of Medicine, 368*(11), 1008–1018.

Jarachovic, M., Mason, M., Kerber, K., & McNett, M. (2011). The role of standardized protocols in unplanned extubations in a medical intensive care unit. *American Journal of Critical Care, 20*(4), 304–312.

Jones, C. M., Stewart, C., & Roszell, S. S. (2015). Beyond best practice: Implementing a unit-based CLABSI project. *Journal of Nursing Care Quality, 30*(1), 24–30.

Perrin, K. O. (2009). *Understanding the essentials of critical care nursing.* Upper Saddle River, NJ: Pearson/Prentice Hall.

Rauen, C. A, Chulay, M., Bridges, E., Vollman, K. M., & Arbour, R. (2008). Seven evidence-based practice habits: Putting some sacred cows out to pasture. *Critical Care Nurse, 28*(2), 98–123.

Riker, R. R., & Fraser, G. L. (2013). The new practice guidelines for pain, agitation, and delirium. *American Journal of Critical Care, 22*(2), 153–157.

Robinson, B., & Branson, R. (2009). Consequences of ventilator asynchrony. *Critical Care Medicine, 37*(10), 2848–2849.

Siela, D. (2010). Evaluation standards for management of artificial airways. *Critical Care Nurse, 30*(4), 76–77.

Tyler, L., Greco, S., Bridges, E., Barnes, S., Brown, L., Green, K. G., & Wolfson, D. (2013). Accuracy of Stop-Cursor Method for determining systolic and pulse pressure variation. *American Journal of Critical Care, 22*(4), 298–305.

U.S. Department of Health and Human Services. (2012). From VAP to VAE: Establishing new definitions for ventilator-associated events in adults. HHS 2012 progress toward eliminating HAI infections meeting summary, 131–134. Retrieved from http://health.gov/hcq/pdfs/2012-hai-progress-meeting-summary.pdf

Vincent, J. L., Rhodes, A., Perel, A., Martin, G. S., Della Rocca, G., Vallet, B., . . . & Singer, M. (2011). Clinical review: Update on hemodynamic monitoring: A consensus of 16. *Critical Care, 15*(4), 229.

Chapter 34
End-of-Life Care

Learning Objectives

34.1 Discuss the stages of the grief process.

34.2 State the main characteristics observed in an individual experiencing grief.

34.3 Identify the factors that influence the outcome of the grieving process.

34.4 Explain three assessment parameters for observing psychological and somatic symptoms that accompany the grief process.

34.5 Describe the stages of grief outlined by Elisabeth Kübler-Ross.

34.6 Explain what is meant by hospice and palliative care.

34.7 Discuss at least two nursing interventions for each stage of grief.

34.8 Explain what is meant by providing emotional care for the dying client.

34.9 Discuss at least four nursing interventions that assist the client during the end-of-life process.

34.10 Describe the three-step analgesic ladder for pain control for the dying client.

34.11 Describe the steps in providing postmortem care.

Chapter Outline

Terminology

Adjuvant drugs drugs that are not primarily designed to control pain, but rather enhance the analgesic efficacy of opioids, treating recurrent symptoms that exacerbate pain and providing independent analgesic effects.

Anorexia loss of appetite occurring from a variety of possible reasons.

Anxiety a troubled or apprehensive feeling; experiencing a sense of dread or fear.

Cope to contend with, strive, or handle.

Counseling giving assistance to or guidance.

Crisis a crucial point or situation in the course of life when previously used coping skills are no longer successful in managing a stressor or stressors; turning point.

Denial refusal to grant the truth of a statement or allegation.

Depression being dispirited, saddened; low in mood.

Empathy objective awareness of an insight into the feelings, emotions, and behavior of another individual.

Fear feeling of fright or dread related to a specific source (e.g., fear of pain or dying).

Grief intense mental anguish, deep remorse, sorrow.

Hospice a multidisciplinary approach that focuses on client care during the last phase of life.

Idealization to regard as ideal; to make or regard someone or something as perfect.

Loss the state of being deprived of or being without something that one has had, for example, the loss of a spouse or friend or natural ability such as sight or hearing.

Opioids drugs that block the transmission of pain messages to the brain such as morphine, methadone, codeine, oxycodone, hydrocodone, and numorphan; they are used to treat severe pain.

Pain an unpleasant sensory and emotional experience arising from actual or potential tissue damage or described in terms of such damage; whatever the experiencing individual says it is, existing whenever he or she says it does.

Palliative care client and family-centered care that focuses on providing clients with relief from the symptoms, pain, and stress of serious illnesses; it optimizes quality of life by anticipating, preventing, and treating suffering throughout the continuum of illness, involving physical, intellectual, emotional, social, and spiritual needs and facilitating client autonomy, access to information, and choice.

Quality Of Life (QOL) in the context of advanced, progressive, incurable illness, the subjective experience of an individual living with the interpersonal psychological and existential or spiritual challenges that accompany the process of physical and functional decline and the knowledge of impending demise. An individual's QOL can range from suffering associated with physical distress and/or a sense of impending disintegration to the completion of developmental work and the mastery of developmental landmarks.

Resolution the state of having made a firm determination; a course decided on.

Restitution a return to a former status.

Somatic referring to the body.

Stress a physically or emotionally disruptive or disquieting influence.

Suffering to feel pain or distress; includes fear of or actual physical distress, fear of dying, changing self-perceptions, relationship concerns, the need to find meaning in any given life experience, and past experiences of witnessing another individual's distress.

Therapeutic having medicinal or healing properties.

Withdrawal pulling back or away.

Loss and Grieving

Loss is part of the experience of dying, both for the individual as well as for family members and significant others. Within the dying experience, several losses can occur including loss of health, possible loss of body parts through surgery or an injury, loss of cognitive functioning, and the like. The individual may be unable to participate in religious activities or rituals that give meaning to life and contribute to the individual's spiritual well-being. The inability to work and provide financially for self and others may lead to impoverishment and financial difficulties. In addition, the individual may experience a loss of control in decision making.

Grief is an emotion experienced in relation to loss; it can also be viewed as a behavioral response to death and dying.

Human beings experience loss as the emotion of grief and must **withdraw** from the painful stimulus to recuperate. Emotions allow us to experience our environment—they are the means of cognition. When we are grieving, we experience the emotion of grief; this experience is accompanied by a definite syndrome with **somatic** and psychological symptoms.

Stages of Grief

George Engle, in a classic article in the *American Journal of Nursing*, 1964, describes progression of the grief process in stages. These stages (Box 34-1 ■) may occur in order, or an individual may skip a stage, become locked in a particular stage, or even return to an earlier stage already worked through.

Box 34-1 STAGES OF GRIEF

According to George Engle	According to Elisabeth Kübler-Ross
• Shock and disbelief	• Denial
• Developing awareness	• Anger
• Restitution	• Bargaining
• Resolution	• Depression
• Idealization	• Acceptance

The first stage is *shock and disbelief*, **denial** and numbness. The first response on learning of a death is shock and a refusal to accept or comprehend the fact. This reaction is followed by a stunned, numb feeling and does not allow the individual to acknowledge the reality of death. This initial phase is characterized by attempts to protect oneself against severe **stress**/distress by blocking recognition of the death.

Developing awareness is the second stage. Within minutes or hours the individual becomes acutely and increasingly aware of the anguish of loss. Anger may be present during this time and may be directed toward individuals or circumstances held to be responsible for the death. Behavior that frequently accompanies this stage is crying and a regression to a more helpless and childlike state. The crying and regression appear to acknowledge the loss, indicating that conscious awareness is now present.

The third stage is **restitution**, in which the various rituals of the culture, such as the funeral, attire, wake, particular folkways, and mores help to initiate the recovery process. These rituals serve the function of emphasizing the reality of death, and the very act of experiencing them assists the mourner to face the loss.

As the reality of death becomes accepted, the **resolution** of the loss begins. This stage involves a number of steps. First, the mourner attempts to deal with the painful void created by the loss of a loved one. At this time, the thoughts of the mourner are occupied almost exclusively with the deceased. Then the mourner becomes more aware of his or her own body and bodily sensations. Finally, the mourner begins to talk about the dead individual, recalling the dead individual's attributes and personality and reminiscing about the memories they shared. Resolving the loss is a long and painful phase that continues until the mourner remembers the positive aspects of the dead individual.

The next stage that is frequently experienced is that of **idealization**. All hostile and negative feelings toward the deceased are repressed. As the process proceeds, two important changes are taking place: The recurring thoughts about the dead individual bring a distinct image of the loss to mind and these memories serve to bring out the more positive aspects of the lost relationship. At the same time, the grieving individual begins to assume certain admired qualities of the dead individual through the mechanisms of identification or incorporation. The mourner may begin to dress, speak, or develop mannerisms or beliefs similar to the individual who was lost. Often, many months are required for this process to be experienced, and as it dissipates, the mourner's preoccupation with the dead individual lessens. It may be at this point that the individual begins to reinvest intimate feelings toward other relationships.

The mourning process usually takes a year or more. The clearest evidence of healing is the ability to remember the deceased comfortably and realistically, with both the pleasures and disappointments of the relationship. At this stage the obsession with the loss is ended and the individual accepts the responsibility of living his or her own life.

Individuals who experience loss move through at least some of these stages as they attempt to **cope** with the loss. The stages of grief are the means human beings have of moving through the loss to resolution.

Elisabeth Kübler-Ross first introduced the five stages of dying in her 1969 book, *On Death and Dying*. It described in five discrete stages a process by which people deal with grief and loss, especially when diagnosed with a terminal illness or catastrophic event. Kübler-Ross originally applied these stages to people **suffering** from terminal illness and later to other forms of emotional trauma or significant life events, such as the death of a loved one, divorce, injury, infertility, or change in financial status. The stages do not necessarily come in the same order, nor are all steps experienced by all individuals. Often, people will experience several stages, going between two or more stages, returning to one or more several times before working through the stages.

The first stage, as Kübler-Ross views this process, is that of denial. The denial may be partial or complete and may occur not only during the first stages of illness or confrontation, but also later on from time to time. This initial denial is usually a temporary defense and is used as a buffer until such time as the individual is able to collect himself or herself, mobilize defenses, and face the inevitability of loss or death.

The second stage is often anger. The individual feels anger and questions why this is happening to him or her. This emotion may be directed toward individuals in the environment or even projected into the environment at random. Kübler-Ross discusses this reaction and the difficulty in handling it for those close to the individual by explaining that we should put ourselves in the client's position and consider how we might feel intense anger at having our life interrupted abruptly, or at experiencing this loss.

The third stage is *bargaining*. The individual attempts to strike a bargain for more time to live or more time to be without pain in return for doing something for God. Often during this stage the individual turns or returns to religion.

Depression is the fourth stage. Usually, when people have completed the stages of denial, anger, and bargaining, they move into depression. Kübler-Ross writes about two kinds of depression. One is preparatory depression: This is a tool for dealing with the impending loss. The second type is reactive depression. In this form of depression, the individual is reacting against the impending loss of life and grieves for himself or herself.

The final stage of grieving is that of *acceptance*. This occurs when the individual has worked through the previous stages and accepts his or her own inevitable death or loss.

With full acceptance of impending death comes the preparation for it; however, even with acceptance, hope is still present and needs to be supported realistically.

Many factors influence how individuals, at the end of life, accept death. Personal values and beliefs about life; views of personal successes, both financial and emotional; the way they look physically during the dying process; their family and friends and their families' attitudes and reactions; their past experiences in coping with difficult or traumatic situations; and, finally, the healthcare staff who are caring for them during this process—all affect an individual's attitude toward dying.

Hospice and Palliative Care

The philosophy of **hospice** and **palliative care** is based on the belief that every individual has the right to die pain-free and with dignity, and that the families should receive the necessary support to ensure this happens (Box 34-2 ■). The word *hospice* comes from the Latin word *hospitium*, which was originally used to describe a place of shelter for weary and sick travelers. The modern hospice movements began in the 1960s by Dr. Cicely Saunders, a British physician. The first hospice in the United States was established in New Haven, Connecticut, in 1974. The National Hospice & Palliative Care Organization (NHPCO) was founded in 1978 as the National Hospice Organization and added palliative care in February 2000. Today there are more than 4,700 hospice programs with 1.5 to 1.6 million Medicare-enrolled people cared for in 2012. Hospice care has expanded around the world with an estimated 10,000 hospice programs internationally to provide palliative care, including specialized palliative care for children. Eighty percent of hospice care is provided in the client's or family member's home and in nursing homes; however, only 25% of clients die at home, with 25% dying in nursing homes and the remainder dying in acute care settings (National Hospice and Palliative Care Organization, 2013).

Hospice focuses on caring, not curing. Hospice is not a place, but a concept of care. Hospice care addresses the needs and opportunities during the last phase of life utilizing a multidisciplinary approach that focuses on the individual's physical symptoms and the emotional and spiritual concerns of the client and his or her family. Hospice care involves a multidisciplinary team collaboration among nurses, doctors, social workers, pastoral care, family, and others. The team works together to develop a plan of care and to provide services that will enhance the **quality of life** and provide support for the individual and family during the terminal phases of the illness and the bereavement period.

Hospice supports the philosophy that death is an integral part of the life cycle. It identifies intensive palliative care focused on pain relief, comfort, and enhanced quality of life as appropriate goals for those at the end of life. Hospice care clients include those with AIDS and amyotrophic lateral sclerosis (ALS) or children with cardiac anomalies or other congenital conditions who have a life expectancy of 6 months. Hospice care is no longer limited to 6 months of care. The healthcare providers still state that in their best judgment the clients have 6 months or less to live when hospice is ordered. However, if the clients are still alive after the six months, the clients can continue care. The clients are recertified that they are still terminal and hospice services are still appropriate. There is no end to the hospice benefit under Medicare if the clients continue to meet the expected 6-month criteria. Hospice can offer any treatment necessary to relieve suffering and allow a client to die peacefully and comfortably. Hospice neither speeds up nor slows down the dying process. It simply focuses on pain relief comfort and enhanced quality of life as appropriate goals for those at the end of life.

Box 34-2 **HOSPICE AND PALLIATIVE CARE INFORMATION**

The National Hospice and Palliative Care Organization
1731 King St.
Suite 100
Alexandria, VA 22314
(703) 837-1500
www.nhpco.org
Nonprofit membership organization representing hospice and palliative care programs and professionals in the United States.

Hospice Foundation of America
1710 Rhode Island Ave. NW
Suite 400
Washington, D.C. 20036
(800) 854-3402
www.hospicefoundation.org
Provides programs for healthcare professionals and the public who cope either personally or professionally with terminal illness, death, and the process of grief.

National Palliative Care Research Center
Brookdale Department of Geriatrics & Adult Development
Box 1070 Mount Sinai Ichan School of Medicine
One Gustave L. Levy Place
New York, NY 10029
(212) 241-7447
www.npcrc.org
E-mail nprc@mssm.edu
NPCRC is a national initiative committed to stimulating, developing, and funding palliative care research directed at improving care for clients with serious illness and their families.

Children's Hospice International
500 Montgomery St.
Suite 400
Alexandria, VA 22314
(703) 684-0330
www.chionline.org
Nonprofit organization to provide a network of support and care for children with life-threatening conditions and their families.

Palliative care is central to the comprehensive treatment of serious or life-threatening illnesses. Palliative care differs from hospice care in that it is appropriate at any point on the illness continuum. The client may receive palliative care at the same time they receive treatments that are meant to improve their health. It does not depend on whether the condition can be cured or not. The purpose of palliative care is to provide relief from distressing symptoms such as **pain**, shortness of breath, fatigue, constipation, loss of appetite, nausea, and many others. The expected outcome of palliative care is the prevention of suffering and improved quality of life.

Clients in hospice always receive palliative care, but hospice focuses on the final months of life. To qualify for hospice programs, clients must no longer be receiving treatments to cure their illness. Most hospice care is provided in the home; however, there are hospice units in hospitals and clinic sites. The care does not vary from site to site.

Core Principles for End-of-Life Care

The Joint Commission and a significant number of specialty medical societies have endorsed, modified, or adopted a consistent set of Core Principles for End-of-Life Care. The overall philosophy was accepted by most societies, but each one amended or expanded certain issues that directly affect their practice.

Note: The Institute of Medicine Committee proposed Core Components of Quality End-of-Life Care in September 2014. There are 12 components in the proposal. (To review the components, go to the Institute of Medicine's website and search "end of life.")

The nurse should follow these basic principles for end-of-life care:

- Respect the dignity of client, family, and caregivers.
- Show sensitivity and respect toward client's and family's wishes.
- Provide for alleviation of pain and other physical symptoms, using measures consistent with client choices.
- Assess and manage psychological, social, and spiritual/religious problems.
- Establish continuity of staff (including primary care and specialist providers) to the greatest extent possible.
- Provide access to palliative care and hospice care.
- Offer access to any therapy that may realistically be expected to improve the client's quality of life, including alternative or nontraditional treatments.
- Respect the client's right to refuse treatment.
- Acknowledge the physician's professional responsibility to discontinue some treatments when appropriate, with consideration for both client and family preferences.
- Actively support clinical and evidence-based research on end-of-life care.

Symptom Management

Management of debilitating symptoms has improved in recent years as a result of clinical research and new pharmacologic and behavioral therapies. Individuals who are dying experience a wide variety of symptoms, including pain, nausea, fatigue, constipation, or diarrhea. Pain and pain control has been identified as the primary concern of clients as they approach the end of life. Inadequate assessment of pain and poor pain control continue to be issues, even though much research on these topics has been done.

Assessment of pain in the dying client relies on the evaluation of level of consciousness and awareness, breathing pattern, and hemodynamics. A method to determine the amount of pain a client has is electroencephalographic signals that assess level of consciousness. This procedure has been used as an adjunctive monitor even though it is not considered an end-of-life technique. Intrusive technology and monitoring are usually discontinued during this stage.

Through routine assessments, planning of care, and administering the appropriate pharmacologic interventions, the nurse plays a critical role in the management of symptoms for clients receiving hospice and palliative care.

The World Health Organization (WHO) developed a model that outlines principles of analgesic selection and titration as well as **adjuvant drugs** that support the effect of the analgesics or counteract adverse side effects. Each step defines the type of pain and analgesic most effective for that level of pain.

In some clients, the pain becomes so severe that even aggressive titration of standard drugs is not sufficient to control the pain. In these cases, sedation should be considered. Sedation for end-of-life clients is considered a comfort measure when there is intractable pain and other symptoms indicate death is near. When sedation is used in this manner, the client usually loses consciousness. Family members, as well as the client, must be informed of this change in client status before sedation is started.

Cultural Awareness
Cross-Cultural Issues at the End of Life

Culture is an important part of how everyone understands their world and makes decisions, especially on healthcare issues. This includes healthcare professionals as well. Culture influences the way people make meaning out of illness and dying; therefore, it also influences how they utilize the medical community at the end of life. Each individual has a perspective that is also influenced by factors such as personal psychology, gender, and life experiences. There is a wide variation of beliefs and behaviors within any ethnic population. This leads us to realize that each client needs to be treated individually. Healthcare professionals must not influence clients with their own beliefs or cultures. Failure to take the client's cultural background seriously means we fail to understand the values held by the client.

Lack of cultural sensitivity and skills can lead to inappropriate clinical outcomes and poor interaction with clients and families at a very crucial point in their end-of-life process. Addressing and respecting cultural differences will increase trust, leading to a more satisfactory end-of-life process for both the client and the family.

Cultural Diversity at the End of Life

The 2012 census revealed that Whites make up about 63% of the U.S. population; 13% are African Americans; 17% are Hispanic; 5.1% are Asian Pacific Islander; and 1.2% are American Indian/Alaskan native. The remaining 2.4% list themselves as bi-ethnic. The makeup of the United States is rapidly moving toward a more ethnically and culturally diverse country in which Whites are expected to account for less than 50% of the population by 2040. The national trends continue to see ethnic minorities dominating the national growth with immigration largely from Latin America and Asia. With this predicted change, healthcare workers must become more aware of how cultural factors influence clients' reactions to serious illness and how they make decisions and cope with end-of-life issues. There are three basic dimensions in end-of-life treatment that vary culturally: communication of "bad news"; locus of decision making; and attitudes toward advance directives and end-of-life care. Many ethnic healthcare workers conceal adverse diagnoses from clients, believing that it is disrespectful, impolite, or even harmful to the client. Decisions on end-of-life care are most often made by the family or the family in consultation with the healthcare provider, not the client. Advance Directives are usually not completed by specific ethnic minority clients because they have a distrust of the U.S. healthcare system.

Source: Coolen (2012)

Death Rituals Vary From One Culture to Another

Death rituals occur in every culture and are practiced in a variety of ways. These rituals may be culturally related or part of a religious practice. An individual affiliated with a particular cultural group may or may not practice rituals from that culture. In providing care to any individual who is dying, it is essential to learn what is important and meaningful to that individual and family as well as how this need can be met. A few general examples related to culture are presented for clarification.

Arab Americans, many of whom are Muslims, do not openly anticipate death or grieve for a dying individual. Most of the Arab American clients prefer to die in the hospital. There are special rituals after the death, such as washing the body and all orifices. The designated head of the family determines how family members will be notified of the death. Organ donation is usually not allowed out of respect for burying the body whole. They will probably not choose a DNR order; in fact, the family may lose trust in the healthcare system if this option is offered to them.

Black Americans vary with respect to dying at home or in the hospital. Many families care for the clients at home until death is imminent, and then bring them to the hospital. Some believe it is bad luck to die at home. There are no rituals associated with care of the body. Cremation is usually not done. Organ donation is usually not done except in cases of immediate family need.

Chinese Americans may be fatalistic when faced with a terminal illness and death. They usually do not talk about it. Some Chinese believe that dying at home brings bad luck, but others believe the spirit will get lost if death occurs in the hospital. Each client and family should be supported in their belief. Organ donation and autopsy are generally not accepted, as they believe the body should be kept intact.

Native Americans embrace the present. Some tribes avoid contact with the dying, while others will want to be present 24 hr a day. Eating, playing games, and making jokes in the hospital are seen as appropriate for some tribes. Many of the tribes will bring healers to attend to the spiritual health of the dying client. Some family members will wrap the body for burial and not allow a mortuary to prepare the body, while others may avoid all contact with the body. Organ donation is generally not accepted.

Within the Mexican American (Hispanic) culture, death is considered a family affair. Family members feel obligated to visit frequently. In the traditional Mexican family, a family member must always be with the dying client. The family members will gather in the home or hospital; therefore, it is necessary to find a place for them to congregate.

Nursing Diagnoses

The following nursing diagnoses are appropriate to include in a client care plan when a client is in the process of grieving or dying.

NURSING DIAGNOSIS	RELATED TO . . .
Death Anxiety	Worry about death's impact on significant others, feeling powerless over issues related to dying, anticipating pain related to death
Compromised Family Coping	Little support by family, alteration in family role
Verbal Communication, Impaired	Family has unresolved questions.
Disabled Family Coping	Surgery, diagnostic tests, treatments, perceived threat to value system, lack of experience in making critical decisions
Fear	Unknown experience related to death; unfamiliarity with environment
Grieving	Loss of significant other, chronic illness, threat of death, perceived loss of biologic integrity
Ineffective Health Maintenance	Lack of motivation, lack of education, religious and cultural beliefs, cognitive impairment
Chronic Pain	Tissue, organ, or skeletal muscle damage as a result of cancer, severe pain at end of life
Spiritual Distress, Risk for	Hospital barriers to practicing spiritual rituals, loss of body part or function, terminal illness, debilitating disease, death or illness of significant other, challenge to belief or value systems

Source: Herdman, T. H. & Kamitsuru, S. (Eds.) *Nursing Diagnoses – Definitions and Classification 2015-2017*. Copyright © 2014, 1994–2014 by NANDA International. Used by arrangement with John Wiley & Sons Limited. Companion website: www.wiley.com/go/nursingdiagnoses. In order to make safe and effective judgments using NANDA-I nursing diagnosis it is essential that nurses refer to the definitions and defining characteristics of the diagnoses listed in this work.

The Grief Process

Nursing Process Data

ASSESSMENT Database

- Observe for presence of psychological symptoms:
  - Weeping
  - Guilt
  - Anger and irritability toward others and the deceased
  - Depression
  - Inability to initiate meaningful activity
- Observe for somatic symptoms:
  - Physical exhaustion
  - Insomnia
  - Restlessness and agitation
  - Digestive disturbance
  - Anorexia or overeating
- Determine client's complaints:
  - Sense of unreality
  - Sense of detachment
  - Lack of strength
- Identify stage of grief client is experiencing:
  - Denial
  - Anger
  - Bargaining
  - Depression
  - Acceptance
  - Outcome of grieving process—positive or negative
- Observe for morbid reaction to grief:
  - Delay of reaction
  - Distorted reaction—acquisition of symptoms of the deceased (e.g., psychosomatic illness or disease)
  - Atypical grief syndrome manifested by distorted pictures of grief

PLANNING Objectives

- To assist the client who is experiencing the grief process
- To intervene therapeutically and provide support
- To allow the client to express feelings of loss openly
- To understand and tolerate client's behavior that is related to loss
- To assist the client to move successfully through stages of the grief process

IMPLEMENTATION Procedures

DOCUMENTATION AND EVALUATION

Expected Outcomes

- Client is able to progress through stages of grief with support of family and nursing staff.
- Client is accepting of loss and eventual outcome of grief process.
- Cultural sensitivity is maintained throughout grief process.

Unexpected Outcomes/Alternative Actions

Pearson Nursing Student Resources

Find additional review materials at
nursing.pearsonhighered.com.
Prepare for success with NCLEX®-style practice questions and Skill Checklists.

Skill 34.1.1 | Identifying Grief

Procedure

1. Understand the importance of the deceased individual as a source of support.
2. Observe the degree of dependency of the relationship between deceased and others. ➤ *Rationale:* The more dependent, the more difficult is the task of resolution.
3. Identify the degree of ambivalence felt toward the deceased. ➤ *Rationale:* When there are persistent hostile feelings, guilt may interfere with the work of mourning.
4. Identify the support system and other relationships the grieving individual has to depend on. ➤ *Rationale:* A client with few other meaningful relationships has a more difficult time and is less willing to give up the attachment to the deceased.
5. Identify client's cultural influence on grieving process.
6. Identify the number and nature of previous grief experiences. ➤ *Rationale:* Losses tend to be cumulative in their effects, and unsuccessfully resolved previous losses only aggravate the current loss.
7. Determine the degree of preparation for the loss. ➤ *Rationale:* In terminal illness, grief work may have begun long before the actual death of the individual.
8. Determine the capacity to cope with loss. The more inner resources the client has available, the better his or her coping ability. ➤ *Rationale:* The physical and psychological health of the mourner at the time of the loss determines capacity.

Skill 34.1.2 | Assisting With Grief

Procedure

1. Become familiar with the grief process, stages of grief, and natural responses to grief.
2. Denial stage:
   a. Allow client denial of grief to give him or her time to move through shock and to mobilize defenses.
   b. Encourage client to talk when he or she is ready to do so.
   c. Understand that shock and disbelief may be first response, and anticipate that behavior may be inappropriate or disturbed.
   d. Accept client's inability to face reality, and allow mood swings and expressions of happier times (which may seem inappropriate at this time).
3. Anger stage:
   a. Allow "acting-out" of feelings and verbalization of anger.
   b. Anticipate expression of anger toward others, loved ones, and the environment.
   c. Understand that unreasonable, insatiable demands are an expression of this stage of grief, and attempt to meet the demands. Anticipate client's needs before demanded.
   d. Encourage client to take as much control as possible over care and environment, allowing the client to make as many decisions as possible. Avoid criticism and negative feedback at this time.
   e. Avoid false reassurance and false cheerfulness, which lead to distrust. Also, avoid diversion by introducing cheerful activities or stories. These actions lead client to believe you do not care about his or her feelings.
   f. Explain and clarify all procedures and treatments to decrease misinterpretation and expansion of **fears**.
4. Bargaining stage:
   a. Allow client to move through bargaining stage; listen to verbal expressions without judgment or pointing out reality.
   b. Encourage client to talk about bargaining with God. This may assist client to cope with guilt and not lose faith.
   c. Assist with contacting spiritual counselor or hospital chaplain.
5. Depression stage:
   a. Encourage verbalizations about loss, its meaning in client's life, and feelings about the loss.
   b. Support client's self-esteem and understand that it is affected by awareness of the loss.
   c. Encourage and reassure as appropriate; do not give false reassurance at this stage but assist client to be realistic.
   d. Be aware of your own feelings of sadness and loss so that they do not interfere with therapy.
   e. Remain with client and share on a nonverbal level.
   f. Verbalize feelings to client when they are appropriate; do not deny yourself of sadness or **empathy** (crying) when appropriate.
   g. Limit association with cheerful, insincere staff, friends, or family.
6. Acceptance stage:
   a. Allow client to express whatever feelings are present, knowing that he or she has moved through the above stages and may now be feeling totally empty of emotion.
   b. Spend quiet time with client, interacting on a nonverbal, nondemanding level.

(continued)

Skill 34.1.2 | Assisting With Grief *(continued)*

c. Encourage client to make preparations for impending death by supporting requests to finish tasks, discussing options for plans to complete areas in his/her life.

d. Encourage client to say the things he or she wants to say to those close to him or her.

e. Honor client's requests to be alone and do not overload client with external information. Client may need a lot of quiet contemplation to prepare for death.

7. Show respect for cultural, religious, and social customs throughout stages of mourning and incorporate client's cultural, religious, and social customs when providing care during the grief process.

8. Offer support and reassurance to family.

Unit 34.1 Documentation and Evaluation

DOCUMENTATION for the Grief Process

- Characteristics of the stage of grief client is experiencing and client's ability to cope
- Behavioral manifestations of grief
- Support systems available to client

- Measures nurse has taken to assist client to cope with grief
- Client's response to psychosocial interventions

EVALUATION/Critical Thinking

Expected Outcomes

- Client is able to progress through stages of grief with support of family and nursing staff.
- Client is accepting of loss and eventual outcome of grief process.
- Cultural sensitivity is maintained throughout grief process.
- Client is able to identify support system.

Unexpected Outcomes	Alternative Actions
• Client experiences a morbid reaction to grief.	• Recognize distorted symptoms and be accepting but firm with client. • Request further assistance from the staff.
• Family cannot support grief of client or handle their own grief.	• Know the general response to death by recognizing the stages of the grief process. • Understand that the behavior of the mourner may be unstable and disturbed. • Request assistance from nursing staff or appropriate community agencies to cope with the family.

Nursing Process Data

ASSESSMENT Database

- Assess current stage of dying.
- Observe the physical symptoms:
  - Evidence of circulatory collapse
  - Variations in blood pressure and pulse
  - Disequilibrium of body mechanisms
  - Deterioration of physical and mental capabilities
  - Absence of corneal reflex
- Observe the client's ability to fulfill basic needs without complete assistance.
- Assess the nature and degree of pain the client is experiencing.
- Observe for impending crisis or emergency situation.
- Observe for psychosocial condition:
  - Need to establish a relationship for support
  - Availability of support systems
  - Grief pattern and stage of grief the client is experiencing
  - Need to express feelings and verbalize fears and concerns
  - Determine client's awareness of terminal nature of disease
  - Identify client's cultural and religious attitudes toward death
- Determine anxiety level, which may be expressed in physical or emotional behavior.
  - Sleep disturbance
  - Palpitations
  - Digestive complaints
  - Anger or hostility
  - Withdrawal
- Determine depression level that client may be experiencing:
  - High fatigue level or lethargy
  - Poor appetite, nausea, or vomiting
  - Inability to concentrate
  - Perception of unfinished business to be completed
  - Expressions of sadness, hopelessness, or uselessness
  - Assess family members' needs during the loss

PLANNING Objectives

- To assist client near the end of life to maintain comfort, if possible
- To assist the dying client to cope with end-of-life experiences
- To handle own feelings of loss and sadness that arise when caring for a client at the end of life

- To provide support for the client and the client's family during the end-of-life process
- To complete the actions necessary to care for the client who has died

IMPLEMENTATION Procedures

DOCUMENTATION AND EVALUATION

Expected Outcomes

- Client is able to progress through stages of grief with support of family and nursing staff.
- Client is accepting of loss and eventual outcome of grief process.
- Client is as pain-free as possible.
- Client's cultural beliefs are considered throughout the dying process.
- Client found internal sources to support acceptance of death.
- Family members are supported throughout the dying process.

Unexpected Outcomes/Alternative Actions

Pearson Nursing Student Resources

Find additional review materials at
nursing.pearsonhighered.com.
Prepare for success with NCLEX®-style practice questions and Skill Checklists.

Skill 34.2.1 | Supporting the Client Near the End of Life

Preparation

1. Determine whether client has a Do Not Resuscitate (DNR) signed form in chart or as part of informed consent. ❶
2. Ensure client has current Advance Directive on file in both the healthcare facility and physician's office. ➤ *Rationale:* Even though the Patient Self-Determination Act of 1991 requires healthcare facilities to inform clients of their right to accept or refuse health care and complete an Advance Directive, this is not always done.

Note: Asian Americans, Hispanic Americans, and African Americans are less inclined to write Advance Directives, whereas 40% of Whites have them. See Advance Directives, Chapter 1.

3. If client is unable to sign form, ensure that legally recognized surrogate healthcare decision maker has signed the request. ➤ *Rationale:* Without signed DNR orders, staff must perform CPR and begin all lifesaving measures.
4. Determine whether hospice or palliative care is appropriate for client.
5. Review agency policies and procedures related to organ procurement. Be prepared to notify the appropriate individual or organization of status of client as death is near. ➤ *Rationale:* Procurement team can be ready to harvest organs and tissues upon client's death.

REQUEST TO FOREGO RESUSCITATIVE MEASURES
(Request Made by Patient)

I, _____ (name of patient) hereby request to forego resuscitative measures. My physician, _____, has explained to me the nature of resuscitative measures, their risks and benefits, the risks and benefits of refusing such resuscitative measures, and the alternatives to such resuscitative measures. I have had all of my questions answered by my physician.
After carefully considering all of the information my physician discussed with me, I request to forego resuscitative measures.

Signature: _____

Date: _____ Time: _____ A.M. / P.M.

Witness: _____

REQUEST TO FOREGO RESUSCITATIVE MEASURES
(Request Made by Legally Recognized Surrogate Decision-maker)

NOTE: *If the patient is determined by his or her physician to be incompetent (that is, unable to understand or appreciate the nature and consequences of the medical decision at issue), a legally recognized surrogate health care decision-maker may sign a request to forego resuscitative measures on behalf of the patient.*

I, _____ (name of legally recognized surrogate health care decision-maker) hereby request to forego resuscitative measures on behalf of _____ (name of patient). The patient's physician, _____, has explained to me the nature of resuscitative measures, their risks and benefits, the risks and benefits of refusing such resuscitative measures, and the alternatives to such resuscitative measures. I have had all of my questions answered by the physician.
After carefully considering all of the information the physician discussed with me, I request to forego resuscitative measures on behalf of the patient named above.

Signature: _____

Relationship to Patient: _____

Date: _____ Time: _____ A.M. / P.M.

Witness: _____

✚ **COMMUNITY HOSPITAL**

PATIENT I.D. #
NAME
SEX   AGE   SS#
BIRTH DATE   MED REC. #   FIN. CLASS

Procedure

Care of Client

1. Introduce yourself to client and family members. Check two forms of identification.
2. Determine whether client has specific needs for comfort. ➤ *Rationale:* Comfort is the primary goal of therapy for dying clients. Provide daily grooming, skin and mouth care, and exercise as client can tolerate.
3. Encourage client to maintain independence by providing remote controls for TV, radio, lights, and fans. Keep ice and water at the bedside within easy reach by client.
4. Provide touch like Reiki or other **therapeutic** touch techniques if culturally appropriate, especially over the area of pain. ➤ *Rationale:* This is soothing and relaxing for client.
5. Incorporate the use of relaxation techniques in your daily nursing care of the client.
6. Serve only small portions of food that client requests. ➤ *Rationale:* Serving large portions only overwhelms client and he or she will not want to attempt to eat. Encourage clients to take in as much fluid as they are able.
7. Keep lemon drops or mint fresheners at bedside and within easy reach for client. ➤ *Rationale:* Breath fresheners make the client feel better, especially if they are not eating.

Interaction With Client and Family Members

1. Determine if and how family members may assist client during this stage and assist family members to provide care as requested. Discuss hospice or palliative care with client and family, if appropriate (Table 34-1 ■).
2. Provide opportunities for client and family to engage in cultural or religious practices. Request a member of the clergy if client or family requests to speak with one.
3. Visiting hours for family or significant others should be unlimited. Assess if client needs rest by observing for signs of **anxiety**, restlessness, and voice trembling. When this occurs, ask the visitors to please leave.
4. Assist with open communication with clients, family, and healthcare providers, regarding any cultural, spiritual, or religious issues they wish to discuss relative to end of life. ➤ *Rationale:* Understanding the client's religious or spiritual concerns will help support client and family during these times.
5. Encourage family members to communicate with clients even if unresponsive. ➤ *Rationale:* Clients reportedly do hear what is being said even though they are unresponsive.

Management of the Environment

1. Move client's bed near window so he or she can see outside vegetation, flowers, sky, and more.
2. Reduce extraneous noise. Client's room may need to be moved to accomplish this. Do not place bed near nurses' station. ➤ *Rationale:* Even a client who is not responding can still hear voices and noises.

❶ DNR form.

Table 34-1 Changes During the Dying Process

Change	Signs and Symptoms
Weakness and fatigue	Inability to move self in bed, unable to perform personal hygiene
Skin breakdown	Erythema surrounding bony prominences, wounds
Decreasing appetite	Poor intake, weight loss, loss of muscle and fat, **anorexia**
Cardiac and renal dysfunction	Oliguria leading to anuria, tachycardia and peripheral cooling, cyanosis, in extremities, hypertension leading to hypotension
Alterations in level of consciousness	Increasing drowsiness leading to unresponsiveness to verbal or tactile stimuli
Delirium	Agitation, moaning, groaning, nonpurposeful movements of limbs
Respiratory dysfunction	Change in respiratory rate, decreasing tidal volume with increased PCO_2 level, abnormal breathing patterns from apnea, Cheyne–Stokes, agonal breaths
Inability to swallow	Coughing, choking, gurgling, loss of gag reflex, dysphagia
Loss of sphincter control	Incontinence of urine or bowel
Pain	Facial grimacing, moaning, agitation, tension in forehead and between eyebrows
Inability to close eyes	Eyelids remain open with only whites of eyes showing

Source: Emanuel, Ferris, von Gunten, & Von Roenn (2010)

3. Display cards, photos, "art work" from children, favorite objects that have special meaning for client in an area where client can see them.
4. Provide room lighting that is muted and soft, not overhead lighting.
5. Eliminate odors: perfume, cigarette smoke.
   a. Open windows when possible.
   b. Turn on fans.
   c. Use air fresheners.
   d. Use aromatherapy (oils or lotion) for massage. Provide massage with aromatherapy products if client agrees.
      ➤ *Rationale:* Massage reduces stress, decreases pain and discomfort, and stimulates blood circulation.
6. Provide soft music according to client's preference for music.
7. Use visualization and guided imagery through audiotapes if client desires.

> ### CLINICAL ALERT
> The goal of care for the dying client changes from curative to palliative care. Helping the client achieve a measure of comfort and knowing that family members and significant others are being supported during this process is a comfort for the client.

Skill 34.2.2 | Providing Pain Management at the End of Life

Procedure

1. Assess client for factors that influence management of pain.
   a. Complete detailed history of the client's condition.
   b. Determine effects of pain relief measures and medications client is currently taking.
   c. Have client explain characteristics of pain and have him or her use pain scale to determine severity of pain (Box 34-3 ■).
   d. Ask client if there are any cultural issues related to pain that should be known by healthcare providers.
   e. Assess client's psychosocial needs.
2. Complete physical assessment of client.
3. Assess client for nonverbal clues indicating pain: restlessness, grimacing, moaning, irritability, furrowed brow, or crying, particularly if the client is sedated.
4. Assess client for physiologic signs of pain: elevated blood pressure and pulse.
5. After determining appropriate drug, dose, and route, administer drug. Observe for effects of medication on pain relief and for potential side effects. ❶

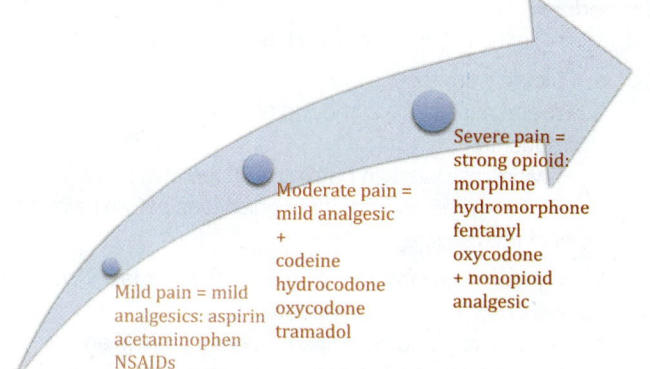

Severe pain = strong opioid: morphine hydromorphone fentanyl oxycodone + nonopioid analgesic

Moderate pain = mild analgesic + codeine hydrocodone oxycodone tramadol

Mild pain = mild analgesics: aspirin acetaminophen NSAIDs

❶ An illustration of analgesic progression for pain management.

Note: When pain is persistent or moderate to severe at the outset, it should be treated by increasing the **opioid** dosage or using a higher potency. Morphine, hydromorphone, methadone, fentanyl, or levorphanol can replace the codeine or hydrocodone when severe pain exists.

(continued)

Skill 34.2.2 | Providing Pain Management at the End of Life *(continued)*

CLINICAL ALERT

Most medications for pain are administered via oral or parenteral routes. The use of continuous subcutaneous opioid infusions in clients with chronic cancer pain is becoming more popular. High-concentration opioid medications are used with this method because the amount of drug administered must be limited to prevent tissue trauma.

Medications for persistent cancer-related pain are administered around the clock for best efficacy, not on a prn basis. Additional prn medications may be administered as needed.

Seventy percent to 90% of clients with advanced cancer experience pain, especially those in long-term care facilities. When properly medicated, more than 95% of the clients gain relief from the pain.

The client's verbal account of his or her pain is accepted for pain measurement. Therefore, it is important to explain the use of the pain scale so the client accurately describes his or her pain because drug therapy is based on the measurement.

6. Assess client frequently for effects of pain management.
7. Maintain around-the-clock sustained-release medications for continuous pain.
8. Treat breakthrough pain with immediate-release medications.
9. Discuss a combination of medications and alternative therapies such as massage for the management of pain.

Box 34-3 WHO ANALGESIC LADDER FOR PAIN CONTROL

Step 1: Nonopioid with or without adjuvant drugs. Acetaminophen, aspirin, or another NSAID for mild to moderate pain.

Adjuvant drugs to enhance analgesic efficacy, treat concurrent symptoms that exacerbate pain, and provide independent analgesic activity for specific types of pain that may be used in this step as well as in the other steps.

Step 2: Opioid for mild to moderate pain and nonopioid drugs; may or may not use adjuvant drugs.

Add codeine or hydrocodone to the NSAID (do not substitute drugs).

Drugs are administered in fixed-dose combinations with acetaminophen or aspirin. This provides additive analgesia.

Dose-related toxicity might occur with the use of acetaminophen or NSAID.

This may limit the drug combination's efficacy.

Step 3: Opioid for moderate to severe pain with or without nonopioid or adjuvant drugs.

This step is used when higher doses of opioids are necessary.

Separate dosage forms of the opioid and nonopioid analgesic are used to avoid exceeding the maximum recommended doses of acetaminophen or NSAID.

Source: World Health Organization
Refer to Chapter 16, Pain Management, for additional information on managing pain.

Skill 34.2.3 | Symptom Management at the End of Life

Procedure

1. Minimize the client's discomfort as much as possible.
   a. Provide warmth.
   b. Provide assistance in moving and position client frequently.
   c. Provide assistance in bathing and personal hygiene.
   d. Administer the appropriate medications before pain becomes severe.
2. Recognize the symptoms of urgency or emergency conditions and seek immediate assistance.
3. Notify the charge nurse or team leader if there is an impending **crisis** and perform emergency actions until help arrives.
4. Encourage dying clients to do as much as they can for themselves so that they do not just give up—a state that only reinforces low self-esteem.
5. Provide emotional nursing care for the client.
   a. Form a relationship with the dying client. Be willing to be involved, to care, and to be committed to caring for a dying client.
   b. Allocate time to spend with the client so that not only physical care is administered.
   c. Recognize the grief pattern and support the client as he or she moves through it.
   d. Recognize that your physical presence is comforting by staying physically close to the client if he or she is frightened. Use touch if appropriate and nonverbal communication.
   e. Respect the client's need for privacy, and withdraw if the client has a need to be alone or to disengage from personal relationships.
   f. Be tuned in to client's cues that he or she wants to talk and express feelings, cry, or even intellectually discuss the dying process.
   g. Accept the client at the level on which he or she is functioning without making judgments.
6. Be aware of your own personal orientation toward the dying process.
   a. Explore your own feelings about death and dying with the understanding that until you have faced the subject of death, you will be inadequate to support the client or the family as they experience the dying process.
   b. Share your feelings about dying with the staff and others; actively work through them so that negativity does not get transferred to the client.

Skill 34.2.4	Supporting the Family or Caregiver

Procedure

1. Introduce yourself to the family or caregiver and explain your role in caring for the client.
2. Support the family of the dying client.
   a. Understand that the family may be going through anticipatory grief before the actual event of dying.
   b. Understand that different family members react differently to the impending death and support the different reactions.
   c. Be aware that demonstrating your concern and caring assists the family to cope with the grief process.
   d. Discuss any cultural diversity differences that would be beneficial for client care.
3. Provide honest answers to questions.
4. Reinforce client's wishes for end-of-life care related to DNR orders, living wills, and advance directive.
5. Explain each procedure or intervention you are providing for client.
6. Ask family members or caregiver how they want to participate in client care.
7. Encourage family or caregiver to take time alone to regroup.
8. Provide or obtain psychosocial support and bereavement **counseling** for family. ➤ *Rationale:* Family members may exhaust much of their energy, develop sleep deprivation, and exhibit signs of depression, anxiety, and even chronic health problems during this stressful time.
9. Encourage family members to build a support group of friends or other family members. ➤ *Rationale:* No one should be alone during this time.
10. Remind family or caregiver to eat properly and maintain an exercise schedule.
11. Refer family members to support groups as needed.
12. Refer family members to social services for help with issues such as insurance, living wills, funeral arrangement, and other financial constraints.
13. Prepare family for client's death.

EVIDENCE-BASED PRACTICE
Critical Care Family Needs Inventory

A meta-analysis of several studies using the Critical Care Family Needs Inventory led to a summary of the 10 most important needs of families of critically ill, dying clients:

1. To be with the individual
2. To be helpful to the dying individual
3. To be informed of the dying individual's changing condition
4. To understand what is being done to the client and why
5. To be assured of the client's comfort
6. To be comforted
7. To ventilate emotions
8. To be assured that their decisions were right
9. To find meaning in the dying of their loved one
10. To be fed, hydrated, and rested

Medical decisions, including those at the end of life, are made using a shared decision-making model. Physicians and other clinicians assist the client to clarify their values and reach consensus about treatment courses consistent with the client. Frequently family members and other surrogates must make end-of-life decisions for the client. They need to keep in mind the client's advance directives and end-of-life wishes.

Source: Luce (2010)

Unit 34.2 Documentation and Evaluation

DOCUMENTATION for the Dying Client

- Client's physical symptoms
- Characteristics of the stage of dying and acceptance by client
- Support systems available to client
- Nursing care measures that make the client comfortable
- Family acceptance and interaction with client
- Comfort or limited support measure provided
- DNR orders in place
- Rituals that are being carried out during care

EVALUATION/Critical Thinking

Expected Outcomes

- Client is able to progress through stages of grief with support of family and nursing staff.
- Client is accepting of loss and eventual outcome of grief process.
- Client is as pain-free as possible.
- Client's cultural beliefs are considered throughout the dying process.
- Client found internal sources to support acceptance of death.
- Family members are supported throughout the dying process.

Unexpected Outcomes	Alternative Actions
• Nurses are unable to care for the dying client due to their own emotional reaction.	• Request that other staff members take over, as the objective is to be able to give good nursing care. • Request assistance from skilled professional so you can work through your own feelings about death in order to be able to cope with the next death experience.
• Client loses confidence in the healthcare team.	• Attempt to ascertain exactly what occurred to cause client to lose confidence in the team. • Report to charge nurse so that staff caring for client may be changed. Be sure to choose experienced personnel who are equipped to cope with a dying client.
• Client lingers on and does not fulfill expectation that death would occur in the near future.	• Report status to staff so arrangements may be made for respite—supportive care for family who is having a difficult time coping. • Discuss hospice care with the client's family.
• Pain cannot be controlled adequately with ordered medication.	• Report to physician so alternative pain relief methods may be used. • Ensure that WHO three-step analysis ladder protocols are being followed. • Ensure that around-the-clock medication administration is occurring. • Assist the client to cope by spending additional time and meeting physical needs.

Postmortem Care

Nursing Process Data

ASSESSMENT Database

- Verify that appropriate documentation is completed by the physician or other healthcare provider as required by state regulations.
- Identify cultural or family needs and desires.
- Identify client by name and client's belongings for labeling.
- Determine organ and tissue donation status.

PLANNING Objectives

- To prepare body for removal from clinical unit
- To acknowledge cultural or family rituals applicable to body preparation
- To protect the condition of the body for the purpose of respect for the deceased and his or her family during final viewing
- To document facts and time relating to death
- To identify and label client and client's belongings

IMPLEMENTATION Procedures

- **Skill 34.3.1** Providing Postmortem Care....................1368
- **Skill 34.3.2** Preparing for Organ and Tissue Procurement..1369

DOCUMENTATION AND EVALUATION

Expected Outcomes

- Postmortem care is completed, maintaining client's dignity.
- Client's family members are supported by staff during grief process.
- Appropriate procedures are carried out for organ and tissue procurement.

Unexpected Outcomes/Alternative Actions

Pearson Nursing Student Resources

Find additional review materials at **nursing.pearsonhighered.com.**
Prepare for success with NCLEX®-style practice questions and Skill Checklists.

Skill 34.3.1 | Providing Postmortem Care

Equipment
Bathing supplies
Shroud or morgue bag
Identification tags
Protective pads, if necessary
Rolls of gauze and abdominal pads, if necessary
Paper bags or plastic bags for personal belongings
Gurney or specialized morgue cart
Clean gloves

Preparation
1. Check client using two forms of identification.
2. Check client's chart to determine appropriate procedure to carry out for postmortem care.

Procedure
1. If previously determined or requested by client or family, notify appropriate clergy or support individual.
2. Determine that client's death has been pronounced per agency policy and determine whether there is going to be an autopsy or a coroner involved.
3. If there are other clients or visitors in the room, carefully explain the situation and ask them to temporarily leave the room if possible. Provide privacy.
4. Collect necessary equipment. Incorporate family requests or cultural preferences when possible.
5. Follow hospital procedure regarding notification of various departments and personnel.
   a. Determine whether client has signed a donor card or has made a decision to donate any organs. ❶
   b. Follow client's advance directive on file at the hospital for donor instructions.

Signed by the donor and the following two witnesses in the presence of each other:

_____   _____
    Signature of Donor   **Date of Birth of Donor**

_____   _____
    Date Signed   **City & State**

_____   _____
      Witness   **Witness**

This is a legal document under the Uniform Anatomical Gift Act or similar laws.

For further information consult your physician or

National Kidney Foundation
116 East 27th Street, New York, N.Y. 10016

❶ To ensure that organs are donated appropriately, instruct client to fill out and keep donor card available at all times.

c. Notify appropriate hospital personnel or local organ-procurement organization (OPO) for assistance with organ donation.
   d. Follow specific procedures for organ transplant according to hospital policy.
6. Maintain proper alignment of the body. Place limbs by client's side. Raise the head of the bed 30 degrees. Place a pillow behind the head. ➤ *Rationale:* If the head is not elevated, the blood will begin to pool around the sides of the face, the earlobes, and the neck leaving it a deep, reddish purple. Place a rolled up washcloth under the chin. ➤ *Rationale:* This will keep the jaw closed until rigor mortis takes place. Rigor mortis sets in within 20 min. Maintain head elevation throughout care and to morgue. ➤ *Rationale:* This is to prevent pooling of fluids in the head or face.
7. Don gloves.
8. Close the eyes. If necessary, use paper tape or gauze pads. You may do this after the family has visited the deceased.
9. Replace dentures and close mouth. ➤ *Rationale:* It is easier to insert dentures before rigor mortis begins, and this maintains the client's natural appearance.
10. Remove any external objects causing pressure or injury to the skin (e.g., oxygen mask).
11. Remove IV lines, catheters, or tubes per agency policy, unless an autopsy is to be done.

Note: Removing catheters and IV lines causes fluid to leak into tissues, resulting in edema and discoloration. Hospital policy may, therefore, direct that all IV lines be converted to hep locks or intermittent infusion devices to prevent fluid leaks. Follow hospital policy.

12. Cleanse the body as needed. A partial bath may be required to remove secretions, wound drainage, or stains. Some facilities provide a complete bath to the deceased client.
13. Place protective incontinent pad under buttocks and between legs in diaper fashion.
14. If family is to visit the deceased, comb hair, place gown on the client, provide clean linen, and leave linens at level of chin with the arms exposed.
15. Remove equipment used for cleansing the client.
16. Allow the family private time to view the body. Allow as much time as they desire.
17. After family and clergy have visited, label the body, attaching ID tags to the big toe, wrist, and morgue bag or as determined by agency policy.
18. Place arms and hands loosely at side or on abdomen. ➤ *Rationale:* This prevents discoloration of hands.
19. Place the body in the shroud or in morgue bag.
20. Label all personal belongings and place them in a bag.
21. Remove gloves and perform hand hygiene.
22. Close doors to client's room and clear hallways in preparation to transfer the body to the morgue.
23. Transfer the body to the morgue on a gurney or a special morgue cart. Keep client's head elevated.

24. Place client's personal belongings in the appropriate place determined by hospital policy.
25. Support family members as needed. Provide for emotional and physical comfort.

Note: Rigor mortis begins about 4 hr after death and reaches its peak about 10 hr later. It passes from the body after 36 hr. It is best to wait until the body passes through this process before embalming. Therefore, it is not a problem to wait for relatives to view the body within a specified time frame.

> **CLINICAL ALERT**
>
> Inform the funeral home if the client has tuberculosis or any other infectious disease so appropriate care can be taken to prevent contamination of the environment.

Skill 34.3.2	Preparing for Organ and Tissue Procurement

Procedure

1. Determine whether organs or tissues are to be "harvested" in a dying client. Check for driver's license information on transplant donor and check for Advance Directives or Living Will.
2. Determine appropriate procedure for securing organs and tissues. Check hospital policy and procedure.
   a. Determine time frame for collecting organs and tissues.
      ➤ *Rationale:* Organs, bones, eyes, skin, and tissues have different time frames for removal in order to preserve them appropriately. If time frame has elapsed, the organs or tissues cannot be used for transplant.
   b. If death is imminent, contact the local organ-procurement organization (OPO) according to hospital policy. Members of the organization or the coordinator will be present during the organ procurement procedures.
   c. If client is not identified as an organ donor, notify physician to determine whether client is a candidate for donation. Contact OPO to alert them about a possibility of organ donation.
   d. After evaluating client's condition, physician should contact family members to determine if they would like to donate organs or tissues. Some organs may not be appropriate for donation, but many times eyes, skin, and tissues are appropriate.
   e. Client is kept hemodynamically stable while decisions about transplantation are made by family members.
   f. When the client has been declared brain dead, the local OPO coordinator, who is a nurse or physician's assistant, will assume responsibility for the donor's management. This does include directing clinical nursing care.

Unit 34.3 Documentation and Evaluation

DOCUMENTATION for Postmortem Care

- The exact time the physician or healthcare professional was informed and death was pronounced
- When family members or significant others were notified
- Time organ procurement team informed, if appropriate
- Consent forms signed
- Condition of the body and postmortem care delivered
- Time the body was sent to the morgue
- Mortuary contacted, if appropriate
- Disposition of client's belongings
- Disposition of organs and tissues

EVALUATION/Critical Thinking

Expected Outcomes

- Postmortem care is completed, maintaining client's dignity.
- Client's relatives are supported by staff during grief process.
- Appropriate procedures are carried out for organ donations.
- Appropriate disposition of client belongings is carried out.

(continued)

Unexpected Outcomes	Alternative Actions
• Client is not identified properly when sent to the morgue.	• Check identification band and shroud label before releasing client to mortician. Request another nurse to check labels.
• Donated organs are needed.	• Provide support to family and give an opportunity for questions. • Obtain signatures for consent form. (Kidneys should be removed within 1 hr after death. Eyes should be removed within 6–24 hr after death.) • Examine reverse side of driver's license, or remind the charge nurse to call mortician if burial plans have been made previously, to check on permission for organ donation through a living will.

Chapter Wrap-Up

GERONTOLOGIC Considerations

Three Out of Four Older Adults Die of Heart Disease, Cancer, or Stroke

- Heart disease is leading cause of death, although it has declined since 1968.
- Death rates from cancer have decreased, but lung cancer has increased in women.
- Death statistics for people in the 65–74 age group: Heart disease accounted for 38%; cancer, 30% of deaths.
- Two-thirds of hospice clients are over 65 years of age.

Death in the Life Cycle

- In American culture, the obsession with youth often results in denial of death as a natural phase of the life cycle, and death is not considered a positive process.
- Older adults may see death as an end to suffering and loneliness.
- Death is usually not feared if the individual has lived a long and fulfilled life, having completed all developmental tasks.
- Spiritual beliefs or philosophy of life are important.

MANAGEMENT Guidelines

Each state legislates a Nurse Practice Act for RNs and LVN/LPNs. Healthcare facilities are responsible for establishing and implementing policies and procedures that conform to their state's regulations. Verify the regulations and role parameters for each healthcare worker in your facility.

Delegation

- Assisting the client to deal with grief may be delegated to another healthcare professional who is trained and experienced in working with grief, such as a social worker or hospice nurse. Assigning staff to work with a dying client will involve similar parameters, with the additional criteria that the nurse has worked through his or her own feelings about dying and can deal directly with the subject of death. If a client wishes to discuss dying or fears related to dying, the nurse must be able to listen and appropriately interact with the client. The nurse assigned to care for the dying client should be aware of the importance of the family in terms of support and communication.
- The nurse is responsible for reviewing the advance directives in the client's chart for organ donation or the living will to determine the appropriate members of the team to care for the client.

- Postmortem care may be provided by the staff. However, if there are organs to be donated, the professional nurse is responsible for carrying out the hospital policies or orders necessary to preserve the organs for organ transplant.

Interprofessional Communication

- Because nonprofessional staff are often assigned to care for the basic needs of a dying client, the RN/LVN/LPN must set up a channel of communication (both written and verbal) so the nurse is constantly aware of the status of the client and the family is informed of the client's status. The professional nurse should also provide the family with opportunities to discuss the condition of the client and plans for the future care of the client (including organ donation and hospice care). It would be inappropriate for nonprofessional staff to be assigned these activities.

CASE STUDY Applications

Scenario 1

You are assigned to care for Mrs. Garcia, an 85-year-old Hispanic client who speaks limited English. Her caregiver at home has been her daughter, who speaks somewhat more English than her mother. A son and grandson visit her often and both of them speak fluent English. Mrs. Garcia has been brought to the hospital in end-stage renal failure. Her BUN and creatinine are both very high. Her blood pressure is 210/110, pulse 110, and respirations 30 and labored. Her skin has a jaundiced appearance and she has many ecchymotic areas throughout her body. She states she "doesn't want to live like this." She is debating asking to be taken off dialysis, but that decision has not yet been made.

1. Considering her condition, what priority interventions should you consider? What is the rationale for your answer?
2. Considering her limited English skills, how will you carry out your priority interventions?
3. Her daughter asks you how long she will live without dialysis. What is your best response? Provide rationale for your response.

4. In the evening after the son has been to visit his mother in the hospital, the family discussed her wishes. It was decided that they would stop dialysis. What steps will you take to provide end-of-life care to Mrs. Garcia?
5. Identify at least four interventions you will use to assist the family in coping with the impending death of their mother and grandmother.
6. During the last day, Mrs. Garcia is complaining about mild to moderate pain. What interventions will you use to make her comfortable?

Scenario 2

You are working with a terminally ill client who is in severe pain. The client's family is considering moving the client to a hospice center.

1. What are some of the advantages for the client if this move is accomplished?
2. What are some of the barriers to hospice care that you would anticipate when discussing this decision with the family?

NCLEX® Review Questions

Unless otherwise specified, choose only one (1) answer.

1. Place the stages of grief, according to Elizabeth Kübler-Ross, in the order in which they progress.
   A. Anger
   B. Depression
   C. Acceptance
   D. Denial
   E. Bargaining

2. How is restitution, the response in Engle's third stage of grief, described?
   A. A time when all feelings of hostility and negative feelings toward the deceased are repressed
   B. The beginning of the recovery process, with the onset of cultural and religious rituals that assist the mourner to face the loss

   C. The stage in which there is a refusal to accept or comprehend the death
   D. The mourner's attempt to deal with the painful void created by the loss of a loved one

3. What do principles for end-of-life care include?
   Select all that apply.
   A. Discontinuing alternative and nontraditional care to allow the client to rest
   B. Allowing the client to refuse treatments
   C. Managing spiritual/religious problems
   D. Encouraging family members to minimize time at the bedside to prevent client and family fatigue
   E. Respecting the dignity of the client and caregivers

4. For which of the following clients is hospice care recommended?

   A. Clients who live alone and require rehabilitation services

   B. Those who have a life expectancy of less than 6 months

   C. Older adults with a short life expectancy

   D. Clients who require comfort care but not treatments

5. What behaviors and/or responses should the nurse tell family members to expect from the client who is in the anger stage of the grief process?

   A. "Inappropriate or disturbed behavior occurs during the stage of denial, so this would not be observed during the anger stage."

   B. "You should not expect acting out of feelings and verbalization of anger at this stage."

   C. "Clients usually yell out at God and blame him for their problems."

   D. "During this time it is helpful if you make as many decisions as possible for the client."

6. What nursing intervention is carried out when clients are near death?

   A. Placing clients in a room near the nurses' station

   B. Displaying a favorite object or children's photos within easy sight

   C. Pulling the curtains around clients so they do not need to look at the activity outside the door

   D. Ensuring that room is well-lit to provide continuous assessment of the client's condition

7. Which cultural group is most likely to have completed advance directives?

   A. Caucasians

   B. Asian Americans

   C. African Americans

   D. Hispanic Americans

8. Using the Three-Step Analgesic Ladder for pain control, which description best illustrates Step 2 of the ladder?

   A. Opioid drugs such as codeine are added to NSAIDs to treat mild to moderate pain.

   B. Nonopioid drugs, such as aspirin, are used for pain without adjuvant drugs.

   C. Opioid drugs such as morphine sulfate are used for moderate pain without adjuvant drugs.

   D. Nonopioid drugs and methadone are used for pain control only in stage II.

9. As the client is dying, what emotional nursing care for the client does the nurse need to provide?

   Select all that apply.

   A. Demonstrating caring and a willingness to be involved in his/her care

   B. Utilizing nonverbal communications and touch, if appropriate, based on cultural and religious beliefs

   C. Coordinating nursing care so it can be completed in a block of time to allow adequate time for communication

   D. Recognizing that your physical presence is comforting, even if you do not talk with the client

   E. Recognizing the grief pattern and supporting the client through the process

10. There are three basic dimensions in end-of-life treatment that vary among different cultures. Which one of the four distracters is not included in these basic dimensions?

    A. Communication between client and physician regarding treatment

    B. Locus of decision making

    C. Attitudes toward advance directives

    D. Communication of "bad news"

QSEN Activity: Postmortem Care Simulation

Domain: Teamwork

KSA: Skills

Activity:

Two to four students will participate in a simulation of providing postmortem care to a deceased client. One of the students should be a family member. The client should be a mannequin.

The other students in class will observe the simulation, using their skills book to evaluate the students participating in the scenario. They will take notes and identify the steps that were taken in providing the care. The scenario will begin with assessing the client to ensure that he/she has died. It will continue to complete the postmortem care as outlined in the skill. At the end of the scenario there will be a discussion of how the students performed the skill, their professionalism while caring for the deceased client, and how the students communicated with the family members and informed others of the situation. At the end of the discussion the students should be asked how they felt about taking care of a deceased client.

Bibliography

Center to Advance Palliative Care. (2012). What is palliative care? Retrieved from http:getpalliativecare.org.

Coolen, P. (May 2012.) Cultural relevence in end-of-life care. Retrieved from https://ethnomed.org/clinical/end-of-life/cultural-relevance-in-end-of-life-care

Emanuel, L., Ferris, F. D., von Gunten, C. F., & Von Roenn, J. H. (2010). The last hours of living: Practical advice for clinicians. *Medscape Nurses.* http://cme.medscape.com/viewprogram/5808.

Institute of Medicine. (2014, Sep.). Dying in America: Improving quality and honoring individual preferences near the end of life. Retrieved from www.iom.edu/endoflife.

Institute of Medicine. (2014, Sep.). Dying in America: IOM committee's proposed core components of quality end-of-life care. Retrieved from www.iom.edu.

Jacques, E. (2014, Apr.) What are adjuvant analgesics? About Health. pain.aboutcom/od/treatment/g/adjuvant.http.

Kübler-Ross, E. (1993). *On death and dying.* New York: Macmillan.

Luce, J. M. (2010). End-of-life decision making in the intensive care unit. *American Journal of Respiratory and Critical Care Medicine, 182*(1), 6–11.

Mazanec, P., & Tyler, M. (2003, Mar.). Cultural considerations in end-of-life care. *American Journal of Nursing, 103*(3), 50–57.

McCurdy, D. (2008, May). Ethical spiritual care at the end of life. *American Journal of Nursing, 108*(5), 11.

National Hospice and Palliative Organization. (2013). Who receives hospice care? Retrieved from http://www.nhpco.org/sites/default/files/public/Statistics_Research/2013_Facts_Figures.pdf

Peiffer, K. (2007, Mar.). Brain death and organ procurement. *American Journal of Nursing, 107*(3), 58–67.

Principles of good end-of-life care. (2012, Sep.). Retrieved from http://www.caresearch.com.au/caresearch/ClinicalPractice/Physical/EndofLifeCare/PrinciplesofGoodEndofLifeCare/tabid/739/Default.aspx

Richardson, P. (2014). Spirituality, religion and palliative care. *Annals of Palliative Medicine, 3*(3), 150–159.

UpToDate. (2014, Oct.). Overview of spirituality in palliative care. Retrieved from www.uptodate.com/overview-of-spirituality-in-palliative-care

World Health Organization. (2015). WHO's cancer pain ladder for adults. Retrieved from http://www.who.int/cancer/palliative/painladder/en/

NCLEX-RN® Answers

CHAPTER 1—PROFESSIONAL NURSING

1. **(B)** Even though nurses do care for clients in all types of settings and they do perform activities of daily living and prepare the clients for home care, these statements do not define nursing (A) and (D). Not all client care is ordered by the physician; nurses have many independent actions (C).

2. **(A)** In both clinical and academic environments, ethical principles are a necessary guide to professional development. This is the rationale for adhering to the code. Answers (B) and (C) are included, but not the most important. Administering medications is not included in the code (D).

3. **(D)** Maintaining the dress code is usually part of the student nurse's responsibility for clinical practice (A). There is no relationship between what staff RNs wear and students' dress code. A professional relationship must be maintained during client care (B). It is unprofessional to call a client by his or her first name (C).

4. **(C, D, E, F)** RN responsibilities cannot be delegated to the LVN/LPN regardless of length of experience (A). (B) CNAs cannot be assigned to a newly admitted client. They cannot complete a health history.

5. **(C)** Nurses in all clinical settings function under the standards, including Advanced Practice Nurses. Each specialty group of nurses develops its specific standards, according to the same protocols. Options (A), (B), and (D) describe smaller groups of nurses.

6. **(A, B, E)** Imprisonment (C) or compensation to cover costs to a facility (D) is not usually associated with professional misconduct cases.

7. **(C)** Examples of malpractice are (A) and (B). (D) is not connected with a legal issue. If the nurse refuses a client assignment after the shift starts, it is considered abandonment of the client and can result in terminating the nurse's employment.

8. **(A)** The first step in providing client care is gathering the appropriate equipment. (D) is an incorrect statement. The client must be identified using two forms of identifiers, such as ID band, asking for date of birth, or asking the client to state his or her name. (B) and (C) are not appropriate actions to determine priority nursing care for a client, which is based on the assessment and on discussion of the client's needs.

9. **(C)** The purpose of the Core Measures is for hospitals to use them as an improvement tool. The information gathered is used to devise methods to improve the client's health care. The Core Measures provide the Hospital's Board of Directors with information that displays an increase in client care outcomes. (A), (B), and (D) are not appropriate as the purpose is not to complete client studies or determine common treatments.

10. **(D)** Soiled linen is never placed on the linen cart. It will contaminate the entire linen cart (A). Alcohol will not decontaminate equipment. Equipment needs to be sterilized in central supply (B). Sharing client equipment is never an accepted practice. Cross-contamination between clients can occur (C).

CHAPTER 2—CRITICAL THINKING AND THE NURSING PROCESS

1. **(D, E, B, C, A)** When planning care, the steps in the nursing process are completed in this order.

2. **(A, B, E)** Nursing care is provided to clients based on their individual care needs. Critical thinking is implemented after collecting data and then determining the needs of the client by priority. In addition to the identified attributes, critical thinkers are realistic, good team players, empathetic, and open-minded. Care is not delivered in the same way for all clients (C, D).

3. **(C)** If you missed the question, review nursing diagnosis statements in this chapter; (D) is a medical diagnosis and (A) and (B) are written incorrectly.

4. **(A, D, F)** These choices represent nursing diagnoses, whereas heart failure (B), cancer of the liver (C), and pulmonary edema (E) are medical. Nursing diagnoses can be treated by a nurse. Medical diagnoses are treated by a physician, or the nurse can collaborate on the treatment. Medical diagnoses require a physician's order before the nurse can provide specific care to the client.

5. **(A)** Nurses should make clinical decisions using the best available research and other evidence that is consistent with policies, procedures, and clinical guidelines. Best practices usually are indicative of the most often used methods of providing client care (B), not used to identify them. They are not necessarily based on research findings. Developing new techniques for providing nursing care (C) and differentiating nursing from medical diagnoses (D) do not describe, nor are they involved in, evidence-based nursing. New techniques may come from evidence-based nursing but would be an offshoot of the research, rather than the goal.

6. **(B)** After a complete assessment of the client, a database of information is then utilized to develop a nursing diagnosis, short- and long-term goals, and appropriate interventions. Developing a nursing diagnosis (A) is not assessment. Identifying short- and long-term goals (C) is planning, and evaluating sources of client data (D) takes place after the assessment is completed.

7. **(C)** Compliance with client care goals is effectively carried out when the client, family, and other individuals who will be participating in the care take an active role. Planning does not identify healthcare needs (A). The care plan is developed as soon as possible after admission but may not be within 1 hour (B); follow hospital policy and procedure on time frame for completion. Teaching plans are best developed using the same group of individuals (D).

8. **(C)** The nurse would collect additional data if needed, and then make the intervention. Gathering data and prioritizing clients' needs (A) are part of the assessment phase of the nursing process. (B) is an action associated with nursing diagnosis phase, and (D) is the last step of the nursing process.

9. **(D)** The major advantage of using the NIC system is that it can be electronically sent to databases nationwide. With the implementation of the electronic health record, standardized nursing languages such as NANDA can be used to provide a broad base of nursing knowledge at the point of care (C); NIC information can also be used as a paper-based document. (A) and (B) are not the best answers.

10. **(C)** LVN/LPNs can assist the RN in revising client care plans. UAPs (A) cannot develop a care plan, and CNAs (B) are not allowed to complete tasks prior to discharge, unless it is in their scope of providing hygienic care, moving, and positioning, etc. (D) Only RNs can develop the plan of care at admission.

CHAPTER 3—MANAGING CLIENT CARE: DOCUMENTATION AND DELEGATION

1. **(A, B, D, E, F)** The only function that is not a purpose of charting is (C), to remind the nurse of the care and treatments given to the client.

2. **(A, C, D)** Computer documentation can give the nurse more time to spend on client care. It provides instant test results and information. It allows nurse to document more client details quickly. These can be considered advantages. It can improve the ability of the nurse to communicate personal aspects of care (B). It does not eliminate the need to provide reports (E).

3. **(C)** The correct method is to draw a single line through the entry and write "mistaken entry" and "wrong chart" above it and initial. It should remain visible. Other options are incorrect.

4. **(C)** Because there may be future legal implications, it is necessary to be very specific and record all of the details, not just those considered major (A) or general (D) details, and not just nursing actions (B).

5. **(B)** A major advantage is that this form is standardized (not individualized) and multidisciplinary. It is a tool developed to encompass all health team members, so it does not allow for complex clients to receive individual goals (options A, C, and D).

6. **(C)** The nurse should make every attempt to provide culturally competent care. This task is suitable to be delegated to a UAP so the nurse would not have to refuse (A), bring it despite an overloaded schedule (B), or say it will get there late (D).

7. **(A)** When making an assignment, the leader should attempt to keep the same nurse with the same client. This allows for better continuity of care. The other choices would help provide continuity of care and stability.

8. **(C)** Proper delegation requires that the nurse delegating tasks must make sure the individual is trained to perform the task, oversees the activity, and evaluates the results. Close supervision will discourage employees and isn't necessary unless a particular problem exists (A). Delegating a task allows the employee to utilize his or her own knowledge (B). It is not done to avoid distasteful tasks (D).

9. **(A)** By witnessing the signing of a surgical consent form, the nurse is merely attesting that the client has signed the form. Answer (B) describes informed consent. Witnessing the form doesn't mean the nurse believes the client is competent (C). The nurse is not in the position to determine the likelihood of success of a procedure (D).

10. **(C)** Some tasks may not ever be delegated, and each state sets its own requirements; for example, total assessment and evaluation may not be delegated. All other statements are correct.

CHAPTER 4—COMMUNICATION AND NURSE–CLIENT RELATIONSHIP

1. **(D)** Aphasia leads to feelings of frustration and discouragement. Clients require frequent praise for their efforts and encouragement to continue to try to communicate. Aphasic clients can best provide information by responding to yes or no questions.

2. **(C)** Termination is an ongoing process, so encouraging the client to follow through with what was learned is a good response. The nurse would *not* encourage the client to stop by, because the relationship was terminated. The last response is *not* encouraging and nontherapeutic.

3. **(D)** A professional relationship must remain on the professional level even though the nurse sets goals with the client, sets limits, and sets boundaries. Hospital policies are not relevant. The nurse will not necessarily maintain a distance, because a degree of emotional involvement is positive. Client needs are important but are not the focus of the relationship.

4. **(C)** This is a reflective response, and it opens up communication and allows the client to express whatever concerns or feelings he or she has without confining the discussion to dying. The other two responses cut the client off and are nontherapeutic.

5. **(C)** This open-ended question allows the client to further comment and expand on the subject. Answers (A) and (B) are closed ended and can be answered by a yes or no. Also, the last response is more focused, so an open-ended question is best.

6. **(B)** This response keeps lines of communication open so that the nurse can hear his fears and clarify any medical lack of knowledge. As he verbalizes, he can begin to more realistically cope with his condition. The remaining responses all close off communication and are nontherapeutic.

7. **(D)** The first intervention is to calmly set limits on the verbally abusive behavior to defuse the situation. Summoning help or sending the client away may escalate the situation. Restraints would only be a last resort.

8. **(A, B, C, F, G)** The age of the client and whether or not he or she believes in God are not components of a cultural assessment.

9. **(A)** The most effective mode of communication if the client is hearing impaired is to use a writing pad and gestures. Speaking, even slowly or loudly, will probably be frustrating and difficult for the client. Nonverbal communication is not as effective as writing.

10. **(D)** The priority is client safety, so whenever caring for a depressed client who is potentially suicidal, the intervention is to assess frequently and place the client on suicide precautions. Encouraging the client to talk about his or her feelings will only deepen the depression. Activity is always useful because mobilizing the client is a goal, but it is not the priority here.

CHAPTER 5—ADMISSION, TRANSFER, AND DISCHARGE

1. **(C)** Only the client has the right to make decisions about resuscitation efforts. This is in compliance with the Client Self-Determination Act. This decision is not a right of the family (A), the advance directive counselor (B), or the client's healthcare provider (D).

2. **(B)** Admitting personnel inquire about advance directives so that documents can be added to the client's record, updated, or executed on admission. A chaplain (A), attorney, (C), or healthcare provider (D) would not be the first to encounter the client at the healthcare facility. Information about advance directives needs to be included in the client's chart from the beginning of care.

3. **(A)** The individual receives an ID bracelet during the admission process and at the point when he or she begins receiving care, at which time he or she becomes a client. The ID cannot be just given out when he or she gets to the nursing unit since he or she may receive care in another department first (B), after assessment (C), or after receiving orders from the healthcare provider (D). Identification of the client at the time in which he or she begins receiving care ensures correct identification and client safety.

4. **(C, D)** The client's date of birth and medical record number are valid identifiers. The Joint Commission requires the utilization of at least two identifiers. Client name, date of birth, and medical record number are all appropriate to use. The client's room number (A), healthcare provider's name (B), and name of hospital (E) are *not* valid forms of identification.

5. **(B)** A strange environment causes anxiety. Familiarity with the room and equipment promotes independence and control. Orientation does not save time (A). It is not done to release the facility from liability (C), and it does not prevent a client from abusing expensive equipment (D).

6. **(A, C, D)** This information on meals, visiting hours, and how to call the nurse is useful and predictable. The client would not use the emergency call system (B); physician visits (E) are unpredictable.

7. **(A, B, C, D):** In order to maintain safety while conducting home care visits, the nurse will wear a name badge, keep a cell phone ready and charged at all times, park in front of the home, and keep valuables locked in the trunk of the car. The nurse will restock supplies at the beginning of each day, not between visits (E).

8. **(C)** Height and weight are the two factors used for calculating BMI. Waist measurement (A), age (B), and gender (D) are not factors for calculating BMI.

9. **(C)** The UAP may escort the client off the unit once the discharge is complete. UAPs may not teach about meds (A), perform assessments (B), or teach about complications to report (D). Only a registered nurse may perform those activities.

10. **(C)** The nurse should notify the healthcare provider first, and then advocate by determining why the client wishes to leave AMA (B), since the client's concerns may be alleviated once identified (e.g., further explanation, social service consult, individualized accommodations). The nurse would not have the client sign the AMA form first (A) or talk about risks of leaving AMA (D).

CHAPTER 6—CLIENT EDUCATION AND DISCHARGE PLANNING

1. **(D)** Nurses are the principal providers of care; therefore, they usually take the leadership role in directing the educational plan. Other health team members may play a major role in the teaching; however, the nurse usually directs and guides the process. (A) Physicians usually do not play a major role in education while the client is hospitalized. A trained health care member would do the teaching (B). (C) Discharge planners are pivotal in determining placement of clients on discharge and in obtaining equipment for the home.

2. **(B)** Clients with multisystem issues usually require education regarding diagnosis, multiple treatments, and medications. (A) Living alone does not necessarily place a client at high risk for discharge. If the client is young, self-sufficient, and has a good support system, the client is not at high risk. Answers (C) and (D), in and of themselves do not place clients in a high-risk category.

3. **(D)** The first three distractors are essential to determine an appropriate educational plan. (A) The educational level determines the level and scope of information that can be presented. (B) Family members should be included in the educational plan. (C) Ethnic and cultural issues need to be taken into account, especially when discussing items such as dietary alterations. The actual employment or occupation in most cases is not necessary in developing the teaching plan.

4. **(B)** The amount of time the family spends at the client's bedside may be dependent on their work schedule, family responsibilities at home, and so on; it does not correlate with willingness and ability to participate in teaching activities. Cognitive ability to understand (A) is important. Once the teaching needs are determined, then it is important to evaluate their active participation (C). The nurse does observe and evaluate interactions between the client and family (D).

5. **(D)** Knowing the lifestyle and usual daily activity can assist with determining the impact of changes on this activity and the emphasis on the teaching plan. (A) This procedure is not considered a major surgical intervention. Most of the listed procedures are done on an outpatient basis; therefore, the home environment would not be evaluated. There is no need for specialized equipment. (B) All clients having outpatient or short-stay surgery must have someone take them home because of the anesthesia. It is not important to determine who will be staying at home with the client or when they return to work (C). The physician will give the client directions on the return-to-work date.

6. **(D)** The initial teaching plan will support the client in respect to the diagnosis, treatment, medications, and expected outcomes. Teaching is a major part of this initial plan. Of course, determining the support system at home will become more essential as the teaching continues

and discharge planning is discussed. **(A)**, **(B)**, and **(C)** are essential components for the teaching plan and will be integrated within the plan.

7. **(A, B, C)** Summarizing the teaching content or clarifying misinformation does not evaluate the effectiveness of the teaching strategies. It does provide information on retention of information, which can play a role in how effective the strategies have been. However, you do want to evaluate the type of strategy utilized in teaching. Basically, what they are doing in **(D)** and **(E)** is reiterating information. You cannot evaluate whether they are able to utilize the information that was covered in the teaching.

8. **(A)** The client will become more agitated with you if you attempt to continue with the teaching. The other responses are all appropriate for this situation. It is best to come back at a different time **(C)**. At that time, you may be able to determine why the client is agitated and hostile **(B)**. Frequently, another nurse is able to establish rapport with a client, and it would be best to ask that nurse for assistance with the client **(D)**.

9. **(A, B, C)** These data are important information for other healthcare workers to have in order to develop an appropriate plan of care for the client. Nursing interventions **(D)** and I&O records **(E)** are not necessary unless there is a specific issue with them. For example, if the client's urine output has been low and he or she is not taking in fluids, it should be included in the discharge summary.

10. **(C)** Older clients frequently have hearing deficits and extraneous noise impairs their hearing. This can lead to perceiving incorrect information and directions. **(B)** Older clients remember about 5% of what they read. **(A)** They remember 50–70% of what they hear and verbalize. **(D)** Usually, older clients do not learn best in groups, because it can be noisy and disruptive.

CHAPTER 7—SAFE CLIENT ENVIRONMENT AND RESTRAINTS

1. **(A)** Characteristics influencing adaptation to the environment are provided in **(B)**, **(C)**, and **(D)**. They must be assessed to determine the client's needs and abilities to safely adjust to his or her immediate surroundings.

2. **(D)** A large percentage of errors occur as a result of either no communication or incomplete communication regarding client care. **(B)** and **(C)** can also lead to sentinel events, but not to the extent of a failure in communication.**(A)**, staffing ratio, is not a major cause.

3. **(B)** The order can be renewed every 4 hours for a total of 24 hours. Children between 9 and 17 must have orders renewed every 2 hours, and every 1 hour for children under 9 years.

4. **(C)** The slipknot allows for a quick release in case of a client requiring release from the restraint. **(D)** The least restrictive method to prevent the client from falling would be the use of sitters. **(A)** and **(B)** are not part of restraint guidelines.

5. **(A)** Keeping the contaminated equipment in the room prevents contamination to other clients. Clients with implants do not usually receive bed baths **(B)**. This protects healthcare workers from unnecessary exposure to radiation. Client care is provided by standing away from the radiation area, but the time for client care is still limited to 15 minutes/shift by one healthcare worker **(C)** and **(D)**.

6. **(D)** Staying with the client is critical to prevent a complication related to the seizure activity. **(A)** The client is turned to the side to protect the airway from tongue occlusion. **(B)** Once a seizure has begun, tongue blades are not inserted in the mouth. **(C)** Clients are not restrained to prevent injury during the seizure activity.

7. **(C)** The priority is to remove the clients, if at all possible. The usual priority for fire safety can be remembered by using the mnemonic RACE. R is remove client, A is activate the fire alarm, C is confine the fire, and E is extinguish the fire if possible.

8. **(A)** Promoting activities of daily living and exercise will increase the clients' strength and mobility. They should be encouraged to get out of bed. **(B)**, **(C)**, and **(D)** are all safety precautions that should be practiced for older adult clients to prevent injury.

9. **(A)** Wedge-roll cushions, use of low-level beds, placing a mat on the floor by the bed can all be used to prevent injury if a client falls. **(C)** Environmental alterations do not include using a geri-chair; **(B)** placing a client near the nurses' desk does not prevent the client from falling. **(D)** Side rails are considered restraints, although if the client is alert and asks that he or she be raised to assist in moving, he or she can be left in the "up" position.

10. **(B, D)** The vest is placed on the client with the zipper to the back. **(C)** After vest tails are crossed in back of the chair, the tails are wrapped around the immovable kickspur. The tails are then tied to the kickspur using a half-bow knot. The zipper is placed in the back, not front **(A)**. A half-bow, not a square knot, is used on the kickspur **(E)**.

CHAPTER 8—BATHING, BEDMAKING, AND MAINTAINING SKIN INTEGRITY

1. **(B)** Tucking the sheet under the bed at the top of the bed and going down to the foot of the bed would take two staff to change the bed. **(A)**, **(C)** Changing only the drawsheet is not considered a complete linen change. **(D)** Linen changes are not made just when the bed is soiled.

2. **(E, B, C, A, D)** A bed bath is completed using the noted sequence. The nurse completes the bath using a head-to-toe approach, working from the front side to the client's back.

3. **(C)** Because the skin of the older adult client is very thin and fragile, it is imperative that it be kept moist. **(B)** and **(D)** are not correct. The bath can be a tub bath or bed bath in addition to a shower. Minimal amounts of mild soap can be used for bathing. **(A)** Fragrant soaps are not recommended as they can cause drying of the skin.

4. **(C)** This is considered a medication and therefore requires a physician's order. **(A)**, **(B)** giving a bath in tepid water does not require an order, nor does using a hydraulic bathtub chair. **(D)** This type of bath is not ordered by the physician. It is the nurse's discretion based on the client's ability to assist with the bath or to ambulate to the tub or shower.

5. **(D)** The client can assist with washing his or her hands and face if the exertion is not too much. **(A)**, **(B)**, and **(C)** would not be appropriate for the client who is short of breath. It would take too much energy to perform any of these tasks.

6. **(A, B)** These activities are considered part of morning care. **(C)**, **(D)**, and **(E)** are considered part of providing evening care. Activities **(C)** and **(D)** are also completed when a bath is provided.

7. **(C)** Maintaining the pH of the skin prevents drying of the skin. **(A)** The cost is less using regular linen in most facilities, but convenience is taken into account when facilities do use disposable systems. **(B)** A wash cloth is also warmed, therefore this is not an advantage of the system. It is not easier or quicker to use.

8. **(C)** Cleansing the eyes first prevents water and particles from entering the lacrimal duct. **(A)** The head and scalp are washed last, after taking the infant out of the bathtub. **(D)** would be completed after the infant's ears and neck are washed.

9. **(B)** Picking up the skin is a good indicator of hydration of the client. If the skin stays tented, the client is dehydrated. **(A)** Checking the temperature of the skin is accomplished by placing the back of your fingers or hand on the client's skin. **(C)** Checking for edema is completed by firmly pressing the finger against the client's skin for several seconds and observing the indentation depth of the skin. **(D)** Checking the color of the skin of the hands might be done to check for peripheral circulation, not hydration.

10. **(B)** Using an adherent dressing will assist the wound to heal. **(A)** The skin is irrigated with normal saline solution, if needed. **(C)** A dry dressing will adhere to the tear and can cause the tear to open up when the dressing is removed. **(D)** It is not necessary to immobilize the arm.

CHAPTER 9—PERSONAL HYGIENE

1. **(A)** Turning the head to the side allows fluids to drain out, facilitates suctioning, and prevents aspiration. **(B)** is important also, but it is not the major safety action. **(C)** Padded tongue blades or a bite lock can be used to separate upper and lower sets of teeth to promote cleaning of inner teeth surface. Gloves are used to prevent spread of infection **(D)**; although important, **(A)** is the major safety action.

2. **(D)** Combing starts at the end of the hair shaft and works toward the scalp. **(A)** It is used to provide routine hair care. **(B)** Oil is used for coarse or curly hair that has dry or flaky areas on the scalp. **(C)** Hair picks are used for hair care when the client has coarse or curly hair.

3. **(B)** Nits within 6 mm of the scalp are usually viable, white in color, and indicate an active infestation. **(A)** Lice are light to dark brown in color, crawl, and feed on blood 3–4 times/day. **(C)** Lice eggs hatch in 7–10 days, not 17 days. **(D)** Lice have six clawed legs and crawl, but do not jump. A fine-toothed comb is necessary to extract the nits from the hair.

4. **(C)** Nits within 6 mm of the scalp are usually viable and indicate an active infestation. **(A)** and **(B)** are incorrect. **(D)** Nits are not easily seen on the hair shaft.

5. **(D)** Clothing can be washed in hot water when nits or lice are found **(A)**. Rid Home Lice Control Spray is used on furniture and mattresses, or any item that cannot be laundered. Family members are treated once lice or nits are found **(B)**. They are usually not treated prophylactically. Launder bedding when nits or lice are found **(C)**.

6. **(B)** Most institutions do not allow nurses to cut the nails of clients with peripheral vascular disease or diabetes **(C)**. Skin lesions can occur with cutting nails and this can lead to infection and poor healing. Physicians, or in some instances nurses, should notify the podiatrist to see the client **(D)**. Documentation is important, but the nurse needs to complete the assessment **(A)**.

7. **(C)** This position prevents the client's knees from buckling. (A) can cause back injury to the nurse if the client loses balance and begins to fall, thus pulling on the nurse. (B) and (D) can lead to the nurse's injury, as it places pressure on back muscles.

8. **(C)** For uncircumcised clients, the foreskin is retracted to expose the glans penis for cleaning (A). Washing begins at the tip of the penis and proceeds to the base (B). The scrotum is washed after the penis, using a clean washcloth (D).

9. **(D)** Only rinsing or saline solution can be used to cleanse contact lenses, so options B and C are incorrect. Daily wear lenses cannot be worn overnight (option A).

10. **(A, B, C, D)** Responses A, B, C, and D are important information when teaching care of hearing aids. Batteries should be replaced when necessary. (E) The hearing aid needs to be repositioned, not cleaned.

CHAPTER 10—VITAL SIGNS

1. **(B)** Loss of peripheral pulses may indicate circulatory collapse, so a further assessment should be made. When peripheral pulses cannot be palpated, a Doppler is used. Thus, the nurse should use a Doppler ultrasound to find the pulse, and then report to the healthcare provider (C) Palpation (A) is less sensitive than auscultation. Administering oxygen (D) would require further assessment data.

2. **(A)** A pulse deficit (when apical is greater than radial rate) occurs when rhythm is irregular and atrial dysrhythmia or premature ventricular beats occur. If a significant pulse deficit is found, assess for other abnormal signs. Bradycardia (B) is slow, not irregular, rate. Tachycardia (C) is fast, not irregular, rate. Pulse deficit is not associated with heart block (D).

3. **(B)** The first intervention is to expand the assessment of vital signs so that you have more data to make a nursing diagnosis. At that point, you may request orders for a cooling blanket (C) because it is more efficient than a cool bath (A). After you report to the physician, there may be an order for a blood culture (D).

4. **(B)** If an unexpected low blood pressure is recorded, the nurse needs to first examine his or her technique. If the cuff is too wide, the blood pressure will be low. If it is too narrow (A), the reading would be high. The client's arm should be supported horizontally at heart level; below heart level (C) would increase BP. The nurse should not notify the healthcare provider as the first step (D).

5. **(A)** The first intervention is to use different equipment because it may be faulty. Then, if it is functioning, validate with another nurse (C). Finally, check his circulatory status (D) and other vital signs, and notify the physician (B).

6. **(A, C, D, E)** These are the breathing patterns considered to be abnormal. Answer (B), respiratory rate 12–20, is normal for an adult.

7. **(A)** A rise in the pulse rate is one of the earliest signs of shock. A blood pressure of 110/70 and a respiratory rate of 24 are normal and do not reflect shock (B), (C). The temperature of 101°F is not associated directly with a sign of shock, but may indicate other problems (D).

8. **(B)** Pressure close to the tympanic membrane seals the ear canal and allows for an accurate reading. Answer (C) is not wrong, but it is not as complete an answer. Answers (A) and (D) are incorrect.

9. **(C)** Because vital signs can be assigned to any healthcare worker as long as their competency has been assessed, it is more manpower effective to have the UAPs start the shift assessment with reporting vital signs, and then have the day's work assigned based on the clients' conditions. The RN and LPN/LVN (A, B, D) would then begin caring for the clients who are most critically ill.

10. **(B)** A proper fitting cuff is required; using a thigh cuff (A) is not acceptable practice. The AHA does not support the use of an extra-long cuff (C), and nurses never adjust readings (D).

CHAPTER 11—PHYSICAL ASSESSMENT

1. **(A, B, C, E)** Costovertebral angle tenderness (D) is a symptom associated with assessment of the renal/kidney system. Curvature of the spine (F) is part of musculoskeletal assessment.

2. **(C)** Rebound tenderness is a symptom of peritoneal irritation such as seen with appendicitis. Hold fingers at 90-degree angle, push fingers deeply in region away from reported tenderness, then rapidly remove fingers. Rebound of structures indented by this maneuver causes a sharp pain on the side of the inflammation. Painful areas should be examined last (A). The client should breathe normally (B). Client should have knees bent to help relax the stomach muscles (D).

3. **(A)** Macules are flat, circumscribed, and show a change in color like first-degree burns, petechiae, and purpura. Wheals are elevated, irregular shaped, and solid (B). Vesicles are elevated and fluid-filled (C). Papules (D) are elevated, firm, and circumscribed, such as a wart or mole.

4. **(C)** +2 is a normal response for deep tendon reflexes. +1 is a diminished, low normal response (A). 0 is no response (B) and +4 is brisk and hyperactive (D).

5. **(C)** IX, glossopharyngeal, is the cranial nerve assessed when testing for the gag reflex. XI, accessory, is the motor nerve that causes contractions of sternocleidomastoid and trapezius muscles (A). VII is the facial, sensory, and motor nerve (B). XII, hypoglossal, is the motor nerve that controls muscles that move the tongue (D).

6. **(D)** The S_1 heart sound can best be heard at the apex of the heart, over the mitral and tricuspid areas. The pulmonic valve is at the left second intercostal space and the aortic valve is at the right second intercostal space (A). S_2 is heard louder over the pulmonic region (B). S_1 is not loudest in the aortic area (C).

7. **(C)** Flexing the neck slightly reduces muscle tension and enhances palpation. Raising the chin tenses the neck muscles, making it more difficult to palpate nodes (A). Lying in a supine position makes it difficult to assess because access is limited (B). Swallowing water is used to assess the thyroid gland and movement of the cartilages (C).

8. **(B)** Examining the adjacent area is the next intervention because pulse locations can differ with clients. The follow-up intervention would be to use a Doppler ultrasound stethoscope to locate the pulse (C). Finally, if no pulse is found, you would notify the healthcare provider (A). It is not correct to move on to the next area of assessment (D) when having difficulty.

9. The normal range of specific gravity is 1.003–1.030. Abnormal specific gravity could indicate dehydration or renal failure.

10. **(C)** You are assessing the client's fund of information, so asking who is the president will reveal deteriorated or impaired cognitive processes. Asking about feelings will not reveal this information (A). With dementia, the client may remember what he did years ago, but cannot remember yesterday (B). Answer (D) is a higher level question that the client may not be able to answer, but it is not as revealing as answer (C).

CHAPTER 12—BODY MECHANICS AND POSITIONING

1. **(D)** The newest method of preventing caregiver injuries is concentrating on handling equipment and devices. (A), (B), and (C) are older common approaches for moving and turning clients that are no longer accepted practices.

2. **(A)** 35 lb is the maximum recommended weight for lifting clients, and this should be done under controlled and limited circumstances. It is preferable to have manual lifting. (D) indicates the average weight of clients in the hospital. (B) and (C) are not correct responses.

3. **(C, D)** Appropriate body mechanics used when moving clients are included in correct answers. (A) is incorrect as the feet are placed flat on the floor to form a strong base of support, with one foot ahead of the other. (B) The abdomen is held firm but the buttocks is tucked in so the spine is in alignment. (E) is incorrect because knees can be flexed if necessary.

4. **(B, C, D, E)** The most comfortable height for working is between the waist and lower level of the hip joint (A).

5. **(C)** It is imperative that you report any injury to your immediate supervisor so that he or she can investigate the situation and provide appropriate support for you. (A) You will need to complete an unusual occurrence form; however, this is done after notifying the immediate supervisor. (D) As with any injury, the nurse is usually taken off any client care assignment and sent to the ER for an evaluation, not sent home to rest and apply ice (B).

6. **(D)** In low-Fowler's position, the client is placed in a 15-degree position. (A) is high-Fowler's position. (B) is Fowler's position, and (C) is semi-Fowler's position.

7. **(C)** The friction-reducing sheet not only assists in turning the client but prevents skin tears. (A) A second nurse is frequently used to assist in turning, but it is not the best method to be used. (B) The lift team is used only when other methods of turning are not safe or the client is too difficult to move. (D) The client is not asked to move up in bed before the turn. This can be accomplished during the lateral move.

8. **(D)** The client turns onto his or her back directly onto the transfer board. (A) The board is placed on the opposite side of the bed before turning the client. (B) The client is placed on his or her back, not in a side-lying position. (C) The client does not roll over the edge of the board to the gurney, maintaining a side-lying position. The client remains on his or her back when using the transfer board.

9. **(C)** Clients with some arm strength and weight-bearing ability can pull themselves up by holding on to the bars. (A) is used for clients who are unable to bear any weight. (B) is used for clients who can bear weight at least on one leg. Client places foot on footrest while a sling is placed under the arms and around the back. (D) assists clients from bed to gurney.

10. **(A, B, D, E)** The client should not determine when he or she will assist in ambulation (C) but rather discuss options for ambulation.

CHAPTER 13 —EXERCISE AND AMBULATION

1. **(D)** Flexion is a movement that decreases the angle between two bones (A). (B) means turning outward. (C) Adduction is a movement of a bone toward the midline of the body.

2. **(A, B, D)** are correct. (C, E) A client on strict bed rest with passive range-of-motion exercises ordered will not be completing the exercises independently.

3. **(C)** Raising the head of the bed slowly several times will stimulate baroreceptors and thus prevent orthostatic hypotension. (A) Client doesn't necessarily need to use a walker. (B) Vital signs are taken, but usually after the client sits up and before standing. (D) Additional assistance may be necessary to help, but this is not directly related to preventing orthostatic hypotension.

4. **(C)** The weaker side of the body is moved first by supporting body weight using the handles and then advancing the weaker leg, not the unaffected leg (B). In (A), the client does push off the bed, but is instructed to grasp the hand grips of the walker before doing so. Motion is forward, not to the center (D).

5. **(D)** Cane is placed on the unaffected side of the body (A). This promotes stability. (B) Cane is placed about 12 inches in front of the foot and slightly to the outside for greater stability. (C) Cane is moved first and then the affected leg.

6. **(D)** When going down stairs, the cane and affected leg are placed on the step first (A). (B) The unaffected leg is moved to the step after the cane and unaffected leg. (C) Cane and affected leg are moved to the next step after the unaffected leg is placed on the step.

7. **(C)** Client stands next to the bed. The measurement is from the axilla to 6–8 in. (15–20 cm) from the heel. (A) If height is incorrect, the axilla could rest on the bar of the crutches, causing skin breakdown or nerve involvement. (B) Measuring while lying in bed will not provide the correct measurement. (D) If the measurement is not taken at a distance of 6–8 in. from the heel, the crutches will be measured at a higher level than can be used appropriately.

8. **(B)** Client can bear weight and move. (A) Three-point gait is used when the client can bear little or no weight on one leg. (C) Client can bear little or no weight on one leg or when the client only has one leg. Gait requires a fast version of the four-point gait. (D) Usually used when client's lower extremities are paralyzed.

9. **(B)** Instructions for clients going upstairs with crutches include: First place the uninjured leg and crutches on the same level. Then place crutches on first step. Next move unaffected leg to step where crutches are placed. (A), (C), and (D) do not follow this sequence.

10. **(C, D)** Applies to a client who sustains axillary nerve pressure resulting in numbness and tingling of the fingers (A). (B) Proficiency is not what is needed to prevent slipping; it is having the tips of the crutches covered with rubber to prevent slipping on floors. (E) The gait belt should only be used if the client is just beginning to use crutches. This would not be an appropriate approach to ensure the client is self-sufficient in use of crutches.

CHAPTER 14—INFECTION CONTROL

1. **(A, C, D)** Interventions A, C, and D require the nurse to make contact with moist body substances. Taking blood pressure (B) and taking temporal temperature (E) do not.

2. **(C)** Soap and water should be used. Hand sanitizers (A) and (D) are not effective against *Clostridium difficile*. Bleach solution (B) is not routinely used for handwashing.

3. **(A, D, C, B)** Put the gown on first, then the mask, face shield or goggles, and then the gloves.

4. **(D)** Hand hygiene before giving care and after all diaper changes is the most important measure in controlling and preventing the spread of infection. Using sterile technique (A) or antibiotics (C) are incorrect for routine care, and ill people should not be allowed near infants in the hospital (B).

5. **(B)** Placing a puncture-resistant container in the home provides the safest means of disposing of contaminated needles. This container needs to be discarded and treated as biohazardous waste when it becomes full or is no longer needed. The needles should not be broken (A), recapped (C), or disposed of in the trash (D), because all of these could lead to inadvertent injury to others.

6. **(D)** An antiseptic solution is an effective cleansing agent for blood or body fluid contamination. This should be readily available to everyone who is at risk for exposure. Recapping the needle will risk repeated injury and exposure and should never be done (A). Breaking the needle will risk repeated injury and exposure (B). The client will not require gamma globulin, because the needle was contaminated after the injection (C).

7. **(B)** Standard Precautions employ using gloves when touching body fluids containing blood. Gloves are not necessary when serving lunch, and the assistant can touch the clients (D). The nurse should continue teaching the nursing assistant by explaining the principles of infection control related to AIDS, not commend the action (A) or suggest the assistant wear a gown also (C).

8. **(B)** There are three primary routes of transmission—contact, droplet, and airborne. HAI (nosocomial) infections such as VRE and MRSA are usually caused by poor hand washing or hand hygiene technique by healthcare workers who move from client to client. Soiled linens (A), medical equipment (C), and food trays (D) are less frequent sources of transmission.

9. **(C, B, D, A)** The first step is to remove your gloves, then your face shield. The third step is to take off your gown; then you would perform hand hygiene.

10. **(C)** Take only needed supplies from bag and place on clean surface, keeping the rest of supplies isolated in the closed bag. It may not be practical to use only disposable items (A) or to leave the supply bag in the car (B). Gloves may be worn (D), but this is not the best answer.

CHAPTER 15—DISASTER PREPAREDNESS

1. **(B)** Research has shown that there is a triangle of safe space beside a car or large piece of furniture. If it collapses, you will not be under it, but it will still provide you with some protection. It will not protect your head if the furniture or car collapses (A). A large piece of furniture could collapse onto you (C). To get beside the item rather than under it is done because it is safer, not easier and quicker (D).

2. **(B)** The correct answer is an event of great magnitude that overwhelms current resources. Options A, C, and D are all characteristics of a disaster.

3. **(D)** Biological agents (bacteria, viruses, or toxins) are the most difficult to identify because they have an insidious onset and symptoms may take days to develop. A nuclear attack (A) and sarin gas (C) would be more readily discovered, and smallpox (B), after an incubation period, would easily be identified by the skin eruptions.

4. **(C)** An individual can absorb anything under 0.75 Gy and not experience radiation poisoning. If a victim absorbs between 0.75 and 8 Gy (option B), he or she may develop acute radiation syndrome (ARS). An individual who absorbs over 8 Gy (A, D) will probably die.

5. **(A, B, D, E)** These are all agents that fall into the category of bacteria, viruses, or toxins that can cause a disease that develops into a mass casualty incident. Radiation poisoning (C) is caused by a nuclear weapon. Sarin gas (F) is a chemical, not a biological, weapon.

6. **(A)** The five-level system of triage decreases ambiguity of the middle level of emergency care where the majority of casualties fall; thus, it is much more effective in handling large numbers of victims. The other answers are inaccurate. The five-level system does not make identification more rapid (B). It does not provide more variety in client conditions (C). It is not more appropriate for large numbers of victims (D).

7. **(B, A, D, C)** When setting up a decontamination site, first be sure it is upwind from the contamination. The next step is to find a downhill slope so that runoff can be captured. Find a source of water. Then supply personnel with protection equipment and begin to decontaminate victims.

8. **(B)** Atropine is the antidote for nerve agents such as sarin, which is an organophosphate. Answer (A), choking agents have no antidote and require physiologic support such as fluids and ventilator management; answers (C) and (D) have specific antidotes such as anti-Lewisite for Lewisite poisoning and sulphur thiosulfate and amyl nitrite for cyanide poisoning.

9. **(B)** Cyanide is a chemical agent, as is chlorine (a pulmonary agent), mustard, and nerve agents (sarin, VX). Tularemia (A), ricin (C), and smallpox (D) are biological agents.

10. **(B)** Smallpox has an asynchronous presentation, appearing first on the face and later on the trunk, rather than arising in bunches on the trunk like varicella. (A), (C), and (D) provide incorrect presentation.

CHAPTER 16—PAIN MANAGEMENT

1. **(C)** The endorphin theory is the most accepted because it explains how the brain produces natural opiates that fit into special cells called receptors. Specificity theory (A) suggests that sensory stimuli send pain impulses to the brain, but this theory only deals with the physiologic, not the psychological, basis for pain. The pattern theory (B) includes

factors not explained by the specificity theory, but is not complete. The gate control theory (D) states that there is transmission of neurologic impulses and gate mechanisms along the nervous system that control the transmission of pain. If the gate is open, pain is experienced. None of these theories, however, adequately explains pain.

2. **(A, B, C, E)** These are the four main factors to measure pain. Pain pathway (D) cannot be measured, and the amount of medication needed (F) is an indication, but not a specific measure, of the degree of pain.

3. **(B)** The rationale for including pain as a vital sign is that it will be assessed and documented at the same time vital signs are taken. This is important, for if the level of pain is neglected, the client's condition/safety is in jeopardy. (A), (C), and (D) may be correct but do not adequately explain the rationale.

4. **(A)** Most of the nonpharmacologic methods are totally noninvasive, and thus are safer and have fewer complications than pharmacologic methods. (B) The methods may not always be better, (C) or faster or (D) preferred, which is why those answers are not correct.

5. **(D)** The priority safety issue is to be sure that the epidural catheter is not mistaken for an IV line. A sign must be posted over the client's bed and the catheter must be labeled clearly as an epidural catheter. All of the other issues are a concern, but they would not result in fatality.

6. **(B)** In order to use this method of pain control, the client must be mentally alert and able to follow the procedure instructions, because the client is in control of the narcotic administration. (A) and (C) will be part of the total assessment criteria, but not the priority assessment. (D) is incorrect because this method is commonly used for chronic pain.

7. **(C)** The correct intervention is to determine that the client is sedated and, because the goal of PCA is to control pain without sedation, notify the healthcare provider for new dose parameters. Assessing the level of medication (A) will become secondary once you determine sedation level; (B) pain relief is not the primary concern here because the client is oversedated; and (D) turning off the PCA may not be necessary; you will need to check agency policies.

8. **(A, B, D, E)** All of these answers are common dangers and should be avoided. Poor pain-relief results (C) are not a common occurrence, because drugs and dosage parameters are designed for individual client pain control with the client administering the narcotic.

9. **(D)** Administration of an epidural must be done by only an RN and may not be delegated to a nonprofessional staff member. In many hospitals, the RN must have special certification because of the safety issues involved with this procedure.

10. **(C)** The preventive approach to pain control includes administration of the medication before or soon after pain begins. Smaller, more frequent doses of medication will control pain better than larger doses taken less often.

CHAPTER 17—ALTERNATIVE THERAPIES AND STRESS MANAGEMENT

1. **(A, B, D, E)** All of the above are signals of stress. Fatigue and eating disorders fall into physiologic signals; anger is a psychological signal, and restlessness is a behavioral indicator. Mouth ulcers (C) are not a signal of stress.

2. **(D)** The most complete definition is to consider all aspects of an individual relating as an open system. (A) and (B) are accurate, but not complete. (C) is inaccurate.

3. **(A)** Herbal medicines are one of the most frequently used alternative treatment modes. They are much more frequently used in other parts of the world than in the United States. Chiropractics (B), energy medicine (C), and homeopathy (D) are used, but not as frequently as herbs.

4. **(A, B, C, E, F)** The only adaptation factor that does not influence how the individual adapts to stress is religion (D). The other factors all influence these patterns.

5. **(B)** Ranking tasks is a positive suggestion for coping with stress. Focusing on unimportant details (A), considering past unpleasant events (C), and anticipating negative outcomes (D) are the opposite of therapeutic suggestions.

6. **(A)** More and more research is showing that diet or nutrition is a major contributor to health and the prevention of disease. Although nutrition may influence how long we live, there is no research proving this (B). (C) and (D) may also be true, but again, there is no research proving it.

7. **(C)** This is the most open–ended response and does not place the nurse in legal jeopardy. (A) and (B) close off communication. (D) may result in legal problems, as it may be viewed as practicing medicine.

8. **(C)** Stress can be controlled and coped with by a variety of methods, including physical activity and relaxation methods such as deep breathing and meditation, not just one, changing thought patterns. (A), (B), and (D) are correct and fit Selye's definition of stress.

9. **(D)** Although there are many signals of stress, including physical, psychological, and behavioral, often they are difficult to identify in the client because many of them are subtle (e.g., lack of interest in life, lack of concentration, irregular heartbeats). (A), (B), and (C) are correct.

10. **(B)** Sitting quietly, clearing the mind, and deep breathing or meditation are the best methods for reducing stress. Counting to ten (A), saying a mantra (D), and jumping on a trampoline (C) may work for certain individuals, but they have not proven to be as effective as meditation and deep breathing.

CHAPTER 18—MEDICATION ADMINISTRATION

1. **(C)** Surveys have found that administering the wrong dose is the most common cause of injury. The client (option A) is generally identified correctly, and the medication (option B) is usually validated. The route (option D) is seldom erroneous.

2. **(B)** The healthcare provider would be the authority to clarify the rationale for the particular medication's use based on the individual client's need or condition. The pharmacist (A) may provide good information but is not the authority; checking the manufacturer (C) only provides information and checking the MAR (D) verifies it is the right medication.

3. **(D)** Systolic pressures less than 90 mm Hg may be associated with decreased cardiac output or orthostatic hypotension and so require that pressure-lowering medication be held. Blood pressures of 110 (A), 100 (B), and 95 (C) are high enough to give the medication.

4. **(C, D)** Alterations for oral medication administration that are acceptable include mixing liquid from capsules with food (C) and administering sublingual tablets to a client who is NPO (D). Capsules can be opened (A). Beads should not be chewed (B) and liquid capsules should not be dissolved (E), as both of those actions might create rapid absorption of the drugs.

5. **(A)** Rapid absorption of drops such as beta blocking agents used for glaucoma can cause serious bradycardia. Pressing the inner canthus helps prevent this adverse effect. Pressing the inner canthus does not prevent burning (B) and is not indicated for infections (D) as it would create contamination. It is not needed for drops that dilate the pupil (C).

6. **(A)** For adults, upward and backward pull straightens the ear canal. Option B is correct for a child under 3 years. Options C and D would close, rather than open, the ear canal.

7. **(B, D)** The anterior superior spine of iliac crest (B) and greater trochanter (D) are identified by using the nurse's right hand for client's left hip, or left hand for client's right hip. The acromion process (A) is a landmark for deltoid injection and the posterior superior spine of iliac crest (C) is used for dorsogluteal injection. The gluteal fold (E) is not a bony landmark and is not used to identify any injection site. The upper outer quadrant of the buttocks (F) relates to soft tissue rather than bony landmarks, is highly variable among clients, and is totally unreliable for predicting location of underlying nerves and blood vessels.

8. **(C)** It is not uncommon for active ingredients to be depleted while propellant remains in the canister, not the opposite (B). The expiration date (A) is not affected by the number of actuations. Becoming drug dependent (D) is an inappropriate answer because this is a drug the client requires.

9. **(B, A, D, C)** The cloudy insulin should never contact the clear insulin, as it would cause the clear insulin remaining in the vial to lose its intended short action. Air is injected first into the cloudy insulin, and then into the clear insulin. Insulin is withdrawn first from the clear insulin vial, and then from the cloudy insulin vial.

10. **(D)** Pump, tubing, or needle malfunction results in failure to deliver insulin and causes risk of diabetic ketoacidosis due to elevated blood sugar. Site infection (A), lipodystrophy (B), and insulin shock (D) are other risks but are not as great.

CHAPTER 19—NUTRITIONAL MANAGEMENT AND ENTERAL INTUBATION

1. **(A)** Trans fats are polyunsaturated and monounsaturated fats that have an additional hydrogen molecule added to make the fat more saturated and that usually come from animal sources. Unsaturated fats (B) come from vegetables, nuts, and seed sources (C), and they are liquid at room temperature (D).

2. **(B)** The kidneys are the major organs for potassium excretion, so potassium intake is restricted in clients with renal failure. Clients with heart failure (A), COPD (C), and burns (D) would all require an increased ingestion of potassium-rich foods or a KCl supplement, because their health conditions are associated with potassium loss.

3. **(C, D)** Drinking thickened liquids and swallowing food without accompanying liquid are helpful for the dysphagic client. Swallowing

liquids (A), ingesting liquids and food together (B), or use of a straw (E) or syringe (F) all increase the dysphagic client's risk of aspiration.

4. **(D)** The blue "pigtail" allows atmospheric pressure to enter the stomach to counteract the negative pressure suction at the NG tube tip. It thus prevents the decompression tube from adhering to the gastric mucosa, which would interfere with gastric content suctioning. The blue lumen does not prevent esophageal reflux (A), nor is it used for siphoning contents (B) or continuous feeding (C).

5. **(B)** Postoperative intestinal motility is regained first by the small intestine. Bowel sounds may be present, but gastric and large bowel motility may be absent. Presence of appetite (A), having flatus (C), and bowel movement (D) are reliable indicators of the return of bowel function.

6. **(C)** Since the pH of aspirate is altered because of formula presence, the best way to verify placement is to note the character of the formula aspirated; it should be curdled or bile tinged. Option A, auscultation of injected air, is no longer recommended. Option B is not reliable, because tube feedings will alter pH. Option D, capnography, is recommended for initial placement of feeding tube.

7. **(D)** Tube feeding may be continued cautiously with close client monitoring if the residual volume is <500 mL and client is not experiencing discomfort. Further client assessment is indicated if the residual volume is >500 mL. The stomach may hold from 10 to 200 mL of gastric fluid normally so 50 mL (A), 100 mL (B), and 150 mL (C) are within normal range.

8. **(C)** The tube should be flushed with warm water every 4–6 hr and before and following medication administration using a gentle push–pull technique. The tube should not require replacement for 4 weeks (D). Cola (A) or acidic juices (B) curdle feeding formula and will increase the incidence of clogging.

9. **(C)** Administration of a prokinetic agent *before* tube insertion is the most effective intervention to promote tube advancement. Positioning (A) and (B) has no beneficial effect on feeding tube advancement. The guide wire (D) should never be replaced once removed.

10. **(C)** Feeding through a surgically created tube enterostomy reduces risk of aspiration, eliminates nasal irritation, is low profile, and facilitates independent feeding. Nasogastric tube feeding (A) and nasointestinal tube feeding (B) are short-term options that will need to be replaced after about 4 weeks or less. Parenteral nutrition (D) carries considerable risk in terms of site infection and hyperglycemia.

CHAPTER 20—SPECIMEN COLLECTION

1. **(A)** The critical factor is to rinse the mouth before obtaining the sample. The best sputum sample is obtained before eating or drinking (B). Several deep breaths, not holding the breath, trigger the cough reflex and raise sputum from the lungs (C). An expectorant could contaminate the sample (D).

2. **(B, C, E)** The skin should be cleansed first with an antimicrobial wipe followed by povidone–iodine swab or use hospital policy. Standard precautions dictate that you should wear gloves during collection of a blood specimen. IV fluid may alter the specimen (A). Contamination of the sample may occur if the needle used to withdraw blood is used to inject the blood specimen into the culture tube (D).

3. **(D)** Ova or cysts may not be revealed in the presence of heavy metals. Barium, oil, or laxatives containing heavy metals, should not be given for 7 days prior to the stool examination. The time of day to collect specimen does not matter (A). Clean catch is used to collect urine, not fecal, samples (B). Sample should be examined within 30 min and kept at body temperature to find organisms in their active state (C).

4. **(C)** Guaiac is used to test for occult blood in the stool that could be a sign of upper GI bleeding or cancer. A stool culture is used to detect bacteria (A). This test does not test for fat in the stool (B). A paddle test is used to determine the presence of pinworms (D).

5. **(C)** Check with the laboratory because, based on the amount lost, time of loss, and the test to be performed, the collection may be able to be completed as scheduled. You would not stop (A) or extend (B) the collection. Reinforcing to the client to save urine would be done if the test is to be repeated (D).

6. **(B)** Urine is normally clear, not cloudy—this could be indicative of an infection. Light yellow is the normal color (A). You require at least 30 mL for an adequate sample (C). Urine is normally odorless (D).

7. **(D)** Cleanse the site with an antimicrobial wipe and allow to dry is the correct technique, because bacteria on the skin surface are reduced if the skin is allowed to dry. The tourniquet should be 8–10 cm (3–4 in.) above the client's elbow (A). The client should relax the fist and the tourniquet should be released before the needle is removed (B). Bending the elbow could cause a hematoma, so this is incorrect (C).

8. **(D)** Allen's test should precede arterial puncture to determine the adequacy of collateral perfusion. Hyperextension, not flexion, of the wrist

will stabilize the radial artery (A). Drawing back on a syringe can cause air bubbles to fill the syringe, and inaccurate ABG results will occur (B). Pressure should be maintained for 5–10 minutes to prevent bleeding after needle withdrawal (C).

9. **(C)** Adding blood to the strip can cause an erroneous reading. If the meter does not show enough blood, remove the strip and begin again. The lancet should be on the lateral side of the finger because it is less painful and prevents bruising (A). Soap and water is best for repeated sticks—alcohol can toughen the skin (B). Stroking gently increases blood flow—squeezing or applying pressure can interfere with blood flow (D).

10. **(B)** Cleanse wounds with normal saline first to avoid contamination. The specimen is collected away from the wound edges (A). Specimens should be sealed in a biohazard bag (C). Specimens should not be refrigerated—they should be transported to the laboratory within 30 min (D).

CHAPTER 21—DIAGNOSTIC PROCEDURES

1. **(B)** The other nursing actions – assisting in preparation for the procedure (A), monitoring VS during the procedure (C), and providing client education (D) are important nursing interventions, but they do not necessarily have to be completed by the nursing staff assisting the physician with interventional radiology.

2. **(A)** Sound waves (B) are related to ultrasound procedures. Scanning with use of an endoscope (C) refers to endoscopic procedures. Use of strong magnetic field and radiofrequency waves (D) describes an MRI.

3. **(C)** Each x-ray has specific restrictions to food or fluids. Determining order of studies (A), signing of informed consent (B), and need for withholding medications (D) would be included during preparation for x-ray studies.

4. **(B, C, D)** These are appropriate instructions to provide for a client having an IVP performed. Fluids are withheld up to 12 hr, so (A) is incorrect. No fluids are to be taken the morning of the study. Monitoring the client is required for 24 hr, not 4 hr, to observe for latent reactions (E).

5. **(C)** It is important to have a baseline value to determine potential bleeding tendencies and kidney function, which are tested with BUN, creatinine, PT/PTT, and APTT. Options (A), (B), and (D) are not baseline lab values before an arteriography.

6. **(A)** Barium falsely increases density of the lumbar spine, therefore an inaccurate reading will be given. Pointing out that the client has had the test before may make him or her feel embarrassed to ask a question(option B). (C) The client is not placed in a scanning machine for the test, so being claustrophobic is not relevant. (D) There are no complications from the test; therefore, the client will not need assistance in getting home.

7. **(B)** There is no need to fast or be NPO for the mammogram (A). (C) Jewelry needs to be removed from around the neck only. (D) Only the upper clothing, including the bra, needs to be removed.

8. **(A)** It is imperative to stop the bleeding with a pressure dressing. Then (C) elevate the extremity. (B) It is not a priority to call the lab at this time. Monitoring peripheral pulses (D) is included in postprocedure care.

9. **(B)** PET scans are very useful to study seizure activity and determine spread of cancer cells because metabolic changes occur before structural changes. Sixty percent of invasive tests or surgeries can be eliminated by using the PET scan. Radioactive chemicals are administered to clients undergoing a PET scan (A). PET scans can take up to 75 min (C). Foods and fluids are restricted for 4–6 hr (D).

10. **(D)** Most clients require only a local anesthetic for the procedure (A). (B) The procedure takes less than 2 hr to complete. (C) Only small incisions, large enough to accommodate the scope, are made around the knee.

CHAPTER 22—URINARY ELIMINATION

1. **(A)** Urine production is directly related to the amount of blood pumped by the heart (cardiac output). A decreased cardiac output decreases renal perfusion and urine production and causes fluid retention and weight gain. It is not directly related to fluid intake (B) but fluid intake will affect cardiac output and indirectly impact renal perfusion. It is not related to bladder capacity (C), or metabolic rate (D).

2. **(B, D)** Pregnancy and the presence of a catheter deflect ultrasound signals, thus interfering with urine volume determination by scanner. Obesity (A), history of hysterectomy (C), male gender (E), and childhood (F) do not affect transmission of ultrasound waves.

3. **(D)** The male urethra is long, so 25–30 cm (10–12 in.) is correct. As the catheter is inserted, some nurses can feel a change as it passes through the prostatic urethra and enters the bladder. Options A, B, and C are not long enough to ensure entry into the male bladder.

4. **(B)** The female urethra is quite short, so 5 cm (2 in.) is correct. This renders females more susceptible to urinary tract infection. One and a quarter centimeters (½ in.) (option A) is too short. Options C and D are too long.

5. **(C)** UTI (as well as bladder spasms) may cause leakage around the indwelling catheter. Use of a larger catheter (option A) only increases bladder spasms and discomfort. The retention balloon (B) should not be overfilled. Leakage would not indicate return of normal urinary function (option D).

6. **(A, B, C, D)** Physicians may need to be reminded that the client has an indwelling catheter and that long-term use is associated with increased risk for UTI. Failure to use aseptic technique during insertion (option B), and to-and-fro movement of a catheter that is not properly secured (option C) promote bacterial growth and UTI, as does an overfull urine drainage bag pulling on the catheter (option D). Cleansing with soap and water (option E) is appropriate. Obtaining urine specimens, if done using aseptic technique through the port in the catheter, should not introduce bacteria (option F).

7. **(A)** Continuous bladder irrigation dilutes postoperative bleed and thus prevents clots from forming and occluding the catheter drainage system. It may help to prevent bladder infection (option B) but this is not the best answer. It may increase bladder spasms (option C). It does not stop postoperative bleeding (option D).

8. **(A)** Protective barriers should be used only when necessary. They contain alcohol and must be removed with a solvent that increases risk of skin irritation to sensitive skin (option B). They may interfere with pouch sealing (options C and D).

9. **(B)** The term *end-stage renal disease* (ESRD) only indicates that the client is receiving renal replacement therapy (dialysis or transplant). It does not mean that the client has no functioning nephrons (A), produces no urine (C), or is uremic (D).

10. **(B, C, E)** The indications for appropriate catheter use are acute urinary retention (E) or bladder outlet obstruction, need for accurate measurement of urinary output in clients who are critically ill, open sacral or perineal wounds in conjunction with incontinence (B), prolonged immobilization, and comfort for clients for end-of-life care, if needed (C). Clients who are postsurgery (A and D) can be intermittently catheterized.

CHAPTER 23—BOWEL ELIMINATION

1. **(A, B, D)** Ultrasonography, electromyography, and colonoscopy are all tests that could be selected for clients with fecal incontinence. The MRI (C) and CAT scan (E) are not usually ordered to rule out issues with fecal incontinence.

2. **(B)** Saying that the client "has to talk to the physician" can upset the client as he or she thinks that something is wrong (A). If you were present when the physician discussed the procedure with the client, you can reiterate the information. Having a drain placed until bowel function returns (C) and having a catheter inserted until the colon has healed (D) are incorrect information.

3. **(A)** There is greater fluid loss with an ileostomy as a result of a more liquid stool. The fluid is not reabsorbed into the body because the ileum is resected, and fluid absorption occurs mainly in the lower part of the bowel. Clients with an ileostomy will also need to wear an appliance (B). Many clients with a colostomy do not need an appliance. An ileostomy is usually performed as a result of Crohn disease or ulcerative colitis, and the ileostomy for these conditions is not reversed (C). There are fluid and food restrictions with either procedure (D).

4. **(C)** Vagal stimulation as a result of fecal removal can lead to decreased pulse rate resulting from decreasing conductivity at the sino atrial node. A consent form is not needed (A). Fluids (B) are infused into the lower colon prior to removal; an enema usually precedes the fecal removal, but it is not done just prior to the removal. Laxatives (D) can be ordered after the removal to prevent another impaction.

5. **(D)** is correct. Placing the pointed end of the suppository 7–10 cm (3–4 in.) beyond the internal sphincter will prevent expulsion of the suppository. The client is not asked to bear down when inserting the suppository. The client is placed in a Sims position and the suppository is inserted beyond the internal, not external, sphincter (A). The pointed, not the flat, end (B) of the suppository is generously lubricated and inserted first for ease in passage through the external and internal sphincters. If the suppository is inserted into fecal material (C), it will not dissolve.

6. **(D, E)** Bananas and white toast should be avoided to prevent odors. Dairy products (A), brown rice (B), and cookies (C) can be eaten; however, they may need to be limited to manage the ostomy.

7. **(A)** is correct. Females require 2.7 L/day, while men require 3.7 L/day. Intake of 2 L/day for women (B) or for men (D) and intake of 2.7 L/day for men (C) is less than optimal.

8. **(B)** The client is placed on the left, not right, side in Sims position (A). The maximum height is 46 cm (18 in.) above the rectal area, not at shoulder height (C). Solution is instilled slowly to prevent cramps; 5–10 min would be too fast (D).

9. **(B)**. The skin and stoma are cleansed with water only. Oily substances and soap can prevent good adhesion of the pouch to the skin. Options (A), (C), and (D) are correct steps in applying a fecal ostomy pouch.

10. **(C)** is correct. Only an RN or an LVN/LPN can administer an enema with medications. Nursing assistants cannot perform a fecal impaction removal (A). The client can have cardiac complications that need to be assessed by an RN or LVN/LPN. Many healthcare facilities do allow UAP to perform enema administration (B). An LVN/LPN cannot develop a teaching plan, but he or she can implement a plan (D).

CHAPTER 24—HEAT AND COLD THERAPIES

1. **(A)** Internal stimuli (pyrogens, cytokines) cause the hypothalamus to alter the body temperature set point; therefore, a *regulated* rise in temperature occurs. Elevation of temperature in fever is not due to (B) injury of the hypothalamus, (C) dehydration, or (D) environment extremes.

2. **(C)** Fever is caused by pyrogens, so an antipyretic is most effective in bringing it down. Physical methods such as (A) tepid sponges (B), cooling blanket, and (D) cool packs to the axillae and groin can aid in fever resolution but are not the best answer.

3. **(C)** Shivering muscle activity increases heat production, thereby counteracting the goal of treatment to reduce body temperature. It does not enhance cooling (A). It increases, not decreases, the metabolic rate (B). It does not affect pyrogens (D).

4. **(C)** Water temperature is regulated to 43.3°C (110°F) as a safety measure. Options (A) and (B) are lower than the regulated temperature; option (D) is too high.

5. **(A)** The surgical client would lose body heat to the environment by radiation because the surgical suite environment is cooler. The cap would not prevent heat loss by evaporation (B), convection (C), or conduction (D).

6. **(A)** Sugar-free and caffeine-free beverages are most appropriate for rehydration due to heat-induced dehydration; in this instance, water is best. IV dextrose (B) and sports drinks (C) have sugar. Sugared cola (D) has both sugar and caffeine, a diuretic.

7. **(B, D, E, F)** Flushing, anesthesia, burning, and numbness are expected effects of cryotherapy applications. Therapy should be discontinued on numbness. Pallor (A) and blister formation (C) are adverse effects.

8. **(A)** The sitz bath causes pelvic vasodilation with diversion of blood flow that could potentially result in orthostatic hypotension on standing. A sitz bath would not cause fungal infection (B) or increased vaginal bleeding (C). It would relieve, not aggravate, hemorrhoids (D).

9. **(D)** Nerves are sensitive to cold application and are most superficial around joints. Reactive vasodilation (A) affects extremities. Joints may become more, not less, flexible with cold application as inflammation is reduced (B). Cold does not induce bleeding (C).

10. **(A)** Tissue metabolic demand increases as it is heated. If circulation is compromised, the tissue's need for oxygen will exceed what the circulation can provide. Heat increases, not decreases, metabolic rate (B). Heat promotes circulation, not inflammation (C). Heat tends to increase sensation, not decrease it (D).

CHAPTER 25—WOUND CARE AND DRESSINGS

1. **(C)** During the regeneration phase of wound healing, there is rapid growth of epithelial cells to produce a protective covering for a wound. The third phase, maturation (A), is the period when wound contraction takes place. The first phase, inflammatory phase (B), occurs immediately after an injury. Wound remodeling (D) is another term for maturation.

2. **(D)** Wounds that heal by being left open, such as an infected wound or one that has dehisced, are referred to as healing by tertiary intention. Healing by granulation (A) refers to secondary intention. Option (B) is primary intention healing. Option (C) refers to a primary intention wound.

3. **(B)** 30–35 Cal/kg/day is required for adequate wound healing. Option (A) is too few calories for adequate healing. Options (C) and (D) are more calories than needed.

4. **(A)** Placing 3-5 mL of antimicrobial soap on the palm of the hand is correct practice for decontaminating hands for surgical asepsis. All surfaces of the hands are rubbed, usually for 20–25 sec. Ten seconds (B) is not sufficient to kill microorganisms; a longer time is required for hand scrubs. Three-minute scrubs (C) are associated with the first OR scrub of the day. The rinse is done in one direction only to prevent recontamination; hands are dried in the OR with a sterile towel (D).

5. **(C)** The last flap of the wrapper is opened toward the nurse to prevent crossing over the sterile field. The first flap of the wrapper is placed away from the sterile field. It is incorrect to reach over the bed (A) because contamination could occur. The package is not held while it is being opened; it is touched as little as possible (B). The sterile dressing tray is not moved once unwrapped (D).

6. **(B)** The knot is grasped with the forceps and lifted away from the skin. Clean gloves are used. It is not necessary to use sterile gloves (A). Curved tip of scissors is used and the cut is next to the knot, not over it (C). Sutures are removed starting at the top or bottom of the incision, not in the middle (D).

7. **(A, B, C)** Transparent adhesive film allows visualization of wound, promotes autolysis of dry eschar, and does not require a secondary dressing. A soothing, cooling effect (D) is an advantage of hydrogel dressings, not of transparent film dressings. It is not intended to warm the wound area (E).

8. **(C)** is correct. Wounds are not cleansed with hydrogen peroxide (A). They are not swabbed in a single line down the middle (B). Cleaning the edge and then swabbing the middle is not a correct method for obtaining a wound culture.

9. **(B)** The nurse fluffs the moist dressings, and then places them over the wound. Dressings are not packed into the wound bed (A). Moist dressings are not placed on top of dry dressings (C). Dry dressings are not placed on top of moistened dressings in the wound (D).

10. **(A, B, C)** For negative pressure wound therapy to be effective, the wound must be surrounded by at least 2 cm (¾ inch) of intact peri-wound tissue, be open enough so the foam dressing can touch all edges, and must already be debrided. Besides these conditions, there must be sufficient circulation to assist in healing. The wound does not need to be on the extremities (D).The therapy needs to be able to be on 22 hr/day to be effective, not 2 (E).

CHAPTER 26—PERIOPERATIVE CARE

1. **(C)** A moderate sedation would not be provided in the preoperative stage. This drug is usually administered during the intraoperative stage. Obtaining a health history (A), identifying a client's allergies (B), and identifying the side and site of the surgical procedure (D) are all activities that will be performed during the preoperative stage.

2. **(D)** The circulating nurse positions the client on the operating table and attaches the grounding pad. The physician and the entire operative team identify the correct side and site, not just the circulating nurse (A). The anesthesiologist inserts the IV if it is not already in place (B). The scrub nurse, not the circulating nurse, assists the physician throughout the surgical procedure (C).

3. **(A)** Both scrub and circulating nurses monitor sponge and instrument counts before, during, and after the procedure. The entire OR staff participates in checking the side and site of the procedure, not just the nurses (B). Burns from incorrectly placed grounding pads (C) and infections at the surgical site postoperatively (D) are not common malpractice actions taken against nurses.

4. **(A, C, D, E)** A, C, D, and E are interventions that can and should be used to reduce anxiety in a preoperative client. The nurse should not promise that everything will be fine (B).

5. **(A)** Sharp pain under the scapula postoperatively is indicative of carbon dioxide irritation of the phrenic nerve in the diaphragm, which causes referred pain. It is very infrequent for a client with a laparoscopy to be hospitalized to monitor pain; this would not happen unless there is some extenuating circumstance (B). (C) Usually a stronger-acting pain medication than acetaminophen is administered for pain following any surgical procedure. (D) Most clients do not return to work the next day; the recovery time for anesthesia is longer than 24 hr, and the usual weight limit may be as low as 5 lb.

6. **(D)** Check for allergies to latex, food, and medications. If the client is allergic, all latex articles must be removed from the OR, and this client should be scheduled as the first OR case for the day. The surgical consent form (B) must be signed before the preoperative medication is given. (C) The medication is usually given at about 45 min, not 2 hr, before the OR transporter arrives to take the client to the OR. Arrangements for home care after discharge (A) are not necessary at this time.

7. **(C, D, E)** "Yes" is written on the surgical checklist line indicating the correct incision site, and final verification of the site is completed in the location where the procedure takes place. The surgical site is marked by the individual performing the procedure, not by the preoperative nurse (A). All members of the surgical team, not just the surgeon, verify the site (B).

8. **(C)** A score of 9 or lower, or a score within 1 point of the preprocedural score on the Aldrete Scale, must be obtained before the discharge is completed. Ramsay (A) and Riker (B) are scales used for sedation assessment parameters during the use of moderate sedation. Glasgow

Coma Scale (D) is used for assessing clients who have head injuries or who are not alert.

9. **(D)** The initial assessment/intervention is to assess for patent airway. If the client is experiencing difficulty breathing, color is pale, skin is cool, oxygen must be administered, and the head of the bed must be slightly elevated. Vital signs (A), type and amount of IV solution (B), and pulse oximetry reading (C) should immediately follow this initial assessment and intervention.

10. **(B)** Onset of signs and symptoms at 24–36 hr postoperatively is correct. Pulmonary complications are usually evident 24–36 hr after surgery. Signs and symptoms of an ileus occur between 36 and 48 hr postoperatively (C). Urinary tract infections occur from the third to the fifth postoperative day. Wound infections can occur from 24 hr (A) to 5 days (D) postoperatively.

CHAPTER 27—ORTHOPEDIC INTERVENTIONS

1. **(A)** Positioning the hand higher than the elbow prevents dependent edema in the hand. Lower than the elbow would promote edema (B). Movement of the shoulder (C) and distal digits (D) maintains joint mobility.

2. **(D)** Natural evaporation allows the cast to dry from inside out. External heat application (A), (B), (C) may cause the cast to dry on the outside but not the inside, causing the cast to weaken.

3. **(A, B, F)** Synthetic casts are more expensive than plaster, dry more quickly, and are more absorbent. Additionally, they are lighter (not heavier) in weight (C). They provide less stability than plaster, not more (D). They can cause skin burns (E) when drying is activated.

4. **(B, D, F)** Pain with passive extension of distal digits, with extremity elevation, and unrelieved by analgesic are early indicators of ischemia. Elevating the extremity worsens ischemia and pain. Pain is out of proportion to the injury and unrelieved by pain medication. Weak or absent distal pulses (A) is a late sign. (C) and (E) are not indications of acute compartment syndrome.

5. **(C)** Peroneal nerve motor function provides dorsiflexion of the foot. Peroneal nerve injury can result in permanent foot drop. Urinary incontinence (A), inability to plantarflex the foot (B), and anesthesia on the sole of the foot (D) would not be results of injury to the peroneal nerve.

6. **(B)** Abduction is correct. Adduction (A) or leg crossing (C or D) may cause implant dislocation.

7. **(A)** Adaptive aids help prevent extremes of flexion that could result in implant dislocation. They do not affect falls (B), hip extension (C), or pain (D).

8. **(A)** Studies show range of motion is reduced if clients do not receive CPM after total knee replacement surgery. Lack of CPM would increase, not decrease, the chance of venous thrombosis (B), edema (C), and wound drainage (D).

9. **(D)** Phantom pain is thought to be a central nervous system response to stored pain sensations from the previously intact limb. It is not associated with drug dependency (A), inadequate stump shrinkage or shaping (B), or traumatic amputation (C).

10. **(C)** Clients have the tendency to abduct and flex the stump postoperatively. Exercises to promote adduction and hip extension help prevent flexion contracture of the stump and help prepare the stump for walking with a prosthesis. Adduction with hip extension is the intent, not hip flexion (A), and not abduction (B) or (D).

CHAPTER 28—INTRAVENOUS THERAPY

1. **(A)** Ringer's lactate solution does not require an in-line filter. TPN (A), PCA (C), and blood platelets (D) require the filters in order to filter out microorganisms and guard against inadvertent infusions of particulate matter and endotoxins.

2. **(D)** Using the distal end of the vein reserves the more proximal areas for future IV sites. Superficial veins are palpated and used for peripheral IVs (A). The antecubital vein is not a primary site for IV placement (B). It is used as a last resort. The catheter can become kinked when placed in this area. (C) IV fluid flow will be affected if the IV is inserted in a site below the same vein that is infiltrated or where phlebitis is present.

3. **(A, E)** The hand is tightened, not held open and loose (B). A warm, not cool, cloth is applied to produce vasodilation that assists with insertion of the IV catheter or needle (C). The arm is placed in a dependent position to prevent venous dilation; it is not elevated (D).

4. **(D)** Chlorhexidine swabs are recommended by the Intravenous Nurses Society to prepare the IV insertion site. Alcohol swabs (A) and beta-dine or iodine swabs (B) and (C) have been used in the past. However, evidence-based nursing practice has identified they are not as effective

as chlorhexidine. Betadine (B) and povidone-iodine (C) are the same thing.

5. **(D)** Blood or blood-product tubing is changed every 4 hr or 2 units. Primary and secondary tubing is changed every 72 hr (A). Primary intermittent tubing is changed every 24 hr, not 96 hr (B). TPN and lipids are changed every 24 hr (C).

6. **(B)** The bevel of the needle is in the up position in order to check the integrity of the end of the catheter (A). (C) The needle is inserted along the side of the needle or about ½inch distal to selected puncture site. (D) After hearing the "pop" sound, check for backflow of blood in the plastic hub.

7. **(B)** The answer is 15 mL. If you did not get this answer, review regulating flow rate to determine the IV drops/min.

8. **(C)** The client's nurse must be notified. The pump needs to be reprogrammed with the scanning device, which requires checking the medication, client's ID, and nurse's ID badge, not just your badge (D) The pump cannot just be restarted when a "hard" alarm sounds (A) or (B), as this indicates that an error in the drug, dose, or equipment has occurred.

9. **(D)** Isotonic solutions are used to expand circulating volume. Hypotonic solutions hydrate cells (A) and are used to correct dehydration (B).. Hypertonic solutions such as dextrose 10% can be used as a nutrient source (C).

10. **(C)** Small amounts of the medication are released at a time to ensure safety. One fourth of the medication is injected over a 20-second time period, so it takes a minimum of 80 seconds to administer the drug (A). Always check the package insert for the time frame. Flushing of the IV tubing is done when an incompatible drug is being administered (B). Check the drug compatibility chart to determine the appropriate IV solution that is acceptable for infusing the drug (D).

CHAPTER 29—CENTRAL VASCULAR ACCESS

1. **(A)** PICC lines and subcutaneous ports and central catheters are termed central vascular access devices. They can be left in place for longer periods of time and with fewer complications than midline catheters (B), peripheral catheters in the basilica vein (C), and long-line catheters threaded into the right atrium (D).

2. **(A)** is the correct statement related to preventing catheter-related bloodstream infections. Catheters are not impregnated with antibiotic agent (B). A solution of 2% chlorhexidine with 70% alcohol, not Betadine or alcohol swabs (C), is used as the antibacterial scrub. A mask is not placed over the client's face (D).

3. **(A)** is the time used when the swab contains chlorhexidine and alcohol. (B) 1 min is incorrect. (C) is the time necessary for drying povidone–iodine, and chlorhexidine alone. (D) is the time when a 70% isopropyl alcohol solution is used.

4. **(C)** The change time for IVs for infusing parenteral nutrition and for primary and secondary IV tubing changes is 72 hr, not 48 hr (B) or 96 hr (D). The time for changing tubing when lipids are infusing is 24 hr (A).

5. **(D)** A plugged filter is the most common problem that occurs when the solution is not infusing at the prescribed rate. If the hyperalimentation flow rate is not infusing at the prescribed time, you do not "catch up" by increasing the flow rate (A). This can lead to hyperglycemia as a result of increasing the amount of glucose from the IV solution. Before notifying the physician (B), a complete assessment of the situation must occur in order to make an informed decision. It is rare that the dressing is tight enough (C) to cause an occlusion of the IV flow.

6. **(A, C, B, D)** These are the steps in obtaining a central venous pressure reading. Refer to Skill 29.1.9 if you missed this question.

7. **(C)** The port is inserted for long-term care, usually for clients receiving chemotherapy intermittently. The port is irrigated monthly and after each use, not daily (B) or every 12 hr (D). Normal saline, not heparin (A), is used in flushing and is followed by heparin infusion.

8. **(B)** After stopping the IV infusion, the next step is swabbing the hub and cap with an antimicrobial swab. Then the cap is removed (C) and the syringe is flushed with normal saline (A) and (D).

9. **(C)** The port is swabbed with chlorhexidine, not Betadine (A). After anchoring the port site, the Huber needle (B) is inserted at a 90-degree angle (D). Check for blood return, and if it is present, the drug can be infused. This is followed by first infusing normal saline and then a heparin solution.

10. **(D)** Positive pressure within the central venous access device prevents blood from being drawn back into the catheter when the syringe is removed. It does not ensure easy blood sampling (A), maintain an accurate drip rate (B), or maintain sterility (C).

CHAPTER 30—RESPIRATORY CARE

1. **(D)** Slow inhalation maximizes volume; holding allows alveoli to open; and exhalation through pursed lips prevents early airway closure. Other options (A), (B), and (C) miss at least one of these important steps.

2. **(B)** Only those with serious retention of secretions have been found to benefit from CPT. Clients with pneumonia (A), clients with acute exacerbation of COPD (C), and clients on ventilators (D) do not necessarily show benefit from CPT.

3. **(B)** The sedated client may not be able to remove the mask in the event of nausea and vomiting, so there is risk of aspiration of emesis. Clients allergic to latex (A) can be fitted with a nonlatex mask. Clients who are asleep (C) and clients who are claustrophobic (D) can use them.

4. **(D)** The nonrebreathing mask with reservoir bag provides the greatest FiO_2 because the client inhales enriched air from the mask as well as the bag and does not rebreathe exhaled air. Other options (A), (B), and (C) provide lesser FiO_2.

5. **(A, C, E)** Pulse oximetry measures are not reliable in anemic clients (A) because the decreased number of RBCs may be fully oxygenated; hypovolemic clients (C) may be vasoconstricted; and circulating contrast (E) can confuse readings. Having high glucose (B) or being hypertensive (D) does not affect readings.

6. **(B)** Intubation provides a patent airway whether or not mechanical ventilation (A) is necessary. It does not prevent aspiration (C) and is not essential for providing oxygenation (D) unless mechanical ventilation is used.

7. **(A, B, C)** The proper inflation of an endotracheal or tracheostomy tube cuff is necessary to prevent complications such as (A) aspiration of food, aspiration of secretions (B), and tube migration (C). It does not prevent but supports mechanical ventilation (D). It prevents communication (E); however, this is not a complication but an expected effect of the cuff inflation.

8. **(A, B, C, E)** Signs and symptoms of hypoxia include A, B, C, and E. Only auditory hallucination (option D) is not a sign.

9. **(B)** The tube cuff must be deflated. If the tube cuff remains inflated (C) and the tube is capped with a speaking valve, the client is unable to inhale air because both the artificial airway and the trachea are occluded. The client does not need mechanical ventilation (A) or a Bivona Fome Cuf (D).

10. **(E, C, A, F, D, H, G, B)** This sequence reflects necessary preparation before sterile steps are taken. Hyperoxygenation is performed before sterile equipment is handled; the catheter is advanced before suction is applied. Finally, the oropharynx is suctioned using the same catheter.

CHAPTER 31—CIRCULATORY MAINTENANCE

1. **(C)** The QRS complex represents the depolarization of the ventricles. Atrial depolarization (A) is represented by the P wave. The PR interval (B) represents the time required for atrial depolarization. The T wave (D) represents ventricular repolarization.

2. **(A)** In an atrial arrhythmia, the SA node sends an abnormal rate of impulse generation. A normal cardiac impulse begins in the sinoatrial node. It is transmitted over myocardium, Bachman's bundle, and internodal pathways to the AV node (B). If there is a disturbance in this transmission, it results in an atrial dysrhythmia. Purkinje fibers (C) and bundle of His (D) are not correct.

3. **(C)** Demand pacemakers are the most frequently used pacemakers. The electrode is triggered to stimulate the heart only when the heart's intrinsic or natural atrial or ventricular pacemaker stimulation fails. They do not alter their rate depending on activity (A). They do not discharge steadily regardless of the underlying HR (B). They do not discharge on ventricular dysrhythmia (D).

4. **(A)** The urine output of 30–40 mL/hr is a normal value. When hemorrhaging occurs, the urine output will decrease because of decreased cardiac output as a result of the hemorrhage. Diastolic pressure of 90 mm Hg for the last 2 hr (B), shallow respirations of 18-20/min (C), and clammy skin with central cyanosis (D) would be observed when hemorrhage occurs.

5. **(A)** Your first priority is to initiate the emergency response system which in this case would be the hospital code team. You would do chest compressions next (B) with rescue breathing using an airway device. The AED (C) is used or placed on the client when it becomes available. You would not check for breathing (D) as a first step after determining the client needs CPR.

6. **(C)** The appropriate thigh-high measurement is from the bottom of the heel to the fold of the buttocks, not the heel to the popliteal fold (B) or

the distance between knee and ankle (D). The circumference is measured at the mid-thigh area, not the largest area of the calf (A).

7. **(B, D, E)** The use of compression devices would be contraindicated in diabetic neuropathy ulcers and arterial ischemia ulcers as well as dermatitis, preexisting pulmonary embolism, and pressure ulcers. Compression devices can be helpful to clients with heart failure (A). These conditions increase venous return to the heart (C).

8. **(C)** If the client can speak, you continue to allow them to cough because they should be able to expel the foreign body. The abdominal thrust is completed (A) if the client cannot talk or if coughing becomes ineffective. CPR (B) is not appropriate in this scenario. Striking the client on the back (D) is not a recommended action.

9. **(A)** Rescue breathing requires a tight seal. The flowmeter (B) is set at 15, not 6, L/min. A backboard (C) helps with compressions, not airway seal. Cricoid pressure (D) is not used.

10. **(A, C, E)** The RRT is utilized when a client meets these criteria. The urine output (B) should be less than a total of 50 mL in 4 hr and the oxygen saturation should be less than 90% *with supplemental oxygen*.

Chapter 32—Neurological Management

1. **(C)** To determine the cerebral perfusion pressure, the ICP is subtracted from the MAP. The MAP is calculated by adding the SBP plus 2 times the DBP, divided by 3 (130 + 160 = 290, divided by 3 = 97). The ICP is 12, so 97 minus 12 = 85. This is an adequate cerebral perfusion pressure. Options (A), (B), and (D) are incorrect.

2. **(C)** An intracranial pressure of 12 is normal. Therefore, there is no increase in any one of the three intracranial components, or normal pressure has been activated by manipulation of one of the components to compensate for an increase in one of the other components (B). It does not indicate severe decrease in pressure (A) or a malfunction of autoregulation (D).

3. **(A)** Frontal lobe dysfunction affects contralateral voluntary motion and causes changes in personality and behavior. These signs are not consistent with tumors in the parietal (B), occipital (C), or temporal (D) lobes.

4. **(D)** Signs of metabolic coma are usually diffuse, rather than unilateral, with coma preceding motor deficits (C) and without orderly rostrocaudal deterioration (A), as seen with structural causes. Pupil reflexes are preserved bilaterally (B), while structural causes of coma are usually associated with a unilateral nonreactive pupil.

5. **(C)** Of the listed options, only hypoxemia (low blood O2) causes cerebral vessels to dilate and increase intracranial pressure, making ventilation a priority. Hypocapnea (hyperventilation) constricts cerebral vessels (A) and may be used briefly to reduce intracranial pressure. Acidemia (rather than alkalemia) causes cerebral vessels to constrict (B). Hypothermia (D) does not affect cerebral vessels, but is used therapeutically to reduce cerebral metabolic demand.

6. **(B)** Pupil response (constriction to light) is controlled by CN III (oculomotor nerve) whose nuclei are attached to the midbrain. The nerve's location at the top of the brainstem is the first to be compressed, as intracranial pressure increases, resulting in sluggish or absent pupil response to light. Pressure on the midbrain does not lead to loss of gag reflex (A), widening pulse pressure (C), or loss of blink reflex (D).

7. **(A)** While changes in respiratory pattern accompany neurologic deterioration, they are not specific to neurologic dysfunction (B). For instance, Cheyne-Stokes respirations occur in clients with heart failure and other systemic disorders. As ICP increases, neurologic deterioration progresses rostrocaudally, the diencephalon (above the brainstem) is compressed, causing impaired consciousness. This occurs before changes due to compression on the midbrain (pupil response C) or alterations of blood pressure and heart rate occur (D). Additionally, changes in vital signs accompany many pathologic conditions.

8. **(B)** The ventriculostomy is the most cost-effective, accurate and reliable method of monitoring ICP. It is the only method that includes an external drainage system and transducer calibrated or zeroed against a known pressure to ensure consistent and accurate pressure measurements. The indwelling ventricular catheter allows CSF drainage to decrease ICP, is used for medication instillation, and provides access to CSF for laboratory testing. (A), (C), and (D) do not describe ventriculostomy.

9. **(D)** The P-1 waveform reflects systolic BP pulsations transmitted through the choroid plexus and is normally the highest of the three waveform components, while the P-3 is the lowest (C). The P-2 waveform (A) reflects relative brain volume and is often elevated in response to compromised intracranial compliance. Waveforms vary in size (B).

10. **(C, D, E, F)** The electroencephalogram is the most commonly used confirmatory test, assessing only cerebral, not brainstem function. The client must have at least 30 min without brainstem electrical activity. With brain death, there is absence of intracerebral blood flow from the carotid arteries and circle of Willis. The EEG (C) is positive if there is no electrical activity throughout 30 min of recording. Cerebral angiography (D), MRI/MRA (E), and brainstem reflexes (F) are other ancillary tests for confirming brain death. Spinal fluid analysis (A), cold caloric test (B), and deep tendon reflexes (G) do not determine brain death.

Chapter 33—Advanced Nursing Skills

1. **(B)** The distal lumen (placed in the pulmonary artery) measures pulmonary artery systolic and diastolic pressures and, when "wedged," indirectly measures the left ventricular end-diastolic pressure. The proximal lumen assists in measuring cardiac output (A), is used to inject solutions (C), and to measure central venous pressure (D).

2. **(F, G)** Because not all chests are equal, this is the most accurate way to determine the level of the right atrium in the supine position. A, B, C, D, and E are not correct landmarks.

3. **(C)** Cannulation of the radial artery can result in inadequate blood flow distally. The Allen Test is used to assess adequacy of distal perfusion through the ulnar artery before radial artery cannulation. (A) Measures are very accurate. (B) Blood sampled is arterial. (D) The readings are blood pressure not heart rate.

4. **(A)** Obtaining arterial blood samples using the conservatory system eliminates the need to waste blood that contains the continuous flush solution, therefore helping to prevent nosocomial anemia. (B) The system still needs to be opened. (C) Alarms still need to be disengaged as the system is disrupted. (D) It can take as much or more time to complete the sampling process.

5. **(B)** Because atrial fibrillation is frequently recurrent (chronic), the client continues anticoagulation therapy (Coumadin) to prevent cardioembolic stroke. (A) Antiarrhymic therapy is not needed if cardioversion is successful. (C) Pacemaker monitoring is used for other treatments. (D) Cardioversion is used when needed, not monthly.

6. **(A, C)** These lethal rhythms require immediate defibrillation to convert to sinus rhythm. The others require cardioversion (B, D) or CPR (E, F).

7. **(C)** A functioning electrical system and a responsive pump in the presence of hypovolemia will produce an ECG without peripheral perfusion (pulseless electrical activity). (A, D) can contribute to heart disease. (B) can cause arrhythmias.

8. **(D)** This mode provides total support. It is used for the client who cannot initiate or who for a clinical situation should not initiate breathing. (A) Provides pressure to open the airways at the end of the delivered ventilated breath. (B) Provides medium level of support. (C) Provides the least amount of support.

9. **(C)** Asynchrony leads to wasted energy; this is especially important in infants. (A) They do not create a state of sleep only paralysis, (B) they do not eliminate the need for restraints and they do not impact pain (D) perception.

10. **(A, B, C, D)** Accumulation of oropharyngeal secretions above the tube cuff is associated with aspiration of secretions that leads to ventilator-associated pneumonia, condensation in the tubing, improper suctioning technique, and lack of mobilization of clients. All contribute to ventilator association pneumonia. (E) Keeping the head of bed elevated 30 degrees is a preventive measure.

Chapter 34—End-of-Life Care

1. **(D, A, E, B, C)** This is the sequencing for the stages of dying. Refer to the "Stages of Grief" in the chapter if you did not get this answer correct.

2. **(B)** In Engle's system, the third stage of grief is the beginning of the onset of cultural and religious rituals that assist the mourner to face the loss. The stage of idealization is (A). (C) is the first stage of shock and disbelief. (D) is the stage of resolution.

3. **(B, C, E)** Nurses continue to provide alternative and nontraditional care to improve the client's quality of life (A). (D) Nurses should be sensitive to the need of family members and should encourage visitation as they desire.

4. **(B)** Clients requiring rehabilitative services are placed in a rehabilitation unit/facility or long-term care facility (A). (C) Unless clients are terminally ill, they would be cared for in a long-term care facility or at home. (D) Treatments can be provided with hospice care.

5. **(C)** Acting out and verbalizing anger is expected to occur during the anger stage of the process (A and B). (D) The client should be

encouraged to take as much control as possible over his/her care and environment during this phase.

6. **(B)** This provides a connection with family members or memories of happy times. Clients should be placed in a calm environment, not near the busy nursing station with all its noises (A). (C) It is best to allow clients to look out windows and see activity around them, unless the client requests that curtains be drawn. (D) Lighting in the room should be muted and soft without overhead lighting being turned on.

7. **(A)** About 40% of Caucasians are more likely to have written advance directives. Other cultures have a distrust of the United States health-care system and will not write advance directives.

8. **(A)** The drugs in (B) are used in Step 1 for pain control that is used for mild to moderate pain. (C) Step 3 utilizes opioid drugs at higher doses for moderate to severe pain. (D) Methadone is used in step 3 for moderate to severe pain.

9. **(A, B, D, E)** Nurses need to allot adequate time not only for physical care, but the dying client (C) will not be able to carry on much conversation.

10. **(A)** Locus of decision making (option B) and attitudes about advance directives (option C) are dimensions that vary among cultures, as is approach to "bad news" (D). Some cultures keep information about adverse diagnoses away from the client. Family members discuss the treatment plan with physicians, without input from the client.

Index

Page numbers followed by a *t* indicate tables.

Index of Skills